Lecture Notes in Computer Science   8673

Commenced Publication in 1973
Founding and Former Series Editors:
Gerhard Goos, Juris Hartmanis, and Jan van Leeuwen

Polina Golland   Nobuhiko Hata
Christian Barillot   Joachim Hornegger
Robert Howe (Eds.)

Medical Image Computing and Computer-Assisted Intervention – MICCAI 2014

17th International Conference
Boston, MA, USA, September 14-18, 2014
Proceedings, Part I

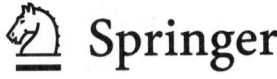 Springer

Volume Editors

Polina Golland
Massachusetts Institute of Technology
Cambridge, MA, USA
E-mail: polina@csail.mit.edu

Nobuhiko Hata
Brigham and Women's Hospital
Harvard Medical School, Boston, MA, USA
E-mail: hata@bwh.harvard.edu

Christian Barillot
IRISA, Rennes, France
E-mail: christian.barillot@irisa.fr

Joachim Hornegger
Friedrich-Alexander University Erlangen-Nuremberg
Erlangen, Germany
E-mail: joachim.hornegger@fau.de

Robert Howe
Harvard University, Cambridge, MA, USA
E-mail: howe@seas.harvard.edu

ISSN 0302-9743   e-ISSN 1611-3349
ISBN 978-3-319-10403-4   e-ISBN 978-3-319-10404-1
DOI 10.1007/978-3-319-10404-1
Springer Cham Heidelberg New York Dordrecht London

Library of Congress Control Number: 2014946218

LNCS Sublibrary: SL 6 – Image Processing, Computer Vision, Pattern Recognition,
and Graphics

Typesetting: Camera-ready by author, data conversion by Scientific Publishing Services, Chennai, India

Printed on acid-free paper

Springer is part of Springer Science+Business Media (www.springer.com)

Preface

The 17th International Conference on Medical Image Computing and Computer-Assisted Intervention (MICCAI 2014) was held in Boston, USA, at the Massachusetts Institute of Technology (MIT) and Harvard Medical School during September 14-18, 2014. We were delighted to welcome the conference back to the location of the very first MICCAI meeting that took place on MIT campus in 1998. Over the last 16 years, the MICCAI conferences have become a premier international event, with papers of high standard addressing open problems in the multidisciplinary fields of biomedical image computing, computer-assisted intervention, and medical robotics. The conference attracts leading scientists, engineers, and clinicians from a wide range of disciplines.

This year, we received a record number of 862 submissions. These covered medical image computing (functional and diffusion image analysis, segmentation, physical and functional modeling, shape analysis, atlases and statistical models, registration, data fusion and multiscale analysis), computer-assisted interventions and robotics (planning and image guidance of interventions, simulation and training systems, clinical platforms, visualization and feedback, robotics and human–robot interaction), and clinical imaging and biomarkers (computer-aided diagnosis, organ/system specific applications, molecular and optical imaging and imaging biomarkers). A careful systematic review process was carried out to create the most exciting scientific program for MICCAI 2014. The Program Committee (PC) of the conference was composed of 52 experts recognized internationally in the main topics of the conference. Each submission was assigned to a primary PC member who recruited between three and four external reviewers for each paper based on their expertise and the topic of the paper. The external reviewers provided double-blind reviews of the papers. Each submission without consensus among the external reviewers was assigned to two secondary PC members and was invited to submit a rebuttal followed by discussion among the external reviewers. Each secondary PC member made recommendations to the PC while taking into account the external reviews, the rebuttal, and the discussion. The list of accepted papers was finalized during a two-day PC meeting held at MIT during May 17-18, 2014, based on the scores and rankings provided by the PC members and external reviewers and on the discussion among the PC members. In all, we accepted 253 papers (29%) to be included in the proceedings of MICCAI 2014 and presented as posters during the meeting. Of these, 36 were selected for podium presentation (4%). We congratulate those who had papers accepted and encourage those who did not to persevere and submit again next year. Selection of papers for MICCAI is a competitive process and with such a strong submission pool it is inevitable that many good papers could not be included in the final program. We sympathize with the authors whose papers were rejected; we had our own share of rejected papers this year!

In addition to the main conference, MICCAI 2014 offered a rich program of workshops, computational challenges, and tutorials. We received a fantastic set of proposals that resulted in an exciting, diverse, and high-quality program. The workshops provided a comprehensive coverage of topics not fully explored during the main conference and of emerging areas of MICCAI; the computational challenges explored empirical solutions to hard open problems; the tutorials provided educational material for training new professionals in the field. We are grateful to all workshop, challenge, and tutorial organizers for making these events a success and to the workshop chairs for creating such a great program.

MICCAI 2014 introduced a completely new Educational Challenge, conceived, organized, and run by the MICCAI Student Board. The long-term goal is to create a video library of educational presentations for students entering the fields. The Educational Challenge was a great step in that direction, and we hope MICCAI will continue to support this effort. Our many thanks go out to the students who organized the challenge. We would also like to thank our invited speaker Neville Hogan (MIT, USA) for his presentation on the use of robots for rehabilitation.

We thank the external reviewers and the PC for volunteering their time and judgement to provide high-quality reviews and ensure a fair paper selection process. The continued improvement in the quality of the conference depends entirely on this tremendous effort. We thank James Stewart of *precisionconference.com* for the efficient organization of the website and amazingly fast responses to our questions and requests for changes. The conference would not be possible without the commitment and hard work of the MIT Conference Services staff that contributed tremendous amount of effort and energy to make sure all the logistics of the meeting ran smoothly. Our special thanks go out to Amy Hansen, who singlehandedly compiled the conference proceedings and conference program brochures, spent many hours in communications with the authors to ensure their papers are properly included in the proceedings, and handling many other aspects of the paper submission process. We also thank all the session chairs for managing and coordinating the presentations during the conference.

We thank the MICCAI Society for providing valuable input and support for the conference. We were delighted to have had a chance to organize a 10th anniversary celebration for the society. Many happy returns! Last but not least, we would like to thank all our sponsors for their kind support. Their generosity ensured the highest quality of the conference and essential support to students and young researchers.

It was our pleasure to welcome MICCAI 2014 participants to Boston. We look forward to seeing you all again next year in Munich, Germany!

September 2014

Polina Golland
Nobuhiko Hata
Christian Barillot
Joachim Hornegger
Robert Howe

Organization

General Chairs

Polina Golland   Massachusetts Institute of Technology, USA
Nobuhiko Hata   Harvard Medical School, USA

Program Chairs

Polina Golland   Massachusetts Institute of Technology, USA
Christian Barrilot   IRISA, France
Joachim Hornegger   Friedrich Alexander University,
                                  Erlangen-Nuremberg, Germany
Robert Howe   Harvard Medical School, USA

Workshop/Tutorial/Challenge Chairs

Georg Langs   Medical University of Vienna, Austria
Mehdi Moradi   University of British Columbia, Canada
Sonia Pujol   Harvard Medical School, USA
Martin Styner   University of Norther Carolina Chapel
                                  Hill, USA

Local Arrangements

MIT Conference Services

Student Liaison

Adrian Dalca   MIT, Cambridge, MA, USA

Program Committee

Purang Abolmaesumi   University of British Columbia, Canada
Stephen Aylward   Kitware, USA
Dean Barratt   University College London, UK
Dorin Comaniciu   Siemens, USA
Christos Davatzikos   University of Pennsylvania, USA
Marleen de Bruijne   Erasmus MC Rotterdam, The Netherlands
James Duncan   Yale University, USA
Randy Ellis   Queen's University, Canada
Gabor Fichtinger   Queen's University, Canada

James Gee	University of Pennsylvania, USA
Guido Gerig	University of Utah, USA
Miguel A. Gonzalez Ballester	ICREA-Universitat Pompeu Fabra, Spain
Leo Grady	HeartFlow, USA
Havit Greenspan	Tel Aviv University, Israel
Gregory D. Hager	Johns Hopkins University, USA
Ghassan Hamameh	Simon Fraser University, Canada
Ameet Jain	Philips, USA
Ron Kikinis	Harvard Medical School, USA
Ender Konukoglu	Harvard Medical School, USA
Hongen Liao	Tsinghua University, China
Huafeng Liu	Zhejiang University, China
Dimitris Metaxas	Rutgers University, USA
Mehdi Moradi	University of British Columbia, Canada
Kensaku Mori	Nagoya University, Japan
Mads Nielsen	University of North Carolina Chapel Hill, USA
Mads Neilsen	University of Copenhagen, Denmark
Wiro Niessen	Eramus MC Rotterdam, The Netherlands
Marc Niethammer	University of North Carolina Chapel Hill, USA
Xenophon Papademetris	Yale University, USA
Xavier Pennec	Inria, France
Joseine Pluim	Univeristy Medical Center Utrecht, The Netherlands
Killian Pohl	SRI International, USA
Francois Rousseau	CNRS, France
Daniel Rueckert	Imperial College London, UK
Mert Rory Sabuncu	Harvard Medical School, USA
Yoshinobu Sato	Osaka University, Japan
Julia Schnabel	University of Oxford, UK
Julia Schnabel	University of Oxford, UK
Dinggang Shen	University of North Carolina Chapel Hill, USA
Li Shen	Indiana University, USA
Kaleem Siddiqi	McGill University, Canada
Lawrence Staib	Yale University, USA
Danail Stoyanov	University College London, UK
Colin Studholme	University of Washington, USA
Gabor Szekely	ETH Zurich, Switzerland
Junichi Tokuda	Harvard Medical School, USA
Koen Van Leemput	Technical University of Denmark, Denmark
Rene Vidal	Johns Hopkins University, USA
Simon Warfield	Harvard Medical School, USA
William (Sandy) Wells	Harvard Medical School, USA
Carl-Fredrik Westin	Harvard Medical School, USA
Alistair Young	University of Auckland, New Zealand

Additional Reviewers

Abu Anas, Emran
Abugharbieh, Rafeef
Acar, Burak
Acosta-Tamayo, Oscar
Afacan, Onur
Afsari, Bijan
Aganj, Iman
Aja-Fernandez, Santiago
Akbari, Hamed
Akhondi-Asl, Alireza
Alavi, Abass
Alberola-Lopez, Carlos
Alexander, Daniel
Aljabar, Paul
Allan, Maximilian
Amini, Amir
Angelini, Elsa
Angelopoulou, Elli
Antani, Sameer
Anwander, Alfred
Arbel, Tal
Arbelaez, Pablo
Ardekani, Siamak
Arimura, Hidetaka
Arteta, Carlos
Ashburner, John
Ashraf, Ahmed
Aubert-Broche, Berengere
Audette, Michel
Auvray, Vincent
Avants, Brian
Avants, Brian
Awate, Suyash
Bach Cuadra, Meritxell
Bach Cuadra, Meritxell
Bagci, Ulas
Baka, Nora
Balicki, Marcin
Baloch, Sajjad
Barbu, Adrian
Barmpoutis, Angelos
Bartoli, Adrien
Bassett, Danielle

Batmanghelich, Kayhan
Bauer, Stefan
Baust, Maximilian
Bazin, Pierre-Louis
Bejar, Benjamin
Ben Ayed, Ismail
Bergeles, Christos
Berger, Marie-Odile
Bernardis, Elena
Betrouni, Nacim
Bharat, Shyam
Bhatia, Kanwal
Bhotika, Rahul
Bilgic, Berkin
Birkfellner, Wolfgang
Biros, George
Biros, George
Bismuth, Vincent
Boctor, Emad
Bogunovic, Hrvoje
Boisvert, Jonathan
Bossa, Matias Nicolas
Bouix, Sylvain
Boukerroui, Djamal
Bourgeat, Pierrick
Bovendeerd, Peter
Brady, Michael
Bron, Esther
Brost, Alexander
Buelow, Thomas
Buhmann, Joachim
Butakoff, Constantine
Caan, Matthan
Cabrera Lozoya, Roco
Cahill, Nathan
Cai, Weidong
Calder, Jeffrey
Camara, Oscar
Carass, Aaron
Cardenes, Ruben
Cardoso, Manuel Jorge
Carmichael, Owen
Caruyer, Emmanuel

Castellani, Umberto
Cathier, Pascal
Cattin, Philippe C.
Cepek, Jeremy
Ceresa, Mario
Cetingul, Hasan Ertan
Chakravarty, M. Mallar
Chang, Ping-Lin
Chaudhry, Rizwan
Chefd'hotel, Christophe
Chen, Elvis C. S.
Chen, Terrence
Chen, Thomas Kuiran
Chen, Ting
Cheng, Jian
Cheng, Jun
Cheriet, Farida
Chinzei, Kiyoyuki
Christensen, Gary
Chung, Albert C. S.
Chung, Moo
Cinquin, Philippe
Ciompi, Francesco
Ciuciu, Philippe
Clancy, Neil T.
Claridge, Ela
Clarkson, Matthew
Clarysse, Patrick
Claus, Piet
Clemmesen, Line
Cobzas, Dana
Collins, D. Louis
Colliot, Olivier
Commowick, Olivier
Cook, Philip
Cootes, Tim
Cordier, Nicolas
Corso, Jason
Counsell, Serena J.
Coupe, Pierrick
Cowan, Brett
Crane, Jason
Criminisi, Antonio
Crum, William
Cuingnet, Remi

Daga, Pankaj
Dalca, Adrian
Darkner, Sune
Das, Sandhitsu
Dauguet, Julien
Dawant, Benoit
De Craene, Mathieu
De Raedt, Sepp
Dehghan, Ehsan
Deligianni, Fani
Delingette, Herve
Demirci, Stefanie
Denney, Tom
Dequidt, Jeremie
Descoteaux, Maxime
Desjardins, Adrien
D'hooge, Jan
Di Battista, Andrew
Dijkstra, Jouke
DiMaio, Simon
Ding, Kai
Dojat, Michel
Donner, Rene
Drew, Mark
Du Bois d'Aische, Aloys
Duchateau, Nicolas
Duchesnay, Edouard
Duchesne, Simon
Duda, Jeffrey
Duits, Remco
Duriez, Christian
Dzyubachyk, Oleh
Eavani, Harini
Ebrahimi, Mehran
Edwards, Philip
Ehrhardt, Jan
Eklund, Anders
El-Baz, Ayman
Elson, Daniel
El-Zehiry, Noha
Erdt, Marius
Erus, Guray
Fahrig, Rebecca
Falco, Alexandre
Fallavollita, Pascal

Fang, Ruogu
Farag, Aly
Fedorov, Andriy
Fenster, Aaron
Feragen, Aasa
Figl, Michael
Fishbaugh, James
Fitzpatrick, J. Michael
Fletcher, P. Thomas
Florack, Luc
Foroughi, Pezhman
Fradkin, Maxim
Freiman, Moti
Freysinger, Wolfgang
Fripp, Jurgen
Fritscher, Karl
Fua, Pascal
Fuerst, Bernhard
Funka-Lea, Gareth
Funke, Jan
Gangeh, Mehrdad
Ganz, Melanie
Gao, Fei
Gao, Mingchen
Gao, Wei
Gao, Yaozong
Gao, Yi
Gaonkar, Bilwaj
Garcia-Lorenzo, Daniel
Garvin, Mona
Gaser, Christian
Ge, Tian
Georgescu, Bogdan
Geremia, Ezequiel
Ghanbari, Yasser
Gholipour, Ali
Ghosh, Aurobrata
Ghosh, Satrajit
Ghosh, Subham
Giannarou, Stamatia
Gibaud, Bernard
Gibson, Eli
Gilbert, Stephen
Gilles, Benjamin
Ginsburg, Shoshana

Giusti, Alessandro
Glocker, Ben
Goh, Alvina
Goksel, Orcun
Goldberger, Jacob
Goni Cortes, Joaquin
Gooya, Ali
Graham, Jim
Grbic, Sasa
Grisan, Enrico
Grova, Christophe
Guetter, Christoph
Guevara, Pamela
Gulsun, Mehmet Akif
Guo, Yanrong
Gur, Yaniv
Gutman, Boris
Hacihaliloglu, Ilker
Haidegger, Tamas
Haj-Hosseini, Neda
Hajnal, Joseph
Hamamci, Andac
Hammers, Alexander
Han, Lianghao
Haneishi, Hideaki
Hastreiter, Peter
Hatt, Chuck
Hauta-Kasari, Markku
Hawkes, David
Haynor, David
He, Huiguang
He, Tiancheng
Heckemann, Rolf
Heimann, Tobias
Heinrich, Mattias Paul
Helmstaedter, Moritz
Heng, Pheng Ann
Hennemuth, Anja
Hermosillo, Gerardo
Hibar, Derrek
Hipwell, John
Ho, Harvey
Holmes, David
Holmes, Jeff
Hong, Byung-Woo

Hontani, Hidekata
Hoogendoorn, Corne
Hu, Chenhui
Hu, Mingxing
Hu, Yipeng
Hu, Zhihong
Hua, Xue
Huang, Heng
Huang, Junzhou
Huang, Xiaojie
Huang, Xiaolei
Huisman, Henkjan
Ibrahim, El-Sayed
Iglesias, Juan Eugenio
Ingalhalikar, Madhura
Iordachita, Iulian
Jacobs, Colin
Jafari-Khouzani, Kourosh
Jagadeesan, Jayender
Jain, Saurabh
Jannin, Pierre
Janoos, Firdaus
Janowczyk, Andrew
Ji, Shuiwang
Jiang, Menglin
Jiang, Yifeng
Jolly, Marie-Pierre
Jomier, Julien
Jones, Geoffrey
Jordan, Petr
Joshi, Anand
Joshi, Gopal Datt
Joshi, Sarang
Joung, Sanghyun
Kabus, Sven
Kachelrie, Marc
Kadoury, Samuel
Kahl, Fredrik
Kainmueller, Dagmar
Kakadiaris, Ioannis
Kapoor, Ankur
Kapur, Tina
Karacali, Bilge
Karssemeijer, Nico
Keeve, Erwin

Kelm, Michael
Kerrien, Erwan
Khallaghi, Siavash
Khan, Ali
Kharazmi, Pegah
Kherif, Ferath
Khurd, Parmeshwar
Kim, Boklye
Kim, Minjeong
Kindlmann, Gordon
King, Andrew
Kiraly, Atilla
Kirisli, Hortense
Kitasaka, Takayuki
Klein, Stefan
Klein, Tassilo
Klinder, Tobias
Knutsson, Hans
Koizumi, Norihiro
Kowalewski, Timothy
Krause, Oswin
Krieger, Axel
Kunz, Manuela
Kwitt, Roland
Kwon, Dongjin
Lotjonen, Jyrki
Ladikos, Alexander
Laine, Andrew
Lam, Fan
Lamata, Pablo
Landman, Bennett
Lang, Pencilla
Langerak, Thomas
Langs, Georg
Lapeer, Rudy
Larsen, Anders Boesen Lindbo
Lartizien, Carole
Lasser, Tobias
Lasso, Andras
Lauze, Francois
Law, Max W.K.
Le, Yen
Lecoeur, Jeremy
Lee, Junghoon
Lee, Su-Lin

Lefevre, Julien
Lefkimmiatis, Stamatis
Le Folgoc, Loc
Lekadir, Karim
Lelieveldt, Boudewijn
Lendvay, Thomas
Lenglet, Christophe
Lepore, Natasha
Lesage, David
Li, Chunming
Li, Fuhai
Li, Gang
Li, Jiang
Li, Quanzheng
Li, Yang
Liao, Rui
Lillholm, Martin
Lin, Henry
Lindner, Claudia
Linguraru, Marius George
Linte, Cristian
Litjens, Geert
Liu, David
Liu, Jiamin
Liu, Jianfei
Liu, Sidong
Liu, Xiaoxiao
Liu, Yixun
Lo, Benny
Lombaert, Herve
Lorenz, Cristian
Lorenzi, Marco
Lu, Le
Lu, Shijian
Lu, Xiaoguang
Luan, K.
Lui, Lok Ming
Luo, Xiongbiao
Lyksborg, Mark
Muller, Henning
Machiraju, Raghu
Maddah, Mahnaz
Madooei, Ali
Mahapatra, Dwarikanath
Mahdavi, Seyedeh Sara

Maier-Hein, Lena
Mailhe, Boris
Majumdar, Angshul
Malandain, Gregoire
Malgouyres, Francois
Manduca, Armando
Manjon, Jose V.
Manniesing, Rashindra
Mansi, Tommaso
Marchal, Maud
Marchesseau, Stephanie
Margeta, Jan
Mari, Jean-Martial
Mariottini, Gian Luca
Marsland, Stephen
Marti, Robert
Martel, Anne
Martin-Fernandez, Marcos
Masamune, Ken
Masutani, Yoshitaka
Mateus, Diana
Mattes, Julian
McClelland, Jamie
McCulloch, Andrew
McIntosh, Chris
Mcleod, Kristin
Medrano-Gracia, Pau
Mendrik, Adrienne
Menze, Bjoern
Metz, Coert
Meyer, Chuck
Michailovich, Oleg
Miga, Michael
Mihalef, Viorel
Miller, James
Miller, Karol
Mirzaalian, Hengameh
Mirzaee, Hanieh
Modat, Marc
Moghari, Mehdi
Mohamed, Ashraf
Mohareri, Omid
Momayyez, Parya
Montillo, Albert
Moore, John

Mountney, Peter
Murphy, Keelin
Nabavi, Arya
Najman, Laurent
Nakamura, Ryoichi
Nakamura, Yoshihiko
Nasiriavanaki, Mohammadreza
Navab, Nassir
Neumuth, Thomas
Ng, Bernard
Nguyen, Hian
Nichols, Thomas
Nicolau, Stephane
Nie, Jingxin
Niederer, Steven
Nielsen, Poul
Noble, Alison
Noble, Jack
Noblet, Vincent
Nolte, Lutz
Nordsletten, David
Nouranian, Saman
Nugroho, Hermawan
Oda, Masahiro
O'Donnell, Lauren
O'Donnell, Thomas
Ofli, Ferda
Oliver, Arnau
Onofrey, John
Orihuela-Espina, Felipe
Otake, Yoshito
Ou, Yangming
Pace, Danielle
Padfield, Dirk
Padoy, Nicolas
Pallavaram, Srivatsan
Pant, Sanjay
Parisot, Sarah
Park, JinHyeong
Parthasarathy, Vijay
Pasternak, Ofer
Patriciu, Alexandru
Paul, Perrine
Paulsen, Rasmus
Pauly, Olivier

Pavlidis, Ioannis
Peitgen, Heinz-Otto
Penney, Graeme
Pernus, Franjo
Peterlik, Igor
Peters, Jochen
Peters, Terry M.
Petersen, Jens
Petersen, Jens
Petersen, Kersten
Petitjean, Caroline
Peyrat, Jean-Marc
Pham, Dzung
Piella, Gemma
Pitiot, Alain
Piuze, Emmanuel
Pizer, Stephen
Plenge, Esben
Poline, Jean-Baptiste
Poot, Dirk
Pop, Mihaela
Poulsen, Catherine
Prasad, Gautam
Prastawa, Marcel
Pratt, Philip
Prevost, Raphael
Price, Brian
Price, True
Prince, Jerry
Punithakumar, Kumaradevan
Qazi, Arish A.
Qi, Jinyi
Qian, Xiaoning
Qian, Zhen
Qiu, Wu
Radeva, Petia
Rafii-Tari, Hedyeh
Raj, Ashish
Rajagopalan, Vidya
Rajchl, Martin
Rajpoot, Nasir
Raju, Balasundar
Ramezani, Mahdi
Rapaka, Saikiran
Rathi, Yogesh

Ravichandran, Avinash
Reader, Andrew
Reiley, Carol
Reinertsen, Ingerid
Reisert, Marco
Reiter, Austin
Reyes, Mauricio
Rhode, Kawal
Richa, Rogrio
Riddell, Cyrill
Riklin Raviv, Tammy
Risholm, Petter
Risser, Laurent
Rit, Simon
Rivaz, Hassan
Riviere, Denis
Robert, Jean-luc
Roche, Alexis
Rohlfing, Torsten
Rohling, Robert
Rohr, Karl
Roth, Holger
Roysam, Badrinath
Russakoff, Daniel
Sorensen, Lauge
Saad, Ahmed
Sakuma, Ichiro
Salcudean, Tim
Salvado, Olivier
San Jose Estepar, Raul
Sanchez, Clarisa
Sands, Greg
Sarrut, David
Sarry, Laurent
Sarunic, Marinko
Savadjiev, Peter
Schaap, Michiel
Scheinost, Dustin
Scherrer, Benoit
Schmidt, Frank
Schmidt-Richberg, Alexander
Schneider, Caitlin
Schroeder, Peter
Schuh, Andreas
Schultz, Thomas

Schweikard, Achim
Seiler, Christof
Seitel, Alexander
Sermesant, Maxime
Seshamani, Sharmishtaa
Shahzad, Rahil
Shamir, Reuben R.
Sharma, Puneet
Shi, Feng
Shi, Kuangyu
Shi, Wenzhe
Shi, Yonggang
Shi, Yonghong
Shinohara, Russell T.
Shou, Guofa
Sijbers, Jan
Simon, Duchesne
Simpson, Amber
Simpson, Ivor
Singh, Nikhil
Singh, Vikas
Singh, Vivek
Sivaswamy, Jayanthi
Smeets, Dirk
Song, Gang
Song, Qi
Sotiras, Aristeidis
Sparks, Rachel
Speidel, Stefanie
Sporring, Jon
Spottiswoode, Bruce
Stuhmer, Jan
Stamm, Aymeric
Staring, Marius
Stetten, George
Stewart, Charles
Stewart, James
Styles, Iain
Styner, Martin
Su, Baiquan
Subramanian, Navneeth
Suinesiaputra, Avan
Suk, Heung-Il
Summers, Ronald
Sundar, Hari

Syeda-Mahmood, Tanveer
Szkulmowski, Maciej
Sznitman, Raphael
Tahmasebi, Amir
Taimouri,Vahid
Tamaki, Toru
Tan, Chaowei
Tanner, Christine
Taquet, Maxime
Tasdizen, Tolga
Taylor, Russell
Taylor, Zeike
Tek, Huseyin
Thirion, Bertrand
Thodberg, Hans Henrik
Thompson, Stephen
Tiwari, Pallavi
Tobon-Gomez, Catalina
Toews, Matthew
Tosun, Duygu
Totz, Johannes
Toussaint, Nicolas
Treeby, Bradley
Troccaz, Jocelyne
Tustison, Nicholas
Twining, Carole
Ukwatta, Eranga
Unal, Gozde
Uzunbas, Mustafa
Vaillant, Regis
Van Assen, Hans
Van de Ven, Wendy
Van Ginneken, Bram
Van Rikxoort, Eva
Van Walsum, Theo
Vannier, Michael
Varoquaux, Gael
Vegas-Sanchez-Ferrero, Gonzalo
Vemuri, Baba
Venkataraman, Archana
Vercauteren, Tom
Vialard, Francois-Xavier
Vignon, Francois
Vik, Torbjorrn
Villard, Pierre-Frederic

Visentini-Scarzanella, Marco
Viswanath, Satish
Vitaladevuni, Shiv
Vitanovski, Dime
Vogelstein, Joshua
Voigt, Ingmar
Von Berg, Jens
Voros, Sandrine
Vos, Pieter
Vosburgh, Kirby
Vrooman, Henri
Vrtovec, Tomaz
Wachinger, Christian
Waelkens, Paulo
Wan, Catherine
Wang, Chaohui
Wang, Hongzhi
Wang, Junchen
Wang, Li
Wang, Liansheng
Wang, Linwei
Wang, Qiu
Wang, Shijun
Wang, Song
Wang, Vicky
Wang, Yalin
Wang, Yinhai
Wang, Yu-Ping
Washio, Toshikatsu
Wassermann, Demian
Wee, Chong-Yaw
Weese, Jurgen
Wei, Liu
Wein, Wolfgang
Wels, Michael
Werner, Rene
Wesarg, Stefan
Whitaker, Ross
Whitmarsh, Tristan
Wiles, Andrew
Wilson, Nathan
Wittek, Adam
Wolz, Robin
Wong, Ken C.L.
Wong, Stephen

Wright, Graham
Wu, Guorong
Wu, John Jue
Wu, Wen
Wu, Xiaodong
Xie, Yuchen
Xing, Fuyong
Xu, Xiao Yun
Xu, Yanwu
Xu, Ziyue
Xue, Zhong
Yan, Pingkun
Yan, Zhennan
Yang, Liangjing
Yang, Lin
Yaniv, Ziv
Yao, Jianhua
Yap, Pew-Thian
Yaqub, Mohammad
Ye, Dong Hye
Yeo, B.T. Thomas
Yin, Youbing
Yin, Zhaozheng
Yokota, Futoshi
Yoshida, Hiro
Yushkevich, Paul
Zeng, Haishan
Zeng, Wei

Zhan, Liang
Zhan, Yiqiang
Zhang, Daoqiang
Zhang, Hui
Zhang, Pei
Zhang, shaoting
Zhang, Zhijun
Zhao, Qian
Zheng, Guoyan
Zheng, Yefeng
Zheng, Yuanjie
Zhou, Jian
Zhou, Jinghao
Zhou, Kevin
Zhou, Luping
Zhou, X. Sean
Zhou, Yan
Zhu, Dajiang
Zhu, Hongtu
Zhu, Yuemin
Zhuang, Xiahai
Zijdenbos, Alex
Zikic, Darko
Zollei, Lilla
Zuluaga, Maria A.
Zwiggelaar, Reyer

Table of Contents – Part I

Microstructure Imaging

Image Reconstruction and Enhancement

Registration

Segmentation I

Intervention Planning and Guidance I

Oncology

Optical Imaging

Segmentation II

Erratum

Table of Contents – Part II

Biophysical Modeling and Simulation

Temporal and Motion Modeling

Computer-Aided Diagnosis

Pediatric Imaging

Endoscopy

Ultrasound Imaging

Machine Learning I

Cardiovascular Imaging

Intervention Planning and Guidance II

Brain I

Table of Contents – Part III

Shape and Population Analysis

Brain II

Diffusion MRI

Machine Learning II

Leveraging Random Forests for Interactive Exploration of Large Histological Images

Loïc Peter[1], Diana Mateus[1,2], Pierre Chatelain[1,3], Noemi Schworm[4],
Stefan Stangl[4], Gabriele Multhoff[4,5], and Nassir Navab[1,6]

[1] Computer Aided Medical Procedures, Technische Universität München, Germany
[2] Institute of Computational Biology, Helmholtz Zentrum München, Germany
[3] Université de Rennes 1, IRISA, France
[4] Department of Radiation Oncology, Technische Universität München, Germany
[5] CCG - Innate Immunity in Tumor Biology, Helmholtz Zentrum München, Germany
[6] Computer Aided Medical Procedures, Johns Hopkins University, USA

Abstract. The large size of histological images combined with their very challenging appearance are two main difficulties which considerably complicate their analysis. In this paper, we introduce an interactive strategy leveraging the output of a supervised random forest classifier to guide a user through such large visual data. Starting from a forest-based pixelwise estimate, subregions of the images at hand are automatically ranked and sequentially displayed according to their expected interest. After each region suggestion, the user selects among several options a rough estimate of the true amount of foreground pixels in this region. From these one-click inputs, the region scoring function is updated in real time using an online gradient descent procedure, which corrects on-the-fly the shortcomings of the initial model and adapts future suggestions accordingly. Experimental validation is conducted for extramedullary hematopoesis localization and demonstrates the practical feasibility of the procedure as well as the benefit of the online adaptation strategy.

1 Introduction

Analyzing histological images is usually an extremely challenging task. Due to the complex appearance of objects of interest, the accuracy of fully-automatic techniques is generally insufficient for clinical use, e.g. in the case of mitosis detection [1] for which a variety of automatic approaches has been recently compared quantitatively [2]. In fact, the accurate identification of patterns within such images is often only achievable by well-trained human experts and remains prone to inter-experts disagreements in some cases [3]. Moreover, histological data are very tedious to process for a human because of their large dimension, which commonly reaches tens of thousands of pixels along each direction. When aiming at finding rare objects within images of this size, a manual search for these instances requires a painstaking exploration of the whole content, and a huge amount of time is spent scrolling through uninteresting background areas.

To overcome this, we propose to leverage fully-automatic pixelwise classification techniques to recover candidate areas of interest (i.e. where positive

P. Golland et al. (Eds.): MICCAI 2014, Part I, LNCS 8673, pp. 1–8, 2014.

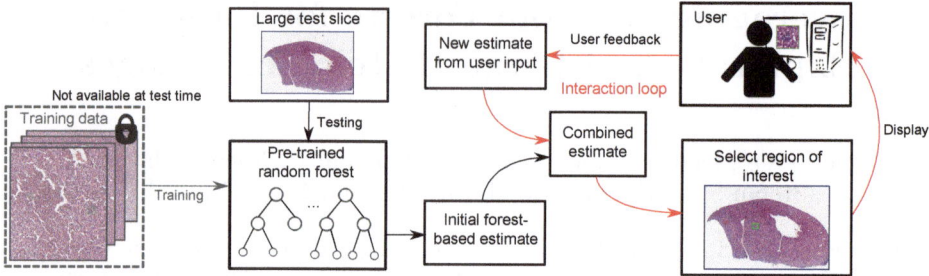

Fig. 1. Summary of our approach

instances are found), leaving the task of interpreting the visual content within these regions to an expert user. To this end, assuming that an available automatic method provides a label confidence at each pixel, an intuitive strategy would be to rank subregions of the images in decreasing order of confidence and display them accordingly one after the other. Having thereby patterns of interest shown early in the process, an exhaustive search would not be necessary anymore. However, such a scenario relies entirely on the accuracy of the automatic detector and can fail if the latter suffers from difficulties on the images at hand. In the case of detectors based on supervised learning procedures, difficulties may arise due to the common mismatches between the training and test data, caused by e.g. differences in noise or illumination. In this context, it would be beneficial to allow the user to interact after each suggestion (in particular after wrong ones) so that the procedure can be adapted to the characteristics of the test data and eventually avoid mistakes for the upcoming region suggestions.

Online transfer learning (OTL) frameworks [4,5] address this problem by combining (i) a kernel-based classifier pre-trained on some source data, and (ii) an online classifier continuously trained on arriving instances from the target data, given by the user input in our case. On the closely related problem of domain adaptation, an unsupervised algorithm based on Gaussian process regression was introduced to adapt the decision boundary of a face detector to a test image [6]. In the case of medical data, random forest classifiers [7,8] demonstrated high accuracy and tractability and are especially used for their ability to handle high amounts of training data and descriptors. Although an online version of random forests exists in the literature [9], replacing the kernel classifiers of the OTL approach by forests is not straightforward: only few samples are available to train the target classifier, and a forest-based OTL scheme would handle the source classifier as a whole, without exploiting the diversity and possibly heterogeneous relevance of its local models on the target data.

In this work, we introduce a regression-based method able to leverage the knowledge carried by a pre-trained random forest classifier to guide the user through the data by suggesting candidate regions of interest. Our approach exploits the multiple partitionings of the feature space defined by the trained forest to perform local updates of the model from one-click inputs provided by the user.

Thereby, characteristics of the test data can be captured and future suggestions are adapted accordingly. These updates are performed in real time between two iterations and do not require the original training data, which makes our method particularly tractable for clinical use. Experimental evaluation is conducted on a high-resolution dataset for hematopoesis identification within mouse liver slices, as well as on synthetic deformations of it, and demonstrates the general feasibility of our approach and the benefit of the adaption scheme.

2 Methods

We first summarize the general scenario of our approach. Let us consider a given set of images composed of pixels. Each pixel $\mathbf{p}$ has a true label $y(\mathbf{p}) \in \{0, 1\}$ and we aim at detecting the positive instances within our images, i.e. the pixels $\mathbf{p}$ such that $y(\mathbf{p}) = 1$. We make the assumption that a random forest classifier has been trained beforehand on some available labeled data and hence provides a probability $P^{\mathrm{RF}}(y(\mathbf{p}) = 1) \in [0, 1]$ for each pixel $\mathbf{p}$. Here, we implicitly assume that this forest has been originally designed for a binary classification task, but any multi-class forest could also be used by grouping as positive the labels considered as interesting for the given application. For tractability, the original training data is not made available during the whole process and is thus only encoded through this forest. In our scenario, a user runs this classifier which is based on prior data on a new set of images that are correlated but potentially slightly different, e.g. because of different imaging conditions. From the resulting pixelwise output, an area of interest, expected to contain positive labels, is then displayed to the user, who provides in return an estimate of the proportion of positive pixels actually observed. In doing so, the bias of the initial model can be progressively assessed and compensated to ultimately increase the relevance of the upcoming region suggestions.

Under these conditions, we can formalize our scenario mathematically. The test images are partitioned into a set of rectangular regions $\mathcal{R} = \{R_1, \ldots, R_n\}$ whose sizes are tractable for a human user. At iteration k, i.e. after the user saw $k - 1$ regions, we proceed as follows:

1. The region $\hat{R} \in \mathcal{R}$, maximizing a scoring function $\phi_k : \mathcal{R} \to \mathbb{R}$ stating the expected relevance of each region, is displayed to the user.
2. The user interacts to provide information about the content observed in $\hat{R}$.
3. Using this feedback, ϕ_k is updated, resulting in a new scoring function ϕ_{k+1}.
4. $\hat{R}$ is removed from the pool of candidate regions $\mathcal{R}$.

The initial scoring function ϕ_1 is based on the initial random forest classifier only. We summarize the random forest model in Sec. 2.1. In Sec. 2.2, we expose our choice of scoring functions ϕ_k and how they can be parametrized. Finally, the update strategy of ϕ_k from the user inputs is described in Sec. 2.3.

2.1 Random Forest Model

Our approach uses a trained random forest classifier as starting point, which provides for each pixel $\mathbf{p}$ a probability of being a positive instance. A random forest is a collection of T decorrelated binary decision trees. Each tree (indexed by $t \in \{1, \ldots, T\}$) is a hierarchical collection of decision rules based on visual features, leading to a partition of the domain into $l(t)$ leaves $\mathcal{L}_{t,1}, \ldots, \mathcal{L}_{t,l(t)}$. Each leaf $\mathcal{L}_{t,i}$ contains a probability model $\pi_{t,i} \in [0,1]$. For each tree t, every newly observed pixel $\mathbf{p}$ reaches exactly one leaf, and we will denote $\pi_t(\mathbf{p})$ the corresponding probabilistic model. Averaging over trees, the final pixelwise probability provided by the random forest for each pixel $\mathbf{p}$ is

$$P^{\text{RF}}(y(\mathbf{p}) = 1) = \frac{1}{T} \sum_{t=1}^{T} \pi_t(\mathbf{p}) \,. \tag{1}$$

We follow the standard procedure [7,8] to train such a classifier, i.e. to infer the decision rules and the leaf models. Starting from a root node, the decision rules are recursively chosen within a set of randomly drawn splitting functions to maximize an information gain criterion. The proportion of positive training samples contained in a leaf defines its probabilistic model.

2.2 Region Scoring Function

In this subsection, we describe our region scoring model. Given a pixelwise estimate $P_k(y(\mathbf{p}) = 1)$ at iteration k, we define the relevance of a region $R \in \mathcal{R}$ as the expectation of the proportion of positive pixels in R. Modeling the pixel labels as independent Bernoulli distributions of success probability $P_k(y(\mathbf{p}) = 1)$, this expectation and hence the scoring function ϕ_k can be written as

$$\phi_k(R) = \frac{1}{|R|} \sum_{\mathbf{p} \in R} P_k(y(\mathbf{p}) = 1) \,, \tag{2}$$

where $|R|$ denotes the number of pixels in the region R. In this work, we would like to define the pixelwise probabilistic model P_k as a combination of (i) the prior knowledge acquired on training data that is encoded by the initial random forest classifier, and (ii) the $k - 1$ inputs provided by the user based on the test data. Therefore, we propose to obtain $P_k(y(\mathbf{p}) = 1)$ from the forest estimate of Eq. 1 by adding to each prior leaf model $\pi_{t,i}$ a signed offset $\epsilon_{t,i}^k \in \mathbb{R}$ whose value will be progressively adapted from the user inputs. Let us denote ϵ_k the vector $(\epsilon_{t,i}^k)_{t,i}$ and rewrite the scoring function $\phi_k(R)$ as $\phi(R|\epsilon_k)$ so that this parametrization clearly appears. Introducing this additive model in Eq. 2 and after some algebraic manipulations, the scoring function can be rewritten as

$$\phi(R|\epsilon_k) = \phi^{\text{RF}}(R) + \phi^{\text{new}}(R|\epsilon_k) \,, \tag{3}$$

where $\phi^{\text{RF}}(R)$ is obtained by using the forest probabilistic output (Eq. 1) as pixelwise model in Eq. 2, and

$$\phi^{\text{new}}(R|\epsilon_k) = \frac{1}{|R|} \frac{1}{T} \sum_{t=1}^{T} \sum_{i=1}^{l(t)} \epsilon_{t,i}^k h_{t,i}(R) = \langle \mathbf{r}, \epsilon_k \rangle \,. \tag{4}$$

In Eq. 4, $h_{t,i}(R)$ denotes the number of pixels $\mathbf{p}$ in R which reached the leaf $\mathcal{L}_{t,i}$, and $\mathbf{r} = (\frac{1}{|R|}\frac{1}{T}h_{t,i}(R))_{t,i}$. Before the user starts providing inputs, the $\epsilon_{t,i}^1$ are set to 0 such that $\phi_1 = \phi^{\text{RF}}$. As the user gives information after each suggestion, the acquired knowledge is encoded through the leaf-dependent $\epsilon_{t,i}^k$ that allow the scoring function ϕ_k to vary around the initial model ϕ^{RF}. The next subsection describes how these $\epsilon_{t,i}^k$ are inferred from the collected user feedbacks.

2.3 Online Model Update

After each suggestion of a region R_j, a feedback $\mathcal{P}^{\text{user}}(R_j) \in [0,1]$ stating the true proportion of positive pixels in R_j is requested from the user. We assume for the sake of formalism that the exact proportion is given, but we will demonstrate in our experiments that providing a discretized approximation of this input does not decrease the performance (Tab. 1). This reduces drastically the necessary amount of interaction, since giving a discrete estimate of this proportion requires only one click from the user, whereas computing the exact value would involve a pixelwise region labeling. Note that this feedback does not provide any information at pixel level and hence excludes a direct update of the leaf statistics [9].

Assuming that k regions $R_1, \ldots, R_k$ have been suggested and their respective user inputs $\mathcal{P}^{\text{user}}(R_1), \ldots, \mathcal{P}^{\text{user}}(R_k)$ collected ($k \geq 1$), we would like to find a new scoring function ϕ_{k+1}, or equivalently a coefficient vector ϵ_{k+1}, which matches with these k user inputs. Considering a squared loss function, we solve the following minimization problem

$$\epsilon_{k+1} = \underset{\epsilon}{\operatorname{argmin}} \sum_{j=1}^{k} (\phi(R_j|\epsilon) - \mathcal{P}^{\text{user}}(R_j))^2 + \lambda \|\epsilon\|^2 \,, \tag{5}$$

which can be rewritten from Eq. 3 and Eq. 4 as a linear ridge regression problem

$$\epsilon_{k+1} = \underset{\epsilon}{\operatorname{argmin}} \sum_{j=1}^{k} (\langle \mathbf{r}_j, \epsilon \rangle - \delta_j)^2 + \lambda \|\epsilon\|^2 \,, \tag{6}$$

where $\delta_j = \mathcal{P}^{\text{user}}(R_j) - \phi^{\text{RF}}(R_j)$. The regularization term aims at keeping the deviation from the initial random forest classifier small and is driven by a hyper-parameter λ. The minimization problem defined by Eq. 6 is equivalent to a linear ridge regression problem with k training instances of feature vectors $\mathbf{r}_1, \ldots, \mathbf{r}_k$ and labels $\delta_1, \ldots, \delta_k$, i.e. a regression problem at the region level. As a consequence, Eq. 6 could be naturally extended to a kernel ridge regression problem if one desires to remove the linearity assumption. The solution ϵ_{k+1} of Eq. 6 can be found in closed form [10]. However, computing this exact value at each iteration involves the computationally expensive inversion of a large matrix, which could force a user to wait between two suggestions of regions. Instead, we adopt an online gradient descent scheme [11] leading to the following incremental update rule:

$$\epsilon_{k+1} = \epsilon_k - \frac{1}{\lambda} (\langle \mathbf{r}_k, \epsilon_k \rangle - \delta_k) \mathbf{r}_k \,. \tag{7}$$

Thereby, the kth user input can be incorporated in real time in our model.

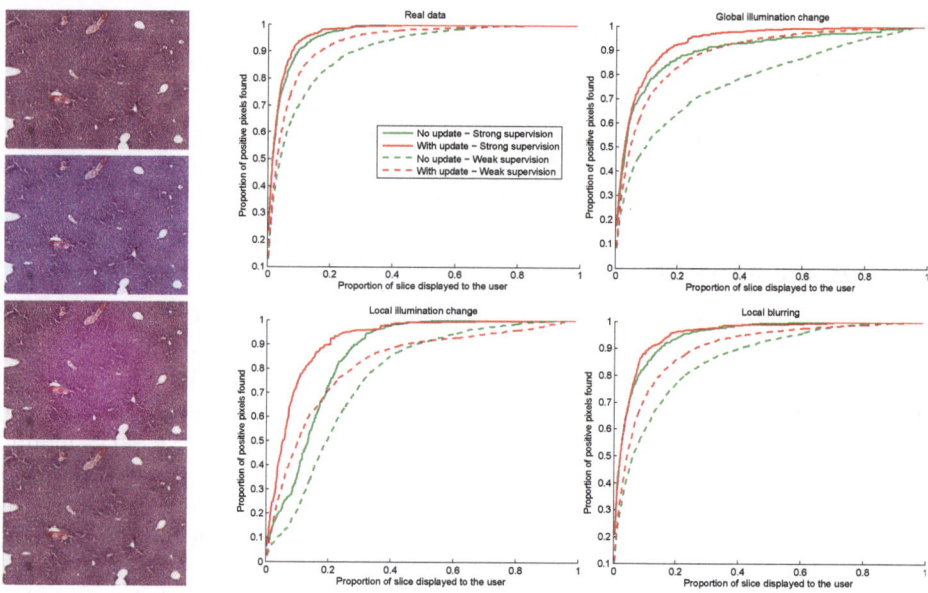

Fig. 2. Results. The curves display the average proportion of recovered positive pixels as a function of the proportion of the slice shown to the user. These experiments are driven under different synthetic conditions, examples of which are shown on the left. From top to bottom: real image, global illumination change, local illumination change, local blurring. The discretized version of the user input was used in these experiments.

3   Experiments

Dataset: Extramedullary hematopoesis, i.e. hematopoesis located outside of the bone marrow, is a rare event in human adults. Yet, in some animals like mice, its presence in the liver can be a reaction to an immense inflammation or to a tumor stimulating extensively the immune system of the organism [12]. Localizing these relatively small lesions as well as estimating their number can be useful to compare the influence of different therapeutic strategies. 34 high-resolution images entirely labeled at pixel level were extracted from 8 mouse liver slices of resolution 0.498 μm/pixel. This restriction to subimages was necessary to obtain accurate labels from a pathologist, since a slice is typically too big (34200×21052 pixels) to be labeled entirely. Since images taken from a same slice share common visual properties, we kept them together for training or testing. Images were downsized by a factor 3 to speed up the training and testing procedures.

Experimental Setup: We performed our experiments at two levels of supervision: (i) a standard leave-one-out strategy (*strong supervision*), where the initial random forest is trained on 7 slices (i.e. approximately 30 images) and tested on the 8th one, and (ii) the inverse setting where one trains only on one slice and tests on the 7 others (*weak supervision*). While the second scenario is plausible

Table 1. Area under the curves in our different settings

	Weak supervision											
	Real data			Global change			Local change			Local blurring		
	Min	Median	Max	Min	Median	Max	Min	Median	Max	Min	Median	Max
No update	82.5	90.9	95.9	63.8	77.0	95.7	56.2	76.4	81.8	78.7	83.7	93.8
Exact input	87.6	92.2	96.1	74.4	87.8	95.7	62.9	82.8	91.6	78.0	86.1	94.1
Discretized input	88.5	92.3	96.1	74.6	87.7	95.9	64.0	83.9	91.6	77.9	86.3	94.1

	Strong supervision											
	Real data			Global change			Local change			Local blurring		
	Min	Median	Max	Min	Median	Max	Min	Median	Max	Min	Median	Max
No update	94.1	96.6	97.7	71.1	93.1	97.1	78.5	85.4	92.7	91.2	95.4	96.0
Exact input	94.7	96.7	98.1	89.1	93.6	97.2	83.2	91.9	95.0	92.4	95.8	97.1
Discretized input	94.8	96.7	98.3	88.9	93.7	97.4	82.8	91.9	95.0	92.4	95.6	97.0

in practical situations due to the difficulty of obtaining pixelwise labels, it also suggests another application of our approach as a way to facilitate collecting hard-to-find positive samples to enrich an existing weak training set. Training samples were collected on a regular grid of step 30, resulting in approximately 500 k instances in the leave-one-out setup. Each pixel was described by its visual content at offset locations. We used the CIELab color space that we enriched with the output of a bank of filters [13]. 40 trees were grown without depth limit but with at least 10 training samples per leaf. The images were partitioned into regions of size 123×123 pixels, which fits to the size of usual hematopoesis patterns. If a hematopoesis pattern is not fully included in a displayed region, the field of view can be extended with a simple click revealing the next adjacent region in the indicated direction. We investigated ways to handle pools of regions of heterogeneous sizes, but this raised issues in terms of scoring function (finding a reliable rule that does not always favor the smallest or the largest regions is not straightforward) and evaluation. The retained solution requires almost no effort from the user and eventually seemed to be the most practical one.

Evaluation: Our approach aims at performing an interactive online adaptation to new imaging conditions, and more generally to mismatches between training and test data. The aforementioned weakly supervised scenario favors naturally such a bias, since training on only one slice is unlikely to generalize well. To go further into this direction, we propose, as additional experiments, to keep the initial training sets and apply three types of synthetic modifications on the test images to simulate classical difficulties occurring in histological imaging: (i) global illumination change, (ii) local illumination change, and (iii) local blurring. These changes were randomly generated on each image. To evaluate our method, we studied the average proportion of positive pixels recovered over time (Fig. 2) and measured the area under these curves (Tab. 1). The results demonstrate that our update framework allows a faster retrieval of interesting areas. As mentioned in Sec. 2.3, we also show that discretizing the user input into 7 predefined bins (i.e. enforcing $P^{\text{user}}(R_j) \in \{0, 0.1, 0.3, \ldots, 0.9, 1\}$) does not reduce the performance and thus lightens the user interaction. Finally, in the leave-one-out setting on real data, we assessed the influence of the parameter λ (Eq. 6). From

Eq. 7, low (resp. high) values of λ are expected to lead to numerical instabilities (resp. negligible updates). These asymptotic behaviors were experimentally observed for $\lambda \leq 0.05$ and $\lambda \geq 100$, respectively. Between these two extremes, a wide range of values of λ led to improvements, and we chose $\lambda = 1$ for simplicity.

4   Conclusion

We proposed an interactive method able to suggest sequentially regions of interest within large data from the output of a pre-trained random forest classifier at pixel level. After each suggestion, one-click user inputs are collected to capture the specificities of the images at hand and update the region scoring function accordingly and in real time *via* an online gradient descent scheme. We evaluated our approach in the context of hematopoesis localization, with and without synthetic deformations simulating common sources of variability in histological imaging. As future work, we would like to extend our method to mitosis detection tasks [2] and generalize it to 2D video sequences and 3D volumes.

Acknowledgments. This work was partially supported by the DFG-funded Collaborative Research Centre 824: "Imaging for Selection, Monitoring and Individualization of Cancer Therapies".

References

1. Veta, M., Pluim, J., van Diest, P., Viergever, M.: Breast cancer histopathology image analysis: A review. IEEE Transactions on Biomedical Engineering (2014)
2. http://amida13.isi.uu.nl/
3. Crowley, R.S., Naus, G.J., Stewart, J., Friedman, C.P.: Development of visual diagnostic expertise in pathology - an information-processing study. Journal of the American Medical Informatics Association 10(1), 39–51 (2003)
4. Zhao, P., Hoi, S.C.: OTL: A framework of online transfer learning. In: Proceedings of the 27th International Conference on Machine Learning, pp. 1231–1238 (2010)
5. Tommasi, T., Orabona, F., Kaboli, M., Caputo, B.: Leveraging over prior knowledge for online learning of visual categories. In: BMVC (2012)
6. Jain, V., Learned-Miller, E.: Online domain adaptation of a pre-trained cascade of classifiers. In: CVPR, pp. 577–584 (2011)
7. Breiman, L.: Random forests. Machine Learning (2001)
8. Criminisi, A., Shotton, J.: Decision Forests for Computer Vision and Medical Image Analysis. Springer (2013)
9. Saffari, A., Leistner, C., Santner, J., Godec, M., Bischof, H.: On-line random forests. In: ICCV Workshops, pp. 1393–1400 (September 2009)
10. Hastie, T., Tibshirani, R., Friedman, J.: The elements of statistical learning: data mining, inference and prediction, 2nd edn. Springer (2009)
11. Shalev-Shwartz, S.: Online learning and online convex optimization. Found. Trends Mach. Learn. 4(2), 107–194 (2012)
12. Tao, K., Fang, M., Alroy, J., Sahagian, G.: Imagable 4t1 model for the study of late stage breast cancer. BMC Cancer 8(1) (2008)
13. Winn, J., Criminisi, A., Minka, T.: Object categorization by learned universal visual dictionary. In: ICCV (2005)

Cell Detection and Segmentation Using Correlation Clustering

Chong Zhang[1], Julian Yarkony[2], and Fred A. Hamprecht[2]

[1] CellNetworks, Heidelberg University, Germany
[2] HCI/IWR, Heidelberg University, Germany

Abstract. Cell detection and segmentation in microscopy images is important for quantitative high-throughput experiments. We present a learning-based method that is applicable to different modalities and cell types, in particular to cells that appear almost transparent in the images. We first train a classifier to detect (partial) cell boundaries. The resulting predictions are used to obtain superpixels and a weighted region adjacency graph. Here, edge weights can be either positive (attractive) or negative (repulsive). The graph partitioning problem is then solved using correlation clustering segmentation. One variant we newly propose here uses a length constraint that achieves state-of-art performance and improvements in some datasets. This constraint is approximated using non-planar correlation clustering. We demonstrate very good performance in various bright field and phase contrast microscopy experiments.

1 Introduction

With recent advances in microscope automation, long-term high-throughput imaging results in a vast amount of data in biological experiments. Consequently, the demand for computer aided microscopy image analysis is high. Cell detection and segmentation are fundamental tasks for further cell-level quantifications. The large diversity of cell lines and microscopy imaging techniques require the development of algorithms for these tasks to perform robustly and equally well in different scenarios. The technique described in this paper is applicable to images that have crowded cell regions acquired from different modalities and cell shapes, as long as they produce intensity changes at cell boundaries. Such patterns result from several microscopy imaging techniques, such as transillumination (e.g. bright field, dark field, phase contrast) and fluorescence (e.g. through membrane or cytoplasmic staining) images. Thus it is specifically suitable for images from which cells are almost transparent (Fig. 1).

Correlation clustering, or multicut, as an image segmentation method has attracted considerable interest in recent years [1,2,6,11]. It finds a partitioning of a weighted region adjacency graph into an arbitrary number of segments such that the set of edges that cohere different segments has minimum total weights. Finding a minimum weight partition is NP-hard for general and planar graphs [4]. Algorithms that can solve NP-hard correlation clustering problems to (near) optimality on instances of practically relevant size are only recently

P. Golland et al. (Eds.): MICCAI 2014, Part I, LNCS 8673, pp. 9–16, 2014.
© Springer International Publishing Switzerland 2014

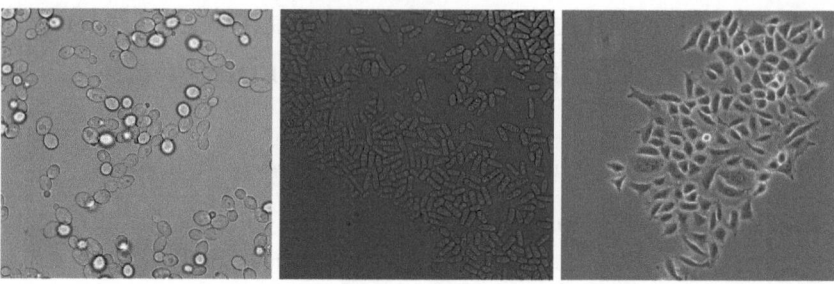

Fig. 1. Example images of (*left-right*): Dataset-a, Bright field image of Diploid yeast cells (1K×1K pix; cell size 40-100 pix). Dataset-b, Bright field image of Fission cells [9] (1K×1K pix; cell size 30-140 pix). Dataset-c, Phase contrast image of cervical cancer cells of the HeLa cell line [3] (400×400 pix; cell size 10-40 pix)

developed [1,11], and their potential for biomedical applications has not yet been explored in depth. Adding cardinality or size constraints makes the problem even harder. Thus, approximate optimization strategies that can give an exact or close to exact solution in short turnaround times are desired. A mathematically sound way to incorporate long-range repulsive interactions while keeping the resulting model tractable has only been discovered very recently [2]. Our work builds on ideas from [2,11] and explores their applicability in cell detection and segmentation. In particular, we leverage this theoretical insight into practice in terms of a length constraint formulation, a sound cue for biological problems.

2   Method

Our method first computes a cell boundary probability map from a trained edge classifier, and then constructs superpixels and builds a weighted superpixel adjacency graph. Segmentation is then reflected from partitioning this graph using a correlation clustering procedure.

Extracting boundary evidence. In our case, we learn the boundary probability from a trained classifier using ilastik [10]. It is an open-source toolkit which relies on a family of generic image features and a robust nonlinear classifier, random forest, to estimate each pixel's probability of belonging to cell boundary. This enables the flexibility of detecting edges from cells of interest (Fig. 2b). We only label very few pixels (<1%) to reduce annotation effort.

Computing superpixels. The obtained boundary probability map is then used to construct a set of initial regions as superpixels. While many computing strategies could be applied, we used the watershed transform. A slightly smoothed probability map helps avoiding tiny non-informative superpixels, while still keeping boundaries with low probability separated from background superpixels. In the test datasets, we relate the amount of smoothing with roughly average cell length l, i.e. a Gaussian filter with filter size $0.3l$ and standard deviation $0.1l$.

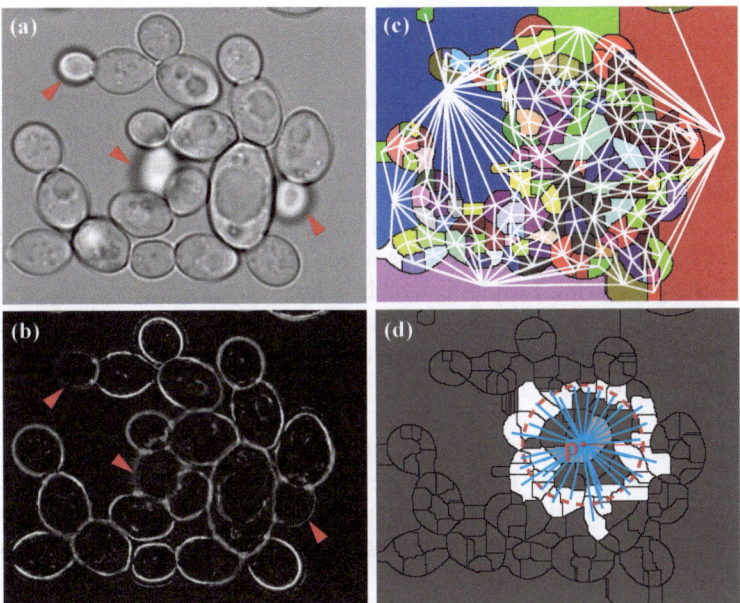

Fig. 2. (a) Example image. (b) Cell boundary pixel probabilities (the brighter the higher probability). The trained classifier gives low boundary probabilities to out-of-focus cells (*arrow*). (c) Superpixels (randomly color-mapped) with an overlay of the corresponding adjacency graph edges (*white*). (d) An illustration of the length constraint for a superpixel p (*light gray*), where non-planar edges (*blue*) indicate the superpixels (*white*) to be separated from p. They lie on the circle (*dashed-red*) of radius d centered at superpixel p's centroid.

Constructing a weighted region adjacency graph. A superpixel adjacency graph $G=(V,E)$ is built (Fig. 2c). Each graph edge e corresponds to an adjacent superpixel pair and is associated with a real valued potential θ_e. Negative potentials forces superpixels to be in separate regions, while positive ones favor to merge them. We first approximate the graph edge probability p_e by the average boundary probability over the pixels separating the corresponding adjacent superpixel pair. Then, the graph edge potential is given by

$$\theta_e = \log\left(\frac{1 - F(p_e + t)}{F(p_e + t)}\right),$$

where $F(x) = \max(\min(x, 0.9999), 0.0001)$, and t is a bias term that adjusts the transform from (non-negative) probabilities to negative/positive potentials. A small bias favors a single region of all superpixels, whereas a large one leads to regions of single superpixels.

Solving the graph partitioning problem. A partition is defined by a binary indicator variable X_e for each edge e. $X_e=1$ if edge e is to be cut and $X_e=0$ otherwise. A valid configuration [11] of labeling $X \in \{0,1\}^E$ of edges gives a possible segmentation. The correlation clustering problem can be expressed as:

$$\min_{X \in C} \theta_e X_e,$$

where C is the set of all possible segmentations. If edges are only between adjacent superpixels and have unrestricted potential values, this results in a planar graph. Given efficient search strategies it can be solved to optimality using an integer linear programming solver using a cutting planes approach [1]; or approximated using dedicated solvers such as PlanarCC [11], which often reaches the global optimum as well (see [5] for a benchmarking). We consider the latter for the cell segmentation problem, which belongs to instances of large sizes (Table 1). Also, given its closed contour property, the application of such models is valuable because cell boundary information is often only partially available and can be inconsistent.

Adding a length constraint. Restricting the size of segments is valid for cell segmentation problems as a specific cell type has a known size prior. This is particularly helpful in situations when cells are largely clustered together and their separation boundaries are missing. Thus, a constraint that no cell has a length (in its major axis) larger than a hyper-parameter d can be imposed. We formulate this to a graph structure that is amenable to a highly efficient approximate (and as it happens often exact) optimization: Semi-PlanarCC [2]. In this model, not only edges between adjacent superpixels have potentials, but also edges between distant non-adjacent superpixels have large negative potentials. To do so, it is sufficient to state that for any two superpixels, if separated by an approximated distance of d, then they must be in separate regions. For every superpixel p, a circle of radius equal to d is drawn at the centroid of p. All superpixels lying on that circle may not be in the same region as superpixel p. An illustration is shown in Fig. 2d. The potentials between these superpixel pairs are set to a large negative value, e.g. $-|\sum_e \theta_e| - 0.001$. This means, it is preferable to cutting all edges with positive potentials rather than missing cutting on edges with negative long-range potentials.

Finally, after removing background segments, each connected component enclosed by the cut edges is considered as an individual cell region. In our case, we currently use two heuristic size filtering steps to remove background: at segments level, consider those larger than $6l^2$ as background, and at superpixel level, consider segments containing superpixel(s) larger than $3l^2$ as background.

3   Experiments and Results

Our aim is to optimize both the detection and segmentation accuracy w.r.t. the ground truth (GT) in each image provided in the form of centroids for every cell and regions of a random subset of cells. Therefore, we evaluate the output of detection based on: A region is considered a true positive (TP) detection if the GT centroid is within this region; Regions that do not cover cell centroids are considered false positives (FP); Missed GT centroids are counted as false negatives (FN). The results are reported in terms of precision P=TP/(TP+FP),

Table 1. Summary of experimetal parameters

Dataset	avg. cell length l	# superpixels	# planar edges	# non-planar edges
a	60	1225±242	3456±701	18025±6791
b [9]	100	3727±2450	10530±7010	147420±160420
c [3]	30	1081±364	3035±1038	26618±12683

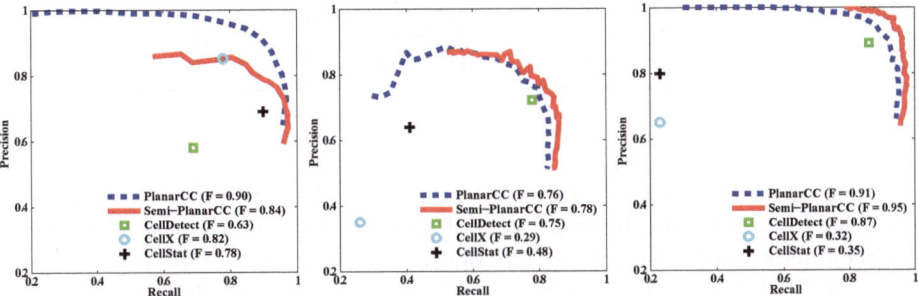

Fig. 3. Precision-Recall plots of detection for the three datasets using various t values. (Results for Dataset-c using CellDetect is reproduced from [3]. Also for CellDetect, detection criteria was the same as in [3] due to the available output.)

recall R=TP/(TP+FN), and F-measure F=2×P×R/(P+R). Due to the high cell density, we randomly selected 10−20% of cells from each image and manually segmented them to provide the GT. The segmentation accuracy is then computed from two area overlap measures between the TP detection regions R_{tpd} and the GT region R_{gt}: $M_1=(R_{tpd}\cap R_{gt})/(R_{tpd}\cup R_{gt})\times100$, $M_2=(R_{tpd}\cap R_{gt})/R_{gt}\times100$.

Three datasets have been used to validate our method (Fig. 1). Dataset-a (15 images with 1768 in-focus cells in total) contains bright field Diploid yeast cells. It is required to detect in-focus cells while discriminating them from out-of-focus cells. The detection task is challenging since the cell boundaries can be partially missing and often exhibit varying contrast patterns even in the same cell. Other challenging issues include poor contrast, partial or changing halo, overlap with out-of-focus cells, and imaging artifacts. Dataset-b (10 images with 2340 cells in total) is from bright field Fission yeast cells in [9], where cells are elongated cylinder like and can be very densely packed as well as in the Dataset-a but having different appearance. Dataset-c (11 images with 1073 cells in total) is from CellDetect [3], which contains phase contrast images of cervical cancer cell colonies of the HeLa cell line. It presents a high variability in cell shapes and sizes. Table 1 summarizes the parameter details.

Detection results are shown in Fig. 3. The detection differences between PlanarCC and Semi-PlanarCC lie on two sides: Semi-PlanarCC splits either large groups of cells or cells from background that would be merged by PlanarCC; It might also split exceptionally large cells or background into multiple segments

Table 2. Results of segmentation in area overlap measures M_1 and M_2 on the TP detected cells (mean±standard deviation). The highest number (100 indicating the best) among the methods is indicated as bold.

Dataset	Meas.	PlanarCC	Semi-PlanarCC	CellX [8]	CellStat [7]
a	M_1	86.3±13.3	86.4±12.0	86.9±16.0	**89.5±13.6**
	M_2	**97.0±1.6**	96.8±3.1	94.8±14.2	91.4±13.9
b [9]	M_1	**74.4±21.8**	74.1±21.3	32.8±23.8	49.3±24.2
	M_2	86.9±23.8	**90.2±21.7**	32.8±23.8	55.7±29.6
c [3]	M_1	**71.4±12.1**	70.1±11.9	42.1±12.7	46.4±8.6
	M_2	93.9±13.3	**94.4±11.4**	42.2±12.7	60.6±14.0

small enough to be rejected. This could be seen in Fig. 3 that Semi-PlarnarCC has achieved higher recall values than PlanarCC for the same t value ranges (i.e. seemingly compressed curve horizontally shifted rightwards). This may suggest that the former is less sensitive to the choice of t. And the lower precision values for Dataset-a are due to the multiple fragmented background segments whose sizes are similar to a cell. This is more likely to happen in microscopy images of cell cultures of medium confluence. This could be alleviated through a post-processing step using e.g. shape or texture features. Table 2 shows the area overlap measures on segmentations from a random subset of TP detected cells, both methods perform similarly in their best F measure cases (Fig. 3).

In Fig. 3 and Table 2, we also show detection and segmentation results of three methods: CellDetect [3], CellX [8], CellStat [7]. PombeX [9] has also been evaluated but the tool does not provide quantifiable output thus not reported. For each method we have tried to optimize their parameters to achieve the best possible results. Reported results for Dataset-c using CellDetect is reproduced from [3]. Also for CellDetect, detection criteria was the same as in [3], since its detection is represented as cell centroids. The overall comparison is favorable to our method over other methods. CellStat is primarily designed for bright field images of round cells, and it looks for contours with consistent profile pattern. This may in part account for their poorer performance for elongated cells and phase contrast images. Similarly, CellX also tries to match boundary profile pattern on cells without extreme shapes. Due to the image appearance variations within each dataset, we expect that these methods would perform better if parameters are tuned for each image individually rather than what we do here: the same set of parameters for the whole dataset. A visual inspection of our segmentation can be seen in Fig. 4 as red contours overlaid on example images. It clearly shows that for Dataset-a, the out-of-focus cells (highly-contrasted and blurred ones) are clustered with the background, i.e. they are excluded from the segmentation.

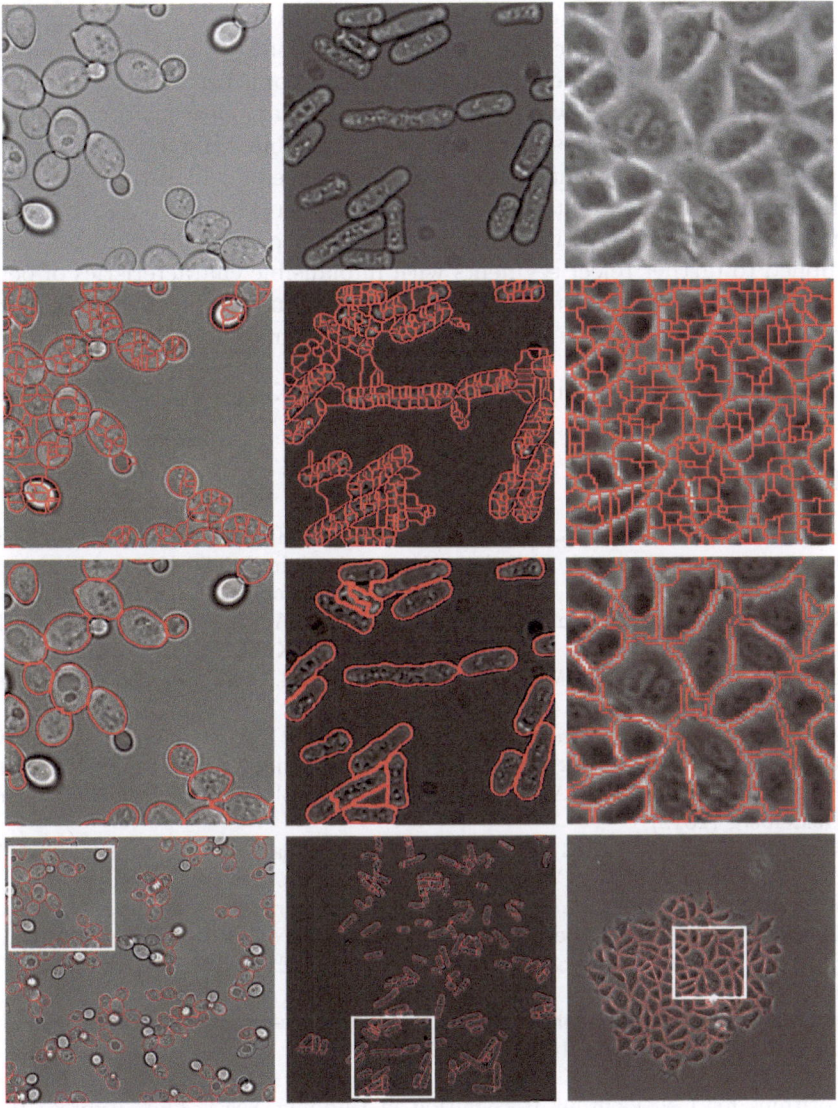

Fig. 4. (*top*) Example original image regions from Datasets a-c (*left* to *right*). Over-laid lines (*red*) on the original images are: superpixel lines (*middle top*), segmentation contours of these regions (*middle bottom*) and the entire example image (*bottom*), with the regions indicated as white frames.

4   Discussion and Conclusions

The technique for cell detection and segmentation presented here is able to achieve state-of-the-art performance across different scenarios. In general PlanarCC and Semi-PlanarCC perform similarly, but for overlapping cells with missing cell boundaries, the latter is more beneficial. The model does not have any specifications about closed region shape and size, which allows for various cell types applications. It has demonstrated that it can also handle large number of superpixels and graphs, which is the case of microscopic cell images. Our method only requires a few sparse labels to train a cell boundary classifier for all images in an experiment. Apart from setting cell length (and bias), further steps are automatic and require no user interaction, thus well suited for high-throughput studies. In addition, the flexibility of training edges from cells of interest allows us to exclude edges from other structures. Deterministic post-processing steps should be applied to further reject segments with implausible characteristics of being a cell, according to e.g. image texture features, or cell morphology features. Here we only focus on evaluating the performance of our technique.

Acknowledgement. We thank F. Huber and M. Knop from ZMBH University of Heidelberg, Germany for sharing Dataset-a.

References

1. Andres, B., Kappes, J.H., Beier, T., Köthe, U., Hamprecht, F.A.: Probabilistic Image Segmentation with Closedness Constraints. In: ICCV (2011)
2. Andres, B., Yarkony, J., Manjunath, B.S., Kirchhoff, S., Turetken, E., Fowlkes, C.C., Pfister, H.: Segmenting Planar Superpixel Adjacency Graphs w.r.t. Nonplanar Superpixel Affinity Graphs. In: Heyden, A., Kahl, F., Olsson, C., Oskarsson, M., Tai, X.-C. (eds.) EMMCVPR 2013. LNCS, vol. 8081, pp. 266–279. Springer, Heidelberg (2013)
3. Arteta, C., Lempitsky, V., Noble, J.A., Zisserman, A.: Learning to Detect Cells Using Non-overlapping Extremal Regions. In: Ayache, N., Delingette, H., Golland, P., Mori, K. (eds.) MICCAI 2012, Part I. LNCS, vol. 7510, pp. 348–356. Springer, Heidelberg (2012)
4. Bachrach, Y., Kohli, P., Kolmogorov, V., Zadimoghaddam, M.: Optimal Coalition Structure Generation in Cooperative Graph Games. In: AAAI (2013)
5. Kappes, J.H., Andres, B., Hamprecht, F.A., Schnörr, C., Nowozin, S., Batra, D., Kim, S., Kausler, B.X., Lellmann, J., Komodakis, N., Rother, C.: A Comparative Study of Modern Inference Techniques for Discrete Energy Minimization Problems. In: CVPR (2013)
6. Kim, S., Nowozin, S., Kohli, P., Yoo, C.D.: Higher-Order Correlation Clustering for Image Segmentation. In: NIPS (2011)
7. Kvarnstrom, M., Logg, K., Diez, A., Bodvard, K., Kall, M.: Image Analysis Algorithms for Cell Contour Recognition in Budding Yeast. Opt. Express 16(17), 1035–1042 (2008)
8. Mayer, C., Dimopoulos, S., Rudolf, F., Stelling, J.: Using CellX to Quantify Intracellular Events. Curr. Protoc. Mol. Biol., Chapter 14, Unit 14.22 (2013)
9. Peng, J.Y., Chen, Y.J., Green, M.D., Sabatinos, S.A., Forsburg, S.L., Hsu, C.N.: PombeX: Robust Cell Segmentation for Fission Yeast Transillumination Images. PLoS One 8(12), e81434 (2013)
10. Sommer, C., Straehle, C., Koethe, U., Hamprecht, F.A.: Ilastik: Interactive Learning and Segmentation Toolkit. In: ISBI (2011)
11. Yarkony, J., Ihler, A., Fowlkes, C.C.: Fast Planar Correlation Clustering for Image Segmentation. In: Fitzgibbon, A., Lazebnik, S., Perona, P., Sato, Y., Schmid, C. (eds.) ECCV 2012, Part VI. LNCS, vol. 7577, pp. 568–581. Springer, Heidelberg (2012)

Candidate Sampling for Neuron Reconstruction from Anisotropic Electron Microscopy Volumes

Jan Funke[1,2], Julien N.P. Martel[1], Stephan Gerhard[1,4], Bjoern Andres[2],
Dan C. Cireşan[3], Alessandro Giusti[3], Luca M. Gambardella[3],
Jürgen Schmidhuber[3], Hanspeter Pfister[2],
Albert Cardona[4], and Matthew Cook[1]

[1] Institute of Neuroinformatics, UZH/ETH Zürich
[2] School of Engineering and Applied Science, Harvard Universiy
[3] IDSIA, Lugano
[4] HHMI Janelia, Ashburn (VA)

Abstract. The automatic reconstruction of neurons from stacks of electron microscopy sections is an important computer vision problem in neuroscience. Recent advances are based on a two step approach: First, a set of possible 2D neuron candidates is generated for each section independently based on membrane predictions of a local classifier. Second, the candidates of all sections of the stack are fed to a neuron tracker that selects and connects them in 3D to yield a reconstruction. The accuracy of the result is currently limited by the quality of the generated candidates. In this paper, we propose to replace the heuristic set of candidates used in previous methods with samples drawn from a conditional random field (CRF) that is trained to label sections of neural tissue. We show on a stack of *Drosophila melanogaster* neural tissue that neuron candidates generated with our method produce 30% less reconstruction errors than current candidate generation methods. Two properties of our CRF are crucial for the accuracy and applicability of our method: (1) The CRF models the orientation of membranes to produce more plausible neuron candidates. (2) The interactions in the CRF are restricted to form a bipartite graph, which allows a great sampling speed-up without loss of accuracy.

1 Introduction

To study the structure and function of nervous systems, neuroscientists need to image volumes of neural tissue that are large enough to contain complete neural circuits, with high enough resolution to resolve individual synapses. Currently, serial section electron microscopy (EM) is the only technique that meets these requirements [1], resulting in multi-terabyte anisotropic image stacks (that is, volumes with high xy-resolution and low z-resolution) even for small organisms like *Drosophila melanogaster*. The biggest bottleneck in the processing of these image stacks is the time needed to manually reconstruct the neuron morphologies. Addressing this issue, automatic reconstruction methods for anisotropic

P. Golland et al. (Eds.): MICCAI 2014, Part I, LNCS 8673, pp. 17–24, 2014.

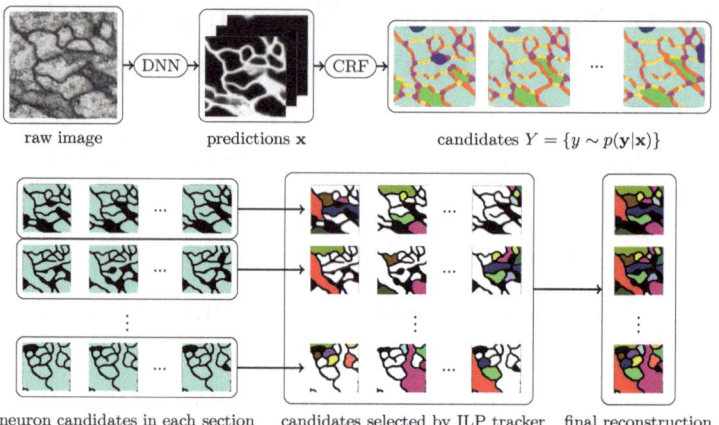

raw image   predictions $\mathbf{x}$ candidates $Y = \{y \sim p(\mathbf{y}|\mathbf{x})\}$

neuron candidates in each section   candidates selected by ILP tracker   final reconstruction

Fig. 1. Overview of the proposed method. **Top:** For each section, 2D neuron candidates are generated by sampling from a CRF. **Bottom:** An integer linear program (ILP) tracker is used to find a consistent subset of the candidates for the whole stack at once.

volumes became the subject of a vivid branch of research at the intersection between computer vision and neuroscience [2–10].

The de facto standard for anisotropic neuron reconstruction methods consists of two steps [7, 8, 10]: In the first step, a set of possible 2D neuron candidates is generated for each section of the stack individually. These candidates are obtained by identifying membranes using predictions of a local image patch classifier like a deep neural network (DNN) [9] or a random forest [7, 8, 10]. Due to ambiguities in the data and imprecisions of the predictions, many plausible and possibly contradictory candidates are extracted for each section to increase the chance that the correct candidates are among them. In the second step, the 2D neuron candidates of the whole stack are fed into an integer linear program (ILP) tracker, which connects them across adjacent sections. The ILP tracker ensures that a non-contradictory subset of candidates is chosen and that the candidates are connected to optimize a global criterion like a smooth continuation.

The accuracy and efficiency of the reconstruction is limited by the quality of the generated 2D neuron candidates. It has been noted that the generation of 2D neuron candidates is responsible for about 50% of the final error [8]. Although the ILP tracker can ignore wrong candidates to some extent, it can not fantasize missing correct candidates. Thus, it is important to generate enough candidates with high variation to make sure that the correct candidates are among them. However, having too many incorrect candidates increases the computational overhead and may lead to spurious results. Therefore, a careful generation of candidates is crucial for accuracy and tractability.

Our Approach.   We are proposing a novel method to generate 2D neuron candidates that greatly improves the reconstruction accuracy. The key of our method is the generation of 2D neuron candidates as samples from a pairwise conditional random field (CRF) that is designed and trained to label 2D sections of neural tissue. An overview of the proposed method is shown in Fig. 1.

Furthermore, we introduce two extensions for pairwise CRFs for image labeling and show that they are essential for the accuracy and applicability of our method: (1) Our CRF explicitly models the orientation of certain labels. We use this to learn shape-related priors for membranes, which are usually thin and elongated. This helps to produce more plausible section labelings, and thus better 2D neuron candidates. (2) We restrict the interactions in the CRF to form a bipartite graph. With this trick, Gibbs sampling [11] on the model can be parallelized and carried out on a GPU with a speed-up factor of 39 compared to a single core CPU implementation. This allows us to model a large number of neighbor interactions for each pixel (improving accuracy) and to use a rich set of biologically relevant labels (cell interior, mitochondria, glia cells, synapses, and different orientations of membranes) while still being fast enough to process large amounts of data.

The following section gives details about our CRF that we use to generate the 2D neuron candidates. In section 3, we show results on a stack of *Drosophila melanogaster* neural tissue, where candidates generated with our method lead to 30% fewer final errors than competing candidate generation methods.

2   2D Neuron Candidate Sampling

To generate 2D neuron candidates, we repeatedly draw samples from a labeling distribution on each section individually and transform them into binary neuron/membrane segmentations. Let $\Omega \subset \mathbb{N}^2$ be the pixel domain of a single EM section. We model the distribution of labelings $\mathbf{y} = \left(y^{(i)} \in K \mid i \in \Omega\right)$ of assigning each pixel in Ω to a label of a discrete set K with a conditional random field (CRF). For the possible values in K, we distinguish between *oriented* labels K_Φ (for membranes) and *non-oriented* labels K_N (for mitochondria, glia cells, *etc.*). Each $k_\alpha \in K_\Phi$ represents a label k at a certain discrete orientation $\alpha \in \Phi$.

The CRF is conditioned on pixel-wise predictions $\mathbf{x} = \left(\mathbf{x}^{(i)} \in \mathbb{R}^F \mid i \in \Omega\right)$ with vectors of size F. We write $y^{(i)}$ or $\mathbf{x}^{(i)}$ to refer respectively to the label or prediction vector of pixel $i \in \Omega$ and $x_f^{(i)}$ to refer to the f$^\text{th}$ prediction component of $\mathbf{x}^{(i)}$. The lateral interactions of each location in the CRF are modeled with pairwise factors to neighbors in different directions Φ (as for the oriented labels) and distances $\Delta = \{d_1, \dots, d_D\}$, approximated to the closest neighbor on the pixel grid (see Fig. 2a for an illustration). We write $\mathcal{N}(i, \alpha, d)$ to denote the closest grid neighbor of i in direction α and distance d. We achieve rotation equivariance by re-using factors of same distance for interactions in different directions to directly model the rotation invariant statistics of our data. Furthermore, the CRF is homogeneous, *i.e.*, the same factors are used at every location. Formally, we model the labeling distribution $p(\mathbf{y}|\mathbf{x})$ as

$$p(\mathbf{y}|\mathbf{x}) = \frac{1}{Z(\mathbf{x})} \exp[-\sum_{i \in \Omega} \langle \boldsymbol{w}^{y^{(i)}}, \mathbf{x}^{(i)} \rangle - \sum_{i \in \Omega} \sum_{\alpha \in \Phi} \sum_{d \in \Delta} R_{\alpha,d}(y^{(i)}, y^{(\mathcal{N}(i,\alpha,d))})], \quad (1)$$

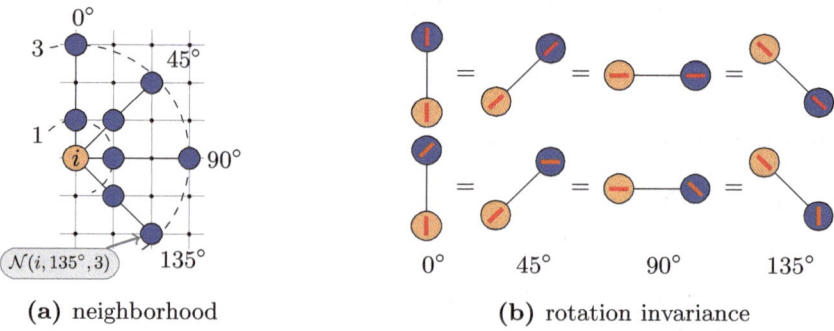

(a) neighborhood   **(b)** rotation invariance

Fig. 2. (a) Neighbors (blue) of a single pixel (i, orange) for orientations $\Phi = \{0°, 45°, 90°, 135°\}$ and distances $\Delta = \{1, 3\}$. Neighbors are approximated to the closest pixel on the grid in the given direction and distance. (b) Illustration of the rotation invariant interactions. The values of rotated interactions are equal for accordingly rotated labels.

where $Z(\mathbf{x})$ is the partition function, the data term (first sum) is a linear combination of the components of the prediction vectors with weights $\boldsymbol{w}^k \in \mathbb{R}^F$ for each label $k \in K$, and the prior (second sum) models the pairwise interactions of each location to its neighbors. For that, $R_{\alpha,d}$ determines the costs for the joint labeling of i and its approximate neighbor $\mathcal{N}(i, \alpha, d)$ in direction α at distance d. These costs are shared across different orientations. Let k^α denote the rotated version of label k by α degrees: oriented labels change their orientation subscript and non-oriented labels do not change at all. Defining $R_{\alpha,d}(k, l) = \tilde{R}_d(k^{-\alpha}, l^{-\alpha})$ ensures that the resulting CRF is rotationally equivariant by treating every pairwise interaction in the same way as the $0°$ interaction (see Fig. 2b for an illustration). Finally, $\tilde{R}_d$ is a lookup table with entries $\tilde{R}_d(k, l) = v_d^{k,l}$ for the joint labeling of neighboring pixels with distance d. The parameters $\mathbf{v} = \{v_d^{k,l}\}$ and $\boldsymbol{w} = \{\boldsymbol{w}^k\}$ of our model are obtained by maximum likelihood learning [12].

Parallelized Sampling. We use Gibbs sampling [11] to draw the samples from $p(\mathbf{y}|\mathbf{x})$ that are needed for the training and generation of 2D neuron candidates. To tackle the slow convergence properties of Gibbs sampling, we restrict the interactions in the CRF to form a bipartite graph. For that, we divide the image domain Ω into "odd" and "even" locations, following a checkerboard pattern on the pixel grid. By modifying $\mathcal{N}$ to find the closest neighbor *of opposite parity* in the given direction and distance, we obtain a bipartite CRF. We write $\mathbf{y}^{(O)}$ and $\mathbf{y}^{(E)}$ to refer to the labeling of the pixels in Ω_O and Ω_E, respectively. It follows that $p(\mathbf{y}^{(E)}|\mathbf{y}^{(O)}, \mathbf{x}) = \prod_{i \in \Omega_E} p(y^{(i)}|\mathbf{y}^{(O)}, \mathbf{x})$, and $p(\mathbf{y}^{(O)}|\mathbf{y}^{(E)}, \mathbf{x}) = \prod_{i \in \Omega_O} p(y^{(i)}|\mathbf{y}^{(E)}, \mathbf{x})$, *i.e.*, labels in one partition are conditionally independent given the labels in the other half [13]. Samples $y^{(i)} \sim p(y^{(i)}|\mathbf{y}^{(E)})$ for $i \in \Omega_O$ and $y^{(i)} \sim p(y^{(i)}|\mathbf{y}^{(O)})$ for $i \in \Omega_E$ can be drawn independently and in parallel. We exploit this property by sampling a whole section in two half-steps, one for

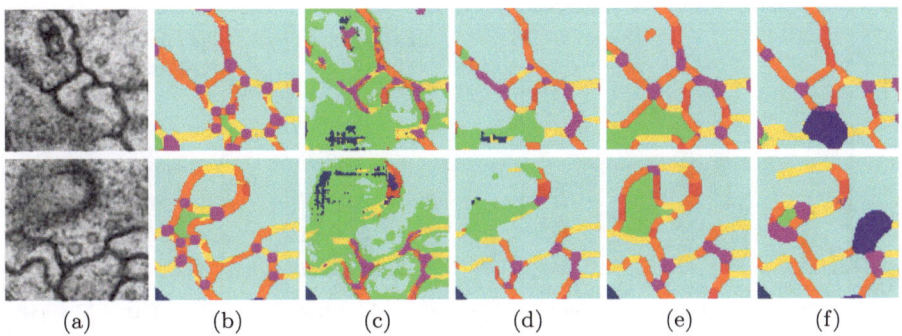

| (a) | (b) | (c) | (d) | (e) | (f) |

Fig. 3. Examples of samples drawn from our CRF for ambiguous cases. The used labels are membrane (four orientations $|,/,-,\backslash$ and junctions $\bullet$), cell interior ($\bullet$), mitochondria ($\bullet$), glia ($\bullet$), and synapse ($\bullet$). (a) shows the raw images, (b) the ground-truth labelings, (c) the plain DNN prediction, (d-f) a representative sample from CRFs D_1, D_4, and D_8, respectively. See Section 3 for details.

$\mathbf{y}^{(E)}$ and one for $\mathbf{y}^{(O)}$, each of which is carried out with our parallelized GPU implementation (source code available at `http://github.com/funkey/prim`).

3   Results

Setup. We evaluate the performance of our 2D neuron candidate generation method on two stacks of 20 EM images of size 1024×1024 from *Drosophila melanogaster* larva neuropil with 4.6nm xy-resolution and 50nm section thickness [14]. These stacks have been selected to capture well the typical variations found in EM images. The first stack was used to train the DNN architecture proposed in [9] to predict the pixel labels (shown in Fig. 3) that are used as features $\mathbf{x}$ in the CRF. The second stack, for which we manually generated ground truth, is used to compare different candidate generation methods. To investigate the effect of different neighborhood sizes, we created three instances of our model with different distance sets: model D_1 (a baseline of our CRF) uses $\Delta = \{1\}$, D_4 uses $\Delta = \{1, 5, 9, 15\}$, and D_8 uses $\Delta = \{1, 3, 5, 7, 9, 15, 21, 31\}$. All models use the same labels (shown in Fig. 3) and the same set of rotations $\Phi = \{0°, 45°, 90°, 135°\}$. From each model, we drew 20 samples per section to generate the 2D neuron candidates. Each sample is the last labeling after 100 Gibbs iterations on the whole section, starting from a random initialization.

Error Measure. We report the accuracy of the reconstruction in terms of an edit distance proposed in [8], since this directly reflects the amount of time needed to fix it. The errors are reported in four categories: "FP" (false positives) are spuriously detected neurons in a section, "FN" (false negatives) are missed neurons in a section, "FS" (false splits) missed links between neurons across

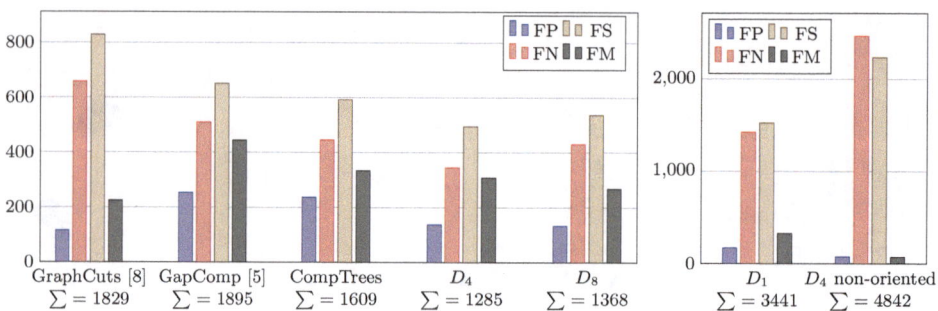

Fig. 4. Reconstruction errors for different 2D neuron candidate generation methods (a). Results are given as false positives (FP), false negatives (FN), false splits (FS), and false merges (FM), see text for details. Our method D_4 produces 30% less errors compared to the best competing approach (GraphCuts). The importance of a rich neighborhood and oriented membranes in the proposed model is shown in (b): Decreasing the neighborhood radius to one (D_1) or ignoring membrane orientations (D_4 non-oriented) dramatically sacrifices reconstruction accuracy.

sections, and "FM" (false merges) are spurious links across sections. Details about this error measure are given in the supplemental material.

Comparison. We compare our model instances D_1, D_4, and D_8 to the current state of the art in neuron candidate generation: A series of graphcuts (Graph-Cuts), applied on the *membrane* predictions of the DNN, as proposed in [8], and gap completion (GapComp) [5] as proposed in [10]. As a baseline, we also generate candidates from component trees (CompTrees) [15], extracted from the same predictions. We reconstructed neurons in the test stack for each candidate generation method using the publicly available ILP tracker SOPNET [8]. The trainable parts of this tracker have been trained and validated for each method individually on the first 10 sections of the test stack. The test results on the last 10 sections are shown in Fig. 4. Model D_4 provides by far the best result, improving the error by 30% compared to the best competing approach (GraphCuts), which is already outperformed by our baseline model (CompTrees). Surprisingly, the larger neighborhood of model D_8 does not lead to better results.

Model Properties. To show the importance of oriented membrane labels, we trained and evaluated a version of D_4 with non-oriented membrane labels (right bars in Fig. 4b). Due to undersegmentation, the model proposed only a few large candidates and thus missed a lot of neurons (high FN and FS). To investigate the effect of the bipartite restriction of our CRF, we also implemented a non-bipartite version of model D_4. The reconstruction errors differ by 1% in favour of the bipartite version and may well be attributed to sampling noise.

Inference Time. Tested on a NVIDIA Quadro 4000, we were able to draw 100 complete samples of size 1024×1024 from D_4 using our GPU implementation

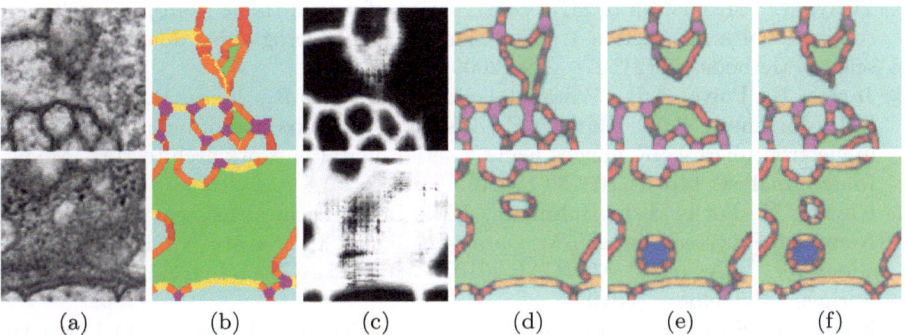

(a)   (b)   (c)   (d)   (e)   (f)

Fig. 5. Demonstration of the candidate generation capabilities of model D_4 (for label legend see caption of Fig. 3). (a) shows the raw image, (b) the ground-truth labeling and (c) the prediction for the class *membrane*. Images (d-f) show three different samples drawn from D_4.

in $4.4s$. A single core CPU Gibbs sampler implementation took $174s$ on a Intel Xeon CPU at 3.47 GHz to achieve the same, resulting in a speed-up factor of 39.

4   Discussion

We showed that replacing fixed sets of 2D neuron candidates with samples drawn from a distribution increases the reconstruction accuracy. Going beyond neuron reconstruction, this scheme might also be applicable to other approaches that rely on the quality of initial candidates, such as super-pixel based algorithms for image segmentation.

In our case, an interesting aspect of our method is the rich labeling in the samples. Besides membrane locations, they also indicate the locations of mitochondria, synapses, and glia cells. These labels are not only of biological relevance, but could also be used to improve the reconstruction accuracy by, for instance, exploiting the fact that mitochondria are surrounded by neuron and synapses are separating neurons.

An open question in our method is how many samples need to be drawn to obtain good results with minimal computational overhead. An interesting solution might be to start with a few initial samples and draw more on demand for locations that are unlikely according to higher level priors, for example where there is a sudden change in direction or an unexpected end of a neural process.

Acknowledgements. We thank Verena Kaynig for training and creating candidates for GapComp. This work was funded by the SNF grant CRSII3 130470.

References

1. Cardona, A.: Towards Semi-Automatic Reconstruction of Neural Circuits. Neuroinformatics 11, 31–33 (2012)

2. Yuriy, M.: Automation of 3D reconstruction of neural tissue from large volume of conventional serial section transmission electron micrographs. Journal of Neuro-science Methods 176(2), 276–289 (2009)
3. Jurrus, E., Paiva, A.R., Watanabe, S., Anderson, J.R., Jones, B.W., Whitaker, R.T., Jorgensen, E.M., Marc, R.E., Tasdizen, T.: Detection of neuron membranes in electron microscopy images using a serial neural network architecture. Medical Image Analysis 14(6), 770–783 (2010)
4. Kaynig, V., Fuchs, T.J., Buhmann, J.M.: Geometrical Consistent 3D Tracing of Neuronal Processes in ssTEM Data. In: Jiang, T., Navab, N., Pluim, J.P.W., Viergever, M.A. (eds.) MICCAI 2010, Part II. LNCS, vol. 6362, pp. 209–216. Springer, Heidelberg (2010)
5. Kaynig, V., Fuchs, T., Buhmann, J.M.: Neuron Geometry Extraction by Perceptual Grouping in ssTEM Images. In: Proceedings of the IEEE Conference on Computer Vision and Pattern Recognition, Los Alamitos, CA, USA, pp. 2902–2909 (2010)
6. Vitaladevuni, S.N.P., Basri, R.: Co-Clustering of Image Segments Using Convex Optimization Applied to EM Neuronal Reconstruction. In: Proceedings of the IEEE Conference on Computer Vision and Pattern Recognition, pp. 2203–2210 (2010)
7. Vazquez-Reina, A., Huang, D., Gelbart, M., Lichtman, J., Miller, E., Pfister, H.: Segmentation Fusion for Connectomics. In: Proceedings of the IEEE International Conference on Computer Vision (ICCV), Barcelona, Spain. IEEE (2011)
8. Funke, J., Andres, B., Hamprecht, F.A., Cardona, A., Cook, M.: Efficient Auto-matic 3D-Reconstruction of Branching Neurons from EM Data. In: CVPR, pp. 1004–1011 (2012)
9. Ciresan, D., Giusti, A., Gambardella, L.M., Schmidhuber, J.: Deep neural net-works segment neuronal membranes in electron microscopy images. In: Pereira, F., Burges, C., Bottou, L., Weinberger, K. (eds.) NIPS, vol. 25, pp. 2843–2851. Curran Associates, Inc. (2012)
10. Kaynig, V., Vazquez-Reina, A., Knowles-Barley, S., Roberts, M., Jones, T.R., Kasthuri, N., Miller, E., Lichtman, J., Pfister, H.: Large-Scale Automatic Recon-struction of Neuronal Processes from Electron Microscopy Images. ArXiv e-prints (March 2013)
11. Geman, S., Geman, D.: Stochastic Relaxation, Gibbs Distributions, and the Bayesian Restoration of Images. IEEE Transactions on Pattern Analysis and Ma-chine Intelligence 6 (6), 721–741 (1984)
12. Sutton, C., McCallum, A.: An Introduction to Conditional Random Fields for Relational Learning. Technical report, Department of Computer Science University of Massachusetts (2006)
13. Gonzalez, J., Low, Y., Gretton, A., Guestrin, C.: Parallel Gibbs Sampling: From Colored Fields to Thin Junction Trees. In: Artificial Intelligence and Statistics (AISTATS), Ft. Lauderdale, FL (May 2011)
14. Gerhard, S., Funke, J., Martel, J., Cardona, A., Fetter, R.: Segmented anisotropic ssTEM dataset of neural tissue (2013), http://dx.doi.org/10.6084/m9.figshare.856713
15. Jones, R.: Component Trees for Image Filtering and Segmentation. In: Proceedings of the 1997 IEEE Workshop on Nonlinear Signal and Image Processing, Mackinac Island (1997)

A Fully Bayesian Inference Framework for Population Studies of the Brain Microstructure

Maxime Taquet, Benoît Scherrer, Jurriaan M. Peters,
Sanjay P. Prabhu, and Simon K. Warfield

Computational Radiology Laboratory, Harvard Medical School, Boston, USA

Abstract. Models of the diffusion-weighted signal are of strong interest for population studies of the brain microstructure. These studies are typically conducted by extracting a scalar property from the model and subjecting it to null hypothesis significance testing. This process has two major limitations: the reported p-value is a weak predictor of the reproducibility of findings and evidence for the absence of microstructural alterations cannot be gained. To overcome these limitations, this paper proposes a Bayesian framework for population studies of the brain microstructure represented by multi-fascicle models. A hierarchical model is built over the biophysical parameters of the microstructure. Bayesian inference is performed by Hamiltonian Monte Carlo sampling and results in a joint posterior distribution over the latent microstructure parameters for each group. Inference from this posterior enables richer analyses of the brain microstructure beyond the dichotomy of significance testing. Using synthetic and in-vivo data, we show that our Bayesian approach increases reproducibility of findings from population studies and opens new opportunities in the analysis of the brain microstructure.

Keywords: Microstructure, Diffusion Imaging, Bayesian Inference.

1 Introduction

Novel models of the microstructure from diffusion-weighted imaging (DWI) provide insights into the cellular architecture of the healthy and diseased brain [4]. Population studies of the brain microstructure are commonly conducted by extracting a property of interest (e.g., diffusivities of a fascicle [8], principal direction of diffusion [7] or fraction of the isotropic compartment [5]) and subjecting it to null hypothesis significance testing (NHST). Because the p-value is uniformly distributed under the null hypothesis, no evidence in favor of the null can be gained in this process [3]. The null hypothesis will thus eventually be rejected if a sufficient number of attempts are made, which significantly hampers the building of scientific knowledge and reduces the reproducibility of results [3]. These limitations are critical in microstructure imaging, wherein reproducibility is a major concern and researchers want evidence for the absence of abnormalities in certain brain regions alongside the detection of abnormalities in other regions.

Bayesian approaches to population studies address these limitations. They proceed by defining a generative model of the data in both populations and

P. Golland et al. (Eds.): MICCAI 2014, Part I, LNCS 8673, pp. 25–32, 2014.

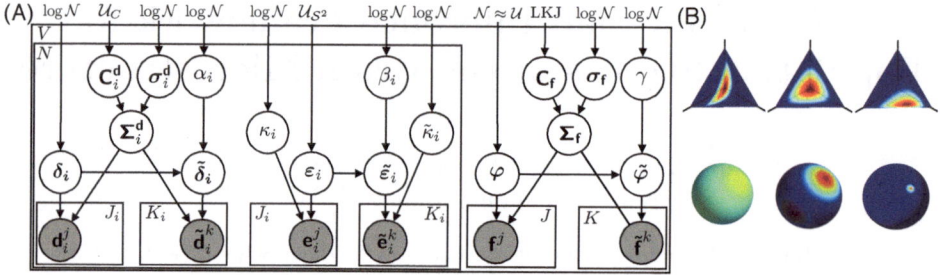

Fig. 1. (A) Generative model of the microstructure at the population level. Circles are random variables and shaded circles have observations. Indices relate to fascicles and superscripts to subject (omitted in the text for clarity). The left box is repeated for the N fascicles in the voxel and the whole is repeated for all V voxels. (B) Instances of logistic-normal distribution over the simplex and Watson distribution over the sphere.

inferring a joint posterior probability over the model parameters. The posterior probability can then be interrogated to answer research questions [1]. Defining a generative model of the microstructure at the population level, however, is challenging due to the geometry of the space of parameters. This paper tackles this challenge and presents a novel Bayesian inference framework for population studies the brain microstructure. Section 2 presents our assumptions. Section 3 and 4 describe our model and its inference. Section 5 shows experimental results.

2   Parameterization and Assumptions

Multi-fascicle models represent the signal from each compartment in each voxel as a separate Gaussian encoded by a tensor $\boldsymbol{D}_i$, weighed by f_i [6]:

$$S(b, \boldsymbol{g}) = S_0 \sum_{i=1}^{N} f_i e^{-b\boldsymbol{g}^T \boldsymbol{D}_i \boldsymbol{g}}, \text{ where } b \text{ is the b-value and } \boldsymbol{g} \text{ is the gradient.}$$

One tensor is isotropic [4,5,6] and the two smallest eigenvalues of each tensor are equated and represent the radial diffusivity [4]. The biophysical properties of this model are: the vector $\mathbf{d}_i = (\mathrm{d}_{\parallel,i}, \mathrm{d}_{\perp,i})$ of axial and radial diffusivities and the principal direction $\mathbf{e}_i$ of Fascicle i, and the vector of fractions $\mathbf{f}$. These variables have observations $\boldsymbol{d}_i^j$, $\boldsymbol{e}_i^j$ and $\boldsymbol{f}^j$ for Subject j. Inter-subject variability in these properties (encoded in the likelihood) is assumed much larger than DWI noise. An extra level in the hierarchical model could otherwise link parameters to DWI [9]. Fascicles are assumed independent from one another. By symmetry, directions are independent from diffusivities and fractions. Signal fractions mostly relate to partial voluming and are thus independent from fascicle properties. Diseases may affect several properties of the microstructure, so that these assumptions are only valid conditional on the diagnoses. In summary, we have:

$$\mathbf{d}_i \hat{=} (\mathrm{d}_{\parallel,i}, \mathrm{d}_{\perp,i}), \mathbf{d}_i \perp\!\!\!\perp \mathbf{d}_{j \neq i}, \quad \mathbf{e}_i \perp\!\!\!\perp \mathbf{e}_{j \neq i}, \quad \mathbf{e}_i \perp\!\!\!\perp \mathbf{d}_i, \quad \mathbf{e}_i \perp\!\!\!\perp \mathbf{f}, \quad \text{and } \mathbf{f} \perp\!\!\!\perp \mathbf{d}_i.$$

3   Model

Fig. 1 shows our hierarchical model for the latent diffusivities $(\boldsymbol{\delta}, \tilde{\boldsymbol{\delta}})$, principal directions $(\boldsymbol{\varepsilon}_i, \tilde{\boldsymbol{\varepsilon}}_i)$ and signal fractions $(\boldsymbol{\varphi}, \tilde{\boldsymbol{\varphi}})$ for the control and patient (tilded) groups respectively. Owing to the biophysical parameterization of the model, the posterior for these variables is of the form (conditioning on diagnoses is implicit):

$$p(\boldsymbol{\delta}, \tilde{\boldsymbol{\delta}}, \boldsymbol{\varepsilon}, \tilde{\boldsymbol{\varepsilon}}, \boldsymbol{\varphi}, \tilde{\boldsymbol{\varphi}}|\boldsymbol{f}, \boldsymbol{D}) = p(\boldsymbol{\varphi}, \tilde{\boldsymbol{\varphi}}|\boldsymbol{f}) \prod_{i=1}^{N} p(\boldsymbol{\delta}_i, \tilde{\boldsymbol{\delta}}_i|d_i) p(\boldsymbol{\varepsilon}_i, \tilde{\boldsymbol{\varepsilon}}_i|e_i).$$

A fully Bayesian hierarchical model is obtained by representing unknowns as random variables and assigning priors over their value [1]. We assign uniform priors for bounded variables, and log-normal priors for unbounded positive-definite variables. The log-normal prior only requires a vague idea about the order of magnitude of the variable, encoded as its mean. Its standard deviation is set to 5 to allow for mistakes in our estimate of the order of magnitude.

Modeling diffusivities. Diffusivities are in $\mathbb{R}^+ \times \mathbb{R}^+$. We represent distributions over their logarithm to assign zero probability to negative values [8]. The inter-subject variability within a group is represented as a normal law:

$$\log \mathbf{d}_i | \boldsymbol{\delta}_i, \boldsymbol{\Sigma}_i^d \sim \mathcal{N}(\log \boldsymbol{\delta}_i, \boldsymbol{\Sigma}_i^d) \quad \text{and} \quad \log \tilde{\mathbf{d}}_i | \tilde{\boldsymbol{\delta}}_i, \boldsymbol{\Sigma}_i^d \sim \mathcal{N}(\log \tilde{\boldsymbol{\delta}}_i, \boldsymbol{\Sigma}_i^d).$$

A prior over $(\boldsymbol{\delta}_i, \tilde{\boldsymbol{\delta}}_i)$ is best expressed conditionally: $p(\boldsymbol{\delta}_i, \tilde{\boldsymbol{\delta}}_i) = p(\tilde{\boldsymbol{\delta}}_i|\boldsymbol{\delta}_i)p(\boldsymbol{\delta}_i)$. The order of magnitude of diffusivities is around 10^{-4}, $10^{-3}\text{mm}^2/\text{s}$, so $\boldsymbol{\delta}_i \sim \log \mathcal{N}(-3.5, 5)$. Given $\boldsymbol{\delta}_i$ and without data from patients, our best guess for $\tilde{\boldsymbol{\delta}}_i$ is $\boldsymbol{\delta}_i$, which we encode as $\tilde{\boldsymbol{\delta}}_i|\boldsymbol{\delta}_i, \alpha_i \sim \log \mathcal{N}(\log \tilde{\boldsymbol{\delta}}_i, \alpha_i^2 \boldsymbol{I}_2)$ for an unknown variance α_i^2. We assign a log-normal hyperprior to α_i with zero mean, to express that $\tilde{\boldsymbol{\delta}}_i$ and $\boldsymbol{\delta}_i$ likely have, a priori, a similar order of magnitude. Regarding $\boldsymbol{\Sigma}_i^d$, the correlation between the axial and radial diffusivities is unknown a priori whereas we have a vague idea of the order of magnitude of the standard deviation of each diffusivity. This prior information is effectively encoded by factorizing $\boldsymbol{\Sigma}_i^d = \text{diag}(\boldsymbol{\sigma}_i^d)\mathbf{C}_i^d\text{diag}(\boldsymbol{\sigma}_i^d)$ [1], where $\boldsymbol{\sigma}_i^d$ is the vector of standard deviations and $\mathbf{C}_i^d$ is a 2×2 correlation matrix. We assign a log-normal prior to $\boldsymbol{\sigma}_i^d$ with zero mean to express that diffusivities likely have the same order of magnitude, and a uniform prior on $[-1, 1]$ for the correlation coefficient in $\mathbf{C}_i^d$.

Modeling directions. Directions are dipoles on the sphere. We model their likelihood as a Watson distribution [7], with unknown concentrations $\kappa_i, \tilde{\kappa}_i$:

$$p(\mathbf{e}_i|\boldsymbol{\varepsilon}_i, \kappa_i) = A(\kappa_i) \exp\left(\kappa_i(\boldsymbol{\varepsilon}_i \cdot \mathbf{e}_i)\right), \quad p(\tilde{\mathbf{e}}_i|\tilde{\boldsymbol{\varepsilon}}_i, \tilde{\kappa}_i) = A(\tilde{\kappa}_i) \exp\left(\tilde{\kappa}_i(\tilde{\boldsymbol{\varepsilon}}_i \cdot \tilde{\mathbf{e}}_i)\right).$$

We express the priors over latent group variables conditionally: $p(\boldsymbol{\varepsilon}_i, \tilde{\boldsymbol{\varepsilon}}_i) = p(\tilde{\boldsymbol{\varepsilon}}_i|\boldsymbol{\varepsilon}_i)p(\boldsymbol{\varepsilon}_i)$. The prior $p(\boldsymbol{\varepsilon}_i)$ is uniform over the sphere and, conditionally on $\boldsymbol{\varepsilon}_i$, we model our prior knowledge about $\tilde{\boldsymbol{\varepsilon}}_i$ as another Watson distribution with mean $\boldsymbol{\varepsilon}_i$ and unknown concentration β_i. At concentrations of 10^{-5}, the Watson is essentially uniform and at 10^5, it is extremely peaky. We therefore assign log-normal hyperpriors to all concentration parameters $\beta_i, \kappa_i, \tilde{\kappa}_i \overset{\text{iid}}{\sim} \log \mathcal{N}(0, 5)$.

Modeling fractions. Fractions belong to an N-simplex: $\{\boldsymbol{f}, f_i \geq 0, \sum_i f_i = 1\}$. The conventional Dirichlet density, with a single parameter for all variances and covariances, is too limited to represent their likelihood. Instead, we apply a change of variables to map $\mathbf{f}$ to an $(N-1)$-vector of unconstrained variables $\mathbf{y}$:

$$\mathbf{y} \hat{=} \boldsymbol{F}(\mathbf{f}) : \quad y_i = F_i(\mathbf{f}) = \text{logit}\left(\frac{f_i}{1 - \sum_{i'=1}^{i-1} f_{i'}}\right) + \log(N - i).$$

The logit maps its argument from $(0,1)$ to $(-\infty, +\infty)$. The second term is added so that $\mathbf{y} = \mathbf{0} \Leftrightarrow f_i = 1/N, \forall i$. We model the likelihood of $\mathbf{y}$ as a multivariate normal distribution with mean $\boldsymbol{F}(\boldsymbol{\varphi})$ for controls, $\boldsymbol{F}(\tilde{\boldsymbol{\varphi}})$ for patients and unknown covariance $\boldsymbol{\Sigma}_{\mathsf{f}}$. This leads to a normal logistic distribution (Fig. 1B) whose expression is derived from the Gaussian density and the Jacobian of $\boldsymbol{F}$:

$$p(\mathbf{f}|\boldsymbol{\varphi}, \boldsymbol{\Sigma}_{\mathsf{f}}) = \frac{\prod_{i=1}^{N} \frac{1}{f_i}}{|2\pi\boldsymbol{\Sigma}_{\mathsf{f}}|^{1/2}} \exp\left[-\frac{1}{2}(\boldsymbol{F}(\mathbf{f}) - \boldsymbol{F}(\boldsymbol{\varphi}))^T \boldsymbol{\Sigma}_{\mathsf{f}}^{-1}(\boldsymbol{F}(\mathbf{f}) - \boldsymbol{F}(\boldsymbol{\varphi}))\right].$$

A non-informative prior on $\boldsymbol{\varphi}$ is obtained by a normal with large variance: $\boldsymbol{F}(\boldsymbol{\varphi}) \sim \mathcal{N}(\mathbf{0}, 1000\boldsymbol{I}_{N-1})$. $\boldsymbol{F}(\tilde{\boldsymbol{\varphi}})|\boldsymbol{F}(\boldsymbol{\varphi})$ is assigned a multivariate normal prior with mean $\boldsymbol{F}(\boldsymbol{\varphi})$ and covariance $\gamma\boldsymbol{I}_{N-1}$ with unknown γ. As for α_i and β_i, γ is assigned a log-normal hyperprior with zero mean. The unknown covariance is decomposed as $\boldsymbol{\Sigma}_{\mathsf{f}} = \text{diag}(\boldsymbol{\sigma}_{\mathsf{f}})\mathbf{C}_{\mathsf{f}}\text{diag}(\boldsymbol{\sigma}_{\mathsf{f}})$. The correlation $\mathbf{C}_{\mathsf{f}}$ is an $(N-1)\times(N-1)$ matrix to which we assign a LKJ($\eta=1$) prior which is uniform over all correlation matrices [1]. As before, $\boldsymbol{\sigma}_{\mathsf{f}}$ is assigned a log-normal prior with zero mean.

4   Inference

The model needs to be estimated in each voxel. Efficient estimation of its posterior is therefore critical to its use in practice. The posterior has no closed-form expression due to interactions between variables and the introduction of non-conjugate priors. Variational Bayes approximations, often used in this case, may introduce biases that would jeopardize the reliability of group differences [2]. We therefore use Markov Chain Monte Carlo (MCMC) sampling. Because our log-posterior is differentiable, we exploit Hamiltonian Monte Carlo (HMC) sampling which converges much faster (in $O(D^{5/4})$ for D dimensions) than conventional Gibbs and Metropolis sampling ($O(D^2)$) [2]. Specifically, we use the No-U-Turn Sampler (NUTS) which automatically optimizes the parameters of the HMC sampling [2]. We draw four Markov chains of 2000 samples and discard the first 1000 burn-in samples. Convergence is monitored by the scale reduction factor $\hat{R}$ [1]. From samples of the joint posterior over the model parameters $\boldsymbol{\theta}$ (all variables in Fig. 1), marginal posteriors of any statistics of interest $\mathsf{T}(\boldsymbol{\theta})$ are simply obtained by computing their values from the posterior samples. Importantly, because the joint posterior is not altered by the computation of $\mathsf{T}(\boldsymbol{\theta})$, many statistics can be simultaneously analyzed without the need to correct for multiple comparisons as in NHST. False discoveries are mitigated by the shrinkage towards the prior. For the validation, we focus on the posterior probabilities

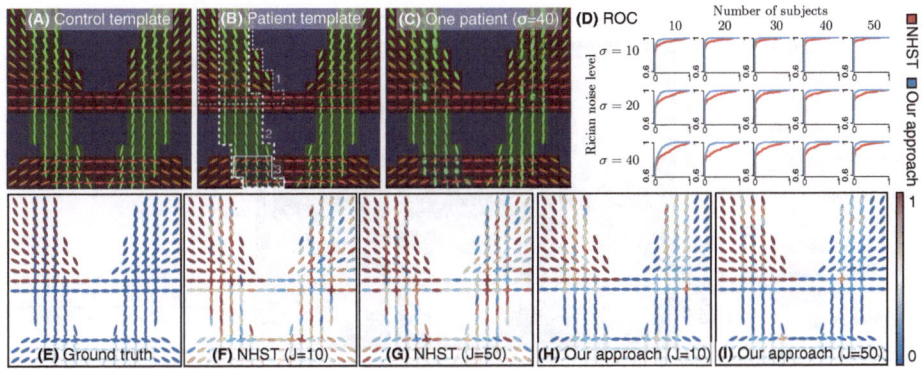

Fig. 2. (A) Template for the control population (fractions encoded as RGB). (B) Template for the patient population with three overlapping affected areas (see text). (C) A simulated patient with noise at level $\sigma = 40$. (D) ROC analysis demonstrates that our approach outperforms NHST for all noise levels and all number of subjects. (E) Ground truth difference in radial diffusivity. (F-G) NHST provides evidence for an alteration in Area 1 but fails to provide evidence that no alteration is present elsewhere. Color encodes $1 - $ p-value. (H-I) Bayesian posterior maps provide both evidence that fascicles in Area 1 are altered (high posterior) and that tensors elsewhere are unaltered (low posterior). This evidence increases as the number of subjects increases.

that the differences in latent group variables fall outside a region of practical equivalence (ROPE):

$$P\left(|\delta_{.,i} - \tilde{\delta}_{.,i}| > \epsilon_d | \text{Data}\right), P\left(|\varphi_i - \tilde{\varphi}_i| > \epsilon_f | \text{Data}\right), P\left(|\text{acos}(\boldsymbol{\varepsilon}_i \cdot \tilde{\boldsymbol{\varepsilon}}_i)| > \epsilon_e | \text{Data}\right).$$

The bounds of ROPE vary with the empirical context. In our experiments, we set $\epsilon_d = 10^{-6} \text{mm}^2/\text{s}$, $\epsilon_f = 0.01$, $\epsilon_e = 1°$. Posterior values close to 1 are strong evidence for the presence of a microstructure abnormality, akin to small p-values in NHST. Posterior values close to zero are strong evidence that the difference between the groups is within the ROPE. This property of the posterior has no equivalent in NHST and has, as will be seen, far-reaching consequences in population studies.

5   Experiments and Results

Implementation. HMC sampling was implemented in Stan 2.2 (`mc-stan.org`), took an average 0.03 sec per chain and always reached full convergence ($\hat{R} = 1$).

Data. Directly simulating multi-fascicle models is biased because the impact of the noise on model parameters is unclear. We therefore simulated the process of estimating models from noisy DWI. We created a control and a patient template with various crossing angles (Fig. 2A-B). The patient template has overlapping areas of microstructural differences: Area 1 has radial diffusivity of oblique fascicles inflated by 10%, Area 2 has in-plane orientation alterations of 10° and Area

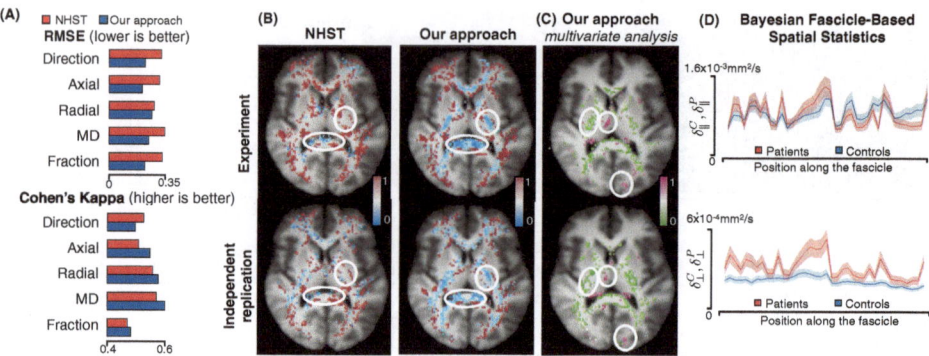

Fig. 3. (A) RMSE and Cohen's κ coefficient both indicate that inference results from the Bayesian approach are more reproducible than those obtained with NHST. (B) The improved reproducibility for the axial diffusivity is explained by the presence of many voxels with low values of the posterior (blue voxels) for which NHST results in uniformly distributed p-values. (C) Our framework can be applied to more complex analyses such as the coupled increase in fraction of isotropic diffusion and radial diffusivity. The resulting posterior map can be interpreted exactly as the others. (D) Augmenting the model with spatial priors enables the analysis of fascicle-wise properties, such as the diffusivity profile along the arcuate fasciculus.

3 has increased fraction of isotropic diffusion by 0.1. For each simulated subject, 90 DWI on 3 shells at b=1,2,3000, were corrupted by Rician noise with scale parameters $\sigma = 10, 20, 40$. Multi-fascicle models were then estimated as in [6] (Fig. 2C). For each σ, groups of K patients and K controls were generated for $K = 10, 20, 30, 40, 50$. The process was repeated 10 times for each pair (σ, K) leading to 150 synthetic populations. In-vivo DWI ($1.7 \times 1.7 \times 2mm^3$, Siemens 3T Trio, 32-channel head coil) were acquired using the CUSP-45 sequence [6] with b-values up to 3000 in 36 patients with Tuberous Sclerosis Complex (TSC), a condition with high prevalence of autism, and 36 age-matched controls. Two-fascicle models with one isotropic compartment were estimated.

Preprocessing. All multi-fascicle models were non-linearly registered to an atlas as in [8]. At each voxel, the tensors of all J controls and K patients were grouped in N clusters using the iterative scheme of [8], where N is the number of fascicles in the atlas. Due to model selection, the number of observations $(J_i + K_i)$ varies between fascicles. The presence or absence of a fascicle may itself be an interesting group contrast and is reflected in the vector of fractions **f** that may contain null values (replaced by an epsilon machine to avoid singularity).

Validation on synthetic phantoms. Population studies were conducted with all 150 simulated populations and for five properties: the radial, axial and mean diffusivities, the orientation of fascicles and the fractions of isotropic diffusion. NHST for log-diffusivities and logit-fractions were performed by independent t-tests as in [8] and NHST for directions used Schwartzman's test for diffusion tensors [7]. For all properties, true positive rates and true negative rates were computed at different thresholds leading to ROC curves (Fig. 2D). Consistently for all noise levels and all number of subjects, our Bayesian approach outperforms NHST. This is also the case independently for each property that presents a group contrast. The improvement of our Bayesian approach over NHST is akin to tripling the number of subjects. This can be attributed to two features of the Bayesian framework. First, the introduction of ROPE avoids the detection of false positives with negligible yet statistically significant magnitude. Second, low values of the Bayesian posteriors is evidence for the absence of a group difference whereas high p-values occur randomly (uniformly) if the null hypothesis is true. This situation is illustrated in Fig. 2E-I for the radial diffusivity. Bayesian posteriors outside of Area 1 takes on small values (Fig. 2H-I) whereas p-values are uniformly distributed in those voxels.

Validation on in-vivo data. In-vivo data were used to assess the reproducibility of results. Patient and control groups were each split in two subgroups, leading to two cohorts each with 18 controls and 18 patients. Population studies for directions, isotropic fraction, radial, axial and mean diffusivities were conducted in each cohort. For each property, the resulting two p-value maps were compared to one another in terms of root mean squared error (RMSE) and so were the two posterior maps. For all five variables of interests, the RMSE was significantly smaller between posterior maps (mean RMSE: 0.23) than between p-value maps (mean RMSE: 0.32; two-sample t-test: $p < 0.0005$) with a mean improvement of 27.5% (Fig. 3A). The largest improvement was observed for the axial diffusivity (reduction of 35%). RMSE directly compares the statistical maps regardless of the decision made from these maps (after thresholding). We therefore also assess reproducibility of inference results based on Cohen's κ coefficient of agreement after thresholding p-values at 0.05 and posteriors at 0.95: $\kappa = \frac{P_a - P_e}{1 - P_e}$ where P_a is the observed agreement probability and P_e is the probability of agreeing by chance. κ was larger with the Bayesian approach for all properties except for the directions (Fig. 3A). The improvement was larger for axial diffusivity (+6.5%). The higher improvement in reproducibility observed for the study of axial diffusivity both in terms of RMSE and κ is elucidated by Fig. 3(B). Strong evidence for the absence of any substantive difference in axial diffusivity can be inferred and reproduced with the Bayesian approach (blue areas in Fig. 3B). In these regions, the p-value is uniformly distributed leading to poor RMSE and κ.

Prospectives. So far, we focused on simple statistics to fairly compare our approach to NHST. But more complex statistics may too be of interest. For instance, the presence of myelin injury with neuroinflammation may result in a coupled increase in fraction of isotropic diffusion due to cell swelling and in radial diffusivity due to demyelination. This association remains hypothetical, but our capability to detect it may increase specificity of microstructure imaging. Detection of these complex responses is not easily framed as an NHST, but is readily computable with our Bayesian approach: $p(\tilde{\varphi}_{\mathsf{iso}} > \varphi_{\mathsf{iso}}, \tilde{\delta}_{\perp,i} > \delta_{\perp,i} | \mathrm{Data})$, depicted in Fig. 3C. Our Bayesian framework also enables incorporation of prior information, such as spatial priors to increase coherence of the posterior. To illustrate this possibility, we augment our model with a Gaussian Markov random field prior over latent diffusivities in adjacent voxels along a fascicle of interest: the median tract of the left arcuate fasciculus (AF). The results are joint posteriors of all diffusivities along the tract, leading to fascicle-wise (rather than voxel-wise) analysis. The profiles in Fig. 3D are maximum a posteriori (lines) and 95% posterior intervals (shades). They indicate that TSC patients have substantially higher radial but unaltered axial diffusivities along the AF.

6   Conclusion

This paper introduced a Bayesian framework to conduct population studies of the brain microstructure. A key property of this framework is its ability to build evidence for the absence of alterations alongside the detection of abnormalities. This key property makes it less prone to false discoveries than NHST and improves reproducibility of findings. By estimating the full posterior distribution over latent variables, our Bayesian framework therefore enables richer and more reliable analyses of the brain microstructure and its alterations in diseases.

Acknowledgments. This work was supported in part by F.R.S.-FNRS, WBI, NIH grants R01 NS079788, R01 LM010033, R01 EB013248, P30 HD018655, and by a research grant from the Boston Children's Hospital Translational Research Program.

References

1. Gelman, A., Carlin, J.B., Stern, H.S., Dunson, D.B., Vehtari, A., Rubin, D.B.: Bayesian data analysis. CRC press (2013)
2. Hoffman, M.D., Gelman, A.: The no-U-turn sampler: Adaptively setting path lengths in Hamiltonian Monte Carlo. Journal of Machine Learning Research (2013)
3. Nuzzo, R.: Scientific method: statistical errors. Nature 506(7487), 150–152 (2014)
4. Panagiotaki, E., Schneider, T., Siow, B., Hall, M.G., Lythgoe, M.F., Alexander, D.C.: Compartment models of the diffusion MR signal in brain white matter: a taxonomy and comparison. Neuroimage 59(3), 2241–2254 (2012)
5. Pasternak, O., Westin, C.F., Bouix, S., et al.: Excessive extracellular volume reveals a neurodegenerative pattern in schizophrenia onset. The Journal of Neuroscience 32(48), 17365–17372 (2012)
6. Scherrer, B., Warfield, S.K.: Parametric representation of multiple white matter fascicles from cube and sphere diffusion MRI. PLoS one 7(11), e48232 (2012)
7. Schwartzman, A., Dougherty, R., Taylor, J.: Cross-subject comparison of principal diffusion direction maps. Magnetic Resonance in Medicine 53(6), 1423–1431 (2005)
8. Taquet, M., Scherrer, B., Commowick, O., Peters, J.M., Sahin, M., Macq, B., Warfield, S.K.: A mathematical framework for the registration and analysis of multi-fascicle models for population studies of the brain microstructure. IEEE Transactions on Medical Imaging 33(2), 504–517 (2014)
9. Taquet, M., Scherrer, B., Boumal, N., Macq, B., Warfield, S.K.: Estimation of a multi-fascicle model from single b-value data with a population-informed prior. In: Mori, K., Sakuma, I., Sato, Y., Barillot, C., Navab, N. (eds.) MICCAI 2013, Part I. LNCS, vol. 8149, pp. 695–702. Springer, Heidelberg (2013)

Shading Correction for Whole Slide Image Using Low Rank and Sparse Decomposition

Tingying Peng[1,3], Lichao Wang[1,4], Christine Bayer[5], Sailesh Conjeti[1,6],
Maximilian Baust[1], and Nassir Navab[1,2]

[1] Computer Aided Medical Procedures (CAMP), Technische Universität München, Germany
[2] Computer Aided Medical Procedures (CAMP), Johns Hopkins University, USA
[3] Department of Nuclear Medicine, Technische Universität München, Germany
[4] Helmholtz Zentrum München, Germany
[5] Department of Radiation Oncology, Technische Universität München, Germany
[6] School of Medical Science and Technology, IIT Kharagpur, India

Abstract. Many microscopic imaging modalities suffer from the problem of intensity inhomogeneity due to uneven illumination or camera nonlinearity, known as shading artifacts. A typical example of this is the unwanted seam when stitching images to obtain a whole slide image (WSI). Elimination of shading plays an essential role for subsequent image processing such as segmentation, registration, or tracking. In this paper, we propose two new retrospective shading correction algorithms for WSI targeted to two common forms of WSI: multiple image tiles before mosaicking and an already-stitched image. Both methods leverage on recent achievements in matrix rank minimization and sparse signal recovery. We show how the classic shading problem in microscopy can be reformulated as a decomposition problem of low-rank and sparse components, which seeks an optimal separation of the foreground objects of interest and the background illumination field. Additionally, a sparse constraint is introduced in the Fourier domain to ensure the smoothness of the recovered background. Extensive qualitative and quantitative validation on both synthetic and real microscopy images demonstrates superior performance of the proposed methods in shading removal in comparison with a well-established method in ImageJ.

1   Introduction

Automated microscopic image processing and analysis are increasingly gaining attention in the field of biological imaging. However, a common artifact that encumbers the use of automatic image processing techniques is intensity inhomogeneity present in microscopic images, also known as shading [1]. Intensity inhomogeneity may originate from non-uniform illumination, uneven sample thickness or camera nonlinearity. As shown in Fig. 1(a), the shading effect manifests itself in whole slide image (WSI) by introducing unwanted seams in stitched mosaics.

In general, shading can be categorized into object-dependent and object-independent shading [2]. A careful prospective calibration process may solve object-independent shading, e.g. by using a calibration slide, which is, however, not always available. More commonly, posteriori (retrospective) image processing algorithms are developed to correct both object-dependent and object-independent shading.

P. Golland et al. (Eds.): MICCAI 2014, Part I, LNCS 8673, pp. 33–40, 2014.
© Springer International Publishing Switzerland 2014

Existing popular retrospective shading correction methods include morphological filtering [3], Gaussian blurring [4], entropy minimization [5] or fitting polynomial surfaces [6]. Some of these methods are not fully automatic, e.g. the control points for the polynomial fitting should not be positioned on the objects, which require either manual interference or object-dependent segmentation. Moreover, it has been shown that the performance of the majority of these methods is strongly affected by the size of the foreground objects [2]. Due to the increased magnification in WSI, the foreground objects in each image tile are enlarged and can therefore negatively affect the performance of conventional shading correction algorithms.

Apart from above mentioned algorithmic limits, there is an additional constraint for shading correction of WSI in practice. The output of currently popular whole slide microscopy scanning devices comes usually in two forms, namely a sequence of tile images that need to be stitched into the WSI or an already-stitched WSI. Shadings exist in both forms. Therefore, we propose two automatic algorithms to remove shading effects of WSI, one for each form of the output image. Both these algorithms are based on approximating the foreground objects and the background illumination field by a sparse and a low rank matrix, respectively. Both algorithms were evaluated qualitatively and quantitatively using synthetic and real microscopic images.

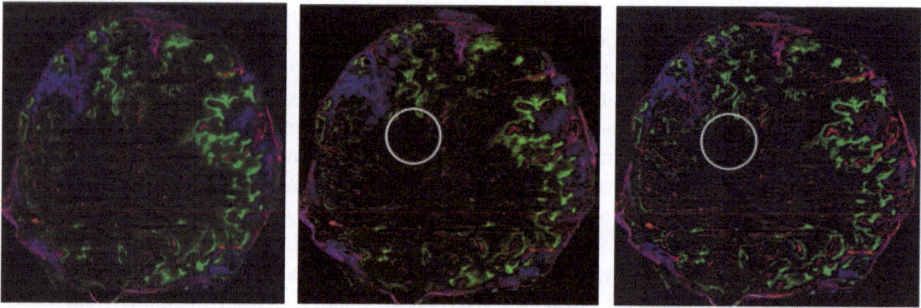

Fig. 1. (Left) the mosaic built using the original (uncorrected) fluorescence image sequences, which reveals strong illumination discontinuity across the stitching borders in the green channel; (middle) shading correction using Algorithm 1 successfully removes this artifact and achieves a seamless mosaicking; (right) artifact remains after "Rolling Ball" correction.

2   Methods

2.1   Modelling the Shading Effect in Microscopy

The effect of shading on microscope image intensities is typically based on either a multiplicative model or an additive model of the artifact [2]:

$$I(x,y) = O(x,y) \cdot S(x,y) \tag{1}$$

$$I(x,y) = O(x,y) + S(x,y) \tag{2}$$

where I and O are the observed and the true stain-related image intensities respectively and S is the distortion caused by shading. By taking the logarithm of the image intensities: $\hat{I}(x,y) = log\big(I(x,y)\big)$, Equation 1 becomes $\hat{I} = \hat{O} + \hat{S}$, thus being the additive model. By taking the exponent of the additive model we can also jump back to the multiplicative one. Hence, although the following proposed illumination correction methods are based on the additive model, it is straightforward to be transferred into a multiplicative one. In the additive model, the shading-free image O is also denoted as the foreground, F, whilst the shading field is denoted as the background, B.

2.2   Shading Correction of WSI Using Multiple Image Tiles

In this subsection the first proposed algorithm (Algorithm 1) is described. In case of the whole slide image, a series of images, $I_1, I_2, ..., I_n$, are collected using the same microscope with the same settings. Hence they share the same background illumination field, $I_i = F_i + B$. Generally, the foreground F_i occupies only a fraction of the image pixels and therefore can be treated as a *sparse* component. If we concatenate each image into a column vector, the observation model can be written as:

$$D \stackrel{\text{def}}{=} [\text{vec}(I_1)| \cdots |\text{vec}(I_n)] = A + E \tag{3}$$

where $A = [\text{vec}(B)| \cdots |\text{vec}(B)] \in \mathbb{R}^{m \times n}$ is a *low rank (rank one)* matrix that models the common background of each image. And $E = [\text{vec}(F_1)| \cdots |\text{vec}(F_n)] \in \mathbb{R}^{m \times n}$ is the sparse signal matrix. Hence, we can solve the following minimization problem:

$$\min_E \|E\|_1, \text{s.t.} \ D = A + E, a_i = a_j \tag{4}$$

where $\|\cdot\|_1$ denotes the l_1-norm (i.e. the sum of the absolute values of matrix elements). a_i is the ith column of matrix A, and $a_i = a_j$ forces the estimated background field from each image to be the same. Moreover, it is also reasonable to assume the background illumination field to be smooth. Smooth functions are typically sparse in the Fourier transformed domain. We could modify the above convex optimization problem (3) as follows to impose this additional smoothness constraint:

$$\min_{W,E} \|W\|_1 + \|E\|_1, \quad \text{s.t.} \ D = A + E, A = \text{repmat}(QWQ^T) \tag{5}$$

where $\text{repmat}(QWQ^T) \stackrel{\text{def}}{=} [\text{vec}(QWQ^T)| \cdots |\text{vec}(QWQ^T)]$ (repeated n times) and Q is chosen to be discrete cosine transform (DCT). W is the matrix of the DCT coefficients and fulfills the sparse constraint.

Solving (4) requires simultaneously minimization of l_1-norm of two matrices, in the original and Fourier spaces respectively. Here we utilize the Linearized Alternating Direction Method (LADM), which is widely used in solving various low-rank and sparse matrix separation and recovery problems (e.g. robust PCA in [7])

$$L(W,E,Y,\mu) = \|W\|_1 + \|E\|_1 + \langle Y, D - \text{repmat}(QWQ^T) - E \rangle \\ + \mu\|D - \text{repmat}(QWQ^T) - E\|_F \tag{6}$$

Here Y denotes the Lagrange multiplier, $\langle \cdot, \cdot \rangle$ is the inner product, $\|\cdot\|_F$ is the Frobenius norm and $\mu > 0$ is a penalty parameter. Incorporating the LADM updating scheme, the proposed Algorithm 1 is described as the following:

Algorithm 1 (Shading correction of WSI using multiple image tiles)

Input: Observation matrix $D \in \mathbb{R}^{m \times n}$, each column of matrix D corresponds to a concatenated vector of each image.

1: $Y_0 = D/J(D)$; $W_0 = 0$; $E_0 = 0$; $\mu_0 > 0$; $\rho > 1$; $k = 0$.

2: **while** not converged **do**

3: $W_{k+1} = T_{\mu_k^{-1}}\{W_k + Q^T[\text{avg}(D - \text{repmat}(QW_kQ^T)) - E_k + Y_k/\mu_k)]Q\}$;

4: $E_{k+1} = T_{\mu_k^{-1}}\{D - \text{repmat}(QW_{k+1}Q^T) + Y_k/\mu_k\}$;

5: $Y_{k+1} = Y_k + \mu_k(D - \text{repmat}(QW_{k+1}Q^T) - E_{k+1})$; $\mu_{k+1} = \rho\mu_k$, $k = k + 1$.

6: **end while**

7: **Output:** (W_k, E_k); QW_kQ^T is the estimated background illumination field.

Where avg$(\cdot)$ is the mean column of the matrix and $T_\varepsilon(x) = \text{sgn}(x)\max(|x| - \varepsilon, 0)$ is the scalar shrinkage operator, $J(x)$ is the dual norm of x (for details refer to [8]).

2.3   Shading Correction of an Already Stitched WSI

In this subsection the proposed Algorithm 2 is described. Instead of providing tile image sequence, many WSI microscopy scanners output only an already-stitched WSI. In such a case, it is generally difficult to recover tile images without the prior knowledge of the detailed microscopy acquisition and stitching protocol and hence Algorithm 1 can no longer be used. We notice in previous studies that the smoothly varying background illumination field is often modeled using limited terms of some basis function, e.g., second-order polynomials [5]

$$B(x, y) = a_0 + a_1 x + a_2 y + a_3 xy + a_4 x^2 + a_5 y^2 \tag{7}$$

It can be seen that the estimated illumination field using polynomials has a low rank ($rank(B) \leq 5$). For a WSI that is stitched from a microscopy sequence, its illumination field is simply a repeating pattern of individual background and hence is also low rank. However, as suggested in [9], being low-rank *does not necessarily imply smoothness*. Therefore, similar to Algorithm 1, we introduce a smoothness constraint, which can be interpreted as the estimated background to be *low rank as well as sparse in the Fourier domain*. In this circumstance, the optimization problem becomes ([9]):

$$\min_{A,E,W} \|A\|_* + \gamma\|W\|_1 + \lambda\|E\|_1, \text{s.t.} D = A + E, A = QWQ^T \tag{8}$$

where $\|\cdot\|_*$ represents the nuclear norm of a matrix (i.e. the sum of the matrix singular values), γ controls the smoothness of the estimated background whilst λ controls the relative sparsity of the foreground. The optimal settings for γ and λ depend on the characteristics of the processed image and will be explained in the results section. Again, we use LADM to solve the optimization problem (Algorithm 2).

3   Experiments and Results

In this section we evaluate the qualitative and quantitative performance of the proposed correction methods on both synthetic and real microscopic images. Further,

---

Algorithm 2 (Shading correction for an already-stitched WSI)

Input: Observation image $D \in \mathbb{R}^{m \times n}$.

1: $Y_{10} = 0$; $Y_{20} = D/J(D)$; $A_0 = 0$; $W_0 = 0$; $E_0 = 0$; $\mu_0 > 0$; $\rho > 1$; $k = 0$.

2: **while** not converged **do**

3: $W_{k+1} = T_{\gamma/\mu_k}\{W_k + Q^T[D + A_k - E_k - 2QW_kQ^T + Y_{1k}/\mu_k + Y_{2k}/\mu_k]Q\}$;

4: $E_{k+1} = T_{\lambda/\mu_k}\{D - QW_{k+1}Q^T + Y_{2k}/\mu_k\}$;

5: $(U, S, V) = \text{svd}(QW_{k+1}Q^T - Y_{1k}/\mu_k)$; $A_{k+1} = UT_{\mu_k^{-1}}(S)V^T$;

6: $Y_{1k+1} = Y_{1k} + \mu_k(A_{k+1} - QW_{k+1}Q^T)$; $Y_{2k+1} = Y_{2k} + \mu_k(D - QW_{k+1}Q^T - E_{k+1})$;

7: $\mu_{k+1} = \rho\mu_k$; $k = k + 1$.

8: **end while**

9: **Output:** (A_k, E_k); A_k is the estimated illumination field and E_k is the corrected image with uniform illumination.

---

we compare our two methods with the "Rolling Ball" shading correction algorithm in ImageJ [10], which achieves the best performance amongst several popular retrospective shading correction methods [11]. For WSI image tiles, "Rolling Ball" is used to estimate a shading field of each image tile separately and the common shading is taken as the median of individually estimated shading fields [12]; for an already-stitched WSI, "Rolling Ball" is used to correct the shading effect of a single image.

3.1   Test on Synthetic Data

Firstly, both the proposed shading correction strategies are tested by using true uniform microscopic images, simulating the shading effect, correcting the images, and comparing the corrected and the original images. For this purpose, 10 synthetic shading-free fluorescence microscopy images (1200x1200 pixels, normalized intensity between 0 and 1) are generated using the simulation tool presented in [13]. For each image, a background illumination field was simulated by the polynomial background model (Eq.8, $a_i \sim \mathcal{U}(0,1)$, maximum amplitude 0.2). The illumination field is used to corrupt the test image according to the additive shading model [13]. The WSI is imitated by dividing an image into multiple tiles using regular grids at a size of $n \times n$, with the same illumination field added to each image tile. Fig. 2 shows a synthetic WSI image without shading (left) and one with shading artifact (right). In the simulation study, we $\gamma = 0.1, \lambda = 0.05$ in Algorithm 2 and the rolling ball radius is set to be 100 pixels, which is about the size of the largest object of interest.

The quantitative performance of the proposed methods is measured by Mean Absolute Error (MAE), defined as the average of the absolute difference between the corrected image and the original shading-free image. Since both image simulation and shading correction are based on the additive model, the MAE of the foreground is equivalent to the error between the estimated and true backgrounds. As shown in Fig. 3, if the image is stitched from a very limited number of image tiles (e.g. 2x2), the Rolling Ball algorithm achieves good performance, which, however, deteriorates rapidly as the stitching size of the WSI increases. This is due to the fact that the Rolling Ball cannot separate the objects of interest if they are similar in size to the variations in the background. In contrast, the two proposed algorithms achieve consistently good results, which demonstrates the effectiveness of the formulation of WSI shading as a low rank matrix in both cases. It is also illustrated that Algorithm 1 using multiple image tiles performs slightly better than Algorithm 2 using a stitched image.

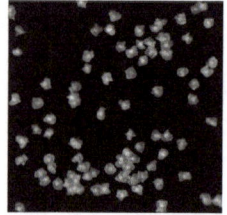 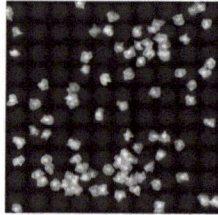

Fig. 2. The synthetic WSI with uniform (left) and uneven (right) illumination

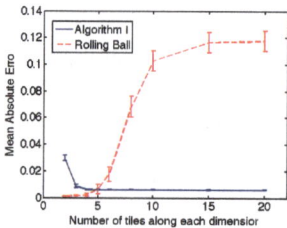 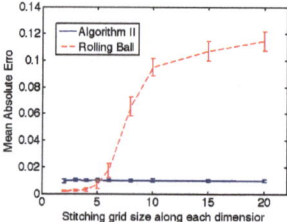

Fig. 3. Mean Absolute Error between the corrected and the reference microscopic image using Algorithm 1 on image tiles (left) and Algorithm 2 on an already-stitched WSI (right)

3.2   Shading Correction in WSI for Seamless Image Mosaic

The proposed algorithms are further evaluated in shading correction of 10 real WSIs (each WSI has a tile size of 50-200). These images were acquired using the MosaiX and Multidimentional acquisition modules of the Axiovision Program (Version 4.8.3.0; Zeiss). The false RGB colors encode AlexaFluor594, FITC-labeled anti-pimonidazole antibody and Hoechst33342 dyes respectively. The strong background shading is presented only in the green channel (Fig .1 left) because of the weak FITC fluorescence as well as its long exposure time. Algorithm 1 is used to perform shading correction, which removes the Moiré pattern artifact originally presented in the green channel completely without corrupting the shading-free red and blue channels (Fig. 1, middle). In contrast, the Rolling Ball algorithm (rolling radius 50 pixels) rejects a part of the red fluorescence (in white circle) as background (Fig.1. right). Besides visual inspection, the quality of our shading correction algorithm is further assessed using root-mean-square error (RMSE) on the overlap regions, a popular criteria to measure the mosaic quality of fluorescence microscopy [1]. As reported in Table 1, a Wilcoxon Signed Rank test indicates that our approach improves over the uncorrected images with high confidence. Although statistical significance is also achieved with the Rolling Ball algorithm, the average improvement (24.2%) is not as good as ours (35.8%).

The second example shown here is a stitched WSI of phase contrast image of neurons. Background non-uniformity is presented in each image tile and between tiles

(Fig. 4 (left)). Shading correction of this image is challenging due to the fact that the light diffraction in the background correlates with the foreground, making it difficult to remove the shading by prospective calibration. Secondly, the foreground consists of both bright and dark objects of difference sizes and hence the fundamental assumption of Rolling Ball algorithm is invalid here (Rolling Ball assumes the foreground is either brighter or darker than the background). By using sparse and low rank decomposition in Algorithm 2 ($\gamma = 0.1, \lambda = 0.005$), the foreground (middle) and background (right) are successfully separated for such a challenging case.

3.3   Discussion of the Results

Amongst the two proposed shading correction methods, Algorithm 1 is a blind method that does not require any user-setting parameters. In Algorithm 2, γ controls the smoothness of the estimated background and we determined that a fixed 0.1 works well for both our synthetic and real microscopy images. In comparison, λ needs to be tuned by users as it is related to the relative proportion of the foreground objects. In practice, this parameter can be fixed for a group of microscopy images collected from a particular experiment, as this proportion does not usually vary by much.

An ideal shading correction algorithm would correct artifact without distorting the underlying biological structures. The synthetic study has quantitatively demonstrated a minuscule error between the corrected image and the ground-truth biology. In the real image study, besides RMSE improvement in the shading-affected green channel, our algorithm does not corrupt the shading-free red and blue channels, which clearly shows that the relevant biological information is preserved. In fact, the low rank and sparse decomposition is completed so that no information is lost. In contrast to a low-rank background, biological structures are unlikely to have a low rank, being falsely removed by our algorithm.

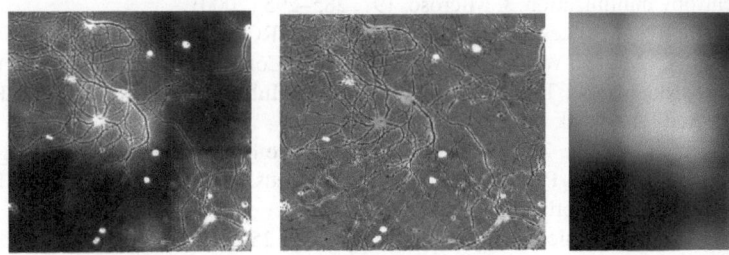

Fig. 4. Part of a WSI without (left) and with (middle) shading correction using Algorithm 2 and the estimated background illumination (right)

Table 1. RMSE on the overlap regions of WSI image tiles with and without shading removal

Mosaic set	Uncorrected	Algorithm 1	Rolling Ball
RMSE	12.0±2.5	7.7±1.4	9.1±1.7
p-value		0.002	0.03
Average Improvement		35.8%	24.2%

4   Conclusion

In this paper we propose two automatic algorithms to correct shading effect in whole slide microscopic imaging. These algorithms decompose a multi-image sequence (Algorithm 1) or an already-stitched image (Algorithm 2) into a background component approximated by a low rank matrix and a foreground component represented by a sparse matrix. In addition, the sparse constraint in the Fourier domain regularizes the smoothness of the recovered background. Both qualitative and quantitative evaluation using synthetic and different types of real microscopic images proves the accuracy of our methods as well as their generality.

Acknowledgement. T. Peng was supported by the Humboldt Research Fellowship (3.5-CHN/1149232 STP). The project was partially supported by SFB824. The authors would also like to thank Christophe Leterrier of Aix Marseille University, France to kindly provide the phase-contrast microscopic image.

References

1. Piccinini, F., Bevilacqua, A., Smith, K., Horvath, P.: Vignetting and photo-bleaching correction in automated fluorescence microscopy from an array of overlapping images. In: 2013 ISBI, pp. 464–467. IEEE (2013)
2. Tomazevic, D., Likar, B., Pernus, F.: Comparative evaluation of retrospective shading correction methods. J. Microsc. 208, 212–223 (2002)
3. Sternberg, S.R.: Biomedical Image Processing. IEEE Comput. 16, 22–34 (1983)
4. Leong, F.J.W.-M., Brady, M., McGee, J.O.: Correction of uneven illumination (vignetting) in digital microscopy images. J. Clin. Pathol. 56, 619–621 (2003)
5. Likar, B., Maintz, J.B., Viergever, M.A., Pernus, F.: Retrospective shading correction based on entropy minimization. J. Microsc. 197, 285–295 (2000)
6. Russ, J.C.: The Image Processing Handbook, 6th edn. CRC Press (2011)
7. Cand, E.J., Li, X., Ma, Y., Wright, J.: Robust Principal Component Analysis? (2009)
8. Lin, Z., Chen, M., Ma, Y.: The Augmented Lagrange Multiplier Method for Exact Recovery of Corrupted Low-Rank Matrices. In: NIPS (2011)
9. Liang, X., Ren, X., Zhang, Z., Ma, Y.: Repairing sparse low-rank texture. In: Fitzgibbon, A., Lazebnik, S., Perona, P., Sato, Y., Schmid, C. (eds.) ECCV 2012, Part V. LNCS, vol. 7576, pp. 482–495. Springer, Heidelberg (2012)
10. Collins, T.J.: ImageJ for microscopy. Biotechniques 43, 25–30 (2007)
11. Babaloukas, G., Tentolouris, N., Liatis, S., Sklavounou, A., Perrea, D.: Evaluation of three methods for retrospective correction of vignetting on medical microscopy images utilizing two open source software tools. J. Microsc. 244, 320–324 (2011)
12. Piccinini, F., Lucarelli, E., Gherardi, A., Bevilacqua, A.: Multi-image based method to correct vignetting effect in light microscopy images. J. Microsc. 248, 6–22 (2012)
13. Lehmussola, A., Ruusuvuori, P., Selinummi, J., Huttunen, H., Yli-Harja, O.: Computational framework for simulating fluorescence microscope images with cell populations. IEEE Trans. Med. Imaging 26, 1010–1016 (2007)

Cell-Sensitive Microscopy Imaging
for Cell Image Segmentation

Zhaozheng Yin[1,*], Hang Su[2], Elmer Ker[3], Mingzhong Li[1], and Haohan Li[1]

[1] Department of Computer Science, Missouri University of Science and Technology
[2] Department of Electronic Engineering, Shanghai Jiaotong University
[3] Department of Orthopedic Surgery, Stanford University

Abstract. We propose a novel cell segmentation approach by estimating a cell-sensitive camera response function based on variously exposed phase contrast microscopy images on the same cell dish. Using the cell-sensitive microscopy imaging, cells' original irradiance signals are restored from all exposures and the irradiance signals on non-cell background regions are restored as a uniform constant (i.e., the imaging system is sensitive to cells only but insensitive to non-cell background). Cell segmentation is then performed on the restored irradiance signals by simple thresholding. The experimental results validate that high quality cell segmentation can be achieved by our approach.

1 Introduction

Phase contrast microscopy imaging [14], a non-invasive technique, has been widely used to observe live cells without staining them. The imaging system consists of a phase contrast microscope and a digital camera to record time-lapse microscopy images on cells to analyze their properties. As shown in Fig.1, the illuminance (L) passes through a Petri dish culturing cells and microscope optics, and generates the irradiance (E) observable by human eyes or digital cameras. The camera captures the irradiance (E) within an exposure duration (Δt) and transforms the accumulated irradiance (X, $X = E\Delta t$) into pixel values (I) in digital images by a CCD sensor response function f, i.e., the pixel value in a microscopy image is a function of irradiance and exposure time: $I = f(E\Delta t)$.

To automatically process cell images by computational algorithms, cell segmentation plays a key role because cells need to be segmented and localized in images first before being tracked and analyzed over time [3,8]. Well-known image segmentation algorithms such as thresholding, morphological operations, watershed, level-set and Laplacian-of-Gaussian filtering, have been explored in various cell image analysis systems [2,5,7,9,11,12]. Since these cell segmentation algorithms overlook the specific image formation process of phase contrast microscopy, recently the imaging model of phase contrast microscope optics and its related features have been exploited to facilitate the cell segmentation [10,13].

* This research is supported by NSF CAREER award IIS-1351049, University of Missouri Research Board, ISC and CBSE centers at Missouri S&T.

P. Golland et al. (Eds.): MICCAI 2014, Part I, LNCS 8673, pp. 41–48, 2014.

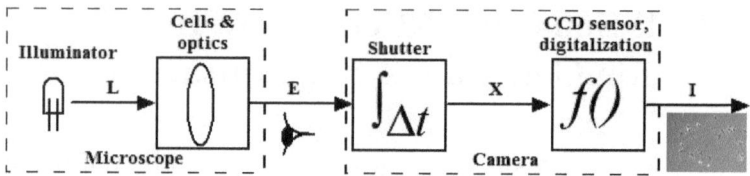

Fig. 1. Microscopy image formation process

However, the work on imaging model of phase contrast optics [13] focuses on the front-end of the entire imaging pipeline but ignores the rear-end (camera) of the pipeline. In fact, different camera settings also affect the cell image analysis. As shown in Fig.2, on the same cell dish, too short or too long exposure duration yields under-exposure (Fig.2(a)) or over-exposure (Fig.2(c)), respectively. Biologists and algorithm developers usually use a single suitable exposure (e.g., Fig.2(b)) to observe cells and analyze their images.

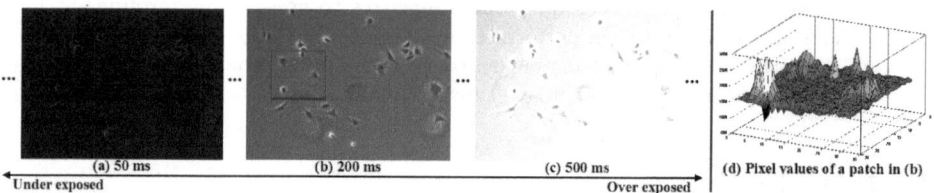

Fig. 2. (a,b,c): Multiple exposures on the same cell dish (ms: millisecond); (d): The pixel values of an image patch in (b) visualized in a surface view

Based on the phase contrast imaging pipeline and observation on differently exposed images, we are motivated to think of two intriguing problems in microscopy imaging and cell image segmentation:

– Biologists and algorithm developers aim to analyze cells' original properties encoded in the irradiance signal E. However, the camera response function f is usually nonlinear [1,4], i.e., the acquired image signal I is not linearly proportional to cells' irradiance E. Therefore, all cell image analysis algorithms directly based on image signal I may deviate from the expected analysis on cells' original physical properties encoded in E. *Can we restore the irradiance signal E from the image signal I for cell signal analysis?*
– During the microscopy imaging, we hope to have high-quality images on cells only without any noise from the culturing dish. But, the pixels of non-cell regions in a dish may exhibit a significant amount of noise as shown in Fig.2(d), causing a nonuniform background and low contrast between cell and background pixels. *Can we create a microscopy imaging system that is only sensitive to cells' irradiance (i.e., insensitive to background, with a constant irradiance signal on non-cell background regions, facilitating the cell segmentation task)?*

We propose to create a *cell-sensitive microscopy imaging* system by considering the rear-end of the imaging pipeline. First, multiple microscopy images with various exposure durations are taken on the same cell dish. Then, the camera response function is estimated from the set of multiple exposed images with a constraint that the irradiance signals of non-cell background pixels should be a constant. Therefore, the imaging system is virtually sensitive to cells only. Finally, the irradiance signal map of cells is restored from all exposures based on the cell-sensitive camera response function. In the restored irradiance signal map, non-cell background region has a constant irradiance different from those of cells, which facilitates cell segmentation by simple thresholding.

2   Methodology

Since cells migrate slowly in a dish, phase contrast images are usually taken every 5 minutes to monitor the cells' proliferation process over weeks. In our cell-sensitive imaging, the process to take multi-exposure images every 5 minutes with a range of known exposure durations ([50, 100, 200, 300, 400, 500]ms, in toal, about 1.55 seconds per set) is very fast compared to the time-lapse interval (5 minutes), hence the irradiance signal for each pixel is stable when capturing a set of multiple exposures and there is no need to do any image registration due to cells' slow motion. Common image acquisition software such as Axiovision 4.7 from Zeiss in our lab can routinely capture the multi-exposures every 5 minutes.

In this section, first we introduce how to estimate the cell-sensitive camera response function, based on which we then describe how to restore the irradiance signal with uniform background. Finally, we present how to perform easy cell segmentation on the restored irradiance signal map by simple thresholding.

2.1   Estimate the Cell-Sensitive Camera Response Function

Let E_i be the irradiance at the i_{th} pixel location in a cell dish. I_{ij}, the intensity of the i_{th} pixel in the j_{th} image with exposure duration Δt_j, is computed by

$$I_{ij} = f(E_i \Delta t_j) \tag{1}$$

where f is the camera response function (monotonic and invertible). Computing the inverse function of Eq.1 and taking the logarithm on both sides, we have

$$\log f^{-1}(I_{ij}) = \log E_i + \log \Delta t_j. \tag{2}$$

We formulate a constrained least square minimization problem to solve the unknown camera response function and irradiance signal

$$O(g, E) = \sum_{i=1}^{N} \sum_{j=1}^{P} \{\omega(I_{ij})[g(I_{ij}) - \log E_i - \log \Delta t_j]\}^2$$

$$+\alpha \sum_{i\in[1,N],\ i\in\Psi} (\log E_i)^2$$

$$+\beta \sum_{I=I_{min}+1}^{I_{max}-1} [\omega(I)g''(I)]^2 \tag{3}$$

where $g = \log f^{-1}$. Note that, we only need to estimate a look-up table for the function g since its input domain is the pixel value range. For a 12-bit TIFF image, the look-up table's length is 4096 with the minimum pixel value $I_{min} = 0$ and the maximum $I_{max} = 4095$. N and P denote the number of pixels and exposed images, respectively. The first term in Eq.3 is the data-fitting cost. The second term in Eq.3 is the regularization cost which enforces the logarithm of background irradiance to zero. Ψ is a set of some background pixel samples (to be explained later). The third term in Eq.3 is a smooth term avoiding overfit on the data, which is defined by curvature approximated by the second order numerical derivative, i.e., $g''(I) = g(I-1) - 2g(I) + g(I+1)$. In phase contrast images, the objects-in-interest (cells) are either dark or bright while the background pixels have a broad value range in the middle. Therefore, we use a weight function $\omega(I)$ to emphasize more on' the two ends of the camera response curve (i.e., sensitive to cells) and less on the middle (i.e., to have a flat background region): $\omega(I) = |I - \frac{I_{min}+I_{max}}{2}|$. α and β in Eq.3 are coefficients to balance the three cost terms. In our experiments, we choose fixed coefficients with $\alpha = 1000$ and $\beta = 100$.

Since the objective function in Eq.3 is quadratic, taking its derivatives regarding to g and E and setting them to zero lead to an overdetermined system of linear equations ($\mathbf{Ax} = \mathbf{b}$) which can be solved using the pseudo inverse or singular value decomposition method. The unknown variable in the linear equation system is $\mathbf{x} = [g(I_{min}), ..., g(I_{max}), \log E_1, ..., \log E_N]$ whose first part is the cell-sensitive camera response function, a look-up table. Given N pixels from P multi-exposed images, we have $(I_{max} - I_{min} + 1) + N$ unknown variables in $\mathbf{x}$. To avoid rank deficiency in the linear equation system, we need $NP > I_{max} - I_{min} + 1 + N$. For our experiments, $P = 6$, $I_{min} = 0$ and $I_{max} = 4095$. We choose $N = 1000$ to satisfy this requirement.

We uniformly divide the image coordinate into 100 rectangular regions (a 10x10 grid). Within each region, we select 10 pixels whose values are evenly distributed from the minimum to the maximum in this region. In total, we obtain 1000 sample pixels some of which will be on the background. Then, we manually pick some (e.g., 50) pixels out of background samples as the set Ψ used in the regularization of Eq.3. Note that, there is no need to select all background pixels for the regularization. A small set of representatives will be enough to estimate the cell-sensitive camera response curve.

Fig.3(a) shows the estimated cell-sensitive camera response function (black curve) from a set of multiple exposed images. The samples from different exposed images (marked by circles with different colors in Fig.3(a)) cover different portions of the camera response curve. Given a fixed camera and culturing dish, the response curve only needs to be estimated once using the first set of multiple exposed images and then it can be applied to successive sets of multi-exposures for time-lapse irradiance signal restoration. As shown in Fig.3(b), the cell-sensitive response curve is estimated every 1 hour using images from a 5-hour time-lapse cell image sequence, and the six curves overlap each other pretty well. Different cameras and culturing dishes may have different cell-sensitive response curves, as shown in Fig.3(c) which includes three slightly different response curves on three different dishes.

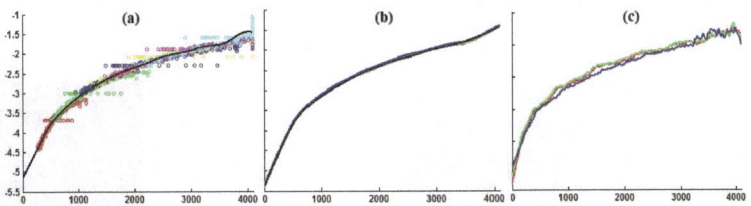

Fig. 3. Camera response curves. (a) The camera response function (black curve) estimated from multi-exposures on the same cell dish. The circles shown with different colors represent samples from different exposed images. (b) The response function of a camera estimated from six sets of multi-exposures captured every 1 hour on the same cell dish. (c) The response function of a camera estimated from three different dishes.

2.2   Restoring the Irradiance Signal

After the cell-sensitive camera response function is estimated from the first set of multi-exposed images, for any other sets in the time-lapse image sequence, we can easily restore their relative irradiance signals from image pixel values by

$$\log E_i = \frac{\sum_{j=1}^{P} w(I_{ij})(g(I_{ij}) - \Delta t_j)}{\sum_{j=1}^{P} w(I_{ij})} \tag{4}$$

where all the exposures are used to restore the irradiance signal robustly.

2.3   Cell Segmentation

Fig.4(a) shows an example of restored irradiance signal map whose surface view (Fig.4(b)) clearly shows that the non-cell background region has uniform background and the contrast between cells and background in the restored irradiance signal map is high. We sort the irradiance values in an ascent order (Fig.4(c)). The majority of the 1.5 million pixels of a 1040x1392 signal map has $E = 1$ (i.e., $\log E = 0$ which is the goal of regularization term in Eq.3).

In phase contrast microscopy imaging there are mainly three types of pixels: background pixels; bright pixels (e.g., mitosis/apoptosis cells or halos [6]); and dark pixels (e.g., migration normal cells [6]). Background pixels are commonly brighter than normal cell pixels but darker than bright pixels, as shown in Fig.4(a) and (b). The three types of pixel patterns are also reflected in Fig.4(c)

where the majority flat region of the curve belongs to background pixels while
the low and high ends of the curve are contributed by the dark and bright cells,
respectively. Two thresholds (T_H and T_L) are sufficient to segment cells out of
the restored irradiance signal: any E signal larger than T_H is a bright pixel and
any E signal lower than T_L is a dark pixel. Fig.4(d) shows the segmentation
results of Fig.4(a). T_H and T_L are determined by basic grid search (comparing
the segmentation accuracy of our method with the ground truth using different
T_H's and T_L's). Given a time-lapse sequence, the thresholds are searched at the
first time instant and then applied to all others.

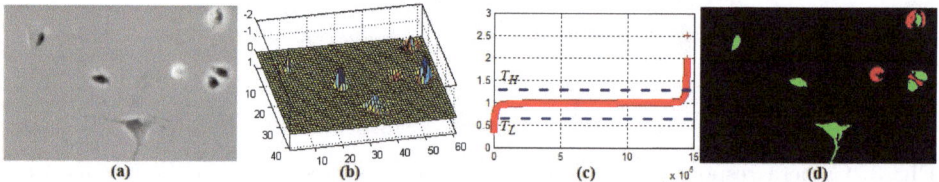

Fig. 4. Cell segmentation. (a) Restored irradiance signal map with constant irradiance
values on the background and high signal contrast; (b) Irradiance map shown in the
surface view. (c) The sorted irradiance signal values (red crosses). (d) Segmentation by
thresholding the irradiance signal (green: dark cell pixels; red: bright cell pixels).

3   Experimental Results

We collected multiple exposed microscopy images on three different cell dishes
with low and high cell densities, and each set has 6 different exposure durations
([50 100 200 300 400 500]ms).

3.1   Qualitative Evaluation

Multi-exposures have been used in Computer Graphics to create High Dynamic
Range (HDR) images [1,4]. Fig.5 (b) shows the HDR image created by using the
code from [1]. Compared to the image with 200ms exposure duration (Fig.5(a)),
the HDR image shows more image details but also amplifies the background
noise largely. However, our cell-sensitive imaging is only sensitive to cells and
enforces the background to have a constant irradiance, showing high contrast
between cells and the uniform background, as shown in Fig.5(c).

Fig.6 shows the qualitative comparison between our segmentation based on
cell-sensitive imaging and two other related methods: (1) the phase contrast
optics based method that considers the front-end of the imaging pipeline [13]
and multi-level Otsu thresholding method [7]. Our restored irradiance signal
map (Fig.6(a)) has uniform background and high contrast between cells and
background regions. Thresholding the irradiance signals can classify both normal
cells and bright cells (Fig.6(b)). The other two methods are ran on the image
with exposure duration 200ms. The phase contrast optics based method can

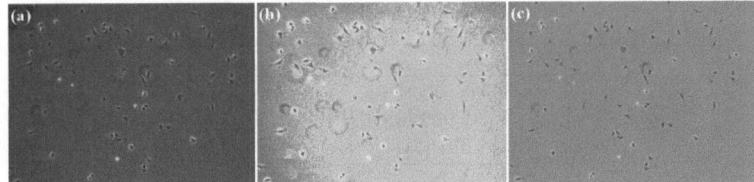

Fig. 5. Comparison with high dynamic range (HDR) image. (a) A phase contrast image captured with exposure duration 200ms. (b) The HDR image created by multi-exposures. (c) Our cell-sensitive imaging where the background is uniform and the image contrast between cells and the background is high.

locate the darkest nuclei regions but the low contrast cells and bright cells are not detected (Fig.6(c)). Considering there are three types of pixels in an image (bright cells, dark cells and background), we use two-level Otsu thresholding to segment the image. Unfortunately, the multi-level Otsu thresholding does not perform well due to the non-uniform background (Fig.6(d)).

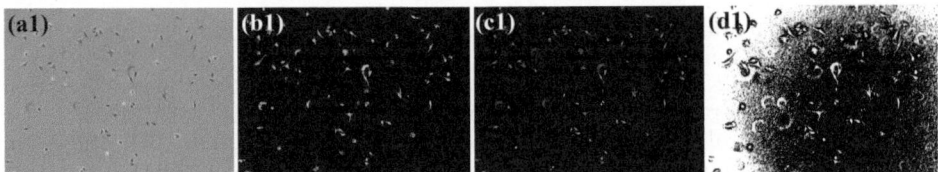

Fig. 6. Three methods on one dish sequence. (a) Restored irradiance signal by our cell-sensitive imaging. (b) The segmentation by thresholding the restored irradiance (red: mitosis/apoptosis cells or halos; green: normal migration cells). (c-d): Segmentation on the image with 200ms exposure duration by the method based on phase contrast optics model [13] and Otsu thresholding [7], respectively.

3.2 Quantitative Evaluation

Two annotators manually labeled cell masks (both mitosis/apoptosis and normal cells but without halos) in all microscopy images with exposure duration 200ms. To reduce the inter-person variability, the intersection of their annotations is used as the ground truth. The segmentation accuracy (ACC) is defined as $ACC = (|TP| + |N_s| - |FP|)/(|N_s| + |P_s|)$ where cell and background pixels are defined as positive (P_s) and negative (N_s) samples, respectively. True positive (TP) stands for cell pixels segmented by our method correctly and false positive (FP) denotes cell pixels segmented by our method mistakenly. Table 1 compares the performance of three segmentation methods on three cell sequences in which our segmentation by cell-sensitive imaging achieves very high accuracy. We did not classify bright halos from bright mitosis/apoptosis cells in this paper, which lowers our cell segmentation performance a bit. In the future work, we will explore cell classification and tracking based on the cell-sensitive imaging.

Table 1. Cell segmentation accuracy of three methods on three dishes

	Dish 1	Dish 2	Dish 3
Our cell-sensitive imaging	0.993	0.994	0.975
Optics model based method [13]	0.974	0.974	0.956
Otsu threshold [7]	0.677	0.665	0.628

4 Conclusion

We propose a novel cell segmentation approach by creating a cell-sensitive microscopy imaging system. A set of variously exposed phase contrast microscopy images on the same cell dish are used to estimate a cell-sensitive camera response function, based on which cells' original irradiance signals are restored from all exposures while the irradiance signals on non-cell background regions are restored as a uniform constant. Therefore, the imaging system is sensitive to cells but insensitive to non-cell background, which greatly facilitates the cell segmentation by simple thresholding. The experimental results show our approach can achieve high cell segmentation accuracy.

References

1. Debevec, P., Malik, J.: Recovering High Dynamic Range Radiance Maps from Photographs. In: SIGGRAPH (1997)
2. House, D., et al.: Tracking of Cell Populations to Understand their Spatio-Temporal Behavior in Response to Physical stimuli. In: Workshop on MMBIA (2009)
3. Kanade, T., et al.: Cell Image Analysis: Algorithms, System and Applications. In: IEEE Workshop on Applications of Computer Vision (WACV) (2011)
4. Larson, G., et al.: A Visibility Matching Tone Reproduction Operator for High Dynamic Range Scenes. IEEE Tran. on Visualization and Computer Graphics 3(4), 291–306 (1997)
5. Li, K., et al.: Cell Population Tracking and Lineage Construction with Spatiotemporal Context. Medical Image Analysis (MedIA) 12(1), 546–566 (2008)
6. Murphy, D.: Fundamentals of Light Microscopy and Electronic Imaging. Wiley (2001)
7. Otsu, N.: A threshold selection method from gray-level histograms. IEEE Transactions on Systems, Man, and Cybernetics 9(1), 62–66 (1979)
8. Rittscher, J.: Characterization of Biological Processes through Automated Image Analysis. Annual Review of Biomedical Engineering 12, 315–344 (2010)
9. Smith, K., et al.: General Constraints for Batch Multiple-Target Tracking Applied to Large-Scale Video Microscopy. In: CVPR (2008)
10. Su, H., et al.: Cell Segmentation in Phase Contrast Microscopy Images via Semi-supervised Classification over Optics-related Features. MedIA 17(7), 746–765 (2013)
11. Wu, K., et al.: Live Cell Image Segmentation. IEEE Tran. on Biomedical Engineering 42(1), 1–12 (1995)
12. Yang, F., Mackey, M.A., Ianzini, F., Gallardo, G., Sonka, M.: Cell Segmentation, Tracking, and Mitosis Detection Using Temporal Context. In: Duncan, J.S., Gerig, G. (eds.) MICCAI 2005. LNCS, vol. 3749, pp. 302–309. Springer, Heidelberg (2005)
13. Yin, Z., et al.: Understanding the Phase Contrast Optics to Restore Artifact-free Microscopy Images for Segmentation. MedIA 16(5), 1047–1062 (2012)
14. Zernike, F.: How I discovered phase contrast. Science 121, 345–349 (1955)

A Probabilistic Approach to Quantification of Melanin and Hemoglobin Content in Dermoscopy Images

Ali Madooei and Mark S. Drew

School of Computing Science
Simon Fraser University, Canada
{amadooei,mark}@cs.sfu.ca
http://www.cs.sfu.ca/~amadooei

Abstract. We describe a technique that employs the stochastic Latent Topic Models framework to allow quantification of melanin and hemoglobin content in dermoscopy images. Such information bears useful implications for analysis of skin hyperpigmentation, and for classification of skin diseases. The proposed method outperforms existing approaches while allowing for more stringent and probabilistic modeling than previously.

1 Introduction

Computer-aided diagnosis of skin cancer is primarily based on analysis of clinical images of skin lesions, such as dermoscopy images[1] Interest in skin image analysis stems from the fact that useful visual information such as lesion colouration, pigmentation, etc. can be obtained via image processing in a computerized and automated fashion.

In this context, one less-studied but potentially interesting topic is quantification of skin's major chromophores (i.e. melanin and hemoglobin) from skin images, and its diagnostic utility. Such measurements are typically obtained through optical analysis of human skin via e.g. diffuse reflectance spectroscopy. This type of analysis is interesting as it offers the possibility of obtaining information about skin physiology and composition in a non-invasive manner. Such information may potentially be useful for diagnosis of skin diseases, screening the state of skin over the course of clinical therapy, and even final evaluation of efficacy of treatment. However, spectrophotometry (and similar techniques) require specific optical instruments. It would be economically and computationally beneficial if this information could be extracted from conventional clinical images. In particular, melanin and hemoglobin content of skin images can aid analysis of skin pigmentation, erythema, inflammation and hemodynamics.

Melanin and hemoglobin strongly absorb light in the visible spectrum and thus are major contributors to skin colouration. This motivates the hypothesis that, through analysis of skin colour, one may extract information about the underlying melanin and hemoglobin content. In this study, we make use of a recently published article by

---

[1] Dermoscopy is a popular [non-invasive] skin imaging technique. With the aid of optical magnification and cross-polarized lighting, it allows enhanced visualization of skin morphological characteristics which are often not discernible by the naked eye.

P. Golland et al. (Eds.): MICCAI 2014, Part I, LNCS 8673, pp. 49–56, 2014.

Madooei et al. [1] which has explored this hypothesis. Their work extends the seminal work of Tsumura et al. [2] who employed independent component analysis (ICA) of skin images for extracting melanin and haemoglobin information. While Tsumura's goal was to develop a computationally efficient model of skin appearance for image synthesis, Madooei et al. employed the extracted information as a feature-space for supervised classification of classes Malignant vs. Benign.[2]

Independent component analysis is a powerful computational method that has been successfully used in many application domains but more specifically for signal processing aimed at solving the "blind source separation problem". It essentially defines a generative model of the observed data as linear mixtures of some underlying (hidden) factors. A variety of techniques have been proposed for this sort of data analysis which differ from each other on the merit of their assumptions, objective, and the constraints which they impose on the decomposition. These include factor analysis, principal component analysis (PCA), sparse component analysis, non-negative matrix factorization (NMF), projection pursuit, etc.

A somewhat related but separate class of techniques has emerged from the research in text/document analysis, known as latent topic models (LTM), which is aimed at identifying the underlying topics that affect the co-occurrence of words in a document. This is a probabilistic approach to model multivariate data (usually in form of histogram counts, i.e. probability distribution) by modeling the distributions of underlying (unobserved) statistical factors (topics) that affect them[3]. The two most popular techniques in this category are probabilistic latent semantic analysis (pLSA) and latent Dirichlet allocation (LDA). These language models (with their many variations) have gradually become an integral part of mainstream computer vision research, with a multitude of applications.

In this paper, we show that latent topic models can be equally effectively employed for quantification of melanin and hemoglobin content in skin lesion images. There are in fact many advantages to do so, as we will explain: Namely, latent topic models allow us to take advantage of their probabilistic framework. Also, as will be shown, the proposed model can overcome shortfalls of ICA-based models, in particular in terms of sign and scale ambiguity. We further demonstrate both qualitatively and quantitatively that probabilistic decomposition indeed results in a superior outcome compared to the state-of-the-art [1].

2   Method

As theoretical underpinning, we begin by adapting the well known dichromatic reflectance model [3] to describe the reflected light $L(\theta, \lambda)$ from skin surfaces:

$$L(\theta, \lambda) = L_{\mathbb{S}}(\theta, \lambda) + L_{\mathbb{B}}(\theta, \lambda) \tag{1}$$

---

[2] Another contribution of [1] over [2] is that a photometric model of image formation is utilized to account for and discard the effects of confounding factors in imagery such as light colour, intensity falloff, shading, and camera characteristics.

[3] This class of probabilistic modeling is more widely known as 'latent variable models' in the literature of mainstream statistical learning theory.

where $L_{\mathbb{S}}$ (specular reflection) is the light reflected immediately at the skin surface, and $L_{\mathbb{B}}$ (body or diffuse reflection) is the radiance caused by the interaction of light with skin tissue. Here, λ denotes wavelength and θ encapsulates geometrical dependencies. We can further expand this model to describe the body reflectance by optical properties of underlying skin layers, such as scattering and absorption of skin's major chromophores.

We consider a simplified skin tissue model composed of three layers from the top: epidermis, dermis and subcutis. The light scattering and absorption properties of epidermis and dermis depend mainly on the distribution and density of melanin and (total, i.e. oxy- & reduced) hemoglobin, respectively[4]; whereas the subcutis mainly contains fat cells which are assumed to diffuse all visible light [4].

By adapting a simple Lambert-Beer type of law for radiance from the multilayer skin tissue similar to that in [4], the body reflectance can be expressed as:[5]

$$L_{\mathbb{B}}(\lambda) \simeq L_e(\lambda) + T_e(\lambda)^2 L_d(\lambda) + T_e(\lambda)^2 T_d(\lambda)^2 L_s(\lambda) \tag{2}$$

where T_e and L_e are the transmittance and diffuse reflectance of epidermis, respectively; T_d and L_d are those of the dermis; and L_s is the diffuse reflectance of subcutis.

For dermoscopy images, the specular reflectance is suppressed by using cross-polarized lighting.[6] Thus, $L_{\mathbb{S}} \simeq 0$. Also, it has been shown [5] that for λ within the visible spectrum (400-700 nm), and for both fair and dark skins, the diffuse reflectance of epidermis and dermis layers are negligible compared to total diffuse reflectance. In other words, $L_{e,d} \ll L_{\mathbb{B}}$. If we assume, therefore, that $L_{e,d}$ both approach zero, then eq.(1) can be simplified as:

$$L \simeq T_e^2 T_d^2 L_s \tag{3}$$

The transmittance of the upper two layers of skin are assumed to bear an exponential relationship to the molar extinction coefficient of melanin and hemoglobin respectively [6] (assuming these are uniformly and randomly distributed, and their dimensions are much less than the thickness of the layers [7]):

$$T_e = \exp(-d_e e_m C_m) \qquad T_d = \exp(-d_d e_h C_h) \tag{4}$$

where d_e and d_d are the thickness of epidermis and dermis respectively; e_m is the extinction coefficient determined by the absorption spectrum of melanin; C_m is the concentration of melanin; and accordingly, e_h and C_h are those quantities for hemoglobin.

By substituting eq.(4) in eq.(3) and taking the logarithm, we arrive at a linear equation which captures the relationship between the radiance entering the camera and the underlying composition of the colour pigments of skin:

$$\log L(\theta, \lambda) \simeq m(\lambda) C_m(\theta) + h(\lambda) C_h(\theta) + l(\lambda) \tag{5}$$

where we have lumped terms: $m(\lambda) = -2d_e e_m(\lambda)$, $h(\lambda) = -2d_d e_h(\lambda)$, and $l(\lambda) = \log L_s(\lambda)$. Note that the diffuse reflectance of subcutis is taken to be spatially uniform (i.e., L_s is not a function of space).

---

[4] Note that scattering of collagen is ignored for simplicity.

[5] Here, reflection of each layer is considered separately and, for simplicity, interreflection inside each layer is ignored.

[6] Also, in general, the specular reflectance in clinical images of skin lesions can be attenuated by using photographic filters or image processing methods.

Assuming a trichromatic colour camera with narrow-band and linear sensor response function $Q_{k \in \{R,G,B\}}(\lambda) = q_k \delta(\lambda - \lambda_k)$ [1], we can adapt eq.(5) to represent skin image data (N.B. for simplicity and without loss of generality we set $q_k = 1$):

$$
\begin{bmatrix} \log R(x,y) \\ \log G(x,y) \\ \log B(x,y) \end{bmatrix} = \begin{bmatrix} m(\lambda_R) & h(\lambda_R) \\ m(\lambda_G) & h(\lambda_G) \\ m(\lambda_B) & h(\lambda_B) \end{bmatrix} \begin{bmatrix} C_m(x,y) \\ C_h(x,y) \end{bmatrix} + \begin{bmatrix} l(\lambda) \\ l(\lambda) \\ l(\lambda) \end{bmatrix} \tag{6}
$$

Eq-6 can be recognized as an instance of the problem of blind source separation (BSS) where the observed data ($\log \mathbf{R}, \mathbf{G}, \mathbf{B}$) is described as linear mixtures of some unknown source signals ($\mathbf{C}_m$ and $\mathbf{C}_h$), and the goal is to recover the source, using minimum assumptions on the mixing procedure (i.e., blindly). The mixing model in Eq-6 can be conveniently rewritten as $\mathbf{Y} = \mathbf{AS}$ where $\mathbf{Y} \in \mathbb{R}^{3 \times p}$ is (mean-subtracted[7]) image data (p = number of pixels); $\mathbf{S} \in \mathbb{R}^{2 \times p}$ is the unknown source matrix which represents (relative) concentration of melanin and hemoglobin at each pixel; $\mathbf{A} \in \mathbb{R}^{3 \times 2}$ is the unknown mixing matrix which defines the contribution of each source in forming the observed data. We will call $\mathbf{S}$ the chromophores density matrix, and $\mathbf{A}$ the chromophores colour matrix. The goal of BSS is to recover these two quantities; however, the decomposition problem is underdetermined and additional assumptions are needed to solve it. Depending on what additional assumptions are considered, there are various methods for solving the BSS.

In [1,2], it is assumed the density of melanin and hemoglobin chromophores (i.e. $\mathbf{C}_m$, $\mathbf{C}_h$) are mutually independent over the image plane. Therefore, ICA [8] was applied to estimate chromophores density and colour matrices[8]. The empirical validity of this assumption is examined in [2], and its utility shown [1] to be useful for skin disease classification.

ICA finds the solution $\mathbf{S} \approx \mathbf{WY}$ where $\mathbf{W} = \mathbf{A}^+$ (where $^+$ denotes pseudoinverse; in case $\mathbf{A}$ is square and invertible, equalling $\mathbf{A}^{-1}$). In this notation, $\mathbf{W}$ is often referred to as *unmixing* or *separating* matrix. Within this framework, once $\mathbf{S}$ is estimated, it can be scaled; negated; and permuted with permutation matrix $\mathbf{P}$ and scaling matrix $\mathbf{M}$ such that new components remain independent: $\mathbf{S}' = \mathbf{MPS} = \mathbf{MPWY}$. So any matrix $\mathbf{W}' = \mathbf{MPW}$ is also a valid separating matrix. This is often referred to as the inherent ambiguity in the ICA model (see Fig-1).

We now move forward from the deterministic nature of classical ICA algorithm to the stochastic treatment of latent topic models, which offers all the advantages of probabilistic frameworks while overcoming some of the limitation of the ICA model. In particular, we utilize probabilistic latent component analysis (PLCA) [9], an extension of the popular pLSA. Unlike ICA, which tries to characterize the observed data directly, PLCA characterizes the underlying distribution that generates the observed data.

We assume, without loss of generality, that observed data $\mathbf{Y}$ is actually a scaled probability distribution $P(x,y,k)_{k \in \{R,G,B\}}$ — or $P(\mathbf{x}, \mathbf{k})$ for brevity. To adapt the data into

---

[7] In eq.(6), the last term is a DC offset and can be easily removed by mean-subtraction.

[8] Note that our model is a more general treatment of image data compared to that in [1,2] where the dimension of observed data was reduced to the number of source signals.

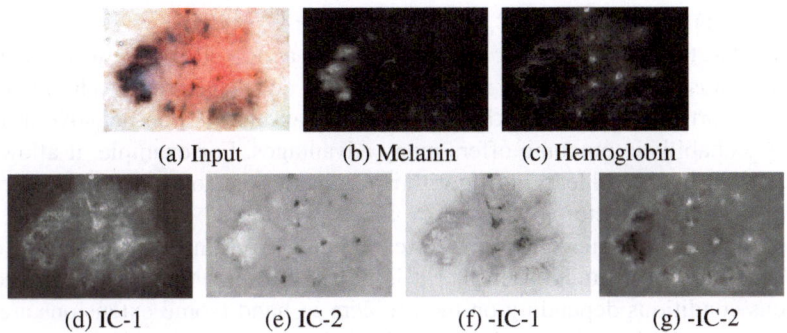

(a) Input   (b) Melanin   (c) Hemoglobin

(d) IC-1   (e) IC-2   (f) -IC-1   (g) -IC-2

Fig. 1. First row: PLCA output. Second row: output of ICA-based model in [1] showing ICA ambiguities (sign and permutation).

this assumption, we normalize $\mathbf{Y}$ to sum to unity[9]. The PLCA model considers a multivariate distribution as a mixture of a number of latent distributions that are specified by their marginals:

$$P(\mathbf{x}, \mathbf{k}) = \sum_{\mathbf{z}} P(\mathbf{z})P(\mathbf{x}|\mathbf{z})P(\mathbf{k}|\mathbf{z}) \tag{7}$$

where $\mathbf{Z}$ is the latent variable that indexes the hidden components, i.e. z_m and z_h for melanin and hemoglobin. The characteristic of eq.(7) is conditional independence, which fits well with the assumption of the ICA model. The goal of PLCA is to discover the marginals $P(\mathbf{x}|\mathbf{z})$ and $P(\mathbf{k}|\mathbf{z})$. These can be considered to be proportional to the probability distributions that generate chromophores density $\mathbf{S}$ and colour $\mathbf{A}$ matrices.

The estimation of marginals is achieved in a modified EM fashion: during the 'expectation' step, we estimate:

$$P(\mathbf{z}|\mathbf{x}, \mathbf{k}) = \frac{P(\mathbf{z})P(\mathbf{x}|\mathbf{z})P(\mathbf{k}|\mathbf{z})}{\sum_{\mathbf{z}} P(\mathbf{z})P(\mathbf{x}|\mathbf{z})P(\mathbf{k}|\mathbf{z})} \tag{8}$$

followed by the 'maximization' step where we update the marginals using:

$$P(\mathbf{x}|\mathbf{z}) = \frac{\sum_{\mathbf{k}} P(\mathbf{x}, \mathbf{k})P(\mathbf{z}|\mathbf{x}, \mathbf{k})}{\sum_{\mathbf{x}} \sum_{\mathbf{k}} P(\mathbf{x}, \mathbf{k})P(\mathbf{z}|\mathbf{x}, \mathbf{k})} \qquad P(\mathbf{k}|\mathbf{z}) = \frac{\sum_{\mathbf{x}} P(\mathbf{x}, \mathbf{k})P(\mathbf{z}|\mathbf{x}, \mathbf{k})}{\sum_{\mathbf{x}} \sum_{\mathbf{k}} P(\mathbf{x}, \mathbf{k})P(\mathbf{z}|\mathbf{x}, \mathbf{k})} \tag{9}$$

$$P(\mathbf{z}) = \frac{\sum_{\mathbf{x}, \mathbf{k}} P(\mathbf{x}, \mathbf{k})P(\mathbf{z}|\mathbf{x}, \mathbf{k})}{\sum_{\mathbf{x}, \mathbf{k}, \mathbf{z}} P(\mathbf{x}, \mathbf{k})P(\mathbf{z}|\mathbf{x}, \mathbf{k})} \tag{10}$$

Estimation of latent components in eq.(7) is obtained by iterating the above EM algorithm to convergence. The resulting decomposition can be expressed as a matrix factorization (cf. eq.(6)):

$$\begin{bmatrix} P(\mathbf{x}, k_R) \\ P(\mathbf{x}, k_G) \\ P(\mathbf{x}, k_B) \end{bmatrix} = \begin{bmatrix} P(k_R|z_m) & P(k_R|z_h) \\ P(k_G|z_m) & P(k_G|z_h) \\ P(k_B|z_m) & P(k_B|z_h) \end{bmatrix} \begin{bmatrix} P(z_M) & 0 \\ 0 & P(z_H) \end{bmatrix} \begin{bmatrix} P(\mathbf{x}|z_m) \\ P(\mathbf{x}|z_h) \end{bmatrix} \tag{11}$$

---

[9] The scaling factor can be multiplied back into the estimated components to avoid e.g. quantization issues.

From eq.(11), we can define $\mathbf{C}_m = P(z_m)P(\mathbf{x}|z_m)$ and $\mathbf{C}_h = P(z_h)P(\mathbf{x}|z_h)$. It is obvious that these quantities are always positive and $\in [0, 1]$ due to the nature of probability (thus we reduced ICA ambiguities). The non-negativity is a highly desired property, in particular when working with image data that is non-negative in nature. Also, the probabilistic outcome offers many advantages. For example, it allows easy integration with statistical learning algorithms; it enables one to evaluate the importance of an underlying factor; etc.

The probabilistic framework of PLCA can benefit from the abundant tools of statistical inference for estimation, in that it is possible to extend the model to account for various conditions depending on the problem in hand (some extensions are shift-invariant PLCA [10], scale-invariant PLCA [11], sparse PLCA [10]). Moreover, it offers the ability to incorporate information known about the problem, or to impose hypothesized structure about the data by e.g. utilizing prior distribution during estimation. Obtaining this flexibility in non-stochastic models such as ICA, if possible, is complex and computationally expensive.

A potentially interesting utilization of PLCA model would be to control the order of separated components through e.g. the imposition of a priori probabilities. We plan to further investigate this. At this stage, however, we recover from permutation ambiguity by a simple post-processing: there is a high correlation between skin's Erythema–Index (redness) and the a* channel of the CIE Lab colourspace [12]. The hemoglobin component, in a sense, embodies a similar meaning, i.e. redness of skin. Therefore, similarity[10] to the a* channel could be used as an indicator of hemoglobin distribution[11].

3   Experiments

In order to verify the validity of the proposed skin colouration model, and the employed probabilistic decomposition approach, we need pathological data associated with skin images. For our dataset, such information is not available. Thus we rely on visual assessment: the proposed method appears to achieve superior results (compared to [1]) in highlighting and isolating hyperpigmented spots (e.g. Fig-1). Some sample outputs are shown in Fig-2.

We demonstrate the utility of our proposed method in application to skin disease classification. In keeping with [1], we applied a Logistic classifier to a set of 500 images taken from [13] with two classes consisting of malignant (melanoma and BCC) vs. all benign lesions (congenital, compound, dermal, Clark, Spitz and blue nevus; dermatofibroma; and seborrheic keratosis). For classification, the same set of features as in [1] are used (details are omitted for space considerations). Table 1 results are averaged over 10 runs of 10-fold cross-validation. We see that our proposed method outperforms [1] in all measures, particularly for malignant lesions, where the results demonstrate up to 5% higher precision and recall for our method. Note that although this improvement is modest, our method achieves the separation of melanin and hemoglobin in a completely automatic fashion, whereas the components were manually labeled in [1].

---

[10] The similarity can be measured by e.g. computing the 2-D correlation coefficient.

[11] N.B. the outcome of the image analysis proposed here is different in general from results simply using CIE Lab values.

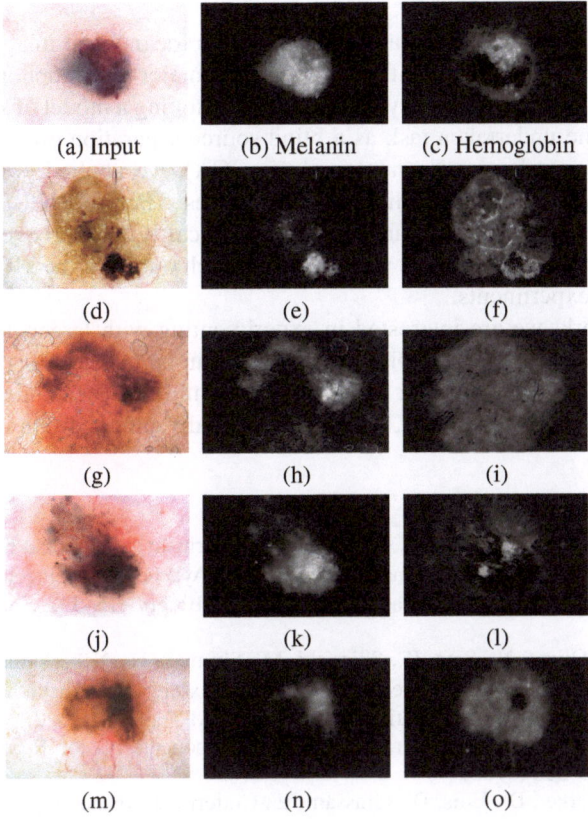

(a) Input   (b) Melanin   (c) Hemoglobin

(d)   (e)   (f)

(g)   (h)   (i)

(j)   (k)   (l)

(m)   (n)   (o)

Fig. 2. Sample outputs – brighter means higher concentration

Table 1. Comparative Results of classifying the dataset in [1]. Since same feature-set & classifier is used, the improvement is the result of using our proposed probabilistic decomposition. Note that Madooei et al. [1] also report classifying using RGB, HSV, and CIELAB colour spaces of which all are outperformed by their proposed colour feature space. We did not repeat those tests. Also, our result is averaged over 10 runs of 10 fold cross-validation. The std of weighted average is 0.043, 0.044, 0.046, 0.041 for precision, recall, f-score, and area under the ROC curve (AUC) respectively.

Colour Space	Class	n	Precision	Recall	F-measure	AUC
	Malignant	135	**0.85**	**0.837**	**0.843**	
Proposed Method	Benign	365	**0.94**	**0.945**	**0.943**	**0.96**
	Weighted Avr.	500	**0.916**	**0.916**	**0.916**	
	Malignant	135	0.806	0.8	0.803	
Method in [1]	Benign	365	0.926	0.929	0.927	0.953
	Weighted Avr.	500	0.894	0.894	0.894	

4   Conclusion

This paper highlights the use of latent topic models for medical image analysis. As a case study, we focused on quantification of skin's major chromophores (i.e. melanin and hemoglobin) from dermoscopy images. By developing a model of skin colouration, we formulated the undertaken task as a blind source separation problem. While prior art relies on independent component analysis (ICA), we applied probabilistic latent component analysis (PLCA) for discovery of sources. The probabilistic framework of PLCA offers many potential advantages over classical ICA. Moreover, when utilized for skin disease classification, the proposed approach outperformed ICA-based model as shown in our experiments.

For future work, we are interested in experimenting with larger datasets; as more data becomes available more ambitious problems can be tackled. Also, we would like to employ the LTM framework for the discovery of mid-level semantic visual concepts such as "asymmetric", "irregular", etc. to automatically annotate skin lesion images.

References

1. Madooei, A., Drew, M., Sadeghi, M., Atkins, M.: Intrinsic melanin and hemoglobin colour components for skin lesion malignancy detection. In: Ayache, N., Delingette, H., Golland, P., Mori, K. (eds.) MICCAI 2012, Part I. LNCS, vol. 7510, pp. 315–322. Springer, Heidelberg (2012)
2. Tsumura, N., Ojima, N., Sato, K., Shiraishi, M., Shimizu, H., Nabeshima, H., Akazaki, S., Hori, K., Miyake, Y.: Image-based skin color and texture analysis/synthesis by extracting hemoglobin and melanin information in the skin. ACM Trans. Graph. 22, 770–779 (2003)
3. Shafer, S.: Using color to separate reflection components. Color Research & Application 10(4), 210–218 (1985)
4. Dawson, J., Barker, D., Ellis, D., Grassam, E., Cotterill, J., Fisher, G., Feather, J.: A theoretical and experimental study of light absorption and scattering by in vivo skin. Physics in Medicine and Biology 25(4), 695–709 (1980)
5. Wan, S., Parrish, J., Jaenicke, K.: Quantitative evaluation of ultraviolet induced erythema. Photochemistry and Photobiology 37(6), 643–648 (1983)
6. Diffey, B., Oliver, R., Farr, P.: A portable instrument for quantifying erythema induced by ultraviolet radiation. The British Journal of Dermatology 111(6), 663–672 (1984)
7. Takiwaki, H.: Measurement of erythema and melanin indices. In: Handbook of Non-Invasive Methods and the Skin, pp. 665–671. Informa Healthcare (1995)
8. Hyvarinen, A.: Fast and robust fixed-point algorithms for independent component analysis. IEEE TNN 10(3), 626–634 (1999)
9. Shashanka, M., Raj, B., Smaragdis, P.: Sparse overcomplete latent variable decomposition of counts data. In: NIPS, vol. 1, p. 2 (2007)
10. Smaragdis, P., Raj, B., Shashanka, M.: Sparse and shift-invariant feature extraction from non-negative data. In: ICASSP, pp. 2069–2072 (2008)
11. Hennequin, R., Badeau, R., David, B.: Scale-invariant probabilistic latent component analysis. In: IEEE WASPAA 2011, pp. 129–132 (2011)
12. Takiwaki, H.: Measurement of skin color: practical application and theoretical considerations. J. of Medical Investigation 44(3-4), 121–126 (1998)
13. Argenziano, G., Soyer, H., De Giorgio, V., Piccolo, D., Carli, P., Delfino, M., Ferrari, A., et al.: Interactive Atlas of Dermoscopy (Book and CD-ROM). Edra Medical Publishing & New Media, Milan (2000)

Automated, Non-Invasive Characterization of Stem Cell-Derived Cardiomyocytes from Phase-Contrast Microscopy

Mahnaz Maddah and Kevin Loewke

Cellogy Inc., Menlo Park, CA 94025, USA

Abstract. Stem cell-derived cardiomyocytes hold tremendous potential for drug development and safety testing related to cardiovascular health. The characterization of cardiomyocytes is most commonly performed using electrophysiological systems, which are expensive, laborious to use, and may induce undesirable cellular response. Here, we present a new method for non-invasive characterization of cardiomyocytes using video microscopy and image analysis. We describe an automated pipeline that consists of segmentation of beating regions, robust beating signal calculation, signal quantification and modeling, and hierarchical clustering. Unlike previous imaging-based methods, our approach enables clinical applications by capturing beating patterns and arrhythmias across healthy and diseased cells with varied densities. We demonstrate the strengths of our algorithm by characterizing the effects of two commercial drugs known to modulate beating frequency and irregularity. Our results provide, to our knowledge, the first clinically-relevant demonstration of a fully-automated and non-invasive imaging-based beating assay for characterization of stem cell-derived cardiomyocytes.

1 Introduction

Stem cell research holds enormous potential for studying and treating a wide range of human diseases [1]. In recent years, there has been significant progress in using induced pluripotent stem cells (iPSCs) for modeling of human disease. A promising and growing application of iPSCs is the generation of patient-specific cardiomyocytes, which can be used in preclinical testing of new drugs that may cause drug-induced arrhythmia or QT prolongation, as well as post-market safety testing or re-purposing of existing drugs [2, 3]. Due to their important clinical applications, beating characterization of stem-cell derived cardiomyocytes is of great interest.

The characterization of iPSC-derived cardiomyocytes is most commonly performed using electrophysiological signals measured through manual or automated patch-clamp systems as well as micro-electrode arrays (MEA)s [4]. While considered the gold-standard for characterization, patch-clamp methods are expensive, laborious and invasive. MEA systems also require high cell plating density, and due to the direct contact between cells and electrodes, may cause undesirable cellular response.

Several image analysis methods have recently been proposed [5–7] using the apparent cell motion, captured by video microscopy, as an alternative to directly measuring the electrophysiology of the cells. These methods have demonstrated the feasibility of non-invasive characterization of cardiomyocyte beating. In [5] and [6] a motion

P. Golland et al. (Eds.): MICCAI 2014, Part I, LNCS 8673, pp. 57–64, 2014.

field is estimated from the intensity images and then a single one-dimensional time-domain signal that captures the essential feature of the beating of the cardiomyocytes is constructed. Motion field estimation, however, is not accurate when the culture lacks enough texture, or contractions are very strong [7]. Moreover, constructing a meaningful temporal beating signal from the full motion field is impossible unless the cell density is high and uniform across the culture. To address these problems, in a subsequent work [7], an alternative approach has been proposed where images are first segmented into a set of regions, each representing a group of cells that beat together, and a set of features are calculated for each region. Their nearly periodic motion feature, however, is based on an explicit assumption that the beating pattern of each region is periodic or nearly periodic, hence limiting the applicability of the method in studying irregularities of cell beating and arrhythmia.

Although the above works show promising results, in order to successfully capture dynamics of cardiomyocyte beating from microscopy images in clinical setting, several challenges need to be addressed. The method should be able to handle variations in the culture density, ranging from sparse single-cell plating to dense monolayer plating, and work for both healthy and diseased cell lines as well as cell cultures treated by drugs. The plating density of cells affects the synchronicity of beating; densely-plated cells usually beat synchronously, while sparsely plated cells can beat asynchronously and with different frequencies for each cell. In addition, the beating pattern for healthy cardiomyocytes is nearly-periodic (but not perfectly periodic), while the beating pattern for unhealthy or perturbed cells can be highly irregular, and with varying contraction forces. Finally, the cardiomyocyte population is not always pure, and can contain other types of cells that proliferate, thereby changing the behavior and appearance of the culture over time.

In this work, we present a new method that can reliably extract and quantify beating signals from cardiomyocyte cell cultures. Our presented pipeline enables, for the first time, automated extraction of quantitative parameters that are of interest in clinical research from cultures with different cell density and with either regular or irregular beating patterns. The robustness of the presented method has been confirmed by successful analysis of more than 500 videos from different cell lines, and culture conditions. As demonstrated in this paper, our method successfully captures the impact of chemical compounds on the beating rate.

2   Method

Figure 1 shows a block diagram depicting the steps of the proposed method. The input is a phase-contrast image sequence $\{I_t\}_{t=1,...,N}$, acquired with high capture frequency (e.g. 24 frames/sec) of a cardiomyocyte cell culture. Images are first segmented into regions that consist of cells that exhibit a cyclic motion (beating cells), regions that consist of cells that do not show a cyclic motion (non-beating cells), and background. The result is a mask, consisting of a group of regions, $R_m, m = 1, ..., M$, where each region represents cells that are spaced close to each other and beat at relatively same time. Next a beating signal is calculated for each region R_m. A raw beating signal $u_m(t)$ is constructed by calculating the correlation coefficient of subsequent frames over R_m. A

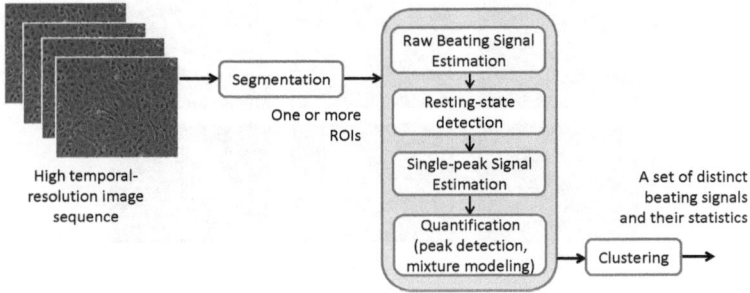

Fig. 1. Block diagram of the proposed method

resting-state reference image is obtained and then a single-peak beating signal $x_m(t)$ is calculated by computing the correlation coefficient of the frames and the resting-state reference image over R_m. Subsequently, features that describe the beating signal, such as its variation of period over time, are extracted. This is achieved by robust peak detection and signal modeling through fitting a mixture of Gaussians to the signal. Finally, a hierarchical clustering algorithm is performed to identify regions with unique beating characteristics and merge adjacent regions that have similar beating characteristics.

2.1   Segmentation

The first step in the proposed image analysis pipeline is segmentation of beating cells from the stationary regions of the image that include non-beating cells and the background. Since there is no difference between beating cells and non-beating cells in terms of their morphology and texture, and there is no clear boundary between the cells in the high density cell cultures, segmentation of individual beating cells is not feasible. Here, we construct a mask of beating regions defined as the intersection of a foreground mask, generated based on the first image in the sequence, and the standard deviation mask, generated over the entire image sequence. Since the cardiomyocyte cells could have a flat structure, the background estimation is done by computing the standard deviation map using a large window. As also proposed in [7], the standard deviation of the image intensity over time is calculated for each location of the image and the resulting standard deviation map is thresholded, followed by morphological operations to fill out holes and remove small segmented regions. The output is a set of M connected regions, $R_m, m = 1, ..., M$. Figure 2 shows two examples of cardiomyocyte image sequences, along with their corresponding computed standard deviation maps and final segmentation.

2.2   Beating Signal Estimation

We estimate a beating signal for each segmented region R_m. We make the assumption that disconnected regions in the image may have different beating signals but each

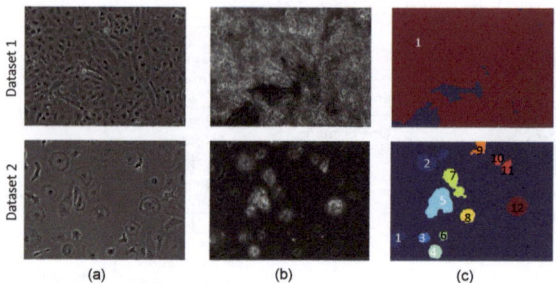

Fig. 2. An example of segmentation of beating regions for two datasets: (a) a frame of the raw image, (b) the corresponding temporal standard deviation map in log scale, and (c) binary segmentation of the beating regions. Top and bottom rows represent an example of high-density and low-density cell plating, respectively.

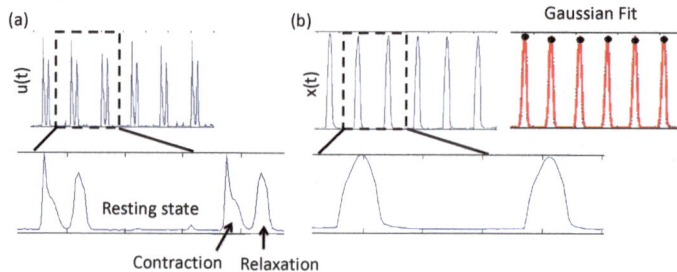

Fig. 3. An example of the beating signal extracted for one of the segmented regions: (a) raw (dual-peak) signal, $u(t)$, and (b) single-peak signal $x(t)$. A zoomed-in version of $u(t)$ and $x(t)$ are shown, along with the Gaussian mixture model fit to $x(t)$ and its peaks.

connected region has a single beating signal. This assumption has worked well in practice. An alternative, without affecting the rest of the pipeline, is to partition each connected region R_m to non-overlapping fixed-sized blocks, derive the beating signal for each block, and then cluster similar beating signals to generate a distinct set of beating signals.

For every image I_t and each segmented region R_m we form a one-dimensional vector of pixel intensities, denoted by $A_m(t)$. Starting from the second image in the sequence ($t = 2$), the correlation coefficient of intensity vectors of the image and its preceding image in the sequence is computed. We denote the beating signal calculated from the correlation of the successive images for each region R_m by $u_m(t)$, i.e.,

$$u_m(t) = 1 - \text{corr}(A_m(t), A_m(t-1)). \tag{1}$$

where $A_m(t)$ and $A_m(t-1)$ are the intensity vectors corresponding to a segmented region R_m at frame t and $t-1$, respectively.

Figure 3 shows an example of a beating signal obtained for cardiomyocyte dataset 1. This raw signal typically exhibits three states: a resting-state, where the correlation of successive images is high, a contraction state, and a relaxation state. Although the beating pattern and frequency can be measured from this signal, automatic identification of beating intervals is challenging due to the presence of double peaks and the lack of prior knowledge on their relative magnitude or distances. To obtain a single-peak signal, we first estimate a reference image by taking the median of resting-state images, identified as the frames that have small $u_m(t)$ and $du_m(t)/dt$. A single-peak signal is then generated by computing the correlation coefficient of the intensity vector of the reference image with those of all images in the sequence:

$$x_m(t) = 1 - \text{corr}(B_m, A_m(t)), \tag{2}$$

where B_m is the intensity vector that corresponds to the resting state of the R_m. Figure 4 shows an example of the resulting signal $x_m(t)$.

2.3 Signal Quantification and Modeling

Once the beating signal is estimated, signal processing techniques in the time and/or frequency domains can be applied to calculate quantitative features that describe the beating signal. To capture irregularity and dynamics of beating over time, we perform the analysis in the time domain. We first identify the peaks of $x_m(t)$. A vector of estimated beating intervals τ_m is constructed by calculating the duration between successive peaks. We define the effective beating rate as $f_m = \text{median}(\tau_m)$ and the irregularity of beating pattern as $f_m(\max(\tau_m) - \min(\tau_m))/2$. In addition to the beating intervals, it is important to measure the duration of each beat as well. For robust estimation of this parameter, we model the beating signal with a mixture of Gaussians, $\sum_i w_i \mathcal{N}(\mu_i, \sigma)$, where μ_i's coincide with the location of the extracted peaks and w_i's and σ's are estimated by minimizing the difference between the Gaussian mixture signal and $x_m(t)$. The duration of each beat is estimated by 6σ.

2.4 Clustering

The aim of clustering routine is to extract a distinct set of beating signals for the image sequence. The definition of "distinct" can be application-dependent: one might be interested in grouping the regions that beat at the same frequency but not necessarily in synchrony. Alternatively, in the case of low-density cell plating, it might of interest to identify groups of cells that are in close proximity and beat synchronously. Furthermore, since the number of clusters is unknown *a priori*, clustering approaches that require the number of clusters, such as k-means, are not suitable. Here, we propose a framework which is flexible to accommodate different applications. First, for each time-series signal, $x_m(t)$, we calculate a descriptor vector that contains the application-dependent parameters that will define similarity between the signals. Here, we use the effective beating rate and the time stamp of the first three peaks. To incorporate spatial information, we first calculate the pairwise distance between the regions, using a distance map for each region for efficient computation. Regions with the spatial distance smaller than a given threshold are identified as potential candidates for synchronous beating. We then calculate the pairwise distance between the descriptive vectors and feed these into

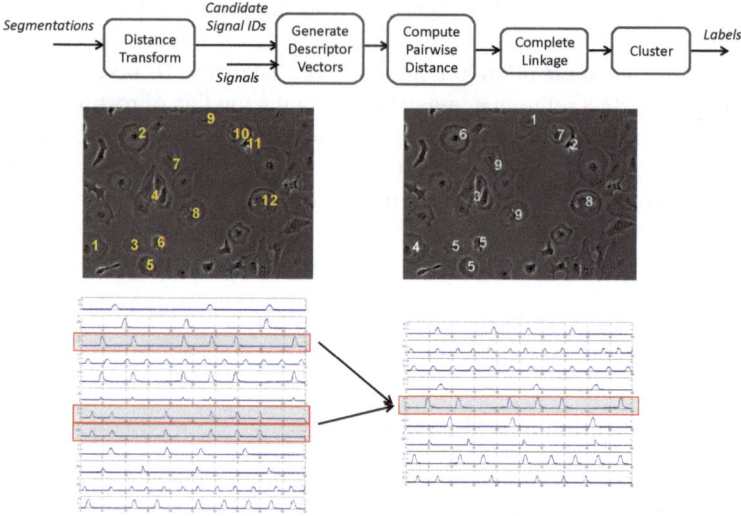

Fig. 4. Clustering of beating regions based on their spatial proximity and similarity of beating signal. The input to the clustering routine is a set of cell segmentations with associated beating signals, some of which may be synchronous, and the output is a set of clusters and associated signals with distinct beating profiles.

an agglomerative hierarchical clustering routine. Figure 4 shows a block diagram of the above flow along with an example of beating regions and their corresponding signals (left) and clustered regions and distinct beating signals (right). As can be seen, regions 3, 5, and 6 are grouped together (cluster 5 on the right) and regions 7 and 8 are grouped together (cluster 9 on the right). Identifying such clusters based on the synchrony of the beating signals provides an indication of the underlying physiological communication between the cells and is of interest for clinical studies.

3   Results

To assess the performance of the presented method, we performed a series of experiments using iPSC-derived cardiomyocytes obtained from commercial vendors. Cardiomyocytes were cultured in multi-well plates following standard culture protocols, with varied plating densities. Imaging data was collected using custom-built 10x phase-contrast microscopes, with capture frequency of 24 frames/sec and typical duration of 15 to 30 seconds. The images were saved in tiff format with 640x480 pixels. The microscopes were constructed using off-the-shelf components, including high-precision multi-well plate scanners, and were configured to work with stage-top incubators that provide precise environmental control during imaging.

We collected and analyzed more than 500 videos of cardiomyocyte cultures from different lines, plated with varied cell culture densities. We observed variation

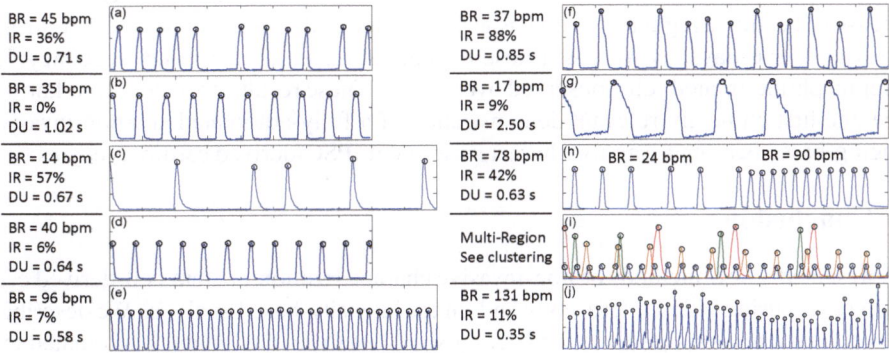

Fig. 5. Examples of estimated beating signals. Effective beat rate (BR), a measure of beating irregularity (IR), and the average beat duration (DU) are automatically measured for each sequence. Signals are extracted from varied cell cultures: Diseased lines (a,h), controls (b,d), after addition of a compound (f), single-cell plating (c, g, i), after media change (e,j).

of beating characteristics over time, after media changes, and with addition of chemical compounds. We used a subset of the videos to experimentally tune parameters such as thresholds for segmentation, peak detection, and cutoff distance in clustering, and the parameters were then fixed for all of our analysis. Figure 5 shows a sample set of beating signals with different profiles, detected and quantified automatically using our method. We confirmed the accuracy of our beating frequency measurements by comparing them to manually derived values from the captured videos. We rendered a movie for each dataset at the frame rate of image capture. A person watched the movie to confirm the number of beating regions and frequencies.

In order to show that our method can characterize the cellular response from different drugs, we performed a set of controlled experiments using Cisapride (a gastrointestinal drug withdrawn from market due to risk of induced arrhythmias) and Norepinephrine (a neurotransmitter used to increase blood pressure and heart rate) applied

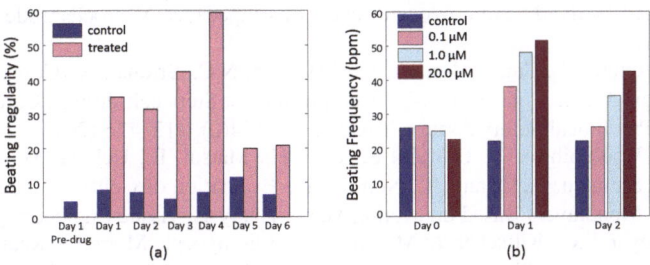

Fig. 6. Characterizing the effect of different compounds: (a) changes in beating irregularity due to addition of Cisapride measured over 6 days, and (b) changes in beating frequency due to addition of Norepinephrine measured over 2 days

to high-confluency cell cultures. As shown in Fig. 6, we measured an average 3-fold increase of beating irregularity with Cisapride-treated cells compared with the controls, observed over 6 days, as well as a dose-dependent increase of beating frequency for Norepinephrine-treated cells, observed over 2 days. These results provide, to our knowledge, the first clinically-relevant demonstration of a fully-automated and non-invasive imaging-based beating assay for characterization of iPSC-derived cardiomyocytes.

4   Conclusion

We presented a new method for non-invasive characterization of stem cell-derived cardiomyocytes using video microscopy and image intensity-based analysis. We described a novel image analysis pipeline for beating signal analysis that enables automated extraction of quantitative parameters that are of interest in clinical research. Our technique accommodates cultures with different cell density and with either regular or irregular beating patterns. We used our method to characterize the effects of two commercial drugs known to modulate beating frequency and irregularity, and showed results for successfully measuring a dose-dependent response. The presented method uses correlation coefficient of images to capture the change in their signal intensity, a simple, yet effective approach in combination with the rest of proposed pipeline in estimating the parameters of interest from varied cardiomyocyte cell cultures. Our future work is focused on estimating additional parameters of interest such as contraction strength, pattern, and accurate shape modeling of the beats.

References

1. Grskovic, M., Javaherian, A., Strulovici, B., Daley, G.: Induced Pluripotent Stem Cells - Opportunities for Disease Modeling and Drug Discovery. Nature Reviews Drug Discovery (2011)
2. Sun, N., Yazawa, M., Liu, J., Han, L., Sanchez-Freire, V., Abilez, O.J., Navarrete, E.G., Hu, S., Wang, L., Lee, A., Chen, R., Hajjar, R.J., Snyder, M.P., Dometsch, R.E., Butte, M.J., Ashley, E.A., Longaker, M.T., Robbins, R.C., Wu, J.C.: Patient-Specific Induced Pluripotent Stem Cells as a Model for Familial Dilated Cardiomyopathy. Science Translational Medicine 4(130) (2012)
3. Navarrete, E.G., Liang, P., Lan, F., Sanchez-Freire, V., Simmons, C., Gong, T., Sharma, A., Burridge, P.W., Patlolla, B., Lee, A.S., Wu, H., Beygui, R.E., Wu, S.M., Robbins, R.C., Bers, D.M., Wu, J.C.: Screening Drug-Induced Arrhythmia Events Using Human Induced Pluripotent Stem Cell-Derived Cardiomyocytes and Low-Impedance Microelectrode Arrays. Circulation (2013)
4. Harris, K., Aylott, M., Cui, Y., Louttit, J., McMahon, N.C., Sridhar, A.: Comparison of Electrophysiological Data from Human-induced Pluripotent Stem cell-derived Cardiomyocytes to Functional Preclinical Safety Assays. Toxicol. Sci. 134(2), 412–426 (2013)
5. Hayakawa, T., Kunihiro, T., Dowaki, S., Uno, H., Matsui, E., Uchida, M., Kobayashi, S., Yasuda, A., Shimizu, T., Okano, T.: Noninvasive Evaluation of Contractile Behavior of Cardiomyocyte Monolayers Based on Motion Vector Analysis. Tissue Engineering 18(1) (2012)
6. Liu, X., Iyengar, S.G., Rittscher, J.: Monitoring Cardiomyocyte Motion in Real Time Through Image Registration and Time Series Analysis. In: ISBI, pp. 1308–1311 (2012)
7. Liu, X., Padfield, D.: Motion-Based Segmentation for Cardiomyocyte Characterization. In: Durrleman, S., Fletcher, T., Gerig, G., Niethammer, M. (eds.) STIA 2012. LNCS, vol. 7570, pp. 137–146. Springer, Heidelberg (2012)

Exploiting Enclosing Membranes and Contextual Cues for Mitochondria Segmentation

Aurélien Lucchi[2,*], Carlos Becker[1], Pablo Márquez Neila[1], and Pascal Fua[1]

[1] Computer Vision Laboratory, EPFL, Lausanne, Switzerland
[2] Department of Computer Science, ETHZ, Zürich, Switzerland

Abstract. In this paper, we improve upon earlier approaches to segmenting mitochondria in Electron Microscopy images by explicitly modeling the double membrane that encloses mitochondria, as well as using features that capture context over an extended neighborhood. We demonstrate that this results in both improved classification accuracy and reduced computational requirements for training.

1   Introduction

In addition to providing energy to the cell, mitochondria play an important role in many essential cellular functions including signaling, differentiation, growth and death. An increasing body of research suggests that regulation of mitochondrial shape is crucial for cellular physiology [1]. Furthermore, localization and morphology of mitochondria have been tightly linked to neural functionality. For example, pre- and post-synaptic presence of mitochondria is known to have an important role in synaptic functioning [2] and mounting evidence also indicates that there is a close link between mitochondrial function and many neuro-degenerative diseases [3, 4].

Since mitochondria range from less than 0.5 to 10 μm in diameter [5], block face scanning microscopes and their ability to image with isotropic resolution of up to $4nm$ are proved invaluable tools to study their exact structure. As a result, new approaches to analyzing the images they produce have begun to appear. For example, in [6] a Gentle-Boost classifier was trained to detect mitochondria based on textural features. In [7], texton-based mitochondria classification in melanoma cells was performed using a variety of classifiers including k-NN, SVM, and Adaboost. While these techniques achieve reasonable results, they incorporate only textural cues while ignoring shape information. More recently, more sophisticated features [8–10] have been successfully used in conjunction with either a Random Forest classifier [11] or a Structured SVM (SSVM) [12, 13]. The latter approach [12, 13] is state-of-the-art in terms of accuracy. In this paper, we show that it can be further improved by

- **Explicitly modeling membranes.** At the resolution we are working with, mitochondria have a clearly visible double membrane, as shown in Figure 1.

* This work was accomplished while the author was in the Computer Vision Lab at EPFL and supported in part by the MicroNano ERC project.

P. Golland et al. (Eds.): MICCAI 2014, Part I, LNCS 8673, pp. 65–72, 2014.
© Springer International Publishing Switzerland 2014

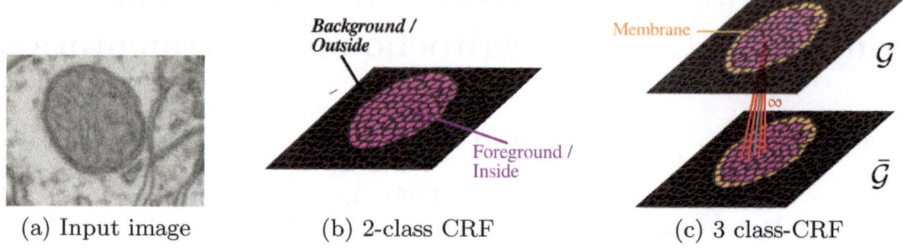

| (a) Input image | (b) 2-class CRF | (c) 3 class-CRF |

Fig. 1. Input image (a slice through a 3D volume) shown in (a). Figure (b) shows the graph used for a standard 2-class CRF commonly used in segmentation [12, 13]. The pink and black colors correspond to the foreground and background classes while the gray color in (b) and (c) shows the boundary of the SLIC supervoxels. The 3-class CRF introduced in Section 2.1 is shown in (c). The outer layer of supervoxels originally labeled as foreground in (b) was converted to a third boundary class shown in orange.

Voxels can therefore be classified as being inside, between the two membranes, or outside. This three-class problem can be formulated so that the membrane class completely encloses the inside and can be solved exactly using the maxflow-mincut approach of [14], which makes it faster than having to rely on Belief Propagation as in [12, 13].

– **Introducing context-based features.** One of the difficulties with mitochondria segmentation is that purely local statistics are not informative enough. As a result, mitochondria voxels are easily confused with others such as those belonging to vesicles and context information has to be used for disambiguation purposes. In [12], this is done by using a linear SSVM with a non-linear transformation applied to the features. However, this approach has a very high worst case computational complexity. We will show that a better result can be obtained at a tenth of the computational cost by exploiting the ability of AdaBoost to process large amounts of training data to learn features that take into account extended neighborhoods around individual voxels [15] and using them to compute the data term of the above maxflow-mincut problem.

We will show on several datasets that this combination allows us not only improve upon the state-of-the-art in terms of accuracy but also to considerably speed-up the training and running times of our algorithms, which is significant when dealing with large amounts of data.

2   Method

As in [9], the first step of our approach is to over-segment the image stack into *supervoxels*, that is, small voxel clusters with similar intensities. The algorithm we use to compute them [16] lets us choose their approximate diameter, which we take to be on the order of the known thickness of the outer mitochondrial membranes. As can be seen in Fig. 1(c), this means that membranes are typically one supervoxel thick. All subsequent computations are performed on supervoxels instead of individual voxels, which speeds them up by several orders of magnitude. Our task is now to classify these supervoxels as being inside the mitochondria, part of the membrane, or outside, as shown in Fig. 1(c). To this end, we introduce a three-class Conditional Random Field (CRF) described below.

2.1   Multi-class Conditional Random Fields

CRF [17] are graphical models used to encode relationships between a set of input and output variables. The one we use here is defined over a graph $\mathcal{G} = (\mathcal{V}, \mathcal{E})$ whose nodes $i \in \mathcal{V}$ correspond to supervoxels and whose edges $(i, j) \in \mathcal{E}$ connect nodes i and j if they are adjacent in the 3D volume. Each node is associated to a feature vector x_i computed from the image data and a label y_i denoting one of the three classes to which a supervoxel can belong. Let Y be the vector of all y_i, which we will refer to as a *labeling*. The most likely labeling of a volume is then found by minimizing an objective function of the form

$$E^{\mathbf{w}}(Y) = \sum_{i \in \mathcal{V}} D_i^{\mathbf{w}}(y_i) + \sum_{(i,j) \in \mathcal{E}} V_{ij}^{\mathbf{w}}(y_i, y_j), \tag{1}$$

where D_i is referred to as the unary data term and V_{ij} as the pairwise term. The superscript denotes the dependency of these two terms to a parameter vector $\mathbf{w}$.

The unary data term D_i is a weighted sum of image features described in Section. 2.2. The pairwise term is a linear combination of a spatial regularization term [12, 13] and a containment term. The spatial term is learned from data and reflects the transition cost between nodes i and j from label y_i to label y_j. The containment term constrains the membrane class to completely enclose the inside class and to be at least one supervoxel thick, as originally proposed in [14]. As shown in Fig. 1(c), this is achieved by duplicating the graph $\mathcal{G}$ to $\bar{\mathcal{G}}$ and adding infinite cost edges emanating from voxels labeled as inside in $\mathcal{G}$ to the neighbors labeled as membrane or inside in $\bar{\mathcal{G}}$ (see red edges in Fig. 1(c)). This infinite cost effectively prohibits inside nodes to be next to outside nodes. The containment term is hand-defined and thus does not depend on any parameters. The set of parameters $\mathbf{w}$ to be learned are therefore the weights given to individual features in the unary term and the spatial regularization term. These parameters are learned with the Structured SVM (SSVM) framework of [13] that requires solving an inference problem on the supervoxel graph. The method of [14] greatly speed-ups this inference step by using graph-cuts instead of Belief-propagation.

2.2   Data term

In this section, we first briefly review the standard features used in the data term of competing approaches [8, 13] before introducing the contextual features we advocate using instead.

Standard Features. As the baseline, we used standard features found in the literature [8, 13] that capture local shape and texture information at each supervoxel. The features extracted are voxel intensity histograms and gradient magnitude, Laplacian of Gaussian, eigenvalues of the Hessian matrix, and eigenvalues of the structure tensor, computed at five different scales. The feature vectors consist of the concatenated features for the supervoxel of interest and those corresponding to its neighbors (adjacent supervoxels in the 3D volume).

Contextual Features. Even though the features described above can be computed efficiently and take surrounding supervoxels into account, this is done in a predetermined manner and over a limited spatial extent.

An early attempt at incorporating contextual information from further afield is found in [9], where Ray Features [18] were used to capture information about the mitochondria shape. Unfortunately, they rely on computing image gradients, which can be noisy. We have found experimentally that adding them into our CRF framework that already contains the standard features described above only had minimal impact.

Instead, we advocate here using the context-aware features first introduced in [15] for synapse segmentation[1] and demonstrate that they can be adapted for a different purpose and are therefore much more generic that initially claimed. These *context cues* capture

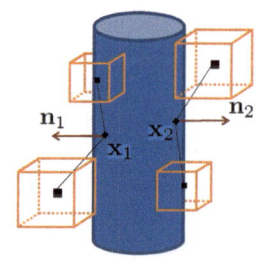

Fig. 2. Contextual Features. Given a mitochondria represented by the blue cylinder, the context surrounding voxels x_1 and x_2 is captured by summing responses of different channels inside cubes whose size and position with respect to the voxel is learned from training data.

context information in an extended neighborhood around voxels of interest by summing responses of different channels inside arbitrary-sized cubes, as depicted in Fig. 2. The extent of the neighborhood is learned by boosting up to a maximum size of 80 voxels. The location of each cube is relative to the voxel of interest and to the orientation estimate $\mathbf{n}$ at that point, computed from the Hessian matrix eigenvectors [15]. These locations and corresponding channels are learned automatically by running AdaBoost on the training data, which requires almost no parameter tuning. Since the number of possible context cue features can be in the order of hundreds of thousands, using AdaBoost is key to selecting a small subset of them based on training data.

To integrate these features into our CRF model, we treat the output of each one of the 1200 weak learners that compose the final AdaBoost classifier as a feature vector component for the unary data term. We then re-learn weights for the weak learners that are optimal when used in conjunction with the pairwise term of Eq. (1).

---

[1] Code publicly available at http://cvlab.epfl.ch/software/synapse

3   Experimental Results

To validate our approach we used the
two large labeled Electron Microscopy
image stacks depicted in Fig. 3. The
first one is publicly available[2] and represents a $1024 \times 1024 \times 165$-voxel volume of 5nm voxel size from the *CA1
hippocampus*. The second stack comes
from the *striatum*, a subcortical brain
region. It is of size $711 \times 872 \times 318$
and of voxel size $6 \times 6 \times 7.8$ nm. Each
stack is divided into two equally-sized
sub-volumes, one for training and the
other one for testing.

CA1 Hippocampus   Striatum

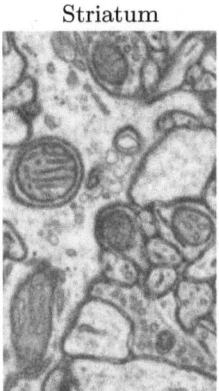

Fig. 3. *EM data sets.* Slices cut from two
EM stacks used for evaluation. Mitochondria are indicated with black arrows.

Performance is measured in terms
of the *Jaccard index*, commonly used
for image segmentation [9, 13, 15, 19].
We report the voxel-based *Jaccard index* for the foreground class, which is
representative for this task since the
mitochondria are the object of inter-
est being segmented. The multi-class CRF returns predictions for the membrane
class which can be of particular interest for biologists. We treat it as part of the
foreground class for quantitative evaluation purposes so as to facilitate comparison with the other methods, which produce only binary foreground/background
labels.

The performance for the different baselines on the test set is summarized in
Table 1. We report results when using standard features from Sec. 2.2 (*Std.*),
their kernelized version (*Kernel.*) introduced in [12], or the context cues of Section 2.2 (*Ccues*). As described in [12], kernelizing means transforming the features non-linearly using a 2-step approach. First, we train a non-structured kernel
SVM using the standard features extracted from $N = 40000$ randomly sampled
supervoxels. This yields a set of support vectors that are then used to compute
new feature vectors whose components are the kernel distances of the original
feature vectors to the support vectors. The three types of features are fed to
different classifiers, either two or three-class SSVM or AdaBoost. The *2-class*
model minimizes the energy as Eq. 1 but without the containment term.

From Table 1 it can be observed that our approach with *3-class* and context cues outperforms the others, especially those that use the 2-class model
and ignore the membrane prior. The next best result is obtained using the *3-
class* model with kernelized features, followed by the *2-class* one with context
cue features. We attribute the good performance of the 3-class model to two
reasons. First, at the 5 nm resolution we are working with, membranes have a

---

[2] http://cvlab.epfl.ch/data/em

Table 1. Segmentation performance measured with the Jaccard index of the foreground class for two EM datasets. We report results for different set of features (*Std.*, *Kernel.*, *Ccues*) and different classifiers (*2-class* CRF, *3-class* CRF and Adaboost).

	Std. + 2-class	Std. + 3-class	Kernel. + 2-class	Kernel. + 3-class	Ccues + AdaBoost	Ccues + 2-class	Ccues + 3-class
Hippocampus	67.6%	68.9%	71.7%	72.3%	69.5%	72.8%	**74.1%**
Striatum	79.3%	82.5%	80.8%	83.4%	79.3%	83.2%	**84.6%**

visible extent and the voxels within them form texture patterns that are different from those inside. Treating the inside and membrane voxels as one single class is therefore a more complex learning task. Furthermore, this specific 3-class problem allows for exact inference and therefore does not incur the penalty of having approximate inference as would have to be done in generic 3-class problems.

As observed in [15], hand-drawn ground truth near mitochondria borders is not always very accurate. As a result, even correctly labeled voxels near the boundary may impact the Jaccard index negatively due to annotation errors. To eliminate this undesirable effect, as in [15], we add an exclusion zone around the mitochondria border for evaluation purposes and report results as a function of its width. The resulting plots for the two top-performing approaches and the 2-class baseline are shown in Fig. 4. Note that our method outperforms the others independently of the exclusion zone width, achieving a difference of up to 10% in Jaccard index with respect to the 2-class approach.

Example segmentation outputs are shown in Fig. 5, where it can be seen that the results of the Ccues + 3-class approach are more accurate than other methods that fail to detect some mitochondria or erroneously insert extra ones.

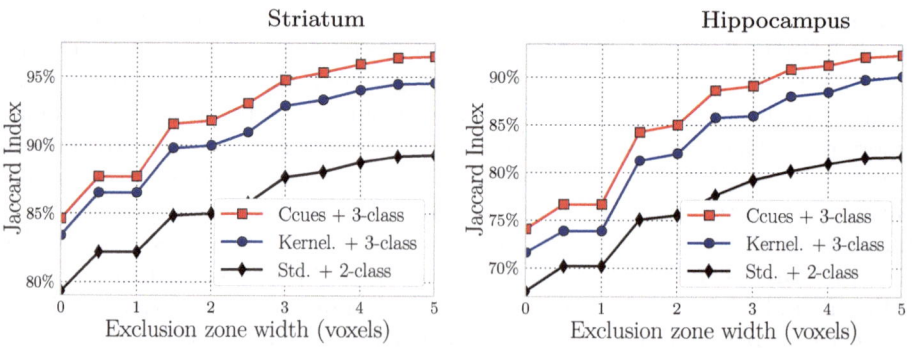

Fig. 4. Jaccard index as a function of the exclusion zone width, used to mitigate annotation errors closer to the mitochondria membrane in the ground truth. Our approach enforcing consistently outperforms the others.

Std. + 2-class   Kernel. + 3-class   Ccues + 3-class   Groundtruth

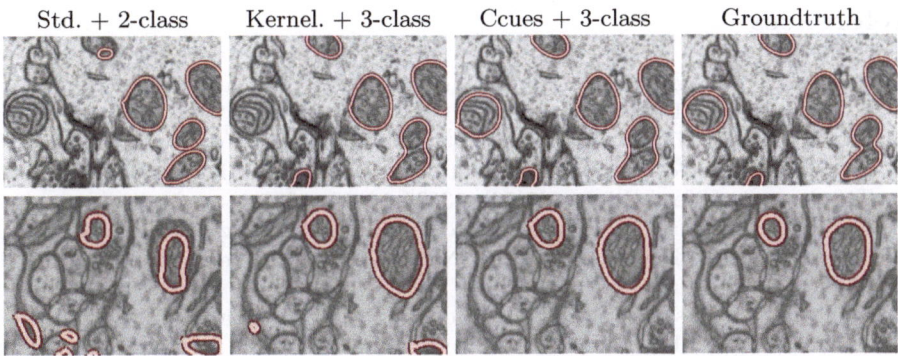

Fig. 5. Segmentation results on the Striatum (top row) and Hippocampus (bottom row) datasets. The Ccues + 3-class method correctly segments all mitochondria in this example, while other methods fail to detect some mitochondria or erroneously insert extra regions. The images above correspond to slices from the test volume and are best viewed in color. The 3D results are shown in the supplementary material.

Table 2. Training time in minutes for $T = 1000$ iterations. Note that using kernelized features increases training time by almost an order of magnitude.

	Std. + 2-class	Std. + 3-class	Kernel. + 3-class	Ccues + AdaBoost	Ccues + 3-class
Hippocampus	3809	275	2365	96	265
Striatum	4530	213	2311	102	282

We conducted a time analysis of the different methods evaluated in this paper. We ran each method on a 8-core Intel Xeon CPU 2.4 GHz machine with 200 GB RAM. As shown in Table 2, the 3-class models are much faster to train than the 2-class models. The total number of training points is of the order of $860K$ and $820K$ for the Hippocampus and Striatum datasets. Yet, we could only use a maximum of $40K$ to train this approach in a reasonable time.

4   Conclusion

We presented a segmentation framework that exploits discriminative contextual features and a CRF model with geometric constraints to model organelles with enclosing membranes. We demonstrated that it produces superior performance in the specific case of mitochondria, though this approach is generic and could be applied to many other biological structures such as the wide array of cells present in all living creatures. The code and datasets used in this paper is available at www.cvlab.epfl.ch.

References

1. Campello, S., Scorrano, L.: Mitochondrial Shape Changes: Orchestrating Cell Pathophysiology. EMBO Reports 11(9), 678–684 (2010)
2. Lee, D., Lee, K., Ho, W., Lee, S.: Target Cell-Specific Involvement of Presynaptic Mitochondria in Post-Tetanic Potentiation at Hippocampal Mossy Fiber Synapses. The Journal of NeuroScience 27(50), 13603–13613 (2007)
3. Knott, A., Perkins, G., Schwarzenbacher, R., Bossy-Wetzel, E.: Mitochondrial Fragmentation in Neurodegeneration. Nature Reviews. Neuroscience 9(7), 505–518 (2008)
4. Poole, A., Thomas, R., Andrews, L., Mcbride, H., Whitworth, A., Pallanck, L.: The Pink1/parkin Pathway Regulates Mitochondrial Morphology. Proceedings of the National Academy of Sciences of the United States of America 105(5), 1638–1643 (2008)
5. Campbell, N., Williamson, B., Heyden, R.: Biology: Exploring Life. Pearson Prentice Hall (2006)
6. Vitaladevuni, S., Mishchenko, Y., Genkin, A., Chklovskii, D., Harris, K.: Mitochondria Detection in Electron Microscopy Images. In: Workshop on Microscopic Image Analysis with Applications in Biology (2008)
7. Narasimha, R., Ouyang, H., Gray, A., McLaughlin, S., Subramaniam, S.: Automatic Joint Classification and Segmentation of Whole Cell 3D Images. PR 42, 1067–1079 (2009)
8. Sommer, C., Straehle, C., Koethe, U., Hamprecht, F.: Interactive Learning and Segmentation Tool Kit. In: Systems Biology of Human Disease, pp. 230–233 (2010)
9. Lucchi, A., Smith, K., Achanta, R., Knott, G., Fua, P.: Supervoxel-Based Segmentation of Mitochondria in EM Image Stacks with Learned Shape Features. TMI 31(2), 474–486 (2011)
10. Kumar, R., Vazquez-Reina, A., Pfister, H.: Radon-Like Features and Their Application to Connectomics. In: Workshop on MMBIA (2010)
11. Kreshuk, A., Straehle, C.N., Sommer, C., Koethe, U., Knott, G., Hamprecht, F.: Automated Segmentation of Synapses in 3D EM Data. In: ISBI (2011)
12. Lucchi, A., Li, Y., Smith, K., Fua, P.: Structured Image Segmentation Using Kernelized Features. In: Fitzgibbon, A., Lazebnik, S., Perona, P., Sato, Y., Schmid, C. (eds.) ECCV 2012, Part II. LNCS, vol. 7573, pp. 400–413. Springer, Heidelberg (2012)
13. Lucchi, A., Li, Y., Fua, P.: Learning for Structured Prediction Using Approximate Subgradient Descent with Working Sets. In: CVPR (June 2013)
14. Delong, A., Boykov, Y.: Globally Optimal Segmentation of Multi-Region Objects. In: ICCV, pp. 285–292 (2009)
15. Becker, C., Ali, K., Knott, G., Fua, P.: Learning Context Cues for Synapse Segmentation. TMI 32(10), 1864–1877 (2013)
16. Achanta, R., Shaji, A., Smith, K., Lucchi, A., Fua, P., Suesstrunk, S.: SLIC Superpixels Compared to State-Of-The-Art Superpixel Methods. PAMI 34(11), 2274–2281 (2012)
17. Lafferty, J., Mccallum, A., Pereira, F.: Conditional Random Fields: Probabilistic Models for Segmenting and Labeling Sequence Data. In: ICML (2001)
18. Smith, K., Carleton, A., Lepetit, V.: Fast Ray Features for Learning Irregular Shapes. In: ICCV, pp. 397–404 (2009)
19. Everingham, M., Van Gool, L., Williams, C., Winn, J., Zisserman, A.: The Pascal Visual Object Classes Challenge (VOC 2010) Results (2010)

Identifying Neutrophils in H&E Staining Histology Tissue Images*

Jiazhuo Wang[1], John D. MacKenzie[2],
Rageshree Ramachandran[3], and Danny Z. Chen[1]

[1] Department of Computer Science & Engineering, University of Notre Dame, USA
[2] Department of Radiology & Biomedical Imaging, UCSF, USA
[3] Department of Pathology & Laboratory Medicine, UCSF, USA

Abstract. Identifying neutrophils lays a crucial foundation for diagnosing acute inflammation diseases. But, such computerized methods on the commonly used H&E staining histology tissue images are lacking, due to various inherent difficulties of identifying cells in such image modality and the challenge that a considerable portion of neutrophils do not have a "textbook" appearance. In this paper, we propose a new method for identifying neutrophils in H&E staining histology tissue images. We first segment the cells by applying iterative edge labeling, and then identify neutrophils based on the segmentation results by considering the "context" of each candidate cell constructed by a new Voronoi diagram of clusters of other neutrophils. We obtain good performance compared with two baseline algorithms we constructed, on clinical images collected from patients suspected of having inflammatory bowl diseases.

1 Introduction

Identifying neutrophils, a major type of immune cells, is a crucial step towards diagnosing acute inflammation diseases; the locations and number of neutrophils with respect to different tissue layers determine whether there is acute inflammation [6]. H&E staining histology tissue image is a very common imaging modality in clinical use. In such imaging modality, neutrophils are characterized as having multiple lobes in nucleus per cell and often hardly visible cytoplasm (in Fig. 1(e)-(f), the lobes are indicated by green arrows).

There are known methods [3,4,10] for identifying neutrophils in blood smear (see [2,5] for complete reviews). But they utilize specific properties of blood smear, which are not valid in H&E staining histology tissue images. For example, in blood smear, immune cells have quite salient colors and are well separated; the lobes of a nucleus are usually distinctive with each other; the cytoplasm is also distinctive from either the nuclei or background, which can help group the lobes of a single cell together. Further, we are not aware of any work that marks

---

* This research was supported in part by NSF Grant CCF-1217906, a grant of the National Academies Keck Futures Initiative (NAKFI), and NIH grant K08-AR061412-02 Molecular Imaging for Detection and Treatment Monitoring of Arthritis.

P. Golland et al. (Eds.): MICCAI 2014, Part I, LNCS 8673, pp. 73–80, 2014.
© Springer International Publishing Switzerland 2014

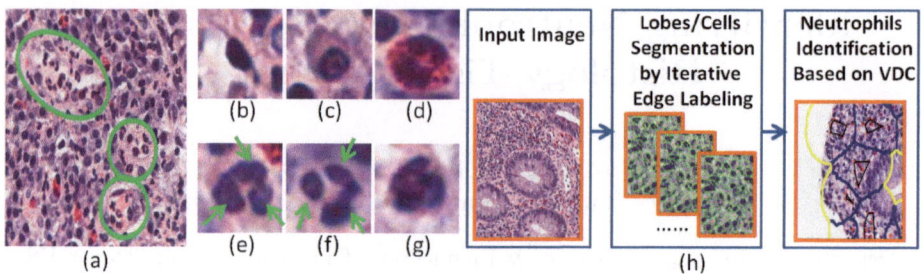

Fig. 1. (a)-(g) Image examples; (h) the framework of our method

neutrophils by a relevant antibody to analyze inflammation, and consequently, no immuno-staining method is known.

There are two main reasons for the lack of effective methods on H&E staining histology tissue images. (a) Identifying cells is inherently challenging [8] here, due to, e.g., non-uniform staining, complex and noisy tissue background, and crowded cells (Fig. 1(a)). (b) Identifying neutrophils is even harder. First, one has to group the lobes of each neutrophil together (otherwise, one may classify each lobe as a single-lobe cell). This is not easy due to the mixture of various types of cells, with either single lobe (e.g., lymphoctyes in Fig. 1(b) and plasma cells in Fig. 1(c)) or multiple lobes (e.g., eosinophils in Fig. 1(d)). Second, the lobes of a neutrophil may not appear perfectly well separated (i.e., lack of multiple-lobes characteristic), but crowded together instead (Fig. 1(g)), which makes grouping these lobes easier but classifying them as a neutrophil harder.

In fact, if based on only the appearance of each individual cell, pathologists are highly/moderately confident at marking roughly half neutrophils (easy cases). They must rely on the *context* of a cell to mark the rest neutrophils (hard cases): They compare a hard case with cells around that they can relatively easily identify, especially clusters of neutrophils (e.g., those inside green circles in Fig. 1(a)). Namely, the ambiguity and the subjectivity on the confidence scale of each annotation of neutrophil can be resolved after considering the context, making pathologists' annotations of all neutrophils still quite robust.

In this paper, we present a new method for identifying neutrophils in H&E staining histology tissue images. Our method combines a lobes/cells segmentation process based on iterative edge labeling and a neutrophils identification process based on Voronoi diagram of clusters (VDC). In segmentation stage (Fig. 1(h)), we seek to group the lobes of each cell (especially, each neutrophil) into one segment, which contains no lobes from other cells, since identification of neutrophils is dependent on the lobes. In identification stage (Fig. 1(h)), we capture quantitatively by VDC how pathologists resolve the ambiguity based on the context when identifying hard cases of neutrophils.

Our most significant contribution is an effective strategy for identifying neutrophils in H&E staining histology tissue images. Also, our iterative edge labeling approach is actually a generally applicable framework for segmenting multiple

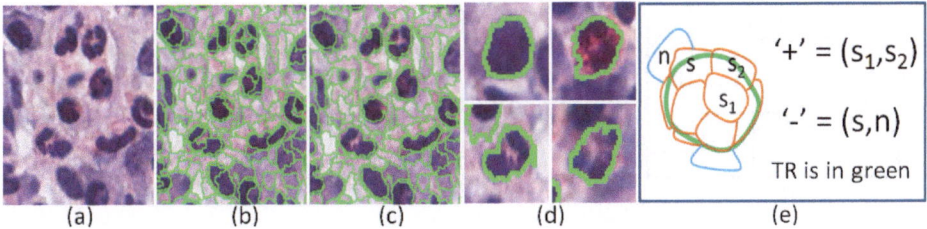

Fig. 2. Segmentation and construction of training examples

objects. Further, our VDC idea provides a new way to model quantitatively the local influence of clusters of objects for identifying objects around such clusters.

2   Method

2.1   Lobes/Cells Segmentation by Iterative Edge Labeling

Our goal of this stage is to obtain a segmentation of the input image, such that the lobes of each cell (especially, each neutrophil) are grouped into one segment, which contains no lobes of other cells. The resulted segments will be used in our later steps for identifying neutrophils.

Our main idea is to apply an iterative edge labeling process, which is essentially based on merging pairs of segments at different scales. At each iteration (i.e., scale), instead of hypothetically designing some criteria for segment merging, we decide to (a) learn such knowledge from training examples of edges in a segment adjacency graph (SAdjG, defined below), and (b) optimally refine it globally by applying MRF [9] to the edge dual graph (EDG, defined below) of SAdjG. By combining learning and refining characteristics exhibited by pairs of segments at different scales, we are able to alleviate or overcome difficulties caused by the high complexity nature of objects and background tissues in our imaging modality. Also, it is actually more natural to obtain segmentation of multiple objects by binary classification based on the *edge* view, rather than the *vertex* view, of SAdjG. This is simply because if two adjacent vertices of SAdjG are both labeled as foreground, one is not able to tell the corresponding two segments (sharing some common border pixels) are one or two objects.

Iterative Edge Labeling. We present steps of our algorithm in detail below.

1. Initialize the segmentation by applying some superpixel segmentation method (e.g., [1]). Tune the parameters of such a method so that the cells are broken into pieces to obtain an over-segmentation. Fig. 2(b) shows the initial segmentation of the image in Fig. 2(a). Let S denote the set of all segments in the current segmentation.

2. Provide training data. For each cell considered as training data, select a group of points in that cell such that the union of the segments (in the **initial segmentation**) each containing at least one such point can roughly represent

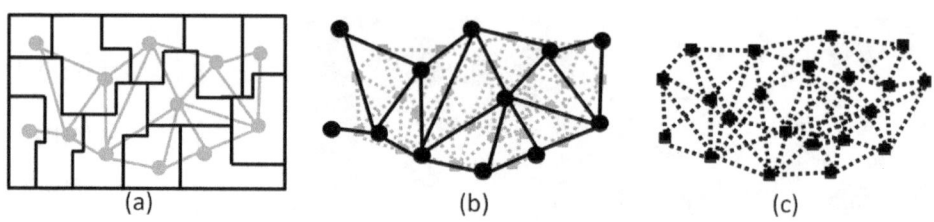

Fig. 3. Segmentation (a) and the corresponding graphs $SAdjG$ (b) and EDG (c)

well the region of that cell. We call the region of a cell thus constructed the training region (TR) of that cell (Fig. 2(d)). It is much easier to provide training data for the region of a cell in this way than delineating each boundary pixel of the cell. We will use the TR's to construct training examples of edges of the graph SAdjG, without making the user provide additional training data at each iteration. Note that the TR's, once constructed, will not change in the algorithm.

3. Construct the graph $SAdjG = (V_{SAdjG}, E_{SAdjG})$ based on S (Fig. 3(b)), where $V_{SAdjG} = \{s \mid s \in S\}$ and $E_{SAdjG} = \{(s_a, s_b) \mid s_a, s_b \in S,$ and they share common border pixels$\}$.

4. Construct weighted training examples for the edges of the graph $SAdjG$. In iterations other than the initial one, segments obtained may cross the boundaries of the TR's, and thus we use the weights to compensate for the potentially noisy knowledge learned in such situations. For TR of each cell provided as training data, let $O = \{s \mid s \in S, s \cap TR \neq \emptyset\}$.

The set of '+' training examples (Fig. 2(f)) based on TR is defined as $PT = \{(s_1, s_2) \mid s_1, s_2 \in O, (s_1, s_2) \in E_{SAdjG}\}$. For each $(s_1, s_2) \in PT$, let

$$weight((s_1, s_2)) = \frac{\frac{(s_1 \cup s_2) \cap TR}{s_1 \cup s_2} + \frac{(s_1 \cup s_2) \cap TR}{TR}}{2}. \tag{1}$$

The set of '-' training examples (Fig. 2(f)) based on TR is defined as $NT = \{(s, n) \mid s \in O, n \notin O, (s, n) \in E_{SAdjG}\}$. For each $(s, n) \in NT$, let

$$weight((s, n)) = \frac{\frac{s \cap TR}{s} + \frac{s \cap TR}{TR}}{2}. \tag{2}$$

5. Build a binary classifier c for the edges of $SAdjG$, which represents our knowledge of what pairs of segments within or not within the same cell usually look like in the current iteration (or at the current scale). Note that we apply Random Forest here, but one can definitely use other classifiers.

6. Construct the edge dual graph $EDG = \{V_{EDG}, E_{EDG}\}$ (Fig. 3(c)), where $V_{EDG} = \{v \mid v = (s_1, s_2) \in E_{SAdjG}\}$ and $E_{EDG} = \{(v_a, v_b) \mid v_a = (s_1, s_2) \in E_{SAdjG}, v_b = (s_1, s_3) \in E_{SAdjG}\}$ (note that s_1 is shared by both v_a and v_b).

7. Apply binary MRF to EDG: Each vertex of EDG (correspondingly, each edge of $SAdjG$) is assigned a value of '1' or '0', representing whether the corresponding pair of segments is within the same cell. By merging the corresponding

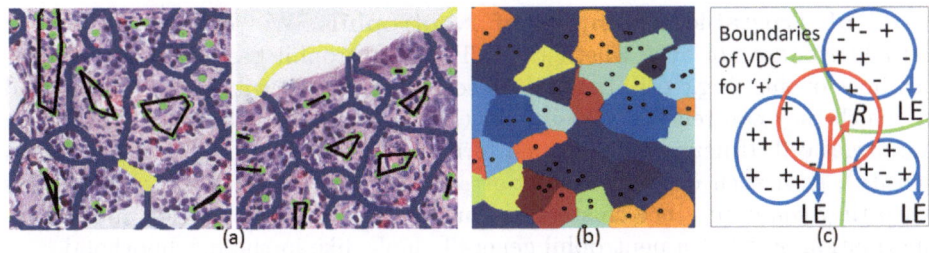

Fig. 4. (a)-(b) Examples of Voronoi diagrams of neutrophil clusters; (c) classifying the ambiguous cases using a VDC-based context

pair of segments for each edge of *SAdjG* labeled as '1' into one segment, we obtain a new segmentation *S* (Fig. 2(c) shows the segmentation of another iteration). The unary cost of MRF comes directly form the probability output of the classifier *c*. We define the pairwise cost between the two labels '1' and '0' as

$$P('0','0') = 0 \qquad P('0','1') = 0.5$$
$$P('1','0') = 0.5 \qquad P('1','1') = 1 \tag{3}$$

Different from the typical usage of pairwise cost as smoothness constraint on labeling, we use it to penalize aggressive merging behavior of the segments (which may result in undesired under-segmentation).

8. Repeat steps 3 to 7, until the resulted segmentation is relatively stable. In practice, we find that 4 or 5 iterations are usually sufficient.

Feature Design. We construct features for the edges of *SAdjG*. They reflect either cues of each individual of the two corresponding segments (e.g., color, texture, compactness, etc), or cues exhibited between the two segments (e.g., color difference, texture difference, the number of common border pixels, etc).

2.2 Neutrophils Identification

Our goal of this stage is to identify neutrophils based on the segmentation results produced by the previous stage. Our main idea is to perform a two-phase process: First identify some "trustable" examples of neutrophils, and then construct a Voronoi diagram of clusters (VDC) based on the trustable neutrophils. We use VDC to extract a local context that can help resolve ambiguous cases of neutrophils around. Intuitively, we aim to capture quantitatively how pathologists identify neutrophils, especially the hard cases, using context information.

Trustable Examples. We first extract trustable examples for both neutrophils and non-neutrophils (i.e., other types of cells, or background tissue), by classifying the obtained segments and examining whether any of the two resulted probabilities, P(neutrophil) and P(non-neutrophil) (note that the sum of the two probabilities is one), is not below a certain threshold *pTrustableT*. The binary classifier (one can apply, e.g., Random Forest) is built based on all training annotations available for neutrophils and non-neutrophils.

VDC of Trustable Examples of Neutrophils. We observed that when pathologists are not sure whether a cell is a neutrophil based on only the appearance of this single cell, they try to compare this cell with some cells around on which they can relatively easily identify the types, to help make decision on the target cell. If neutrophils around form some clusters (i.e., in relatively high density), then such clusters usually attract more attention of the pathologists when they compare, since clusters of neutrophils often may provide appearance information on what a neutrophil generally looks like in the neighborhood.

Based on the observation above, first, we apply density-based clustering (DBC) [11] to the trustable examples of neutrophils, to capture the potential clustering behavior of neutrophils. In Fig. 4(a), the convex hull of each such cluster is colored in black, and trustable examples of neutrophils are in green.

Second, we compute a Voronoi diagram (VD) of these clusters (the VDC boundaries are colored in blue or yellow in Fig. 4(a)). Different from the common VD [7] whose sites are each a single point only, every site of our VDC can be a set of points (i.e., the center locations of the neutrophils in a cluster). The distance between a point p and a cluster $C = \{p_1, p_2, \ldots, p_m\}$ is defined as

$$D(p, C) = \sum_{i=1}^{m} F(p, p_i), \qquad F(p, p_i) = \begin{cases} \frac{w(p_i)}{d(p, p_i)^2}, & \text{if } d(p, p_i) \leq dist_T \\ 0, & \text{otherwise} \end{cases} \qquad (4)$$

where $F(p, p_i)$ is a function measuring the "influence" of a point $p_i \in C$ on p, which depends on both the weight $w(p_i)$ (measuring the importance of p_i, and set as 1 here) and the Euclidean distance $d(p, p_i)$. We assume no influence is from p_i if $d(p, p_i)$ is larger than a threshold $dist_T$ (set as 160 pixels). Essentially, $D(p, C)$ measures the amount of collective influence of a cluster C on any point p. Thus, suppose there are k clusters, then a point p belongs to the (geometric) VD cell C_{VD} (i.e., not a biological cell, see Fig. 4(b)) associated with cluster C, if $D(p, C) = max\{D(p, C_i) \mid i = 1, 2, ..., k\}$ (i.e., with the biggest influence). Note that since $F(p, p_i)$ is truncated by a Euclidean distance threshold $dist_T$, there may exist points far away from all clusters that do not lie in any VD cell (e.g., in Fig. 4(a), points in regions bounded by only yellow curves).

Third, as shown in Fig. 4(c), for each VD cell C_{VD}, we build a binary classifier (such as Random Forest) such that its '+' and '-' training examples are trustable examples for respectively neutrophils and non-neutrophils whose center locations lie in C_{VD}. We call this classifier a *Local Expert* (LE) for C_{VD}, which represents our knowledge of what neutrophils and non-neutrophils look like around the corresponding cluster of neutrophils of C_{VD}.

Finally, for each ambiguous segment s, we define its *context* as the set of all VD cells overlapped with the circle with a radius R (set as 60 pixels; see Fig. 4(c)) centered at the center of s (note that it is possible for an ambiguous segment to have an empty context, and we take the segment as non-neutrophil in such cases). The probability outputs of the segment s is the average of the probability outputs by *LE* of each VD cell in its *context*, weighted by normalized distance $D(p, C)$ between the center point p of the segment s and the corresponding

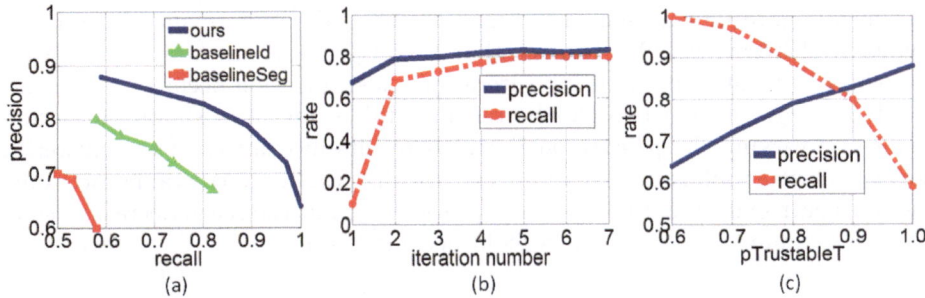

Fig. 5. (a) Precision and recall curves of identifying neutrophils by different methods; (b)-(c) analysis of influence of each algorithm stage

cluster C of each such VD cell. We take s as a neutrophil if such probability output for neutrophil is above a certain threshold p_T (set as 0.5).

3   Experiments and Evaluation

Clinical Data Sets. We collected images scanned at 40x magnification from patients suspected of having inflammatory bowl diseases. Pathologists annotated 339 neutrophils (not a small set, considering neutrophils do not infiltrate as prevalently as some other immune cells), and based just on appearance of each individual cell, they were highly/moderately confident at marking only about half of them (nevertheless, our method is blind to such confidence scales because such ambiguity to pathologists is finally resolved by considering the context).

Performance Evaluation. Since no direct effective method was known before (we have actually tried out related methods for blood smear on our images, but the results are quite poor to be used as a fair comparison), to show the necessity and effectiveness of both our segmentation and identification stage, we compare our method with two baselines: *baselineSeg* and *baselineId*, constructed by us in a structured manner. *BaselineSeg* applies superpixel segmentation [1] followed by the same VDC identification process as in our method. *BaselineId* applies the same segmentation process as in our method followed by directly thresholding the classification results for segments, without using VDC.

To measure the performance, we compute $precision = \frac{TP}{TP+FP}$ and $recall = \frac{TP}{TP+FN}$ for neutrophils, using 10-fold cross validation on ground truth data. Fig. 5(a) presents the precision and recall curves, obtained by varying key parameters (specifically, number of superpixels for *baselineSeg*, thresholding value for *baselineId*, and *pTrustableT* for our method) respectively for each method. One can see that both our segmentation and identification processes help improve the overall performance significantly compared with the baselines.

Analysis of Influence of Each Algorithm Stage. We examine the influence of each stage of our method on the final performance, by varying key parameters to which final results are sensitive. Fig. 5(b) shows the performance for different numbers of iterations. One can see that at early iterations, bad segmentation leads to bad identification; at later iterations, identification becomes better and stable as segmentation becomes better and stable. Fig. 5(c) shows the performance by varying the $pTrustableT$, which results in changes of the clustering settings of neutrophils in VDC. One can see that the more trustable the examples for neutrophils are, the higher the precision is; but the recall decreases, since trustable examples above the threshold become fewer.

4   Conclusions

We presented a new and effective method for identifying neutrophils in H&E staining histology tissue images, based on iterative edge labeling and VDC. This lays a crucial foundation for successful acute inflammation analysis.

References

1. Achanta, R., Shaji, A., Smith, K., Lucchi, A., Fua, P., Susstrunk, S.: SLIC superpixels compared to state-of-the-art superpixel methods. TPAMI 34(11), 2274–2282 (2012)
2. Gurcan, M., Boucheron, L., Can, A., Madabhushi, A., Rajpoot, N., Yener, B.: Hitopathological image analysis: A review. IEEE Rev. Biomed. Eng. 2, 147–171 (2009)
3. Hiremath, P., Bannigidad, P., Geeta, S.: Automated identification and classification of white blood cells (leukocytes) in digital microscopic images. IJCA, Special Issue on RTIPPR (2), 59–63 (2010)
4. Huang, D.C., Hung, K.D., Chan, Y.K.: A computer assisted method for leukocyte nucleus segmentation and recognition in blood smear images. J. Syst. Software 85, 2104–2118 (2012)
5. Jatti, A., Urs, V.M.: Review paper of conventional analysis of cell smear under a microscope. IJIRD 3(2) (2013)
6. Naini, B.V., Cortina, G.: A histopathologic scoring system as a tool for standardized reporting of chronic (ileo) colitis and independent risk assessment for inflammatory bowel disease. Human Pathology 43, 2187–2196 (2012)
7. Okabe, A., Boots, B., Sugihara, K., Chiu, S.N.: Spatial Tessellations: Concepts and Applications of Voronoi Diagrams. Wiley (2000)
8. Saraswat, M., Arya, K.: Leukocyte classification in skin tissue images. In: Bansal, J.C., Singh, P.K., Deep, K., Pant, M., Nagar, A.K. (eds.) BIC-TA 2013. AISC, vol. 201, pp. 65–73. Springer, Heidelberg (2013)
9. Szeliski, R., Zabih, R., Scharstein, D., Veksler, O., Kolmogorov, V., Agarwala, A., Tappen, M., Rother, C.: A comparative study of energy minimization methods for Markov random fields. In: Leonardis, A., Bischof, H., Pinz, A. (eds.) ECCV 2006. LNCS, vol. 3952, pp. 16–29. Springer, Heidelberg (2006)
10. Theera-Umpon, N., Dhompongsa, S.: Morphological granulometric features of nucleus in automatic bone marrow white blood cell classification. IEEE Trans. Inf. Technol. Biomed. 11, 353–359 (2007)
11. Xu, B., Chen, D.Z.: Density-based data clustering algorithms for lower dimensions using space-filling curves. In: Zhou, Z.-H., Li, H., Yang, Q. (eds.) PAKDD 2007. LNCS (LNAI), vol. 4426, pp. 997–1005. Springer, Heidelberg (2007)

Active Graph Matching for Automatic Joint Segmentation and Annotation of *C. elegans*

Dagmar Kainmueller[1], Florian Jug[1], Carsten Rother[2], and Gene Myers[1]

[1] Max Planck Institute of Molecular Cell Biology and Genetics, Germany
[2] Computer Vision Lab Dresden, Technical University Dresden, Germany
kainmueller@mpi-cbg.de

Abstract. In this work we present a novel technique we term *active graph matching*, which integrates the popular active shape model into a sparse graph matching problem. This way we are able to combine the benefits of a global, statistical deformation model with the benefits of a local deformation model in form of a second-order random field. We present a new iterative energy minimization technique which achieves empirically good results. This enables us to exceed state-of-the art results for the task of annotating nuclei in 3D microscopic images of *C. elegans*. Furthermore with the help of the generalized Hough transform we are able to jointly segment and annotate a large set of nuclei in a fully automatic fashion for the first time.

1 Introduction

A frequently used model organism in developmental biology is the worm *C. elegans*. Since *C. elegans* is highly stereotypical it is well suited for comparative developmental studies. A common and time consuming problem in such studies is the segmentation and annotation of cell nuclei with their unique biological names in 3D microscopic images [1,2,3,4]. This work presents a fully automated joint segmentation and annotation method for this task.[1]

Previous approaches for automatic annotation of nuclei in *C. elegans* [2,3,4] build an average atlas of nuclei locations, and annotate new target worms by mapping the atlas to the target. One approach finds a globally optimal one-to-one mapping but is agnostic to covariances between nucleus positions [2,3]. Another approach incorporates heuristic prior knowledge on relative positions of nuclei in the form of a local deformation model, but does not tackle local deformation and mapping of nuclei jointly in a globally optimal way [4].

While these approaches are in principle capable of performing segmentation and annotation of nuclei in a fully automatic manner in images that show all nuclei of *C. elegans* L1 larvae, none of them has been evaluated quantitatively in this respect: Only the annotation of given, correct segmentations is evaluated quantitatively in [2], and only images which exclusively show the 80 widely spaced *body wall muscles* of *C. elegans* L1 larvae are considered in [4].

---

[1] We work exclusively with *disentangled, straightened* images of *all 558 nuclei* of *L1 larvae*. Disentangling and straightening are not topics of this paper. See e.g. [5,6].

P. Golland et al. (Eds.): MICCAI 2014, Part I, LNCS 8673, pp. 81–88, 2014.

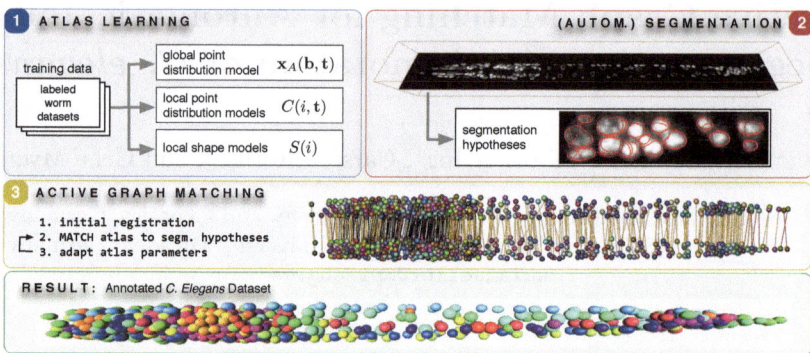

Fig. 1. A sketch of the proposed pipeline. First, a statistical atlas is learned from annotated data. New, straightened images are then segmented automatically. Subsequently, the body axes of atlas and segmentation are aligned. *Active Shape Matching* then alternates between graph matching and optimization of atlas parameters.

We propose to *learn* from training data a global-plus-local deformation model of *C. elegans*. The global model serves as a "backbone" of plausible nuclei constellations, while the local model penalizes deviations from this backbone. We use an *active shape model* [7] as a global model, and exploit the 2nd moments of the learned distribution of relative locations of nuclei for a local model.

We achieve a one-to-one mapping between atlas and target nuclei which is *approximately globally optimal* w.r.t. the local deformation model with an advanced *graph matching* method [8]. However, our overall goal is to find a one-to-one mapping which is optimal w.r.t. the local *as well as the global* deformation model. Our main technical contribution is a strong optimization technique for this problem. It can be seen as a generalization of the Iterative-Closest-Points method, where "Closest" (referring to local, point-wise measures) is replaced by "Best Matching" in terms of a global 2nd order matching energy. To the best of our knowledge only one work [9] has presented a related idea, but active shape models are not considered.

To summarize, our main contributions are (*i*) a new model we term *active graph matching* with an associated optimization technique, and (*ii*) an experimental validation that such a complex model can be optimized successfully for fully automatic segmentation and annotation of nuclei in *C. elegans* L1 larvae. Our method is, to our knowledge, the first fully automatic method ever evaluated quantitatively for this problem. Furthermore it considerably outperforms the state-of-the-art for annotation of given manual segmentations [2]. Finally, a small contribution is the idea of *in-painting* missing nuclei into the training set.

2   Method and Data

Figure 1 sketches the proposed pipeline. It builds upon a *statistical atlas* of *C. elegans* learned from training data. (cf. Sec. 2.1). Given a new target image,

(a)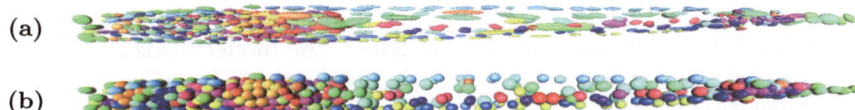

(b)

Fig. 2. Two types of local statistical models in our *C. elegans* atlas. **(a)** Local point distribution models per nucleus: Respective covariance matrices $C(i, I)$ represented as ellipses. **(b)** Average shape $s_A(i)$ of each nucleus in the atlas. Note that the local shape models also contain the respective covariances. Figures show the *in-painted* atlas.

first, a set of segmentation hypotheses is generated (cf. Sec 2.2). Then the *body axes* of the worm are determined for rough initial alignment of the atlas (cf. Section 2.3). An *objective function* encodes the problem of matching the atlas to the segmentation hypotheses. We optimize the objective by *Active Graph Matching* (cf. Sec. 2.3), a novel "iterative best matching points" method that alternates between optimal graph matching and optimal adaptation of global atlas parameters. The matching selects a subset of segmentation hypotheses, while simultaneously annotating them with their biological names.

We use a set of *training worms* also used in [2].[2] All nuclei that can be distinguished by eye were segmented manually in 30 images of *C. elegans* L1 larvae. Per worm 357 nuclei were annotated manually. See [2] for more details on the data. Let n_W denote the number of training worms, and n_A the number of annotated nuclei. Per worm, index i, with $1 \leq i \leq n_A$, represents the i-th annotated nucleus. Nuclei are sorted consistently by their biological names.

2.1   Atlas

Our statistical atlas of *C. elegans* consists of (i) a global model of the variability of the *point clouds* formed by each worm's nuclei center points, (ii) local models of the variability of single nucleus locations (cf. Figure 2a), (iii) local models of the variability of the shape of each nucleus (cf. Figure 2b), and (iv) local models of the variability of offsets between any two nucleus locations.

Global Point Distribution Model. From the set of training worms we extract locations of nuclei center points. We denote the center point location of nucleus $i \leq n_A$ in training worm $w \leq n_W$ as $x(i, w) \in \mathbf{R}^3$, the concatenation of all locations of worm w as $\mathbf{x}_w := (\dots, x(i, w)^T, \dots)^T \in \mathbf{R}^{3n_A}$, and the matrix of all training vectors as $\mathcal{X} := (\dots, \mathbf{x}_w, \dots)$. From the set of training vectors $\mathbf{x}_w$, we build a point distribution model [7] of nuclei locations. Therefore we align all training vectors via Procrustes analysis, and then perform principle component analysis, yielding the eigenvectors $\mathbf{p}_k \in \mathbf{R}^{3n_A}$ of the covariance matrix $(1/(n_W - 1))(\mathcal{X} - \bar{\mathcal{X}})(\mathcal{X} - \bar{\mathcal{X}})^T$, where $\bar{\mathcal{X}}$ denotes a matrix with the average nuclei location vector $\bar{\mathbf{x}}_A := (1/n_W) \sum_w \mathbf{x}_w$ in every column. We denote the matrix assembled from the eigenvectors as $P := (\dots, \mathbf{p}_w, \dots)$. The point distribution model can then be formulated as $\mathbf{x}_A(\mathbf{b}, \mathbf{t}) := \mathbf{t}(\bar{\mathbf{x}}_A + P \cdot \mathbf{b})$ with $\mathbf{b}$ denoting a vector of global

---

[2] We thank H. Peng, F. Long, X. Liu and S. Kim for providing the data.

shape parameters, and $\mathbf{t} : \mathbf{R}^3 \to \mathbf{R}^3$ an affine transformation. $\mathbf{t}$ consists of a 3x3 matrix R, and an offset vector $\mathbf{o}$. Per nucleus i, the model reads $x_A(i, \mathbf{b}, \mathbf{t}) := R(\bar{x}_A(i) + P(i) \cdot \mathbf{b}) + \mathbf{o}$, with $\bar{x}_A(i)$ denoting the average location of nucleus i, and $P(i)$ denoting rows $3i - 2$, $3i - 1$ and $3i$ of P. Each training vector can be represented by some global shape parameter vector: $\exists \mathbf{b}_w : \bar{\mathbf{x}}_A + P \cdot \mathbf{b}_w = \mathbf{x}_w$. In our global shape model we confine the shape parameters to the min/max respective values that appear in training data.

Local Models. As for our local point distribution model: Let $\mathcal{X}(i)$ denote the matrix with all training locations of nucleus i as columns. The covariance matrix per nucleus location, $C(i, R) := (1/n_W)R(\mathcal{X}(i) - \bar{\mathcal{X}}(i))(\mathcal{X}(i) - \bar{\mathcal{X}}(i))^T R^T \in \mathbf{R}^{3 \times 3}$, allows us to measure the distance of some point $x \in \mathbf{R}$ to location i in the atlas: $\text{locDiff}(x, i, \mathbf{b}, \mathbf{t}) := (x - x_A(i, \mathbf{b}, \mathbf{t}))^T \cdot C(i, R)^{-1} \cdot (x - x_A(i, \mathbf{b}, \mathbf{t}))$.

We describe the shape of an individual nucleus by means of the radii of an ellipsoid fit to the nucleus volume, sorted by value. We denote the shape of nucleus i in training worm w as $s(i, w) \in \mathbf{R}^3$. From the training data, we derive the average shape per nucleus, $s_A(i)$, as well as the respective covariance matrix $S(i)$. Thus we can measure the distance of some shape s to the shape of atlas nucleus i as $\text{shapeDiff}(s, i) := (s - s_A(i))^T \cdot S(i)^{-1} \cdot (s - s_A(i))$.

In addition to nucleus-individual statistics, we also perform statistics on offset vectors between any two nuclei: Let $d(i, j, w) := x(i, w) - x(j, w)$ denote a training offset vector. We retrieve the average offset $\bar{d}_A(i, j) := (1/n_W) \sum_w d(i, j, w)$ as well as the respective covariance matrix $D(i, j, R)$. Let $d_A(i, j, \mathbf{b}, R)$ denote an offset vector in an instance of the global point distribution model. Then, we can measure the distance of some offset d w.r.t. nuclei i and j in the atlas: $\text{offsetDiff}(d, i, j, \mathbf{b}, R) := (d - d_A(i, j, \mathbf{b}, R))^T \cdot D(i, j, R)^{-1} \cdot (d - d_A(i, j, \mathbf{b}, R))$.

Furthermore the determinant of the covariance of offsets, $\det D(i, j, R)$, lets us measure how closely two nuclei locations correlate, and thus lets us define a K-neighborhood on the atlas, denoted as $\mathcal{N}_K$. This neighborhood contains all pairs of atlas nuclei (i, j) for which nucleus j is among the K "closest" to i in terms of $\det D(i, j, R)$, or vice-versa i is among the K "closest" to j.

Inpainting. Nuclei that are "missing" in our 357-nuclei-atlas, mainly in the brain region, pose a challenge to the annotation problem: The atlas region posterior to the brain can freely match to target nuclei within the brain, taking the posterior body part with them. Therefore we *inpaint* the missing 201 nuclei into the training worms by taking one complete manual segmentation as reference and warping it to all the other training point clouds by means of Thin Plate Spline Warps. We inpaint the missing nuclei shapes by assigning the shape of the closest not-annotated nucleus in the respective manual segmentation.

2.2 Segmentation Hypotheses

For nuclei segmentation we use the Generalized Hough Transform (GHT) [10] with an ellipsoid as a template. We run GHT multiple times with a range of differently scaled and oriented templates. One GHT run yields one segmentation hypothesis per voxel, namely the template with highest *scoring* scale/orientation at the respective voxel position, where the score, $GHT(x) \in [0, 1]$, measures how well the template fits the image gradient. From this abundant pool, per GHT run, we greedily select the n best-scoring hypotheses which do not overlap. Our final set of hypotheses is the union of sets of selected from the different GHT runs. Note that hypotheses from different GHT runs do, in general, overlap. This way we reduce the risk of missing nuclei. Figure 1 shows examples.

2.3   Active Graph Matching

Objective. Let n_T denote the number of segmentation hypotheses. An *assignment* $a_{i,j} \in \{0,1\}$ encodes whether atlas index $i \le n_A$ is assigned to target index $j \le n_T$. We denote the matrix of assignments as $\mathcal{A} := (a_{i,j})_{i=1,j=1}^{n_A,n_T}$. A bipartite matching is a matrix $\mathcal{A}$ which satisfies $\forall i \le n_A : \sum_{j=1}^{n_T} a_{i,j} \le 1$ and $\forall j \le n_T : \sum_{i=1}^{n_A} a_{i,j} \le 1$. I.e., an atlas nucleus can be matched to at most one target nucleus, and vice-versa. We define the energy of matching the atlas to the target with affine transformation $\mathbf{t}$, shape parameters $\mathbf{b}$, and matching $\mathcal{A}$, as

$$E(\mathcal{A}, \mathbf{b}, \mathbf{t}) := \sum_{i \le n_A, k \le n_T} \phi(i,k,\mathbf{b},\mathbf{t}) \cdot a_{i,k} + \sum_{(i,j) \in \mathcal{N}_K, k,l \le n_T} \psi(i,j,k,l,\mathbf{b},\mathbf{t}) \cdot a_{i,k} \cdot a_{j,l}$$

$$(1)$$

where $\mathcal{N}_K$ is the neighborhood relation we defined on the atlas, cf. Section 2.1. *Unary potentials* $\phi(i,k,\mathbf{b},\mathbf{t})$ encode the cost per assignment $a_{i,k}$. We define

$$\phi(i,k,\mathbf{b},\mathbf{t}) := \lambda_1 \cdot \mathrm{locDiff}(x_T(k),i,\mathbf{b},\mathbf{t}) + \lambda_2 \cdot \mathrm{shapeDiff}(s_T(k),i) + \lambda_3 \cdot \mathrm{cost}(k) + c$$

$$(2)$$

where $x_T(k) \in \mathbf{R}^3$ is the center point of the k-th hypothesis, $k \le n_T$, $s_T(k) \in \mathbf{R}^3$ is the target shape descriptor, $\mathrm{cost}(k) := 1 - GHT(x_T(k))$ encodes how well the image data supports the k-th hypothesis, and c is a negative constant that serves as an incentive to make matches. Terms are weighted by positive constants λ. *Binary potentials* $\psi(i,j,k,l,\mathbf{b},\mathbf{t})$ encode costs per pair of assignments, $a_{i,k}, a_{j,l}$:

$$\psi(i,j,k,l,\mathbf{b},\mathbf{t}) := \lambda_4 \cdot \mathrm{offsetDiff}(d_T(k,l),i,j,\mathbf{b},\mathbf{t}) \qquad (3)$$

where $d_T(k,l)$ denotes the offset between target nuclei k,l, namely $x_T(k) - x_T(l)$.

Optimization. To minimize (1) we first estimate initial parameters, $\mathbf{b}, \mathbf{t}$, and then alternate between minimization w.r.t. $\mathcal{A}$ (matching) and w.r.t. $\mathbf{b}, \mathbf{t}$.

Initial Atlas Parameters: We initialize the global shape parameters $\mathbf{b}$ to zero. As for an initial affine transformation $\mathbf{t}$, we align the first eigenvector of the point cloud given by all segmentation hypotheses with the anterior-posterior axis of the atlas such that the centers of gravity line up. We identify the correct rotation around this axis via the fact that nuclei are distributed asymmetrically along the dorso-ventral axis, while symmetrically along the left-right axis.

Optimal Matching: For fixed $\mathbf{b}, \mathbf{t}$ we minimize (1) w.r.t. the matching $\mathcal{A}$ with the Dual-Decomposition-based method of Torresani et al. [8]. In practice, considering all entries of $\mathcal{A}$ is intractable. Hence we only consider assignments $a_{i,k}$ for which $\mathrm{locDiff}(x_T(k),i,\mathbf{b},\mathbf{t})$ falls below a fixed threshold.

Table 1. Evaluation of annotation accuracy on 30 worms. Measures: median/mean(std), all in %. See text for description of scenarios (rows) and algorithms (columns). *Results presented as plot in [2], but numbers not given. **Results presented as plot in [2], but error measure not described and numbers not given.

	ActiveGM	**ActiveIGM**	ActiveHungarian	Long et al.
Synthetic	95/94(7)	-	93/88(12)	-
SemiAuto	92/90(8)	**93/92**(7)	79/77(9)	*/86(*)
Automatic	86/82(12)	**86/83**(11)	62/60(12)	**

Optimization of Atlas Parameters: For a fixed matching, the objective is the sum of squared residuals of an overdetermined system of equations which is linear in the global parameters **b** and **t**, as described in the following. In the objective, only the terms locDiff and offsetDiff depend on atlas parameters. For locDiff each matched nucleus i entails three equations, namely

$$S \cdot R^{-1} x_T(k) - S \cdot \bar{x}_A(i) - S \cdot P(i)\mathbf{b} - S \cdot R^{-1}\mathbf{o} = (0,0,0)^T \qquad (4)$$

where S satisfies $S^T \cdot S = C(i,I)^{-1}$. Such an S exists in case $C(i,I)$ is symmetric and positive definite, which is the case in our practical setting. The equations are linear in the entries of R^{-1}, **b**, and $\tilde{\mathbf{o}} := R^{-1}\mathbf{o}$, respectively. For offsetDiff, each pair of matched neighbors i,j entails the following three equations:

$$G \cdot R^{-1}(x_T(k) - x_T(l)) - G \cdot (\bar{x}_A(i) - \bar{x}_A(j)) - G \cdot (P(i) - P(j))(b) = (0,0,0)^T \quad (5)$$

where G satisfies $G^T \cdot G = D(i)^{-1}$. Analogous to S, such a G exists in our practical setting. Overall we have, in practice, far more equations than parameters. Hence we can solve for optimal R, **o** and **b** with the method of least squares.

3   Results and Discussion

We run our method in a leave-one-out fashion on the 30 datasets used for atlas training (cf. Sec. 2). We consider three different scenarios. (1, *Synthetic*): We match the 357-nuclei atlas to the corresponding 357 target nuclei, which requires these 357 to be tagged in the manual segmentation. (2, *SemiAuto*): We match the atlas to all manually segmented target nuclei. (3, *Automatic*): We run fully automatic joint segmentation and annotation.

We run our algorithm in three different ways: (1, *ActiveGM*) with the 357-nuclei atlas, (2, *ActiveIGM*) with the inpainted 558-nuclei atlas, and (3, *Active-Hungarian*) without binary potentials. We run ActiveIGM only for the real-world scenarios. We run ActiveHungarian without in-painting in the synthetic scenario, and with in-painting in the real-world scenarios.

As for the parameters of our method, we always set: $\lambda_2 := 1$, $c := -150$, $K := 6$, and as optimization steps 3 times the sequence $\mathcal{A}, \mathbf{t}$, followed by 3 times $\mathcal{A}, \mathbf{b}$. We consider the first two modes of variation in **b**. As for locDiff we set $\lambda_1 := 0$ for ActiveGM, and $\lambda_1 := 1$ for ActiveHungarian. As for offsetDiff we

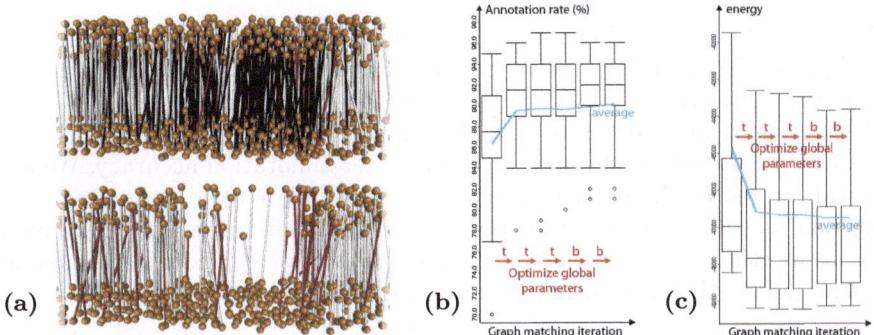

Fig. 3. (a) Close-up to matching results in the head of an exemplary worm. Top: inpainted atlas; bottom: partial atlas. Inpainting leads to better matching performance. White lines: correct annotation; black lines: inpainted nuclei, no ground truth available; red lines: annotation errors (fewer on top). (b) Evolution of annotation accuracy for semi-automatic matching scenario. X-axis: matching iteration. Y-axis: fraction of correctly annotated nuclei. (c) Evolution of the respective matching energy.

set $\lambda_4 := 1$ for ActiveGM, but $\lambda_4 := 0$ for ActiveHungarian since it cannot handle binary potentials. As target cost weight we set $\lambda_3 := 0$ in all but the fully automatic scenario, where we set $\lambda_3 := 10$. All parameter values were chosen heuristically.

To measure annotation accuracy, in case of manual segmentations, we count the fraction of correctly annotated nuclei. For the fully automatic scenario, we count the fraction of matched segmentation hypotheses whose center points lie within the respective ground truth nucleus, or are at most one average nucleus radius apart from the true center point. Table 1 lists the results for all experiments described above. For reference we also include the result of Long et al. [2].

Apart from annotation accuracy we analyzed the optimality of matching in terms of the gap between lower bound and found energy: In the synthetic and the semi-automatic scenario, lower bounds are tight, i.e. here we find the globally optimal matching. As for the fully automtatic scenario, the matching problem is solved approximately with an average duality gap of about $2c$.

Discussion. For the task of annotating manual segmentations of nuclei our average annotation rate of 92% considerably outperforms the result of Long et al. who report an average of 86%. Note that furthermore Long et al. need an additional image channel which our method does not. For the fully automatic task our median/average annotation rate of 86/83% approaches the rate that Long et al. achieved in the much simpler partly manual scenario.

Employing 2nd order graph matching instead of just the Hungarian algorithm makes a huge difference: ActiveHungarian works relatively well *only* in the synthetic scenario, while the inferiority as compared to ActiveGM increases as the matching problem gets more sophisticated: In the order of complexity of the matching problem (top to bottom in Table 1), ActiveGM is on average 6%, 15%, and 23% better than ActiveHungarian, respectively.

Figure 3(a) shows the benefit of using the in-painted atlas instead of the 357-nuclei-atlas. Figure 3(b,c) shows how the annotation rate and the respective value of the objective evolve during Active Graph Matching iterations.

Neglecting location differences in the 2nd order energy, i.e. $l_1 := 0$ instead of $l_1 := 1$ for ActiveGM, yields considerably better annotation accuracy. We argue that this is due to the respective much more flexible local deformation model. Note that locDiff $= 0$ means that the objective is invariant w.r.t. **o**. However, in practice we still need **o** for selecting the assignments we consider in the matching problem (cf. Section 2.3), hence we always derive it via locDiff.

Conclusion. We have presented *active graph matching*, a method that combines active shape models with graph matching in one objective and provides an approach for global optimization. With this method we do not only outperform the current state of the art in annotating manual segmentations of nuclei in *C. elegans* L1 larvae, but furthermore define the state of the art in solving both segmentation and annotation simultaneously in a fully automatic fashion. We hypothesize that our method will be highly beneficial for the equally relevant task of nuclei annotation in later stages of *C. elegans* development, where nuclei are more numerous and more densely packed.

Acknowledgments. We thank Vladimir Kolmogorov and Stephan Saalfeld for inspiring discussions.

References

1. Sarov, M., et al.: A Genome-Scale Resource for In Vivo Tag-Based Protein Function Exploration in C. Elegans. Cell 150(4), 855–866 (2012)
2. Long, F., Peng, H., Liu, X., Kim, S.K., Myers, E.: A 3D Digital Atlas of C. Elegans and its Application to Single-Cell Analyses. Nature Methods 6, 667–672 (2009)
3. Aerni, S.J., Liu, X., Do, C.B., Gross, S.S., Nguyen, A., Guo, S.D., Long, F., Peng, H., Kim, S.S., Batzoglou, S.: Automated Cellular Annotation for High-resolution Images of Adult C. Elegans. Bioinformatics 29(13), i18–i26 (2013)
4. Qu, L., Long, F., Liu, X., Kim, S., Myers, E., Peng, H.: Simultaneous Recognition and Segmentation of Cells. Bioinformatics 27(20), 2895–2902 (2011)
5. Riklin Raviv, T., Ljosa, V., Conery, A.L., Ausubel, F.M., Carpenter, A.E., Golland, P., Wählby, C.: Morphology-guided graph search for untangling objects: C. elegans analysis. In: Jiang, T., Navab, N., Pluim, J.P.W., Viergever, M.A. (eds.) MICCAI 2010, Part III. LNCS, vol. 6363, pp. 634–641. Springer, Heidelberg (2010)
6. Peng, H., Long, F., Liu, X., Kim, S.K., Myers, E.: Straightening Caenorhabditis Elegans Images. Bioinformatics 24(2), 234–242 (2008)
7. Cootes, T.F., Taylor, C.J., Cooper, D.H., Graham, J.: Active Shape Models - Their Training and Application. CVIU 61(1), 38–59 (1995)
8. Torresani, L., Kolmogorov, V., Rother, C.: A dual decomposition approach to feature correspondence. IEEE TPAMI 35(2), 259–271 (2013)
9. Zhou, F., De La Torre, F.: Deformable graph matching. In: CVPR, pp. 2922–2929 (2013)
10. Khoshelham, K.: Extending Generalized Hough Transform to Detect 3D Objects in Laser Range Data. In: ISPRS Workshop Laser Scanning, p. 206 (2007)

Semi-automated Query Construction for Content-Based Endomicroscopy Video Retrieval

Marzieh Kohandani Tafreshi[1,2,*], Nicolas Linard[2,*], Barbara André[2],
Nicholas Ayache[1], and Tom Vercauteren[2]

[1] Inria Asclepios Project-Team, Sophia Antipolis, France
[2] Mauna Kea Technologies, Paris, France

Abstract. Content-based video retrieval has shown promising results to
help physicians in their interpretation of medical videos in general and
endomicroscopic ones in particular. Defining a relevant query for CBVR
can however be a complex and time-consuming task for non-expert and
even expert users. Indeed, uncut endomicroscopy videos may very well
contain images corresponding to a variety of different tissue types. Using
such uncut videos as queries may lead to drastic performance degradations for the system. In this study, we propose a semi-automated methodology that allows the physician to create meaningful and relevant queries
in a simple and efficient manner. We believe that this will lead to more
reproducible and more consistent results. The validation of our method is
divided into two approaches. The first one is an indirect validation based
on per video classification results with histopathological ground-truth.
The second one is more direct and relies on perceived inter-video visual
similarity ground-truth. We demonstrate that our proposed method significantly outperforms the approach with uncut videos and approaches
the performance of a tedious manual query construction by an expert. Finally, we show that the similarity perceived between videos by experts is
significantly correlated with the inter-video similarity distance computed
by our retrieval system.

1 Introduction

Probe-based Confocal Laser Endomicroscopy (pCLE) enables the endoscopist
to acquire real-time *in situ* and *in vivo* microscopic images of the epithelium
during an endoscopy. As shown in [3], content-based retrieval (CBR) methods
may provide interpretation support for the endoscopist, helping him or her in
making an informed decision and establishing a more accurate pCLE diagnosis.
However, the selection of adapted query can be quite challenging and time-
consuming for the user of such a CBR system. Also, because of the complexity
of such manual query construction, the CBR system may not have a sufficient
reproducibly and may be subject to large intra and inter-observer variability.

The approach presented in this paper allows physicians to efficiently create
reproducible queries in a semi-automated fashion. This allows to boost retrieval

---

* Authors have contributed equally to the paper.

P. Golland et al. (Eds.): MICCAI 2014, Part I, LNCS 8673, pp. 89–96, 2014.

performance when compared to using uncut videos as queries. It also allows us to approach the performance of carefully constructed queries by an expert. To achieve this, our query construction approach is decomposed in two steps.

In the first step, we perform an automated temporal segmentation of the original video into a set of subsequences of interest. The segmentation is based on kinematic stability assessment. Since endomicroscopy is a handheld interventional modality, users often swipe a region of interest to look for diagnostically relevant criteria. In this work we leverage the observation that spatial stability across time is related to the informativeness of the images to design a first video stream temporal segmentation algorithm dedicated to endomicroscopy.

The second step consists in a fast user selection of a subset of the segmented subsequences. The physician is simply asked to keep or discard the subsequences provided by the first step. Although each of the possible subsequences may still contain images of different tissue type, the segmentation step makes each subsequence much more self-consistent than the original uncut video.

Once a query has been constructed, our method relies on the video CBR method presented in [2]. This system is based on the Bag-of-Visual-Words (BoW), a review of which can be found in [15]. Instead of relying on salient features, [2] uses a regular grid of descriptors at a fixed scale to construct a visual signature. This signature is then used to index and query a database of annotated cases.

Evaluation of CBR systems is known to be a difficult task. In our work, similarly to [3], two validation methodologies with different strengths are used. The first indirect one uses the retrieval results and a k-nearest neighbors (k-NN) voting scheme to classify each video. This approach benefits from the fact that, in most clinically validated databases, each video is associated with a histopathologically validated diagnosis. The k-NN classification is more a quantitative evaluation and serves only as a CBR evaluation proxy. The second validation methodology compares the inter-video distances computed by the CBR method with the perceived visual similarities experienced by experts.

2   A Temporal Segmentation with User Selection Pipeline

As illustrated in Fig. 1, our approach to query construction and CBR works as follows. During a procedure, the physician acquires pCLE videos in real time. The acquired frames are stored in a bounded circular FIFO buffer. At any moment during the intervention the user may want to consult the annotated database to provide him or her with visually similar cases that have been confirmed by histopathology examination. At this point, the acquisition is paused and our software displays the image buffer with a timeline that shows the automatic temporal segmentation. The user is then asked to briefly review each segmented subsequence and click on the ones that are of interest to him. This simplified interaction allows the user to construct a fast and reproducible query with sufficient visual similarity within and between the selected subsequences. Because all this happens during the procedure, our temporal segmentation needs to be running in real-time. Then, the user-chosen subset of subsequences is used to

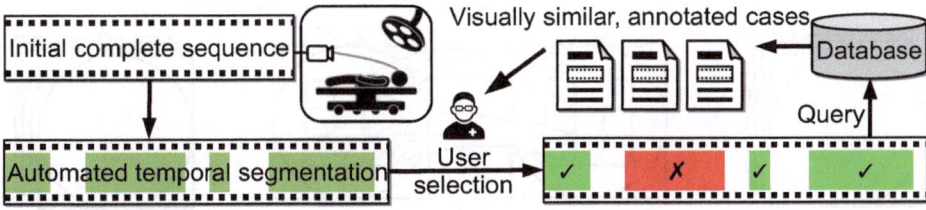

Fig. 1. An overview of our semi-automated query construction algorithm as used in a clinically relevant CBR pipeline

create a single visual signature to query the database. The most visually similar cases are presented to the physician along with their annotations.

3   Temporal Segmentation from Kinematic Stability

As outlined in [6,7], temporal video segmentation is a key step in most existing video management tools. Many different types of algorithms have been developed to perform temporal video segmentation. Early techniques focused on cut-boundary detection or image grouping using pixel differences, histogram comparisons, edge differences, motion analysis and the like, while more recent methods such as presented in [5] have also used image similarity metrics, classification and clustering to achieve the same goal. In some applications as in [11,12], the problem of temporal video segmentation may be reformulated as a classification problem that distinguishes between informative and noise images.

Our approach in this work relies on the observation that, during an pCLE procedure, the user will navigate the imaging probe across the region of interest and will typically stay longer and remain more stable onto areas that catches his or her interest. As such, in our application, kinematic stability may serve as a proxy to characterize the interest of an image within a sequence.

Image registration-based approaches can be used to identify kinematically stable temporal regions. This can be done by actually registering temporally consecutive images and then analyzing the quality of the spatial transformation. For exemple, [13] relies on real-time registration algorithms. Kinematic stability assessment may also be done by using only a subset of the steps of an image registration algorithm and analyze the quality of the results provided by this subset. In this paper, feature matches are analyzed in terms of *local* spatial consistency so as to obtain a result that is more robust to modeling error and to tissue deformation than looking for an accurate spatial transformation.

In [2], the authors have shown that, although the typical feature detectors from computer vision described in [15,8] are not suitable for endomicroscopy, one may rely on a regular grid of Scale Invariant Feature Transform (SIFT) descriptors for the purpose of defining visual signatures. Because our method requires features both to assess kinematic stability and to create visual signatures, we propose to rely on the same set of SIFT descriptors so as to reduce the computational

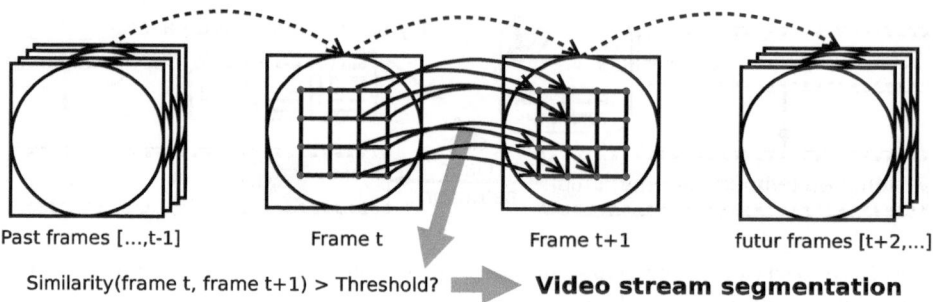

Past frames [...,t-1]   Frame t   Frame t+1   futur frames [t+2,...]

Similarity(frame t, frame t+1) > Threshold? ➡ **Video stream segmentation**

Fig. 2. Our temporal segmentation algorithm based on kinematic stability assessment

requirements. In the field of computer vision, regular grids of descriptors have also recently been used for image matching and video analysis with compelling results [9,14]. However, to the best of our knowledge, our work is the first to rely on such regular grids of descriptors to evaluate kinematic stability by looking at the local consistency of feature matches.

As illustrated in Fig. 2, our method starts by decomposing each frame into a grid of SIFT descriptors and matching the descriptors between consecutive frames. Local consistency of the matches is assessed by making each match vote for a translation in a vote map. A kinematic stability criterion is then computed from the vote map and a threshold on this criterion is used to discriminate kinematically stable and unstable frame transitions.

In more detail, we associate a grid point at time t with one at $t+1$ by minimizing the Euclidean distance between the corresponding descriptors. Although other distances may be used, Euclidean distance allows for the use of efficient approximate nearest neighbor algorithms. Similarly to [10], we filter out bad matches by comparing, for each source grid point, the best match with subsequent ones. When working with sparsely located features, one may simply compute the ratio of the distances for the first and second best match and use a threshold on this ratio. However, in the case of a regular grid, the regions covered by adjacent descriptors may show a large overlap. This implies that the first and second best match will often be very close in terms of descriptors distance. We therefore propose to compute the distance ratio between the first and n^{th} best matches. We choose n such that the description regions associated with a grid point and with its nth spatial neighbor grid point have no overlap.

From the set of filtered matches, our goal is not to find an accurate spatial transformation as in [9], but to define a computationally efficient kinematic stability criterion. For this purpose, and although we know that pCLE videos suffer from motion distortions and tissue deformation, we rely on a local translation model that was proven to work in [13]. As such, we build a map where each match votes for its translation. It should however be noted that not all translations can receive the same maximum number of votes. To account for this potential bias, the vote map is weighted according to the maximum number of potential voters per voting bin. This normalization is computed by the autocorrelation of a mask image that represent the spatial organization of the description grid.

For a simple translation across two frames, we observe a single main peak in the normalized vote map. However, in the standard case of more complex transformations, we may observe several peaks, blobs or ridges in the vote map, all of them corresponding to locally consistent translations. To account for this effect, we define our kinematic stability criterion by adding up all votes that are above a predefined consistency threshold. Finally, a frame transition is considered kinematically stable if the kinematic stability criterion is above a predefined stability threshold. This stability threshold was obtained by optimizing the correlation between automatic and manual segmentation results.

4   Video Retrieval Based on Bag of Visual Words

Given a temporal segmentation and a user selection within the subsequences, our aim now is to query a database with the selected video parts. In our study we rely on the approach of [2] but do not use their mosaicing strategy for computational reasons. The Bag of Visual Words method is adapted to pCLE retrieval by working with a regular grid of SIFT descriptors at a fixed scale. Avoiding scale invariance is a requirement for pcLE videos, where for example, in colonic polyps, a mesoscopic crypt and a microscopic goblet cell have both a rounded shape, but have different sizes. From the sets of SIFT descriptors, each image within the selected video part gets associated with a visual signature. By averaging these signatures, each subsequence and each video are associated with a visual signature that can be used for retrieval purposes.

5   Results: Classification and Perceived Similarity

To evaluate the relevance of our retrieval results, two procedures are used: an indirect one based on classification and a direct one based on perceived similarity. In both cases, we rely on a pCLE database of colonic polyps sequences that were retrospectively collected from pCLE procedures performed in the Mayo Clinic in Jacksonville, Florida, USA. This database is composed of 118 pCLE videos (35 benign, 83 neoplastic) that were acquire from 66 patients [4]. The length of these videos ranges from 1 second to 4 minutes and their median duration is 28.2 secs. Long videos may contain different tissues, however as such most videos are sufficiently short to display a single tissue type. The parameters of the retrieval method we used are the one provided in [2].

For the classification evaluation, a straightforward k-NN classification is performed and its accuracy is estimated. Two classes are considered, benign and neoplastic. For these videos, the pCLE diagnosis is matched to the *gold standard* established by a pathologist after the histological review of biopsies acquired on the pCLE imaging spots. Given the small number of videos contained in the database, each of the videos is used for both training and testing. A leave-one-patient-out (LOPO) cross-validation allows us to respect the independence

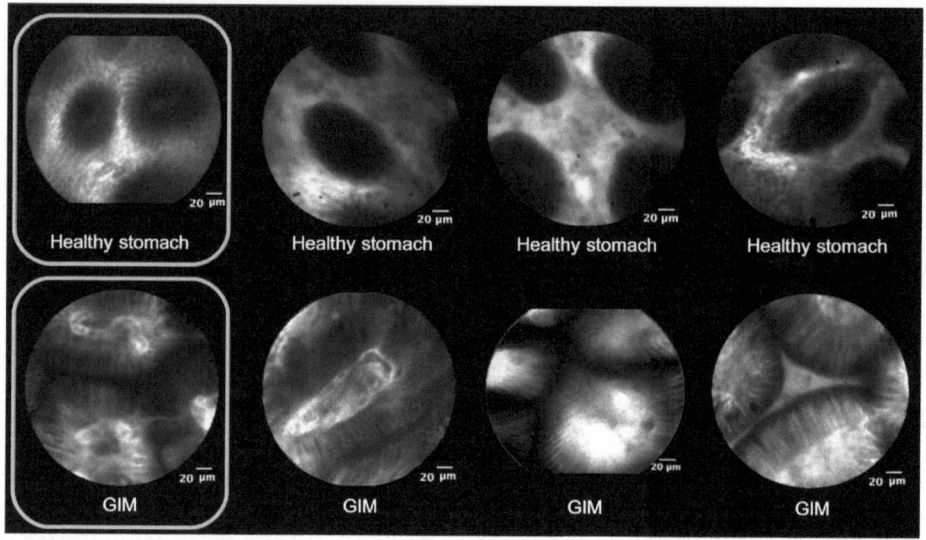

Fig. 3. Retrieval examples of our colonic polyps datasets. The query video is on the left and its 3 most similar videos represented by single frames are on the right. B. indicates Benign and N. Neoplastic.

assumption that is challenged by the fact that several videos are acquired from the same patient. Although an indirect evaluation, these experiments allow for quantitative evaluation of our method and rely on an objective ground truth.

For the perceived similarity experiments, we rely on the database of [1]. Using an online survey tool, a pairwise similarity ground-truth between pCLE videos was estimated by 17 human observers, ranging from middle expert to expert in establishing pCLE diagnosis, who are completely ignorant to the video metadata such as the pCLE diagnosis. Each video couple gets assigned a score from the following four-points Likert scale: *very dissimilar, rather dissimilar, rather similar* and *very similar*. In total 4,836 similarity scores were given for 2,178 distinct video couples. Thus 16,2% of all 13,343 distinct video couples were scored. We can then compare the visual similarity distance computed by our method with the perceived one. These results shed a different light on the evaluation. They reflect our target application better but rely on a more subjective ground truth with high inter-observer variability.

In this paper, four different methods are compared. The first one is that of [3], without the mosaicing part, in which an expert carefully constructs the queries. The second one relies on uncut videos. The third one uses the entire set of subsequences generated by the automated temporal segmentation algorithm. Finally, the fourth one is our proposed semi-automated method. For each compared method, the same number of sequences is used. To enable a fair comparison between the methods, the following procedure was used for the selection of the subsequences in the semi-automated approach. Instead of asking an expert to

Table 1. Evaluation of the performance of our proposed semi-automated approach in comparison to state of the art methods. The evaluation is performed both indirectly in terms of classification and directly in terms of correlation with perceived similarity.

Method	Classification results			Perception
	Accuracy	Sensitivity	Specificity	Spearman ρ
Complete uncut sequences	72.9 %	72.3 %	74.3 %	35.9 %
Fine expert temporal segmentation	94.1 %	96.4 %	88.6 %	52.8 %
Automated temporal segmentation	61.9 %	56.6 %	74.9 %	31.6 %
Proposed semi-automated method	89.9 %	90.4 %	88.6 %	48.8 %

perform the selection, we re-used the careful query construction from the first method. For each temporal segment, if it contains at least one frame that was chosen in the careful query construction, the temporal segment is marked as selected. This allows for an unbiased comparison of both methods.

In all cases, to ensure strong self-consistency within the annotated database, only the carefully constructed sequences by the expert were used in the training phases. For each step, different experts from different clinical trials were consulted. Particularly, 17 observers participated to create the visual similarity ground-truth using the online VSS tool. We believe that the fact that these steps are performed by different experts leads to unbiased results.

As shown in Table 1, our semi-automated method significantly outperforms the two automated ones and approaches to performance of the reference manual one. The accuracies with uncut sequences and automated temporal segmentation are indeed low, but even with these baselines, the correlation between the computed and the perceived similarity is higher than chance with statistical significance. A McNemar's test show that, with statistical significance, our proposed semi-automated method is better than the uncut sequences method (p-value < 0.0005 for $k = 10$) and than the automated temporal segmentation method (p-value $< 10^{-6}$ for $k = 10$) in terms of classification. We also observe that the difference between our method and the fine expert temporal segmentation method is not statistically significant.For the correlation with perceived similarity, we performed a Steiger's Z-test applied to the Spearman ρ correlation coefficient. This test indicates that the improvement of our method over the uncut sequences method and over the automated temporal segmentation method is statistically significant (p-value $< 10^{-6}$). Unsurprising, the fine expert temporal segmentation statistically outperforms our method.

6   Discussion

This study proposes a fast and semi-automated approach to constitute a relevant and informative query to submit to the retrieval system. Our results have demonstrated that the classification results and the perceived similarity remain consistent in comparison with the results obtained using queries which are manually selected by an expert. Future work will improve the selection of the query, and aim at achieving better fully automated query construction. Nonetheless, we believe that the proposed methodology makes content-based retrieval techniques closer to clinical utility.

References

1. André, B., Vercauteren, T., Buchner, A.M., Wallace, M.B., Ayache, N.: Retrieval evaluation and distance learning from perceived similarity between endomicroscopy videos, 289–296 (2011)
2. André, B., Vercauteren, T., Buchner, A.M., Wallace, M.B., Ayache, N.: A smart atlas for endomicroscopy using automated video retrieval 15(4), 460–476 (2011)
3. André, B., Vercauteren, T., Buchner, A.M., Wallace, M.B., Ayache, N.: Learning semantic and visual similarity for endomicroscopy video retrieval 31(6), 1276–1288 (2012)
4. Buchner, A.M., Shahid, M.W., Heckman, M.G., Krishna, M., Ghabril, M., Hasan, M., Crook, J.E., Gomez, V., Raimondo, M., Woodward, T., Wolfsen, H.C., Wallace, M.B.: Comparison of probe-based confocal laser endomicroscopy with virtual chromoendoscopy for classification of colon polyps 138(3), 834–842 (2010)
5. Cooper, M., Liu, T., Rieffel, E.: Video segmentation via temporal pattern classification 9(3), 610–618 (2007)
6. Gargi, U., Kasturi, R., Strayer, S.H.: Performance characterization of video-shot-change detection methods 10(1), 1–13 (2000)
7. Hu, W., Xie, N., Li, L., Zeng, X., Maybank, S.: A survey on visual content-based video indexing and retrieval 41(6), 797–819 (2011)
8. Li, B., Meng, M.H.: Capsule endoscopy video boundary detection, 373–78 (June 2011)
9. Liu, C., Yuen, J., Torralba, A.: SIFT flow: Dense correspondence across scenes and its applications 33(5), 978–994 (2011)
10. Lowe, D.G.: Distinctive image features from scale-invariant keypoints 60, 91–110 (2004)
11. Oh, J., Hwang, S., Lee, J., Tavanapong, W., Wong, J., de Groen, P.C.: Informative frame classification for endoscopy video 11(2), 110–127 (2007)
12. Sun, Z., Li, B., Zhou, R., Zheng, H., Meng, M.H.: Removal of non-informative frames for wireless capsule endoscopy video segmentation, 294–299 (August 2012)
13. Vercauteren, T., Meining, A., Lacombe, F., Perchant, A.: Real time autonomous video image registration for endomicroscopy: Fighting the compromises. In: Conchello, J.A., Cogswell, C.J., Wilson, T. (eds.) Proc. SPIE BIOS - Three-Dimensional and Multidimensional Microscopy: Image Acquisition and Processing XV. SPIE, San Jose (2008)
14. Wang, H., Kläser, A., Schmid, C., Liu, C.L.: Dense trajectories and motion boundary descriptors for action recognition 103(1), 60–79 (2013)
15. Zhang, J., Lazebnik, S., Schmid, C.: Local features and kernels for classification of texture and object categories: a comprehensive study 73, 213–238 (2007)

Optree: A Learning-Based Adaptive Watershed Algorithm for Neuron Segmentation

Mustafa Gökhan Uzunbaş*, Chao Chen, and Dimitris Metaxas

CBIM, Rutgers University, Piscataway, NJ, USA

Abstract. We present a new algorithm for automatic and interactive segmentation of neuron structures from electron microscopy (EM) images. Our method selects a collection of nodes from the watershed merging tree as the proposed segmentation. This is achieved by building a conditional random field (CRF) whose underlying graph is the merging tree. The maximum a posteriori (MAP) prediction of the CRF is the output segmentation. Our algorithm outperforms state-of-the-art methods. Both the inference and the training are very efficient as the graph is tree-structured. Furthermore, we develop an interactive segmentation framework which selects uncertain regions for a user to proofread. The uncertainty is measured by the marginals of the graphical model. Based on user corrections, our framework modifies the merging tree and thus improves the segmentation globally.

Keywords: Conditional Random Field, Watershed, EM Segmentation, User Interaction.

1 Introduction

The *watershed transform* [9] partitions a given image into *segments* by simulating a water flooding of the landscape of a given scalar function, e.g. the gradient magnitude or the likelihood of each pixel being the boundary (Fig. 1(c)). In order to mitigate the over-segmentation effect, one often merges neighboring segments when the minimal function value along the boundary between them (called the *saliency*) is below certain threshold. Considering all saliency thresholds, a hierarchical merging tree is constructed [9] in which each leaf node is a segment of the original watershed and each non-leaf node is a merged segment. A *height* function can be assigned to each node according to the minimal saliency threshold at which it disappears (is merged with others). The watershed segmentation at any given threshold can be computed by cutting all tree nodes below the threshold and taking all leaf nodes of the remaining tree. In Fig. 1(d) and 1(e), we show the original watershed result and a thresholded one.

The watershed method and its variations have been used on EM images [4,2,8]. However, running watershed using a certain threshold usually leads to

---

* This grant was partially supported based on funding from the following grants NIH-R01-HL086578, NIH-R21-HL088354 and NSF-MRI-1229628.

P. Golland et al. (Eds.): MICCAI 2014, Part I, LNCS 8673, pp. 97–105, 2014.

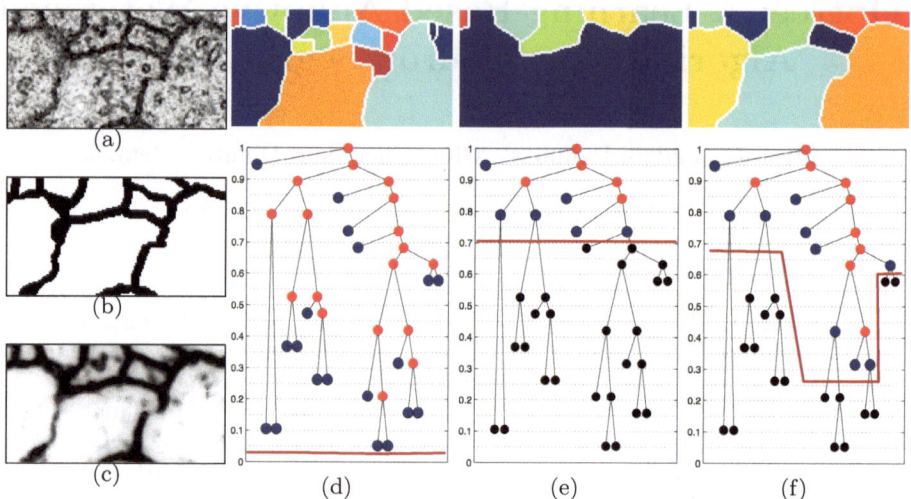

Fig. 1. (a) The EM image patch; (b) the ground truth; (c) the boundary likelihood map (dark pixels have high values); (d) the watershed segmentation and its tree, built using the boundary likelihood map as the landscape function; (e) the watershed segmentation with a higher threshold; (f) the result of our algorithm.

accurate segments at certain area yet over/under-segmentation at other areas (see Fig. 1(d) and 1(e)). In this paper, we propose a CRF-based learning algorithm which finds a segmentation of higher quality by selecting different saliency thresholds at different areas of the image. Essentially, our algorithm learns from training data how to cut a hierarchical tree adaptively to achieve a better result. See Figure 1(f) for an example of our result. We train our algorithm to construct a tree-structured graphical model for each image and its hierarchical tree. The (MAP) probability of this graphical model gives a segmentation. Our method outperforms state-of-the-art in automatic segmentation of high resolution 2D (ssTEM) [3] and 3D (FIBSEM) [7] EM images.

Our CRF model leads to a novel interactive segmentation framework. Connectomics requires extremely accurate partitioning of EM images into distinct neuron cells. In order to achieve a satisfying quality, human experts have to *proofread*, namely, to manually correct the segmentation results [12,4]. It is a difficult and tedious task due to the huge data size (500^3 voxels and more than 1000 cells). Fig. 4(a) shows what a human expert is facing in proofreading. Our interactive interface only highlights a small set of locations for human experts to verify, namely, the locations at which our graphical model has very low confidence. When a user fixes a mistake at one of these locations, our framework modifies the merging tree accordingly and recomputes the segmentation. The improvement to the segmentation is global. Our experiments show that under the new framework, within fifteen user inputs, the segmentation is improved to the optimal quality, much faster than classical user interaction frameworks.

Related Work. The closest works to us are [2,8], which also start with an initial watershed segmentation. The problem is formulated as a labeling problem of boundaries under certain topological constraints. The problem is solved using multicut integer linear programming. Another recent work [10] which also uses an initial watershed segmentation and performs agglomeration, learns how to merge watershed segments via active learning methods.

Kiran *et al.* [11] compute cuts of the hierarchical tree optimizing certain pre-defined energy. However, their energy is not learned in a supervised fashion as we did. Turaga *et al.* [13] learn to construct a hierarchical tree so that the water-shed cut at a certain threshold produces a high quality segmentation. There are many other learning based methods for Connectomics segmentation task. See [6] and references therein.

2   Background

Suppose we are given a graph, e.g. a hierarchical merging tree. Denote by $\mathcal{V}$ and $\mathcal{E} \subseteq \mathcal{V} \times \mathcal{V}$ the set of nodes and the set of edges respectively. Each node can take a label from a label set $\mathcal{L}$. We call each label configuration of all nodes a *labeling*. Denote by $\mathcal{Y} = \mathcal{L}^{\mathcal{V}}$ the space of all labelings. Given an observation x and a parameter vector w, the conditional probability of a labeling y is $P(y|x, w) = \exp(-E(y|x, w) - \log Z(x, w))$, where $Z(x, w) = \sum_{y \in \mathcal{Y}} \exp(-E(y|x, w))$ is the *partition function*. The energy is often defined as the negative inner product $E(y|x, w) = -\langle w, \phi(x, y) \rangle$, in which $\phi(x, y)$ is the concatenation of features of all nodes and edges. Note that the feature vector also depends on y.

In prediction, one computes the *maximum a posteriori (MAP)*,

$$\text{argmax}_y\, P(y|x, w) = \text{argmin}_y\, E(y|x, w). \tag{1}$$

It is also very useful to compute the *marginals*, $P(y_i = \ell|x, w) = \sum_{y: y_i = \ell} P(y|x, w)$. Since our graph is tree-structured, computing MAP and marginals can be solved exactly and efficiently using dynamic programming algorithms. For more general graphs, the inference tasks are NP-hard and have to be solved approximately, e.g. using loopy belief propagation.

We train the parameter vector w from a given set of training data $\{(x^n, y^n)\}$, $n = 1, \ldots, N$. This can be achieved by minimizing the convex loss function $\text{loss}(w) = \|w\|^2 + c \sum_{n=1}^{N} [\log Z(x^n, w) - \langle w, \phi(x^n, y^n) \rangle]$. We can find the opti-mal w efficiently using gradient descent. The gradient can be computed effi-ciently as long as the marginals can be computed efficiently. We use the UGM package by Mark Schmidt for the training[1].

Factorization and Labeling Constraints. Assuming the Markov properties, the energy E can be factorized into the summation of unary potentials and pairwise potentials, $E(y|x, w) = \sum_{(i,i') \in \mathcal{E}} E_{i,i'}(y_i, y_{i'}|x, w) + \sum_{i \in \mathcal{V}} E_i(y_i|x, w)$. For a node/edge, one can forbid a certain label/label combination by forcing the

---

[1] http://www.di.ens.fr/~mschmidt/Software/UGM.html

corresponding potential to be infinite. Thus we can compute MAP and marginals only over the set of feasible labelings $\mathcal{Y}' \subseteq \mathcal{Y}$. This makes it possible to do training and inference only over $\mathcal{Y}'$, as we will do in this paper.

3   Computing Tree-Derived Segmentation

For any given image, we construct a watershed merging tree by running on a boundary likelihood map, namely, the likelihood of whether a pixel belonging to the boundaries between neuron cells (Figure 1(c)). Next, we construct a tree-structured graphical model whose underlying graph is the same as the hierarchical tree. The problem of computing the optimal segmentation is transformed into the problem of computing the optimal labeling of this graphical model (Equation (1)). In order to achieve the transformation, we need to build a correspondence between segmentations and labelings.

The Correspondence between Segmentations and Labelings. Denote by $\mathcal{P} = \{p_1, \ldots, p_M\}$ the set of all regions corresponding to the leaf nodes of the tree. We call these regions the *superpixels*. A *segmentation* is a decomposition of the set of superpixels into a disjoint set of *segments*. Formally, a segmentation $S = \{s_1, \ldots, s_m \mid s_i \subseteq \mathcal{P}, \forall i; \bigcup_{i=1}^{m} s_i = \mathcal{P}\}$.

Denote by $\mathcal{S}$ the space of all possible segmentations. For a given image I, we would like to find the most probable segmentation $\mathrm{argmax}_{S \in \mathcal{S}} P(S|I)$, with a suitably defined posterior probability $P(S|I)$. Since $\mathcal{S}$ is too large to search through, we restrict the solution space to a smaller subset. Given a hierarchical tree, T, a segmentation S is T-*derived* if and only if each segment $s_i \in S$ is a node of T. We call such segmentations *tree-derived* and our algorithm search through the space of all T-derived segmentations, denoted by $\mathcal{S}_T \subseteq \mathcal{S}$. The correspondence between tree-derived segmentations and the labelings of T is provided as follows. Let the label set $\mathcal{L} = \{-1, 0, 1\}$, represent whether each tree node is an under-segment, a segment or an over-segment. An under-segment node is the ascendant of a set of segment nodes. An over-segment node is the descendant of a segment node. For each labeling y, we take the set of zero-labeled nodes as the corresponding segmentation. In Figure 1(f), the tree represents a labeling. Red, blue and dark colors correspond to -1, 0 and $+1$ labels respectively. The corresponding segmentation is shown in the top row.

We are only interested in labelings that derive legit segmentations. Therefore we enforce certain restrictions on the labelings. For a labeling y and a node v, let $\Gamma_v(y)$ be the sequence of labels along the path from v to the root.

Theorem 1. *There is an one-to-one correspondence between $\mathcal{S}_T$ and the set of labelings $\mathcal{Y}_T$, such that for any leaf node v, (1) $\Gamma_v(y)$ is monotonically non-increasing; (2) The zero label appears exactly once in $\Gamma_v(y)$; (3) The first label (label of v) cannot be -1 and the last label (label of the root node) cannot be $+1$.*

We defer the proof to the supplemental material.

We call labelings within $\mathcal{Y}_T$ *segmentation labelings*. Conditions in Theorem 1 can be translated into restrictions on labels of nodes and edges. In particular, a labeling y is a segmentation labeling if and only if (1) the root has label $y_{root} \in \{-1, 0\}$; (2) any leaf node, v, has label $y_v \in \{0, 1\}$; (3) for any child-parent pair, (c, p), $y_c \geq y_p \geq y_c - 1$; (4) if $y_p = y_c$, $y_c \neq 0$.

Prediction and Training. For any given image and hierarchical tree, we construct a graphical model.[2] Let the posterior probability of a tree-derived segmentation $S \in \mathcal{S}_T$ be $P(S|I) = P(y^S|I, w)$, where y^S is the corresponding segmentation labeling of S. Recall that we can enforce all aforementioned label constraints by setting certain potentials to infinity. Therefore, we can restrict the set of feasible solutions of the graphical model to be $\mathcal{Y}_T$ and compute the MAP, $\mathrm{argmax}_{y \in \mathcal{Y}_T} P(y|I, w)$. The corresponding segmentation is the predicted segmentation. At the training stage, for each data, we construct the graphical model similarly so that the marginals are computed within $\mathcal{Y}_T$. It remains to show how to compute the ground truth labeling for each training data.

Computing the Optimal Tree-Derived Segmentation. For each training data, we are given a ground truth segmentation $\widehat{S}$, which may not be tree-derived. In order to find a ground truth labeling of this data, we find the tree-derived segmentation that best approximates $\widehat{S}$, $S^* = \mathrm{argmax}_{S \in \mathcal{S}_T} \mathrm{score}(S, \widehat{S})$. For EM images, there are two popular score functions, the random index and the variation of information. Notice that both functions can be decomposed into a summation of scores of elements of S, $\mathrm{score}(S) = \sum_{s_i \in S} f(s_i)$. Based on this observation, we provide a polynomial algorithm to compute S^* using standard dynamic programing techniques. See the supplemental material for the pseudocode.

4   Interactive Segmentation

Our interactive algorithm works as follows. For a given test image, we compute an automatic segmentation using the algorithm presented in the previous section. Based on marginals of the graphical model, we suggest the user a few locations to proofread. When a user finds a mistake in the segmentation, he/she clicks and corrects it. The boundaries that have been corrected would not be highlighted during the remaining iterations. We modify the merging tree accordingly and recompute the segmentation on the modified tree. This process is repeated until the user is satisfied. Recall that to construct a graphical model, we need a parameter vector w. Throughout the user interaction, we use the same w which is learned in the training stage. See Figure 2(a) for the flowchart.

Boundaries and Their Marginals. The basic elements for a user to handle are boundaries between superpixels. Recall superpixels form a bottom layer watershed segmentation. We collect the set of all boundaries (curves for 2D images and surface patches for 3D images). For a given segmentation, we say a boundary is labeled *merged* if the two adjacent superpixels belong to a same segment. Otherwise, it is labeled *split*. In other words, the boundary will appear (not appear)

---

[2] See the supplemental material for details of extracting features $\phi(x, y)$ in Eq. 1.

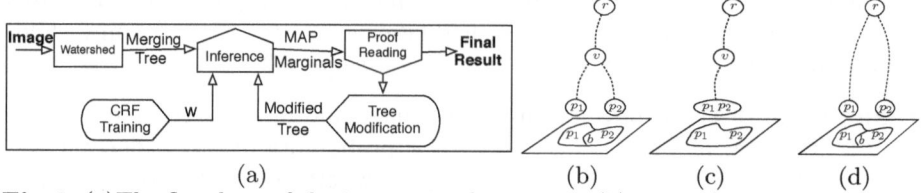

(a)   (b)   (c)   (d)

Fig. 2. (a)The flowchart of the interactive framework; (b) a tree (nodes on the curved paths are not shown for clarity); (c) b is labeled merged; (d) b is labeled split

in the segmentation if it is labeled split (merged). The task of segmentation is equivalent to finding an optimal split/merged labeling to all the boundaries. Our CRF generates marginals for nodes of the tree. However, we can easily translate node marginals into marginals of whether each boundary being split or merged. For a given boundary b and its two adjacent superpixels, p_1, p_2, we find the least common ancestor of the leaf nodes containing p_1 and p_2. We call this node, v, the *containing node* of b, because b is in the interior of v and all its ancestors (Fig. 2(b)). The boundary b is split if and only if v is an under-segment, i.e. has label -1. Therefore, the probability of b being split is equal to the marginal $P(y_v = -1|x, w)$. At each iteration of the segmentation, we show the predicted segmentation and highlight the boundaries that we have low confidence of being either merged or split. This gives a user a small number of options to proofread (see Fig. 4(a)). After the user corrected a boundary, the system will update the tree accordingly and present the low marginal boundaries again.

Modifying Trees. We conclude this section by explaining how to update the tree according to user inputs. When a user specifies a boundary between two superpixels to be merged, we merge the paths from the two leaf nodes containing the two superpixels to their common ancestor node into a single path. When user specifies a boundary to be split, we split the path from v to the root into two paths, nodes along the original path are assigned to either of the two new paths, depending on the situation. Also we enforce an extra constraint that the raised containing node could only have label -1. These operations will ensure the boundary is merged/split in any tree-derived segmentation of the modified tree. In Fig. 2, we illustrate the two operations on a same tree.

5   Experiments

2D Experiments. We applied our method to neuron EM images from the ISBI 2012 EM image segmentation challenge [3]. The data contains 30 2D sections of ssTEM images, each of which has 512×512 pixels. We used the boundary likelihood map from [5]. We submitted our result on test data to the challenge website and our method achieved the 2nd place overall in the competition, with an adjusted Rand Index Error of 0.023, Warping Error 0.0008 and Pixel Error 0.11. [1]. Note that our group name is "optree-idsia". The training took 167 seconds and the MAP computation during testing per image was 0.05 seconds.

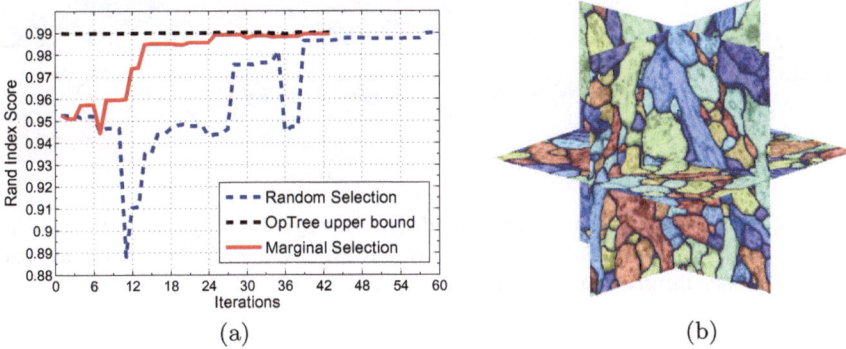

Fig. 3. (a) Interaction Simulation; (b) 3D Result

To demonstrate the necessity of all structural constraints that we enforce in our algorithm, we ran a holistic experiment. We compared our method with three baseline approaches: watersheds (WS); node classifier (NC); unconstrained CRF (UNC). WS is the the classical watershed using the best threshold. In NC we trained a random forest classifier to predict node labels. In UNC, we used CRF on trees without constraints defined in Theorem 1. We used post-processing to ensure the final results of these methods are legit segmentations. Note that NC and UNC are both supervised training methods, like ours.

In the table, Optree outperforms all baselines in the Adjusted Rand Index (ARI). We also present the optimal tree-derived segmentation result (Optimal)

	WS	NC	UNC	Optree	Optimal
ARI	0.05	0.14	0.10	0.023	0.015

for reference, which is achieved when the ground truth is known. This is the theoretical upper-bound of our tree-derived segmentations. We observe that UNC outperforms NC, justifying the significance of the tree structure in the model.

3D Experiments. We applied our method to a $500 \times 500 \times 500$ 3D EM image from [7]. We used the boundary likelihood map from "Ilastik" [12]. To reduce the watershed tree size, we removed all nodes with height less than 0.05. We divided the initial volume into 8 250x250x250 sub-volumes. We run experiments for 8 times. Each time we use one sub-volume for training and the rest for testing. Training took 465 seconds and MAP computation took 0.9 seconds on average. The average Rand Index score (one minus the Rand Index Error) is 0.9837. Our method performs better than state-of-the-art [8,2]. The optimal score of tree-derived segmentations (Optimal) is 0.9923. There is still room for improvement over the optree segmentation result. In the next section, we show the result can be improved to the optimal via user interactions, as explained in Section 4.

Interactive Experiments. Our interactive system suggests a few boundaries for users to proofread at each iteration. Users judge by observation whether a boundary is mislabeled and correct it. We run experiments to show how this

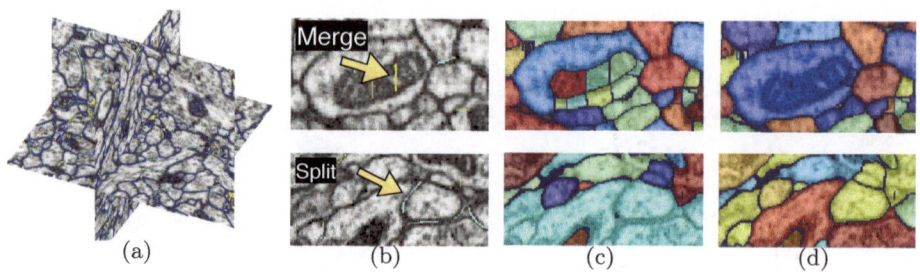

Fig. 4. (a): boundaries a user has to proofread; (b): our system only shows boundaries with low marginals (yellow if labeled split, cyan if labeled merged); (c): before user input; (b): after user input, many boundaries are fixed

method could improve the efficiency of proofreading. We simulate a user interaction process on a particular 250^3 sub-volume on which our automatic method has the worst score. We start from the automatic algorithm result and correct mislabeled boundaries iteratively. At each iteration, the simulated user (robot) selects one mislabeled boundary based on certain strategy. The merging tree is modified accordingly. We implemented two strategies (1) always select the mislabeled boundary with the least confidence (least marginal); (2) randomly select a mislabeled boundary. In Figure 3(a), correcting low-marginal boundaries (red curve) clearly improves the results much faster than correcting randomly selected boundaries (blue curve). The former takes about 14 iterations to reach the accuracy > 98.7 while the latter takes 39 iterations to reach the same accuracy. We also show the optimal result (black curve) of tree-derived segmentation as a theoretical upper bound.

We illustrate how one user input can improve the segmentation globally. In Figure 4(a), a user has to verify all colored boundaries. However, in our system, she only needs to pay attention to boundaries with low marginals (yellow and cyan). Boundaries of yellow (resp. cyan) color are labeled split (resp. merged). After a selected boundary (yellow arrow) is corrected, many other boundaries are automatically corrected (Figure 4(b), 4(c) and 4(d)). Our interactive segmentation framework is very efficient. In average, each iteration takes around 1.9 second. This includes modifying the tree and recomputing MAP and marginals.

6   Conclusion

This paper presents a CRF-based algorithm for neuron segmentation. The tree-structured graphical model allows us to compute accurate segmentation of 500^3 dataset within a second. Furthermore, we develop an interactive segmentation framework that takes advantage of the marginals of the graphical model. The new framework improves the segmentation to the optimal quality within a small number of user inputs.

References

1. ISBI Challenge, http://brainiac2.mit.edu/isbi_challenge/leaders-board
2. Andres, B., Kroeger, T., Briggman, K.L., Denk, W., Korogod, N., Knott, G., Koethe, U., Hamprecht, F.A.: Globally optimal closed-surface segmentation for connectomics. In: Fitzgibbon, A., Lazebnik, S., Perona, P., Sato, Y., Schmid, C. (eds.) ECCV 2012, Part III. LNCS, vol. 7574, pp. 778–791. Springer, Heidelberg (2012)
3. Cardona, A., Saalfeld, S., Preibisch, S., Schmid, B., Cheng, A., Pulokas, J., Tomancak, P., Hartenstein, V.: An integrated micro-and macroarchitectural analysis of the drosophila brain by computer-assisted serial section electron microscopy. PLoS biology 8(10) (2010)
4. Chklovskii, D.B., Vitaladevuni, S., Scheffer, L.K.: Semi-automated reconstruction of neural circuits using electron microscopy. Current Opinion in Neurobiology 20(5), 667–675 (2010)
5. Ciresan, D., Giusti, A., Schmidhuber, J., et al.: Deep neural networks segment neuronal membranes in electron microscopy images. In: Advances in Neural Information Processing Systems, vol. 25, pp. 2852–2860 (2012)
6. Jain, V., Seung, H.S., Turaga, S.C.: Machines that learn to segment images: a crucial technology for connectomics. Current Opinion in Neurobiology 20(5), 653–666 (2010)
7. Knott, G., Marchman, H., Wall, D., Lich, B.: Serial section scanning electron microscopy of adult brain tissue using focused ion beam milling. The Journal of Neuroscience 28(12), 2959–2964 (2008)
8. Kroeger, T., Mikula, S., Denk, W., Koethe, U., Hamprecht, F.: Learning to segment neurons with non-local quality measures. In: Mori, K., Sakuma, I., Sato, Y., Barillot, C., Navab, N. (eds.) MICCAI 2013, Part II. LNCS, vol. 8150, pp. 419–427. Springer, Heidelberg (2013)
9. Najman, L., Schmitt, M.: Geodesic saliency of watershed contours and hierarchical segmentation. PAMI 18(12), 1163–1173 (1996)
10. Nunez-Iglesias, J., Kennedy, R., Parag, T., Shi, J., Chklovskii, D.B.: Machine learning of hierarchical clustering to segment 2d and 3d images. PLoS ONE 8 (2013)
11. Ravi Kiran, B., Serra, J.: Global–local optimizations by hierarchical cuts and climbing energies. Pattern Recognition 47(1), 12–24 (2014)
12. Sommer, C., Straehle, C., Koethe, U., Hamprecht, F.A.: Ilastik: Interactive learning and segmentation toolkit. In: 8th IEEE Int. Symposium (ISBI) (2011)
13. Turaga, S.C., Briggman, K.L., Helmstaedter, M., Denk, W., Seung, H.S.: Maximin affinity learning of image segmentation. In: NIPS, pp. 1865–1873 (2009)

Application-Driven MRI:
Joint Reconstruction and Segmentation from Undersampled MRI Data

Jose Caballero[1], Wenjia Bai[1], Anthony N. Price[2],
Daniel Rueckert[1], and Joseph V. Hajnal[2]

[1] Department of Computing, Imperial College London, UK
[2] Division of Imaging Sciences and Biomedical Engineering Department, King's
College London, St. Thomas' Hospital, London, UK
{jose.caballero06,w.bai,d.rueckert}@imperial.ac.uk,
{anthony.price,jo.hajnal}@kcl.ac.uk

Abstract. Medical image segmentation has traditionally been regarded
as a separate process from image acquisition and reconstruction, even
though its performance directly depends on the quality and characteristics of these first stages of the imaging pipeline. Adopting an integrated
acquisition-reconstruction-segmentation process can provide a more efficient and accurate solution. In this paper we propose a joint segmentation
and reconstruction algorithm for undersampled magnetic resonance data.
Merging a reconstructive patch-based sparse modelling and a discriminative Gaussian mixture modelling can produce images with enhanced
edge information ultimately improving their segmentation.

1 Introduction

Magnetic resonance imaging (MRI) produces highly detailed images with excellent soft tissue contrast. In some cases images are not an end in themselves, but
rather a means of access to clinically relevant parameters which are obtained as
post-processing steps, such as segmentation or tissue characterisation. Acquiring the data necessary to produce images is a time consuming process that can
impose significant demands on the patient, but at the same time a lot of information is discarded during post-processing. In cases where the clinically relevant
parameters sought are known a priori, the design of image acquisition and reconstruction would ideally be application-driven, such that they are tailored to
the information necessary to determine them within some reliability standards.

Compressed sensing (CS) [5, 9] has emerged as an effective way of reducing
acquisition time. Incoherently acquiring a fraction of the data normally needed,
perfect recovery is possible imposing a sparsity condition on the image, hence
allowing scan acceleration without disrupting quantitative analysis. However, it
is possible that better measurements could be achieved from fast acquisition
data by directly focusing on the final analysis to be performed and treating any
reconstruction as an enabling step rather than a distinct endpoint to be achieved
first.

P. Golland et al. (Eds.): MICCAI 2014, Part I, LNCS 8673, pp. 106–113, 2014.
© Springer International Publishing Switzerland 2014

This concept of application-driven MRI is broad, given that each imaging design is dependent on the information required from the image. This paper focusses on the case of image segmentation, which is central to many applications of medical image analysis. Segmentation enables the extraction of parameters such as hippocampal volume from brain scans to diagnose or monitor Alzheimer's disease, or ventricular morphology from cardiac cine data revealing cardiac function or ventricular mass.

The problem of segmentation from undersampled measurements has been studied for images that are easily represented in a low dimensional labelled space. Examples are hyperspectral images, which can be described by a few distinct spectral signatures [15], and tomography, where images are well represented as piece-wise constant elements [8, 12]. In the case of MRI it is more challenging to provide a simple description of different regions. An arsenal of segmentation methods is available, based amongst others on region-growing [7], atlas registration [4] or deformable models [10], but the vast majority assume a fully acquired image, despite the growing interest on fast MRI acquisition supported by CS.

We propose a joint optimisation which balances reconstruction fidelity and segmentation performance using a patch-based dictionary sparsity model and a Gaussian mixture model (GMM) on intensity values. Patch-based dictionary sparsity has been proposed as an effective way of exploiting MRI redundancy for reconstruction, notably enabling the use of adaptive dictionaries [2,11]. The GMM term promotes simpler reconstructions by penalising deviations from the mean values of a few Gaussian distributions. Using 2D brain phantom images and cardiac cine scans, we show that reconstructed images benefit from enhanced edges ultimately improving their segmentation. The paper focusses on a reconstruction-segmentation process but eventually anticipates expanding this to consider optimal sampling strategies for the acquisition.

The paper is organised as follows: Section 2 introduces the necessary background on CS for MRI using patch-based dictionaries and GMM segmentation, and describes the joint reconstruction-segmentation method proposed. Section 3 presents experiments performed on MRI data, visually and quantitatively analysing the benefits of jointly segmenting while reconstructing.

2   Methods

2.1   Patch-Based Compressed Sensing MRI

CS targets perfect data recovery from incomplete samples. Provided incoherent sampling, perfect reconstruction can in theory be guaranteed with the assumption that the data is redundant when represented in a sparsity transform domain [5]. For MRI, transforms such as total variation, wavelets or temporal Fourier transforms apply depending on the imaging modality [9]. Recently, the use of redundant patch-based dictionaries in the image domain has been proposed to sparsely represent images [11] and dynamic data [2,3], and have gained particular attention for their additional ability of becoming adaptive through dictionary learning (DL) algorithms [6,13].

Let $\mathbf{y}$ be an undersampled acquisition from a scan of size N. Given a dictionary $\mathbf{D}$ with N_a atoms of size N_p, a CS reconstruction $\mathbf{x}$ is given by

$$\min_{\mathbf{x},\boldsymbol{\Gamma}} \ \|\mathbf{F}_u\mathbf{x} - \mathbf{y}\|^2 + \frac{\lambda}{N_p} \sum_{n=1}^{N} \|\mathbf{R}_n\mathbf{x} - \mathbf{D}\boldsymbol{\gamma}_n\|^2 \ \text{s.t.} \ \|\boldsymbol{\gamma}_n\|_0 \leq T \ \forall n, \qquad (1)$$

where $\mathbf{F}_u$ is an undersampled Fourier transform, $\mathbf{R}_n$ is a patch extraction operator, λ is a weighting parameter, T is a sparsity threshold, and $\boldsymbol{\gamma}_n$ is the sparse representation of patch $\mathbf{R}_n\mathbf{x}$ organised as column n of matrix $\boldsymbol{\Gamma}$. The dictionary can be a non-adaptive sparsifying dictionary (e.g. discrete cosine transform (DCT) or wavelets), or can be included as a free variable in the problem letting it become adaptive [2,3,11]. Solving this problem directly is difficult as it is non-convex in both variables, but they can be individually updated as a least-squares and orthogonal matching pursuit (OMP) problem iteratively [3,11].

Although CS reconstructions have demonstrated great potential, in practice images can only be assumed to be approximately sparse. Problems are typically encountered at high acceleration rates in regions of the image that do not adhere to the sparse model, generally resulting in lost fine details and smoothed edges [14]. These reconstruction errors are prone to propagate into post-processing stages, compromising the accuracy of quantitative measurements.

2.2 Gaussian Mixture Model Segmentation

Image segmentation based on a GMM assumes image features that are randomly generated from an underlying mixture of Gaussian distributions [1]. In some cases, similar pixel intensities correspond to the same tissue class, and can therefore be used to label data. This typically applies for brain scans, where grey matter, white matter and cerebrospinal fluid show different intensities, or cardiac cine data, where blood pool regions have a characteristic high intensity.

Assuming $\mathbf{x}$ to be MRI data, each pixel x_n can be expressed by a mixture of K Gaussians as $\mathrm{P}(x_n) = \sum_{k=1}^{K} \pi_k \mathcal{N}(x_n|\mu_k, \sigma_k)$, denoting $\boldsymbol{\mu}$, $\boldsymbol{\sigma}$ and $\boldsymbol{\pi}$ as the means, standard deviations and mixture weightings of all Gaussians. The GMM is formally found by maximising the log-likelihood of the posterior distribution

$$\max_{\boldsymbol{\mu},\boldsymbol{\sigma},\boldsymbol{\pi}} \ \ln \mathrm{P}(\mathbf{x}|\boldsymbol{\mu},\boldsymbol{\sigma},\boldsymbol{\pi}) = \max_{\boldsymbol{\mu},\boldsymbol{\sigma},\boldsymbol{\pi}} \ \sum_{n=1}^{N} \ln\left(\sum_{k=1}^{K} \pi_k \mathcal{N}(x_n|\mu_k,\sigma_k)\right). \qquad (2)$$

The solution of this maximisation is complicated by the sum inside the logarithm, but the Expectation-Maximisation (EM) [1] algorithm can iteratively find it by alternating the update of the model ($\boldsymbol{\mu}$, $\boldsymbol{\sigma}$, $\boldsymbol{\pi}$) and a latent variable $r_{nk} \equiv \mathrm{P}(z_k = 1|x_n)$. This term provides a labelling of pixels with an associated uncertainty as the probability that Gaussian k generated data point x_n.

2.3 Segmentation-Driven MRI (SegMRI)

The following task formulates reconstruction imposing a model on the data that weights the deviation from a patch-based sparse and a GMM representation:

$$\min_{\substack{\mathbf{x},\boldsymbol{\Gamma} \\ \boldsymbol{\mu},\boldsymbol{\sigma},\boldsymbol{\pi}}} \quad \|\mathbf{F}_u\mathbf{x} - \mathbf{y}\|^2 + \frac{\lambda}{N_p}\sum_{n=1}^{N}\|\mathbf{R}_n\mathbf{x} - \mathbf{D}\boldsymbol{\gamma}_n\|^2 - \beta\ln\mathrm{P}(\mathbf{x}|\boldsymbol{\mu},\boldsymbol{\sigma},\boldsymbol{\pi})\ \text{s.t.}\ \|\boldsymbol{\gamma}_n\|_0 \le T \ \forall n.$$

$$(3)$$

If the new tuning parameter is set to $\beta = 0$, the problem is the same as in (1) and is purely reconstructive as the GMM model is not used. For $\beta > 0$, the reconstructed intensities need to be consistent with the GMM emerging as a by-product of the reconstruction. The larger the penalisation of this term is, the closer intensities are to the means of Gaussians, so effectively it homogenises intensities within a region and reduces the number of intensities sitting around the boundaries of two regions. At the extreme $\beta \to \infty$, each pixel intensity is set to the mean of the Gaussian that is the most likely to have generated it.

Problem (3) is also non-convex, but can be solved alternating a conjugate gradient (CG) update of image $\mathbf{x}$, OMP coding of the sparse modelling $\boldsymbol{\Gamma}$, and the EM update of the GMM parameters. The method is summarised in algorithm 1. At each iteration the uncertainty in segmentation is reduced as r_{nk} tends to an indicator function for each n pulling intensities closer to their attributed Gaussian mean. The EM step can eventually become unstable ($\sigma_k \to 0$) as a result, so a minimum variance that the Gaussians in the GMM can achieve is set to prevent this. Global convergence is not proven, but small K and constrained variances reduce the chance of EM local minima, and patch-based MRI reconstruction is empirically robust [2, 3, 11]. The computational bottleneck is OMP ($\sim 2NT(N_p + N_a)$ operations/iteration), although patch coding is parallelisable.

Algorithm 1. SegMRI reconstruction

Input: Acquisition $\mathbf{y}$, number of Gaussians K, sparse model parameters (T, N_p, N_a).
Output: Reconstructed k-space $\mathbf{x}$, GMM parameters $(\boldsymbol{\mu}, \boldsymbol{\sigma}, \boldsymbol{\pi})$.
Initialise: $\mathbf{x}_0 = \mathbf{F}_u^H\mathbf{y}, \boldsymbol{\Gamma}_0 = 0, t = 0, \sigma_{0,k} = 0.5\ \forall k, \boldsymbol{\mu}_0$ randomly chosen from $\mathbf{x}$.
repeat

> **1.** $t \leftarrow t + 1$
> **2.** Update sparse coding with OMP using $\mathbf{x}_{(t-1)}$:
> $$\boldsymbol{\Gamma}_t \leftarrow \arg\min_{\boldsymbol{\Gamma}} \sum_{n=1}^{N}\|\mathbf{R}_n\mathbf{x}_{(t-1)} - \mathbf{D}\boldsymbol{\gamma}_n\|^2\ \text{s.t.}\ \|\boldsymbol{\gamma}_n\|_0 \le T$$
> **3.** Update GMM parameters with EM using $\mathbf{x}_{(t-1)}$:
> $$\{\boldsymbol{\mu}_t, \boldsymbol{\sigma}_t, \boldsymbol{\pi}_t\} \leftarrow \arg\max_{\boldsymbol{\mu},\boldsymbol{\sigma},\boldsymbol{\pi}} \ln\mathrm{P}\left(\mathbf{x}_{(t-1)}|\boldsymbol{\mu},\boldsymbol{\sigma},\boldsymbol{\pi}\right)$$
> **4.** Update reconstruction given the GMM and sparse coding:
> $$\mathbf{x}_t \leftarrow \arg\min_{\mathbf{x}} \ \|\mathbf{F}_u\mathbf{x} - \mathbf{y}\|^2 + \frac{\lambda}{N_p}\sum_{n=1}^{N}\|\mathbf{R}_n\mathbf{x} - \mathbf{D}\boldsymbol{\gamma}_n\|^2 - \beta\ln\mathrm{P}\left(\mathbf{x}|\boldsymbol{\mu},\boldsymbol{\sigma},\boldsymbol{\pi}\right)$$

until $\frac{\|\mathbf{x}_{t-1} - \mathbf{x}_t\|^2}{\|\mathbf{x}_t\|^2} \le 10^{-4}$;

---

3   Experiments and Results

In order to assess the benefits of jointly segmenting while reconstructing images, accelerated data is reconstructed with the SegMRI method in (3) and the CS method in (1). The latter reconstruction is segmented with a GMM as a separate step and both results are compared with a GMM segmentation of the fully sampled data. All tests use real-valued images, but the extension to complex-valued data is possible with complex-valued dictionaries [2, 11] and GMMs [1]. Parameters are fixed throughout using DCT dictionaries with $N_p = 8^2$ and $N_p = 4^3$ for 2D and cine tests respectively, $N_a = 196$, $T = 5$, $\lambda = 10^{-3}$ and $\beta = 10^{-9}$. The minimum standard deviation to prevent instability in EM is set to $\sigma_k > 10 \times \sigma_{min}$, with σ_{min} the lowest standard deviation from the fully sampled image GMM, which can be known from prior scans. Experiments were performed on Matlab, Intel Core i72600 CPU, 3.4 GHz, 8 GB RAM.

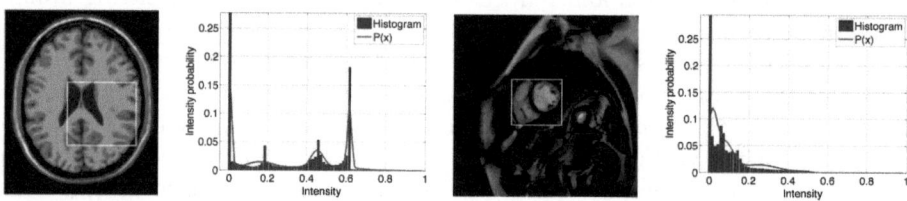

Fig. 1. Test data examples. From left to right: 2D phantom image, its histogram and GMM, one frame from a cardiac cine scan, and its histogram and GMM.

3.1   2D Brain Phantom Experiments

In this experiment the method is evaluated for 2D image reconstruction using sagittal, axial and coronal slices from a brain phantom[1]. A test image is shown in figure 1 alongside its histogram. Notice that the histogram has 4 distinct peaks and that it is well fitted by a 5 component GMM (including one for outliers).

Consider a 5-fold accelerated acquisition of this image. Performing a patch-based CS reconstruction recovers coarse structure but misses fine details and edges as shown in figure 2. When this reconstruction undergoes GMM segmentation, these errors propagate resulting in significantly more partial volume effects compared to the the fully sampled image segmentation. The result from SegMRI is more accurate, for instance at locations highlighted by arrows in figure 2(e). A stable result was found after 30 iterations of 2 seconds each.

Table 1 presents the mean and standard deviation of total misclassified pixels using 18 test images (6 from each plane) at several acceleration factors. As expected, the segmentation accuracy tends to decrease in both cases with increasing acceleration. However, notice that the SegMRI result outperforms the segmentation from the CS reconstruction, which reaffirms the visual inspection of figure 2. We use these percentages in a paired t-test and display the mean difference between CS+GMM and SegMRI errors (μ), t-values (t) and p-values (p). The very low p-value of the full set reveals high statistical significance.

---

[1] Phantom from BrainWeb (`http://brainweb.bic.mni.mcgill.ca/brainweb/`)

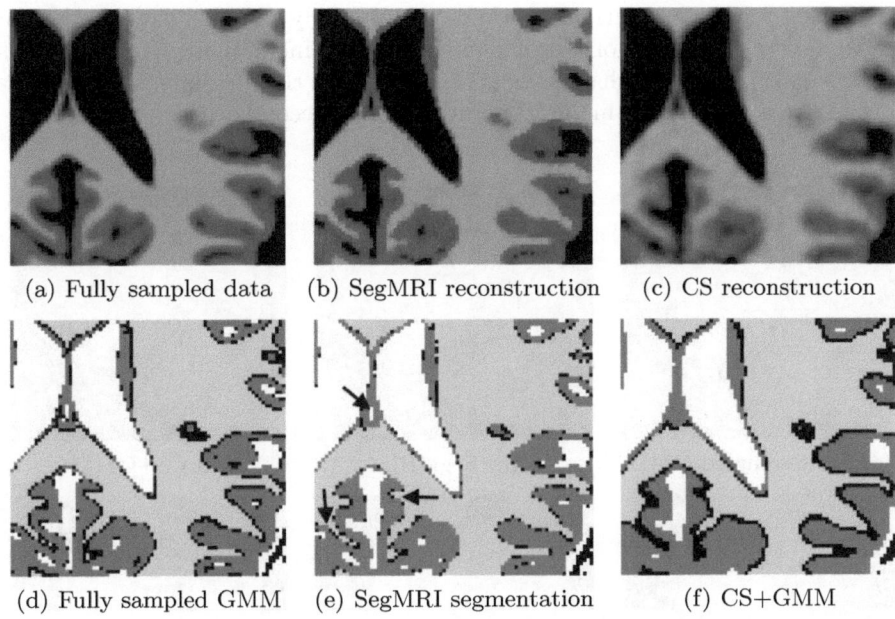

(a) Fully sampled data   (b) SegMRI reconstruction   (c) CS reconstruction

(d) Fully sampled GMM   (e) SegMRI segmentation   (f) CS+GMM

Fig. 2. Brain phantom reconstruction and segmentation.

Table 1. Pixel misclassification (mean±std%) and t-test for brain phantom

Acceleration	2	4	6	8	10	12	14	Full set
CS+GMM	5.1±0.9	10.2±1.4	12.8±1.7	14.6±1.9	15.5±2.1	16.3±2.3	17.0±2.4	**13.1 ± 4.3**
SegMRI	3.8±1.0	8.3±1.7	10.8±1.9	12.4±2.2	13.4±2.3	14.0±2.3	14.5±2.4	**11.0 ± 4.1**
μ	1.25	1.93	2.07	2.20	2.10	2.28	2.52	**2.05**
t	11.12	10.70	12.19	11.34	11.13	13.53	10.47	**27.59**
p ($\times 10^{-9}$)	3.2	5.7	0.8	2.4	0.8	0.2	7.8	**5.3×10^{-46}**

3.2 Cardiac Cine Experiments

The same experiment is performed on 7 cardiac cine MRI data, a frame of which is shown in figure 1, using 3D (2D+t) dictionaries. Considering left ventricular structure analysis, the choice $K = 3$ for all tests ensures a clear left ventricle segmentation due to the high intensity difference between blood pool and myocardium. We perform CS reconstruction followed by GMM segmentation on 10-fold accelerated scans and compare them with SegMRI segmentation.

Table 2 shows the 7 patient dataset results of pixel classification for the left ventricle. Again, SegMRI consistently outperforms the disjoint segmentation procedure. Although quantitative differences are small, visual inspection shows that SegMRI is able to capture fine details also revealed in the segmentation run on the fully sampled data. An example is given in figure 3 with the boundaries of the left ventricle segmentations overlaid onto the fully sampled data on the slice plane and across the temporal profile of the dashed line in figure 3(a). The t-test performed also implies high statistical significance in these results. For cine data, convergence was attained in 20-30 iterations of 60 seconds each.

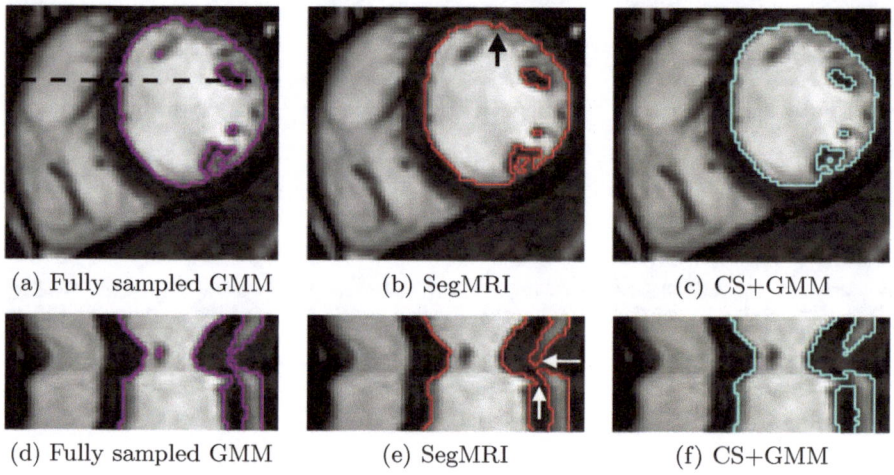

(a) Fully sampled GMM	(b) SegMRI	(c) CS+GMM
(d) Fully sampled GMM	(e) SegMRI	(f) CS+GMM

Fig. 3. Left ventricle segmentation overlaid onto fully sampled data

Table 2. Pixel misclassification (mean±std%) and t-test for left ventricle structure

Acceleration	2	4	6	8	10	12	14	Full set
CS+GMM	2.5±1.5	4.8±3.0	6.0±3.9	6.8±4.2	7.3±4.5	7.8±4.7	7.9±4.9	**6.2 ± 4.4**
SegMRI	2.0±1.1	4.0±2.6	5.1±3.4	5.9±3.8	6.3±4.2	6.8±4.4	7.0±4.7	**5.3 ± 4.0**
μ	0.49	0.78	0.88	0.88	0.90	1.04	0.86	**0.83**
t	3.87	4.55	4.64	4.70	5.68	6.45	5.72	**13.3**
p ($\times 10^{-3}$)	8.3	3.9	3.6	3.3	1.3	0.6	1.2	**9.5×10^{-15}**

4   Conclusion

We have proposed a joint reconstruction-segmentation framework for undersampled fast acquisitions of MRI data. Imposing a GMM term in the reconstruction provides a segmentation that degrades less with increasing undersampling compared to a separated reconstruction and segmentation processing. Extensions of this work could look at natural additions to GMM segmentations such as Markov random fields and spatial priors for improved robustness. An interesting direction could also further integrate segmentation and reconstruction by performing region specific dictionary learning informed by intermediate segmentations.

The traditional analysis pipeline is burdened with high amounts of data that is time-consuming and expensive to acquire and process, and in scenarios where the information needed from the images is not the images themselves, but information derived from them, an application-driven scan could provide a more efficient and accurate solution. Image analysis tools, other than the segmentation example discussed in this paper, might also benefit from symbiotically combining post-processing with acquisition and reconstruction.

References

1. Bishop, C.M.: Pattern recognition and machine learning. Springer, New York (2006)
2. Caballero, J., Price, A.N., Rueckert, D., Hajnal, J.V.: Dictionary learning and time sparsity in dynamic MR data reconstruction. IEEE Trans. Med. Imag. 33(4), 979–994 (2014)
3. Caballero, J., Rueckert, D., Hajnal, J.V.: Dictionary learning and time sparsity in dynamic MRI. In: Ayache, N., Delingette, H., Golland, P., Mori, K. (eds.) MICCAI 2012, Part I. LNCS, vol. 7510, pp. 256–263. Springer, Heidelberg (2012)
4. Cabezas, M., Oliver, A., Lladó, X., Freixenet, J., Cuadra, M.B.: A review of atlas-based segmentation for magnetic resonance brain images. Comput. Meth. Prog. Bio. 104(3), 158–177 (2011)
5. Candès, E.J., Romberg, J., Tao, T.: Robust uncertainty principles: Exact signal reconstruction from highly incomplete frequency information. IEEE Trans. Inf. Theory 52(2), 489–509 (2006)
6. Elad, M., Aharon, M.: Image denoising via sparse and redundant representations over learned dictionaries. IEEE Trans. Image Process. 15(12), 3736–3745 (2006)
7. Haralick, R.M., Shapiro, L.G.: Image segmentation techniques. Comput. Vision Graph. 29(1), 100–132 (1985)
8. Hsiao, I.T., Rangarajan, A., Gindi, G.: Joint-MAP reconstruction/segmentation for transmission tomography using mixture-models as priors. IEEE Nucl. Sci. Symp. Conf. Rec. 3, 1689–1693 (1998)
9. Lustig, M., Donoho, D., Pauly, J.M.: Sparse MRI: The application of compressed sensing for rapid MR imaging. Magn. Reson. Med. 58(6), 1182–1195 (2007)
10. McInerney, T., Terzopoulos, D.: Deformable models in medical image analysis: A survey. Med. Image Anal. 1(2), 91–108 (1996)
11. Ravishankar, S., Bresler, Y.: MR image reconstruction from highly undersampled k-space data by dictionary learning. IEEE Trans. Med. Imag. 30(5), 1028–1041 (2011)
12. de Sompel, D.V., Brady, M.: Simultaneous reconstruction and segmentation algorithm for positron emission tomography and transmission tomography. In: ISBI 2008, pp. 1035–1038. IEEE (2008)
13. Tosic, I., Frossard, P.: Dictionary learning. IEEE Signal Process. Mag. 28(2), 27–38 (2011)
14. Virtue, P., Uecker, M., Elad, M., Lustig, M.: Predicting image quality of undersampled data reconstruction in the presence of noise. In: Proc. 21st Annual Meeting ISMRM, Salt Lake City, Utah, USA, p. 2668 (2013)
15. Zhang, Q., Plemmons, R., Kittle, D., Brady, D., Prasad, S.: Joint segmentation and reconstruction of hyperspectral data with compressed measurements. Appl. Opt. 50(22), 4417–4435 (2011)

Joint Parametric Reconstruction and Motion Correction Framework for Dynamic PET Data

Jieqing Jiao[1,*], Alexandre Bousse[2,*], Kris Thielemans[2], Pawel Markiewicz[1],
Ninon Burgos[1], David Atkinson[3], Simon Arridge[1],
Brian F. Hutton[2], and Sébastien Ourselin[1,4]

[1] Translational Imaging Group, Centre for Medical Image Computing, UCL, UK
[2] Institute of Nuclear Medicine, University College London, UK
[3] Centre for Medical Imaging, University College London, UK
[4] Dementia Research Centre, Institute of Neurology, University College London,
Queen Square, WC1N 3BG, UK

Abstract. In this paper we propose a novel algorithm for jointly performing data based motion correction and direct parametric reconstruction of dynamic PET data. We derive a closed form update for the penalised likelihood maximisation which greatly enhances the algorithm's computational efficiency for practical use. Our algorithm achieves sub-voxel motion correction residual with noisy data in the simulation-based validation and reduces the bias of the direct estimation of the kinetic parameter of interest. A preliminary evaluation on clinical brain data using [18F]Choline shows improved contrast for regions of high activity. The proposed method is based on a data-driven kinetic modelling method and is directly applicable to reversible and irreversible PET tracers, covering a range of clinical applications.

Keywords: Dynamic PET, direct parametric reconstruction, motion correction, optimisation transfer, kinetic analysis.

1 Introduction

Dynamic Positron Emission Tomography (PET) imaging in conjunction with appropriate tracer kinetic models allow for the estimation of biological parameters that are essential for disease understanding, clinical diagnosis and drug development. Conventionally, the raw PET data in the form of photon counts recorded by the detectors are first reconstructed to provide the temporal images of the spatial distribution of the PET tracer (activity), and a selected kinetic model is then applied to the time activity curves on a voxel/region basis to derive the biological parameters of interest. However, subject motion and photon count statistics are two of the fundamental issues in PET imaging and, if not accounted for, may lead to significant errors in the kinetic quantification for any clinical decision making. To address the uncertainties in photon emissions, direct parametric reconstruction approaches [1,2] have been developed to derive

---

* These authors contributed equally to this work.

P. Golland et al. (Eds.): MICCAI 2014, Part I, LNCS 8673, pp. 114–121, 2014.
© Springer International Publishing Switzerland 2014

the kinetic parameters directly from the raw PET data, with the incorporation of kinetic modelling. This improves the reconstruction by utilising the complete spatio-temporal information rather than inappropriately ignoring the temporal dependencies within the data. To address the subject motion, a framework is proposed in [3] to estimate subject motion in PET data with steady activity from simultaneous PET-MR reconstruction. In [4], the motion correction approach has been developed for reconstructed dynamic PET images using kinetic model based registration. To the best of our knowledge, so far there has not been any work yet to address both the kinetics and motion in a unified framework.

In this work, we propose a joint motion correction and parametric reconstruction framework for dynamic PET data, in which the subject motion and tracer kinetics are estimated directly from the raw photon counts, by maximising a penalised log-likelihood with respect to the motion parameters and the kinetic parameters. The problem of head movements in brain imaging is addressed here, thus a rigid transformation model is used and the motion parameters are updated by a trust region algorithm [5]. For modelling tracer kinetics, the data-driven basis function based approach is applied for generality, and we derive here a closed form update for the kinetic parameters in the penalised log-likelihood, by applying the optimisation transfer technique to decouple the dependencies between the voxels and also to separate each kinetic parameter for every voxel. This greatly improves the algorithm's convergence speed and also leads to a parallelisable solution of this problem. The simulation-based validation shows that the proposed method achieves a sub-voxel size motion correction residual in noisy data, and that the parametric reconstruction is improved with reduced bias. We also apply the proposed algorithm to real clinical [18F]Choline data, and the results show that it enhances the detection of a [18F]Choline hot spot in the brain which is otherwise difficult to identify due to motion and noise.

2   Method

Discretising the continuous 3-D+t PET activity $f(x,t)$, $x \in \mathbb{R}^3$, $t \in \mathbb{R}^+$, on a regular spatial grid $\boldsymbol{x} = [x_1, \ldots, x_{n_v}] \in \mathbb{R}^{n_v \times 3}$, and discrete temporal time $\boldsymbol{t} \in \mathbb{R}^{n_t}$ obtains $\boldsymbol{f} = f(\boldsymbol{x}, \boldsymbol{t}) \in \mathbb{R}^{n_v \times n_t}$, where n_v and n_t are the numbers of voxels and time frames respectively. Denote the PET system detected photon counts by $\boldsymbol{g} \in \mathbb{R}^{n_d \times n_t}$ where n_d is the number of detector pairs. Given the activity distribution $\boldsymbol{f}$, $\boldsymbol{g}$ is a Poisson random vector with parameter $\bar{g}(\boldsymbol{f}) = \boldsymbol{P}\boldsymbol{f} + \boldsymbol{r}$ where $\boldsymbol{P} \in \mathbb{R}^{n_d \times n_v}$ is the system matrix i.e. $[\boldsymbol{P}]_{i,j} = p_{i,j}$ is the probability that an event occurring in voxel j is detected by the detector pair i, and $\boldsymbol{r} \in \mathbb{R}^{n_d \times n_t}$ is the expected scattered and random events. The dynamic activity $\boldsymbol{f} = [\boldsymbol{f}_1, \ldots, \boldsymbol{f}_{n_t}]$, $\boldsymbol{f}_l \in \mathbb{R}^{n_v}$ being the activity at frame l, can be described by the tracer kinetic model $\mathcal{F}$ parameterised by $\boldsymbol{\vartheta} = \vartheta(\boldsymbol{x})$, $\boldsymbol{\vartheta} \in \mathbb{R}^{n_v \times n_k}$ where n_k is the number of kinetic parameters in the model, so that $\boldsymbol{f} = \mathcal{F}(\boldsymbol{\vartheta}) = [\mathcal{F}_1(\boldsymbol{\vartheta}), \ldots, \mathcal{F}_{n_t}(\boldsymbol{\vartheta})]$, $\mathcal{F}_l(\boldsymbol{\vartheta}) \in \mathbb{R}^{n_v}$ for all l. The kinetic model is assumed to be applied at each voxel independently i.e. $[\mathcal{F}_l(\boldsymbol{\vartheta})]_j = \mathcal{F}_l(\boldsymbol{\vartheta}_j)$, $\boldsymbol{\vartheta}_j \in \mathbb{R}^{n_k}$ being the kinetic parameter vector at voxel j. When the subject motion is present, the activity $\boldsymbol{f}$ is warped.

The motion can be modelled as a warping operator $\mathcal{W}$ parameterised by $\boldsymbol{\alpha} = [\boldsymbol{\alpha}_1, \ldots, \boldsymbol{\alpha}_{n_t}] \in \mathbb{R}^{n_w \times n_t}$ where n_w is the number of transformation parameters. Thus the activity at frame l is redefined as $\boldsymbol{f}_l = \mathcal{W}_{\boldsymbol{\alpha}_l} \mathcal{F}_l(\boldsymbol{\vartheta})$. The warping operator $\mathcal{W}_{\boldsymbol{\alpha}_l}$ is determined by the interpolation and its motion function $\varphi_{\boldsymbol{\alpha}_l} : \mathbb{R}^3 \to \mathbb{R}^3$, so that $\boldsymbol{f}_l = \mathcal{W}_{\boldsymbol{\alpha}_l} \mathcal{F}_l(\boldsymbol{\vartheta}) = \mathcal{F}_l \circ \vartheta(\varphi_{\boldsymbol{\alpha}_l}(\boldsymbol{x}))$. For kinetic model $\mathcal{F}$ and warping operator $\mathcal{W}$, the expected photon counts can be written as

$$\bar{g}(\boldsymbol{\vartheta}, \boldsymbol{\alpha}) = [\boldsymbol{P}\mathcal{W}_{\boldsymbol{\alpha}_1} \mathcal{F}_1(\boldsymbol{\vartheta}), \ldots, \boldsymbol{P}\mathcal{W}_{\boldsymbol{\alpha}_{n_t}} \mathcal{F}_{n_t}(\boldsymbol{\vartheta})] + \boldsymbol{r}. \qquad (1)$$

Omitting the constant terms, the log-likelihood of the detected events $\boldsymbol{g}$ is

$$L(\boldsymbol{g}|\boldsymbol{\vartheta}, \boldsymbol{\alpha}) = \sum_{l=1}^{n_t} \sum_{i=1}^{n_d} (g_{i,l} \log \bar{g}_{i,l}(\boldsymbol{\vartheta}, \boldsymbol{\alpha}_l) - \bar{g}_{i,l}(\boldsymbol{\vartheta}, \boldsymbol{\alpha}_l)),$$

where $\bar{g}_{i,l}(\boldsymbol{\vartheta}, \boldsymbol{\alpha}_l) = \sum_{j=1}^{n_v} p_{i,j} [\mathcal{W}_{\boldsymbol{\alpha}_l} \mathcal{F}_l(\boldsymbol{\vartheta})]_j + r_{i,l}$. Since the penalties $\boldsymbol{\vartheta}$ and $\boldsymbol{\alpha}$ are independent, the penalised log-likelihood (PL) function is $\Phi(\boldsymbol{\vartheta}, \boldsymbol{\alpha}) = L(\boldsymbol{g}|\boldsymbol{\vartheta}, \boldsymbol{\alpha}) - \beta U(\boldsymbol{\vartheta}) - \gamma V(\boldsymbol{\alpha})$, where $U(\boldsymbol{\vartheta})$ and $V(\boldsymbol{\alpha})$ are penalty functions, β and γ are hyperparameters. $\boldsymbol{\vartheta}$ and $\boldsymbol{\alpha}$ can then be estimated as $(\hat{\boldsymbol{\alpha}}, \hat{\boldsymbol{\vartheta}}) \in \arg\max_{\boldsymbol{\vartheta}, \boldsymbol{\alpha}} \Phi(\boldsymbol{\vartheta}, \boldsymbol{\alpha})$. Here we find a maximum by updating $\boldsymbol{\vartheta}$ and $\boldsymbol{\alpha}$ in alternation.

Given the measured photon counts $\boldsymbol{g}$ and current estimation of kinetic parameters $\boldsymbol{\vartheta}$, $\boldsymbol{\alpha}$ is updated by maximising $E(\boldsymbol{\alpha}) = L(\boldsymbol{g}|\boldsymbol{\vartheta}, \boldsymbol{\alpha}) - \gamma V(\boldsymbol{\alpha})$. The gradient of log-likelihood part, $\nabla_{\boldsymbol{\alpha}} L$ can be derived by applying the chain rule, as $\frac{\partial L}{\partial \alpha_{q,l}} = \sum_{i=1}^{n_d} (\frac{g_{i,l}}{\bar{g}_{i,l}} - 1) \frac{\partial \bar{g}_{i,l}}{\partial \alpha_{q,l}}$, with $\frac{\partial \bar{g}_{i,l}}{\partial \alpha_{q,l}} = \sum_{j=1}^{n_v} p_{i,j} \langle \nabla_{\varphi_{\boldsymbol{\alpha}_l}(x_j)} \mathcal{F}_l \circ \vartheta(\varphi_{\boldsymbol{\alpha}_l}(x_j)), \frac{\partial \varphi_{\boldsymbol{\alpha}_l}(x_j)}{\partial \alpha_{q,l}} \rangle$ where $\langle \cdot, \cdot \rangle$ is the inner product in $\mathbb{R}^3$. Furthermore, an approximated second order Taylor expansion gives

$$L(\boldsymbol{\alpha} + \Delta \boldsymbol{\alpha}) \approx L(\bar{g}(\boldsymbol{\vartheta}, \boldsymbol{\alpha})) + \nabla_{\bar{g}} L^\top \boldsymbol{J}_{\boldsymbol{\alpha}}(\bar{g}) \Delta \boldsymbol{\alpha} + \frac{1}{2} \Delta \boldsymbol{\alpha}^\top \boldsymbol{J}_{\boldsymbol{\alpha}}^\top(\bar{g}) [\nabla_{\bar{g}}^2 L] \boldsymbol{J}_{\boldsymbol{\alpha}}(\bar{g}) \Delta \boldsymbol{\alpha} \qquad (2)$$

where $\boldsymbol{J}_{\boldsymbol{\alpha}}(\bar{g}) \in \mathbb{R}^{(n_d \times n_t) \times (n_w \times n_t)}$ is the Jacobian of $\bar{g}$ w.r.t. $\boldsymbol{\alpha}$ and $\Delta \boldsymbol{\alpha}$ is a small perturbation on $\boldsymbol{\alpha}$ (reshaped into a vector). Therefore the Hessian matrix can be approximated by $H_{\boldsymbol{\alpha}}(L) \approx \boldsymbol{J}_{\boldsymbol{\alpha}}^\top(\bar{g}) [\nabla_{\bar{g}}^2 L] \boldsymbol{J}_{\boldsymbol{\alpha}}(\bar{g})$. Adding the gradient and Hessian of V allows to maximise Φ with respect to $\boldsymbol{\alpha}$ using a trust region algorithm [5]. Here the rigid brain motion is addressed, and no prior V is considered on $\boldsymbol{\alpha}$.

With the estimated $\boldsymbol{\alpha}$, the direct parametric reconstruction with motion compensation is performed to update $\boldsymbol{\vartheta}$ as the maximiser of the penalised log likelihood $G(\boldsymbol{\vartheta}) = L(\boldsymbol{g}|\boldsymbol{\vartheta}, \boldsymbol{\alpha}) - \beta U(\boldsymbol{\vartheta})$. Each warping operator $\mathcal{W}_{\boldsymbol{\alpha}_l}$ is replaced by its discrete version $\boldsymbol{W}_{\boldsymbol{\alpha}_l} \in \mathbb{R}^{n_v \times n_v}$. The composition $\boldsymbol{P}\mathcal{W}_{\boldsymbol{\alpha}_l}$ in (1) becomes a matrix product $\boldsymbol{P}\boldsymbol{W}_{\boldsymbol{\alpha}_l} = \boldsymbol{P}^l$ which represents the motion-compensated system matrix at frame l. We considered a quadratic prior $U(\boldsymbol{\vartheta}) = \frac{1}{8} \sum_{l,j} \sum_{m \in \mathcal{N}_j} \omega_{j,m} (\mathcal{F}_l(\boldsymbol{\vartheta}_j) - \mathcal{F}_l(\boldsymbol{\vartheta}_m))^2$, where $\mathcal{N}_j$ denotes the 26 voxels neighbourhood of voxel j and $\omega_{j,m}$ is the weighting factor equal to the inverse distance between voxels j and m.

To separate the voxels in $G(\boldsymbol{\vartheta})$, the optimisation transfer technique used in [1] was first applied on $L(\boldsymbol{g}|\boldsymbol{\vartheta}, \boldsymbol{\alpha})$ and $U(\boldsymbol{\vartheta})$ to derive surrogate functions $Q^L(\boldsymbol{\vartheta}|\boldsymbol{\vartheta}^{[k]})$ and $Q^U(\boldsymbol{\vartheta}|\boldsymbol{\vartheta}^{[k]})$, where $\boldsymbol{\vartheta}^{[k]}$ is the estimation at iteration k. For the log-likelihood, the surrogate function is $Q^L(\boldsymbol{\vartheta}|\boldsymbol{\vartheta}^{[k]}) = \sum_l \sum_j p_j^l (f_{j,l}^{\mathrm{em},[k]} \log(\mathcal{F}_l(\boldsymbol{\vartheta}_j)) - \mathcal{F}_l(\boldsymbol{\vartheta}_j))$, where $f_{j,l}^{\mathrm{em},[k]} = \frac{\mathcal{F}_l(\boldsymbol{\vartheta}_j^{[k]})}{p_j^l} \sum_i p_{i,j}^l \frac{g_{i,l}}{\bar{g}_{i,l}(\boldsymbol{\vartheta}^{[k]})}$, $p_{i,j}^l = [\boldsymbol{P}^l]_{i,j}$ and $p_j^l = \sum_i p_{i,j}^l$. For the quadratic penalty, $Q^U(\boldsymbol{\vartheta}|\boldsymbol{\vartheta}^{[k]}) = \frac{1}{2}\sum_{l,j}\omega_j(f_{j,l}^{\mathrm{reg},[k]} - \mathcal{F}_l(\boldsymbol{\vartheta}_j))^2$, where $\omega_j = \sum_{m\in\mathcal{N}_j}\omega_{j,m}$, and $f_{j,l}^{\mathrm{reg},[k]} = \frac{1}{2\omega_j}\sum_{m\in\mathcal{N}_j}\omega_{j,m}(\mathcal{F}_l(\boldsymbol{\vartheta}_j^{[k]}) + \mathcal{F}_l(\boldsymbol{\vartheta}_m^{[k]}))$. The resulting surrogate separates the voxels so that each $\boldsymbol{\vartheta}_j$ can be obtained independently by maximising $q_j(\boldsymbol{\vartheta}_j|\boldsymbol{\vartheta}^{[k]}) = q_j^L(\boldsymbol{\vartheta}_j|\boldsymbol{\vartheta}^{[k]}) - \beta q_j^U(\boldsymbol{\vartheta}_j|\boldsymbol{\vartheta}^{[k]})$, where $q_j^L(\boldsymbol{\vartheta}_j|\boldsymbol{\vartheta}^{[k]}) = \sum_l p_j^l(f_{j,l}^{\mathrm{em},[k]}\log(\mathcal{F}_l(\boldsymbol{\vartheta}_j)) - \mathcal{F}_l(\boldsymbol{\vartheta}_j))$ and $q_j^U(\boldsymbol{\vartheta}_j|\boldsymbol{\vartheta}^{[k]}) = \sum_l \frac{1}{2}\omega_j(f_{j,l}^{\mathrm{reg},[k]} - \mathcal{F}_l(\boldsymbol{\vartheta}_j))^2$.

Generally, maximising $q_j(\boldsymbol{\vartheta}_j|\boldsymbol{\vartheta}^{[k]})$ can be solved by a non-linear optimisation algorithm at each voxel j. Note that the activity depends on the form of the kinetic model $\mathcal{F}$, and both linear and non-linear models can be used. In this work, a closed-form solution to update $\boldsymbol{\vartheta}_j^{[k]}$ was derived with linear kinetic models $\mathcal{F}(\boldsymbol{\vartheta}) = \boldsymbol{\vartheta}B$, where $B \in \mathbb{R}^{n_k \times n_t}$ is the temporal basis matrix.

With $\mathcal{F}_l(\boldsymbol{\vartheta}_j) = \sum_q \vartheta_{j,q}b_{q,l}$, $b_{q,l} = [B]_{q,l}$, the optimisation transfer can be applied again on the log part $q_j^L(\boldsymbol{\vartheta}_j|\boldsymbol{\vartheta}^{[k]})$ and the quadratic part $q_j^U(\boldsymbol{\vartheta}_j|\boldsymbol{\vartheta}^{[k]})$ to separate each of the n_k parameters $\vartheta_{j,q} \in \mathbb{R}^+$. A separable surrogate function for $q_j(\boldsymbol{\vartheta}_j|\boldsymbol{\vartheta}^{[k]})$ at sub-iteration r is

$$\tilde{q}_j(\boldsymbol{\vartheta}_j|\boldsymbol{\vartheta}_j^{[k,r]}) = \sum_{q=1}^{n_k} \tilde{b}_{j,q}(\vartheta_{j,q}^{\mathrm{em},[k,r]}\log(\vartheta_{j,q}) - \vartheta_{j,q}) - \beta\frac{1}{2}\omega_j a_q\left(\vartheta_{j,q} - \vartheta_{j,q}^{\mathrm{reg},[k,r]}\right)^2$$

$$= \sum_{q=1}^{n_k} \ell_{j,q}^{[k,r]}(\vartheta_{j,q}), \tag{3}$$

$$\vartheta_{j,q}^{\mathrm{em},[k,r]} = \tilde{b}_{j,q}^{-1}\vartheta_{j,q}^{[k,r]}\sum_l \frac{p_j^l b_{q,l} f_{j,l}^{\mathrm{em},[k]}}{\mathcal{F}_l(\boldsymbol{\vartheta}_j^{[k,r]})} \text{ and } \vartheta_{j,q}^{\mathrm{reg},[k,r]} = \vartheta_{j,q}^{[k,r]} - \frac{\sum_l b_{q,l}(\mathcal{F}_l(\boldsymbol{\vartheta}_j^{[k,r]}) - f_{j,l}^{\mathrm{reg},[k]})}{a_q}$$

are the intermediate parametric values at voxel j, $\tilde{b}_{j,q} = \sum_l p_j^l b_{q,l}$, and $a_q = \sum_l b_{q,l}\sum_{q'} b_{q',l}$. The quadratic surrogate was obtained using De Pierro's technique [6]. Note that $\vartheta_{j,q}^{\mathrm{em},[k,r]}$ corresponds to the nested EM update from [7] whereas $\vartheta_{j,q}^{\mathrm{reg},[k,r]}$ is a quasi-Newton update of $\vartheta_{j,q}^{[k,r]}$ to minimise $\sum_l(\mathcal{F}_l(\boldsymbol{\vartheta}_j^{[k,r]}) - f_{j,l}^{\mathrm{reg},[k]})^2$. Each $\ell_{j,q}^{[k,r]}$ in (3) has a unique maximiser which corresponds to the $r+1$ inner-update of the optimisation w.r.t. $\boldsymbol{\vartheta}$ with the current $f_{j,l}^{\mathrm{em},[k]}$ and $f_{j,l}^{\mathrm{reg},[k]}$:

$$\vartheta_{j,q}^{[k,r+1]} = \frac{1}{2\beta\omega_j a_q}\left(\beta\omega_j a_q\vartheta_{j,q}^{\mathrm{reg},[k,r]} - \tilde{b}_{j,q} + \sqrt{\Delta_{j,q}(\vartheta_{j,q}^{\mathrm{em},[k,r]}, \vartheta_{j,q}^{\mathrm{reg},[k,r]})}\right), \tag{4}$$

where $\Delta_{j,q}(\vartheta_{j,q}^{\mathrm{em},[k,r]}, \vartheta_{j,q}^{\mathrm{reg},[k,r]}) = (\beta\omega_j a_q\vartheta_{j,q}^{\mathrm{reg},[k,r]} - \tilde{b}_{j,q})^2 + 4\beta\omega_j a_q\tilde{b}_{j,q}\vartheta_{j,q}^{\mathrm{em},[k,r]}$. For given $\boldsymbol{\alpha}$, the penalised likelihood function is concave and a monotonic convergence is guaranteed for $\boldsymbol{\vartheta}$ [1]. The overall scheme is summarised in Algorithm 1.

To relate the linear coefficients $\boldsymbol{\vartheta}$ directly with the transport rate constants in the compartmental model to represent the tracer kinetics, the temporal basis B is defined as in spectral analysis [8], which is able to describe differing tracer behaviour across all voxels in the image, as $b_{q,l} = \int_{t_{l,s}}^{t_{l,e}} e^{-\phi_q\tau} \star C_p(\tau)d\tau$, where $\star$ is the convolution, $t_{l,s}$, $t_{l,e}$ are the starting and ending times of frame l, $\phi = [\phi_1, \ldots, \phi_q, \ldots, \phi_{n_k}]$ are the pre-chosen kinetic rate constants from a physiologically plausible range, and $C_p(t)$ is the plasma input function. Note that if needed, the blood component can be added to the temporal basis to account for the blood volume in the measured PET data as $b_{0,l} = \int_{t_{l,s}}^{t_{l,e}} C_B(\tau)d\tau$ where $C_B(t)$ is the activity in blood. To ensure the sufficient representation of the kinetics, usually the temporal basis $\boldsymbol{B}$ is over-complete. The under-determined problem is constrained by the non-negativity of $\boldsymbol{\vartheta}$, which represents the transport rate constants so intrinsically $\boldsymbol{\vartheta} \geq \boldsymbol{0}$.

Algorithm 1. Joint 4-D parametric reconstruction and motion correction

---

Input: PET projection data $\boldsymbol{g}$, the basis function $\boldsymbol{B}$, regularisation parameter β
Output: Motion-corrected parametric images $\boldsymbol{\vartheta}$ and the motion estimate $\boldsymbol{\alpha}$.
Initialisation $\boldsymbol{\alpha} = \boldsymbol{0}$, $\boldsymbol{\vartheta} = 0.01$;
while *not converged* **do**
  $\boldsymbol{\vartheta}^{[0]} = \boldsymbol{\vartheta}$;
  for $k=1,\ldots,K$ **do**
    Compute $f_{j,l}^{\mathrm{em},[k]}$ and $f_{j,l}^{\mathrm{reg},[k]}$ from $\boldsymbol{\vartheta}^{[k-1]}$ for all j,l ;
    $\boldsymbol{\vartheta}^{[k,0]} = \boldsymbol{\vartheta}^{[k-1]}$;
    for $r=1,\ldots,R$ **do**
      Compute $\vartheta_{j,q}^{\mathrm{em},[k,r]}, \vartheta_{j,q}^{\mathrm{reg},[k,r]}$ from $\boldsymbol{\vartheta}_j^{[k,r-1]}$ for all j,q ;
      Update $\boldsymbol{\vartheta}^{[k,r]}$ by (4) ;
    end
    $\boldsymbol{\vartheta}^{[k]} = \boldsymbol{\vartheta}^{[k,R]}$;
  end
  $\boldsymbol{\vartheta} = \boldsymbol{\vartheta}^{[K]}$;
  Optimise $\boldsymbol{\alpha}$ using the trust region algorithm with the gradient and Hessian derived from (2) and the current estimate of $\boldsymbol{\vartheta}$;
end

---

3 Results

3.1 Simulation-Based Validation

The proposed algorithm was firstly validated using simulated [11C]Raclopride data. 60-min dynamic PET scans were generated based on the Zubal brain phantom, with various kinetics defined on background, grey matter, white matter, cerebellum, putamen and caudate nucleus. The time activity curves were generated based on the two-tissue compartment model using kinetic parameters derived from clinical studies in conjunction with a population input function. Rigid head movements were introduced by transforming the activity images at various time points (Fig. 1), in accordance with the expected amplitude and frequency of head motion that happens within a brain scan. In practice, detection of such motion events can be performed by applying the PCA technique proposed in [9] with a moving time window for dynamic PET data. The activity images were defined on a grid of $128 \times 128 \times 80$ voxels and then used to generate PET projections (5 mm FWHM resolution). Poisson noise was added to the projections and reconstruction was then performed with ideal pre-reconstruction correction for randoms, scatter and attenuation (e.g. derived from the simultaneous CT or MRI [10]). For comparison, the direct parametric reconstruction without motion correction (*direct*) [1] and the indirect parametric reconstruction with motion correction (*indirect+MC*) [4] were also performed in addition to the proposed algorithm (*direct+MC*). In all the methods we used spectral analysis [8] for kinetic modelling with the same temporal basis functions $\boldsymbol{B}$ for which $n_k = 16$,

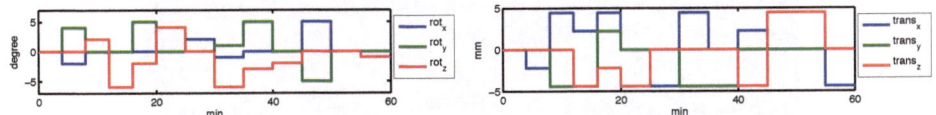

Fig. 1. Simulated random rigid head movements

and ϕ_q is spaced logarithmically in the range of $[0.0001s^{-1}, 1s^{-1}]$. Different β values were applied to each reconstruction. For the *indirect+MC* method, the quadratic penalty with β was applied to reconstructing the activity images by MLEM [6]. Motion correction accuracy was quantified by the target registration error (TRE) [11] averaged over time, shown in Fig. 2. For the parametric recon-

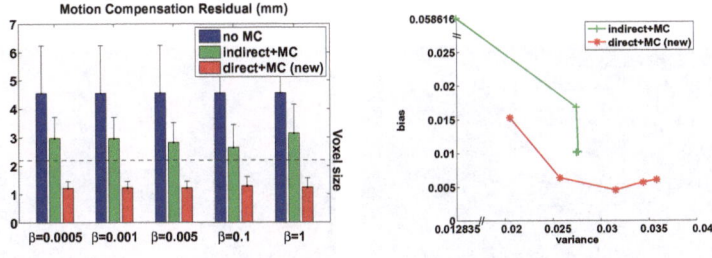

Fig. 2. Left: Motion correction performance quantified by time-averaged target registration error (TRE). The proposed *direct+MC* achieves sub-voxel size(< 2.2 mm) MC accuracy with noisy data, the β range has little impact on the motion correction performance due to the low smoothing level; Right: Bias versus variance trade-off of the volume of distribution (V_T) images of [^{11}C]Raclopride reconstructed by *indirect+MC* and *direct+MC (new)*. Data points from left to right correspond to β values of 1, 0.1, 0.005, 0.001 and 0.0005. The proposed *direct+MC* algorithm achieves lower bias.

struction, the outcome measures of interest, which is the volume of distribution V_T for [^{11}C]Raclopride was calculated using ϑ, by $V_T = \sum_q \frac{\vartheta_q}{\phi_q}$ [12]. The corresponding bias and variance plots of the parametric reconstruction of V_T are shown in Fig. 2, and Fig. 3 shows the ground truth and reconstructed V_T images by all these methods from one simulated scan.

3.2   Clinical Data

The proposed algorithm was also applied to reconstruct clinical [^{18}F]Choline data from a patient scanned for 44 mins using a Siemens Biograph mMR scanner. The reconstruction was performed by the proposed algorithm integrated with STIR [13]. The attenuation correction was conducted during the iterations using the attenuation map repositioned by the current motion estimate to account for the mismatch caused by motion. The kinetic parameter of interest

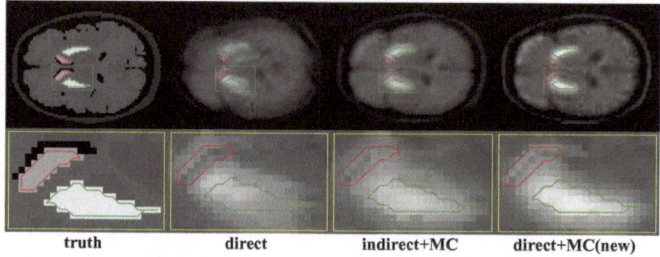

Fig. 3. Selected slice ($z : 45/80$) of the reconstructed V_T images of [^{11}C]Raclopride when the penalty weight $\beta = 0.005$. The direct reconstruction with no motion correction (*direct*) results in severely blurred images. The indirect reconstruction with post MC in the image space (*indirect+MC*) loses the spatial contrast due to inadequate MC. The proposed joint direct reconstruction with motion correction (*direct+MC*) better preserves the ROIs (e.g. putamen).

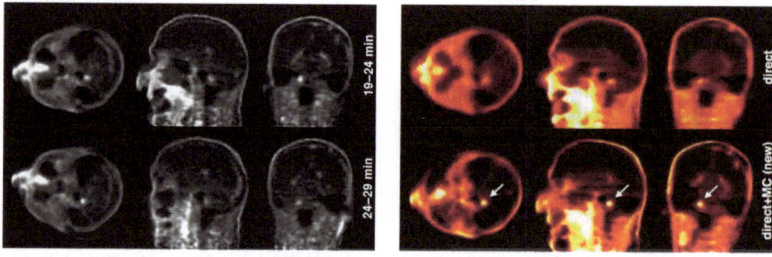

Fig. 4. Left: Two [^{18}F]Choline time frames reconstructed by MLEM to illustrate the data. Right: The K_I images reconstructed by the *direct* method without motion correction, and by the proposed *direct+MC* algorithm. The identification of the [^{18}F]Choline hot spot is greatly enhanced by the proposed method.

K_I was calculated for [^{18}F]Choline, which is the irreversible uptake rate constant from plasma defined by $K_I = \vartheta_{n_k}$ (corresponds to $\phi_{n_k} = 0$) [12]. For the temporal basis functions $\boldsymbol{B}$, $n_k = 16$ and ϕ_q is logarithmically in the range of $[0.000001s^{-1}, 0.01s^{-1}]$. Fig. 4 shows the reconstruction of K_I by the *direct* method without motion correction and by the proposed *direct+MC* algorithm. The result demonstrates that, by applying the proposed method, the reconstructed K_I image shows the [^{18}F]Choline hot spot which is otherwise difficult to identify due to motion or noise.

4   Discussion and Conclusion

This work proposed a novel algorithm for joint motion correction and parametric reconstruction of dynamic PET data, which addresses two of the fundamental issues in PET imaging in a unified framework. In particular, a parallelisable closed form solution of a sub-problem derived here has greatly enhanced the computational efficiency for practical use. Initial evaluation on clinical data has shown improved identification of the kinetic activity in the regions of interest. The proposed method can adapt to different PET tracers without the need of reimplementation, and future evaluation over a range of clinical applications will determine the full utility of the method.

Acknowledgement. EPSRC (EP/H046410/1, EP/J020990/1, EP/K005278), the MRC (MR/J01107X/1), the NIHR Biomedical Research Unit (Dementia) at UCL and the National Institute for Health Research University College London Hospitals Biomedical Research Centre (NIHR BRC UCLH/UCL High Impact Initiative), Roger Gunn and Graham Searle from Imanova Ltd (kinetic analysis).

References

1. Wang, G., Qi, J.: An optimization transfer algorithm for nonlinear parametric image reconstruction from dynamic PET data. IEEE. Trans. on Med. Imag. 31(10), 1977–1988 (2012)
2. Cheng, X., Navab, N., Ziegler, S.I., Shi, K.: Direct Parametric Image Reconstruction of Rapid Multi-tracer PET. In: Mori, K., Sakuma, I., Sato, Y., Barillot, C., Navab, N. (eds.) MICCAI 2013, Part III. LNCS, vol. 8151, pp. 155–162. Springer, Heidelberg (2013)
3. Pedemonte, S., Bousse, A., Hutton, B.F., Arridge, S., Ourselin, S.: 4-D generative model for PET/MRI reconstruction. In: Fichtinger, G., Martel, A., Peters, T. (eds.) MICCAI 2011, Part I. LNCS, vol. 6891, pp. 581–588. Springer, Heidelberg (2011)
4. Jiao, J., Searle, G.E., Tziortzi, A.C., Salinas, C.A., Gunn, R.N., Schnabel, J.A.: Spatio-temporal pharmacokinetic model based registration of 4D PET neuroimaging data. Neuroimage 84, 225–235 (2014)
5. Madsen, K., Nielsen, H.B., Tingleff, O.: Methods for non-linear least-squares problems. Technical report, Technical University of Denmark (2004)
6. De Pierro, A.R.: A modified expectation maximization algorithm for penalized likelihood estimation in emission tomography. IEEE Trans. on Med. Imag. 14(1), 132–137 (1995)
7. Wang, G., Qi, J.: Acceleration of the direct reconstruction of linear parametric images using nested algorithms. Phys. Med. Biol. 55, 1505–1517 (2010)
8. Cunningham, V.J., Jones, T.: Spectral analysis of dynamic PET studies. J. Cereb. Blood Flow Metab. 13(1), 15–23 (1993)
9. Thielemans, K., Schleyer, P., Dunn, J., Marsden, P.K., Manjeshwar, R.M.: Using PCA to detect head motion from PET list mode data. In: IEEE Nucl. Sci. Syp. & Med. Im. Conf. (2013)
10. Burgos, N., Cardoso, M.J., Modat, M., Pedemonte, S., Dickson, J., Barnes, A., Duncan, J.S., Atkinson, D., Arridge, S.R., Hutton, B.F., Ourselin, S.: Attenuation correction synthesis for hybrid PET-MR scanners. In: Mori, K., Sakuma, I., Sato, Y., Barillot, C., Navab, N. (eds.) MICCAI 2013, Part I. LNCS, vol. 8149, pp. 147–154. Springer, Heidelberg (2013)
11. Fitzpatrick, J., West, J., Maurer Jr., C.R.: Predicting error in rigid-body point-based registration. IEEE Trans. on Med. Imag. 17(5), 694–702 (1998)
12. Gunn, R.N., Gunn, S.R., Cunningham, V.J.: Positron emission tomography compartmental models. J. Cereb. Blood Flow Metab. 21(6), 635–652 (2001)
13. Thielemans, K., Tsoumpas, C., Mustafovic, S., Beisel, T., Aguiar, P., Dikaios, N., Jacobson, M.W.: STIR: software for tomographic image reconstruction release 2. Phys. Med. Biol. 57(4), 867–883 (2012)

Deformable Reconstruction of Histology Sections Using Structural Probability Maps

Markus Müller[1], Mehmet Yigitsoy[1], Hauke Heibel[3], and Nassir Navab[1,2]

[1] Computer Aided Medical Procedures, Technische Universität München, Germany
[2] Computer Aided Medical Procedures, Johns Hopkins University, USA
[3] microDimensions GmbH, München, Germany

Abstract. The reconstruction of a 3D volume from a stack of 2D histology slices is still a challenging problem especially if no external references are available. Without a reference, standard registration approaches tend to align structures that should not be perfectly aligned. In this work we introduce a deformable, reference-free reconstruction method that uses an internal structural probability map (SPM) to regularize a free-form deformation. The SPM gives an estimate of the original 3D structure of the sample from the misaligned and possibly corrupted 2D slices. We present a consecutive as well as a simultaneous reconstruction approach that incorporates this estimate in a deformable registration framework. Experiments on synthetic and mouse brain datasets indicate that our method produces similar results compared to reference-based techniques on synthetic datasets. Moreover, it improves the smoothness of the reconstruction compared to standard registration techniques on real data.

1 Introduction

With a high resolution up to $0.25\,\mu m$, microscopy histology is an important technique to study anatomy on cellular level. Histology slices are created by cutting a tissue sample into ultra thin slices. These slices are then stained with certain chemicals in order to highlight different structures and finally the results are observed under a microscope. This process, however, introduces structural inconsistencies between slices: especially the stress put on the sample during cutting leads to deformations and artifacts such as holes, tears or foldings. Such artifacts make the reconstructing of a 3D volume from the individual slices very challenging. Nevertheless, such a reconstruction is very useful when assessing the progression of structures over several slices or creating atlases on micron level.

There are various techniques for reconstructing a histology volume. While global rigid/affine approaches are not able to correct for the local deformations resulting from the cutting procedure [1,2], a common approach applies several rigid/affine transformations on successive smaller subdivision of each image [3]. While this approach produces good results with a reasonable runtime, a local deformable registration is more suited to model the deformation of the cutting precedure and therefore improve the consistency between consecutive pairs. On the other hand this will also perfectly align structures that are not supposed to be

P. Golland et al. (Eds.): MICCAI 2014, Part I, LNCS 8673, pp. 122–129, 2014.

aligned anatomically, therefore straightening all features in stack direction and deviating from the original shape of underlying structures. Literally speaking, a deformable registration of a stack forming a cone would turn it into a cylinder which is not desirable.

One common approach to avoid this drift problem is to register each slice to an external reference. Either 3D in-vivo images such as Magnetic Resonance Images (MRI) [4] or so called block-face images, acquired by taking an image of the tissue block-face before cutting each histology slice [5], can be used as external references. While these methods provide excellent results, a reference is often not available. To circumvent the need for external references, Gaffling et al. [6] introduced a reference-free method that uses the regression of manually extracted landmarks to restrict the deformation. By using a polynomial regression over corresponding landmark positions, they obtain a smooth and consistent reconstruction of histology slices. Although the results of this method seem promising, given the large size of histology slices, manual extraction of landmarks is not feasible in practice and the author does not reference any method for automatic detection. Another reference-free method was proposed in [7] which extracts vessel structures from each slice and performs a rigid- followed by a deformable registration, that are both based on the extracted features. While this seems to produce very promising results on a liver sample, it is difficult to extend to samples that do not contain washed out vessel structures, like brain datasets.

In this paper, we propose two new, reference-free methods for 3D histology reconstruction that use the structural coherency of the histology data as an internal regularization. Our methods do not require any landmark extraction or blockface image acquisition processes. Inspired by [8], we employ the tensor voting framework [9] to extract a structural probability map (SPM), which contains a rough estimate of the original structures of the stack that should be retained by the registration. For structures that were destroyed in one slice, SPM can still be estimated from the surrounding slices. Coupled with the intensity similarity and the deformation regularization, SPM is used as a structural regularization constraint in the registration framework.

2   Methods

2.1   Structural Probability Map

Tensor voting is a conceptual grouping method that is employed for the inference of salient structures from a set of incoherent input points [9]. Inference is based on a communication scheme where every point, *voter*, casts its information that is encoded as a second order symmetric tensor, $\mathbf{T}$, to other sites, *votee*, over a hypothesized smooth curve with low total curvature. The strength of the vote cast depends on the voter's perceptual salience, the voter-to-votee distance, as well as the curvature of presumed curve connecting them. A votee at $\mathbf{y}$ accumulates incoming votes from all voters $\mathbf{x}$, using tensor addition $\mathbf{T}(\mathbf{y}) = \sum_{\mathbf{x} \in \mathcal{P}} \mathbf{A}^{\mathbf{x}}(\mathbf{y})$ where $\mathcal{P}$ is the set of voters and $\mathbf{A}^{\mathbf{x}}(\mathbf{y})$ is a tensor vote that $\mathbf{x}$ casts at $\mathbf{y}$. A tensor is represented as $\mathbf{T} = \sum_{d=1}^{\mathcal{D}} \lambda_d \hat{e}_d \hat{e}_d^T$ which can be decomposed as

$$\mathbf{T} = \sum_{d=1}^{\mathcal{D}-1} (\lambda_d - \lambda_{d+1}) \sum_{k=1}^{d} \hat{e}_k \hat{e}_k^T + \lambda_{\mathcal{D}} \sum_{k=1}^{\mathcal{D}} \hat{e}_k \hat{e}_k^T \tag{1}$$

$$= \sum_{d=1}^{\mathcal{D}} s_d \mathcal{N}_d \quad \text{with} \quad s_d = \begin{cases} \lambda_d - \lambda_{d+1} & , d < \mathcal{D} \\ \lambda_{\mathcal{D}} & , d = \mathcal{D} \end{cases} \quad \text{and} \quad \mathcal{N}_d = \sum_{k=1}^{d} \hat{e}_k \hat{e}_k^T$$

where $\lambda_1 \geq \ldots \geq \lambda_{\mathcal{D}} \geq 0$ are eigenvalues, $\hat{e}_1 \ldots \hat{e}_{\mathcal{D}}$ are eigenvectors of $\mathbf{T}$, s_d is the salience, $\mathcal{N}_d$ is the d-D normal space, and $\mathcal{D}$ is the dimensionality of the space [10]. Every structure type is identified by the dimensionality, d, of its normal space, $\mathcal{N}_d$ and its strength is determined by the magnitude of its salience, s_d. Similar to the above decomposition, a tensor vote $\mathbf{A}^{\times}(\mathbf{y})$ can be written as

$$\mathbf{A}^{\times}(\mathbf{y}) = \sum_{d=1}^{\mathcal{D}} s_d^{\times} \mathbf{A}_d^{\times}(\mathbf{y}) \quad \text{with} \quad \mathbf{A}_d^{\times}(\mathbf{y}) = \sum_{j=1}^{d} \mathbf{S}_{d,j}^{\times}(\mathbf{y}) \tag{2}$$

where $\mathbf{A}_d^{\times}(\mathbf{y})$ is a vote for structure type d that consists of stick votes, $\mathbf{S}_{d,j}^{\times}(\mathbf{y})$, for each basis vector of $\mathcal{N}_d^{\times}$. Due to the limited space, we refer the reader to [9,8] for the details regarding the stick vote and communication scheme.

Let $I = (I_1, ..., I_n)$ be a stack of 2D images. We consider this stack as a volumetric image. We further define structural probability map images $SPM = (SPM_1, ..., SPM_n)$ where $SPM_i(\mathbf{y})$ is the structural saliency at $\mathbf{y}$. In this paper, we consider strong edges in images I_i detected by a standard 2D edge detector as the set of voters $\mathcal{P} = (\mathcal{P}_1, ..., \mathcal{P}_n)$ and every point in the SPM as votees. Inference is done by performing a voting for each votee and then extracting surface saliences from the accumulated tensors $\mathbf{T}(\mathbf{y})$ using Eq.1, which are set as scalar values for $SPM(\mathbf{y})$.

2.2 Consecutive Registration

We assume that the histology stack was already roughly pre-aligned by a standard rigid registration, thus our method aims to improve the smoothness by performing a modified deformable registration based on 2D Free-Form Deformations (FFDs). We model the deformations as a discrete optimization problem using Markov Random Fields (MRFs) [11]. A 2D FFD grid G^i is assigned to every slice I_i, thus each control point $\mathbf{p}$ resembles a node in the MRF. In order to model the actual displacement of control points we designate a labeling l of discrete values to all nodes. Each label $l_{\mathbf{p}}$ therefore describes the displacement $\mathbf{d}_{l_{\mathbf{p}}}$ of the control point $\mathbf{p}$ (see Fig. 1). The labeling problem can then be solved with a quadratic pseudo-boolean optimization (QPBO) algorithm [12].

In our first approach the labeling is solved consecutively for each slice I_i in the stack:

$$E_i(l) = \sum_{\mathbf{p} \in G^i} \left(E_{data}(I_i, I_{i+1}, l_{\mathbf{p}}) + \gamma E_{SPM}(\mathcal{P}_i, SPM_i, l_{\mathbf{p}}) + \rho R(\mathbf{d}_{l_{\mathbf{p}}}) \right) \tag{3}$$

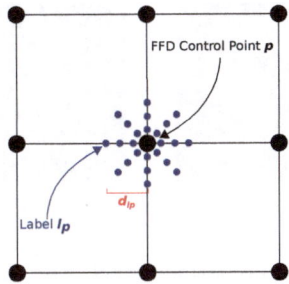

Fig. 1. Example for MRF labeling around a control point

γ and ρ weight the contribution of the regularization. E_{data} compares the deformed slice with the undeformed neighbour with a Normalized Cross Correlation (NCC), that yields robust results with lower computational cost. Other similarity measures like Mutual Information are possible but have not been tested yet.

$$E_{data}(I_i, I_{i+1}, l_{\mathbf{p}}) = \sum_{\mathbf{x}} NCC(I_i(\mathbf{x} + \mathbf{d}_{l_{\mathbf{p}}}), I_{i+1}) \tag{4}$$

We are not registering to the deformed neighbouring slice because this would accumulate deformations and therefore introduce a strong drift. Therefore this term alone can only align the slices roughly, because the deformations of two neighboring slices are not connected. However, the smoothness is improved by E_{SPM} that aligns the edges with the estimated structure map. Since the SPM represents the 3D structure of the stack, it also contrains the 2D FFDs in order to respect the global consistency of the structures and avoid clustering.

$$E_{SPM}(\mathcal{P}_i, SPM_i, l_{\mathbf{p}}) = \sum_{\mathbf{x}} NCC(\mathcal{P}_i(\mathbf{x} + \mathbf{d}_{l_{\mathbf{p}}}), SPM_i) \tag{5}$$

The energy R penalizes implausible or unnatural deformations and, in our case, depends only on the distance of all in-plane neighbours $N(\mathbf{p})$ of each control point $\mathbf{p}$:

$$R(l_{\mathbf{p}}) = \sum_{r \in N(\mathbf{p})} ||\mathbf{d}_{l_{\mathbf{p}}} - \mathbf{d}_{l_r}||^2 \tag{6}$$

The consecutive registration method has the advantage of being fast and performs well when the stack does not involve too complex structures or deformations (e.g. the synthetic data used in section 3.1). However, because the deformations are not directly connected between slices, its performance deteriorates when the tissue deformations are complicated which is often the case in real histology data.

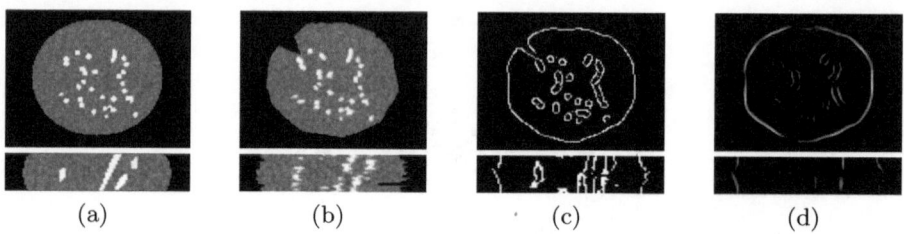

(a)   (b)   (c)   (d)

Fig. 2. Synthetic dataset: (a) undeformed stack, (b) corrupted stack, (c) edge map, (d) structural probability map

2.3   Simultaneous Registration

Therefore, we extended our algorithm to register the whole stack simultaneously, which is computational more expensive but also produces better results. For this we employ a method similar to the one proposed in [5], which splits the MRF energy into one pair-wise term and two unary ones.

$$E(l) = \sum_{i=1}^{n-1} \sum_{\substack{\mathbf{p} \in G^i \\ \mathbf{q} \in G^{i+1}}} E_{data}(I_i, I_{i+1}, l_{\mathbf{p}}, l_{\mathbf{q}}) + \sum_{i=1}^{n} \sum_{\mathbf{p} \in G^i} \left(\gamma E_{SPM}(\mathcal{P}_i, SPM_i, l_{\mathbf{p}}) + \rho R(l_{\mathbf{p}}) \right)$$

(7)

In this formulation, the unary terms E_{SPM} and R stay the same as Eqs. 5 and 6 respectively and act as in-plane regularizations. However, to make the model better, we recapitulate the data term E_{data} in a pair-wise manner by coupling the deformations of neighboring slices.

$$E_{data}(I_i, I_{i+1}, l_{\mathbf{p}}, l_{\mathbf{q}}) = \sum_{\mathbf{x}} NCC(I_i(\mathbf{x} + \mathbf{d}_{l_{\mathbf{p}}}), I_{i+1}(\mathbf{x} + \mathbf{d}_{l_{\mathbf{q}}})) \tag{8}$$

Contrary to Eq. 4, the term now connects the control points (or more accurately its labels) of neighboring slices, thus significantly increasing their possible alignment. This also means that the weighting γ should be treated differently in the simultaneous case (Eq. 7) than in the consecutive one (Eq. 3), because E_{SPM} is now only responsible for the regularization and no more for the smoothness itself. For the consecutive one we empirically found out that $\gamma = 1.0$ is good overall value but can be increased if the structure map is of good quality. Whereas for the simultaneous registration, a lower value around 0.5 usually produces regularized but still structurally consistent results.

3   Experimental Validation and Results

3.1   Synthetic data

We performed experiments on synthetic and real data. The synthetic data consists of a stack of 20 slices with a resolution of 128x96 and a pixel spacing of

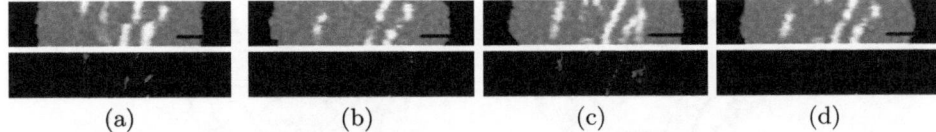

(a)   (b)   (c)   (d)

Fig. 3. Reconstruction results in the first row and absolute difference with Fig. 2(a) in the second. (a) Consecutive Registration w/o SPM, (b) Consecutive Registration w/ SPM, (c) Simultaneous Registration w/o SPM, (d) Simultaneous Registration w/ SPM.

1mm. An example of an original slice is shown in Fig. 2(a). The slices contain a circular tissue which grows to the middle and several skewed vascular structures. Each slice is deformed by a random FFD with a maximum displacement of 5mm and the deformation field is saved as ground truth. Additional tears are introduced in randomly selected slices to simulate the real histology cutting process. Distorted slices are shown in Fig. 2(b).

In order to quantify the results of our method, we calculated the absolute end point error (EE) and the relative angular error (AE) between the resulting deformation fields and the ground truth fields [13]. Table 1 shows the errors after the application of different reconstruction approaches discussed here.

Table 1. End point error (EE) and angular error (AE) of the presented methods

Method	EE		AE	
	Error (mm)	STD (mm)	Error (°)	STD (°)
Consecutive Registration w/o SPM	2.91	1.78	60.31	31.41
Consecutive Registration w/ SPM	1.69	1.25	45.39	26.63
Simultaneous Registration w/o SPM	2.37	1.27	57.31	33.17
Simultaneous Registration w/ SPM	1.68	1.13	45.95	26.89

For the registration we used a grid spacing of 15mm and 2 grid levels. In the consecutive case both ρ and γ were set to 1.0 in order to put more emphasis on the structural map. For the simultaneous method, we used 0.5 for both instead. The results in Fig. 3 show the same coronal slice as Fig. 2.

The consecutive registration without the SPM regularization performs worst in terms of the error but also in it's visual appearance (c.f. Fig. 3(a)). All curvilinear structures get straightened in stack direction and especially two vessel structures on the right side cluster into four distinctive structures. Extending this with our SPM maintains the outer round shape but also preserves the curvilinearity of the vessels inside (Fig. 3(b)). This is similiar for the simultaneous method: while the unregularized registration (Fig. 3(c)) does perform significantly better than the unregularized consecutive method from a visual perspective, it still produces a high error which can be again compensated with the use of our SPM. Since the

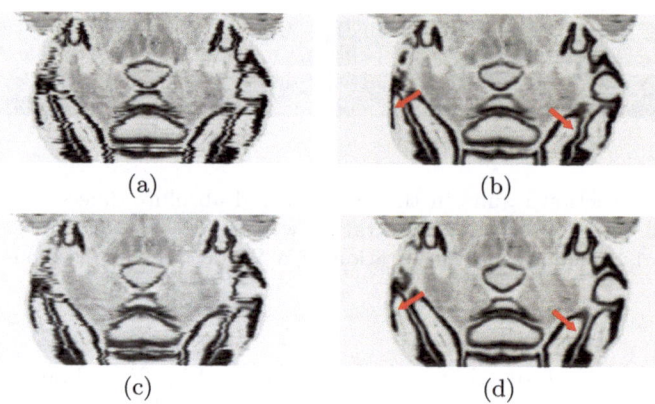

(a)   (b)

(c)   (d)

Fig. 4. Coronal view of the reconstructed mouse brain dataset: (a) rigidly aligned source stack, (b) simultaneous registration w/o SPM, (c) consecutive registration w/ SPM, (d) simultaneous registration w/ SPM.

simultaneous methods put more emphasis on aligning the actual image data, the reconstructed stacks have a slightly smoother appearance (Fig. 3(c)). However, without the regularization through a structure map, there is a drift error. Also the results of both of our methods are visually closer to the original stack in Fig. 2(a) than the unregularized methods.

3.2 Mouse Brain

We also performed experiments on a mouse brain dataset of 100 slices with 213x168 pixel that was provided online by [14]. Since the spacing was missing, we assumed it to be 1mm. The FFD grid size was therefore set to 20mm and subdivided on 3 grid levels. γ and ρ were set to 0.5 again. The slices were aligned rigidly before hand (see Fig. 4(a)). Since there is no ground truth available, only visual results are provided. As indicated before, the consecutive method (Fig. 4(c)) improves the stack consistency over the source stack but the result is less smooth than the unregularized simultaneous method (Fig. 4(b)). Our simultaneous method (Fig 4(d)), however, improves the results significantly over the other two approaches. It especially corrects drift errors that are present on the highlighted structures in Fig. 4(b). The overall simultaneous reconstruction including the tensor voting took around 20 minutes while the consecutive one only needs around 7 minutes which is a potential advantage on big datasets.

4   Discussion and Conclusion

In this work we presented a new, reference free method for histology stack alignment. We make use of tensor voting technique as a means to recover structural information that has been corrupted by the histology cutting process. Our experiments show that the proposed algorithm can improve upon conventional method. However, our method can only maintain structures that are still present in the corrupted stack and is therefore not meant as a replacement for reference-based methods but in the case when no reference is available. Due to the FFD formulation, the proposed method is unable to correctly close tears, a problem that should be addressed in future work. In order to use the algorithm on full resolution histology stack, the implementation also requires a more sophisticated memory management and subdivision of the data both for the tensor voting and the registration itself. This project has been partially supported by SFB 824.

References

1. Malandain, G., Bardinet, E., Nelissen, K., Vanduffel, W.: Fusion of autoradiographs with an mr volume using 2-d and 3-d linear transformations. NeuroImage 23(1), 111–127 (2004)
2. Cifor, A., Bai, L., Pitiot, A.: Smoothness-guided 3-d reconstruction of 2-d histological images. NeuroImage 56(1), 197–211 (2011)
3. Likar, B., Pernuš, F.: Registration of serial transverse sections of muscle fibers. Cytometry 37(2), 93–106 (1999)
4. Bardinet, E., Ourselin, S., Dormont, D., Malandain, G., Tandé, D., Parain, K., Ayache, N., Yelnik, J.: Co-registration of histological, optical and mr data of the human brain. In: Dohi, T., Kikinis, R. (eds.) MICCAI 2002, Part I. LNCS, vol. 2488, pp. 548–555. Springer, Heidelberg (2002)
5. Feuerstein, M., Heibel, H., Gardiazabal, J., Navab, N., Groher, M.: Reconstruction of 3-d histology images by simultaneous deformable registration. In: Fichtinger, G., Martel, A., Peters, T. (eds.) MICCAI 2011, Part II. LNCS, vol. 6892, pp. 582–589. Springer, Heidelberg (2011)
6. Gaffling, S., Daum, V., Hornegger, J.: Landmark-constrained 3-D histological imaging: A morphology-preserving approach. In: VMV, pp. 309–316 (2011)
7. Schwier, M., Böhler, T., Hahn, H.K., Dahmen, U., Dirsch, O.: Registration of histological whole slide images guided by vessel structures. Journal of Pathology Informatics 4(suppl.) (2013)
8. Yigitsoy, M., Navab, N.: Structure propagation for image registration. IEEE Transactions on Medical Imaging 32(9), 1657–1670 (2013)
9. Medioni, G., Tang, C., Lee, M.: Tensor voting: Theory and applications. In: Proceedings of RFIA, Paris, France (2000)
10. King, B.: Range data analysis by free-space modeling and tensor voting. ProQuest (2008)
11. Glocker, B., Komodakis, N., Tziritas, G., Navab, N., Paragios, N.: Dense image registration through mrfs and efficient linear programming. Medical Image Analysis 12(6), 731–741 (2008)
12. Kolmogorov, V., Rother, C.: Minimizing nonsubmodular functions with graph cuts-a review. TPAMI 29(7), 1274–1279 (2007)
13. Baker, S., Scharstein, D., Lewis, J., Roth, S., Black, M.J., Szeliski, R.: A database and evaluation methodology for optical flow. IJCV 92(1), 1–31 (2011)
14. Ju, T., Warren, J., Carson, J., Bello, M., Kakadiaris, I., Chiu, W., Thaller, C., Eichele, G.: 3d volume reconstruction of a mouse brain from histological sections using warp filtering. Journal of Neuroscience Methods 156(1), 84–100 (2006)

Optimally Stabilized PET Image Denoising Using Trilateral Filtering*

Awais Mansoor, Ulas Bagci**, and Daniel J. Mollura

Department of Radiology and Imaging Sciences
National Institutes of Health (NIH), Bethesda, MD 20892
ulas.bagci@nih.gov

Abstract. Low-resolution and signal-dependent noise distribution in positron emission tomography (PET) images makes denoising process an inevitable step prior to qualitative and quantitative image analysis tasks. Conventional PET denoising methods either over-smooth small-sized structures due to resolution limitation or make incorrect assumptions about the noise characteristics. Therefore, clinically important quantitative information may be corrupted. To address these challenges, we introduced a novel approach to remove signal-dependent noise in the PET images where the noise distribution was considered as *Poisson-Gaussian* mixed. Meanwhile, the generalized Anscombe's transformation (GAT) was used to stabilize varying nature of the PET noise. Other than noise stabilization, it is also desirable for the noise removal filter to preserve the boundaries of the structures while smoothing the noisy regions. Indeed, it is important to avoid significant loss of quantitative information such as standard uptake value (SUV)-based metrics as well as metabolic lesion volume. To satisfy all these properties, we extended bilateral filtering method into trilateral filtering through multiscaling and optimal Gaussianization process. The proposed method was tested on more than 50 PET-CT images from various patients having different cancers and achieved the superior performance compared to the widely used denoising techniques in the literature.

Keywords: Positron emission tomography, trilateral filtering, generalized variance stabilizing transformation, denoising.

1 Introduction

Positron emission tomography (PET) is a 3-D non-invasive technique that uses radioactive tracers to extract physiological information. Like other low-photon counting applications, the reconstructed image in PET scanners has low signal-to-noise ratio (SNR), which can affect the diagnosis of disease through quantification of clinically relevant quantities such as standardized uptake value (SUV) and metabolic lesion volume. Therefore, a denoising mechanism for PET images has to be adopted as a preprocessing step for accurate quantification [1, 2].

---

* This research is supported by CIDI, the intramural research program of the National Institute of Allergy and Infectious Diseases (NIAID) and the National Institute of Biomedical Imaging and Bioengineering (NIBIB).
** Corresponding author.

P. Golland et al. (Eds.): MICCAI 2014, Part I, LNCS 8673, pp. 130–137, 2014.

Current approaches in PET denoising are mostly inherited from optical imaging where primary criteria for denoising is qualitative rather than quantitative. Among the effective methods derived from other biomedical imaging modalities, Gaussian smoothing [3], anisotropic diffusion [4], non-local means [5], and bilateral filtering approaches [6] either over-smooth the edges or violates the Poisson statistics of the data; hence, corrupting vital information. Recently, multiscale denoising approaches such as [7] and soft-thresholding methods [8] have been adapted for PET images to avoid over-smoothing of the edges. These methods have shown improvement in SNR compared to the conventional methods due to their superiority in preserving edges. However, multiscale methods do not perform well in the vicinity of weak boundaries because they fail to eliminate point-singularities. Soft thresholding approach, on the other hand, is promising and shown to be superior to others since the noise is modeled in more realistic way and boundaries of small-sized objects are preserved; however, optimal transformation of noise characteristics has not been addressed yet [8].

Parametric denoising methods in the literature consider the noise in PET images to be additive Gaussian [3]. However, Gaussian assumption in PET images may result in the further loss of already poor resolution, increased blurring, and altered clinically relevant imaging markers. Recent attempts such as [8] used a more realistic Poisson-distributed noise assumption in PET images where authors first "Gaussianize" the Poisson measurement followed by unbiased risk estimation based denoising filtering. Gaussianization is achieved by applying a linear transformation such as a square-root and known as variance stabilizing transformation (VST) [9]. However, the algebraic inverse VST used by this denoising method may be sub-optimal. Regarding these difficulties, we proposed a novel approach in this paper to denoise PET images using the optimal noise characteristics and a 3-D structure preserving noise removal filtering.

2   Methods

We consider the noise in PET images as a mixed distribution of Poisson and Gaussian. Our assumption stems from the *Poisson* nature of photon-counting and *Gaussian* nature of the reconstruction process. In our proposed methodology, a linear transformation (i.e., GAT) was first used to stabilize the noise variation optimally. Second, trilateral denoising filter (TDF) was developed and applied to the variance stabilized image. Finally, optimal exact unbiased inverse GAT (IGAT) was applied to obtain denoised PET images.

2.1   Generalized Anscombe Transformation (GAT)

Let $x_i, i \in 1, \ldots, N$ be the observed voxel intensity obtained through the PET acquisition system. Poisson-Gaussian noise distribution models each observation as an independent random variable p_i, sampled from Poisson distribution with mean λ_i, and scaled by a constant $\alpha > 0$, and corrupted by Gaussian noise η_i^* (with mean μ_i and variance σ_i^2) as

$$x_i^* = \alpha p_i + \eta_i^*, \tag{1}$$

where $x_i^* \sim P(\lambda_i)$ and $n_i^* \sim N(\mu_i, \sigma_i^2)$.

A variance stabilization transformation (GAT) assumes the existence of a function f_σ that can approximately stabilize the variation of x (i.e., var $(f(x_i^*) | p_i) \approx$ constant). Mathematically, for the Poisson-Gaussian noise model $x_i^* = \alpha p_i + n_i^*$, $f_\sigma(x)$ gives the optimal variance stabilization when f_σ is piecewise linear and having the following form [10]:

$$f_\sigma(x) = \begin{cases} \frac{2}{\alpha}\sqrt{\alpha x + \frac{3}{8}\alpha^2 + \sigma^2} - \alpha\mu & \text{if } x > -\frac{3}{8} - \sigma^2 \\ 0 & \text{otherwise.} \end{cases} \tag{2}$$

Note that GAT equals to the traditional Anscombe transformation when noise is considered Poisson only ($\alpha = 1$, $\sigma = 0$, and $\mu = 0$):

$$f_\sigma(x) = \begin{cases} 2\sqrt{x + \frac{3}{8} + \sigma^2} & \text{if } x > -\frac{3}{8} - \sigma^2 \\ 0 & \text{else,} \end{cases} \tag{3}$$

where $x = \frac{x^* - \mu}{\alpha}$ and $\sigma = \frac{\sigma^*}{\alpha}$.

2.2 Trilateral Denoising Filter (TDF)

Trilateral denoising filter (TDF) is an extension to bilateral filter, and similar to the bilateral filters, TDF belongs to an edge preserving Gaussian filtering family. Herein, we briefly describe the principal of TDF.

Let the GAT transformed image $f_\sigma(x)$ be f_G. A bilateral filter is an edge preserving filter defined as:

$$g_f(i) = \frac{1}{k(i)} \int f_G(i + \mathbf{a}) w_1(\mathbf{a}) w_2(\mathbf{a}) (\|f_G(i + \mathbf{a}) - f_G(i)\|) d\mathbf{a},$$

$$k(i) = \int w_1(\mathbf{a}) w_2(\|f_G(i + \mathbf{a}) - f_G(i)\|) d\mathbf{a}, \tag{4}$$

where $\mathbf{a}$ is an offset vector (i.e., defines a small neighborhood around the voxel i). The weight parameters w_1 and w_2 respectively measure the geometric and photometric similarities within a predefined local neighborhood N_x and are designed as Gaussian kernels with standard deviations σ_1 (geometric range) and σ_2 (photometric range), the size of the neighborhood is adjusted using σ_1 and σ_2. Function $k(i)$ is the normalization factor.

A trilateral filter is a gradient preserving filter. It preserves the gradient by applying bilateral filter along the gradient plane. Let ∇f_G be the gradient of the GAT transformed image f_G, the trilateral filter is initiated by applying a bilateral filter on ∇f_G,

$$g_f(i) = \frac{1}{\nabla k(i)} \int \nabla f_G(i + \mathbf{a}) w_1(\mathbf{a}) w_2(\mathbf{a}) (\|\nabla f_G(i + \mathbf{a}) - \nabla f_G(i)\|) d\mathbf{a},$$

$$\nabla k(i) = \int w_1(\mathbf{a}) w_2(\|\nabla f_G(i + \mathbf{a}) - \nabla f_G(i)\|) d\mathbf{a}. \tag{5}$$

For refinement, subsequent second bilateral filter is applied using the g_f. Assuming $f_G(i, a) = f_G(i + \mathbf{a}) - f(x) - ag_f(x)$ and let a neighborhood weighting function be

$$N_i = \begin{cases} 1 & \text{if } |g_f(i + \mathbf{a}) - g_f(i)| < c, \\ 0 & \text{otherwise,} \end{cases} \tag{6}$$

where c specifies the size of adaptive region. Ultimately, the final trilateral smoothed image is given as

$$S_{TDF}(f_G(i)) = f_G(i) + \frac{1}{\nabla k(i)} \int \nabla f_G(i, \mathbf{a}) w_1(\mathbf{a}) w_2(\nabla f_G(i, \mathbf{a})) N(i, \mathbf{a}) da$$

$$\nabla k(i) = \int w_1(\mathbf{a}) w_2(\nabla f_G(i, \mathbf{a})) N(i, \mathbf{a}) da. \tag{7}$$

For TDF, σ_1 (geometric range) is the only input parameter to trilateral filter, σ_2 (photometric range) can be defined as (see [11] for the justifications)

$$\sigma_2 = 0.15 \left| \max_i \overline{g}_f(i) - \min_i \overline{g}_f(i) \right| \tag{8}$$

and $\overline{g}_f(i)$ is the mean gradient of the GAT transformed image.

2.3 Optimal Exact-Unbiased Inverse of Generalized Anscombe Transformation (IGAT)

After obtaining the $f_\sigma(x)$, we can treat the denoised data $\mathcal{D} = S_{TDF}(f_G)$ as the expected value $E\{f_\sigma(x)|\lambda, \sigma\}$. The closed form of optimal exact unbiased IGAT is given as,

$$\mathcal{I} = E\{f_\sigma(x)|\lambda, \sigma\} = \int_{-\infty}^{+\infty} f_\sigma(x) p(x|\lambda, \sigma) dx$$

$$= \int_{-\infty}^{+\infty} 2\sqrt{x + \frac{3}{8} + \sigma^2} \sum_{k=0}^{+\infty} \left(\frac{\lambda^k e^{-\lambda}}{k!\sqrt{2\pi\sigma^2}} e^{-\frac{(x-k)^2}{2\sigma^2}} \right) dx. \tag{9}$$

The optimal inverse $\mathcal{I}$ (in maximum likelihood sense) is applied to the denoised data $\mathcal{D}$ followed by scaling and translation (i.e., $\alpha\mathcal{I}(\mathcal{D}) + \mu$) for obtaining the denoised PET image.

3   Experiments and Results

We performed a comprehensive analysis and comparison of our approach with widely used denoising methods (i) Gaussian filter, (ii) bilateral filter [6], (iii) anisotropic diffusion filter [4], and (iv) our presented trilateral filter; without noise stabilization, with Poisson noise stabilization (VST, eq. 3), and Poisson-Gaussian noise stabilization (GAT, eq. 2).

Data: We used both phantoms as well as clinical data for evaluation of the denoising algorithms.

Phantoms: Data for the SNM Germanium Phantom were acquired using a GE DSTE-16 PET/CT scanner (16-row MDCT) [12]. A total of 6 scans were acquired consisting of 5, 7, and 30 minute acquisitions using both 3D (no septa) and 2D (with septa) modes. A total of 36 reconstructions were completed consisting of 3 OSEM and 3 filtered back projection (FBP) reconstructions per scan. Both OSEM and FBP images were reconstructed using smoothing filters of 7, 10, and 13 mm (Fig. 2). The resulting activity concentrations were also converted into target-to-background (T/B) ratios, and SUVs.

Clinical Data: With the IRB approval, PET-CT scans from 51 patients pertaining to various cancer diseases were collected retrospectively. All patients underwent PET-CT imaging (on Siemens Biograph 128 scanners) such that patients were instructed to fast for a minimum of 6-hours before scanning. At the end of the 6 hour period, 3.7-16.3 mCi (median=10.1 mCi, mean=9.45 mCi) of ^{18}F-FDG was administered intravenously to the patients depending on the body weight. PET images were obtained in two dimensional mode. The intrinsic spatial resolution of the system was 678.80 mm. CT was performed primarily for attenuation correction with the following parameters: section thickness, 3 mm; tube voltage, 120 kVp; tube current, 26 mAs; field of view, 500 × 500 mm.

3.1   Qualitative and Quantitative Evaluations

We qualitatively performed a comparison of our proposed method with above mentioned methods with different combinations of variance stabilization (no stabilization, VST, GAT). Results of GAT+anisotropic filter, GAT+bilateral filter, VST+TDF, and GAT+TDF are presented in Fig. 1. As pointed out with arrows, the boundary contrast is the highest in the proposed GAT+TDF; whereas other methods either over-smoothed or over-saturated the noisy areas. This is ensured using the TDF by employing an iterative approach coupled with narrow spatial window to preserve edges at finer scales. Also VST+TDF result (Fig. 1) verifies that Poisson noise assumption is more realistic than Gaussian but suboptimal with respect to the Poisson-Gaussian assumption.

To evaluate the potential loss of resolution and enhanced blurring after the denoising procedure, we employed *line profiling* through lesion ROIs in phantom image (shown in Fig. 2). Superiority of GAT+TDF can be readily depicted from the figure.

For quantitative evaluation of PET imaging markers, we manually drew the region of interest (ROI) around lesions/tumors and large homogeneous regions such as liver and lung in the PET scans. Quantitative information including SNR was then extracted from these ROIs as shown in the boxplot (Fig. 3(a)). The SNR of the image from selected ROIs was defined as

$$SNR_i = 20\log_{10}\left(\frac{m_i}{\sigma_i}\right), \tag{10}$$

where m_i is the mean and σ_i is the variance of the ith ROI. In addition, the relative contrast (RC) of the ROIs (Fig. 3(b)) was calculated using the following relationship [8]

$$RC_i = \frac{|m_i - M_B|}{\sqrt{\sigma_i \sigma_B}} \tag{11}$$

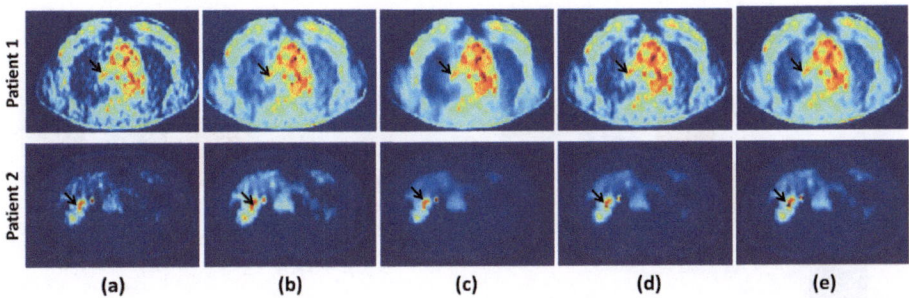

Fig. 1. Qualitative evaluation of the proposed method with current methods. Each row shows PET scans from different subjects. Each row shows different patient. (a) original noisy image, (b) GAT+anisotropic filter, (c) GAT+bilateral filter, (d) VST+trilateral filter, and (e) GAT+trilateral filter (proposed). *Black* arrows indicate the object of interest where edge information is preserved.

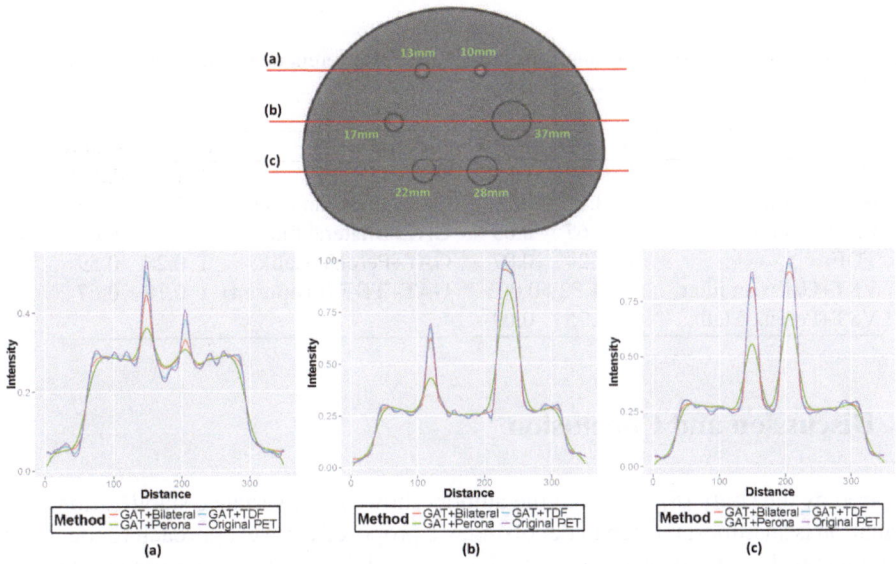

Fig. 2. Profile plots on all six spheres for simulated phantom dataset

In clinics, an optimal denoising method is expected to reduce the noise and increase the SNR whilst preserving the clinically significant information such as SUV_{max}, SUV_{mean}, metabolic tumor volume, etc. To assess how these values were affected from the denoising process, we measured significance of the percentage change in SUV_{max} and SUV_{mean} in different ROIs using Kruskal-Wallis test, a non-parametric *one-way analysis of variance*. The results of the test for SUV_{mean} and SUV_{max} together for our method in comparison other methods is presented in Table 1. As shown in the table, the change in SUV matrices are not statistically significant with our approach. Other imaging markers (SUV_{max} and metabolic tumor volume) have shown similar trends.

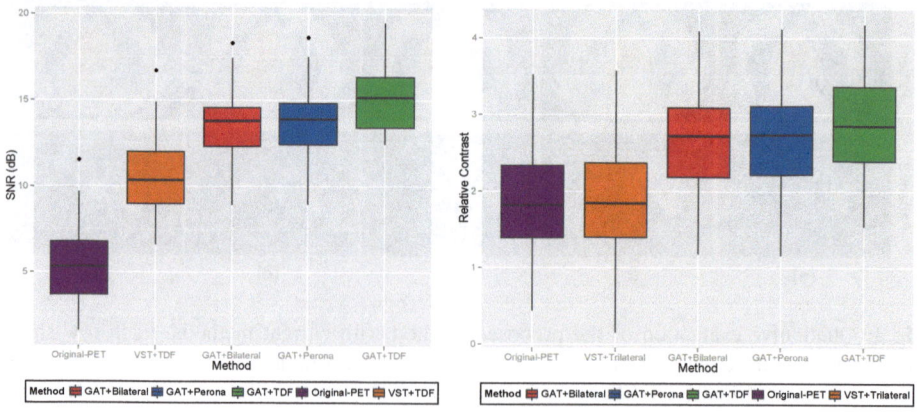

Fig. 3. Box-plots for (a) SNR (eq. 10) and (b) relative contrast (eq. 11) are demonstrated

Table 1. Kruskal-Wallis one-way analysis of variance for different denoising methods of SUV_{mean} and SUV_{max} together. df=Degrees-of-freedom.

Method	df	χ^2	p-value	Method	df	χ^2	p-value
Gaussian filter	1	18.86	0.001	VST+TDF	1	1.12	0.289
Bilateral filter	1	3.77	0.05	GAT+Gaussian filter	1	2.34	0.12
Perona-Malik	1	3.67	0.05	GAT+Bilateral filter	1	0.27	0.60
TDF	1	3.24	0.07	GAT+Perona-Malik	1	0.28	0.59
VST+Gaussian filter	1	11.32	0.001	**GAT+TDF (proposed)**	1	0.18	0.67
VST+Perona-Malik	1	2.75	0.09				

4   Discussion and Conclusion

Inspired by the study [8], in which the authors showed that variance stabilization transformation is an important step in denoising, we proposed a novel approach for denoising PET images. In particular, we presented an optimal formulation for variance stabilization transformation and its inverse. Furthermore, a more realistic noise distribution of PET images (i.e., Poisson-Gaussian) was considered. For smoothing of PET images after Gaussianizing the noise characteristics, we extended bilateral filtering into trilateral denoising filter that is able to preserve the edges as well as quantitative information such as SUV_{max} and SUV_{mean}. Experimental results demonstrated that our proposed method: (i) effectively eliminate the noise in PET images, (ii) preserve the edge and structural information, and (iii) retain clinically relevant details. As an extension to our approach, we plan to integrate our algorithm with partial volume correction step in order to study the impact of the combined method on object segmentation. We are also determined to compare our algorithm with the trending soft-thresholding and non-local means based algorithms in a larger evaluation platform where objective comparison and assessment of the denoising steps will be possible.

References

1. Foster, B., Bagci, U., Mansoor, A., Xu, Z., Mollura, D.J.: A review on segmentation of positron emission tomography images. Computers in Biology and Medicine 50, 76–96 (2014)
2. Sandouk, A., Bagci, U., Xu, Z., Mansoor, A., Foster, B., Mollura, D.J.: Accurate quantification of brown adipose tissue through PET-guided CT image segmentation. Society of Nuclear Medicine Annual Meeting Abstracts 54(suppl. 2), 318 (2013)
3. Chatziioannou, A., Dahlbom, M.: Detailed investigation of transmission and emission data smoothing protocols and their effects on emission images. IEEE Transactions on Nuclear Science 43(1), 290–294 (1996)
4. Demirkaya, O.: Anisotropic diffusion filtering of PET attenuation data to improve emission images. Physics in Medicine and Biology 47(20), N271 (2002)
5. Dutta, J., Leahy, R.M., Li, Q.: Non-local means denoising of dynamic PET images. PloS One 8(12), e81390 (2013)
6. Hofheinz, F., Langner, J., Beuthien-Baumann, B., Oehme, L., Steinbach, J., Kotzerke, J., van den Hoff, J.: Suitability of bilateral filtering for edge-preserving noise reduction in PET. EJNMMI Research 1(1), 1–9 (2011)
7. Turkheimer, F.E., Boussion, N., Anderson, A.N., Pavese, N., Piccini, P., Visvikis, D.: PET image denoising using a synergistic multiresolution analysis of structural (mri/ct) and functional datasets. Journal of Nuclear Medicine 49(4), 657–666 (2008)
8. Bagci, U., Mollura, D.J.: Denoising PET images using singular value thresholding and stein's unbiased risk estimate. In: Mori, K., Sakuma, I., Sato, Y., Barillot, C., Navab, N. (eds.) MICCAI 2013, Part III. LNCS, vol. 8151, pp. 115–122. Springer, Heidelberg (2013)
9. Anscombe, F.J.: The transformation of poisson, binomial and negative-binomial data. Biometrika 35(3-4), 246–254 (1948)
10. Starck, J.L., Murtagh, F.D., Bijaoui, A.: Image processing and data analysis: the multiscale approach. Cambridge University Press (1998)
11. Wong, W.C., Chung, A.C., Yu, S.C.: Trilateral filtering for biomedical images. In: IEEE International Symposium on Biomedical Imaging: Nano to Macro, pp. 820–823. IEEE (2004)
12. Doot, R., Kinahan, P.: SNM lesion phantom report. Technical report, University of Washington (2007)

Real Time Dynamic MRI with Dynamic Total Variation

Chen Chen[1], Yeqing Li[1], Leon Axel[2], and Junzhou Huang[1]

[1] Department of Computer Science and Engineering, University of Texas
at Arlington, TX, USA 76019
[2] Department of Radiology, New York University, New York, NY 10016

Abstract. In this study, we propose a novel scheme for real time dynamic magnetic resonance imaging (dMRI) reconstruction. Different from previous methods, the reconstructions of the second frame to the last frame are independent in our scheme, which only require the first frame as the reference. Therefore, this scheme can be naturally implemented in parallel. After the first frame is reconstructed, all the later frames can be processed as soon as the k-space data is acquired. As an extension of the convention total variation, a new online model called dynamic total variation is used to exploit the sparsity on both spatial and temporal domains. In addition, we design an accelerated reweighted least squares algorithm to solve the challenging reconstruction problem. This algorithm is motivated by the special structure of partial Fourier transform in sparse MRI. The proposed method is compared with 4 state-of-the-art online and offline methods on in-vivo cardiac dMRI datasets. The results show that our method significantly outperforms previous online methods, and is comparable to the offline methods in terms of reconstruction accuracy.

1 Introduction

Dynamic magnetic resonance imaging (dMRI) is an important medical imaging technique that widely used in hospitals for medical diagnosis and medical research. In general, there is a trade-off between the spatial resolution and temporal resolution, due to the acquisition speed of MR scanner. The undersampling often results in aliasing artifacts if the inverse Fourier transform is directly applied. Fortunately, the MR image sequence often provides redundant information in both spatial and temporal domains, which makes the use of compressive sensing (CS) theory repeatedly successful in MRI [1–4].

Based on the reconstruction schemes, the dMRI reconstruction methods can be online or offline. Most of existing methods are offline as they require the data of all frames to be collected before reconstruction. These methods applies sophisticated techniques that exploit the redundancies of the whole dataset, such as motion correction [5–7], dictionary learning [8], group clustering [9] and low rank approximation [10]. By these offline methods, the MR images can be reconstructed accurately but the drawbacks are their relatively slow speeds.

P. Golland et al. (Eds.): MICCAI 2014, Part I, LNCS 8673, pp. 138–145, 2014.
© Springer International Publishing Switzerland 2014

Online reconstruction means that the reconstruction of one frame only relies on the previous frames but not the later frames. Therefore, it is possible to reconstruct each frame once the corresponding k-space data is acquired. Of course, online reconstruction is much more difficult due to the lack of entire information as well as the concerns of reconstruction speed. Previous online methods usually assume that the difference between two adjacent frames are very small, either in the image or wavelet domain [11–13]. The difference can be reconstructed by sparsity regularization and the images are then updated by these changes. However, due to the lack of entire information, these methods have been shown to be less accurate than the state-of-the-art offline methods. And they all suffer from error accumulation, which makes them not feasible for relatively long sequences. Moreover, it is difficult for these methods to achieve real time reconstruction (i.e. the ideal case of online reconstruction), as they have to wait for the reconstruction of previous frame.

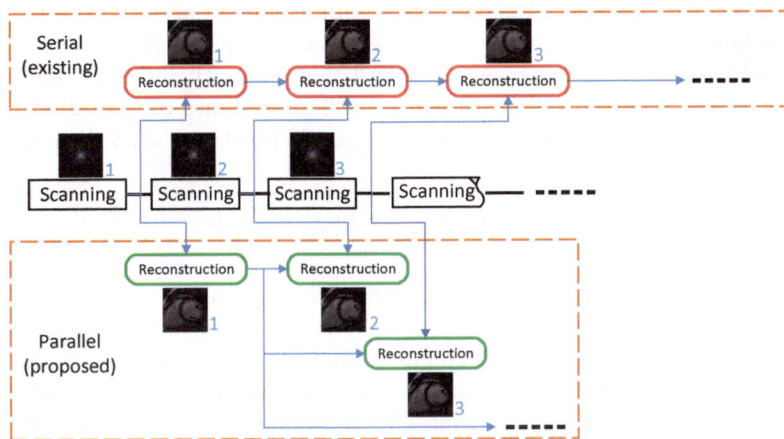

Fig. 1. Comparison between the proposed scheme and the existing online scheme

The data acquisition speed can be very fast with some recent developed techniques [14], e.g. 20ms, while real time MRI is still limited by the speed of iterative reconstruction methods. To bridge this gap, we propose a new online reconstruction scheme in this study, where the first frame is used to guide all the later reconstructions to exploit the temporal redundancy. A comparison with previous online methods is shown in Fig. 1. In contrast to previous serial system, our scheme is parallel and can naturally avoid error accumulation. After the first frame is reconstructed, all the later frames can be processed as soon as the data is acquired. In this new scheme, the sparsity assumptions in previous online methods may not hold any more. To address this issue, we extend the conventional spatial total variation (TV) to dynamic total variation (dTV), to exploit the sparsity in both spatial and temporal domains. An accelerated reweighted least squares algorithm is proposed to solve the dTV reconstruction by observing the diagonally dominant prior in CS-MRI. Finally, the proposed method is validated on in-vivo cardiac MR sequences with comparisons to the state-of-the-art online and offline methods. Our contributions are from the novel scheme, the robust modeling to the efficient algorithm, which make real time dMRI much more feasible than before.

2   Modeling with Dynamic Total Variation

Dynamic MR images are significantly similar in the temporal domain, that the same organ(s) is contained through the whole image sequence. After the first frame is obtained, intuition tells that the later frames should be very close to it. This motivates us to design a new online reconstruction scheme, which has been presented in Fig. 1. With the prior information in the first frame, it is possible to guide the later reconstructions with fewer k-space measurements. As we always use the first frame but not the previous frame as reference, the reconstruction problem becomes more challenging. The assumptions in previous online method may not hold any more, e.g. the difference image is sparse [12].

To address this problem, we propose a new sparsity inducing norm called dynamic total variation (dTV) to utilize both spatial and temporal correlations in online reconstruction. For an image x with N pixels, its dTV is defined as:

$$dTV(x,r) = \sum_{i=1}^{N} \sqrt{(\nabla_x(x-r)_i)^2 + (\nabla_y(x-r)_i)^2} \tag{1}$$

where r denotes a reference image (the first frame in this work) that has similar boundaries as x, ∇_x and ∇_y denote the gradients along the x and y directions. It means that the sparsity in gradient domain is not fixed but dynamic to a reference image. When there is no reference image, i.e. r is a zero image, it is identical to the conventional spatial TV. A similar idea of residual coding has been successfully applied in image registration [15].

We denote x_t as the frame at time t and $X = [x_1, x_2, ..., x_T]$ denotes the whole T images to be reconstructed. The dMRI reconstruction is therefore to solve x_t from an inverse problem $b_t = R_t F x_t$, where b_t is the measurement vector that may contain noise; R_t is a submatrix of the identity matrix that indicates undersampling, F denotes the Fourier transform. With the proposed dTV, the dMRI reconstruction is formulated as:

$$\min_{x_t} dTV(x_t, x_1), \text{ s.t. } ||R_t F x_t - b_t||_2 \leq \epsilon \text{ for } t = 2, ..., T \tag{2}$$

Same as that in existing online methods [11–13], the first frame should be reconstructed accurately with more k-space sampling. From this formulation, our scheme can be clearly observed. The reconstruction of each frame (except the first frame) only depends on the first one, but not the previous one. Therefore, it can be implemented in parallel to avoid waiting in the serial scheme.

Here, we only have a mild assumption, that the motions of organs are bounded. This assumption is quite natural because the cardiac motion is near periodic in breath-hold imaging. If we divide the cardiac motion into several phases, the frame with the closest phase to the first frame should have minimum reconstruction error, and vice versa. One of the advantages of the proposed dTV is that it can always sparsify the images even in the worst case.

3   Preconditioning in Fast MRI Reconstruction

The reconstruction speed of offline methods is often not of big concern. However, fast reconstruction is essential to online methods. In this section, we proposed a new algorithm to efficiently minimize (2). Let $z = x_t - x_1$, and the problem (2) can be written as the Lagrange relaxed form of TV minimization:

$$\min_z \{\frac{1}{2}||Az - y||_2^2 + \lambda||z||_{TV}\} \tag{3}$$

where $A = R_t F$, $y = b_t - R_t F x_1$ and λ is a parameter. There are many methods to solve (3) in the literature of convex optimization. Some of them have very fast convergence rate (e.g. [16]), but the computational cost in each iteration is very high. Some other methods are less computationally expensive in each iteration, such as that in [17], while they converge relatively slower. We expect to design an algorithm with both fast convergence and low computational cost.

Our algorithm is based on the reweighted least squares framework [16, 18], which can converge exponentially fast. Let D_1, D_2 be two N-by-N two first-order finite difference matrices in vertical and horizontal directions. The TV can be re-formulated as $||z||_{TV} = |||[D_1 z, D_2 z]||_{2,1}$, where the $\ell_{2,1}$ norm is the summation of the ℓ_2 norm of each row, $[x, y]$ denotes concatenating two vectors x, y horizontally. With this notations, the problem (3) can be solved by iteratively updating the weight matrix W and the solution z [16, 18]. W is a diagonal matrix with the i-th diagonal entry:

$$W_i^k = 1/\sqrt{(\nabla_x z_i^k)^2 + (\nabla_y z_i^k)^2}, \text{ for } i = 1, 2, ..., N, \tag{4}$$

where k is the iteration counter. z^{k+1} is updated by solving the following linear equation:

$$(A^*A + \lambda D_1^* W^k D_1 + \lambda D_2^* W^k D_2)z = A^*y. \tag{5}$$

where * denotes the conjugate transpose. This step dominates the computational cost of the whole algorithm. There is close form solution $z^k = S^{-1} A^* y$ for (5), where $S = A^*A + \lambda D_1^* W^k D_1 + \lambda D_2^* W^k D_2$ denotes the system matrix. However, the exact inversion is often not computationally feasible. In [16], this subproblem is solved by the conventional conjugate gradient method. Besides, a faster version called preconditioned conjugate gradient (PCG) method [18] can be used here. It requires a preconditioner P that is close to S and the inverse can be obtained efficiently. The design of good preconditioner P is problem-dependent and not easy due to the tradeoff between accuracy and computational cost.

We observe that the matrix $R_t^* R_t$ is diagonal, and more importantly, $A^* A = F^* R_t^* R_t F$ is therefore diagonally dominant. Thus, an accurate approximation could be made by removing the non-diagonal elements. Due to the properties of the Fourier transform, all the diagonal elements of $A^* A$ is equal to the mean of diagonal elements of $R^* R$, i.e. the sampling ratio s. Motivated by this, we define a new preconditioner $P = sI + \lambda D_1^* W^k D_1 + \lambda D_2^* W^k D_2$ to accelerate the whole algorithm, where I is the identity matrix.

The proposed preconditioner P is a symmetric penta-diagonal matrix, which has no closed form inverse. Fortunately, P is diagonally dominant as the regularization parameter λ is often very small in CS-MRI. It is not hard to find the incomplete LU decomposition of such penta-diagonal matrix $P \approx LU$, where L and U are a lower triangle matrix and an upper triangle matrix, respectively. The time complexity for the decomposition and inversion is $\mathcal{O}(N)$. To our best knowledge, this is the first study to accelerate MRI reconstruction with such preconditioner. We summarize the whole algorithm to solve (3) in Algorithm 1. All N-by-N matrices can be efficiently stored using sparse matrices in MATLAB.

Algorithm 1. dTV Reconstruction

Input: $A = R_t F$, x_1, $y = b_t - R_t F x_1$, z^1, λ, $k = 1$
Output: z, $x_t = z + x_1$.
while not meet the stopping criterion **do**
   Update W^k by (4)
   Update $S = A^* A + \lambda D_1^* W^k D_1 + \lambda D_2^* W^k D_2$
   Update $P = sI + \lambda D_1^* W^k D_1 + \lambda D_2^* W^k D_2 = LU$, $P^{-1} \approx U^{-1} L^{-1}$
   while not meet the PCG stopping criterion **do**
      Update z^{k+1} by PCG for $Sz = A^* y$ with preconditioner $P \approx LU$
   end while
   Update $k = k + 1$
end while

---

4   Experiments

We compare our method with two online method modified CS (MCS) [13], the approach based on difference image (DI) [12] and two state-of-the-art offline methods k-t SLR [10] and the dictionary learning based method DLTG [8]. The codes are downloaded from each author's website and we use their default parameter settings for all experiments. For our method, we set $\lambda = 0.001$ for all experiments. In-vivo breath-hold cardiac perfusion and cine datasets are used here, which contains image sequences of $192 \times 192 \times 40$ and $256 \times 256 \times 24$, respectively. The proposed reconstruction method can be combined with the fast acquisition hardware radial FLASH [14] for real time imaging. Therefore, the radial sampling mask is used to simulate undersampling. The root-mean-square error (RMSE) is used as the metric for result evaluation. The ground-truth image is obtained by inverse FFT with full sampling.

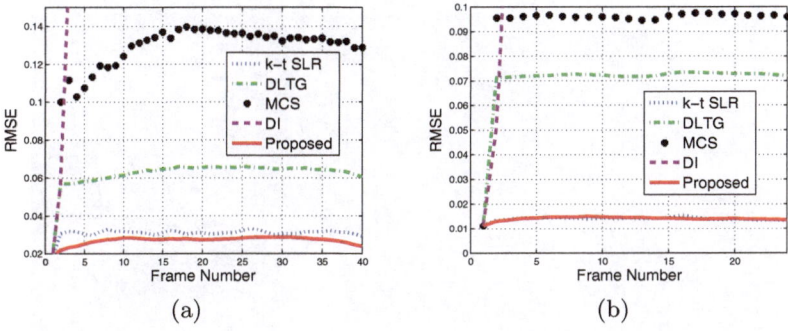

Fig. 2. Reconstruction accuracy comparisons of different methods. (a) On the perfusion dataset. (b) On the cine dataset. Our method and k-t SLR almost overlap on the second dataset.

The first frame is often required to be reconstructed very accurately for all online methods [13, 12]. Therefore, we use 1/2 sampling for the first frame and 1/6 sampling for the rest frames. The reconstruction RMSEs are shown in Fig. 2. From these results, it is obvious that the previous online methods [13, 12] have larger reconstruction errors than the offline methods [8, 10], while the proposed real time method is comparable or even better than the k-t SLR [10] on both datasets. The DLTG is currently designed for real-valued images [8], and it seems less effective on the complex-valued data here. DI does not perform as good as that presented in the paper [12]. From the 4th and 5th frame, it starts to fail. However, in [12], the curve of DI is often between those of k-t SLR and MCS. We found that it used the full sampling for the first frame, while the reconstruction error occurs at the first frame here with 1/2 sampling. With the same setting in [12], we conduct additional experiments for DI. It shows that DI starts to fail after 20-30 frames. These results demonstrate that DI is very sensitive to error accumulation.

A frame of the reconstructed perfusion sequence is shown in Fig. 3. Visible artifacts can be obviously observed on the images reconstructed by MCS and DI. The image reconstructed by DLTG tends to be blurry. In contrast, the reconstruction results of k-t SLR and the proposed method are similar to the ground-truth image, and less noisy.

We vary the sampling ratios of the second frame to the end frame and compare the average reconstruction errors of all frames. Those results are presented in Fig. 4, which demonstrates the comparable performance of our method to the state-of-the-art offline methods. At a low sampling ratio that we are interested, the proposed method seems to be even better. As the previous online methods [13, 12] are much less accurate, they are not compared in these experiments. For the $192 \times 192 \times 40$ perfusion sequence, the average reconstruction speed of our method is 0.71 seconds for each frame on a desktop with Intel i7-3770 CPU.

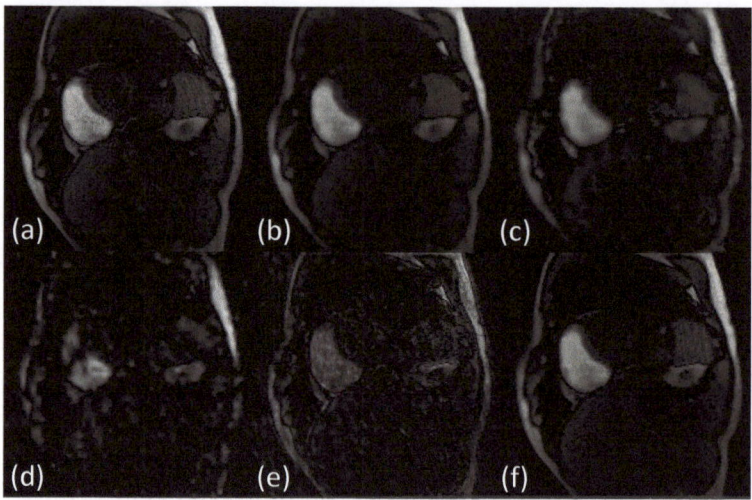

Fig. 3. Results of the third frame of the perfusion sequence at sampling ratio 1/6. (a) The ground-truth image with full sampling. The rest images are reconstructed by (b) k-t SLR; (c) DLTG; (d) MCS; (e) DI; (f) the proposed method.

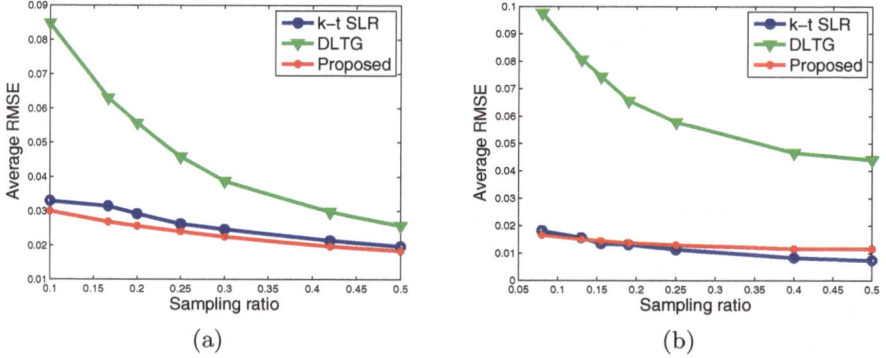

Fig. 4. Comparisons with the offline methods k-t SLR and DLTG at different sampling ratios. (a) On the perfusion dataset. (b) On the cine dataset.

5   Conclusion

In this paper, we have proposed a novel scheme for parallel reconstruction, a robust model to exploit both spatial and temporal redundancies, and an accelerated reweighted least squares algorithm to solve the reconstruction problem. Experiments on in-vivo cardiac perfusion and cine datasets have validated the efficiency and effectiveness of our method over the state-of-the-arts. These contributions make real time dMRI much more feasible than before. We will combine our method in parallel imaging as future work [19].

References

1. Lustig, M., Donoho, D., Pauly, J.: Sparse MRI: The application of compressed sensing for rapid MR imaging. Magn. Reson. Med. 58(6), 1182–1195 (2007)
2. Huang, J., Zhang, S., Metaxas, D.: Efficient MR image reconstruction for compressed MR imaging. Medical Image Analysis 15(5), 670–679 (2011)
3. Huang, J., Chen, C., Axel, L.: Fast Multi-contrast MRI Reconstruction. In: Ayache, N., Delingette, H., Golland, P., Mori, K. (eds.) MICCAI 2012, Part I. LNCS, vol. 7510, pp. 281–288. Springer, Heidelberg (2012)
4. Chen, C., Huang, J.: The benefit of tree sparsity in accelerated MRI. Medical Image Analysis 18(6), 834–842 (2014)
5. Gupta, V., van de Giessen, M., Kirişli, H., Kirschbaum, S.W., Niessen, W.J., Lelieveldt, B.: Robust motion correction in the frequency domain of cardiac MR stress perfusion sequences. In: Ayache, N., Delingette, H., Golland, P., Mori, K. (eds.) MICCAI 2012, Part I. LNCS, vol. 7510, pp. 667–674. Springer, Heidelberg (2012)
6. Xue, H., Guehring, J., Srinivasan, L., Zuehlsdorff, S., Saddi, K., Chefdhotel, C., Hajnal, J.V., Rueckert, D.: Evaluation of rigid and non-rigid motion compensation of cardiac perfusion MRI. In: Metaxas, D., Axel, L., Fichtinger, G., Székely, G. (eds.) MICCAI 2008, Part II. LNCS, vol. 5242, pp. 35–43. Springer, Heidelberg (2008)
7. Jung, H., Sung, K., Nayak, K.S., Kim, E.Y., Ye, J.C.: k-t FOCUSS: A general compressed sensing framework for high resolution dynamic MRI. Magn. Reson. Med. 61(1), 103–116 (2009)
8. Caballero, J., Rueckert, D., Hajnal, J.V.: Dictionary learning and time sparsity in dynamic MRI. In: Ayache, N., Delingette, H., Golland, P., Mori, K. (eds.) MICCAI 2012, Part I. LNCS, vol. 7510, pp. 256–263. Springer, Heidelberg (2012)
9. Usman, M., Prieto, C., Schaeffter, T., Batchelor, P.: k-t group sparse: A method for accelerating dynamic MRI. Magn. Reson. Med. 66(4), 1163–1176 (2011)
10. Lingala, S.G., Hu, Y., DiBella, E., Jacob, M.: Accelerated dynamic MRI exploiting sparsity and low-rank structure: k-t SLR. IEEE TMI 30(5), 1042–1054 (2011)
11. Sümbül, U., Santos, J.M., Pauly, J.M.: A practical acceleration algorithm for real-time imaging. IEEE TMI 28(12), 2042–2051 (2009)
12. Majumdar, A., Ward, R., Aboulnasr, T.: Compressed sensing based real-time dynamic MRI reconstruction. IEEE TMI 31(12), 2253–2266 (2012)
13. Vaswani, N., Lu, W.: Modified-CS: Modifying compressive sensing for problems with partially known support. IEEE Trans. Signal Process. 58(9), 4595–4607 (2010)
14. Zhang, S., Block, K.T., Frahm, J.: Magnetic resonance imaging in real time: advances using radial FLASH. J. Magn. Reson. Imaging 31(1), 101–109 (2010)
15. Myronenko, A., Song, X.: Intensity-based image registration by minimizing residual complexity. IEEE TMI 29(11), 1882–1891 (2010)
16. Rodrıguez, P., Wohlberg, B.: Efficient minimization method for a generalized total variation functional. IEEE Trans. Image Process 18(2), 322–332 (2009)
17. Huang, J., Zhang, S., Li, H., Metaxas, D.: Composite splitting algorithms for convex optimization. Comput. Vis. Image Und. 115(12), 1610–1622 (2011)
18. Chen, C., Huang, J., He, L., Li, H.: Preconditioning for accelerated iteratively reweighted least squares in structured sparsity reconstruction. In: Proceedings of CVPR (2014)
19. Chen, C., Li, Y., Huang, J.: Calibrationless parallel MRI with joint total variation regularization. In: Mori, K., Sakuma, I., Sato, Y., Barillot, C., Navab, N. (eds.) MICCAI 2013, Part III. LNCS, vol. 8151, pp. 106–114. Springer, Heidelberg (2013)

Improved Reconstruction of 4D-MR Images by Motion Predictions*

Christine Tanner, Golnoosh Samei, and Gábor Székely

Computer Vision Laboratory, ETH Zurich,
Sternwartstrasse 7, 8092 Zurich, Switzerland
tannerch@vision.ee.ethz.ch

Abstract. The reconstruction of 4D images from 2D navigator and data slices requires sufficient observations per motion state to avoid blurred images and motion artifacts between slices. Especially images from rare motion states, like deep inhalations during free-breathing, suffer from too few observations.

To address this problem, we propose to actively generate more suitable images instead of only selecting from the available images. The method is based on learning the relationship between navigator and data-slice motion by linear regression after dimensionality reduction. This can then be used to predict new data slices for a given navigator by warping existing data slices by their predicted displacement field. The method was evaluated for 4D-MRIs of the liver under free-breathing, where sliding boundaries pose an additional challenge for image registration.

Leave-one-out tests for five short sequences of ten volunteers showed that the proposed prediction method improved on average the residual mean (95%) motion between the ground truth and predicted data slice from 0.9mm (1.9mm) to 0.8mm (1.6mm) in comparison to the best selection method. The approach was particularly suited for unusual motion states, where the mean error was reduced by 40% (2.2mm vs. 1.3mm).

1 Introduction

Minimal invasive radiation therapies for the abdomen during free-breathing require guidance for keeping the beam on the moving target. For proton and focused ultrasound therapies, the position of other structures, like bones or vessels, passed through by the beam are also of great importance for accurate calculation of the Bragg Peak, and avoidance of hot and cold spots. Real-time observation and tracking of all structures of interest during therapy is currently not possible. Motion models, which predict the motion of the remaining structures from partial observations have been proposed [1, 2]. For capturing respiratory irregularities, these rely on learning the motion patterns from 4D-MRIs, which allow in comparison to 4D-CTs, for long term observations.

* We acknowledge funding from the EU's Seventh Framework Program (FP7/2007-2013) under grant agreement n° 270186 (FUSIMO) and n° 611889 (TRANS-FUSIMO). We thank Prof. S. Kozerke and Dr. J. Schmidt (Institute for Biomedical Engineering, University and ETH, Zurich) for their help with the MRI acquisitions.

P. Golland et al. (Eds.): MICCAI 2014, Part I, LNCS 8673, pp. 146–153, 2014.

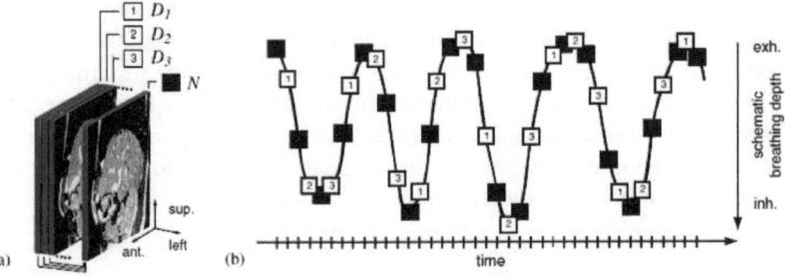

Fig. 1. Illustration of MR sequence with alternating navigator (N) and data slices (D_1,...,D_3). (Courtesy von Siebenthal [3])

4D-MRIs can be created by an interleaved acquisition of 2D navigator and data slices and retrospective sorting [3], as illustrated in Fig. 1. Per data slice, a whole 3D image was created by stacking data slices, which are enclosed by a similar navigator pair as the current one. Similarity was measured by the difference in displacements to a reference navigator slice [3] or by the difference in intensities of the navigators after manifold embedding [4]. To improve SNR of the reconstruction, the mean of the T most similar data slices was employed. 2D navigator-free 4D-MRI reconstruction methods have been proposed, relying for example on external breathing signals [5] or the consistency between neighbouring data slices after manifold embedding [6]. However, we focus here on the 2D navigator-based 4D-MRI liver reconstructions, as the additional information from continuously observing the liver motion at the same position has the potential to provide superior reconstructions and allows for quantitative evaluation.

Currently 4D-MRI reconstructions are based on selecting the most similar images. For unusual motion states, like large inhalations, this leads to blurry images and motion artifacts between slices since the most similar images are quite different. The problem is emphasised for reconstructions from shorter sequences, as fewer motion states are available. In this work, we propose to actively create more similar images by learning the relationship between navigator and data-slice motion, predict for a given navigator motion the data-slice motion and then use this predicted motion to warp the data slice to a more similar position. Additionally, this was compared to using navigator intensities instead of motion.

Mean images have previously been sharpened by image registration in the field of superresolution [7, 8] and atlas creation e.g. [9–11]. In the former application, SNR and image resolution is generally improved for an existing image by registering images of additional observations to it. This task is much simpler than our problem due to the existence of a reference image. Early works in atlas creation by registration also used one of the subjects as representative image to which all others were registered. Nowadays the benefit of avoiding this bias is known and atlases are generated for an interpolated state from a group of images. Important concepts for realistic interpolation between images from spatial transformations are geodesic rather than linear averaging for large deformations and ensuring that transformations are diffeomorphic [12]. Unfortunately enforcing the latter will introduce errors when registering whole abdominal images due to discontinuities at sliding boundaries. Furthermore our problem requires extrapolation and generation of unusual images, which is much harder than interpolation. We will employ dimensionality reduction and linear functions for regularization to avoid over-fitting and hence badly predictive models.

2   Material

MR images of the abdomen during free-breathing were acquired for 10 healthy volunteers according to the method proposed by von Siebenthal et al. [3]. These consisted of a sequence of interleaved 2D sagittal navigator and data slices, where the navigator slice is positioned in the center of the right liver lobe and the sagittal data slices cover the whole abdomen. The 2D images were acquired on a Philips Achieva 1.5T whole body MR system with a balanced turbo field echo sequence, a flip angle of 70°, a TR=2.3ms, an in-plane resolution of 1.3x1.3mm^2, a slice thickness of 5mm and a temporal resolution of 163-226ms. To cover the abdomen, 53-65 data slices with a size of 224×224-240×240 pixels were required. To simulate short 4D-MRIs, only the first K=30 observations per data slice were processed, which would require a total acquisition time of 9-12min.

3   Method

The inter-leaved MR sequences, used for reconstructing the 4D-MRIs, consist of alternating acquisitions of a navigator slice N at the same liver position and a data slice D^a at changing positions $a = 1, ..., A$ to cover the whole abdomen, see Fig. 1. The problem of 4D reconstruction is to find for a given data slice D^a the remaining data slices $D^{b \neq a}$ which show the same liver motion state.

Selection Methods. So far, this problem has been approached by selecting data slices which are enclosed by most similar navigator images [3, 4]. The selection criteria has been based on the similarity of either the liver motion [3] or the image intensities [4] of the navigators.

In the former approach [3], the 2D navigator images were registered to a reference navigator image within the liver region using a B-Spline based registration method [13]. Then for each navigator image (N_i), the 2D displacement vectors at the C control points which lie within the liver ($\mathbf{u}_{c,i}^T = [u_{1,c,i} \; u_{2,c,i}]$ for $c = 1, 2...C$) are extracted. Finally for data slice D_i^a, with enclosing navigator images (N_i, N_{i+1}), D_j^b (with enclosing navigators (N_j, N_{j+1})) is selected for slice position b if it minimizes the overall dissimilarity measure $d_{i,j}^u$, i.e. $\arg\min_j d_{i,j}^u = \frac{1}{C} \sum_{c=1}^C |\bar{\mathbf{u}}_{c,i} - \bar{\mathbf{u}}_{c,j}|_2$, where $\bar{\mathbf{u}}_{c,i} = (\mathbf{u}_{c,i} + \mathbf{u}_{c,i+1})/2$. We also tested the selection performance after dimensionality reduction of the $K \times 2C$ dimensional dissimilarity matrix $\mathbf{M}^{u,i}$, which is given by $\mathbf{M}_{j,c}^{u,i} = \bar{u}_{1,c,i} - \bar{u}_{1,c,j}$ and

$\mathbf{M}_{j,C+c}^{u,i} = \bar{u}_{2,c,i} - \bar{u}_{2,c,j}$ for $c = 1, 2...C$ and $j = 1, 2, ...K$. Using Principle Component Analysis (PCA), Laplacian Eigenmaps or Neighbourhood Preserving Embedding (NPE), dissimilarity matrix $\mathbf{M}^{u,i}$ was transformed to a $K \times L$ dimensional matrix $\tilde{\mathbf{M}}^{u,i}$ and the optimal D_j^b determined by $\arg\min_j \tilde{d}_{i,j}^u = \frac{1}{L}\sum_{l=1}^{L}|\tilde{\mathbf{M}}_{j,l}^{u,i}|_2$.

In the intensity-based approach [4], each navigator image was first normalized to have an intensity distribution with zero mean and unit standard deviation. The $K \times R$ dissimilarity matrix $\mathbf{M}^{N,i}$ was then defined by $\mathbf{M}_{j,r}^{N,i} = N_{r,i} - N_{r,j}$ for $r = 1, 2, ...R$ and $j = 1, 2, ...K$, where $N_{r,i}$ is the normalized intensity of navigator N_i at pixel r. Laplacian Eigenmaps were used for dimensionality reduction of $\mathbf{M}^{N,i}$ to a $L=3$ dimensional manifold. The data slice with the smallest Euclidean distance in this 3D space ($\arg\min_j \tilde{d}_{i,j}^N = \frac{1}{L}\sum_{l=1}^{L}|\tilde{\mathbf{M}}_{j,l}^{N,i}|_2$) was then selected.

Prediction Methods. We propose to actively predict data slices instead of only selecting from the pool of available data slices. The aim is to predict the motion required to warp an existing data slice (D_j^b) to a similar liver position as the observed data slice (D_i^a) from the dissimilarity of the associated navigators ($\mathbf{M}^{u,i}$ or $\mathbf{M}^{N,i}$ denoted as $\mathbf{M}^i$). Our approach consists of the following steps:

- Pre-processing
  - (S1) Determine dissimilarity $\mathbf{M}^i$ for all navigator images
  - (S2) Determine data-slice displacement fields ($\mathbf{V}^j$) by registering all K data slices from the same position to each other
  - (S3) Dimensionality reduction of $\mathbf{M}^i$ and $\mathbf{V}^j$
- For each data slice D_i^a, with enclosing navigator images (N_i, N_{i+1}), and for all slice positions $b = 1...B$
  - (S4) Select most similar data slices D_j^b based on minimizing $\tilde{d}_{i,j}^u$ (or $\tilde{d}_{i,j}^N$)
  - (S5) Determine linear function parameters $\mathbf{Q}$ from $\tilde{\mathbf{M}}^i$ and $\tilde{\mathbf{V}}^j$
  - (S6) Predict D_j^b motion from zero dissimilarity ($\mathbf{M}_{j,c}^i = 0 \ \forall \ c$) and $\mathbf{Q}$

For step S1, the dissimilarity between navigators ($\mathbf{M}^{u,i}$ or $\mathbf{M}^{N,i}$) was determined in the same way as for the selection method.

For registering the data slices (step S2) we used the deeds registration method [14, 15], as we want to register the whole images and it is currently one of the most accurate methods for registering images with sliding boundaries. Furthermore it is fast (≈ 0.5s per slice) and publically available. It was configured to provide displacement vectors at every 4th pixel in the image. We denote the displacement field from registering D_j^b to D_k^b by $\mathbf{v}_{j,k}^T = [v_{1,1,j,k} \ \cdots \ v_{1,P,j,k} \quad v_{2,1,j,k} \ \cdots \ v_{2,P,j,k}]$, with $P=R/16$. Including zero displacements for $\mathbf{v}_{j,j}^T$ and collecting all results for D_j^b in $\mathbf{V}^j = [\mathbf{v}_{j,1}...\mathbf{v}_{j,K}]^T$ provides a $K \times 2P$ matrix.

Dimensionality reduction methods were applied in step S3 to $\mathbf{M}^{u,i}$ (or $\mathbf{M}^{N,i}$) and $\mathbf{V}^j$ to avoid underdetermined systems in step S5. The low-dimensional projections are denoted as $\tilde{\mathbf{M}}^i$ and $\tilde{\mathbf{V}}^j$, with dimensions $2C$ (or R) and $2P$ being reduced to L_m and L_v respectively. We used $L_m=L_v=3$ and employed PCA or NPE as these allow, in contrast to Laplacian Eigenmaps, construction of the full displacement field in step S6.

During the reconstruction, we first selected in step S4 the most similar data slice D_j^b by one of the previously described selection methods.

In step S5, the system of linear equations $\tilde{\mathbf{V}}^j = [\tilde{\mathbf{M}}^i \ \mathbf{1}]\mathbf{Q}$ was then solved in the least squares sense for the $(L_\mathbf{m} + 1) \times L_\mathbf{v}$ parameter matrix $\mathbf{Q}$.

In the final step (S6), we want to determine motion $\mathbf{v}_{j,i}$ such that the resulting transformed image $(\check{D}_j^b)$ should have the liver in a similar motion state as data slice D_i^a. So far we have learned how the dissimilarity in navigators $(\tilde{\mathbf{M}}^i)$ relate to motion between data slices $(\tilde{\mathbf{V}}^j)$. This learned function is now used to predict the required data slice motion for the given navigator pair, i.e. for a zero dissimilarity. In details, motion $\tilde{\mathbf{v}}_{j,i}$ was predicted by $\tilde{\mathbf{v}}_{j,i}^T = [\tilde{\mathbf{z}}^T \ 1]\mathbf{Q}$, where $\tilde{\mathbf{z}}$ is the L_m dimensional zero vector mapped to the low-dimensional space. The predicted motion $\tilde{\mathbf{v}}_{j,i}$ was then mapped back to the high-dimensional $(2P)$ space and applied to data slice D_j^b to get $\check{D}_j^b$.

To improve SNR, steps S4 to S6 were performed for the $T=5$ most similar data slices and the resulting transformed images were averaged to $\bar{D}^b$. Finally the 3D image, associated with data slice D_i^a, was formed by stacking the mean images $\bar{D}^b$ for $b = 1, ..., B$.

4   Results

Quantitative evaluation was performed by leaving out a data slice (which serves as ground truth (GT)), predicting it from the other available data slices and measuring the mean residual motion within the liver between the predicted and the GT data slice by image registration (deeds method [14, 15]). In this way the impact of the reconstruction errors on extracting the liver motion from 4D-MRIs can be measured. We evaluated the mean residual motion per subject for 25 liver slices and 30 temporal samples, and summarized this distribution by its mean and 95th percentile. We also assess the performance at the end-inhalation state and for the most unusual data slices. The latter were selected based on the GT data slice having navigators with a mean displacement difference $(d_{i,j}^u)$ of 3mm or more to all other navigators for this slice.

Fig. 2 shows an example where the GT image is very dissimilar to the available data slices according to the corresponding navigator motion (Fig. 2b, $d_{i,j}^u=4.2$mm). Selecting the 5 most similar data slices leads not only to a blurry reconstruction but also to a misaligned liver (Fig. 2c). The prediction method is able to estimate most of this unseen motion (Fig. 2d).

Table 1 shows that higher accuracies were achieved when using the displacement information of the navigators rather than their intensities. PCA performed well against the other tested dimensionality reduction methods. Highest accuracies were achieved with predictions from navigator displacements and PCA, which provided a substantial mean improvement over the best selection method for end-inhalation states (23%) and for unusual positions (40%).

A coronal slice from a reconstruction example is shown in Fig. 3. An improved consistency across slices can be observed at the diaphragm, and for lung and liver vessels for the prediction method (Fig. 3b).

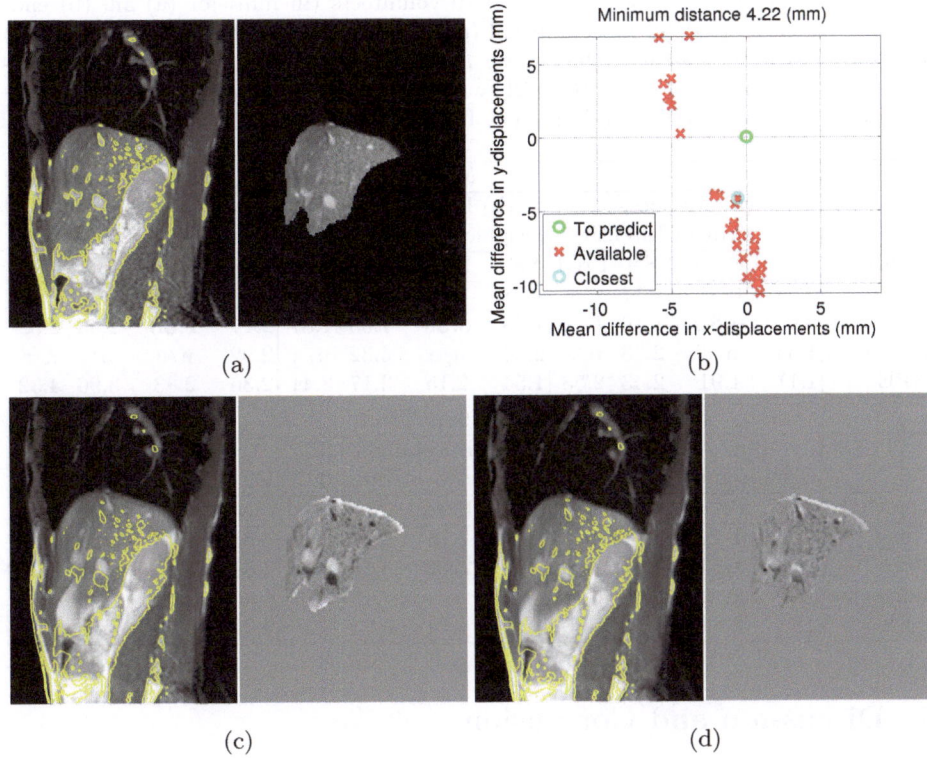

(a)   (b)

(c)   (d)

Fig. 2. (a) Ground-truth (GT) image (right: liver region) to predict, (b) 2D dissimilarity of available data slices (red crosses) to GT (green circle) based on difference in navigator displacements, (c,d) reconstructed slice (right: its difference to GT within liver) based on (c) selecting the 5 closest observations (meanError: 8.1mm), or (d) predicting the motion of 5 data slices from the navigator displacements after dimensionality reduction by PCA (meanError: 2.4mm). All yellow contours are from GT.

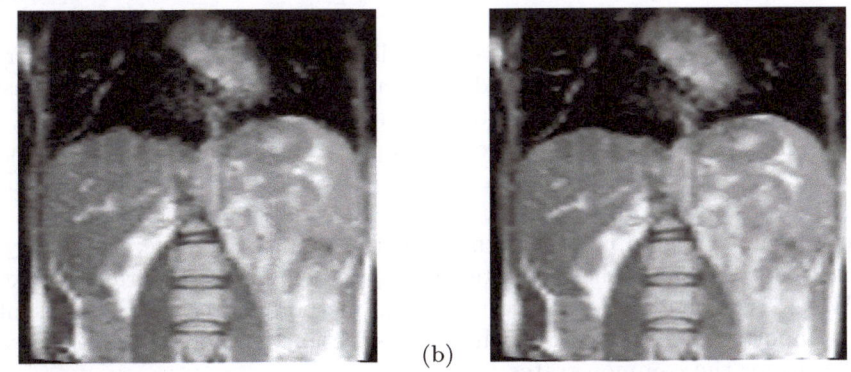

(a)   (b)

Fig. 3. Example of 3D reconstruction from 30 observations for (a) baseline selection method [3] and (b) proposed prediction method (navigator displacements, PCA)

Table 1. Mean performance results for 10 volunteers (in mm) for (a) all, (b) end-inhalation (10.8%) and (c) most unusual ($d_{i,j}^u \geq 3$mm, 16.4%) data slices when (Sel) selecting or (Pred) predicting the closest $T=5$ data slices from navigator (right) displacements or (left) intensities. Rows show results for dimensionality reduction methods. Best results are marked in bold. The baseline approach [3] is underlined.

	Mean Error											
	(a) All slices				(b) End-inhalation				(c) Most unusual			
	Displacement		Intensity		Displacement		Intensity		Displacement		Intensity	
DimRed	Sel	Pred	Sel	Pred	Sel	Pred	Sel	Pred	Sel	Pred	Sel	Pred
None	<u>0.93</u>	0.87	1.17		<u>1.28</u>	1.15	1.56		<u>2.16</u>	1.79	2.43	
PCA	0.94	**0.80**	1.19	1.43	1.28	**0.98**	1.55	1.87	2.17	**1.30**	2.43	2.52
Laplacian	1.54	n/a	2.53	n/a	2.24	n/a	3.32	n/a	2.92	n/a	4.11	n/a
NPE	1.11	1.91	2.43	2.53	1.54	2.15	3.17	3.41	2.36	2.83	3.96	4.32

	95% Error											
	(a) All slices				(b) End-inhalation				(b) Most unusual			
	Displacement		Intensity		Displacement		Intensity		Displacement		Intensity	
DimRed	Sel	Pred	Sel	Pred	Sel	Pred	Sel	Pred	Sel	Pred	Sel	Pred
None	<u>1.94</u>	1.79	2.71		<u>3.26</u>	2.76	3.70		<u>4.61</u>	4.08	4.84	
PCA	1.96	**1.57**	2.71	3.02	3.26	**2.02**	3.65	4.13	4.60	**2.99**	4.70	5.17
Laplacian	4.33	n/a	5.85	n/a	6.34	n/a	7.19	n/a	6.96	n/a	7.72	n/a
NPE	2.71	3.82	5.38	5.60	4.16	4.74	6.75	7.35	4.92	6.07	7.50	8.07

5 Discussion and Conclusion

We proposed a method for improving 4D-MRI reconstruction of rare motion states, by actively predicting the unseen motion rather than only selecting from the available data. The method is based on learning the relationship between the motion of the navigator images and the motion of the data slices by linear regression after dimensionality reduction. It is most powerful for unusual motion states where a 40% improvement in mean accuracy can be achieved. Where enough similar samples are available it is less needed, but also does no harm as it is well constrained.

Using navigator intensities rather than displacements was clearly inferior. Initial test with extrapolations showed that non-linear functions or high-dimensional spaces leading to high errors due to the limited number of samples.

Currently every data slice prediction is optimized independently, without considering the gathered information across slices or over time. Such a combined framework would certainly benefit to make the predictions more robust, as currently improvements for extreme motion states can be of different quality and hence reduce the data slice consistency despite being more accurate on average.

We envision that the proposed prediction method is used for the unusual but very important motion states, while the selection method, which is faster, is sufficient for the common states.

References

1. Tanner, C., Boye, D., Samei, G., Székely, G.: Review on 4D models for organ motion compensation. Critical Reviews in Biomedical Engineering 40(2), 135–154 (2012)
2. McClelland, J.R., Hawkes, D.J., Schaeffter, T., King, A.P.: Respiratory motion models: A review. Medical Image Analysis 17(1), 19–42 (2013)
3. Von Siebenthal, M., Székely, G., Gamper, U., Boesiger, P., Lomax, A., Cattin, P.: 4D MR imaging of respiratory organ motion and its variability. Phys. Med. Biol. 52, 1547 (2007)
4. Wachinger, C., Yigitsoy, M., Rijkhorst, E.J., Navab, N.: Manifold learning for image-based breathing gating in ultrasound and MRI. Medical Image Analysis 16(4), 806–818 (2012)
5. Tryggestad, E., Flammang, A., Han-Oh, S., Hales, R., Herman, J., McNutt, T., Roland, T., Shea, S.M., Wong, J.: Respiration-based sorting of dynamic MRI to derive representative 4D-MRI for radiotherapy planning. Medical Physics 40(5), 051909 (2013)
6. Baumgartner, C.F., Kolbitsch, C., McClelland, J.R., Rueckert, D., King, A.P.: Groupwise simultaneous manifold alignment for high-resolution dynamic MR imaging of respiratory motion. In: Gee, J.C., Joshi, S., Pohl, K.M., Wells, W.M., Zöllei, L. (eds.) IPMI 2013. LNCS, vol. 7917, pp. 232–243. Springer, Heidelberg (2013)
7. Fransens, R., Strecha, C., Van Gool, L.: Optical flow based super-resolution: A probabilistic approach. Computer Vision and Image Understanding 106(1), 106–115 (2007)
8. Wu, G., Wang, Q., Lian, J., Shen, D.: Estimating the 4D respiratory lung motion by spatiotemporal registration and building super-resolution image. In: Fichtinger, G., Martel, A., Peters, T. (eds.) MICCAI 2011, Part I. LNCS, vol. 6891, pp. 532–539. Springer, Heidelberg (2011)
9. Hamm, J., Ye, D.H., Verma, R., Davatzikos, C.: Gram: A framework for geodesic registration on anatomical manifolds. Medical Image Analysis 14(5), 633–642 (2010)
10. Gerber, S., Tasdizen, T., Fletcher, T., Joshi, S., Whitaker, R.: Manifold modeling for brain population analysis. Medical Image Analysis 14(5), 643–653 (2010)
11. Wu, G., Jia, H., Wang, Q., Shen, D.: Sharpmean: Groupwise registration guided by sharp mean image and tree-based registration. NeuroImage 56(4), 1968–1981 (2011)
12. Avants, B., Gee, J.C.: Geodesic estimation for large deformation anatomical shape averaging and interpolation. Neuroimage 23, S139–S150 (2004)
13. Hartkens, T., Rueckert, D., Schnabel, J.A., Hawkes, D.J., Hill, D.L.G.: VTK CISG registration toolkit: An open source software package for affine and non-rigid registration of single-and multimodal 3D images. In: Bildverarbeitung für die Medizin 2002, pp. 409–412 (2002)
14. Heinrich, M.P., Jenkinson, M., Brady, S.M., Schnabel, J.A.: Globally optimal deformable registration on a minimum spanning tree using dense displacement sampling. In: Ayache, N., Delingette, H., Golland, P., Mori, K. (eds.) MICCAI 2012, Part III. LNCS, vol. 7512, pp. 115–122. Springer, Heidelberg (2012)
15. Heinrich, M., Jenkinson, M., Brady, M., Schnabel, J.A.: MRF-based deformable registration and ventilation estimation of lung CT. IEEE Transactions on Medical Imaging 32(7), 1239–1248 (2013)

Tensor Total-Variation Regularized Deconvolution for Efficient Low-Dose CT Perfusion

Ruogu Fang[1], Pina C. Sanelli[2,3], Shaoting Zhang[4], and Tsuhan Chen[1]

[1] Department of Electrical and Computer Engineering, Cornell University, Ithaca, NY
[2] Department of Radiology, Weill Cornell Medical College, New York, NY
[3] Department of Public Health, Weill Cornell Medical College, New York, NY
[4] Department of Computer Science, University of North Carolina at Charlotte, Charlotte, NC

Abstract. Acute brain diseases such as acute stroke and transit ischemic attacks are the leading causes of mortality and morbidity worldwide, responsible for 9% of total death every year. 'Time is brain' is a widely accepted concept in acute cerebrovascular disease treatment. Efficient and accurate computational framework for hemodynamic parameters estimation can save critical time for thrombolytic therapy. Meanwhile the high level of accumulated radiation dosage due to continuous image acquisition in CT perfusion (CTP) raised concerns on patient safety and public health. However, low-radiation will lead to increased noise and artifacts which require more sophisticated and time-consuming algorithms for robust estimation. We propose a novel efficient framework using tensor total-variation (TTV) regularization to achieve both high efficiency and accuracy in deconvolution for low-dose CTP. The method reduces the necessary radiation dose to only 8% of the original level and outperforms the state-of-art algorithms with estimation error reduced by 40%. It also corrects over-estimation of cerebral blood flow (CBF) and under-estimation of mean transit time (MTT), at both normal and reduced sampling rate. An efficient computational algorithm is proposed to find the solution with fast convergence.

1 Introduction

As the second leading cause of death worldwide, stroke is responsible for 4.4 million (9 percent) of the total 50.5 million deaths each year [1]. It affects more than 700,000 individuals annually in the United States (approximately one person every 45 seconds). It is also the No. 1 cause of disability among adults in US. Fast and accurate diagnosis and treatment for acute stroke is critical for the survival rate and life quality. Computed tomography perfusion (CTP) is the most widely used imaging modality for acute cerebrovascular disease diagnosis and detection, due to its widespread availability, rapid acquisition time, high spatial resolution and low cost. However, the elevated radiation dosage issue has raised significant public concerns regarding its potential biological effects, such as hair loss, skin damage, cataract formation, very small but definite increase of cancer risk [2].

The low-dose protocols, on the other hand, are leading to higher photon and imaging noise, which is compensated by more complicated and time-consuming algorithms with spatial smoothing, reduced matrix reconstruction and/or thick-slices, with the cost

P. Golland et al. (Eds.): MICCAI 2014, Part I, LNCS 8673, pp. 154–161, 2014.

of longer processing time, lowering spatial resolution and accuracy [3, 4]. While edge-preserving filtering algorithms are relatively slow in computation, HighlY constrained back-PRojection (HYPR) and Markov Random Fields (MRF) require motion-free images across the scan duration. Furthermore, these algorithms attempt to reduce the noise in the reconstructed CT image series, instead of improving the deconvolution process or the quantification of perfusion maps.

In this work, we propose an efficient and accurate deconvolution algorithm to improve the perfusion parameter estimation at low dose by tensor total variation (TTV) regularized deconvolution. All the previously mentioned noise reduction algorithms for CT image sequences can complement our model to further reduce the noise and improve the image quality. Total variation has been proposed for low-dose CT image reconstruction [5], while here we address a different problem of deconvolution to estimate the perfusion parameters.

The contribution of our work is three-fold. First, we propose to regularize the impulse residue functions instead of the perfusion parameter maps. Second, the optimization is performed globally on the entire spatio-temporal data, instead of each patch individually. Third, total variation regularizer is extended into the three dimensional sequence to consider the regional effect and temporal correlation of the tissue. The method reduces the necessary radiation dose to only 8% of the original level and outperforms the state-of-art algorithms with estimation error reduced by 40%. It also corrects over-estimation of cerebral blood flow (CBF) and under-estimation of mean transit time (MTT), at both normal and reduced sampling rate. An efficient computational algorithm is proposed to find the solution with fast convergence.

2 Tensor Total Variation Regularized Deconvolution

2.1 CT Perfusion Convolution Model

The physiological model of blood flow in CTP is built on tracing the intravenously injected contrast agent using X-ray scans. For a volume under consideration V_{voi}, let AIF (arterial input function) be the contrast agent concentration at the artery inlet, and C_{voi} be the average contrast agent concentration in V_{voi}. ρ_{voi} is the mean density of the volume V_{voi}. The residue function $R(t)$ quantifies the relative amount of contrast agent that is still inside the volume V_{voi} of interest at time t after a contrast agent bolus has entered the volume at the arterial inlet at time $t = 0$.

CBF is defined as the blood volume flow normalized by the mass of the volume V_{voi} and is typically measured in mL/100g/min. MTT, usually measured in seconds, is defined as the first moment of the probability density function $h(t)$ of the transit times.

The convolution model can be expressed as follows:

$$C_{voi}(t) = (AIF \otimes K)(t) \tag{1}$$

where the flow-scaled residue function $K(t)$ is introduced:

$$K(t) = CBF \cdot \rho_{voi} \cdot R(t) \tag{2}$$

By forming the matrix-vector notation, the convolution can be formulated as matrix multiplication. For a volume of interest with N voxels, we have

$$C = AK \tag{3}$$

where $C = [c_1, \ldots, c_N] \in \mathbb{R}^{T \times N}$, $K = [k_1, \ldots, k_N] \in \mathbb{R}^{T \times N}$ represent the contrast agent concentration and scaled residue function for the N voxels in the volume of interest. To overcome the inaccuracies due to delay and dispersion of the contrast agent, block-circulant version of A and C are adopted [6] to make the algorithm insensitive to the tracer arrival time. The perfusion parameters CBF and MTT can be determined from K [7].

2.2   Tensor Total Variation Regularized Deconvolution

The least square solution of Eq. (3) is equivalent to minimizing the squared Euclidean residual norm of the linear system given by Eq. (3) as

$$K_{ls} = \underset{K \in \mathbb{R}^{T \times N}}{\arg \min} (\|AK - C\|_2^2) \tag{4}$$

However, for the ill-conditioned Toeplitz matrix A, the least-square solution K_{ls} does not represent a proper solution. A small change in C (e.g. due to projection noise or low-dose scan) can cause a large change in K_{ls}. Regularization is necessary to avoid the strong oscillation in the solution due to small singular values of matrix A.

Since the voxel dimensions in a typical CTP image are much smaller than tissue structures, changes in perfusion are regional effects rather than single voxel effects. Our assumption is that within extended voxel neighborhoods the perfusion parameters will be constant or of low-variation. Meanwhile, it is also important to identify edges between different regions where tissues undergo perfusion changes, particularly ischemic regions. In the temporal dimensional, the residue functions are continuous, while the rapid rise and slow decay of contrast agent should also be preserved. We introduce the tensor total variation regularizer to the data fidelity term in Eq. (4) as

$$K = \underset{K \in \mathbb{R}^{T \times N}}{\arg \min} (\frac{1}{2} \|AK - C\|_2^2 + \gamma \|K\|_{TV}) \tag{5}$$

where γ is a positive parameter. It is based on the assumption that the piecewise smooth residue functions in CTP should have small total variation in both the temporal and spatial domain. Here we use a same $\gamma = 1$ for the spatial and temporal dimension, which yields satisfactory results. The tensor total variation term is defined as

$$\|K\|_{TV} = \sum_{t,i,j,k} (|\tilde{K}_{t+1,i,j,k} - \tilde{K}_{t,i,j,k}| + |\tilde{K}_{t,i+1,j,k} - \tilde{K}_{t,i,j,k}| \\ + |\tilde{K}_{t,i,j+1,k} - \tilde{K}_{t,i,j,k}| + |\tilde{K}_{t,i,j,k+1} - \tilde{K}_{t,i,j,k}|) \tag{6}$$

where $\tilde{K} \in \mathbb{R}^{T \times N_1 \times N_2 \times N_3}$ is the 4-D volume obtained by reshaping matrix K based on the spatial and temporal dimensions. Here $N = N_1 \times N_2 \times N_3$ and T is the time

Algorithm 1. The framework of TTV algorithm.

Input: Regularization parameters γ
Output: Flow-scaled residue functions $K \in \mathbf{R}^{T \times N_1 \times N_2 \times N_3}$.
$K^0 = 0$
$t^1 = r^1 = K^0$
for $n = 1, 2, \ldots, N$ **do**
   (1) Steepest gradient descent: $K_g = r^n + s^{n+1}(A^T(C - Ar^n))$
   where $s^{n+1} = \frac{Q^T Q}{(AQ^T)(AQ)}$, $Q \equiv A^T(Ar^n - C)$
   (2) Proximal map: $K^n = prox_\gamma(2\|K\|_{TV})(K_g)$,
   where $prox_\rho(g)(x) := \arg\min_u \left\{ g(u) + \frac{1}{2\rho}\|u - x\|^2 \right\}$
   (3) Update t, r: $t^{n+1} = (1 + \sqrt{1 + 4(t^n)^2})/2$, $r^{n+1} = K^n + ((t^n - 1)/t^{n+1})(K^n - K^{n-1})$
end for

duration. The tensor total variation term here uses the forward finite difference operator with L_1 norm. The regularization parameter γ controls the regularization strength, and the larger the γ, the more smoothed the residue functions. Since the TV term is non-smooth, this problem is difficult to solve. Conjugate gradient (CG) and partial differential equation (PDE) methods could be used to attack it, but they are very slow and impractical for real CTP images. Motivated by the effective acceleration scheme in Fast Iterative Shrinkage-Thresholding Algorithm (FISTA) [8, 9], we propose a total variation regularization algorithm (Algorithm 1) to efficiently solve the problem in Eq. (5). We extended the 2-dimensional TV regularizer in [8] to 4-dimensional and adapted the algorithm to tensor total variation, to impose both temporal and spatial edge-preserving regularization.

2.3 Implementation Details

All algorithms were implemented using MATLAB 2013a (MathWorks Inc, Natick, MA) on a MacBook Pro with Intel Core i7 2.8G Hz Duo CPU and 8GB RAM. Four baseline methods were compared: standard truncated singular value decomposition (sSVD) [7], block-circulant truncated SVD (bSVD) [6], Tikhonov regularization (Tikh) [10] and sparse perfusion deconvolution (SPD)[11]. Perfusion maps are computed on the high-dose 190 mA and the simulated low-dose 15 mA images by adding correlated statistical noise [12] with standard deviation of $\sigma_a = 25.54$, which yields PSNR=40. The maps calculated using bSVD from the 190 mA high-dose CTP data is regarded as the "gold standard" or reference images in clinical experiments. A threshold value λ is empirically chosen as 0.1 (10% of the maximum singular value) to yield optimal performance for SVD-based algorithms. One-tail student test is used to determine whether there is significant difference between the evaluation metrics of the comparing algorithms. A α level of .05 is used for all statistical tests to indicate significance. Two metrics were used to evaluate the image fidelity to the reference: Root mean-squared-error (RMSE) and Lin's Concordance Correlation Coefficient (CCC). Low RMSE and high Lin's CCC indicate high accuracy for the perfusion maps.

3   Experiments

3.1   Synthetic Studies

Because the clinical CTP does not have ground truth perfusion parameter values for comparison, we first use synthetic data to evaluate the proposed algorithm, following the synthetic experiment setup in [13].

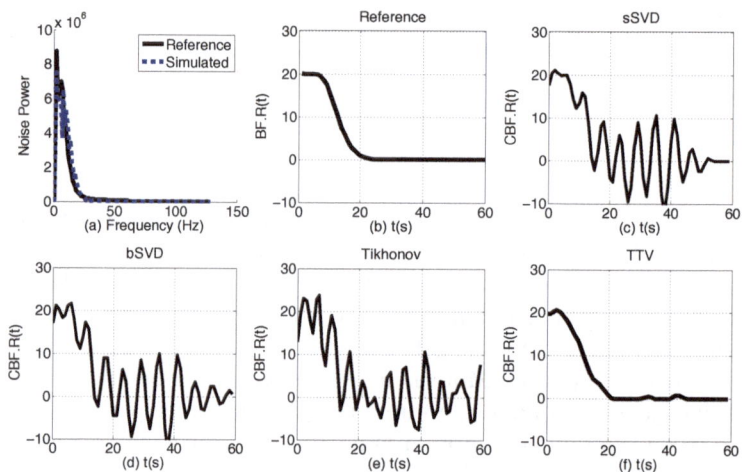

Fig. 1. The Noise power spectrum and the recovered residue functions by baseline methods and TTV. (a) The noise power spectrum is of the scanned phantom image at 15 mA and simulated statistical correlated Gaussian noise at 15 mA. (b)-(f) The parameters used for residue function recovery are the simulation is CBV = 4 mL/100 g, CBF = 20 mL/100 g/min, PSNR=25. SPD is not included since it optimizes the perfusion maps directly.

Residue Recovery: The simulated noise power spectrum (NPS) at 15 mA is compared with the NPS of the real scanned phantom image at 15 mA, as shown in Figure 1(a). The residue function recovered by the baseline methods and TTV are shown in Figure 1(b-f). The baseline methods show severe oscillation and elevated peak value, while the residue function recovered by TTV is in agreement with the reference.

Uniform Region Estimation: From the recovered residue function, perfusion parameters CBF and MTT can be estimated. We generate a small region containing 40×40 voxels with the same perfusion characteristics, and compute the mean and standard deviation of the perfusion parameters over this region. 1) Fig. 2 (a)-(b) show the estimated CBF and MTT values when the true perfusion parameter values vary. All the baseline methods overestimate the CBF values and under-estimate the MTT values while TTV yields accurate CBF and MTT estimations. 2) To explore the effect of noise levels on the performance of perfusion parameter estimation, we simulate different levels of noise (PSNR varies from 5 to 60) and fix CBF at 20 mL/100 g/min and MTT at 12 s. Fig. 2 (c)-(d) show the estimation results. When the accuracy of the baseline methods degrades

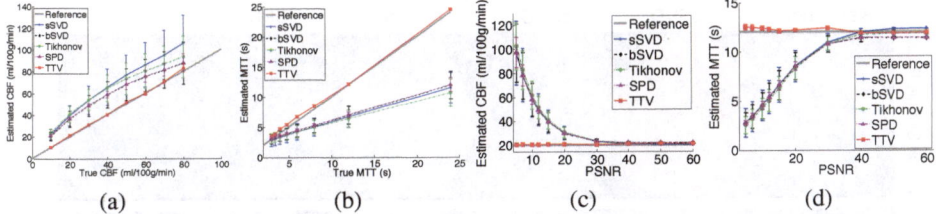

Fig. 2. Comparison of the accuracy in estimating CBF and MTT by sSVD, bSVD, Tikhonov, SPD and TTV deconvolution methods. True CBV = 4 mL/100 g. The error bar denotes the standard deviation. (a) Estimated CBF values at different true with PSNR=15. (b) Estimated MTT values at different true MTT with PNSR=15. (c) Estimated CBF values at different PSNRs with true CBF=20 mL/100 g/min. (d) Estimated MTT values at different PSNRs with true MTT = 12 s.

Table 1. Quantitative evaluation of the perfusion parameters in Fig. 2. 'Estimated' mean the perfusion parameter to be estimated. 'Condition' means the varying condition. The best performance is highlighted in bold font.

Estimated	CBF			MTT		
Varying	CBF		PSNR	MTT		PSNR
Method/Metric	RMSE	Lin's CCC	RMSE	RMSE	Lin's CCC	RMSE
sSVD	23.52	0.6878	52.07	6.056	0.4283	6.278
bSVD	15.05	0.8129	52.01	5.827	0.4567	6.309
Tikhonov	19.94	0.7198	43.92	5.64	0.4748	6.015
SPD	15.02	0.8294	44.36	5.804	0.4586	3.3323
TTV	**0.993**	**0.9991**	**0.7954**	**0.6847**	**0.9945**	**0.294**

Table 2. Quantitative comparison of five methods on ten patients in terms of RMSE, Lin's CCC and linear regression. The best performance is highlighted in bold font. * $P < .001$ in one-tail student test compared to the four baseline methods.

Method	RMSE	Lin's CCC
sSVD	25.69	0.049
bSVD	7.60	0.185
Tikhonov	11.27	0.161
SPD	6.03	0.267
TTV	**3.63***	**0.505***

dramatically as the noise level increases, TTV method appears to be more robust. Table 1 shows the quantitative evaluation of the different methods in terms of RMSE and Lin's CCC while the ground truth parameter or the PSNR varies.

3.2 Clinical Studies

Retrospective review of consecutive CTP exams performed on aneurysmal subarachnoid hemorrhage patients enrolled in an IRB-approved and HIPAA-compliant clinical trial from August 2007-July 2013 was used. Ten consecutive patients (9 women, 1 men) admitted to the Weill Cornell Medical College, with mean age (range) of 54 (35-83) years were included. 5 patients had brain deficits shown in the CTP images and the other 5 patients had normal brain images.

Visual Comparison: At normal sampling rate, Fig. 3 shows significant differences visually between the CBF maps of the different deconvolution methods, where sSVD, bSVD, Tikhonov and SPD overestimate CBF, while TTV estimates accurately. At reduced temporal sampling rate by downsampling 2 times, the errors in the four baseline methods increase, while TTV maintains accurate estimation, with the potential to further minimize the radiation dosage level by increasing sampling intervals.

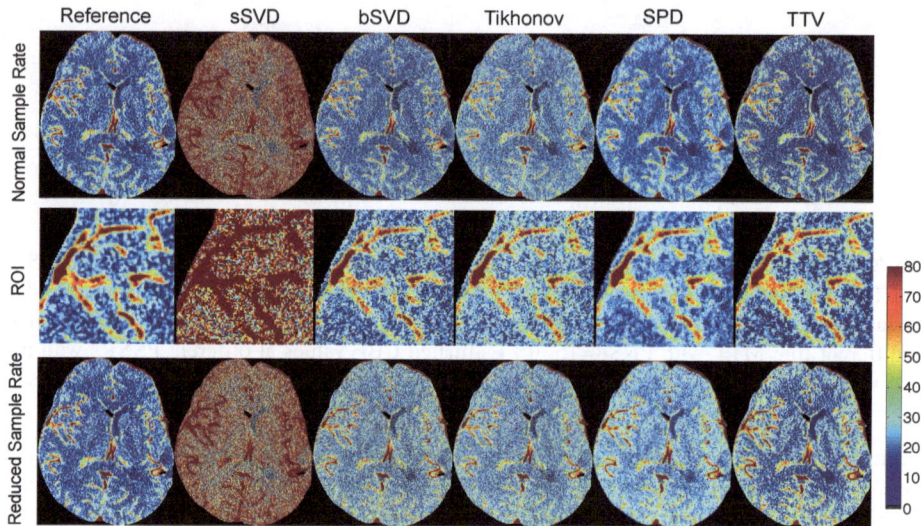

Fig. 3. The CBF maps with zoomed ROI regions of a patients calculated using different methods at normal sampling rate (first two rows) and reduced rate by downsampling 2 times (bottom row). Baseline methods sSVD, bSVD and Tikhonov overestimate CBF values, while SPD and TTV correspond with the reference. At reduced rate, the difference is more significant. (Color image)

Quantitative Comparison: There is significant improvement in image fidelity between the low-dose CBF maps and the high-dose CBF maps by using the TTV algorithm compared to the baseline methods. On average, the RMSE decreases by 40%, Lin's CCC increases by 89% from the best performance by using the baseline methods (Table 2).

Computation Time: It takes approximately 25 s to process a clinical dataset of $512 \times 512 \times 118$ by TTV method with 5 iterations, and approximately 0.83 s, 2.04 s and 1.35 s for sSVD, bSVD and Tikhonov algorithms. For SPD, it takes 80.6 s for the whole image. The TTV algorithm usually converges within 5 iterations. Though SVD and Tikhonov based methods are faster, the over-estimation, low spatial resolution, less differentiable tissue types and graining in the image in the perfusion maps generated by these baseline methods for the low-dose data are not acceptable. SPD reduces the variation in the smooth region to certain extent, however, TTV takes only 30% of the computation time compared to the time for SPD and yields more accurate estimation.

4   Conclusion

In this study, a new tensor total variation regularized deconvolution algorithm is proposed to improve the quality and quantification of the low-dose CTP perfusion maps and extensively compared with the existing widely used algorithms, e.g. sSVD, bSVD and Tikhonov regularization, as well as SPD for low-dose deconvolution. Synthetic evaluation with accurate ground truth data is used to compare the quality of the residue functions, uniform regions, sensitivity to hemodynamic conditions and noise levels. Clinical evaluation using high-dose perfusion maps as the reference image is conducted to show the visual quality and data fidelity at normal and reduced sampling rate. The proposed TTV method is able to achieve both high accuracy and computational efficiency to save critical time for the clinical diagnosis.

References

[1] Feigin, V.L., Lawes, C.M., Bennett, D.A., Barker-Collo, S.L., Parag, V.: Worldwide stroke incidence and early case fatality reported in 56 population-based studies: a systematic review. The Lancet Neurology 8(4), 355–369 (2009)

[2] Wintermark, M., Lev, M.: FDA investigates the safety of brain perfusion CT. American Journal of Neuroradiology 31(1), 2–3 (2010)

[3] Saito, N., Kudo, K., Sasaki, T., Uesugi, M., Koshino, K., Miyamoto, M., Suzuki, S.: Realization of reliable cerebral-blood-flow maps from low-dose CT perfusion images by statistical noise reduction using nonlinear diffusion filtering. Radiological Physics and Technology 1(1), 62–74 (2008)

[4] Supanich, M., Tao, Y., Nett, B., Pulfer, K., Hsieh, J., Turski, P., Mistretta, C., Rowley, H., Chen, G.H.: Radiation dose reduction in time-resolved CT angiography using highly constrained back projection reconstruction. Physics in Medicine and Biology 54(14), 4575 (2009)

[5] Tian, Z., Jia, X., Yuan, K., Pan, T., Jiang, S.B.: Low-dose ct reconstruction via edge-preserving total variation regularization. Physics in Medicine and Biology 56(18), 5949 (2011)

[6] Wu, O., Østergaard, L., Weisskoff, R.M., Benner, T., Rosen, B.R., Sorensen, A.G.: Tracer arrival timing-insensitive technique for estimating flow in MR perfusion-weighted imaging using singular value decomposition with a block-circulant deconvolution matrix. Magnetic Resonance in Medicine 50(1), 164–174 (2003)

[7] Østergaard, L., Weisskoff, R.M., Chesler, D.A., Gyldensted, C., Rosen, B.R.: High resolution measurement of cerebral blood flow using intravascular tracer bolus passages. Part I: Mathematical approach and statistical analysis. Magnetic Resonance in Medicine 36(5), 715–725 (1996)

[8] Beck, A., Teboulle, M.: A fast iterative shrinkage-thresholding algorithm with application to wavelet-based image deblurring. In: IEEE International Conference on Acoustics, Speech and Signal Processing, ICASSP 2009, pp. 693–696. IEEE (2009)

[9] Huang, J., Zhang, S., Metaxas, D.: Efficient MR image reconstruction for compressed MR imaging. Medical Image Analysis 15(5), 670–679 (2011)

[10] Fieselmann, A., Kowarschik, M., Ganguly, A., Hornegger, J., Fahrig, R.: Deconvolution-based CT and MR brain perfusion measurement: theoretical model revisited and practical implementation details. Journal of Biomedical Imaging 2011, 14 (2011)

[11] Fang, R., Chen, T., Sanelli, P.C.: Towards robust deconvolution of low-dose perfusion ct: Sparse perfusion deconvolution using online dictionary learning. Medical Image Analysis 17(4), 417–428 (2013)

[12] Britten, A., Crotty, M., Kiremidjian, H., Grundy, A., Adam, E.: The addition of computer simulated noise to investigate radiation dose and image quality in images with spatial correlation of statistical noise: an example application to x-ray ct of the brain. British Journal of Radiology 77(916), 323–328 (2004)

[13] He, L., Orten, B., Do, S., Karl, W.C., Kambadakone, A., Sahani, D.V., Pien, H.: A spatio-temporal deconvolution method to improve perfusion ct quantification. IEEE Transactions on Medical Imaging 29(5), 1182–1191 (2010)

Speckle Reduction in Optical Coherence Tomography by Image Registration and Matrix Completion

Jun Cheng[1], Lixin Duan[1], Damon Wing Kee Wong[1], Dacheng Tao[2], Masahiro Akiba[3], and Jiang Liu[1]

[1] Institute for Infocomm Research, Agency for Science, Technology and Research, Singapore
{jcheng,duanlx,wkwong,jliu}@i2r.a-star.edu.sg
[2] University of Technology, Sydney, Australia
[3] Topcon Corporation, Tokyo, Japan

Abstract. Speckle noise is problematic in optical coherence tomography (OCT). With the fast scan rate, swept source OCT scans the same position in the retina for multiple times rapidly and computes an average image from the multiple scans for speckle reduction. However, the eye movement poses some challenges. In this paper, we propose a new method for speckle reduction from multiply-scanned OCT slices. The proposed method applies a preliminary speckle reduction on the OCT slices and then registers them using a global alignment followed by a local alignment based on fast iterative diamond search. After that, low rank matrix completion using bilateral random projection is utilized to iteratively estimate the noise and recover the underlying clean image. Experimental results show that the proposed method achieves average contrast to noise ratio 15.65, better than 13.78 by the baseline method used currently in swept source OCT devices. The technology can be embedded into current OCT machines to enhance the image quality for subsequent analysis.

Keywords: Speckle, matrix completion, bilateral random projection.

1 Introduction

Optical coherence tomography (OCT) is a micrometer-scale, cross-sectional imaging modality for biological tissue. In OCT images, the structures are often obscured due to speckle noise. Recently, Topcon has developed DRI OCT-1, a swept source OCT for posterior imaging of the eye, utilizing a wavelength sweeping light source at 1,050nm wavelength range. It has a fast scanning speed of 100,000 A-scans/second. In DRI OCT-1, the speckle noise in a single raw B-scan image often makes it challenging to examine the detailed structure. Fig. 1 shows an example of raw slice. Thus, speckle noise reduction is important to improve the image quality in the DRI OCT-1.

Besides OCT, speckle reduction has also been an important research topic in many other imaging modalities such as ultrasound, sonar, remote sensing, etc. In

P. Golland et al. (Eds.): MICCAI 2014, Part I, LNCS 8673, pp. 162–169, 2014.

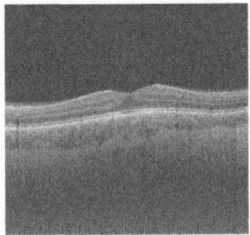

Fig. 1. A raw slice (*B*-scan) of OCT image captured by DRI OCT-1

these fields, many speckle reduction algorithms have been proposed such as enhanced Lee filter [1], adaptive Wiener filter [2], anisotropic diffusion [3], speckle reduction anisotropic diffusion (SRAD) [4], etc. Although these methods are efficient in removing speckle noise, they often remove some details simultaneously. Therefore, their practical usage is limited.

With the fast imaging speed, DRI OCT-1 utilizes a new strategy for speckle reduction by scanning the same or approximately the same position for multiple times. For example in a line scan mode in DRI OCT-1, a maximum of 96 scans can be obtained for the same line. Then an average image is computed from the 96 scans to generate a *B*-scan image. The averaging strategy expects the cancelling out of speckle noise from the different scans. It has been shown that averaging successfully reduces the noise [5]. However, it has limitations. Firstly, the actual locations scanned are often shifted due to eye movement in the capture. This may lead to some changes in the underlying image. Although the changes are normally small, they hardly cancel out with each other. Secondly, the multiply-scanned slices are often not well aligned due to eye movement and image registration is required. However, the high amount of speckle may dominate the registration. In DRI OCT-1, a rigid sub-pixel registration algorithm [6] is used to register the slices. It minimizes the mean square intensity difference between one slice and its reference mainly through translation. However, it is not robust in presence of large speckle noise.

In this paper, we propose a new method for speckle reduction from multiple OCT slices. In this method, a preliminary speckle reduction is first applied on the raw unprocessed slices. Then, a non-rigid two-step registration is proposed to align the slices. After that, low rank matrix completion is proposed to compute the clean image. Because the multiple scans are usually obtained from very close but different locations, it is inevitable that the underlying images have some slight differences. The basic idea of low rank matrix completion is to formulate the kth OCT slice I_k as a sum of its underlying clean image part l_k, a sparse part s_k due to eye movement and a noise part n_k due to speckle noise:

$$I_k = l_k + s_k + n_k \qquad (1)$$

Define $X = [\tilde{I}_1, \tilde{I}_2, \cdots, \tilde{I}_m]$, $L = [\tilde{l}_1, \tilde{l}_2, \cdots, \tilde{l}_m]$, $S = [\tilde{s}_1, \tilde{s}_2, \cdots, \tilde{s}_m]$, and $N = [\tilde{n}_1, \tilde{n}_2, \cdots, \tilde{n}_m] \in \mathbb{R}^{n \times m}$, where m is the number of slices, n is the number of pixels in each slice, $\tilde{I}_k$, $\tilde{l}_k$, $\tilde{s}_k$, and $\tilde{n}_k$ are strung out of I_k, l_k, s_k and n_k into column vectors, $k = 1, 2, \cdots, m$. Although each $\tilde{I}_k$ can be significantly different from others because of the different noise $\tilde{n}_k$, $\tilde{l}_k$ is expected to be the same for all k. The rank of L is thus low. In low rank matrix completion, we want to solve L from given X. Instead of relying on the cancel out of the noise by averaging, our low rank approach estimates the noise and relies on the estimation accuracy.

The rest of paper is organized as follows. In Section 2, we introduce the method including the preliminary speckle reduction using SRAD, the image registration by global and local alignment based on iterative diamond search, and the image recovery by low rank matrix completion. Section 3 shows the experimental results and is followed by conclusions in the last section.

2   Method

2.1   Denoising

Because of the inevitable eye movement, the raw OCT slices are usually not well aligned and registration is required. However, they are affected by large speckle noise which may dominate the image registration. In this paper, we propose to use SRAD [4] to have a preliminary noise reduction. Our tests show that SRAD is able to remove the noise though some details are removed. The basic principle of SRAD is as follows. Given an intensity image $I_0(x, y)$, the output image $I(x, y, t)$ is evolved according to following partial differential equations in SRAD:

$$\begin{cases} \partial I / \partial t = div[c \cdot \nabla I] \\ I(t = 0) = I_0, \end{cases} \tag{2}$$

where c denotes the diffusion coefficient computed from I.

2.2   Image Registration

In this paper, we propose to register the raw OCT slices based on their de-noised version obtained using the above SRAD algorithm. The image registration or alignment between two slices is done by a global alignment followed by a local alignment. In the global alignment step, a translation $(\Delta x, \Delta y)$ including both horizontal and vertical directions is applied on the entire slice. Taking I_i as a reference, for each $I_j, j = 1, 2, \cdots, m$ and $j \neq i$, we find the alignment $(\Delta x_j, \Delta y_j)$ between I_i and I_j such that their difference is minimized.

In the local alignment step, an A-scan line (i.e., a column) or a group of neighboring A-scan lines from one B-scan slice are translated vertically (up or down) for best matching to the corresponding A-scan lines in a reference B-scan slice. As illustrated in Fig. 2, we divide a B-scan slice B_j to non-overlapping A-scan group $A_{j,k}, k = 1, 2, \cdots, P$, where P is the number of A-scan groups in B_j. Each group has l A-scan lines. For $A_{i,k}$ and $A_{j,k}$ from B_i and B_j, find the vertical translation $\Delta x_{j,k}$ between them such that their error is minimized. In this paper, we use $l = 8$. Since the eye movement is expected to be smooth, a

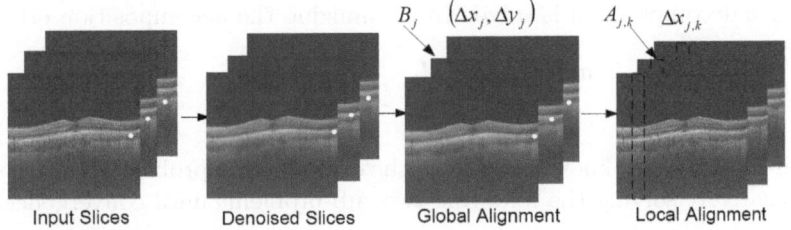

Fig. 2. Illustration of Image Registration

smoothing process is applied to the vertical translations for lines in the same slice. The local alignment is done based on A-scans instead of other patches because each column is an outcome of an A-scan and the eye movement during the capture of one A-scan is minimal and ignored. By applying vertical alignment on A-scans, we protect the integrity of each A-scan.

In the above, a full search of the matching can be time consuming. In this paper, we use the iterative diamond search strategy [7] because of its efficiency and easy implementation. In the searching procedure, the algorithm iteratively searches among the neighboring points for the alignment between current and reference slice until the error in between is no longer decreasing. In the global alignment, the searching is done in both horizontal and vertical neighbors. In the local alignment, the searching is done in vertical neighbors only.

2.3 Image Recovery

After the image registration, a set of registered slices are obtained. Then they are vectorized and stacked to form matrix X, where $X = L + S + N$ as illustrated in Fig. 3. Low rank matrix completion is applied to compute the underlying clean image.

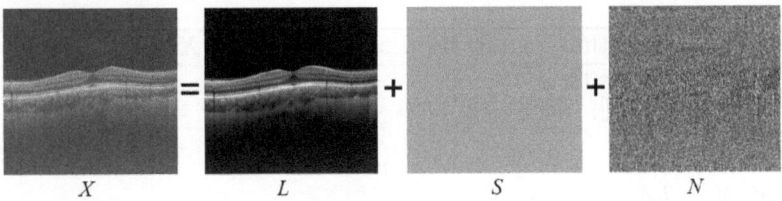

Fig. 3. Illustration of the model: each image shown here corresponds to a column in the matrix X, L, S, N, reshaped to a 2D image

Ideally, the clean images for all the slices are identical. In low rank approximation, X is modelled as:

$$X = L + S + N, s.t., \texttt{rank}(L) \leq r, \texttt{card}(S) \leq k$$

The above decomposition is solved by minimizing the decomposition error:

$$\min_{L,S} \|X - L - S\|_F^2 \tag{3}$$
$$s.t., \quad \mathbf{rank}(L) \le r, \mathbf{card}(S) \le k$$

Since there are two unknowns L and S, the optimization problem above is solved by alternatively solving the following two sub-problems until convergence.

$$L_t = \arg \min_{\mathbf{rank}(L) \le r} \|X - L_{t-1} - S_{t-1}\|_F^2 \tag{4}$$

$$S_t = \arg \min_{\mathbf{card}(S) \le k} \|X - L_{t-1} - S_{t-1}\|_F^2 \tag{5}$$

The problem in (4) can be solved using a singular value decomposition of $(X - S_{t-1})$ as in robust principle component analysis (RPCA) [8]. However, RPCA is very slow. In this paper, we solve it using the power scheme modified bilateral random projection (BRP) [9],[10]. We calculate the BRP of a matrix $\tilde{X} = ((X - S_{t-1})(X - S_{t-1})^T)^q (X - S_{t-1})$. The BRP of $\tilde{X}$ is:

$$Y_1 = \tilde{X} A_1, Y_2 = \tilde{X}^T A_2, \tag{6}$$

where $A_1 \in \mathbb{R}^{m \times r}$ and $A_2 \in \mathbb{R}^{n \times r}$. The approximation of $(X - S_{t-1})$ with rank r is then computed by

$$L = Q_1 [R_1 (A_2^T Y_1)^{-1} R_2^T]^{\frac{1}{2q+1}} Q_2^T, \tag{7}$$

where Q_1, R_1, Q_2, R_2 are obtained by QR decompositon of Y_1 and Y_2.

The problem in (5) is solved by updating S_t via entry-wise hard thresholding of $X - L_t$:

$$S_t = \wp_\Omega (X - L_t), \tag{8}$$

where $\wp_\Omega(Z)$ is a mapping to keep the largest k entries of $|Z|$ and assign the rest as 0. Detailed computation steps are summarized in the algorithm below.

Algorithm 1. Algorithm for solving L and S in model $X = L + S + N$

$t := 0, L_0 := X, S_0 = 0, r = 2;$
while $\|X - L_t - S_t\|_F^2 / \|X\|_F^2 > \epsilon$ and $t < t_{max}$ **do**
$t := t + 1;$
$\hat{L} = [(X - S_{t-1})(X - S_{t-1})^T]^q (X - S_{t-1});$
Compute $Y_1 = \hat{L} A_1, A_2 = Y_1;$
Compute $Y_2 = \hat{L}^T A_2 = Q_2 R_2, Y_1 = \hat{L} Y_2 = Q_1 R_1;$
    if $rank(A_2^T Y_1) \le r$ **then** $r = rank(A_2^T Y_1)$, go to the first step;
    end if;
$L_t = Q_1 \left[R_1 (A_2^T Y_1)^{-1} R_2^T) \right]^{1/(2q+1)} Q_2^T;$
$S_t = \wp_\Omega (X - L_t);$
end while

---

3   Experimental Results

In this paper, we conducted tests using 20 different subject eyes. For each subject eye, a line mode scan with 96 repeated slices are obtained. Each slice is an image with $992 \times 1024 = 1015808$ pixels. The matrix X is a 1015808×96 dimensional matrix.

It is important to have an objective measurement to evaluate the performance of speckle noise reduction. As we do not have the ground truth image or original image for comparison, traditional measurement such as peak signal to noise ratio cannot be computed here. In this paper, we compute the contrast to noise ratio (CNR) that is commonly used in similar tasks [5],[11]. It measures the contrast between a set of regions of interest and a background region:

$$CNR = \frac{1}{R} \sum_{r=1}^{R} \frac{\mu_r - u_b}{\sqrt{(\sigma_r^2 + \sigma_b^2)}} \tag{9}$$

where μ_b and σ_b are the mean and variance of the same background region, and μ_r and σ_r are the mean and variance of all the regions of interest. In this paper, we randomly obtain 20 ($R = 20$) regions of interest with 5×5 pixels from the retina layers in each image and one 5×5 background region.

To evaluate the performance of the proposed method, two methods denoted as 'Baseline' and 'Motion+Average' are compared with the proposed method. The 'baseline' denotes the state-of-the-art method which uses the sub-pixel registration and averaging approach as that in the current DRI OCT-1. In 'Motion+Average', we replace the sub-pixel registration in the 'Baseline' with the proposed registration while maintaining the averaging step. In the proposed method, we further replace the averaging with the BRP-based low rank matrix completion. Table 1 shows the average CNR computed from 20 images with the number of re-scanned slices $m = 96$. With a preliminary speckle reduction, the proposed diamond search based registration helps improve the CNR. The proposed method further improves the CNR by replacing averaging with low rank matrix completion. This is because the low rank reconstruction model is less sensitive to large noise from one or several slices compared with averaging as the latter cannot avoid it while the former is able to handle it better by estimation.

Table 1. Performance (CNR) by various methods

Method	Baseline	Motion + Average	Proposed
CNR	13.78	14.07	15.65

To evaluate the robustness of the proposed methods for different number of slices, we further conducted tests for the number of slices m from 16 to 96 with a step of 16. Fig. 4 plots the average CNRs for the three methods. The results show that the proposed method outperforms the baseline method consistently

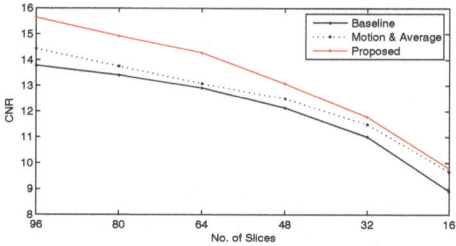

Fig. 4. Performance comparison for different number of reference images

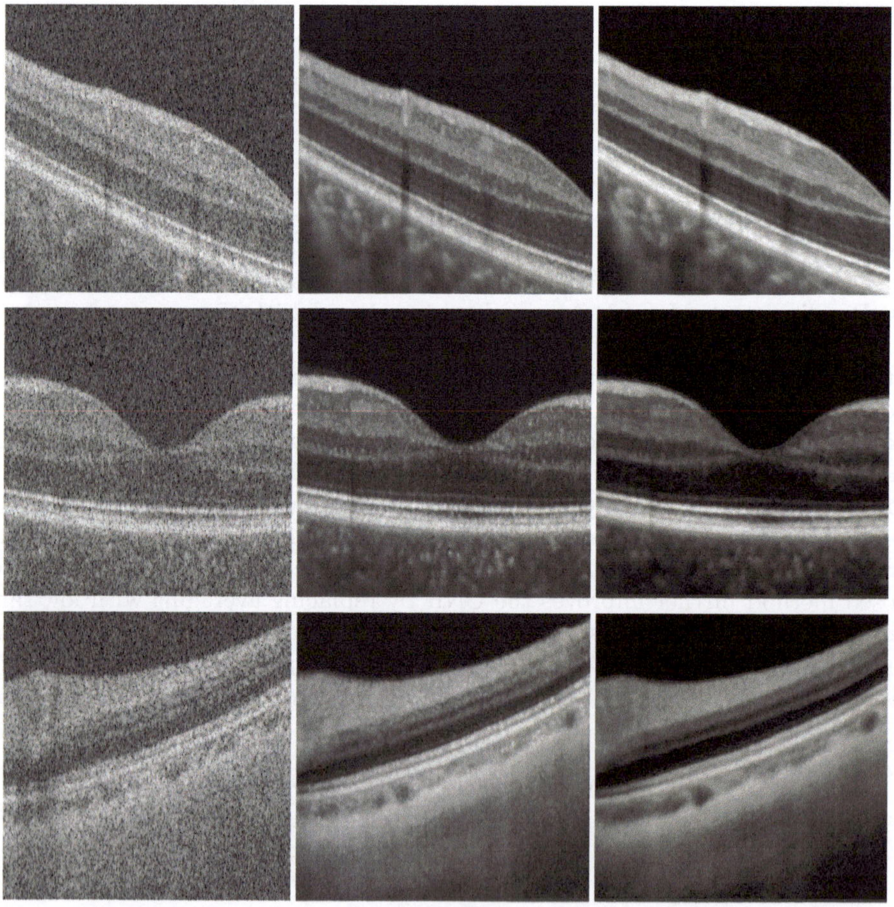

(a) Raw slice	(b) Baseline	(c) Proposed

Fig. 5. Sample results: (a) 300 × 300 regions cropped from raw slices for highlight, (b) and (c) are the corresponding portion of images obtained by the baseline and proposed method

but the improvement decreases with m. In addition, Fig. 5 shows three sample results to visualize the difference between the baseline and proposed method. As we can see, the images obtained from the proposed method show less speckle noise and better structure details than those from the baseline method.

In this paper, we solve the low rank matrix completion using power scheme modified BRP. It is faster than traditional algorithms such as RPCA with similar recovered results. It takes about 5s for one iteration of L_t to recover a image of 992×1024 pixels from 96 slices in a dual core 3.0 GHz PC with 3.25 GB RAM in MATLAB. For the same task, RPCA [8] requires 100s.

4   Conclusions

In this paper, we propose a novel algorithm for specke noise reduction in swept source OCT images. Instead of using a sub-pixel registration algorithm that minimizes the mean square intensity difference, we propose to register the raw OCT slices using fast diamond search from speckle reduced slices. In addition, averaging is replaced by low rank matrix completion using power scheme modified BRP. The main difference is that the former averaging approach relies on the cancelling out of speckle noise while the later low rank algorithm estimates the noise and relies on its accuracy in the estimation. Our experimental results show that the proposed method outperforms the currently used baseline method. The limitation of current method is that it requires a number of repeated scans from the same location.

References

1. Lopes, A., Touzi, R., Nesby, E.: Adaptive speckle filter and scene heterogeneity. IEEE Trans. Geosci. Remote Sens. 28, 992–1000 (1990)
2. Lim, S.J.: Two-Dimensional Signal and Image Processing. Prentice Hall (1990)
3. Perona, P., Malik, J.: Scale space and edge detection using anisotropic diffusion. IEEE Trans. Pattern Anal. Machine Intell. 12 (1990)
4. Yu, Y., Acton, S.T.: Speckle reducing anisotropic diffusion. IEEE Trans. Image Processing 11, 1260–1270 (2002)
5. Szkulmowski, M., Wojtkowski, M.: Averaging techniques for oct imaging. Opt. Express 21, 9757–9773 (2013)
6. Thévenaz, P., Ruttimann, U.E., Unser, M.: A pyramid approach to subpixel registration based on intensity. IEEE Trans. Image Processing 7, 27–41 (1998)
7. Zhu, S., Ma, K.: A new diamond search algorithm for fast block-matching motion estimation. IEEE Trans. Image Processing 9, 287–290 (2000)
8. Candès, E., Recht, B.: Exact matrix completion via convex optimization. Commun. ACM 55, 111–119 (2012)
9. Zhou, T., Tao, D.: Bilateral random projections. In: IEEE Int. Symp. on Information Theory, pp. 1286–1290 (2012)
10. Zhou, T., Tao, D.: Godec: Randomized low-rank & sparse matrix decomposition in noisy case. In: Proc. of the 28th Int. Conf. on Machine Learning, pp. 33–40 (2011)
11. Rogowaka, J., Brezinski, M.E.: Evaluation of the adaptive speckle suppression filter for coronary optical coherence tomography imaging. IEEE Trans. Medical Imaging 19, 1261–1266 (2000)

Signal Decomposition for X-ray Dark-Field Imaging

Sebastian Kaeppler[1], Florian Bayer[2], Thomas Weber[2], Andreas Maier[1],
Gisela Anton[2], Joachim Hornegger[1], Matthias Beckmann[3], Peter A. Fasching[3],
Arndt Hartmann[3], Felix Heindl[3], Thilo Michel[2], Gueluemser Oezguel[3],
Georg Pelzer[2], Claudia Rauh[3], Jens Rieger[2], Ruediger Schulz-Wendtland[3],
Michael Uder[3], David Wachter[3], Evelyn Wenkel[3], and Christian Riess[1]

[1] Pattern Recognition Lab
[2] Erlangen Centre for Astroparticle Physics
[3] University Hospital of Erlangen

Friedrich-Alexander-University Erlangen-Nuremberg, Erlangen, Germany
sebastian.kaeppler@fau.de

Abstract. Grating-based X-ray dark-field imaging is a new imaging
modality. It allows the visualization of structures at micrometer scale
due to small-angle scattering of the X-ray beam. However, reading dark-
field images is challenging as absorption and edge-diffraction effects also
contribute to the dark-field signal, without adding diagnostic value. In
this paper, we present a novel – and to our knowledge the first – algorithm for isolating small-angle scattering in dark-field images, which
greatly improves their interpretability. To this end, our algorithm utilizes the information available from the absorption and differential phase
images to identify clinically irrelevant contributions to the dark-field image. Experimental results on phantom and ex-vivo breast data promise
a greatly enhanced diagnostic value of dark-field images.

1 Introduction

Absorption X-ray imaging is the standard modality for a wide range of applications. Recently, *phase-sensitive* X-ray imaging attracted much attention. Different measurement principles have been proposed to obtain phase-sensitive images,
most notable are propagation-based systems [1], diffraction-enhanced systems [2]
and grating-based interferometers [3]. One particular benefit of grating-based
systems is that three output images are obtained, containing per pixel complementary information on absorption (i.e., overall intensity attenuation), differential phase shift of the X-ray wavefront, and dark-field (i.e., the contrast reduction
of the grating pattern due to the object).

While the differential phase shift contrast (DPC) can significantly increase
soft-tissue contrast over absorption imaging [4], the contrast loss of the grating
pattern, referred to as dark-field signal (DFI), reveals unique information about
structural tissue variations at micro and nano meter scale [5], often subsumed

P. Golland et al. (Eds.): MICCAI 2014, Part I, LNCS 8673, pp. 170–177, 2014.

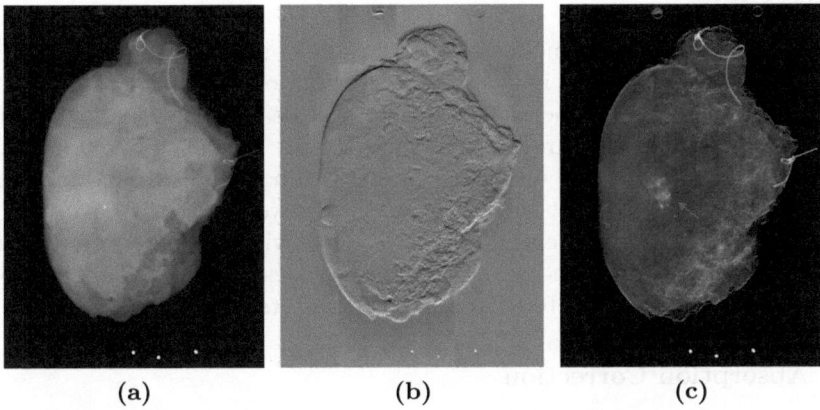

(a)   (b)   (c)

Fig. 1. Images of a cancerous mastectomy sample acquired using X-ray interferometry. (a) Absorption image. (b) Differential phase image. (c) Dark-field image. Note the visualization of the tumor in the dark-field image (red arrow).

as small-angle scattering. Such structures are well below the resolution limit of conventional X-ray imaging systems, and hence difficult to detect. First studies concluded that DFI yields important insights, and might be particularly useful for detecting microcalcifications in mammography (see, e.g., [6]).

However, for medical purposes, interpreting DFI images is difficult, as not only small structure variations contribute to the dark-field image. While its image formation process has not been fully understood yet, it has been empirically observed that scattering and beam hardening effects within the object create an absorption-like contribution to the dark-field signal. Additionally, diffraction effects at material edges also produce a dark-field signal. Fig. 1 shows an example for the absorption, differential-phase and dark-field image of a cancerous mastectomy sample. Note that the microcalcifications, although present in DFI, appear within a large amount of disturbing structural information.

In this work, we propose a method to greatly enhance the interpretability of dark-field images by removing or weakening these disturbing effects from the DFI image. For this task, we exploit the observations that a) disturbing influences in the dark-field signal often arise from the absorption or phase signal, and are hence correlated between these images, while b) small-angle scattering is contained only in the dark-field signal. We demonstrate on mammographic data that the result of this separation is a clean dark-field signal, in which microcalcifications can be readily detected.

Previous work on the post-processing of data obtained using interferometric X-ray imaging is scarce and has only dealt with image fusion in combination with denoising [7] or visualization [8]. To our knowledge, this is the first algorithm which allows to isolate the unique small-angle scattering information contained within dark-field X-ray images.

2   Methods

As no complete physical model of the dark-field image formation process is available, we assume three independent contributions to the dark-field image: absorption-based effects, such as scattering and beam hardening; edge diffraction and small-scale structure variations. Since only the signal due to the small-scale structure variations is unique to the DFI signal (and, for our application, a strong indicator of breast microcalcifications), we seek to remove the other two contributions by decorrelating the DFI image with the absorption and DPC signal. First, the absorption-based contribution is estimated and subtracted. In a second stage, signals due to edge diffraction effects are suppressed.

2.1   Absorption Correction

In a first examination of the images, we noted that most unwanted DFI signals occur due to absorption effects. To remove these influences, we propose a method that is inspired by water correction for CT-reconstruction. There, a polynomial correction factor is commonly used to rescale the recorded intensities to account for the effects of scatter in homogeneous materials. For our task, we assume that there exists a transfer function f_{abso} which maps pixel intensities of the absorption image to their corresponding contribution to the dark-field image. We further assume that this function is constant over the image (and thus for all materials in the object). We model this function as a polynomial of degree p. Let $\boldsymbol{A}$ be the absorption image and $\boldsymbol{D}$ be the dark-field image. We obtain a first estimate f_{abso}^0 of the transfer function by solving the least-squares problem

$$f_{abso}^0 = \underset{f_{abso}}{\arg\min} \| f_{abso}(\boldsymbol{A}) - \boldsymbol{D} \|_2^2 \ . \tag{1}$$

This global estimation is only valid if – as initially observed – most of the DFI signal co-occurs in the absorption image. Still, the initial estimate is biased by the pixels of the DFI images which contain signals due to edge diffraction and structure variations. To address this issue, the estimates of f_{abso} are iteratively refined. At each refinement step i, a thresholding map $\boldsymbol{T}^i$ is computed as

$$\boldsymbol{T}^i(n) = \begin{cases} 1 & \text{if } f_{abso}^i(\boldsymbol{A}(n) - \boldsymbol{D}(n)) < (t_{thresh} \cdot \max(\boldsymbol{D})) \\ 0 & \text{otherwise} \end{cases} . \tag{2}$$

The threshold operator selects pixels of the dark-field image that arise only from absorption effects for estimating the transfer function. Refinements of the transfer function f_{abso}^i, $1 \le i \le i_{max}$ are estimated by

$$f_{abso}^{i+1} = \underset{f_{abso}}{\arg\min} \| \boldsymbol{T}^i \cdot (f_{abso}(\boldsymbol{A}) - \boldsymbol{D}) \|_2^2 \ . \tag{3}$$

Finally, the absorption-corrected dark-field image $\boldsymbol{D}_{abso}$ is computed as

$$\boldsymbol{D}_{abso} = \boldsymbol{D} - \max(f_{abso}^{i_{max}}(\boldsymbol{A}), 0) \ , \tag{4}$$

where the maximum operator ensures the non-negativity of the estimated absorption contribution. An example of the absorption correction is shown in Fig. 2.

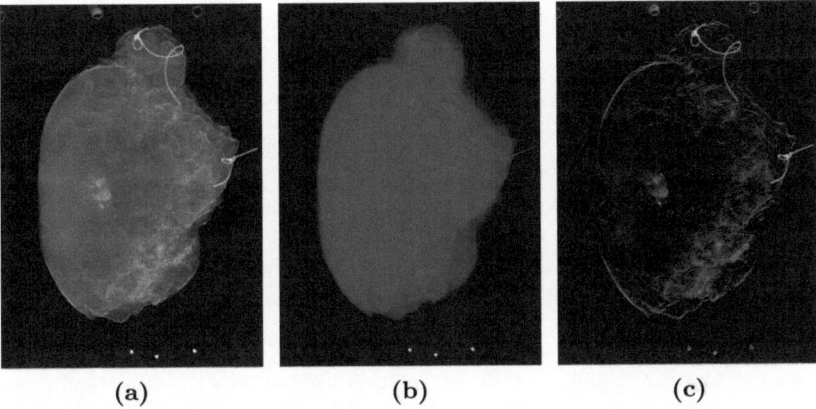

Fig. 2. Example of the absorption correction. (a) Input dark-field image $\boldsymbol{D}$. (b) Estimated absorption contribution $f_{\text{abso}}^{i_{\max}}(\boldsymbol{A})$. (c) Absorption-corrected dark-field image $\boldsymbol{D}_{\text{abso}}$.

2.2   Edge Diffraction Correction

After obtaining the absorption-corrected dark-field image $\boldsymbol{D}_{\text{abso}}$, the second stage of our algorithm attempts to correct for the signal contribution due to diffraction effects at object edges. We utilize the fact that the differential phase image $\boldsymbol{P}$ shows a significantly increased edge contrast compared to the absorption image. Thus, we assume that a signal $\boldsymbol{D}(n)$ at a pixel n is likely due to edge diffraction if the corresponding magnitude of the DPC image, $\text{abs}(\boldsymbol{P}(n))$ is high. We've experimented with several methods about how to utilize this information. Using the information of the DPC image directly is difficult due to scaling variations of individual edges. Local methods, such as cross-correlation maps, suffer from noise amplification problems, as the dark field image typically shows a low signal-to-noise ratio. We found that Independent Component Analysis (ICA) is a useful preprocessing step of the edge information. To this end, we compute the two resulting independent components of the absorption-corrected dark-field image and the absolute value, $\text{abs}(\boldsymbol{P})$, of the differential phase image. To obtain the independent components we utilize the FastICA algorithm [9], using the *deflation* method with the tanh function as nonlinearity measurement. Only one of the two independent components $\boldsymbol{I}_1$ and $\boldsymbol{I}_2$ corresponds to the edge map. Additionally, the data scaling after ICA can be arbitrary. Thus we compute rescaled components $\boldsymbol{I}_1^R$ and $\boldsymbol{I}_2^R$ to fit the DPC image in a least squares sense:

$$\boldsymbol{I}_j^R = \arg\min_{a,b} \|(a \cdot \boldsymbol{I}_j + b) - \text{abs}(\boldsymbol{P})\|_2^2 \ . \tag{5}$$

We then select the component as edge map $\boldsymbol{E}$ that fits the DPC image best:

$$\boldsymbol{E} = \begin{cases} \max(\boldsymbol{I}_1^R, 0) & \text{if } \|\boldsymbol{I}_1^R - \text{abs}(\boldsymbol{P})\|_2 < \|\boldsymbol{I}_2^R - \text{abs}(\boldsymbol{P})\|_2 \\ \max(\boldsymbol{I}_2^R, 0) & \text{otherwise} \end{cases} . \tag{6}$$

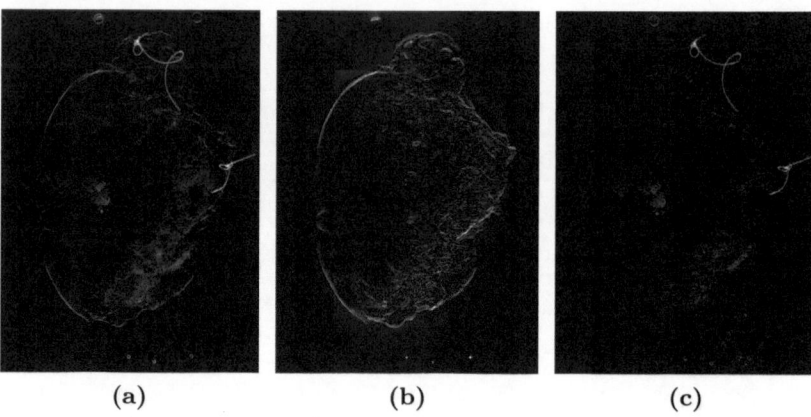

(a)   (b)   (c)

Fig. 3. Example of the edge correction. (a) Absorption-corrected dark-field image D_{abso}. (b) Computed edge map E. (c) Final image D_{corr}. Edge contributions are well suppressed, except for the specimen cutting edge at the bottom right.

Again, we enforce the non-negativity of the edge map. After determining the edge map, the edge- and absorption-corrected dark-field image D_{corr} is computed using soft shrinkage

$$D_{\mathrm{corr}} = \max(D_{\mathrm{abso}} - t_{\mathrm{shrink}} \cdot E, 0) \ . \qquad (7)$$

The shrinkage factor t_{shrink} can be used to tune the balance between edge removal and signal preservation. Finally, negative intensities are set to zero and the resulting image is normalized to the interval $[0; 1]$ for the purpose of visualization. Fig. 3 illustrates the edge removal step.

3   Evaluation and Results

Evaluation of our processing scheme is challenging. As the DFI formation is not yet fully understood, it is difficult to obtain accurate simulations that include the absorption and edge-diffraction effects that we seek to remove. Thus, we were not able to use synthetic evaluation data. Additionally, performing a reader study is non-trivial, as radiologists are not yet familiar with the reading of dark-field images. Hence, we evaluate our approach in two parts. First, we present a quantitative evaluation of the algorithm on a phantom. Second, we display qualitative results of applying our algorithm to cancerous mastectomy samples. All images were acquired using our experimental setup of a three-grating Talbot-Lau interferometer. Details on the setup are reported in [6]. As no ground truth data is available to optimize the parameters of our algorithm, we determining them heuristically. To this end, we used an extensive database of 76 data sets, comprising various objects. For the absorption correction, we set the polynomial degree $p = 4$, the number of iterations $i_{\mathrm{max}} = 2$ and the threshold $t_{\mathrm{thresh}} = 0.05$. For the edge correction, we set the shrinkage factor $t_{\mathrm{shrink}} = 1.0$.

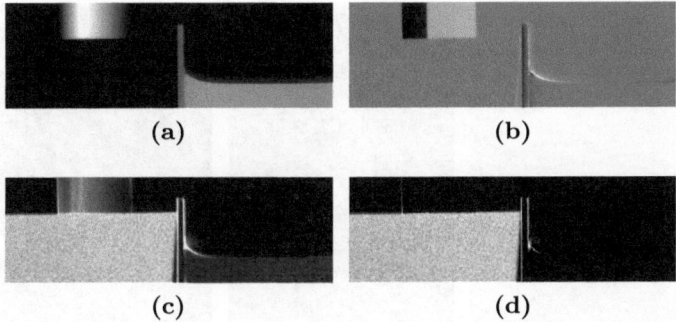

Fig. 4. The test phantom consisting of a teflon wedge on top of a foam block, next to a basin filled with water. (a) Absorption image. (b) Differential phase image. (c) Dark-field image. (d) Processed dark-field image.

3.1 Phantom Data

The test phantom for the quantitative evaluation, depicted in Fig. 4, consisted of a foam block with a teflon wedge on top (left side) and a basin filled with water (right side). As expected, the foam block is invisible in the absorption image, yet is clearly visible on the dark-field image due to its porous structure causing small-angle scattering. The water and the wedge also show some dark-field signal due to absorption effects. After processing with our algorithm, the foam block remains clearly visible, while the signals of the wedge and the water are suppressed.

For quantitative evaluation, we calculated the correlation of the intensities between the original and the processed dark-field image within and outside of the foam block. For the pixels belonging to the foam block, the correlation is 0.946. For the outside pixels, the correlation is 0.588. In addition to the correlation coefficient, we computed the average contrast between the foam block and the other two objects before and after processing. The contrast increased from 5.23 : 1 in the unprocessed image to 46.56 : 1 in the processed image.

3.2 Mastectomy Data

For qualitative evaluation, we examined 12 cancerous mastectomic specimen. In Fig. 5, we present two representative examples. Visual inspection of the resulting processed images reveals that absorption-based contributions are effectively suppressed. Within the specimens, edge effects have been almost completely removed. At the border of the objects, especially at the cutting edges, some residual edge signals remain. Signals due to small-angle scattering caused by microcalcification at the tumors have been well preserved. Also, the marking strings remain visible in the dark-field image due to their fiber structure. However, we notice some loss of signal at pixel-level. We attribute this to noise in the dark-field signal and our edge map used for shrinking the signal.

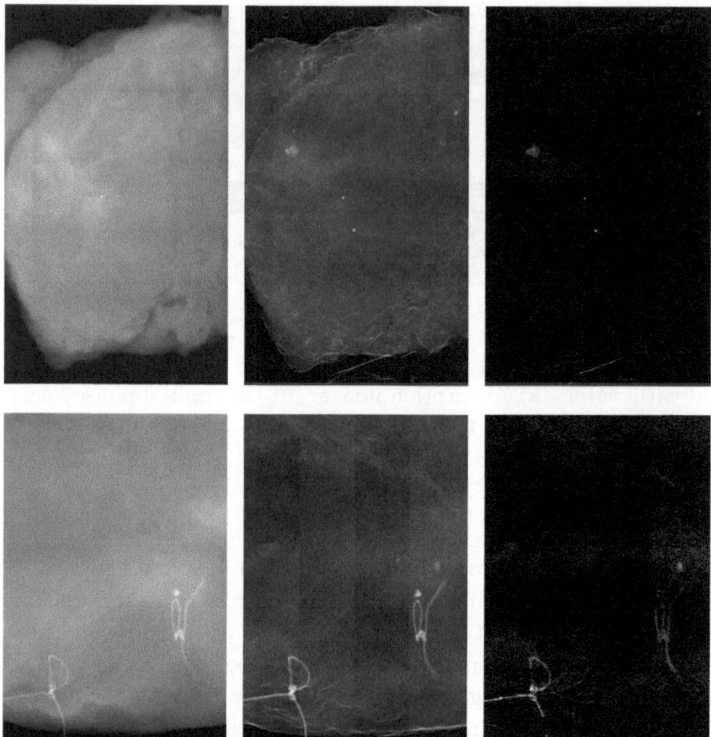

Fig. 5. Two additional examples of cancerous mastectomy samples processed using the proposed algorithm. From left to right: absorption, dark-field and processed dark-field images. Note the improved differentiability between the tumor and surrounding tissue.

4   Discussion and Conclusions

We presented an algorithm to determine the influence of small-scale structure variations to dark-field images, using a two-step decorrelation approach. To our knowledge, this is the first algorithm proposed for this purpose. We have shown a quantitative evaluation using a test phantom and a qualitative evaluation using mastectomic breast images. Overall, we observe a good suppression of absorption- and phase-related signals in the DFI image. The resulting images have the potential to provide greatly enhanced diagnostic value for, e.g., early detection of breast cancer lesions and DFI interpretation in general.

Possibilities for future research are vast. Due to broadening of the edge responses in the dark-field image, some edge diffraction effects are not fully removed. A physically or learning-based edge model could account for this effect. Also, we currently do not utilize prior information about the structure of the dark-field signal, which could be used to devise more effective task-specific algorithms. Finally, we aim to perform a radiologist reader study to assess the clinical impact of the proposed algorithm.

Acknowledgments. This work was funded by the German Ministry for Education and Research (BMBF), project grant No. 13EX1212B and the cluster of excellence Medical Valley EMN and Siemens Healthcare. The authors thank Dr. Jürgen Mohr and Jan Meiser from the Karlsruhe Institute of Technology and the Karlsruhe Nano Micro Facility (KNMF) for manufacturing the gratings used in the experiments. Patient consent and approval of the local ethics committee were obtained before the experiments involving the breast samples.

References

1. Wilkins, S.W., Gureyev, T.E., Gao, D., Pogany, A., Stevenson, A.W.: Phase-contrast imaging using polychromatic hard x-rays. Nature 384(6607), 335–338 (1996)
2. Parham, C., Zhong, Z., Connor, D.M., Chapman, L.D., Pisano, E.D.: Design and implementation of a compact low-dose diffraction enhanced medical imaging system. Academic Radiology 16(8), 911–917 (2009)
3. Pfeiffer, F., Weitkamp, T., Bunk, O., David, C.: Phase retrieval and differential phase-contrast imaging with low-brilliance x-ray sources. Nature Physics 2(4), 258–261 (2006)
4. Momose, A., Yashiro, W., Takeda, Y.: Sensitivity of x-ray phase imaging based on talbot interferometry. Japanese Journal of Applied Physics 47(10), 8077–8080 (2008)
5. Yashiro, W., Terui, Y., Kawabata, K., Momose, A.: On the origin of visibility contrast in x-ray talbot interferometry. Optics Express 18(16), 16890–16901 (2010)
6. Michel, T., Rieger, J., Anton, G., Bayer, F., Beckmann, M., Durst, J., Fasching, P., Haas, W., Hartmann, A., Pelzer, G., Radicke, M., Rauh, C., Ritter, A., Sievers, P., Schulz-Wendtland, R., Uder, M., Wachter, D., Weber, T., Wenkel, E., Zang, A.: On a dark-field signal generated by micrometer-sized calcifications in phase-contrast mammography. Physics in Medicine and Biology 58(8), 2713–2732 (2013)
7. Wang, Z., Clavijo, C.A., Roessl, E., van Stevendaal, U., Koehler, T., Hauser, N., Stampanoni, M.: Image fusion scheme for differential phase contrast mammography. Journal of Instrumentation 8(7), C07011 (2013)
8. Haas, W., Polyanskaya, M., Bayer, F., Gödel, K., Hofmann, H., Rieger, J., Ritter, A., Weber, T., Wucherer, L., Durst, J., Michel, T., Anton, G., Hornegger, J.: Image fusion in x-ray differential phase-contrast imaging. In: Proc. SPIE 8314 Medical Imaging, p. 83143U (2012)
9. Hyvarinen, A.: Fast and robust fixed-point algorithms for independent component analysis. IEEE Transactions on Neural Networks 10(3), 626–634 (1999)

Iterative Most Likely Oriented Point Registration

Seth Billings and Russell Taylor

Johns Hopkins University, Department of Computer Science, Baltimore, MD, USA
{sbillin3,rht}@jhu.edu

Abstract. A new algorithm for model based registration is presented that optimizes both position and surface normal information of the shapes being registered. This algorithm extends the popular Iterative Closest Point (ICP) algorithm by incorporating the surface orientation at each point into both the correspondence and registration phases of the algorithm. For the correspondence phase an efficient search strategy is derived which computes the most probable correspondences considering both position and orientation differences in the match. For the registration phase an efficient, closed-form solution provides the maximum likelihood rigid body alignment between the oriented point matches. Experiments by simulation using human femur data demonstrate that the proposed Iterative Most Likely Oriented Point (IMLOP) algorithm has a strong accuracy advantage over ICP and has increased ability to robustly identify a successful registration result.

Keywords: point cloud registration, Fisher distribution, PD tree.

1 Introduction

The need to register multiple representations of anatomy is a problem frequently encountered in the medical imaging and computer assisted intervention domains. As an example, computer assisted total hip replacement may involve sampling points from a femur bone during surgery and registering those points with a surface model derived from preoperative CT images. For such clinical applications, the Iterative Closest Point (ICP) algorithm has been extensively applied with many variants [1] since its introduction by Besl and McKay [2]. Surface normals could also be acquired in this context from range imaging techniques, surface probing, etc., enabling use of points and orientations as proposed in this paper.

1.1 Iterative Closest Point (ICP) Algorithm

Consider a source shape represented by a set of n points $X = \{x_i\}$ and a target shape represented by Ψ (typ. another point cloud or a mesh). The ICP algorithm seeks to compute the rigid body transformation T that minimizes the sum of square distances between the two shapes

$$T = \operatorname*{argmin}_{T} \sum_{i=1}^{n} \|y_i - T(x_i)\|_2^2 \tag{1}$$

P. Golland et al. (Eds.): MICCAI 2014, Part I, LNCS 8673, pp. 178–185, 2014.

where $\boldsymbol{y}_i$ is the point on the target shape closest to $T(\boldsymbol{x}_i)$ as defined by the closest point correspondence operator

$$\boldsymbol{y}_i = \mathrm{C}_{\mathrm{CP}}(T(\boldsymbol{x}_i), \varPsi) = \underset{\boldsymbol{y} \in \varPsi}{\operatorname{argmin}} \|\boldsymbol{y} - T(\boldsymbol{x}_i)\|_2 \;. \tag{2}$$

The ICP algorithm may be summarized as an iteration of two key steps:

1. Compute correspondences between the source and target shapes.
2. Compute the transformation T that minimizes the sum of square distances between the correspondences.

The first step has an efficient implementation using a KD tree search, while the second step has a closed form solution via Arun's method [3].

In this paper we present a novel variant of ICP that incorporates surface orientations alongside position data. In [4] surface normals were considered in the correspondence phase of an ICP method by limiting match orientation differences to within 45 degrees. Lara et al. [5] extended this approach by adaptively computing allowable bounds on the match orientation errors. In [6] contour normals were used in an expectation maximization (EM) framework for 3D-2D registration involving single X-ray images. Other ICP variants are found in [1].

Rather than using orientations to narrow the range of permitted matches, as in [4,5], our method combines orientation and position information in a cohesive probabilistic framework within both the correspondence and registration phases of the algorithm in order to directly compute the most probable matches and optimize match alignment. Thus, we name our method the Iterative Most Likely Oriented Point (IMLOP) algorithm. Our probabilistic model is similar to that of [6], though [6] is not a 3D-3D method. For the correspondence phase, we devise a novel tree search strategy that efficiently computes the most likely oriented point correspondences. We also incorporate a closed-form solution to the match alignment subproblem of the registration phase that optimizes alignment of both match positions and orientations, which was previously addressed in [7]. Our methods are summarized in Algorithms 1-3 to follow.

2   Methods

In this section, we present the proposed IMLOP algorithm, beginning with an overview of the method and then describing in detail the computations of the correspondence and registration sub-phases of the algorithm. For the purposes of this section, consider a source shape represented by a set of n oriented sample points $X = \{(\boldsymbol{x}_{\mathrm{p}i}, \boldsymbol{x}_{\mathrm{n}i})\}$ where $\boldsymbol{x}_{\mathrm{p}i}$ is a position vector and $\boldsymbol{x}_{\mathrm{n}i}$ is an orientation unit vector associated with oriented sample point $\boldsymbol{x}_i$. Also consider a target shape represented by $\varPsi$, such as a surface mesh or a second oriented point cloud.

2.1   Iterative Most Likely Oriented Point (IMLOP) Algorithm

The IMLOP algorithm incorporates a probabilistic framework formulated using Fisher and Gaussian distributions to model the measurement errors of orientation and position, respectively. Since the Fisher distribution is the analogue of

Gaussian on the unit sphere, pairing them to model oriented point measurement error is both natural and analytically convenient. Assuming unbiased, iid error and independence of orientation and position, the PDF describing the probability that a measured oriented point $x = (x_{\mathrm{p}}, x_{\mathrm{n}})$ corresponds to $y = (y_{\mathrm{p}}, y_{\mathrm{n}})$ has the form

$$f_{\mathrm{match}}(x, y) = \frac{k}{(2\pi\sigma^2)^{3/2} \cdot 2\pi(e^k - e^{-k})} \cdot e^{k y_{\mathrm{n}}^T x_{\mathrm{n}} - \frac{1}{2\sigma^2}\|y_{\mathrm{p}} - x_{\mathrm{p}}\|_2^2} \tag{3}$$

where k is a concentration parameter for orientation error and σ^2 is the variance of positional error. The correspondence phase of IMLOP selects the most probable match for each $T(x_i)$ via the most likely point correspondence operator

$$y_i = \mathrm{C}_{\mathrm{MLP}}(T(x_i), \Psi) = \operatorname*{argmax}_{y \in \Psi} f_{\mathrm{match}}(T(x_i), y) \tag{4}$$

and the registration phase solves a new transformation T to maximize the correspondence likelihood over all point pairs, which reduces to solving

$$T = \operatorname*{argmin}_{T} \left(\frac{1}{2\sigma^2} \sum_{i=1}^{n} \|y_{\mathrm{p}i} - T(x_{\mathrm{p}i})\|_2^2 - k \sum_{i=1}^{n} y_{\mathrm{n}i}^T R x_{\mathrm{n}i} \right) \tag{5}$$

where R is the rotation component of T. The IMLOP algorithm is summarized in Algorithm 1.

Algorithm 1. Iterative Most Likely Oriented Point (IMLOP)

---

    input : Source shape X and target shape Ψ
              Initial noise parameters k_0 and σ_0^2
              Initial transformation T_0
    output: Final transformation T that aligns X and Ψ
1 Initialize: $T \leftarrow T_0$, $k \leftarrow k_0$, $\sigma^2 \leftarrow \sigma_0^2$
2 **while** *not converged* **do**
3   Compute oriented point correspondences: $y_i = \mathrm{C}_{\mathrm{MLP}}(T(x_i), \Psi)$, $i = 1..n$
4   Register oriented point correspondences:

$$T = \operatorname*{argmin}_{T} \left(\frac{1}{2\sigma^2} \sum_{i=1}^{n} \|y_{\mathrm{p}i} - T(x_{\mathrm{p}i})\|_2^2 - k \sum_{i=1}^{n} y_{\mathrm{n}i}^T R x_{\mathrm{n}i} \right)$$

5   Update noise parameters: $k = \frac{\bar{R}(3 - \bar{R}^2)}{1 - \bar{R}^2}$, $\sigma^2 = \frac{1}{n} \sum_{i=1}^{n} \|y_{\mathrm{p}i} - T(x_{\mathrm{p}i})\|_2^2$
6 **end**

The noise parameters k and σ^2 are estimated from the residual match errors at each iteration. The variance of position error (σ^2) is simply estimated as the mean square distance between matches. The concentration of orientation error (k) is estimated by an approximation to its maximum likelihood estimate [8,9]

$$k \approx \frac{\bar{R}(3 - \bar{R}^2)}{1 - \bar{R}^2}, \quad \bar{R} = \frac{1 - w}{n} \sum_{i=1}^{n} y_{\mathrm{n}i}^T R x_{\mathrm{n}i} + \frac{w}{\alpha} \sum_{i=1}^{n} y_{\mathrm{p}i}'^T R x_{\mathrm{p}i}', \tag{6}$$

$$x_{\mathrm{p}i}' = x_{\mathrm{p}i} - \frac{1}{n} \sum_{i=1}^{n} x_{\mathrm{p}i}, \quad y_{\mathrm{p}i}' = y_{\mathrm{p}i} - \frac{1}{n} \sum_{i=1}^{n} y_{\mathrm{p}i}, \quad \alpha = \sum_{i=1}^{n} (\|y_{\mathrm{p}i}'\| \cdot \|R x_{\mathrm{p}i}'\|) \; .$$

For a continuous surface, it is often possible to find a nearly perfect orientation match for any given orientation. Thus, estimating k based on the matched orientation differences alone may tend to progressively over-estimate k's value until positional differences would no longer be relevant. To prevent this, we consider the rotational misalignment represented in both match orientations and match positions when computing $\bar{R}$ in (6), which balances k at reasonable values. In our implementation, we equally weight each term using $w = 0.5$. In light of the above, one may also wish to restrict the effect of position errors to only decrease orientation confidence. In this case, the following alternative for $\bar{R}$ may be used

$$\bar{R} = \min\left(\frac{1}{n} \sum_{i=1}^{n} \boldsymbol{y_{ni}}^T R\boldsymbol{x_{ni}}, \frac{1-w}{n} \sum_{i=1}^{n} \boldsymbol{y_{ni}}^T R\boldsymbol{x_{ni}} + \frac{w}{\alpha} \sum_{i=1}^{n} \boldsymbol{y'_{pi}}^T R\boldsymbol{x'_{pi}} \right) . \quad (7)$$

2.2 Computing Most Likely Oriented Point Correspondences

This section describes an efficient method for implementing the most likely point correspondence operator of (4). Our implementation is based on a modified principal direction (PD) tree search, though the method is equally suited to modifying the more standard KD tree. The idea is to construct a tree search structure around the target shape using positional data in the standard manner. During tree construction, a minimal bounding box enclosing the shape is computed for each node. The average surface orientation ($\boldsymbol{N}_{\mathrm{avg}}$) and the maximum angular deviation from the average orientation ($\theta_{\max}$) is also computed within each node.

$$\boldsymbol{N}_{\mathrm{avg}} = \frac{\sum_{j \in Node} \boldsymbol{y_{nj}}}{\| \sum_{j \in Node} \boldsymbol{y_{nj}} \|}, \quad \theta_{\max} = \max_{j \in Node} \{ \mathrm{acos}\left(\boldsymbol{N}_{\mathrm{avg}}^T \boldsymbol{y_{nj}} \right) \} \quad (8)$$

Equivalent to maximizing the match probability of (3), the most likely point correspondence operator computes a match to minimize the match error equation

$$\mathrm{E}_{\mathrm{match}}(\boldsymbol{x}, \boldsymbol{y}) = \frac{1}{2\sigma^2} \| \boldsymbol{y}_\mathrm{p} - \boldsymbol{x}_\mathrm{p} \|_2^2 + k(1 - \boldsymbol{y}_\mathrm{n}^T \boldsymbol{x}_\mathrm{n}) \quad (9)$$

which is always positive, unlike the form in (5).

When performing a correspondence search for a given oriented point $\boldsymbol{x}$, we begin with a current guess for the best correspondence (such as the match from the previous iteration), which has some match error E_{best}. At each node in the tree we require a fast test whether any point within the node may produce a lower match error than the current guess. Noting that lower match error is obtained for smaller orientation differences, we compute a lower bound on the difference in orientation between $\boldsymbol{x}_\mathrm{n}$ and any orientation $\{ \boldsymbol{y_{nj}} \}$ within the node as

$$\theta_{\min} = \max\left(0, \mathrm{acos}\left(\boldsymbol{N}_{\mathrm{avg}}^T \boldsymbol{x}_\mathrm{n} \right) - \theta_{\max} \right) . \quad (10)$$

It follows that for match errors lower than E_{best} there is an upper bound on the positional match distance given by

$$d_{\max} = \sqrt{2\sigma^2 \left[E_{\mathrm{best}} - k(1 - \cos(\theta_{\min})) \right]} . \quad (11)$$

Thus, if x_p lies at a distance greater than d_{max} from a node bounding box, then the node must not contain a better match and may be skipped. This PD tree search strategy is summarized in Algorithm 2.

Algorithm 2. PD Tree Node Search for Oriented Point Correspondences

---

    input : Oriented source point: x
             Current noise parameters: k and σ^2
             Best match so far: y_{best}, E_{best}
             This node object: $\mathcal{N}$
    output: Updated best match: y_{best}, E_{best}

1 Compute θ_{min} and d_{max} for this node
2 $\mathcal{B} \leftarrow$ bounding box of $\mathcal{N}$ expanded by d_{max} in all directions
3 **if** $\mathcal{B}$ *contains* x_p **then**
4   **if** $\mathcal{N}$ *is a leaf node* **then**
5   **foreach** $y_j \in \mathcal{N}$ **do**
6   Compute match error: $E_j \leftarrow E_{match}(x, y_j)$
7   **if** $E_j < E_{best}$ **then** Update best match: $y_{best} \leftarrow y_j$, $E_{best} \leftarrow E_j$
8   **end**
9   **else**
10   Search left and right child nodes
11   **end**
12 **else** Skip node

Note that when the target shape is a mesh (rather than point cloud) the tree is constructed by representing each triangle in the mesh as a single point (such as the triangle center). After building the tree, the node bounding boxes are expanded as necessary to fully enclose all vertices of the triangles represented. Then in line 6 of Algorithm 2 the procedure for searching a leaf node is to first compute the point on the triangle represented by y_j that is closest to x_p and then incorporate the triangle normal to compute the full match error.

2.3 Registering Oriented Point Correspondences

This section presents a closed-form solution to the subproblem of computing the rigid body transformation T, composed of a rotation R and translation t, that solves the minimization of (5). This minimization turns out to be a special case of a more general form and solution proposed in [7]. For completeness sake, we present the solution for this special case as Algorithm 3.

Recentering the point positions (line 1 of Algorithm 3) enables factoring the translation component of T out of (5). Rotation R is then found by minimizing

$$E = \frac{1}{2\sigma^2} \sum_{i=1}^{n} \|y'_{pi} - Rx'_{pi}\|_2^2 - k \sum_{i=1}^{n} y_{ni}{}^T R x_{ni} \qquad (12)$$

$$= \frac{1}{2\sigma^2} \left[\sum_{i=1}^{n} \|y'_{pi}\| - 2 \sum_{i=1}^{n} y'_{pi}{}^T R x'_{pi} + \sum_{i=1}^{n} \|Rx'_{pi}\| \right] - k \sum_{i=1}^{n} y_{ni}{}^T R x_{ni}$$

which is equivalent to maximizing

$$F = \frac{1}{\sigma^2} \sum_{i=1}^{n} {y'_{pi}}^T R x'_{pi} + k \sum_{i=1}^{n} {y_{ni}}^T R x_{ni} \qquad (13)$$

which is solved by modifying the SVD method of Arun [3] as shown in line 2.

Algorithm 3. Register Oriented Point Correspondences

---

   input : Corresponding oriented point sets: $X = \{x_i\}$ and $Y = \{y_i\}$
             Noise parameters: k and σ^2
   output: Transformation T that aligns X and Y
1 Compute new positions: $x'_{pi} \leftarrow x_{pi} - \bar{x}_p$, $y'_{pi} \leftarrow y_{pi} - \bar{y}_p$
    where $\bar{x}_p = \frac{1}{n} \sum_{i=1}^{n} x_{pi}$, $\bar{y}_p = \frac{1}{n} \sum_{i=1}^{n} y_{pi}$
2 Compute covariance matrix: $H \leftarrow kH_1 + \frac{1}{\sigma^2} H_2$
    where $H_1 = \sum_{i=1}^{n} x'_{pi} {y'_{pi}}^T$, $H_2 = \sum_{i=1}^{n} x_{ni} {y_{ni}}^T$
3 Compute rotation from SVD of H: $R \leftarrow VU^T$ where $H = USV^T$
4 **if** $\det(R) = -1$ **then** $R \leftarrow V'U^T$ where $V = [v_1, v_2, v_3]$, $V' = [v_1, v_2, -v_3]$
5 Compute translation: $t \leftarrow \bar{y}_p - R\bar{x}_p$
6 $T \leftarrow [R, t]$

---

3 Experiments

In this section, a simulation study (motivated by the introductory clinical scenario) is presented using a human femur segmented from CT imaging to evaluate the performance of IMLOP relative to ICP under known ground truth. A common termination condition is applied for both ICP and IMLOP, requiring the magnitude of change in the transformation T to be less than 0.001 mm and 0.001 degrees for two consecutive iterations. A triangular mesh of the femur surface is used as the target shape (Fig. 1). The source shape is constructed by randomly sampling oriented points from a subregion of the target shape (identified as a dark patch in Fig. 1). Registrations are performed after adding random noise to the oriented point positions and orientations and after applying a random misalignment selected uniformly from $[10, 20]$ degrees and $[10, 20]$ millimeters. Registrations are performed for different source shape sample sizes of 10, 20, 35, 50, 75 and 100 points and for different noise levels of 0, 0.5, 1 and 2 millimeters (degrees) standard deviation of Gaussian (wrapped Gaussian) noise applied to the sample positions (orientations). Three-hundred randomized trials are performed for each sample size / noise level pair. The accuracy of registration is evaluated using 100 validation points selected randomly from the mesh, with the average distance between registered and ground truth position forming the positional target registration error (TRE). An orientation TRE is similarly defined.

Figure 2 compares "success" TRE results and "failure" rates of ICP and IMLOP for various sample sizes at two noise levels. Registration failures are automatically detected using a threshold on the average of final match distances. For

IMLOP, the failure test is extended by an "or" condition to include a threshold on the final match orientation errors as well, enabling a more robust determination of registration success as may be appreciated by inspection of Fig. 1, which provides a detailed look at all registration trials for one sample size and noise level. In order to better appreciate the relationship between the final match errors and true registration error for each algorithm, trials along the x-axis in Fig. 1 are sorted by their positional TRE. For Fig. 2, we have set the match error threshold for registration failure at twice the standard deviation of applied noise. Plots of the remaining two noise levels and plots using different match error thresholds to flag success show similar results.

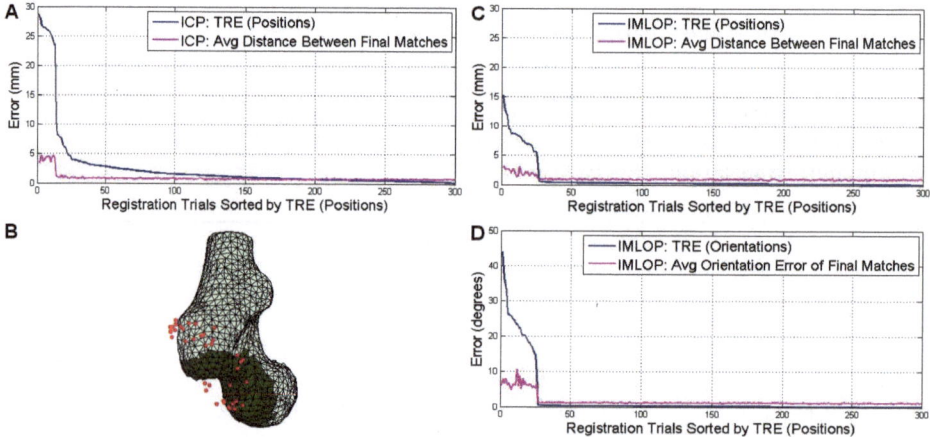

Fig. 1. Femur mesh and an example misaligned source shape point cloud (B); TRE and average final match error for the test case involving 75 samples and 1 mm (degree) noise level. Trials are sorted by positional TRE for both ICP (A) and IMLOP (C,D).

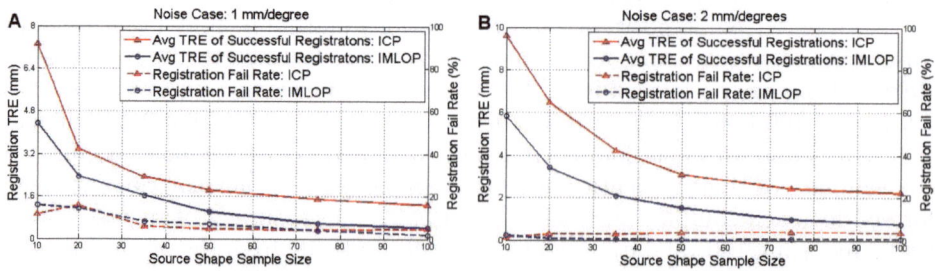

Fig. 2. Average TRE of successful registrations and registration failure rates across all sample sizes for noise level 1 mm (degree) (A) and 2 mm (degrees) (B)

4   Discussion and Conclusion

We have presented a novel algorithm for 3D-3D shape registration that extends the popular ICP method using a probabilistic framework to incorporate both position and orientation information. In addition, we have devised an efficient search strategy for computing the most probable oriented point correspondences and incorporated an efficient, closed-form solution for computing the optimal alignment of corresponding oriented points in the registration phase. As shown in the experimental results, the proposed IMLOP algorithm achieves significantly higher accuracy and has the advantage of a more robust mechanism for detecting registration failure by added criterion that is not avialable in ICP. Figure 1 shows that the registration errors of IMLOP decrease sharply when terminating close to the correct alignment, whereas ICP errors remain widely distributed. We have observed that IMLOP computes a solution in less than half the runtime of a similarly programmed ICP implementation, which demonstrates both a rate of convergence advantage for our method as well as the efficiency of our search strategy for computing the most probable oriented point correspondences.

Acknowledgments. Funded by the National Science Foundation Graduate Research Fellowship Program and Johns Hopkins University internal funds.

References

1. Rusinkiewicz, S., Levoy, M.: Efficient variants of the icp algorithm. In: Proceedings of the Third International Conference on 3-D Digital Imaging and Modeling, pp. 145–152 (2001)
2. Besl, P., McKay, N.D.: A method for registration of 3-d shapes. IEEE Transactions on Pattern Analysis and Machine Intelligence 14, 239–256 (1992)
3. Arun, K., Huang, T.S., Blostein, S.D.: Least-squares fitting of two 3-d point sets. IEEE Transactions on Pattern Analysis and Machine Intelligence 9, 698–700 (1987)
4. Pulli, K.: Multiview registration for large data sets. In: Proceedings of the Second International Conference on 3-D Digital Imaging and Modeling, pp. 160–168 (1999)
5. Lara, C., Romero, L., Calderón, F.: A robust iterative closest point algorithm with augmented features. In: Gelbukh, A., Morales, E.F. (eds.) MICAI 2008. LNCS (LNAI), vol. 5317, pp. 605–614. Springer, Heidelberg (2008)
6. Kang, X., Armand, M., Otake, Y., Yau, W.P., Cheung, P., Hu, Y., Taylor, R.: Robustness and accuracy of feature-based single image 2D-3D registration without correspondences for image-guided intervention. IEEE Transactions on Biomedical Engineering 61, 149–161 (2014)
7. Liu, X., Cevikalp, H., Fitzpatrick, J.M.: Marker orientation in fiducial registration. In: Medical Imaging 2003, International Society for Optics and Photonics, pp. 1176–1185 (2003)
8. Banerjee, A., Dhillon, I.S., Ghosh, J., Sra, S., Ridgeway, G.: Clustering on the unit hypersphere using von mises-fisher distributions. Journal of Machine Learning Research 6 (2005)
9. Mardia, K., Jupp, P.: Directional Statistics. Wiley Series in Probability and Statistics. Wiley (2009)

Robust Anatomical Landmark Detection for MR Brain Image Registration

Dong Han, Yaozong Gao, Guorong Wu, Pew-Thian Yap, and Dinggang Shen

Department of Radiology and BRIC,
University of North Carolina at Chapel Hill, NC, USA
dgshen@med.unc.edu

Abstract. Correspondence matching between MR brain images is often challenging due to large inter-subject structural variability. In this paper, we propose a novel landmark detection method for robust establishment of correspondences between subjects. Specifically, we first annotate distinctive landmarks in the training images. Then, we use regression forest to simultaneously learn (1) the optimal set of features to best characterize each landmark and (2) the non-linear mappings from local patch appearances of image points to their displacements towards each landmark. The learned regression forests are used as landmark detectors to predict the locations of these landmarks in new images. Since landmark detection is performed in the entire image domain, our method can cope with large anatomical variations among subjects. We evaluated our method by applying it to MR brain image registration. Experimental results indicate that by combining our method with existing registration method, obvious improvement in registration accuracy can be achieved.

1 Introduction

Accurate matching of anatomical structures is a key step in many medical image processing and analysis tasks [1]. However, anatomical structures can vary significantly across different individuals, thus posing huge challenges for accurate correspondence detection. Current methods typically perform local searching to determine anatomical correspondences between images [2,3]. Such approach is limited in two aspects: (1) Due to large inter-subject variability, even after affine registration, corresponding structures could be distant and exhibit different appearances, thus leading to inaccurate matching. (2) The similarity between corresponding points is often measured using predefined local image features that do not necessarily respect the local structural variations.

In this paper, we propose two ways to improve correspondence detection: (1) a global correspondence detection mechanism that can deal with large anatomical differences, and (2) development of feature descriptors that are unique and discriminative for correspondence detection. Specifically, a robust detector is learned for each landmark by using regression forest [4]. Note that a regression forest is an ensemble of randomly-trained binary decision trees that can map a complex input space to continuous output parameters [4]. In our framework, regression forest is used to simultaneously learn the optimal set of features that can

P. Golland et al. (Eds.): MICCAI 2014, Part I, LNCS 8673, pp. 186–193, 2014.

best characterize the annotated landmarks and also a set of complex non-linear mappings from the local appearances of image points to their 3D displacements towards each landmark. The learned forests are then used to detect the corresponding landmarks in a new image based on the displacements predicted from each point in the image. Since landmark detection is performed in the entire image domain, our method is able to handle large structural variations. Moreover, since a unique detector is learned for each landmark, more discriminative features can be used to distinguish a landmark from other points in the image.

We evaluate our method by applying it to provide robust initial correspondences and subsequently the initial deformation field for MR brain image registration. The initial deformation field can be refined with a non-rigid registration method such as HAMMER [5]. Experimental results show that these learned landmark detectors are robust to large inter-subject anatomical variability. By combining these detectors with HAMMER, more accurate and robust results can be obtained, especially for the cases with large anatomical differences.

2   Methods

2.1   Multi-resolution Regression-Guided Landmark Detection

In this paper, landmark detection is formulated as a multivariate non-linear regression problem. Specifically, given a point $p \in \mathbb{R}^3$ in the image, we want to predict the displacement $d \in \mathbb{R}^3$ from p to the latent landmark $v \in \mathbb{R}^3$ based on the local image appearance of p. This highly non-linear mapping between p and d is learned by using regression forest, which belongs to random forest family and is specialized for non-linear regression problems. A regression forest consists of a set of binary decision trees. Each tree contains a number of split and leaf nodes. A split node is associated with a split function, which directs an incoming data item to either the left or right child based on a single feature and the learned threshold. A leaf node stores a statistical distribution of outputs of training data items that fall into it, which will be used to determine the output of an unseen data item. In the following, we will introduce (1) in the training stage how the regression forest is learned to capture non-linear relationship between p and d, and (2) in the application stage how the learned regression forest can be used to predict the location of the corresponding landmark in a new image.

In the training stage, the training dataset consists of a set of linearly aligned MR brain images $\{I_j\}$. Each image is associated with the annotated location of a corresponding landmark $\{v_j \in \mathbb{R}^3\}$. For each image I_j, we sample a set of training image points $\{p_j^i \in \mathbb{R}^3\}$ in a spherical region Ω_j centered at v_j. The output of each p_j^i is calculated as $d_j^i = v_j - p_j^i$. Here, we use $\mathfrak{P}$ and $\mathfrak{D}$ to denote the training points from all images and their corresponding outputs, respectively. The features used to characterize each point are Haar-like features [4], i.e., displaced intensity patch differences. When training a specific tree, we first randomly generate a set of Haar-like features to form a specific feature pool $F = \{f_k\}$. Then, we push $\mathfrak{P}$ and $\mathfrak{D}$ through the tree starting at the root.

At each split node n, we randomly generate one set of thresholds T_k for each feature f_k based on the distribution of the feature responses $f_k(\mathfrak{P}_n)$, where $\mathfrak{P}_n$ denotes the training points reaching node n. Then, we perform exhaustive search to find the best feature f_n^* and threshold t_n^* that maximize the information gain $G_n(f,t) = E(\mathfrak{D}_n) - w_L E(\mathfrak{D}_n^L) - w_R E(\mathfrak{D}_n^R)$ after splitting, where $\mathfrak{D}_n$ denotes the set of outputs of training points reaching node n, $\mathfrak{D}_n^L = \{d \in \mathfrak{D}_n | f(d) \le t\}$ and $\mathfrak{D}_n^R = \{d \in \mathfrak{D}_n | f(d) > t\}$ are the output sets for the left and right children after splitting, $w_L = |\mathfrak{D}_n^L|/|\mathfrak{D}_n|$, $w_R = |\mathfrak{D}_n^R|/|\mathfrak{D}_n|$, $E(\mathfrak{D}_n) = \text{Trace}(\text{Cov}(\mathfrak{D}_n))$ computes the consistency of $\mathfrak{D}_n$, Trace denotes matrix trace, and Cov denotes covariance matrix. The best f_n^* and t_n^* are saved in node n and will be used in the application stage. For each leaf node, we can save the posterior probability $g(d|p)$ by summarizing the outputs of all training points reaching this leaf node. Here, we assume that the outputs in each leaf node obey Gaussian distribution. In this case, only mean $\bar{d}$ and covariance C of the outputs need to be saved. The training of the entire tree continues until all training paths reach the leaves.

In the application stage, when a new image comes, we can use the learned forest to predict the displacement from any image point p to the latent landmark. Specifically, for each tree in the forest, we push p through it starting at the root. At each split node n, we compute the feature response $f_n^*(p)$ and compare it with threshold t_n^*. If $f_n^*(p) \le t_n^*$, p is passed to the left child; otherwise, it is passed to the right child. When p reaches a leaf, the saved $\bar{d}$ in this leaf is regarded as the prediction result of this tree. The final prediction $\widehat{d}$ of a forest is computed as the average over predictions of all trees in the forest. When performing landmark detection, we can adopt the idea of majority voting [4]. Specifically, for each p in the image, we can use the forest to estimate $\widehat{d}$. Then, a vote is given to the point nearest to $p + \widehat{d}$. After voting from all image points, the point that receives the most votes is regarded as the landmark location. However, the major limitation of such voting strategy is that when large anatomical variations exist near the landmark, image points far away from the landmark will not be informative about that and their votes will be less reliable, which may eventually lead to false landmark detection. *To make the prediction more robust to anatomical structure variations, a "point jumping" strategy is adopted in our method.* The basic idea is that instead of directly using $p + \widehat{d}$ as the predicted landmark location [6,7], we repeatedly use the forest to estimate a pathway from p to the landmark, and during this procedure the landmark prediction is iteratively refined. Specifically, given the current location of p, we can estimate its displacement $\widehat{d}$. Then, we let p jump to the new location $p + \widehat{d}$. After several such jumps, the final location of p is regarded as the predicted landmark location from p. Given a set of image points, we can use "point jumping" to obtain one predicted landmark location from each point. Then, the predicted location with the smallest $||\widehat{d}||$ is regarded as the landmark location. Because the prediction from each point is iteratively refined via "point jumping", a small set of sampled points is generally enough for successful landmark detection, which makes this approach very efficient.

To further improve the robustness of our landmark detection method, we adopt *multi-resolution strategies* in both training and application stages. Specifically, in the training stage, we train one regression forest for each resolution. In the coarsest resolution, we sample the training points all over the image in order to ensure the robustness of the detector; in the finer resolutions, we only sample the training points near the annotated landmark to increase the specificity of the detector. During the application stage, in the coarsest resolution we sparsely sample a set of points from the entire image. Using the "point jumping" on these sampled points, we can obtain an initial guess of the landmark location. In a finer resolution, we take the predicted location in the previous resolution as the initialization and then sample points only near the initialization, thus improving the specificity of landmark detection. In this way, the detected landmark will be gradually refined from coarse to fine resolutions.

2.2   Application of the Proposed Method to Image Registration

We evaluate our landmark detection method by applying it to MR brain image registration. Ideally, to achieve this goal, we can learn a large number of detectors that are densely distributed in the whole brain. However, for typical MR brain images, thousands of landmark detectors are needed to model sufficiently the high-dimensional deformation field between two images, which is computationally infeasible. To resolve this issue, we choose an alternative way. Specifically, we learn a relatively small set of landmark detectors (located at distinctive brain regions) to provide robust initial correspondences between two images. Then, a dense deformation field can be interpolated from the initial correspondences on the landmarks, and is used to initialize the deformable image registration. Since the most important and challenging correspondences can be well established by our landmark detectors, the subsequent refinement of deformation field becomes much easier than the direct registration between two images. In this way, the conventional image registration can be divided into two sub-tasks, i.e., (1) accurate initial correspondence establishment by robust landmark detectors and (2) efficient deformation refinement by an existing image registration method. Next, we will describe the landmark-based initialization method in detail.

For detector training, given a group of training MR brain images, we annotate a small set of corresponding landmarks in each image. These landmarks should cover the entire brain, in order to effectively drive the whole deformation field. After landmark annotation, a unique detector is learned for each landmark by using the method described in Subsection 2.1.

When registering two new MR brain images, landmark detection is first performed in each image by using the learned landmark detectors. Then, sparse correspondences can be established between the two images based on the detected corresponding landmark pairs. Next, thin plate spline (TPS) method can be used to interpolate an initial dense deformation field from these sparse correspondences [8]. The generated initial deformation field can be further refined by existing deformable registration algorithms.

3 Experimental Results

3.1 Image Dataset and Parameter Setting

For evaluation, 62 MR adult brain images were selected from the ANDI dataset with large inter-subject variability. The dimensions of these images are 256 × 256 × 256, and the voxel size is 1 × 1 × 1mm. All images were first linearly aligned by using FLIRT in FSL package [9]. Then, 44 images were selected as the training set and the other 18 images as the testing set. To learn a landmark detector, the training of regression forest was performed on 3 image resolutions. For each resolution, 10 trees were trained. To train a single tree, 6,000 points were sampled from each training image and 1,500 Haar-like features were randomly selected. At each split node, 1,000 thresholds were randomly generated for each feature. The maximum tree depth was 12. In this setting, training one tree costs about 15 minutes. The detection of a single landmark costs about 0.5 second.

3.2 Validation of the Proposed Method

In this subsection, the performance of the proposed method is evaluated by training detectors for a few specified landmarks and comparing the detection results with the manually annotated landmark locations in the testing images. Specifically, in this experiment, we manually annotated 6 specific landmarks on the corners/edges of the ventricular regions in both training and testing images. Fig. 1 shows the 6 annotated landmarks in one training image. Then, one detector was trained for each of the 6 landmarks.

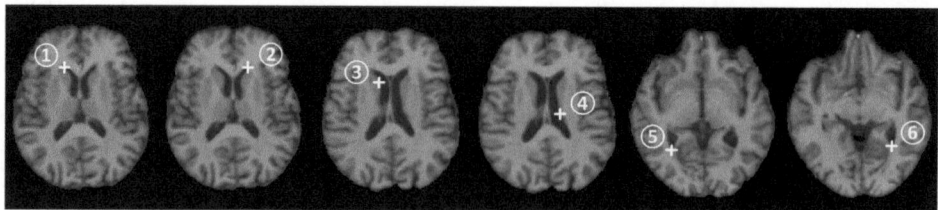

Fig. 1. The six manually annotated landmarks on the corners/edges of the ventricular region in one training image. The white cross marks denote the landmark locations.

After training, the detectors were used to detect the corresponding landmarks in each testing image. Then, the detection results were compared with the annotated landmark locations. To better evaluate our method, we compared it with the voting-based method. Table 1 presents the detection errors for the 6 landmarks from both methods. For the first four landmarks, both methods achieve reasonable detection accuracy with good stability. However, for landmarks 5 and 6, the performance of the voting-based method is far worse. This is mainly because the inter-subject variability of these two landmarks is much larger than

Table 1. The detection errors for the six landmarks from both voting-based method and our proposed method, respectively. Both mean errors and corresponding standard deviations are shown. (Unit: mm)

No.	1	2	3	4	5	6
Voting-Based	2.69 ± 1.14	1.94 ± 1.15	2.36 ± 1.21	1.38 ± 0.93	8.60 ± 9.25	5.38 ± 4.94
Proposed	2.62 ± 1.26	2.40 ± 1.08	1.73 ± 1.29	1.48 ± 0.77	2.34 ± 1.53	2.77 ± 1.24

that of the other four landmarks. In this case, the prediction from the voting-based method is more likely to be dominated by the wrong votes. However, our method is much more robust to anatomical variability among individuals.

3.3   Evaluation of the Proposed Method in Image Registration

In this experiment, the proposed method was further evaluated by applying it to assist MR brain image registration, where a set of landmark detectors were learned to provide a good initial deformation field between the two images. Further refinement of the remaining deformation field was performed by the HAMMER algorithm. In this experiment, each MR brain image was further segmented into white matter (WM), gray matter (GM), ventricle (VN), and cerebrospinal fluid (CSF) regions by FAST in FSL package [10]. Here, we regard these segmentations as the ground truth for evaluating the accuracy of the registration results by comparing the tissue overlap ratio.

In this experiment, 1,350 landmarks were annotated that covered the whole brain. After training all the landmark detectors, these detectors were used to establish rough initial correspondences between the two images. Here, one testing image was selected as the fixed image, and all other testing images were warped to it. Registration results from the landmark-based initialization, HAMMER, and the combination of these two methods were obtained and compared. The Dice ratios [11] (and their standard deviations) of these methods, computed for CSF, VN, GM and WM, are reported in Table 2. It can be observed that using landmark-based initialization increases the Dice ratios (and decreases the standard deviations) for all tissue types. This indicates that the correspondences established by the landmark detectors are accurate and robust. Refinement using HAMMER further improves the registration accuracy to a level that is better than the original HAMMER. To better illustrate the advantage of our approach, we select 5 images from the testing set that are substantially different in appearance from the fixed image. Fig. 2 presents the registration results for the 5 images. From Fig. 2 we can see that after landmark-based initialization, the inter-subject anatomical differences of these images are reduced significantly, which makes further refinement much easier than directly registering two images from scratch. The improvements in registration accuracy from the Landmark+HAMMER approach can be easily observed from these results.

Table 2. The Dice ratios and the corresponding standard deviations of CSF, VN, GM and WM regions before and after registration by using (1) the landmark detectors only, (2) the Landmark+HAMMER approach, and (3) the original HAMMER algorithm

Region	Before Reg.	Landmark	Landmark+HAMMER	HAMMER
CSF	$40.3\% \pm 2.32\%$	$48.6\% \pm 2.28\%$	$62.7\% \pm 1.95\%$	$61.1\% \pm 2.16\%$
VN	$54.7\% \pm 10.5\%$	$78.6\% \pm 3.36\%$	$85.9\% \pm 1.51\%$	$76.8\% \pm 11.1\%$
GM	$45.2\% \pm 2.06\%$	$50.4\% \pm 1.87\%$	$66.1\% \pm 1.58\%$	$65.1\% \pm 1.85\%$
WM	$60.0\% \pm 2.65\%$	$67.0\% \pm 1.39\%$	$79.9\% \pm 1.28\%$	$77.8\% \pm 2.09\%$

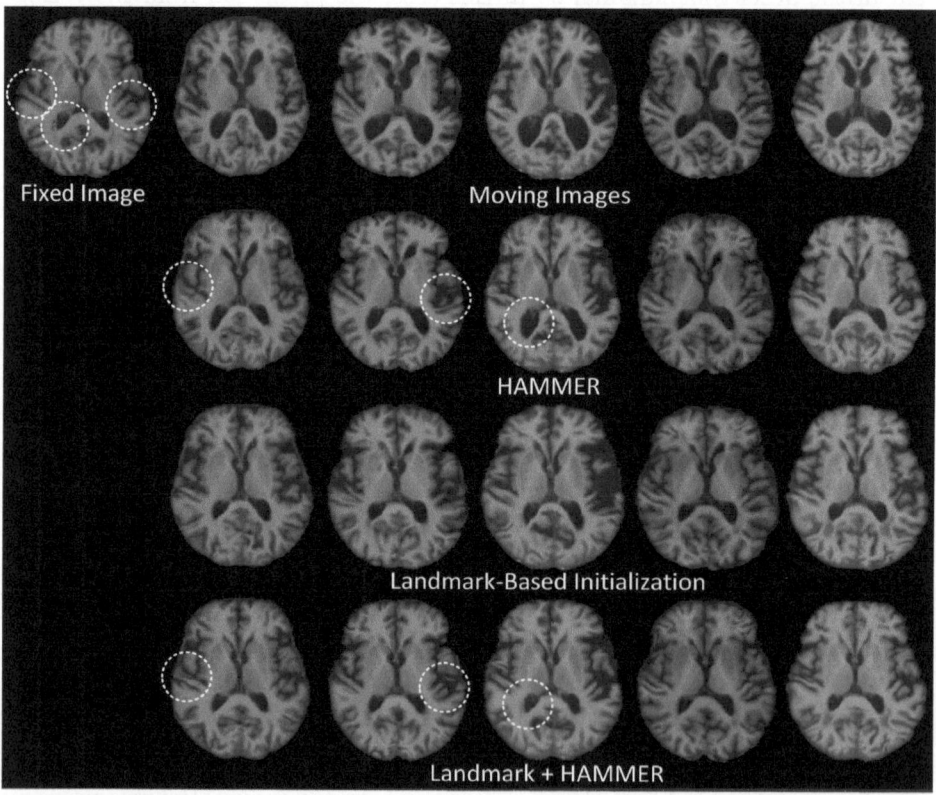

Fig. 2. Registration results on 5 testing images that are substantially different in appearance from the fixed image. Row 1: The fixed image and the original moving images. Row 2: Registration results given by HAMMER alone. Row 3: Registration results given by landmark-based initialization. Row 4: Registration results given by further refinement using HAMMER.

4   Conclusion

In this paper, we analyze the limitations of conventional anatomical correspondence detection methods, and then propose a multi-resolution regression-guided landmark detection method to overcome these limitations. In our method, regression forest is employed to learn the complex non-linear mappings from local patch appearances of image points to their 3D displacements towards the landmarks. The learned regression forest is used to predict the locations of the corresponding landmarks in new images. We evaluate the proposed landmark detection method by applying it to assist MR brain image registration. Experimental results show that, with the help of reliable initial correspondences established by the proposed method, structural differences between two images can be reduced significantly. By refining the initial correspondences with the HAMMER algorithm, the final registration results are more accurate and robust than those given by HAMMER alone. Our future research will include (1) further improving landmark detection accuracy and (2) incorporating our landmark detection method with other non-rigid registration algorithms to further evaluate the advantage of our method in helping initialize image registration algorithms.

References

1. Prastawa, M., Gilmore, J.H., Lin, W., Gerig, G.: Automatic Segmentation of MR Images of the Developing Newborn Brain. Med. Image Anal. 9, 457–466 (2005)
2. Shen, D.: Fast Image Registration by Hierarchical Soft Correspondence Detection. Pattern Recogn. 42, 954–961 (2009)
3. Wu, G., Kim, M., Wang, Q., Shen, D.: S-HAMMER: Hierarchical Attribute-Guided, Symmetric Diffeomorphic Registration for MR Brain Images. Hum. Brain Mapp. 35, 1044–1060 (2014)
4. Criminisi, A., Robertson, D., Konukoglu, E., Shotton, J., Pathak, S., White, S., Siddiqui, K.: Regression Forests for Efficient Anatomy Detection and Localization in Computed Tomography Scans. Med. Image Anal. 17, 1293–1303 (2013)
5. Shen, D., Davatzikos, C.: HAMMER: Hierarchical Attribute Matching Mechanism for Elastic Registration. IEEE Trans. Med. Imaging 21, 1421–1439 (2002)
6. Zhou, S.K., Comaniciu, D.: Shape Regression Machine. In: Karssemeijer, N., Lelieveldt, B. (eds.) IPMI 2007. LNCS, vol. 4584, pp. 13–25. Springer, Heidelberg (2007)
7. Zhou, S.K., Zhou, J., Comaniciu, D.: A Boosting Regression Approach to Medical Anatomy Detection. In: IEEE Conference on Computer Vision and Pattern Recognition, CVPR (2007)
8. Bookstein, F.L.: Principal Warps: Thin-Plate Splines and the Decomposition of Deformations. IEEE Trans. Pattern Anal. Mach. Intell. 11, 567–585 (1989)
9. Jenkinson, M., Smith, S.M.: A Global Optimisation Method for Robust Affine Registration of Brain Images. Med. Image Anal. 5, 143–156 (2001)
10. Zhang, Y., Brady, M., Smith, S.: Segmentation of Brain MR Images Through a Hidden Markov Random Field Model and the Expectation-Maximization Algorithm. IEEE Trans. Med. Imaging 20, 45–57 (2001)
11. Van Rijsbergen, C.J.: Information Retrieval, 2nd edn. Butterworth-Heinemann, London (1979)

Free-Form Deformation Using Lower-Order B-spline for Nonrigid Image Registration

Wei Sun[1], Wiro J. Niessen[1,2], and Stefan Klein[1]

[1] Biomedical Imaging Group Rotterdam, Erasmus MC, Rotterdam, The Netherlands
{w.sun,w.niessen,s.klein}@erasmusmc.nl
[2] Department of Image Science and Technology, Faculty of Applied Sciences,
Delft University of Technology, Delft, The Netherlands

Abstract. In traditional free-form deformation (FFD) based registration, a B-spline basis function is commonly utilized to build the transformation model. As the B-spline order increases, the corresponding B-spline function becomes smoother. However, the higher-order B-spline has a larger support region, which means higher computational cost. For a given D-dimensional nth-order B-spline, an mth-order B-spline where $(m \leq n)$ has $(\frac{m+1}{n+1})^D$ times lower computational complexity. Generally, the third-order B-spline is regarded as keeping a good balance between smoothness and computation time. A lower-order function is seldom used to construct the deformation field for registration since it is less smooth. In this research, we investigated whether lower-order B-spline functions can be utilized for efficient registration, by using a novel stochastic perturbation technique in combination with a postponed smoothing technique to higher B-spline order. Experiments were performed with 3D lung and brain scans, demonstrating that the lower-order B-spline FFD in combination with the proposed perturbation and postponed smoothing techniques even results in better accuracy and smoothness than the traditional third-order B-spline registration, while substantially reducing computational costs.

1 Introduction

The B-spline based FFD registration is a popular approach for nonrigid registration. In general, the third-order B-spline is utilized to model the transformation in B-spline FFD method. B-spline functions with different orders are a series of convolutional basis functions. The nth-order B-spline function is n times convolution of the zeroth-order B-spline. As the n goes to infinity, B-splines converge to a Gaussian function with an infinite support. The smoothness is improved as the growth of B-spline order. However, this improvement is accompanied by the increasing computational cost because of a larger support which means more control points have to be involved in computation.

Our previous work [1] has initially investigated by using the randomly shifted second-order B-spline with uniform distribution to simulate third-order B-spline method. In this work, we extend the whole theoretical framework into a statistical view, go down to the first and zeroth orders of B-splines, and introduce

P. Golland et al. (Eds.): MICCAI 2014, Part I, LNCS 8673, pp. 194–201, 2014.
© Springer International Publishing Switzerland 2014

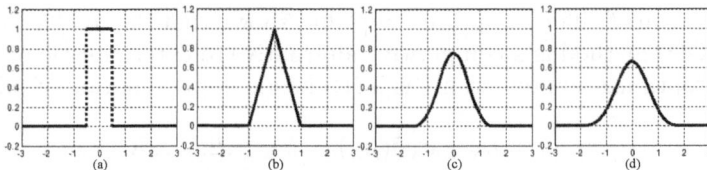

Fig. 1. One-dimensional B-splines with four different orders: (a) $\beta^0(x)$; (b) $\beta^1(x)$; (c) $\beta^2(x)$; (d) $\beta^3(x)$

the Gaussian perturbation to the framework. The performances of lower-order B-splines for nonrigid registration were evaluated in terms of registration accuracy, smoothness and efficiency.

2 Method

2.1 B-spline Basis Functions

In B-spline FFD registration method, B-spline functions are equally placed on a D-dimensional uniform control-point grid. The nth-order B-spline function is obtained by n times convolution of the zeroth-order B-spline functions,

$$\beta^n(x) = \beta^0(x) \underbrace{* \cdots * \beta^0(x)}_{n \text{ times}}, \tag{1}$$

where $\beta^0(x)$ is fixed to be 1 when $(-0.5 \leq x < 0.5)$ and the operator '$*$' denotes the convolution operation. Figure 1 presents the curves of $\beta^0(x)$, $\beta^1(x)$, $\beta^2(x)$, and $\beta^3(x)$. With increasing spline order, the smoothness improves, but the support (nonzero domain) becomes larger. For a D-dimensional transformation model, the tensor product of $\beta^n(x)$ is used to span a multidimensional B-spline basis function $\Phi_D^n(\mathbf{x})$.

2.2 Registration Framework

B-splines based FFD registration is a parametric intensity-based type of registration method. The D-dimensional fixed and moving images are denoted as $F(\mathbf{x}) : \Omega_F \subset \mathcal{R}^D \to \mathcal{R}$ and $M(\mathbf{x}) : \Omega_M \subset \mathcal{R}^D \to \mathcal{R}$ where $\mathbf{x} \in \mathcal{R}^D$ represents an image coordinate. Then, the registration problem is defined as:

$$\hat{\boldsymbol{\mu}} = \arg\min_{\boldsymbol{\mu}} \mathcal{C}(F, M(\mathbf{T}_{\boldsymbol{\mu}}(\mathbf{x}))), \tag{2}$$

where $\mathcal{C}$ represents the dissimilarity measurement between the fixed image and the transformed moving image, $\mathbf{T}_{\boldsymbol{\mu}}(\mathbf{x}) : \Omega_F \to \Omega_M$ is a coordinate transformation, and $\boldsymbol{\mu}$ represents the parameter vector of the transformation model.

A comparison of different optimizers [2] has shown that the stochastic gradient descent (SGD) method is a competitive alternative to deterministic methods. In SGD, the "optimization direction" is a stochastic approximation of $\partial \mathcal{C}/\partial \boldsymbol{\mu}$,

$$\boldsymbol{\mu}_{k+1} = \boldsymbol{\mu}_k - a_k \tilde{\boldsymbol{g}}(\boldsymbol{\mu}_k), \quad k = 1, 2, \ldots, K \tag{3}$$

where $\tilde{\boldsymbol{g}}(\boldsymbol{\mu}_k)$ represents the approximate derivative of the cost function evaluated at the current optimization position $\boldsymbol{\mu}_k$. In [2] the stochastic approximation was calculated by evaluating the cost function derivative on a small random subset $\widetilde{\Omega}_F \subset \Omega_F$ of image samples, newly selected in each iteration k, thus reducing the computation time per iteration. To guarantee the convergence of stochastic optimization, step size a_k is defined as a decaying function of k in most theoretical work. In [3] an adaptive strategy for automatically setting a_k was proposed. This adaptive SGD (ASGD) optimizer is used in this work.

2.3 B-spline FFD

The traditional FFD transformation model [4] is defined as

$$\mathbf{T}_{\boldsymbol{\mu}}^n(\mathbf{x}) = \mathbf{x} + \sum_{\boldsymbol{\xi} \in \Xi} \mathbf{c}_{\boldsymbol{\xi}} \Phi_D^n(\mathbf{x}/\eta - \boldsymbol{\xi}), \tag{4}$$

where $\Xi \subset \mathcal{Z}^D$ denotes a D-dimensional uniform control-point grid, η is the grid spacing, $\mathbf{c}_{\boldsymbol{\xi}}$ represents the coefficient vector for a control point $\boldsymbol{\xi}$, and the vector of transformation parameters $\boldsymbol{\mu}$ is constructed from the elements of all coefficient vectors ($\boldsymbol{\mu} = \{\mathbf{c}_{\boldsymbol{\xi}} \mid \boldsymbol{\xi} \in \Xi\}$). As described in Section 2.2, a stochastic approximation of the derivative $\partial \mathcal{C}/\partial \boldsymbol{\mu}$ is calculated in the SGD based registration, which requires evaluation of transformation and its derivative.

Therefore, the size of the support of B-spline function has a significant influence to the computational cost of registration.

2.4 Random Perturbation and Postponed Smoothing

Random perturbation and postponed smoothing techniques are derived from the convolutional property of B-spline function. If the nth-order B-spline function is utilized to model the transformation, the number of control points considered in each dimension is $n + 1$ inside the support region. Then, the number of control points for a D-dimensional transformation is $(n+1)^D$. In practical medical image registration tasks, the input images F and M are usually 3D images. Thus, the numbers of control points which need to be considered around one image coordinate are 64, 27, 8, and 1 for $\beta^3(x)$, $\beta^2(x)$, $\beta^1(x)$, and $\beta^0(x)$, respectively. As introduced in Section 2.3, the computational cost of nonrigid registration is dominated by evaluating the transformation and its derivative. Therefore, the computational cost could be significantly reduced if lower-order B-spline function could replace the commonly used third-order B-splines.

From Eq.(1) and the convolution operation, we derive

$$\beta^n(x) = (\beta^m * \beta^{n-m-1})(x) = \int_{-\infty}^{\infty} \beta^m(x-t)\beta^{n-m-1}(t)dt = \int_{-\infty}^{\infty} \beta^m(x-t)p(t)dt,$$

(5)

where $m \leq n$ and $p(t)$ represents the probability density function (PDF) corresponding to $\beta^{n-m-1}(t)$. For example, $p(t)$ is a uniform PDF as the box function $\beta^0(t)$ when $m = n - 1$, or $p(t)$ is a Dirac delta PDF for the conventional non-perturbed FFD registration. Therefore, $\beta^n(x)$ can be considered as a mathematical expectation of $\beta^m(x - t)$ with the given PDF $p(t)$, and $\beta^m(x - t)$ is a shifted $\beta^m(x)$. Inspired by this relation, we propose to construct an expected B-spline FFD by randomly shifting lower-order B-splines $\beta^m(x - t)$ with $p(t)$.

This leads to the following definition of random perturbation transformation model

$$\widetilde{\mathbf{T}}_{\mu}^m(\mathbf{x}, \mathbf{t}) = \mathbf{x} + \sum_{\xi \in \Xi} c_{\xi} \Phi_D^m(\mathbf{x}/\eta - \xi - \mathbf{t}),$$

(6)

where m is the order of lower-order B-spline, $\mathbf{t} = [t_1, t_2, \cdots, t_D]^T$ denote the random shifts in each dimension. Through this way, the entire B-spline control point grid is thus shifted by vector $\mathbf{t}$ but the grid layout is kept.

As introduced in Section 2.1, a higher-order B-spline is convolved from lower-order B-splines. Therefore, to smooth the transformation field recovered by a lower-order B-spline function with a higher-order B-spline, the postponed smoothing technique is further proposed.

The new random perturbation and postponed smoothing techniques fit naturally in the framework of stochastic gradient descent optimization. For the computation of $\partial \mathcal{C}/\partial\mu$, we use $\widetilde{\mathbf{T}}_{\mu}^m(\mathbf{x}, \mathbf{t})$ instead of $\mathbf{T}_{\mu}^n(\mathbf{x})$, with a perturbation $\mathbf{t}$ randomly chosen in each iteration k of optimization. We thus obtain a stochastic approximation of the true derivative, at a lower computational cost. It is worth to note that this approximation comes on top of the approximation by randomly subsampling the image as explained in Section 2.2. The optimization procedure therefore can be described as

$$\mu_{k+1} = \mu_k - a_k \tilde{g}(\mu_k, \mathbf{t}_k),$$

(7)

where $\mathbf{t}_k$ is the realization of $\mathbf{t}$ in iteration k. The computationally efficient mth-order B-spline function is utilized only during the optimization process. The postponed smoothing approach is applied to the lower-order transformation field once the stochastic gradient descent optimization has finished. Through this way, the estimated parameters $\hat{\mu}$ are directly plugged into a higher-order B-spline FFD to obtain the final transformation. Please note that the random perturbation and postponed smoothing techniques can be used separately or combined together in a sequential way for later comparison.

In the present work, we focused on B-splines with the highest order $n = 3$. The standard third-order B-spline registration method is defined as the reference method. For a clear comparison, the whole registration process with lower-order B-spline is divided into three components (Perturbation-Optimization-Postponed smoothing) which are denoted as ($< p(t) > - < m > - < n >$) where $p(t) \in$ {Uniform, Gaussian, Dirac delta}, $m \in \{0, 1, 2\}$ and $n \in \{0, 1, 2, 3\}$. If the perturbation process is used, $p(t)$ can be assigned with uniform PDF ($\beta^0(t)$) or its corresponding truncated Gaussian PDF. The options of these components should be combined together to create a candidate registration method under the restriction that only higher or equal order ($n \geq m$) is allowed for postponed smoothing. Besides the conventional third-order B-spline, we compared 27 possible combinations in the experiments. In the following parts, the naming rule ($< p(t) > - < m > - < n >$) is used for shorthand notation for each registration method. For example, Dirac-3-3 denotes the conventional third-order B-spline registration method. Algorithm 1 provides an overview of the proposed registration method.

Input: $F \leftarrow$ fixed image, $M \leftarrow$ moving image, $K \leftarrow$ number of iterations,
$S \leftarrow$ number of samples $|\widehat{\Omega}_F|$, $m \leftarrow$ B-spline order for optimization,
$n \leftarrow$ B-spline order for final transformation, and
$p(\mathbf{t}) \leftarrow$ Uniform, Gaussian or Dirac delta
Output: Registered moving image $M\left(\mathbf{T}_{\hat{\mu}}^n(\mathbf{x})\right)$

1 Initialize transformation parameters $\boldsymbol{\mu} \leftarrow \mathbf{0}$
2 **for** $k \leftarrow 1$ **to** K **do**
3   Initialize random samples $[\mathbf{x}_1 \ldots \mathbf{x}_S]$, $\tilde{g} = \mathbf{0}$ and step size a_k
4   Draw random perturbation $\mathbf{t}_k \leftarrow p(\mathbf{t})$
5   **for** $\mathbf{x} \leftarrow \mathbf{x}_1$ **to** $\mathbf{x}_S$ **do**
6   Evaluate $F(\mathbf{x})$, and $\mathbf{y} \leftarrow \widetilde{\mathbf{T}}_{\mu}^m(\mathbf{x}, \mathbf{t}_k)$
7   Interpolate moving image value $M(\mathbf{y})$, and calculate gradient $\nabla M(\mathbf{y})$
8          $\partial \widetilde{\mathbf{T}}_{\mu}^m(\mathbf{x}, \mathbf{t}_k)/\partial \boldsymbol{\mu}$, and calculate contribution to $\tilde{g}$
9   **end**
10   Update transformation parameters $\boldsymbol{\mu} \leftarrow \boldsymbol{\mu} - a_k \tilde{g}$
11 **end**
12 $\hat{\mu} \leftarrow \boldsymbol{\mu}$
13 Instantiate nth-order FFD transformation $\mathbf{T}_{\hat{\mu}}^n(\mathbf{x})$,and **return** $M\left(\mathbf{T}_{\hat{\mu}}^n(\mathbf{x})\right)$

Algorithm 1. Proposed registration method

---

3 Experiments

The open source image registration package `elastix` [5] was used to implement all registration methods. For lung and brain data, similarity measures sum of squared differences (SSD), normalized correlation coefficient (NCC) were used as dissimilarity terms, respectively. For the ASGD optimizer, the numbers of random samples S and iterations K were set to 2000 in all experiments. To create 4 image resolution levels of input images, a Gaussian filter using $\{\sigma_1, \ldots, \sigma_4\} = \{4, 2, 1, 0.5\}$ voxels was applied. During the registration, the transformation of a finer scale was initialized by the transformation estimated at the coarser scale. The grid schedules $\{\eta_1, \eta_2, \eta_3, \eta_4\} = \{64, 32, 16, 8\}$mm and $\{64, 38, 22, 13\}$mm were used on lung data. On the brain data, the grid schedule $\{40, 20, 10, 5\}$mm was utilized. For the perturbation process, the standard deviation σ_U of uniform PDF changes with grid spacing η_i, but for the σ_G of Gaussian PDF we restricted it to be the σ_U on the finest grid spacing η_4.

Since the Gaussian PDF is not compactly supported, we truncated the Gaussian PDF using $min(\eta_i, 4 \times \sigma_G)$.

We used 10 pairs of DIR-Lab 3D chest CT scans with 300 manually annotated landmarks on the lung structure. The voxel and dimension sizes of lung data are around $1 \times 1 \times 2.5$mm and around $256 \times 256 \times 110$. Lung masks were created to constraint the registration on the lung region. For all cases, the exhale phase (moving image) was registered to the inhale phases (fixed image). The mean target registration error (mTRE) which calculates the distance between the transformed and ground truth landmarks was used to measure the registration accuracy. To evaluate the transformation smoothness of registration, the standard deviation of the determinant of spatial Jacobian D_{SJ} was calculated inside lung mask. The standard deviation of D_{SJ} represents the fluctuation of the estimated transformation field, and therefore gives an indication of the smoothness of a transformation.

The Internet Brain Segmentation Repository (IBSR v2.0), which contains 18 T1-weighted MRI 3D brain scans, was also used to evaluate the registration methods with inter-subject registration. The volumes of these images are $256 \times 256 \times 128$. The voxel sizes are around $1 \times 1 \times 1.5$mm. To evaluate the registration accuracy, overall mean overlap which measures the overlap between the transformed and ground truth atlases over all labels was used. To measure the smoothness of the transformation, we used the same standard deviation of D_{SJ} which was calculated inside a brain mask. The same affine registrations were used to roughly align the data first for each registration method.

4   Results

Figure 2 (a) plots a 2D average rank in terms of accuracy and smoothness based on the results from the 20 test cases for each methods on lung data. The X-axis and Y-axis indicate the ranking in registration accuracy and smoothness ,and the lower ranking number means better performance. From Figure 2 (a), both $m = 2$ and $m = 1$ methods can produce better accuracy and smoothness than the traditional third-order B-spline method with proper perturbation and postponed smoothing techniques. The green line in Figure 2 (a) shows the trace of improved rank by uniform perturbation and followed by the third-order postponed smoothing. Similarly, the blue line indicates the trace of improved ranks in both accuracy and smoothness by only the postponed smoothing technique.

On the lung data, the results of several typical methods using the finest grid spacings 13mm and 8mm were pooled and shown as box plots in Figure 3 (a) and (b). Overall, the lower-order B-spline registration can generate better accuracy and smoothness than the conventional third-order registration method (Dirac-3-3). Since the calculation of spatial Jacobian on Dirac-0-0 is impossible, its blank position is marked as black cross in Figure 3 (b).

The 2D ranks of 28 registration methods on the brain data are shown in Figure 2 (b). Compared with the rank of third-order B-spline, the lower-order B-spline can also generate better accuracy and smoothness on brain data. Because the overlap measurement is less sensitive to the smoothness, the first-order

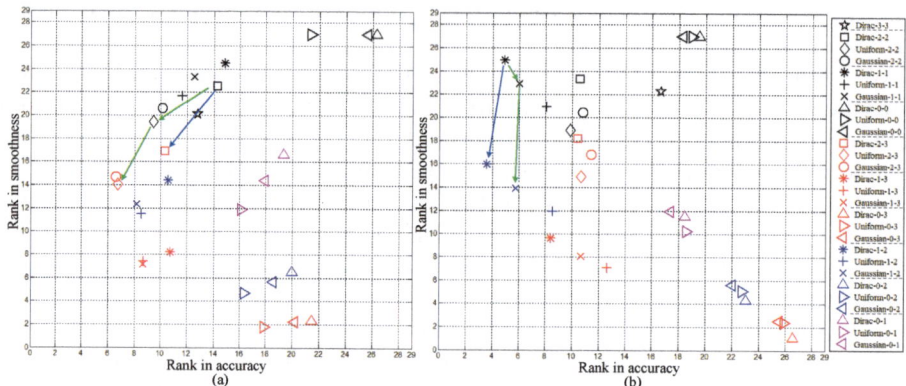

Fig. 2. Two dimensional averaged ranking number of different methods: (a) lung data; (b) brain data

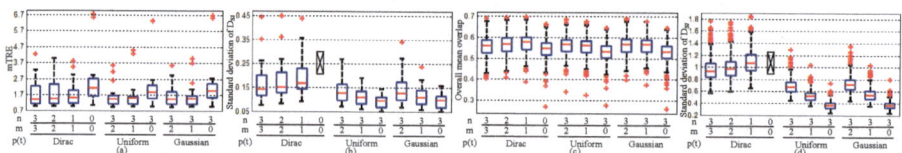

Fig. 3. Registration results by different methods: (a) accuracy on lung data (mTRE, in mm, lower values are better); (b) smoothness on lung data (standard deviation of D_{SJ}, lower values are better); (c) accuracy on brain data (overall mean overlap, higher values are better); (d) smoothness on brain data (standard deviation of D_{SJ}, lower values are better)

B-spline is more favorable on brain data than the second-order B-spline on lung data. The green and blue lines indicate the trace of rank change after the random perturbation and postponed smoothing technique. By applying these two techniques, more adjacent image information is considered during registration. Therefore, the smoothness is improved more significantly than accuracy. The detailed registration results of several typical methods are provided in Figure 3 (c) and (d).

Experimentally, the computation time on lung (subject No.3) using an Intel Core i7-2720QM with 8G memory were 149.4 ± 1.7 seconds, 90.1 ± 1.1 seconds, 64.9 ± 0.9 seconds, and 53.5 ± 0.5 seconds (mean $\pm$ standard deviation over 10 runs) for the methods with B-spline orders third, second, first, and zeroth during optimization, respectively. On the brain data (registering subject No.6 to subject No.8) were 223.7 ± 1.3 seconds, 145.0 ± 0.7 seconds, 115.5 ± 1.6 seconds, and 103.7 ± 0.7 seconds for B-spline orders from third to zeroth, respectively.

5   Discussion

The improvements on accuracy and smoothness show that both random perturbation process and postponed smoothing technique are essential for good registration performance. According to the accuracy and smoothness on lung and brain data, Gaussian-1-3, Uniform-1-3 and Dirac-1-3 produced consistently better registration results. There are two possible explanations for the improved registration results. First, in perturbation process, a new stochastic dynamic is introduced to the stochastic gradient descent optimization. The stochastic perturbations may help to avoid the local minima as has been previously reported in the literature on stochastic approximation optimization [6]. Second, due to the disproportionate B-spline weighting of the control points [7], the traditional B-spline FFD can lead to ill-conditioned optimization spaces. In current work, the influences of different control points to the cost function are randomly changed in each iteration by randomly shifting the control point grid. Thus, the disadvantage of the disproportionate control point weighting might be alleviated by the perturbation process. The current stochastic perturbation process was derived from the convolutional property of B-spline functions. In the future, we could also test the potential of the perturbation process on other basis functions.

6   Conclusions

In this work, the potential of FFD registration based on lower-order B-spline was investigated. With the proposed random perturbation and postponed smoothing approaches, the lower-order B-spline FFD method produced better registration accuracy and smoothness than the popular third-order B-spline registration method. Because less control points are involved in the lower-order B-spline registration, the method is computationally less expensive than the traditional approach.

References

1. Sun, W., Niessen, W.J., Klein, S.: Randomly perturbed free-form deformation for nonrigid image registration. In: Ourselin, S., Modat, M. (eds.) WBIR 2014. LNCS, vol. 8545, pp. 62–71. Springer, Heidelberg (2014)
2. Klein, S., et al.: Evaluation of optimization methods for nonrigid medical image registration using mutual information and B-splines. IEEE Trans. Image Process. 16(12), 2879–2890 (2007)
3. Klein, S., et al.: Adaptive stochastic gradient descent optimisation for image registration. Int. J. Comput. Vis. 81(3), 227–239 (2009)
4. Rueckert, D., et al.: Nonrigid registration using free-form deformations: Application to breast MR images. IEEE Trans. Med. Imag. 18(8), 712–721 (1999)
5. Klein, S., et al.: Elastix: a toolbox for intensity-based medical image registration. IEEE Trans. Med. Imag. 29(1), 196–205 (2010)
6. Maryak, J., et al.: Global random optimization by simultaneous perturbation stochastic approximation. IEEE Trans. Automat. Contr. 53(3), 780–783 (2008)
7. Tustison, N.J., et al.: Directly manipulated free-form deformation image registration. IEEE Trans. Image Process. 18(3), 624–635 (2009)

Multispectral Image Registration Based on Local Canonical Correlation Analysis

Mattias P. Heinrich[1], Bartłomiej W. Papież[2],
Julia A. Schnabel[2], and Heinz Handels[1]

[1] Institute of Medical Informatics, University of Lübeck, Germany
[2] Institute of Biomedical Engineering,
Department of Engineering, University of Oxford, UK
heinrich@imi.uni-luebeck.de
http://www.mpheinrich.de

Abstract. Medical scans are today routinely acquired using multiple
sequences or contrast settings, resulting in multispectral data. For the
automatic analysis of this data, the evaluation of multispectral similarity
is essential. So far, few concepts have been proposed to deal in a principled way with images containing multiple channels. Here, we present
a new approach based on a well known statistical technique: canonical
correlation analysis (CCA). CCA finds a mapping of two multidimensional variables into two new bases, which best represent the true underlying relations of the signals. In contrast to previously used metrics, it
is therefore able to find new correlations based on linear combinations
of multiple channels. We extend this concept to efficiently model local
canonical correlation (LCCA) between image patches. This novel, more
general similarity metric can be applied to images with an arbitrary number of channels. The most important property of LCCA is its invariance
to affine transformations of variables. When used on local histograms,
LCCA can also deal with multimodal similarity. We demonstrate the performance of our concept on challenging clinical multispectral datasets.

Keywords: multichannel, canonical correlation, multimodal, MRI.

1 Introduction

Multispectral imaging, in particular multi-sequence magnetic resonance imaging
(MRI), is increasingly becoming available in clinical practice. Image registration
forms an integral part in the analysis pipeline for computer aided diagnosis and
interventions based on medical imaging. However, to this date, few algorithms
have been proposed to explicitly handle multichannel image data [1,2]. A further
difficulty arises when not all exact same sequences are available for all patients
in a study. In order to establish correspondences across multichannel scans of
different patients (or with respect to an atlas), image registration relies on a
robust similarity metric. For different MRI sequences, such as T1-weighted, T2-
weighted or fluid attenuated inversion recovery (FLAIR), a certain degree of

P. Golland et al. (Eds.): MICCAI 2014, Part I, LNCS 8673, pp. 202–209, 2014.
© Springer International Publishing Switzerland 2014

correlation across channels can be expected, since they are all based on the same physical principle of the magnetisation of water protons. It is however difficult to establish a priori which channels correlate best with each other and represent a true correspondence based on the underlying physiology.

In order to deal with similarity of multichannel images one approach is to average the cross-correlations [3] calculated for each channel individually. This, however, disregards all cross-channel correlation. Generalised correlation coefficients for diffusion tensor images have been proposed in [4], which are used to calculate a scalar correlation value (but also ignore cross-channel correlations). This concept was extended to multi-tensor images in [5] using the matrix logarithm of diffusion matrices. The linear correlation of linear combination (LC^2) metric [6], captures the similarity of a multichannel and a scalar image. Image synthesis based on aligned training data [7], or general polynomial models [8] have been used to predict the appearance of a different modality or contrast. Multichannel demons [1], use squared intensity differences as force fields derived independently from multiple channels. Multi-variate mutual information has been proposed in e.g. [2], but certain approximations have to be made to overcome the large complexity. In [9], image registration is performed by choosing the optimal subset of Gabor wavelet features of multichannel images, using independent component analysis and a 'choose max' fusion strategy.

In this work, we overcome the challenges of multispectral image similarity using a established statistical technique: canonical correlation analysis (CCA) [10]. CCA has been previously used in the context of medical image analysis, e.g. to detect neural activity in functional MRI [11]. It has also been used as a metric in [12] for log tensor images, calculated over disjunct blocks, and was called generalised correlation coefficient in that work. CCA measures the linear relationships between two multi-dimensional random variables (see Sec. 2.1). We apply CCA to define similarity across multichannel images, because it allows us to find a mapping of the images into a new space where they maximally correlate. The canonical correlation is invariant to affine transformations or permutations of the input variables. Since linear relations between channels in medical images do not hold globally, we propose an efficient scheme to evaluate the **local** canonical correlation (LCCA). For this purpose, we extend the recently proposed guided filter [13], which uses a (multichannel) image as a guidance to filter a second scalar input image (in our work both images have multiple channels). The filter can be implemented using box filters, with a computational complexity independent of the local neighbourhood size. We make a further contribution by applying LCCA to local histogram images enabling multimodal registration. In Sec. 3, we demonstrate the state-of-the-art performance of our approach for two challenging clinical multispectral datasets, evaluated with manual segmentations.

2   Methods

Let us consider two general 3D multichannel images $\mathbf{I}$ and $\mathbf{J}$, where each location x is represented by an intensity vector of length m and n respectively. Given a neighbourhood radius r, image patches $\mathbf{X}(x)$ (in $\mathbf{I}$) and $\mathbf{Y}(x)$ (in $\mathbf{J}$) are defined at every x within a spatial window Ω_x with a size of $(r \times 2 + 1)^3$. The individual channels of each patch are denoted by a subscript: $X_1, \ldots, X_m$ and $Y_1, \ldots, Y_n$. The similarity at location x between two patches can be defined for the most trivial case of two scalar images as the normalised correlation coefficient (NCC):

$$\rho^2(X_1, Y_1, x) = \frac{(\sum_{\Omega_x}(X_1 - \bar{X}_1)(Y_1 - \bar{Y}_1))^2}{\sum_{\Omega_x}(X_1 - \bar{X}_1)^2 \sum_{\Omega_x}(Y_1 - \bar{Y}_1)^2} \tag{1}$$

where $\bar{X}_i = \frac{1}{|\Omega_x|}\sum_{\Omega_x} X_i$ represents the mean intensity of an image patch. The scalar NCC is invariant to any affine intensity transform $X' = aX + b$ of the image patches. It can be extended to multichannel images (MC-NCC), defining a vectorial correlation coefficient $\boldsymbol{\rho}$:

$$\boldsymbol{\rho}^2(\mathbf{X}, \mathbf{Y}, x) = \{\rho^2(X_1, Y_1, x), \ldots, \rho^2(X_{d_{\min}}, Y_{d_{\min}}, x)\} \tag{2}$$

where $d_{\min} = \min(m, n)$ is the minimal channel dimensionality. We note that $\boldsymbol{\rho}$ is not well adapted to images with differing numbers of channels $m \neq n$, since a choice of which extra channel to drop has to be made. Furthermore, it is not invariant to arbitrary linear transformations of the input variables.

2.1   Canonical Correlation Analysis (CCA)

CCA is able to overcome these limitations by finding the two bases $\mathbf{w}_X$ and $\mathbf{w}_Y$, which maximise the sum over $\boldsymbol{\rho}$ for the transformed variables $\mathbf{X} \cdot \mathbf{w}_X$ and $\mathbf{Y} \cdot \mathbf{w}_Y$. In order to find the canonical basis vectors, we first need to construct a full correlation matrix D. Let us define a $m \times n$ cross-covariance matrix $\boldsymbol{\Sigma}_{\mathbf{XY}}$, where the entry in the kth row and lth column is defined to be:

$$\Sigma_{X_k Y_l} = \frac{1}{|\Omega_x|} \sum_{\Omega_x} (X_k - \bar{X}_k)(Y_l - \bar{Y}_l). \tag{3}$$

The variance matrices $\boldsymbol{\Sigma}_{\mathbf{XX}}$ and $\boldsymbol{\Sigma}_{\mathbf{YY}}$ are defined analogously. The full correlation matrix D then becomes:

$$D(\mathbf{X}, \mathbf{Y}) = \boldsymbol{\Sigma}_{\mathbf{XX}}^{-1} \boldsymbol{\Sigma}_{\mathbf{XY}} \boldsymbol{\Sigma}_{\mathbf{YY}}^{-1} \boldsymbol{\Sigma}_{\mathbf{XY}}^T \tag{4}$$

The basis vectors can be obtained by performing an eigendecomposition, where $\mathbf{w}_X$ is build up from the eigenvectors of $D(\mathbf{X}, \mathbf{Y})$ and $\mathbf{w}_Y$ from the eigenvectors of $D(\mathbf{Y}, \mathbf{X})$. The canonical correlations are the eigenvalues $\boldsymbol{\lambda}_{\mathbf{XY}} = \{\lambda_1, \ldots, \lambda_{d_{\min}}\}$ of D. A scalar similarity metric $\mathcal{S}(\mathbf{X}, \mathbf{Y})$ of two patches can now be defined based on the sum over $\boldsymbol{\lambda}_{\mathbf{XY}}$ divided by $d_{\min}$. Note, that even though the number of non-zero eigenvalues is limited by $\min(rank(m), rank(n))$ every image channel has the same influence weight on calculating the eigenvalues. Another simplification can be obtained, based on the fact that for any matrix the sum of eigenvalues equals the trace of that matrix. So finally we get:

$$\mathcal{S}(\mathbf{X}, \mathbf{Y}, x) = 1 - \frac{1}{d_{\min}} trace(D(\mathbf{X}, \mathbf{Y}, x)) \tag{5}$$

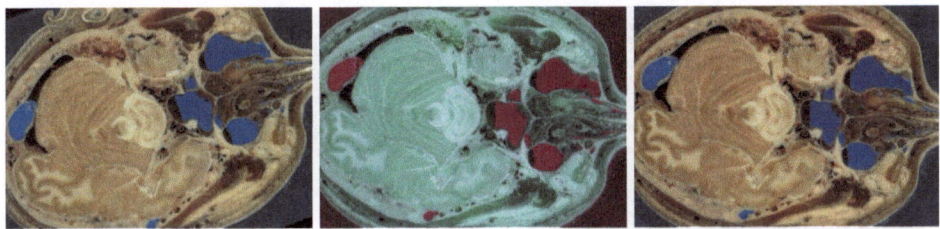

Fig. 1. Visual example of (global) canonical correlation analysis applied to colour images. Left: **I** slice of the visible human dataset with its original colour, but rotated by $20°$. Centre: **J** same slice without rotation, but with cyclically shifted hue. Right: **J**′ reconstructed true slice estimated using CCA (of **I** and **J**) and $\mathbf{J}' = \mathbf{w}_Y \mathbf{w}_Y^{-1} \mathbf{J}$.

In contrast, to Eq. 2 the canonical correlation is invariant to affine intensity mappings of multichannel images. Figure 1 demonstrates the capabilities of finding an intensity mapping, which affects all image channels simultaneously even when one image is geometrically transformed. S is symmetric and also independent of the order of **X** and **Y**. When one of the images is scalar $n = 1$, the correlation matrix D becomes a scalar, and it can be shown that LCCA is equivalent to the linear correlation of linear combination (LC^2) metric [6] for this special case.

Local Canonical Correlation (LCCA) Computation: Linear correlations rarely hold for the whole image, yet to get a point-wise local evaluation of the similarity metric, we have to calculate D for every voxel, using all $(2r+1)^3$ voxels within the patch Ω_x. Fortunately, the calculation can be simplified without loss of accuracy using box filters, following the ideas of guided image filtering [13]. The similarity has to be evaluated for every voxel, so the complexity is greatly reduced and independent of the patch-size by first rearranging Eq. 3:

$$\sum_{\Omega_x}(X - \bar{X})(Y - \bar{Y}) = \sum_{\Omega_x} XY - \bar{X}\bar{Y} \tag{6}$$

and then replacing the summation in Eq. 6 by a convolution kernel K_r. The moving average kernel has a constant complexity independent of kernel size and the local means $\bar{X}$ and $\bar{Y}$ can be precomputed (again by convolution). For the purpose of image registration, where multiple displacements have to be evaluated, we can furthermore pre-calculate the inverse variance matrices $\mathbf{\Sigma}_{\mathbf{XX}}^{-1}$ and $\mathbf{\Sigma}_{\mathbf{YY}}^{-1}$ once (per iteration). Thus only mn box filter convolutions (for the whole image) and two matrix multiplications (for every voxel) are required. For a typical dual channel image with one million voxels this enables us to process the patch-wise similarity for every voxel and up to 40 displacements per second.[1]

Non-functional Intensity Mappings Using Local Histograms: A limitation of NCC for medical image registration is that it is usually not applicable to multimodal images. We present an interesting second application of LCCA to address this shortcoming. Given a pair of scalar images I and J from different

---

[1] Source code for LCCA will be made public at
`http://www.mpheinrich.de/software.html`

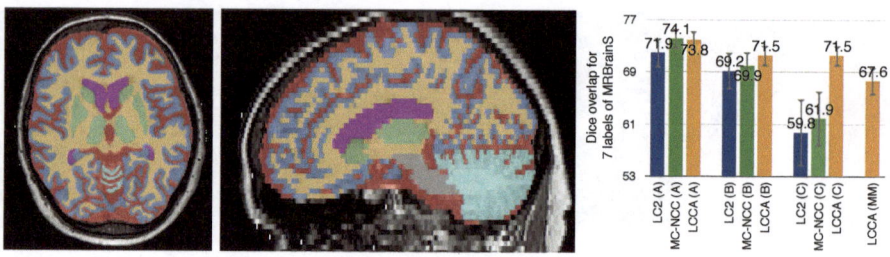

Fig. 2. Left-centre: MRBrainS dataset with manual segmentations: ■ Cortical gray matter, ■ Basal ganglia, ■ White matter and White matter lesions, ■ Cerebrospinal fluid in the extracerebral space, ■ Ventricles, ■ Cerebellum, ■ Brainstem. Right: Quantitative results of 4 multi-spectral registration experiments on training set of 5 patients. MC-NCC and LCCA both outperform LC^2 for experiment A, while LCCA yields higher accuracy for all other tests (descriptions see text) than MC-NCC or LC^2.

modalities, they can be transformed into multichannel images $\mathbf{I} = \{I_1, \ldots, I_m\}$ and $\mathbf{J} = \{J_1, \ldots, J_m\}$, where each channel represents the distance from a range of m quantised intensity value $\mathbf{v} = \{v_1, \ldots, v_m\}$, with $I_k = \exp(-(I - v_k)^2/\sigma^2)$. Here, σ represents the uncertainty in image intensity similar to the Parzen window in mutual information calculation. This representation enables LCCA to model even non-functional intensity mappings. In practice a very low number m of histogram channels is sufficient. For this application the invariance of LCCA to permutations of the channels is of great importance.

Regularisation and Optimisation: LCCA is employed in a discrete non-rigid registration framework, which we have recently published in [14]. An explicit search is performed over a discrete displacement space $\mathbf{d} \in \mathcal{L} = \{0, \pm q, \ldots, \pm q_{max}\}^3$ (with quantisation step q) using the patch-wise formulation of CCA as similarity metric. Starting from an initial estimate using the argmin $\mathbf{v}$ of the discrete search, a globally smooth displacement field $\mathbf{u}$ is iteratively estimated by two alternating steps. First, a Gaussian smoothing $\mathbf{u} \leftarrow K_\sigma \mathbf{v}$ of the current field is performed. Second, an auxiliary term $\frac{1}{\theta}(\mathbf{u} - \mathbf{v})^2$ is added to the local similarity distributions and a new argmin $\mathbf{v}$ selected. When the parameter θ is subsequently reduced, a convergence ($\mathbf{u} = \mathbf{v}$) is reached after few iterations.

3   Experiments

We compare the performance of the presented canonical correlation analysis based similarity metric (LCCA) to multichannel NCC (MC-NCC) and the LC^2 metric on two different multispectral image datasets.

Multispectral Brain Image Registration: First, we employ data from the multispectral brain segmentation challenge (MRBrainS) held at MICCAI 2013 [15]. The organisers provided training datasets of five patients with T1-weighted, T1 with inversion recovery (IR) and FLAIR MRI modalities. The scans have a resolution of 1x1x3 mm, are rigidly aligned (to the FLAIR sequence) and manually segmented into 8 labels (since white matter lesions cannot be detected using atlas-based segmentation, we merge labels 3 and 4). Pair-wise registrations between all five patients are performed using a three-level approach of our registration framework and the following parameters: down-sampling factors of $\{3, 2, 1\}$, maximal displacement range of $q_{max} = \{6, 2, 1\}$ and patch-radius $r = 2$ voxels. The Dice overlap before registration is on average 45.5%. We perform four different experiments using all of the three metrics, whenever they are applicable on dual-channel MRI scans (within the same optimisation framework):

- **A**: both channels are of the same modality for both moving and target image and in the right order (e.g. $\mathbf{I} = \{T1, T2\}, \mathbf{J} = \{T1, T2\}$)
- **B**: one channel is of the same modality for both images the other channel is from two different modalities (e.g. $\mathbf{I} = \{T1(IR), T1\}, \mathbf{J} = \{T1(IR), T2\}$)
- **C**: analogous to **B**, but the order of the channels is swapped for one image (e.g. $\mathbf{I} = \{T2, T1\}, \mathbf{J} = \{T1(IR), T2\}$)
- **MM** (multimodal registration): only one MR sequence is used for the target image and a different one for the moving image. Three histogram channels are constructed for both single channel MR images.

MC-NCC performs best when the exact same two channels are available, closely followed by LCCA. Both methods improve significantly over LC^2 ($p < 0.01$ for Wilcoxon rank sum test), which can only utilise one multichannel image. When only one channel is of common modality across scans, LCCA achieves significantly better registration accuracy than MC-NCC or LC^2 ($p < 0.01$), which demonstrate that it correctly finds new relationships between different multispectral channels. When using local histograms for multimodal registration (T1→FLAIR) LCCA nearly reaches its performance from experiments **B** and **C**. However, further experiments and comparisons are necessary to confirm its suitable for other multimodal registration tasks. We also tested, if a combination of global and local CCA would be beneficial, but found no improvements.

Canine Muscle Segmentation: To facilitate further comparison, we perform registration experiments on the canine dataset (22 training subjects) from the MICCAI SATA challenge [16] for which SyN [3] was used to provide standardised registrations using both MRI channels (T2 and T2 with fat suppression). Manual segmentations of seven proximal leg muscles have been provided (see Fig. 3) to study muscular dystrophy. The significant differences in size and appearance of the studied dogs render this a very challenging registration task. We include an affine alignment step (using block matching with LCCA and trimmed least squares [17]) and increase the patch-radius r to 3 voxels. Our registration approach significantly outperforms SyN (both use affine+deformable transformations) with an improvement in overlap of 15% ($p < 0.01$). When initialising SyN using the affine transforms obtained for LCCA, the results improve to $D=52.4\pm15\%$, which is still significantly ($p = 0.008$) inferior to our results of $D=55.5\pm13\%$. These results for single-atlas segmentation can be further improved using label fusion [16]. Already a simple majority voting results in a Dice overlap of $D=73.0\pm14\%$ for our approach (compared to 55.1% for SyN in [16]). Our algorithm is with a runtime of ≈40 sec. several times faster than SyN.

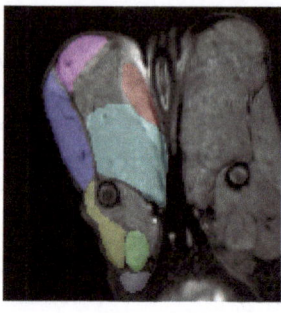 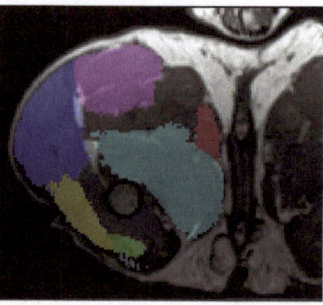 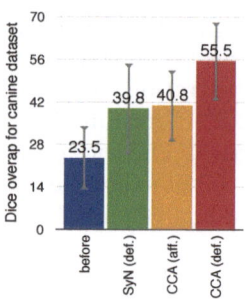

Fig. 3. Results of registration of canine dataset with LCCA. Left: Slice of atlas scan with manual segmentation. Centre: Target scan with automatically transferred labels. Right: Quantitative evaluation of Dice overlap shows improvement using our approach with deformable (def.) registration (D=55.5 %) compared to ANTs SyN (D=39.8 %). When applying majority voting, LCCA achieves a segmentation accuracy of D=73.0%.

4   Conclusion

We have presented a novel similarity metric for registration of multispectral images. Local canonical correlation analysis (LCCA) is based on an established statistical concept for multivariate variables. An efficient computational scheme inspired by guided image filtering is used to calculate dense patch-wise similarities. The main benefit of LCCA is its ability to find new linear relationships **across** channels. Our new metric generalises established techniques, such as NCC [3] and LC^2 [6], and works for images with an arbitrary number of channels. When applied to local histograms it is able to deal with multimodal data. The validation results demonstrate its advantages over current state-of-the-art methods especially for challenging multispectral data.

LCCA can be very useful in clinical practice where not always the same sequences are acquired for every patient and scanner parameters (e.g. repetition time, flip angle) may vary. In future work, we plan to apply this concept within an ongoing clinical study to improve the detection and segmentation of stroke lesions in multispectral MRI. A further application is its use to analyse sequences, where time-points are not necessarily temporally aligned [1]. LCCA can also be used to achieve rotational invariance for multidimensional orientated image descriptors [18], removing the need for recalculation/reorientation of them. It could also be used to find optimal correlations across feature-based image representations. The metric can easily be applied to multi-atlas based label fusion and extend it to multichannel images. Future work may investigate whether selecting only the strongest correlations (akin to dimensionality reduction) and/or the calculation of the eigenvector mapping on a coarser scale are beneficial.

Acknowledgements. B.W.P. and J.A.S. would like to acknowledge funding from the CRUK/ EPSRC Cancer Imaging Centre, Oxford. M.P.H. thanks Adrian Dalca and Ramesh Sridharan for fruitful discussions, which initiated this article.

References

1. Peyrat, J.M., Delingette, H., Sermesant, M., Xu, C., Ayache, N.: Registration of 4D cardiac CT sequences under trajectory constraints with multichannel diffeomorphic demons. IEEE Transactions on Medical Imaging 29(7), 1351–1368 (2010)
2. Rohde, G., Pajevic, S., Pierpaoli, C., Basser, P.: A comprehensive approach for multi-channel image registration. In: Gee, J.C., Maintz, J.B.A., Vannier, M.W. (eds.) WBIR 2003. LNCS, vol. 2717, pp. 214–223. Springer, Heidelberg (2003)
3. Avants, B.B., Epstein, C.L., Grossman, M., Gee, J.C.: Symmetric diffeomorphic image registration with cross-correlation: evaluating automated labeling of elderly and neurodegenerative brain. Med. Imag. Anal. 12(1), 26–41 (2008)
4. Ruiz-Alzola, J., Westin, C., Warfield, S., Alberola, C., Maier, S., Kikinis, R.: Non-rigid registration of 3D tensor medical data. Med. Imag. Anal. 6(2), 143–161 (2002)
5. Taquet, M., Macq, B., Warfield, S.K.: A generalized correlation coefficient: Application to DTI and multi-fiber DTI. In: MMBIA 2012, pp. 9–14. IEEE (2012)
6. Wein, W., Brunke, S., Khamene, A., Callstrom, M.R., Navab, N.: Automatic CT-ultrasound registration for diagnostic imaging and image-guided intervention. Med. Imag. Anal. 12(5), 577–585 (2008)
7. Iglesias, J.E., Konukoglu, E., Zikic, D., Glocker, B., Van Leemput, K., Fischl, B.: Is synthesizing MRI contrast useful for inter-modality analysis? In: Mori, K., Sakuma, I., Sato, Y., Barillot, C., Navab, N. (eds.) MICCAI 2013, Part I. LNCS, vol. 8149, pp. 631–638. Springer, Heidelberg (2013)
8. Guimond, A., Roche, A., Ayache, N., Meunier, J.: Three-dimensional multimodal brain warping using the demons algorithm and adaptive intensity corrections. IEEE Transactions on Medical Imaging 20(1), 58–69 (2001)
9. Li, Y., Verma, R.: Multichannel image registration by feature-based information fusion. IEEE Transactions on Medical Imaging 30(3), 707–720 (2011)
10. Hotelling, H.: Relations between two sets of variates. Biometrika 28(3-4), 321–377 (1936)
11. Friman, O., Cedefamn, J., Lundberg, P., Borga, M., Knutsson, H.: Detection of neural activity in functional MRI using canonical correlation analysis. Magnetic Resonance in Medicine 45(2), 323–330 (2001)
12. Suarez, R.O., Commowick, O., Prabhu, S.P., Warfield, S.K.: Automated delineation of white matter fiber tracts with a multiple region-of-interest approach. NeuroImage 59(4), 3690–3700 (2012)
13. He, K., Sun, J., Tang, X.: Guided image filtering. IEEE Transactions on Pattern Analysis and Machine Intelligence 35(6), 1397–1409 (2013)
14. Heinrich, M.P., Papież, B.W., Schnabel, J.A., Handels, H.: Non-parametric discrete registration with convex optimisation. In: Ourselin, S., Modat, M. (eds.) WBIR 2014. LNCS, vol. 8545, pp. 51–61. Springer, Heidelberg (2014)
15. Mendrik, A.: Evaluation framework for MR brain image segmentation. In: MICCAI Grand Challenge (2013), http://mrbrains13.isi.uu.nl
16. Landman, B., Warfield, S.: Segmentation: Algorithms, theory and applications. In: MICCAI SATA (2013), https://masi.vuse.vanderbilt.edu/workshop2013
17. Ourselin, S., Roche, A., Prima, S., Ayache, N.: Block matching: A general framework to improve robustness of rigid registration of medical images. In: Delp, S.L., DiGoia, A.M., Jaramaz, B. (eds.) MICCAI 2000. LNCS, vol. 1935, pp. 557–566. Springer, Heidelberg (2000)
18. Heinrich, M.P., Jenkinson, M., Papież, B.W., Brady, S.M., Schnabel, J.A.: Towards realtime multimodal fusion for image-guided interventions using self-similarities. In: Mori, K., Sakuma, I., Sato, Y., Barillot, C., Navab, N. (eds.) MICCAI 2013, Part I. LNCS, vol. 8149, pp. 187–194. Springer, Heidelberg (2013)

Topology Preservation and Anatomical Feasibility in Random Walker Image Registration

Shawn Andrews, Lisa Tang, and Ghassan Hamarneh

Medical Image Analysis Lab, Simon Fraser University, Canada

Abstract. The random walker image registration (RWIR) method is a powerful tool for aligning medical images that also provides useful uncertainty information. However, it is difficult to ensure topology preservation in RWIR, which is an important property in medical image registration as it is often necessary for the anatomical feasibility of an alignment. In this paper, we introduce a technique for determining spatially adaptive regularization weights for RWIR that ensure an anatomically feasible transformation. This technique only increases the run time of the RWIR algorithm by about 10%, and avoids over-smoothing by only increasing regularization in specific image regions. Our results show that our technique ensures topology preservation and improves registration accuracy.

1 Introduction

Medical image registration (MIR), which is finding a spatial transformation that maps anatomical objects in one image to corresponding objects in another image, is a key step in many medical analysis tasks, including tracking disease progression, multi-modal fusion, shape analysis, and atlas construction. To encourage anatomical feasibility, regularization is imposed on the transformation to encourage smoothness and topology preservation (TP). However, regularizing sufficiently to ensure anatomical feasibility without over-smoothing and losing accuracy can be difficult   or computationally expensive. A variety of techniques have been proposed to ensure TP, including implicitly, e.g. by expressing transformations as integrals over vector fields [1], or explicitly, e.g. by penalizing the lack of TP in the regularization objective term [9].

Recently, registration approaches that represent transformations in the discrete domain have arisen [4,3,11,12]. In discrete approaches every pixel (or voxel) is assigned a displacement vector from a predefined set, referred to as a *discrete transformation*, allowing the image registration energy to be formulated as a Markov random field (MRF) and well established optimization techniques such as graph cuts [2] to be utilized.

The discrete random walker image registration (RWIR) algorithm [3] uses a globally optimizable Gaussian MRF energy for regularization and has been shown to achieve results comparable to other state-of-the-art registration schemes [3,10,7]. RWIR provides a probabilistic registration that can be leveraged to calculate uncertainty. Registration uncertainty can be utilized to direct clinicians to possible registration errors or image abnormalities, and can influence diagnostic and therapeutic decisions. [8,6].

A useful feature of RWIR is that it seamlessly allows for spatially adaptive regularization weights, which have been shown to improve registration accuracy compared to

P. Golland et al. (Eds.): MICCAI 2014, Part I, LNCS 8673, pp. 210–217, 2014.

a constant regularization weight [11]. However, it is not clear a priori how much regularization is required in RWIR to ensure topology preservation. One option to deal with this is time consuming trial and error. Alternatively, post-processing techniques such as scaling and squaring [1] can convert a transformation to one that preserves topology, but such methods discard the uncertainty information provided by RWIR.

In this paper, we introduce a technique that determines if a set of regularization weights for RWIR will result in a topology preserving transformation without having to run the RWIR algorithm. We use our technique to iteratively increase regularization in regions where topology is not preserved, avoiding over-smoothing in other regions.

2 Anatomical Feasibility in RWIR

2.1 RWIR Review

In RWIR, we wish to align two images, I_1 and I_2, defined over Ω, a set of n pixels (or voxels). We define $\hat{\Omega}$ as the n by d matrix of pixel locations, where d is the dimensionality of the images. Transformations are represented using a discrete set of K displacements, $V = [\mathbf{v}_1, \ldots, \mathbf{v}_K]$, where $\mathbf{v}_k \in \mathbb{R}^d$. A *probabilistic transformation* assigns, to each pixel a, probabilities for the displacement vectors, $\mathbf{u}^a = [u_1^a, \ldots, u_K^a] \in \mathbb{P}_K$. $\mathbb{P}_K \subset \mathbb{R}^K$ is the unit simplex of positive vectors that are normalized to sum to one. $\mathbf{u}_k$ denotes a vector of length n of the probabilities of $\mathbf{v}_k$ at each pixel.

The first step in RWIR is to calculate *prior probabilities* for each pixel a and displacement $\mathbf{v}_k$ from a data similarity term $f_{sim}(I_1, I_2, a, \mathbf{v}_k)$. The prior probabilities at a are given by $\mathbf{p}^a = [p_1^a, \ldots, p_K^a] \in \mathbb{P}_K$, $p_k^a = f_{sim}(I_1, I_2, a, \mathbf{v}_k)/Z^a$, where Z_a normalizes.

The second step is to construct a weighted image graph, with a node for each pixel and a weighted edge between neighboring pixels, and use it to regularize the displacement labels. The edge weights are stronger for pixels of similar intensities; for pixels a and b, and $\beta = 50$, we use edge weight $w_{a,b} = \exp(-\beta|I(a) - I(b)|)$. Defining W as the n by n matrix of edge weights and D as the n by n diagonal matrix of the row sums of W, then $L = D - W$ is known as the combinatorial Laplacian of the image graph. The probabilities $\mathbf{u}_k$ are then calculated by minimizing the energy:

$$E_{RW}(\mathbf{u}_k) = \mathbf{u}_k^\top L \mathbf{u}_k + (\mathbf{u}_k - \mathbf{p}_k)^\top \Gamma^{-1}(\mathbf{u}_k - \mathbf{p}_k), \quad k \in \{1, \ldots, K\}, \tag{1}$$

where Γ is an n by n diagonal matrix of spatially varying weights $\gamma_1, \ldots, \gamma_n$, controlling the trade-off between regularization and image similarity. We note the larger the value for γ_a, the more regularization is applied at pixel a. We must solve (1) for every $k \in \{1, \ldots, K\}$, but denoting $U = [\mathbf{u}_1, \ldots, \mathbf{u}_K]$ and $P = [\mathbf{p}_1, \ldots, \mathbf{p}_K]$, n by K matrices, we can combine the K problems into one linear system of equations, which we solve for U to get the RWIR probabilistic transformation:

$$(L + \Gamma^{-1})U = \Gamma^{-1}P. \tag{2}$$

2.2 Anatomical Feasibility for Probabilistic Transformations

TP primarily requires that the Jacobian[1] of T, $J(T)$, is positive everywhere. We adopt the convention that a probabilistic transformation is TP if its *expected transformation*,

---

[1] For brevity, we refer to the Jacobian determinant as simply the Jacobian.

with the expected displacement taken at each pixel, has a positive Jacobian everywhere. Formally, the expected transformation corresponding to a probabilistic transformation U is given by:

$$T^* = \hat{\Omega} + UV^\top . \tag{3}$$

T^* is a discrete transformation, whose a^{th} row corresponds to the location pixel a is mapped to. $J(T)$ is defined in the continuous case as a function of the derivatives of the components of T. So, to discretize the Jacobian, we must choose a discrete approximation of the derivative operators. It has been shown that if all combinations of forward and backward difference operators along the d axis directions, Δ_i^F and Δ_i^B, $i \in \{1, \ldots, d\}$, are used to construct 2^d approximate Jacobians, and if they are all positive everywhere, then the continuous bi- or tri-linear interpolated version of T^* will also have positive Jacobian everywhere [5]. We thus define the discrete Jacobian at pixel a, $J_a(T)$, to be the minimum of the 2^d approximate Jacobians.

We note that while TP is often a necessary condition for anatomical feasibility, it is not always sufficient: transformations exhibiting excessive stretching may be anatomically infeasible. These conditions can be identified by pixels with very large or small (but still positive) Jacobians.

Our goal in the following sections is to choose spatially adaptive weights $\gamma_1, \ldots, \gamma_n$ in such a way that U, calculated from (2), corresponds to an anatomically feasible expected transformation T^* with respect to its Jacobian values.

2.3 Efficient Jacobian Calculation

In this section, we introduce a technique for calculating the Jacobian of the expected transformation $J(T^*)$ *without* needing to calculate the probabilistic transformation U. This technique is orders of magnitude faster than the calculation of U via (2), allowing regularization to be increased where needed, *prior* to running the RWIR algorithm.

In order to calculate $J(T^*)$, where $T^* = [\mathbf{t}_1^*, \ldots, \mathbf{t}_d^*]$, we must calculate $\Delta_i \mathbf{t}_j^*$ for $i, j \in \{1, \ldots, d\}$, where $\Delta_i \in \{\Delta_i^F, \Delta_i^B\}$. Combining (2) and (3) gives

$$\Delta_i \mathbf{t}_j^* = \Delta_i \left(\hat{\Omega} \mathbf{e}_j + \left(L + \Gamma^{-1}\right)^{-1} \Gamma^{-1} PV^\top \mathbf{e}_j \right) , \tag{4}$$

where $\mathbf{e}_j$ is the jth standard basis vector for $\mathbb{R}^d$. We define $\mathbf{b}_j = \Gamma^{-1} PV^\top \mathbf{e}_j$ and $\mathbf{x}_j = \left(L + \Gamma^{-1}\right)^{-1} \mathbf{b}_j$, and note that $\mathbf{x}_j$ can be calculated without performing an expensive matrix inversion by solving the system of equations

$$\left(L + \Gamma^{-1}\right) \mathbf{x}_j = \mathbf{b}_j . \tag{5}$$

We note the similarity between (2) (used to solve for U) and (5). The difference is that in (5), the right hand side has 1 column, whereas in (2) the right hand side has K columns, which is on the order of hundreds or even thousands in 3D registration.

Solving for $\mathbf{x}_j$ allows us to rewrite (4) as:

$$\Delta_i \mathbf{t}_j^* = \Delta_i \hat{\Omega} \mathbf{e}_j + \Delta_i \mathbf{x}_j . \tag{6}$$

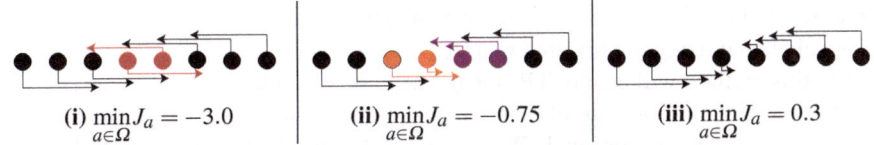

(i) $\min_{a\in\Omega} J_a = -3.0$ **(ii)** $\min_{a\in\Omega} J_a = -0.75$ **(iii)** $\min_{a\in\Omega} J_a = 0.3$

Fig. 1. A 1D example with circles representing pixels, unit distance apart, and arrows representing their displacement vectors. (*i*) The red pixels have crossing displacements and thus a negative Jacobian. (*ii*) After increasing regularization at the red pixels, the orange and purple pairs of pixels now have crossing displacements instead. (*iii*) Increasing the regularization of pixels based on their proximity to the location of the negative Jacobian in (*i*) results in a TP transformation.

Once (6) is solved for each (i, j) pair, we can calculate $J(T^*)$. By repeating this process for each combination of forward and backward operators, we will determine if and where the discrete Jacobian of the expected transformation is negative.

The calculations in this section consist mainly of efficient multiplications between sparse matrices, with the exception being the need to solve (5) for each $j \in \{1, \dots, d\}$; this is the computational bottleneck. Since d is usually only 2 or 3, this bottleneck is still orders of magnitude faster than the full RWIR algorithm. This leads us to the strategy of repeatedly calculating $J(T^*)$ with different settings for Γ until we determine how much regularization is needed at each pixel in order to ensure an anatomically feasible Jacobian, as we detail in the next section.

2.4 Determining Regularization Weights

Using the technique from the previous section, one could increase regularization slightly wherever the Jacobian is negative, recalculate the Jacobians, and iterate. This would ensure TP and avoid over-regularization, but may require many iterations. We reduce the number of iterations by using larger increases in regularization each iteration and preemptively increasing regularization in a neighborhood around pixels with negative Jacobian (as the non-invertibility may be "pushed out" to nearby pixels, see Fig. 1).

To make this concept concrete, we define a function $\phi_1 : \Omega \to \mathbb{R}^+$ evaluating how much additional regularization each pixel needs:

$$\phi_1(a) = \lambda_1 \max_{b\in\Omega} \left(\underbrace{\max(0, -J_b(T^*))}_{\text{Amount of Violation}} - \lambda_2 \underbrace{\|a - b\|_2}_{\text{Proximity}} \right), \tag{7}$$

where λ_1 and λ_2 are positive scalar parameters. Larger values for λ_1 and λ_2 speed convergence, but may result in over-regularization if too large. We found $\lambda_1 = 0.3$ and $\lambda_2 = 5$ provide a good trade-off. We increase the regularization at pixel a by updating the trade-off weight γ_a:

$$\gamma_a \leftarrow \gamma_a \cdot (1 + \phi_1(a)) . \tag{8}$$

The update values for each pixel can be efficiently computed using dynamic programming. With the updated Γ, $J(T^*)$ can be recalculated, and the update (8) performed again until all Jacobian values are positive. A TP probabilistic transformation U can then be calculated using the updated matrix Γ.

While this method will ensure TP, it can easily be extended to enforce other restrictions on the Jacobian. For example, one may want a volume preserving transformation that has Jacobian values close to 1. We can use $J(T^*)$ to identify pixels with Jacobians that are deemed too small or too large, e.g. outside of the range $[\lambda_3, \lambda_4]$, $\lambda_3 < \lambda_4$. We define a second function to capture this idea:

$$\phi_2(a) = \lambda_1 \max_{b \in \Omega} \left(\max\left(0, \underbrace{\lambda_3 - J_b(T^*)}_{J \text{ Too Small}}, \underbrace{J_b(T^*) - \lambda_4}_{J \text{ Too Large}} \right) - \lambda_2 \underbrace{\|a - b\|_2}_{\text{Proximity}} \right). \quad (9)$$

By replacing ϕ_1 with ϕ_2 in (8) we not only regularize away negative Jacobian values, but also Jacobian values that we deem anatomically infeasible. This targeted approach avoids over-regularizing regions that already have feasible transformations, allowing those regions to stay loyal to their prior probabilities.

3   Results

In this section, we perform experiments to demonstrate the benefits of our spatially adaptive regularization scheme. We compare registration results from RWIR with and without our technique for choosing Γ. We also establish the correlation between uncertainty and error in probabilistic transformations, indicating that uncertainty information should not be discarded by post-processing techniques designed for non-probabilistic transformations. We focus on comparisons to RWIR instead of other techniques for ensuring TP since previous MICCAI papers [3,10,7] have shown RWIR to be comparable to other state-of-the-art techniques, and this comparison removes confounding factors.

Our experiments are performed on 40 T1-MR volumetric thigh images of dimension $250 \times 250 \times 40$, each segmented into 16 regions, including 11 different muscles (Fig. 3). This data set was used because it contains regions with rich details leading to accurate priors (e.g. around the bone) and other regions that are largely devoid of detail (e.g. the homogeneous thigh muscles), so we expect well chosen spatially adaptive regularization weights to be important for accurate registration. f_{sim} is defined as the negative exponential of the sum of squared intensity differences in a patch of size $5 \times 5 \times 5$. We used unoptimized MATLAB code run on a machine with 2 Quad Core Intel Xeon 2.33 GHz CPUs.

3.1   Synthetic Warpings

We applied known warps to each image and attempted to recover these warps using RWIR. We generated 5 warps for each image by randomly displacing B-spline control points, spaced 30 mm apart, where the displacements were sampled uniformly from vectors up to 8 mm in magnitude.

For each of the 200 image/warp pairs, we compare the results of RWIR run using 3 different matrices Γ. First, we use a spatially constant $\Gamma = cI$, where I is the identity

Table 1. The results of running RWIR with different regularization matrices. RWIR-TP achieves less error than the other registrations while also ensuring topology preservation, while only requiring marginally longer computation time.

	TRE (mm)	% of Pixels with $J \leq 0$	Run Time (sec)
Priors P	2.83 ± 0.18	16.6 ± 1.0	–
RWIR-C	2.56 ± 0.24	1.67 ± 0.54	4957 ± 533
RWIR-U	1.70 ± 0.19	0.36 ± 0.11	5056 ± 561
RWIR-TP	1.64 ± 0.19	0.0 ± 0.0	5657 ± 577

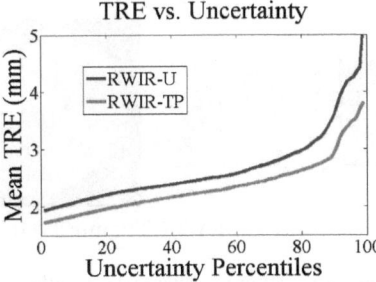

Fig. 2. Mean TRE for different uncertainty percentiles. The mean TRE of the top $k\%$ most uncertain pixels was calculated, for $k = \{1, \dots, 99\}$. The mean TRE consistently increases across percentiles, indicating uncertainty could be used to identify errors in a registration. Particularly, we see a sharp increase in TRE for the top 10% most uncertain pixels.

matrix and c is a scalar. We refer to the results of this registration as RWIR-C. Second, we use uncertainty information from the prior probabilities P to construct Γ (based on an idea presented in previous works [10]):

$$\gamma_a = c \cdot \exp\left(\frac{-H(\mathbf{p}^a)}{H_{max}}\right) \, , \quad H(\mathbf{p}^a) = \sum_{k=1}^{K} \sum_{\ell=1}^{K} p_k^a p_\ell^a \|\mathbf{v}_k - \mathbf{v}_\ell\|^2 \, , \quad (10)$$

where H is a measure of uncertainty found to correlate well with registration error [6], and H_{max} is the maximum possible value for H. Using (10) results in stronger regularization for pixels with uncertain prior probabilities. We refer to the results of this registration as RWIR-U. Third, we use (8) with ϕ_2 to iteratively update Γ, initialized using (10) and iterating 10 times, which was found to be sufficient to ensure TP. We refer to the results of this registration as RWIR-TP. In both RWIR-C and RWIR-U, c was empirically set to minimize target registration error (TRE). The Jacobian is restricted to the range $[0.5, 1.5]$, chosen based on the minimum and maximum Jacobian values of a random synthetic warping, constructed as stated above.

A comparison of the results achieved by the 3 registrations is shown in Table 1. The regularization used in RWIR-TP ensures a positive Jacobian, while only requiring about 10% longer to run. Further, RWIR-TP achieves less error than RWIR techniques.

To demonstrate the benefits of a probabilistic registration, for each test we calculated uncertainty values for each pixel by applying H from (10) to the displacement probabilities generated by RWIR-U and RWIR-TP. We found a Pearson correlation coefficient between the uncertainty and the TRE of 0.45 for RWIR-U and 0.50. Fig. 2 demonstrates the relationship between uncertainty and TRE by taking the top $k\%$ most uncertain pixels, for $k = \{1, \dots, 99\}$, and calculating their mean error. We see that error

Table 2. TOs from registering pairs of images, averaged across all regions and tests. RWIR-TP and RWIR-U achieve similar TOs, but RWIR-TP provides TP transformations. Note the target overlap of RWIR-U is slightly higher than RWIR-TP because TO is only an approximate measure of accuracy - an erroneous displacement (e.g. one causing negative Jacobian) may still map a voxel to the correct label.

	Original	Priors P	RWIR-U	RWIR-TP
Target Overlap (TO)	0.632 ± 0.108	0.762 ± 0.134	0.841 ± 0.071	0.833 ± 0.062
% of Pixels with $J \leq 0$	–	38.2 ± 8.10	3.37 ± 0.88	0.0 ± 0.0

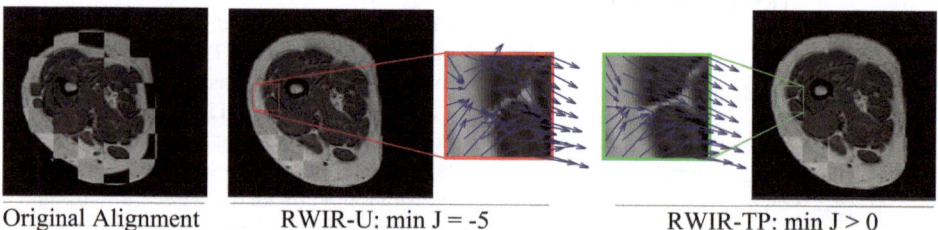

Original Alignment   RWIR-U: min J = -5   RWIR-TP: min J > 0

Fig. 3. An example on real data demonstrating how our technique increases regularization locally where necessary without over-regularizing other areas. While the registration results are unchanged in most areas, RWIR-TP smooths out certain problem areas in the RWIR-U registration.

steadily increases for more uncertain pixels, and that the top 10% most uncertain pixels have significantly more error than an average pixel. Using post-processing techniques to ensure topological invertibility would discard these uncertainty values.

3.2   Real Data

In this section, we demonstrate the usefulness of our method in a real medical imaging application by taking each pair of thigh images and registering them to each other, using both RWIR-U and RWIR-TP with the same bounds on the Jacobian as in Sec. 3.1. We evaluate registration results using the target overlap, the number of correctly mapped foreground pixels divided by the total number of foreground pixels. We evaluate anatomical feasibility by looking at the number of pixels with negative Jacobian.

The results of this experiment are summarized in Table 2, and an example slice of the registered 3D images is seen in Fig. 3. We see that while the transformations resulting from RWIR-U and RWIR-TP have very similar target overlaps, the RWIR-U transformations have 3.37 ± 0.88% of pixels with negative Jacobian on average, and thus are not anatomically feasible transformations, whereas none of the RWIR-TP transformations have negative Jacobians, and thus represent anatomically feasible alignments (again, with only about 10% increased run time).

4 Conclusion

Properly selecting regularization parameters is often key to accurate registration, yet in general can be very difficult without expensive trial and error approaches, involving a registration being performed multiple times and the results examined. Our method efficiently adjusts spatially adaptive regularization in order to provide explicit guarantees regarding topology preservation without over-regularizing regions with accurate prior probabilities. For future work, we will more rigorously examine how the values of λ_1 and λ_2 affect the speed and accuracy of the registration for different applications.

References

1. Arsigny, V., Commowick, O., Pennec, X., Ayache, N.: A log-Euclidean framework for statistics on diffeomorphisms. In: Larsen, R., Nielsen, M., Sporring, J. (eds.) MICCAI 2006, Part I. LNCS, vol. 4190, pp. 924–931. Springer, Heidelberg (2006)
2. Boykov, Y., Veksler, O., Zabih, R.: Fast approximate energy minimization via graph cuts. IEEE TPAMI 23(11), 1222–1239 (2001)
3. Cobzas, D., Sen, A.: Random walks for deformable image registration. In: Fichtinger, G., Martel, A., Peters, T. (eds.) MICCAI 2011, Part II. LNCS, vol. 6892, pp. 557–565. Springer, Heidelberg (2011)
4. Glocker, B., Komodakis, N., Tziritas, G., Navab, N., Paragios, N.: Dense image registration through MRFs and efficient linear programming. MedIA 12(6), 731–741 (2008)
5. Karaçalı, B., Davatzikos, C.: Topology preservation and regularity in estimated deformation fields. In: Taylor, C.J., Noble, J.A. (eds.) IPMI 2003. LNCS, vol. 2732, pp. 426–437. Springer, Heidelberg (2003)
6. Lotfi, T., Tang, L., Andrews, S., Hamarneh, G.: Improving probabilistic image registration via reinforcement learning and uncertainty evaluation. In: Wu, G., Zhang, D., Shen, D., Yan, P., Suzuki, K., Wang, F. (eds.) MLMI 2013. LNCS, vol. 8184, pp. 187–194. Springer, Heidelberg (2013)
7. Popuri, K., Cobzas, D., Jägersand, M.: A variational formulation for discrete registration. In: Mori, K., Sakuma, I., Sato, Y., Barillot, C., Navab, N. (eds.) MICCAI 2013, Part III. LNCS, vol. 8151, pp. 187–194. Springer, Heidelberg (2013)
8. Risholm, P., Pieper, S., Samset, E., Wells III, W.M.: Summarizing and visualizing uncertainty in non-rigid registration. In: Jiang, T., Navab, N., Pluim, J.P.W., Viergever, M.A. (eds.) MICCAI 2010, Part II. LNCS, vol. 6362, pp. 554–561. Springer, Heidelberg (2010)
9. Rohlfing, T., Maurer Jr., C.R., Bluemke, D.A., Jacobs, M.A.: Volume-preserving nonrigid registration of MR breast images using free-form deformation with an incompressibility constraint. IEEE TMI 22(6), 730–741 (2003)
10. Tang, L., Hamarneh, G.: Random walks with efficient search and contextually adapted image similarity for deformable registration. In: Mori, K., Sakuma, I., Sato, Y., Barillot, C., Navab, N. (eds.) MICCAI 2013, Part II. LNCS, vol. 8150, pp. 43–50. Springer, Heidelberg (2013)
11. Tang, L., Hamarneh, G., Abugharbieh, R.: Reliability-driven, spatially-adaptive regularization for deformable registration. In: Fischer, B., Dawant, B.M., Lorenz, C. (eds.) WBIR 2010. LNCS, vol. 6204, pp. 173–185. Springer, Heidelberg (2010)
12. Tang, T., Chung, A.: Non-rigid image registration using graph-cuts. In: Ayache, N., Ourselin, S., Maeder, A. (eds.) MICCAI 2007, Part I. LNCS, vol. 4791, pp. 916–924. Springer, Heidelberg (2007)

DR-BUDDI: Diffeomorphic Registration for Blip Up-Down Diffusion Imaging

M. Okan Irfanoglu[1,2], Pooja Modi[1], Amritha Nayak[1,2], Andrew Knutsen[1,2], Joelle Sarlls[1], and Carlo Pierpaoli[1]

[1] National Institutes of Health, Bethesda, MD, USA
[2] Center of Neuroregenerative Medicine, Bethesda, MD, USA

Abstract. In this work we propose a novel method to correct echo planar imaging (EPI) distortions in diffusion MRI data acquired with reversed phase encoding directions ("blip-up blip-down" acquisitions). The transformation model is symmetric, diffeomorphic and capable of capturing large deformations. It can take advantage of a structural MRI target and include the contribution of diffusion weighted images, in addition to EPI images acquired without diffusion sensitization. The proposed correction significantly outperform existing strategies, assuring anatomically accurate characterization of the orientation, mean diffusivity, and anisotropy of white matter structures in the human brain.

1 Introduction

Susceptibility and concomitant field distortions in echo planar images (EPI) have been shown to affect diffusion MRI tractography findings [7]. Correction methods have typically involved B_0 field maps [8] or anatomical image targets [12]. The corrections achieved with these methods, however, are suboptimal in areas of large field inhomogeneities, with associated large distortions and large signal pile-ups or expansions. More recently, a methodology which involves the acquisition of the same EPI image twice with reversed phase-encoding gradient originally proposed by [5,4] has been revisited, due to its potential ability to better handle regions of severely piled-up or expanded signals. The original implementation of this method employed the *"line-integral"* principle, which stated that the cumulative signal along a phase encoding line between corresponding points in the up and down image should be equal and that these points should be equidistant to the true anatomical location. The original correction method suffered from numerical instabilities and non-smooth deformation fields because of its $1D$ nature. Andersson et al. proposed a different strategy [1], which aimed to estimate the B_0 map from up and down images together in an image restoration framework. This method, has been released as the *"topup"* tool within the popular FSL package. Elastic or diffemorphic registration based approaches have also been proposed [6,10].

Tools that utilize blip up - blip down acquisitions generally show the potential for superior performance compared to methods using only a single phase encoding direction. However, in many applications to real clinical data, the correction can still be unsatisfactory. This is likely due to inconsistencies between the real data and the underlying physical model, which assumes a stable B_0 field regardless of subject motion, magnetic

P. Golland et al. (Eds.): MICCAI 2014, Part I, LNCS 8673, pp. 218–226, 2014.

drift or heating. Additional artifacts not accounted for, such as Gibbs ringing, ghosts, gradient non-linearities, phase cancellations and the effects of hitting the noise floor, further complicates the problem. In this work, our aim is to propose a robust correction framework for blip-up blip-down acquisitions that suffer less from these limitations.

2 Methodology

The main distinctive properties of the proposed registration framework include:

- *Deformations*: The transformation model is symmetric, diffeomorphic and capable of capturing large deformations with its time varying velocity based model [2].
- *Two deformations*: Instead of one deformation field (and its inverse), we employ two co-dependent deformation fields, which are still almost inverses of each other but with enough flexibility to account for differences in B_0 field between blip up and down acquisitions.
- *Structural image information*: Constraining the flow of the velocity fields composing the deformation fields to pass through a distortion-free structural image at the middle time point is hypothesized to significantly improve registration accuracy.
- *Diffusion image information*: In typical blip-up blip-down correction frameworks, regions homogeneous in $b = 0$ images tend to be freely deformable with insufficient spatial constraints. With other methods, we observed that even with near-perfect alignment between the $b = 0 \ s/mm^2$ images and the structural image, DTI-derived directionally encoded color (DEC) maps sometimes reveal anatomically inaccurate corrections. Therefore, the proposed method also employs information extracted form blip up blip down diffusion weighted images to improve anatomical accuracy.
- *Anisotropic deformation regularization*: A new form of deformation regularization is employed to prevent bleeding of small structures into others. Instead of using traditional Gaussian or B-Splines kernels, this method employs a PDE based regularization that results in locally anisotropic smoothing of the deformation fields.

An illustration of the complete correction pipeline is presented in Figure 1. This manuscript will focus on the "DR-BUDDI correction" phase of this pipeline.

2.1 Blip-Up Blip Down Correction

The symmetric registration idea employed in this work originates from the SyN algorithm of Avants used in the popular ANTS registration toolkit [2,3]. The original SyN optimization function formulation aims to register the fixed (I_{up}) and moving image (I_{down}) onto a middle image at $t = 0.5$ as: (without the regularization term)

$$\xi_0 = \int_\Omega CC(\bar{I}_{up}(\phi_1(\mathbf{x}, 0.5)), \bar{I}_{down}(\phi_2(\mathbf{x}, 0.5)), \mathbf{x})d\Omega \tag{1}$$

where Ω signifies the image domain, CC is the cross-correlation metric, $\bar{I}_{up}$ is the mean subtracted version of I_{up}, $\phi_1(\mathbf{x}, t)$ the displacement field that maps the up image to down and $\phi_2(\mathbf{x}, t)$ the field mapping the down image to up. Even though theoretically ϕ_1 and ϕ_2 should be of equal norm, the middle images $\bar{I}_{up}(\phi_1(\mathbf{x}, 0.5))$ and $\bar{I}_{down}(\phi_2(\mathbf{x}, 0.5)$ can lie anywhere on the hyperplane between the original images and do not necessarily have to be the distortion-free images, which is a single point on this hyperplane.

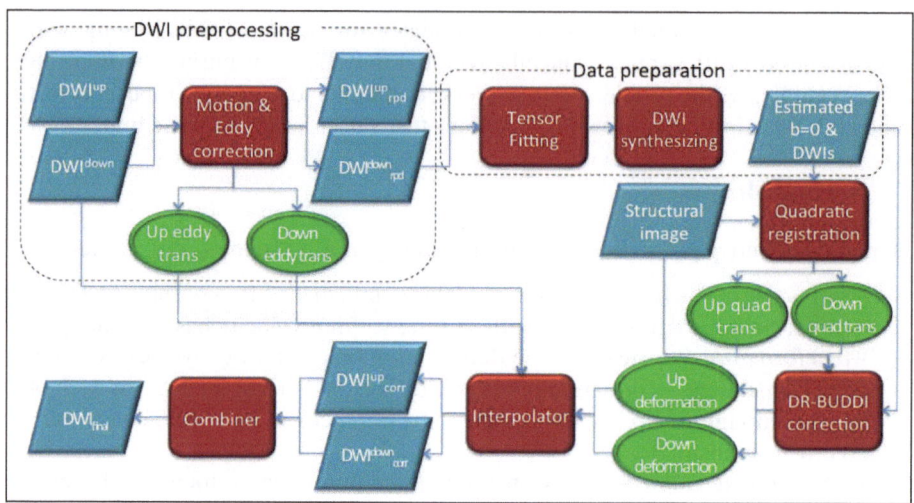

Fig. 1. DWIs are first corrected for motion&eddy currents distortions, then a quick tensor fitting is performed to computed the estimated $b = 0$ images and synthetic DWIs. Quadratic registration is performed with the $b =$ and the structural images to estimate the concomitant fields. Subsequently, the blip up-down correction is performed. All transformations are combined to yield the distortion-free up and down data, which are later combined to produce the final "signal corrected" dataset.

2.2 Metric 1 - Incorporating Geometrical Structural Information

To constrain the flow of displacement velocity fields, the middle images are constrained to pass through a distortion-free structural image $\mathscr{S}$ at the middle time point as:

$$\xi_1 = \int_\Omega \left(CC \left(\overline{I}_{up} \left(\phi_1 \left(\mathbf{x}, 0.5 \right) \right), \mathscr{S} \right) + CC \left(\mathscr{S}, \overline{I}_{down} \left(\phi_2 \left(\mathbf{x}, 0.5 \right) \right) \right) \right) d\Omega \qquad (2)$$

This metric encourages the similarity between the structural image and the middle images. Note that it is different from registering the two images to the structural because the displacement fields ϕ_1 and ϕ_2 are of the same norm and can be inter-related (Section 2.4). Therefore, this formulation enforces the up image to go through the structural image at $t = 0.5$ during registration. Displacements can be computed as decribed in [2]:

$$\frac{\partial \xi_1}{\partial \phi_1} (\mathbf{x}) = \frac{2 < I'_{up}, \mathscr{S} >}{< I'_{up}, I'_{up} >< \mathscr{S}, \mathscr{S} >} \times \left(\overline{\mathscr{S}} - \frac{< I'_{up}, \mathscr{S} >}{< I'_{up}, I'_{up} >} \overline{I'_{up}} \right) | \mathscr{J} (\phi_1) | \nabla \overline{I'}_{up} \qquad (3)$$

where I'_{up} is $\overline{I}_{up}(\phi_1(\mathbf{x}, 0.5))$ and $< A, B > = \sum_x (A(x) - \mu_A)(B(x) - \mu_B)$. This metric is suitable for calculating geometric displacements but it does not take into account the signal redistribution that should accompany the deformation.

2.3 Metric 2 - Addressing Signal Redistribution

As described by Bowtell [4], once a correspondence between the up and down images is established, signal redistribution can be computed with geometric average as:

$$K = 2 \frac{I'_{up} \cdot I'_{down}}{I'_{up} + I'_{down}} \qquad , \qquad \xi_2 = \int_\Omega CC(\overline{K}, \overline{S}, \mathbf{x}) d\Omega \qquad (4)$$

This metric optimizes the similarity between the anatomical and the final signal-redistributed images. Displacements can then be computed with chain-rule as: $\frac{\partial \xi_2}{\partial \phi_1} = \frac{\partial \xi_2}{\partial K} \frac{\partial K}{\partial \phi_1}$.

$$\frac{\partial \xi_2}{\partial K} = \frac{2 < K', \mathscr{S} >}{< K', K' >< \mathscr{S}, \mathscr{S} >} \left(\dot{\mathscr{S}} - \frac{< K', \mathscr{S} >}{< K', K' >} K \right) \tag{5}$$

$$\frac{\partial K}{\partial \phi_1} = 2 \left(\frac{I'_{down}}{I'_{up} + I'_{down}} \right)^2 |\mathscr{I}(\phi_1)| \nabla I'_{up} \quad , \quad \frac{\partial K}{\partial \phi_2} = 2 \left(\frac{I'_{up}}{I'_{up} + I'_{down}} \right)^2 |\mathscr{I}(\phi_2)| \nabla I'_{down} \tag{6}$$

Metric 2 ensures proper signal redistribution only for the combined image K. The correction of the individual images I_{up} and I_{down} may not be optimal. Therefore, in our algorithm we use a (equally) weighted combination of Metric 1 and 2.

2.4 Constraints and Other Properties of the Registration

Phase Encoding Direction ($\vec{pe}$): The gradient formulations of Equations 3 and 5 result in free-deformations, which need to be constrained along $\vec{pe}$ to physically model the system. Let $\mathscr{R}_{up}$ and $\mathscr{R}_{down}$ be the rotational components of the quadratic registration that maps the up and down images to the structural image respectively. Because the diffeomorphic registration is performed on the structural space, $\vec{pe}$ become oblique. For simplicity, let $\vec{pe}$ be the y-axis, then the gradients are projected as:

$$\vec{pe}_{up} = \mathscr{R}_{up}^{\mathbf{T}} \begin{bmatrix} 0 \\ 1 \\ 0 \end{bmatrix} \quad , \quad \{\frac{\partial \xi_i}{\partial \phi_1}\}_{\vec{pe}_{up}} = \left(\frac{\partial \xi_i}{\partial \phi_1} \cdot \vec{pe}_{up} \right) \vec{pe}_{up}$$

Enforcing Deformation Equality: Theoretically, only one deformation field ϕ_1 and its inverse ϕ_1^{-1} would be sufficient to correct the up and down images. Because of the reasons mentioned in Section 2, we found that employing two co-dependent fields ϕ_1 and ϕ_2 with soft-constraints outperforms the former model. Another term is added to the cost function as: $\xi_i^f = \xi_i + \beta \|\phi_1 - \phi_2^{-1}\|$. Then displacements can be rewritten as:

$$\frac{\partial \xi_i}{\partial \phi_1}^f (\mathbf{x}) = \frac{\partial \xi_i}{\partial \phi_1} (\mathbf{x}) + \frac{\beta}{2} \left(\mathscr{R}_{up}^{\mathbf{T}} \mathscr{R}_{down} \left(\frac{\partial \xi_i}{\partial \phi_2} \right)^{-1} (\mathbf{x}) - \frac{\partial \xi_i}{\partial \phi_1} (\mathbf{x}) \right) \tag{7}$$

where β is a continuous user-defined parameter that forces ϕ_1 and ϕ_2^{-1} to be identical when set to one and leave them unconstrained when zero.

2.5 Image Modality for I_{up} and I_{down}

Other methods compute the deformation fields using only non-diffusion weighted $b = 0$ images. Having T_2 contrast, $b = 0$ images are homogeneous in regions such as the brain stem, where different tracts are in close proximity. Using only $b = 0$ images may cause improper distortions of different pathways, sometimes even merging them into a single tract. To address this problem, we perform a vector-image based registration, using synthesized DWIs in addition to the $b = 0$ image. The displacements are computed as a weighted sum over different channels. The number of diffusion weighted images used in registration is a user defined parameter (default=6) with DWIs synthesized with $b = 1000 \, s/mm^2$ and gradients generated from electro-static repulsion algorithm.

2.6 Deformation Regularization

Traditionally, regularization of displacement fields have been achieved with convolution of Gaussian or B-Splines kernels. In this work, we preferred to employ an anisotropic filter to avoid blending of neighboring regions such as the brain stem and the surrounding cerebro-spinal fluid. For this purpose, vector valued image regularization framework proposed by Tschumperlé [11] is employed as: $\partial\phi_1^{xyz}/\partial t = trace(\mathbf{TH}^{xyz})$. The Hessian matrix $\mathbf{H}$ is computed from the x, y and z components of the deformation field ϕ_1 and the structure tensor field $\mathbf{T}$ is computed directly from the vector images I'_{up}. Five smoothing iterations are performed for regularizing the fields.

3 Experiments

High-quality, good spatial resolution data (matrix size=128×128, 2mm isotropic, $SNR >$ 30) with very large distortions were collected from one subject on a GE $3T$ scanner with no parallel imaging. Diffusion scans consisted of 10 $b = 0$ and 60 $b = 1100 \, s/mm^2$ images. The acquisition was repeated for both phase encode directions; Anterior-Posterior (AP) and Right-Left (RL) with both blips, yielding four datasets: AP_p, AP_m, RL_p, RL_m. The assessment of the quality of the correction was based on the assumption that better corrections should lead to higher similarity between tensor quantities computed from corrected AP and RL data. This assesment was performed both by visual inspection of the corrected $b = 0$ images to the structural image and the directionally encoded color (DEC) maps [9] and analysis of difference images of Fractional Anisotropy (FA) maps. Results from two existing methods, topup and Holland method, were also generated. To validate our hypotheses of Section 2, we also performed tests to show the contributions of using a structural image, using DWIs v.s. using just the $b = 0$ image and using only a single deformation field.

4 Results

Figure 2 displays the distorted up and down $b = 0$ images at two slice levels.

The corrected images with the proposed and existing methods for the first slice level can be found in Figure 3. The proposed algorithm produces very sharp tissue interfaces, an anatomically accurate shape and very similar AP_{corr} and RL_{corr} compared to the other methods. The Holland method does not converge because the phase encode direction of the AP and PA were not collinear in this dataset due to subject motion. The agreement between the FA maps of the corrected AP and RL data is high with the proposed method (Figure 4.a).

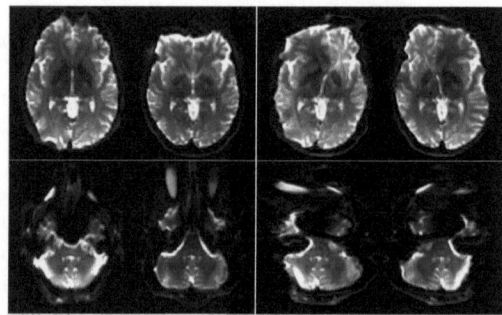

a) Up&down images from AP data b)Up&down images from RL data

Fig. 2. The original distorted blip up and blip down images for two slice levels, for both the AP and RL data. The distortions in this dataset are very large.

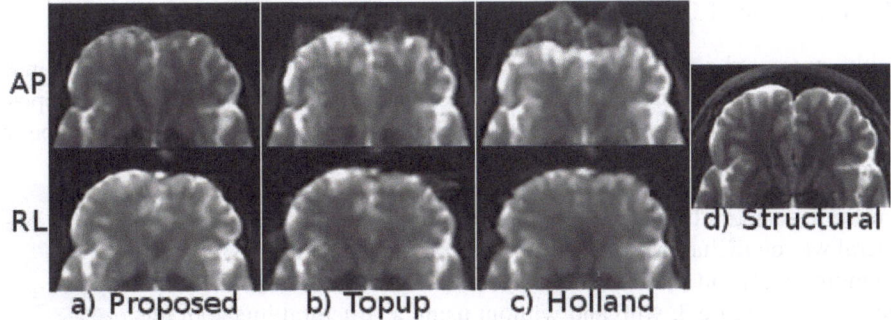

Fig. 3. Corrected b=0 images for a) proposed , b) Topup and c) Holland methods along with the structural image (d), with AP_{corr} (top) and RL_{corr} (bottom), for the first slice level

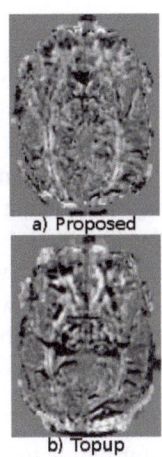

No structures are present in the AP_{corr}–RL_{corr} difference maps whereas the *topup* method shows misalignement especially around the genu of the Corpus Callosum and internal capsule (Figure 4.b). The median of the absolute value of all brain voxels in the difference image was significantly lower for DR-BUDDI compared to "topup" ($p \simeq 0$ with non-parametric Wilcoxon test).

Figure 5 displays the corrections for the brain stem level. At this level, CSF surrounding the brain stem bleeds into the white matter with all methods with varying degrees. Figure 6 displays the enlarged RL_{corr} DEC maps of this region. With the proposed method, CST and inferior cerebellar peduncles are clearly distinct and show high anisotropy, whereas with the topup method, the two lateral CST bundles are split into three with an artifactual bundle created at the mid-sagittal line. The transverse pontine fibers also bleed into CSF. With Holland's method, the two CST bundles are instead merged into one.

Fig. 4. FA differences

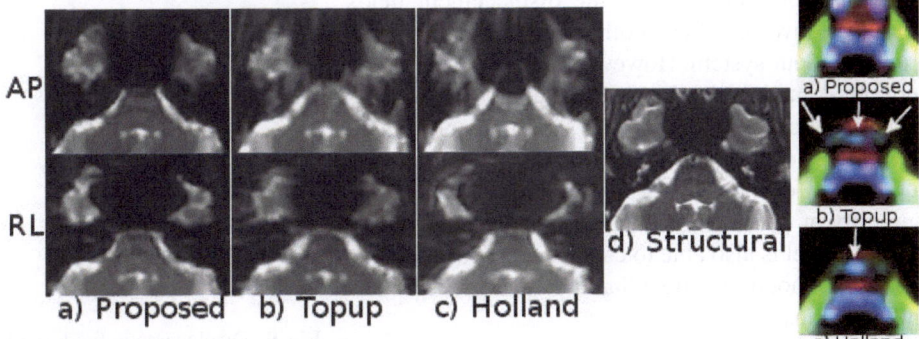

Fig. 5. Corrected images for a) proposed , b) Topup and c) Holland methods along with the structural image for the second slice level

Fig. 6. DEC maps

4.1   Validation of Distinctive Properties

Results presented so far indicates that the proposed method performs better than existing techniques. In this section, we will focus on specific properties of the proposed method and analyze their independent contributions to the overall DR-BUDDI pipeline.

Effect of Using the Structural Image: We analyzed the contribution of using a structural image to guide the flow of the velocity fields. In general we found that the use of the structural image makes the registration more robust and anatomically correct. In Figure 7 we show the same brain used in Figure 3, with and without using a structural image in the registration. The correction obtained without using the structural image shows imperfect correction in the frontal areas.

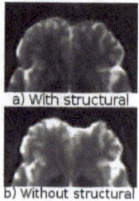

Fig. 7. Structural effect

Effect of Using DWIs: Figure 8 displays the effect of using DWIs with the $b = 0$ image for correction. The Pons is homogeneous in T_2W and using only the $b = 0$ may not contain enough information for a correct registration of pathways within the Pons. In fact, Figure 8.b shows that the Trans-

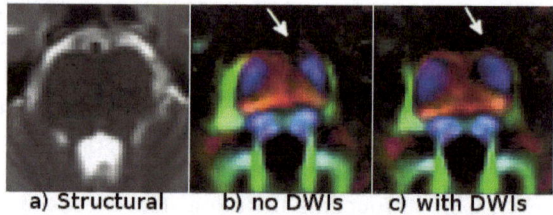

Fig. 8. Effects of using DWIs for correction

verse pontine fibers in the ventral aspect of the Pons (arrows) appear broken. Including DWIs within a vector-image registration framework solves this issue (Figure 8.c).

Effect of Two Deformations: The effect of using two deformation fields v.s. one was tested by setting β to 1 in Equation 7. Figure 9 displays the displacement fields obtained, at the first slice level, with one and two deformation models. The initial observation is that even with the two deformation model, the displacement fields are almost inverses of each other, which is an implicit property of our system. However, there are differences between ϕ_1 and ϕ also between ϕ_2 and ϕ^{-1}. Two deformation model is able to model a larger displacement with ϕ_1 in the orbito-frontal regions, whereas this was not needed for the moving image as indicated by the similarity of ϕ_2 and ϕ^{-1} in this region. The two deformation model is also able to capture more local details due to the smoothing effect that the other model inherently contains.

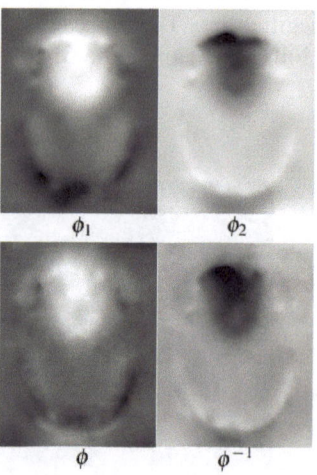

Fig. 9. Displacement fields with two deformation model (top row) and single deformation model (bottom row)

5   Conclusions

In this work, we proposed a novel blip-up blip-down correction method for diffusion MRI. Our method is based on a symmetric, diffeomorphic registration framework, robust at dealing with common issues such as Gibbs ringing, ghosts and motion artifacts. One of our main observations is that it is not sufficient to quality assess only the $b = 0$ s/mm^2 images for diffusion MRI as the DEC maps could reveal spurious, anatomically incorrect features that are not apparent on the former. Therefore, we decided that it was of fundamental importance to make use of DWIs for correction. Using DWIs improved correction quality throughout the white matter but the effects were more pronounced in the brain stem. All the other factors such as the use of a structural MRI, anisotropic regularization and the deformation model also contributed significantly to the overall performance. Future work involves the acquisition of phantom data and creation of simulated models to systematically analyze the limitations of the assumptions underlying blip up/down strategies, such as hitting the noise floor in high q regimes, and phase cancellations in k-space, which invalidate the mass preservation principle.

References

1. Andersson, J.L., Skare, S., Ashburner, J.: How to correct susceptibility distortions in spin-echo echo-planar images: application to diffusion tensor imaging. NeuroImage 20(2), 870–888 (2003)
2. Avants, B., Epstein, C., Grossman, M., Gee, J.: Symmetric diffeomorphic image registration with cross-correlation: Evaluating automated labeling of elderly and neurodegenerative brain. Medical Image Analysis 12(1), 26–41 (2008)
3. Avants, B., Tustison, N.J., Song, G., Cook, P.A., Klein, A., Gee, J.C.: A reproducible evaluation of ANTs similarity metric performance in brain image registration. NeuroImage 54(3), 2033–2044 (2011)
4. Bowtell, R.W., McIntyre, D.J.O., Commandre, M.J., Glover, P.M., Mansfield, P.: Correction of geometric distortion in echo planar images. In: Proceedings of 2nd Annual Meeting of the SMR, San Francisco, p. 411 (1994)
5. Chang, H., Fitzpatrick, J.M.: A technique for accurate magnetic resonance imaging in the presence of field inhomogeneities. IEEE TMI 11(3), 319–329 (1992)
6. Holland, D., Kuperman, J.M., Dale, A.M.: Efficient correction of inhomogeneous static magnetic field-induced distortion in echo planar imaging. Neuroimage 50, 175–183 (2010)
7. Irfanoglu, M.O., Walker, L., Sarlls, J., Marenco, S., Pierpaoli, C.: Effects of image distortions originating from susceptibility variations and concomitant fields on diffusion MRI tractography results. Neuroimage 15(61), 275–288 (2012)
8. Jezzard, P., Balban, R.: Correction for geometric distortion in echo planar images from B0 field variations. Magnetic Resonance in Medicine 34, 65–73 (1995)
9. Pajevic, S., Pierpaoli, C.: Color schemes to represent the orientation of anisotropic tissues from diffusion tensor data: application to white matter fiber tract mapping in the human brain 42, 526–540 (1999)
10. Ruthotto, L., Kugel, H., Olesch, J., Fischer, B., Modersitzki, J., Burger, M., Wolters, C.H.: Diffeomorphic susceptibility artifact correction of diffusion-weighted magnetic resonance images. Physics in Medicine and Biology 57(18), 5715 (2012)

11. Tschumperlé, D., Deriche, R.: Vector-valued image regularization with PDEs: A common framework for different applications. IEEE Trans. PAMI 27(4), 506–517 (2005)
12. Wu, M., Chang, L.-C., Walker, L., Lemaitre, H., Barnett, A.S., Marenco, S., Pierpaoli, C.: Comparison of EPI distortion correction methods in diffusion tensor MRI using a novel framework. In: Metaxas, D., Axel, L., Fichtinger, G., Székely, G. (eds.) MICCAI 2008, Part II. LNCS, vol. 5242, pp. 321–329. Springer, Heidelberg (2008)

Spatially-Varying Metric Learning for Diffeomorphic Image Registration: A Variational Framework[*]

François-Xavier Vialard[1] and Laurent Risser[2]

[1] Université Paris Dauphine, CEREMADE (UMR 7534), France
[2] CNRS, Institut de Mathématiques de Toulouse (UMR 5219), France

Abstract. This paper introduces a variational strategy to learn spatially-varying metrics on large groups of images, in the Large Deformation Diffeomorphic Metric Mapping (LDDMM) framework. Spatially-varying metrics we learn not only favor local deformations but also correlated deformations in different image regions and in different directions. In addition, metric parameters can be efficiently estimated using a gradient descent method. We first describe the general strategy and then show how to use it on 3D medical images with reasonable computational ressources. Our method is assessed on the 3D brain images of the LPBA40 dataset. Results are compared with ANTS-SyN and LDDMM with spatially-homogeneous metrics.

1 Introduction

Diffeomorphic image registration often consists in minimizing an objective function which contains a similarity term and a regularization term. In this work, we focus on the regularization term which can be seen as a prior when approximating the biomechanical properties of the registered structures (*e.g.* deformation smoothness, magnitude, ...). In the context of *Large Deformation Diffeomorphic Metric Mapping* (LDDMM) different works have addressed this question. Sum of kernels strategies were proposed in [7,13] to account for multi-scale effects and therefore obtain plausible deformations while still preserving good matchings. Other approaches do not learn the metric but a distribution on initial momenta which defines the optimal deformations between a template and a learning set of images [12]. Such approaches however require to first choose a metric and the momenta distribution or their PCAs strongly depend on this choice.

To overcome these limitations, the Bayesian approach is often the method of choice, allowing to learn parameters distribution [14]. Full Bayesian approaches require the use of stochastic optimization methods which are slow. Sometimes approximations such as variational Bayes are preferred. For small deformations,

[*] This work was supported by the ANR DEMOS grant, the *Chaire Havas-Dauphine Économie des nouvelles données*, and the AO1 grant MALAC3D from Université Paul Sabatier. The authors also thank the reviewers for their constructive and insightful comments.

P. Golland et al. (Eds.): MICCAI 2014, Part I, LNCS 8673, pp. 227–234, 2014.

[1] estimates the covariance matrix of the deformations parametrized by a set of points. The approach has been extended to large deformations in [4] by reducing the metric learning to a set of control points. In a non-diffeomorphic context, variational Bayes methods were also introduced in [11,10] to perform image registration with the automatic tuning of global or spatially-varying regularisation parameters. The motivation of this method is however to be flexible and not to learn optimal metrics on large groups of images, which differs from our goal.

Spatially-varying metrics have recently been introduced in LDDMM by changing the Eulerian point of view on the regularization strategy to a Lagrangian point of view [8]. Although this strategy is appealing, its practical use is limited, as the tuning of a large amount of metric parameters is made manually. To overcome this issue, we propose in this paper a fully variational approach to estimate a kernel matrix M, which parametrizes the regularization term.

We present the variational approach to learn M in section 2. Strategies to reduce the problem dimensionality are developed in section 3. Results are finally given in section 4.

2   Mathematical Model

2.1   LDDMM Registration

Our model is based on the LDDMM framework. Let $(I_n)_{n=1,...,N}$ be a population of N images and T be a given template. Registering the template T onto the image I_n consists in minimizing:

$$\mathcal{J}_{I_n}(v, K) = \frac{1}{2} \int_0^1 \|v(t)\|_V^2 \, dt + E(\phi(1) \cdot T, I_n) \, , \tag{1}$$

where the path $\phi(t)$, $t \in [0,1]$ is encoded by the velocity field $v(t)$, $t \in [0,1]$: $\phi(0) = Id$ and $\partial_t \phi(t) = v(t) \circ \phi(t)$. Importantly, the optimal diffeomorphism depends on a smoothing kernel K which defines the metric V. In LDDMM, K is usually translation and rotation invariant so that the Fourier transform can be used to write the metric as $\|\mathbf{v}_t\|_V^2 = < \mathcal{F}(\mathbf{v}_t)\mathcal{F}(K)^{-1}, \mathcal{F}(\mathbf{v}_t) >_{L^2}$, where $\mathcal{F}(.)$ is the Fourier transform and $< ., . >_{L^2}$ is the L^2 inner product [3]. Following [3], the energy can be minimized using a gradient descent with $\nabla_v E_t = \mathbf{v}_t - K \star P_t$, where $P_t = \text{Det } J_{\phi_{t,1}} \nabla T_t (T_t - I_t)$ is the momentum at time t and $\star$ denotes the convolution operator. Images T_t and I_t are also T and I_n transported at time t by $\phi(t)$: $T_t = \phi(t) \cdot T$ and $I_t = \phi(t) \cdot \phi^{-1}(1) \cdot I_n$.

2.2   Spatially Varying Metrics

A mathematical interpretation of spatially-varying metrics in LDDMM has recently been given by [8], opening the opportunity to design metrics adapted to the different structures contained in the template T. Based on this interpretation, we design a set of kernels expressing spatially-varying metrics. More specifically, we use (symmetric) positive definite matrices M as a parametrization of this set of kernels. In order to ensure smoothness of the deformations, any kernel of this set has to satisfy the constraint that the Hilbert space of vector fields is embedded in the Banach space of C^1 vector fields. To enforce this constraint, we propose the following parametrization,

$$\mathcal{K} = \{\hat{K} M \hat{K} \mid M \text{ SDP operator on } L^2(\mathbb{R}^d, \mathbb{R}^d)\}, \qquad (2)$$

where $\hat{K}$ is a spatially-homogeneous smoothing kernel (typically Gaussian). Instead of using K as in section 2.1, $\mathcal{K}$ smoothes the vector field P_t as follows:

1. P_t is first convoluted with $\hat{K}$: $\Gamma_t = \hat{K} \star P_t$.
2. Matrix M multiplies the values of the 3D vector field Γ_t as follows: We suppose that Γ_t has a size (N_x, N_y, N_z) and denote $\Gamma_t(x_i, y_i, z_i, d_i)$ the value of Γ_t at point (x_i, y_i, z_i) and in direction d_i. Γ_t is first reshaped as a vector, so that $\Gamma_t(x_i, y_i, z_i, d_i)$ is located at the index $\nu_i = x_i + y_i N_x + z_i N_x N_y + d_i N_x N_y N_z$ of the vector. The vector is first multiplied with M and then reshaped as a 3D vector field.
3. The vector field resulting from step 2 is finally convoluted with $\hat{K}$.

By construction $M(\nu_i, \nu_j)$ therefore correlates the velocities of Γ_t at points (x_i, y_i, z_i) and (x_j, y_j, z_j) and in directions d_i and d_j, respectively. Remark that if $M = Id$ and $\hat{K}$ is a Gaussian kernel of standard deviation σ, then $\mathcal{K}$ is a Gaussian kernel of standard deviation $\sqrt{2}\sigma$. If M has non-null and heterogeneous values on its diagonal only, the metric will *favor* the deformations at specific locations and in specific directions. More interestingly, if M contains non-null terms outside of its diagonal, it will *favor* deformations in correlated locations and/or directions. Of course, this correlation can be non-local.

2.3   Learning Optimal Metrics

To shorten the notations, we use $\mathcal{J}_{I_n}(v, M)$ instead of $\mathcal{J}_{I_n}(v, \hat{K} M \hat{K})$. The variational model consists in minimizing the functional, with β a positive real:

$$\mathcal{F}(M) = \frac{\beta}{2} d_{S++}^2(M, Id) + \frac{1}{N} \sum_{n=1}^{N} \min_{v} \mathcal{J}_{I_n}(v, M), \qquad (3)$$

The first term is a regularizer of the kernel parameters so that that the minimization problem is well posed. Here, it favors parametrizations of M close to the identity matrix but other a priori correlation matrix could be used. The term $d_{S++}^2(Id, M)$ can be chosen as the squared distance on the space of positive definite matrices given by $\|\log(M)\|^2$. Here again, other choices of regularizations could have been used such as the log-determinant divergence. We simply remark that this distance comes from a Riemannian metric denoted by g on S^{++} which makes it complete [6,2]: namely we consider S^{++} endowed with the inner product at S given by $tr(S^{-1} dS S^{-1} dS)$ where tr is the standard trace operator. The variational problem would have been ill-posed if the standard L^2

metric (Frobenius norm) had been used. Note that the energy term in $\mathcal{J}_{I_n}$ is linear in M^{-1}. A direct calculation shows that the gradient of $\mathcal{F}$ with respect to the metric g denoted by $\nabla_g \mathcal{F}$ is

$$\nabla_g \mathcal{F}(M) = \beta M \log(M) - \frac{1}{N} \sum_{n=1}^{N} \int_0^1 (M\hat{K} \star P_n(t)) \otimes (M\hat{K} \star P_n(t))dt, \quad (4)$$

where $A \otimes B$ is the tensor product and is defined by $A \otimes B(f) = \langle B, f \rangle_{L^2} A$ for $A, B \in L^2(\mathbb{R}^d, \mathbb{R}^d)$. Momenta $P_n(t)$ are obtained at convergence of the diffeomorphic matching algorithm on $\mathcal{J}_{I_n}(v, M)$. Note that this tensor product is performed in the space of vectorized vector fields defined in step 2 of the algorithm section 2.2. We now develop a brief proof of how Eq. (4) is obtained: The second term is a minimization over v of each term independently and therefore can be rewritten as a function of M: $\sum_{n=1}^{N} \min_v \mathcal{J}_{I_n}(v_n(M), M)$, so that at convergence we have $\partial_1 \mathcal{J}_{I_n}(v_n(M), M) = 0$ for each $n = 1, \ldots, N$, where ∂_1 is the partial derivative w.r.t. v. Thus, $\nabla_{L^2} \mathcal{F}(M)$ equals $\frac{\beta}{2} \nabla_{L^2} d_{S++}^2(M, Id) + \frac{1}{N} \sum_{n=1}^{N} \min_v \partial_M \mathcal{J}_{I_n}(v, M)$. Using the linearity w.r.t. M^{-1} and the chain rule formula, we obtain $\partial_2 \mathcal{J}_{I_n}(v, M) = -\int_0^1 (\hat{K} \star P_n(t)) \otimes (\hat{K} \star P_n(t)) \, dt$. We then derive the Riemannian gradient using the formula $\nabla_g f(S) = S \nabla_{L^2} f(S) S$. The differentiation of the first term is standard on a Riemannian manifold and its gradient is given by the tangent vector of the geodesic between Id and M evaluated at M. Then the geodesic starting at identity and ending at M is given by $t \to e^{t \log(M)}$ (see [6,2]). As a consequence, $\nabla_g \frac{1}{2} d_{S++}^2(M, Id) = M \log(M)$.

After initializing M to identity, the algorithm is a simple gradient descent which iterates: (1) Register T on the images I_n, $n = 1, \ldots, N$ to obtain the momenta $P_n(t)$; (2) Compute the gradient $\nabla_g \mathcal{F}(M)$ using formula (4); (3) Update $M := M - \varepsilon \nabla_g \mathcal{F}(M)$, where ε is the chosen step length.

3   Reducing the Problem Dimension

In this section, we propose two straightforward solutions to make the learning problem of section 2 usable on most computers when treating 3D medical images. Other dimensionality reduction methods could be applied as discussed in section 5. Considering that the registered 3D images have N voxels, matrix M has a size $3N \times 3N$ which may be a huge amount of information to store.

3.1   Diagonal Matrix M

A straightforward solution to reduce the problem's dimension is to constrain M to have diagonal terms only. As explained in section 2, matrix M will only favor deformations in specific locations and directions. The amount of parameters to store and to estimate is however $3N$ instead of $3N \times 3N$, which makes it usable in 3D medical imaging with resonable computational ressources. Moreover, Eq. (4) becomes numerically obvious to compute as the logarithm of $3N$ scalars is computed instead of the logarithm of a $3N \times 3N$ matrix.

3.2   Basis Projection

Another solution, which allows to model long distance and inter-axes correlations, is to project Γ_t on a 3D basis. In this work, we use a 3D B-spline basis, with elements denoted by ψ_l, $l \in \{1, \cdots, L\}$. Each element has its origin at point $p_l = (p_l^x, p_l^y, p_l^z)$ and we suppose the p_l sampled on a spatially homogeneous grid with a larger step size than the image resolution. We also associate the vector $\alpha_l = (\alpha_l^x, \alpha_l^y, \alpha_l^z)$ to element l of the basis. We denote $\hat{\Gamma} = (\alpha_1^x, \cdots, \alpha_L^x, \alpha_1^y, \cdots, \alpha_L^z)$ the vector of size $d = 3L$ which will be used to learn M. A dense vector field v can be constructed from $\hat{\Gamma}$ using:

$$v(p) = \sum_{l=1}^{L} \alpha_l \psi(p - p_l), p \in \Omega \tag{5}$$

Projecting Γ_t on the basis only would induce a loss of information related to deformations at a finer scale than the grid step size. To address this issue, we perform the orthogonal projection of Γ_t on a closed subspace, $\Pi : L^2(\mathbb{R}^d, \mathbb{R}^d) \mapsto W$, to learn parameters only on this subspace:

$$\mathcal{K} = \{\hat{K}M\Pi\hat{K} + \hat{K}(Id - \Pi)\hat{K} \mid M \text{ SDP operator on } L^2(\mathbb{R}^d, \mathbb{R}^d)\}. \tag{6}$$

Let us interpret how Eq. (6) reduces the problem dimensionality. Instead of step 2 in the pseudo-algorithm of section 2.2: (1) We compute $\hat{\Gamma}_t$ ($\hat{\Gamma}$ at time t) by projecting Γ_t on the basis. (2) A vector field Q_1 is constructed using Eq. (5) with $\hat{\Gamma}_t$ and we define the residual vector field $R_t = \Gamma_t - Q_1$. (3) Another vector field Q_2 is constructed using Eq. (5) with $M\hat{\Gamma}_t$, the product of M and $\hat{\Gamma}_t$. (4) The vector field $Q_2 + R_t$ is finally the result of this modified step 2. The interest of this strategy is twofold: Spatially-varying metric can be learnt using the information projected on $\hat{\Gamma}_t$. Residue R_t which is related to deformations at a finer scale than the grid step size also ensures that all information, and not only the one projected on $\hat{\Gamma}_t$, is used to register the images. In addition to these modified steps, the gradient of Eq. (4) is now computed using the projected values of Γ_t and not the values of Γ_t directly.

4   Results

We assessed our method on the 40 subjects of the LONI Probabilistic Brain Atlas (LPBA40) [9]. All 3D images were affinely aligned to subject 5 using ANTS[1] and then resampled to a resolution of 2 mm. We then learnt different matrices M using the strategies of sections 3.1 and 3.2: T was the probability tissue map (TM) of subject 5, the I_n were the TM of subjects 1 to 30 (except 5) and $\hat{K}$ was a Gaussian kernel of width $\sigma = 10$. For the strategy of section 3.2, we used a regular 3D grid sampled with a step size of 20mm. The parameter ε was semi-empirically tuned so that ε equals 0.01 divided by the

---

[1] http://stnava.github.io/ANTs/

Axial	Coronal	Sagittal	Axial	Coronal	Sagittal

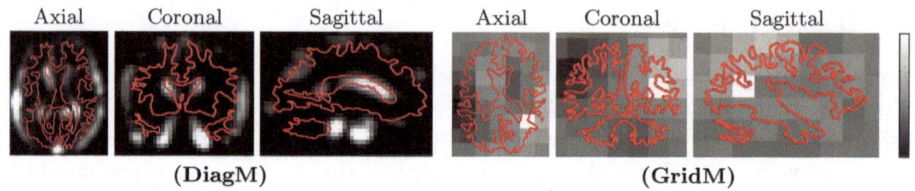

(DiagM)   (GridM)

Fig. 1. Values out of M after the two learning steps of section 4. The values are represented at their corresponding location in the template image T. **(DiagM):** Values $M(j, j)$ for $j \in [1, \cdots, N]$. Color bar ranges from 1 (black) to 1.04 (white). **(GridM):** $M(i, j)$ for a fixed i and $j \in [1, \cdots, L]$. White point corresponds to $i = j$ and has an intensity of 1.03. Color bar ranges from -0.05 (black) to 0.05 (white) for other points. Red curves represent the boundary between white and grey matter in T.

maximum of $\left| \sum_{n=1}^{N} \int_0^1 (M\hat{K} \star P_n(t)) \otimes (M\hat{K} \star P_n(t)) dt \right|$ at the first iteration of the algorithm. Parameter β is also equal to $0.025\hat{\beta}$ divided by the maximum of $|\varepsilon M \log(M)|$ at the second algorithm iteration. We used four values of $\hat{\beta}$ to test different regularization levels of M.

We can see in Fig. 1(DiagM) the location of the deformations favored by the diagonal matrix M learnt with $\hat{\beta} = 1$ on the x-axis. For M learnt on a grid with $\hat{\beta} = 1$, Fig. 1(GridM) also indicates how the motion on the x-axis at point i is empirically correlated with the motion at other locations j on the same axis. Note that this information is computed for all grid nodes and not only i.

We then compared different registration strategies by registering the TM of subject 5 on those of subjects 31 to 40: **(DiagM)** and **(GridM)** LDDMM registration with the kernels learnt using the strategies of sections 3.1 and 3.2, respectively. **(K_{ref})** Same as (DiagM) or (GridM) with M equals identity (nothing learnt). This is equivalent to LDDMM registration using a Gaussian kernel with $\sigma = 10\sqrt{2}$. **(K_σ)** To compare (GridM) with results obtained using stronger spatially-homogeneous regularizations than in (K_{ref}), we also performed LDDMM registration with different values of σ. Finally, to compare our results with state of the art strategies we finally performed ANTS-SyN registration with the regularisation parameters of [5] **(SyN)** and LDDMM registration with the multiscale strategy of [7][2] with σ sampled between 2 and 20mm **(K_{fine})**. After registration, we computed the target overlaps (TO) between the segmented cortical regions (given in LPBA40) to measure the matching quality and the determinant of the Jacobians (DetJ) to quantify the deformation smoothness. We also performed Kruskal-Wallis rank tests, where $p \leq 0.05$ was chosen as significance threshold, to compare different strategies.

As shown Table 1, we obtained more accurate TO using (SyN) and (K_{fine}) than other methods. This is because other methods derive from (K_{ref}) and are then constrained to register the images at a relatively large scale, as shown by the DetJ of Table 1. Note that the relatively large kernel of (K_{ref}) was chosen to

---

[2] http://sourceforge.net/projects/utilzreg/

emphasize the effect of M with the grid of (GridM). Learning M on finer grids would allow to learn multiscale kernels derived from (K_{fine}) for instance. On 3D brain images this would however either require more advanced dimensionality reduction techniques than those of section 3 or a very large amount of memory. Comparing (K_{ref}) with the methods using M shows the effect of our strategy, as (K_{ref}) is strictly equivalent to the other methods if M is identity: Remark first that, in our tests, no significant difference was found between (K_{ref}) and the different (DiagM). We also did not found significant differences between (K_{ref}) and (GridM) close to identity (eg: (GridM1) in Table 1) or (K_σ) with σ close to $10\sqrt{2}$ (eg: (K_{20}) in Table 1). No significant difference is also found between (GridM1) and (K_{20}). Significantly different TO and maximum DetJ to those of (K_{ref}) were found using stronger spatial regularization, e.g. (GridM2) and (K_{30}) in Table 1. Comparing these two strategies leads to our key result: For a similar TO, (GridM2) has significantly lower $DetJ_{Max}$ and $DetJ_{Std}$ than (K_{30}). Remark finally that the average $DetJ_{Std}$ of (K_{30}) is higher than the one of (K_{20}) although the one of (GridM2) is lower than the one of (GridM1). The spatially-varying kernel therefore seems to take advantage of the learnt information with non-local correlations to estimate smoother meaningful deformations.

Table 1.   Average results obtained on the 3D brain images of the LPBA40 dataset

	No Reg	SyN	K_{fine}	K_{ref}	DiagM	GridM1	GridM2	K_{20}	K_{30}
TO	0.665	0.750	0.732	0.712	0.711	0.710	**0.704**	0.710	**0.704**
$DetJ_{Max}$	1	3.17	4.65	1.66	1.66	1.61	**1.41**	1.62	**1.50**
$DetJ_{Min}$	1	0.047	0.46	0.67	0.68	0.70	0.67	0.73	0.66
$DetJ_{Std}$	0	0.17	0.11	0.063	0.062	0.059	**0.049**	0.056	**0.063**

5   Discussion

In this paper, we addressed the problem of regularization in diffeomorphic registration using a new variational approach to learn spatially-varying metrics in the LDDMM setting. We parametrized the space of spatially-varying metrics with positive definite matrices M and used the logarithm norm on this space as a Tychonov regularizer to make the variational problem well posed. We also gave a semi-analytical expression of the minimized energy gradients relative to M, as well as two strategies to keep the problem's dimensionality resonable, making our learning strategy doable on standard computers. Note that the proposed method has a natural *maximum a posteriori* interpretation and thus, Bayesian methods could be developed in coherence with this variational model. We obtained encouraging results showing that the spatially-varying metrics we learnt allowed to register 3D brain images with smoother deformations than by using a spatially-homogeneous metric, for similar structure overlaps.

Future work will focus on dimensionality reduction methods to learn M. Our goal is to learn multiscale smoothing kernels, making our strategy more pertinent on large 3D medical images. An exciting perspective of this work would also be the statistical analysis of the spatially-varying metric parameters defined here.

References

1. Allassonnière, S., Amit, Y., Trouvé, A.: Towards a coherent statistical framework for dense deformable template estimation. J. R. Statist. Soc. B 69(1), 3–29 (2007)
2. Arsigny, V., Fillard, P., Pennec, X., Ayache, N.: Geometric means in a novel vector space structure on symmetric positive-definite matrices. SIAM Journal on Matrix Analysis and Applications 29(1), 328–347 (2007)
3. Beg, M.F., Miller, M.I., Trouvé, A., Younes, L.: Computing large deformation metric mappings via geodesic flows of diffeomorphisms. IJCV 61(2), 139–157 (2005)
4. Durrleman, S., Allassonnière, S., Joshi, S.: Sparse adaptive parameterization of variability in image ensembles. IJCV 101(1), 161–183 (2013)
5. Klein, A., Ghosh, S.S., Avants, B.B., Yeo, B.T.T., Fischl, B., Ardekani, B.A., Gee, J.C., Mann, J.J., Parsey, R.V.: Evaluation of volume-based and surface-based brain image registration methods. NeuroImage 51(1), 214–220 (2010)
6. Moakher, M., Zerai, M.: The Riemannian Geometry of the Space of Positive-Definite Matrices and Its Application to the Regularization of Positive-Definite Matrix-Valued Data. JMIV 40(2), 171–187 (2011)
7. Risser, L., Vialard, F.X., Wolz, R., Murgasova, M., Holm, D.D., Rueckert, D.: Simultaneous Multi-scale Registration Using Large Deformation Diffeomorphic Metric Mapping. IEEE Transactions on Medical Imaging 30(10), 1746–1759 (2011)
8. Schmah, T., Risser, L., Vialard, F.X.: Left-invariant metrics for diffeomorphic image registration with spatially-varying regularisation. In: Mori, K., Sakuma, I., Sato, Y., Barillot, C., Navab, N. (eds.) MICCAI 2013, Part I. LNCS, vol. 8149, pp. 203–210. Springer, Heidelberg (2013)
9. Shattuck, D.W., Mirza, M., Adisetiyo, V., Hojatkashani, C., Salamon, G., Narr, K.L., Poldrack, R.A., Bilder, R.M., Toga, A.W.: Construction of a 3D probabilistic atlas of human cortical structures. NeuroImage 39, 1064–1080 (2008)
10. Simpson, I., Schnabel, J., Groves, A., Andersson, J., Woolrich, M.: Probabilistic inference of regularisation in non-rigid registration. NeuroImage 59(3) (2012)
11. Simpson, I.J.A., Woolrich, M.W., Cardoso, M.J., Cash, D.M., Modat, M., Schnabel, J.A., Ourselin, S.: A bayesian approach for spatially adaptive regularisation in non-rigid registration. In: Mori, K., Sakuma, I., Sato, Y., Barillot, C., Navab, N. (eds.) MICCAI 2013, Part II. LNCS, vol. 8150, pp. 10–18. Springer, Heidelberg (2013)
12. Singh, N., Fletcher, P.T., Preston, J.S., King, R.D., Marron, J., Weiner, M.W., Joshi, S.: Quantifying anatomical shape variations in neurological disorders. Medical Image Analysis (2014)
13. Sommer, S., Lauze, F., Nielsen, M., Pennec, X.: Kernel bundle EPDiff: Evolution equations for multi-scale diffeomorphic image registration. In: Bruckstein, A.M., ter Haar Romeny, B.M., Bronstein, A.M., Bronstein, M.M. (eds.) SSVM 2011. LNCS, vol. 6667, pp. 677–688. Springer, Heidelberg (2012)
14. Zhang, M., Singh, N., Fletcher, P.T.: Bayesian estimation of regularization and atlas building in diffeomorphic image registration. In: Gee, J.C., Joshi, S., Pohl, K.M., Wells, W.M., Zöllei, L. (eds.) IPMI 2013. LNCS, vol. 7917, pp. 37–48. Springer, Heidelberg (2013)

Sparse Bayesian Registration

Loïc Le Folgoc[1], Hervé Delingette[1], Antonio Criminisi[2], and Nicholas Ayache[1]

[1] Asclepios Research Project, INRIA Sophia Antipolis, France
[2] Machine Learning and Perception Group, Microsoft Research Cambridge, UK

Abstract. We propose a Sparse Bayesian framework for non-rigid registration. Our principled approach is flexible, in that it efficiently finds an optimal, sparse model to represent deformations among any preset, widely overcomplete range of basis functions. It addresses open challenges in state-of-the-art registration, such as the automatic joint estimate of model parameters (*e.g.* noise and regularization levels). We demonstrate the feasibility and performance of our approach on cine MR, tagged MR and 3D US cardiac images, and show state-of-the-art results on benchmark datasets evaluating accuracy of motion and strain.

1 Introduction

Non-rigid image registration is the ill-posed task of inferring a deformation u from a pair of observed (albeit typically noisy), related images I and J. Classical approaches propose to minimize a functional which weighs an image similarity criterion $\mathcal{D}$ against a regularizing (penalty) term $\mathcal{R}$:

$$\arg\min_{u} \mathcal{E}(u) = \mathcal{D}(I, J, u) + \lambda \cdot \mathcal{R}(u) \tag{1}$$

Prior knowledge to precisely model the space of plausible deformations or the regularizing energy is generally unavailable. Adequate choices thus result from a compromise between computational efficiency, numerical stability of the optimization schemes and extent of the spanned space. Furthermore, the optimal regularizing trade-off λ is unknown. Cross-validation presupposes availability of either a set of ground-truth transforms or a criterion to measure the 'goodness' of a transform. Even then, high variability in images of the same modality can render the use of any single value of λ unsuitable. In the end, user expertise acquired via lengthy trial-and-error processes often remains necessary to improve the quality of registration.

Recent advances pave the way to go beyond this state of things. Bayesian formulations of registration allow to infer from the data ([1]) or to integrate over ([2,3]) such parameters as the regularization penalty λ. Such probabilistic frameworks additionally let us derive uncertainty estimates over the solution, which may prove instrumental in improving the accuracy and robustness of downstream medical imaging applications. These methods remain computationally intensive, and typically achieve tractability *via* a sound use of theoretical or numerical approximations; they also introduce a number of additional user-defined hyperparameters. On a different note, sparsity-inducing priors provide a venue for the use of rich, over-complete representations of deformations,

P. Golland et al. (Eds.): MICCAI 2014, Part I, LNCS 8673, pp. 235–242, 2014.

at little added computational cost, while preserving the stability of solvers. L_1 regularizers were recently proposed in the context of registration [4]; as a drawback, they so far render both the joint estimation of model parameters and the uncertainty estimation impractical.

In this paper, we further build on the tools from the Sparse Bayes and Automatic Relevance Determination fields so that we retain the computational and numerical advantages of sparse formulations, while jointly estimating the most adequate deformation model and its parameters thanks to a probabilistic setting. As a result, the need for manual interaction and expertise is reduced. Our contributions are as follows:

1. We extend a state-of-the-art tool for sparse regression [5,6] in scope, so that it may now handle multivalued outputs and generic quadratic priors.
2. We develop a registration framework that makes use of sparse regression to jointly select the most appropriate deformation model and estimate its parameters.
3. We demonstrate our approach by tracking the cardiac motion on cine MR, tagged MR and $3D$-US images.

2   Registration Setting

At a high-level, our approach casts the registration process into two easier sub-tasks: the search for (voxel) pairwise correspondences, followed by the estimate of a smooth displacement *via* the tools of statistical regression. This can be interpreted as minimizing the quadratic approximation of (1) w.r.t. the displacement field u, near a local minimum of the similarity term.

This two-step process is in turn embedded in a multi-resolution pyramidal scheme: each resolution level runs on a smoothed, subsampled version of the images at the previous level.

2.1   Data-Matching Strategy

The similarity energy $\mathcal{D}(I, J, u)$ relates a fixed image I and a moving image J warped according to some candidate displacement field u. Defining an image as a set of intensity measurements regularly sampled at points x_i, $1 \leq i \leq N$, and taking the quadratic approximation of $\mathcal{D}(I, J, u)$ around one of its local minima yields:

$$\arg\min_{u} \sum_{1 \leq i \leq N} (\bar{u}_i - u(x_i))^\mathsf{T} \mathbf{H}_i (\bar{u}_i - u(x_i)) + \lambda \cdot \mathcal{R}(u) \qquad (2)$$

$$\text{s.t.} \quad \partial_u \mathcal{D}(I, J, u)\big|_{\bar{u}} = 0.$$

$\bar{u}$ is a local minimizer of $\mathcal{D}(I, J, u)$ and $\bar{u}_i \triangleq \bar{u}(x_i)$. $\mathbf{H}_i$ is the Hessian of $\mathcal{D}(I, J, u_i)$ evaluated at $\bar{u}$. In this paper, we use the sum of squared differences (SSD) as a similarity energy and thus approximate $\mathbf{H}_i$ with the structure tensor at $y_i = x_i + \bar{u}_i$, that is to say $\mathbf{H}_i = \sum_{p \in \mathcal{W}} \nabla I(y_i+p) \nabla I(y_i+p)^\mathsf{T}$. To compute the local estimate of displacement $\bar{u}$, we adopt a block matching strategy where the optimization is done using the L-BFGS-B algorithm independently for each voxel, which is highly parallelizable. The structure matrix $\mathbf{H}_i$ captures local structures such as boundaries and edges. $n^\mathsf{T} \mathbf{H}_i n$ relates to our confidence in $\bar{u}_i$ along the direction n. These 'weights' $\mathbf{H}_i$ naturally account for the inhomogeneous spread of informative features in the image.

2.2   Representation of Displacements

For this work, we constrain the displacement field $u(x)$ to be expressed over a dictionary of radial basis functions $\{\phi_k, 1 \leq k \leq M\}$, specifically Gaussian kernels $\phi_k(x) = K_{S_k}(x_k, x)\,\mathbf{I}$, of varying variance S_k and centered at a given voxel x_k:

$$u(x) = \sum_{1 \leq k \leq M} \phi_k(x)\boldsymbol{w}_k \tag{3}$$

The kernel width S_k spans a user-predefined set of values, which allows for a redundant, multiscale representation. Therefore we benefit both from a compact representation *via* larger kernels, and from the ability to capture finer local details *via* smaller kernels.

2.3   Regularization Framework

While any quadratic energy $\mathcal{R}(u)$ suits our framework, we specifically consider those that exploit the R.K.H.S. structure of the space $\mathcal{H}$ spanned by Gaussian kernels of width $S \leq \min_k \{S_k\}$; namely $\mathcal{R}(u) = \|Du\|_{\mathcal{H}}^2$, with Du a(ny) differential operator acting on u. Indeed, mathematical bridges between the theory of translation invariant kernels and that of Fourier analysis allow us to derive *analytic* expressions for quantities of the form

$$(D\phi_k | D\phi_l)_{\mathcal{H}} = \int_{\xi} \widehat{D\phi_k}(\xi)^* \widehat{D\phi_l}(\xi)\, \widehat{K}_S^{-1}(\xi) d\xi. \tag{4}$$

The properties of Gaussian kernels under Fourier transform, multiplication (by Gaussian kernels) and summation reduce (4) to an analytic expression evaluated *via* basic calculus operations and exponentiation. In other words, our framework comes with a computationally efficient, analytic implementation of *e.g.* a thin-plate energy ($D = \nabla$), a bending energy ($D = \nabla^2$) or a 'compressibility' penalty ($D = \mathrm{div}$).

3   Sparse Bayes Regression

Solving (2) w.r.t. u constitutes a canonical regression problem: from a finite set of noisy observations $\bar{u}_i$ at points x_i (with confidence $\beta \mathbf{H}_i$), and further assuming a prior over u proportional to $\exp -\lambda \mathcal{R}(u)$, find an optimal reconstruction of the complete signal u. To introduce sparsity in such a formulation, we resort to a mechanism first suggested in the seminal work [5,6]. We hereby present the few core ideas of our algorithm, whereas additional details are left to the electronic appendix. Consider the effect of adding a penalty term $\boldsymbol{w}^\mathsf{T}\mathbf{A}\boldsymbol{w} \triangleq \sum_k \boldsymbol{w}_k^\mathsf{T}\mathbf{A}_k\boldsymbol{w}_k$ on the magnitude of the $\boldsymbol{w}_k$'s in Eq. (2). The problem remains quadratic with additional diagonal weights:

$$\underset{\boldsymbol{w}}{\arg\min}\, (\bar{u} - \Phi\boldsymbol{w})^\mathsf{T} \beta\mathbf{H}\,(\bar{u} - \Phi\boldsymbol{w}) + \boldsymbol{w}^\mathsf{T}\,(\lambda\mathbf{R} + \mathbf{A})\,\boldsymbol{w} \tag{5}$$

where we resorted to block notations: $\boldsymbol{w}$ and $\bar{u}$ are respectively the concatenation of the $\boldsymbol{w}_k$ and $\bar{u}_i$, $\Phi_{ik} \triangleq \phi_k(x_i)$, $\mathbf{H} \triangleq \mathrm{diag}(\mathbf{H}_i)$ and $\mathbf{A} \triangleq \mathrm{diag}(\mathbf{A}_k)$. The minimizer of (5) is given by $\mu = \Sigma\Phi^\mathsf{T}\beta\mathbf{H}\bar{u}$, with $\Sigma = (\Phi^\mathsf{T}\beta\mathbf{H}\Phi + \lambda\mathbf{R} + \mathbf{A})^{-1}$. In fact μ coincides with the expectation of the posterior distribution of w conditionally to the model $\mathbf{A}, \beta, \lambda, \mathbf{R}$, and Σ with its covariance.

Sparsity will ultimately stem from the fact that if a penalty $\mathbf{A}_k$ becomes 'infinite', the corresponding coefficients in w and Σ will in turn be null, effectively pruning the corresponding basis from the solution. Automatic selection of the optimal basis penalties $\mathbf{A}_k$ and of the model parameters β, λ can be achieved either by maximizing the evidence $l(\mathbf{A}) \triangleq \log p(\bar{u}|\mathbf{A}, \beta, \lambda)$; or *via* an Expectation-Maximization (EM) scheme, by maximizing $\mathbb{E}_{w \sim \mathcal{N}(\mu, \Sigma)}[\log p(\bar{u}, w|\mathbf{A}, \beta, \lambda)]$. Tipping proposed an efficient *evidence*-based procedure to estimate the $\mathbf{A}_k$'s for his Relevance Vector Machine [6], in the case of *scalar* regression with $\lambda = 0$, which we extend to the fully general setting.

3.1 Automatic Determination of A_k

We maximize the evidence $l(\mathbf{A}) = \int_w p(\bar{u}|w, \beta)p(w|\mathbf{A}, \lambda)dw$. The distribution of $\bar{u}$ conditionally to the model is a zero-mean Gaussian with covariance $\mathbf{C}$ given by (6). The evidence thus reduces to the sum of two antagonistic terms, $-1/2\{\log|\mathbf{C}| + \bar{u}^{\mathsf{T}}\mathbf{C}^{-1}\bar{u}\}$, that respectively induce complexity control (sparsity) and data fidelity.

$$\mathbf{C} = (\beta\mathbf{H})^{-1} + \Phi(\mathbf{A} + \lambda\mathbf{R})^{-1}\Phi^{\mathsf{T}} \tag{6}$$

The process of setting the $\mathbf{A}_k$'s can be seen as fitting a covariance model $\mathbf{C}$ to the data $\bar{u}$: since part of the data is explained 'for free' by the contribution $(\beta\mathbf{H})^{-1}$ of the noise to $\mathbf{C}$, only a few degrees of freedom need be active and sparsity is achieved.

3.2 A Fast Greedy Iterative Scheme

The procedure relies on efficient updates *via* rank-one matrix identities to iteratively build a solution starting with no base (all $\mathbf{A}_k$'s set to ∞): at each iteration, we take a single action among the addition of a previously inactive basis, or the update or deletion of an active one. The contribution of a given basis to the evidence can be singled out in the form of Eq. (7). We leave the maximization of $l(\mathbf{A}_k)$ to the technical appendix.

$$l(\mathbf{A}_k) = \log|\mathbf{A}_k + \kappa_k| - \log|\mathbf{A}_k + \kappa_k + s_k| + q_k^{\mathsf{T}}\{\mathbf{A}_k + \kappa_k + s_k\}^{-1}q_k \tag{7}$$

The action that leads to the largest gain in evidence is implemented, and the current estimate of the solution $w^* = \mu$ is in turn updated. The evidence therefore increases monotonically: convergence towards a local minimum is guaranteed, and monitored *via* the gain in evidence. The asymptotic complexity of the algorithm is of the same order as the specific case of the regular RVM [6] ($\lambda = 0$).

3.3 Automatic Determination of the Model Parameters

We jointly estimate the model parameters *via* an EM algorithm. For the regularizing trade-off λ, this leads to the maximization problem (8), which involves a single SVD of $\mathbf{A}^{-1/2}\mathbf{R}\mathbf{A}^{-1/2}$ followed by a Newton optimization in log-scale.

$$\lambda^* = \arg\max_{\lambda} -\frac{\lambda}{2}\mathrm{tr}(\Sigma\mathbf{R}) + \frac{1}{2}\log|\mathbf{A} + \lambda\mathbf{R}| - \frac{\lambda}{2}\mu^{\mathsf{T}}\mathbf{R}\mu \tag{8}$$

For the estimation of the noise level β^{-1} in the context of registration, we follow Simpson *et al* [1] in introducing a virtual decimation factor α that accounts for the local covariance in image measurements. We thus estimate both the virtual decimation and the noise level (9) from the residual image, once per resolution level in the pyramid.

$$N \cdot \beta^{*-1} = \|I - J \circ (\mathrm{Id} + \mathrm{u})^{-1}\|^2 + \mathrm{tr}(\Sigma \Phi^\intercal \mathbf{H} \Phi) \tag{9}$$

4   Experimental Results

For all of our experiments, the multiscale representation consists of three levels of progressively finer, isotropic Gaussian kernels, of respective variance $S_1 = 18^2$ mm^2, $S_2 = 9^2$ mm^2 and $S_3 = 4^2$ mm^2. The pyramidal scheme starts with only the coarsest bases at the coarsest pyramid level; a finer basis type is added for each subsequent pyramid level. Therefore at the finest level in the pyramid, all scales S_k are available and jointly optimized upon. Gaussian basis centers coincide with the voxel centers. Furthermore, we use the compressibility penalty as a regularizer (section 2.3) for the 3DTAG dataset, and a bending energy for the other modalities. Note also that our registration scheme does not make use of pre-segmentations of regions of interest, that can be challenging or otherwise impractical to obtain.

4.1   Synthetic 3D Ultrasound Cardiac Dataset

We first demonstrate our approach on synthetic 3D US data from the STACOM 2012 registration challenge [7]. The datasets consist of 4 B-mode image sequences generated from the same mechanical simulation at varying signal-to-noise ratios (SNRs). A dense ground truth, in terms of motion and strain, is available from the simulated meshes.

Fig. 1b evidences a slight tendency to underestimate the radial strain that is consistent with the level of accuracy reported in Fig. 1a. Of note for this dataset is that part of the mesh of interest falls outside of the image domain (around 1.5cm beyond); yet our regularization strategy ensures that the visible portion of the motion drives the part of the mesh left-out: this typically yields a maximum error of 6mm and a median error

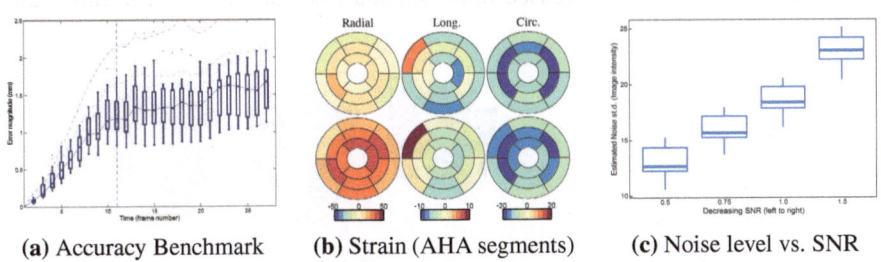

(a) Accuracy Benchmark   (b) Strain (AHA segments)   (c) Noise level vs. SNR

Fig. 1. (Left) Accuracy over time for decreasing SNRs, from blue to cyan, green and red. (Middle) Strain at End-Systole averaged over AHA segments: estimated (top) and ground truth (bottom). (Right) Boxplots of the estimated noise level per SNR dataset.

of 2.5mm for this unseen region. Fig. 1c reveals a consistent increase in the (automati-cally) estimated noise level as the signal-to-noise ratio worsens. Lastly, we believe that the impact of temporal and spatial speckle patterns with regard to the Block Match-ing procedure would be worth investigating thoroughly, so as to improve the quality of voxel-wise correspondences in 3D US imaging prior to the regularization.

4.2   Tagged Magnetic-Resonance Imaging Benchmark

Next we validate our approach on real data from the STACOM 2011 registration chal-lenge [8], consisting of 3D+T tagged MR sequences. Ground-truth is available in the form of 2 sets of 12 landmarks manually followed over time (by 2 observers), equally distributed on the 4 walls at 3 ventricular levels. The median accuracy at End-Systole (ES) was benchmarked for state-of-art contestants. Fig.2a summarizes challengers' re-sults along with ours; our approach achieves best on this benchmark.

The Block Matching strategy appears to adequately capture the texture of the tags and provides good voxel-wise correpondences. As evidenced in Fig.2b, the regression step in turn estimates an appropriate regularity level, which results in smooth deforma-tions and strain maps: longitudinal, circonferential and radial strain values are consistent with the literature and reveal a thickening of the myocardium along the radial orienta-tion, and contraction in other directions. Note that strain values are simply computed from the analytical expression of the transform (Eq. (3)) without resorting to finite dif-ferences approximations.

4.3   Cardiac Cine Magnetic-Resonance Imaging Dataset

The STACOM 2011 challenge [8] additionally provides cine MR (3D+T) cardiac volun-teer data, along with End-Diastole (ED) segmentations of the Left Ventricle. For every volunteer, the motion is tracked over the cardiac cycle and resulting mesh deformations and volume curves are reported in Fig. 3. Cine MR cardiac sequences typically include basal slices, with visible outflow tracts and apparent topology changes which make the estimation of a regular motion difficult. To cope with this challenge, we allow the noise level β^{-1} to vary spatially along the long-axis, and derive independent estimates per slice according to Eq. (9). Fig 3a shows that our algorithm properly captures this speci-ficity of basal slices via an increased noise standard deviation, which in turns allows

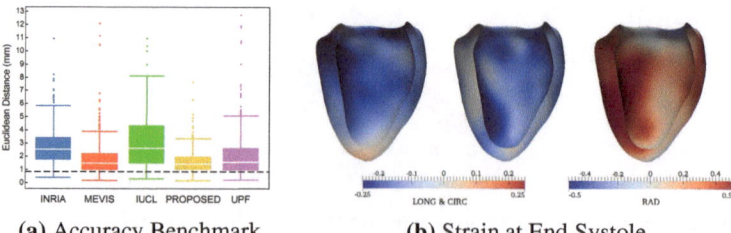

(a) Accuracy Benchmark   (b) Strain at End Systole

Fig. 2. (Left) Box-plots of tracking errors. Doted black line represents average inter-observer variability. (Right) Strain computed from the 3DTAG data of volunteer V9.

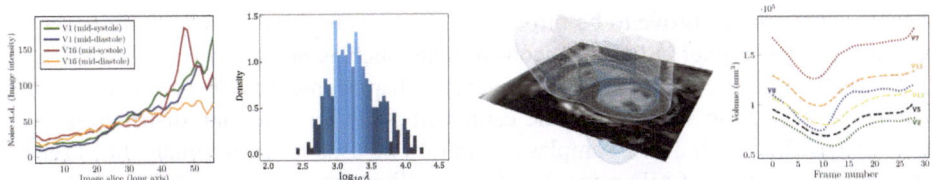

Fig. 3. (From Left to Right) Spatial and inter-image variability of the noise level estimate. Variability in the estimated regularization, illustrated as a density plot over all the datasets. Example 2D slice at ES, obtained by propagating the reference segmentation from ED *via* the registration output. Example volume curves for volunteers.

to preserve the smoothness of the estimated displacement without affecting the overall accuracy of the tracking. Moreover, Fig 3a and Fig. 3b attest to the high variability of the optimal model parameters β^{-1} and λ, both within an image sequence or between different volunteer datasets, which otherwise render their manual estimation via a trial-and-error approach cumbersome.

4.4 Uncertainty Estimates

Our regression framework provides us not only with a pointwise estimate of the displacement field, parameterized by the weights $w^* = \mu$, but also a covariance matrix Σ interpretable in terms of uncertainty over w. What is more, such information can be translated into a spatially meaningful estimate of variance in the registration.

Fig 4 (Right) displays such variance estimates in the form of a tensor map, where each single tensor fully captures directional information about the uncertainty at a given point in space. The color scheme encodes the orientation of the second eigenvector of the tensor. Indeed, the first principal direction of uncertainty is, to an overwhelming majority over the image, oriented approximately along the long-axis. This observation is in agreement with the drastically lower resolution of cine MR sequences in this direction. The direction of lowest uncertainty roughly coincides with the gradient of intensity, as

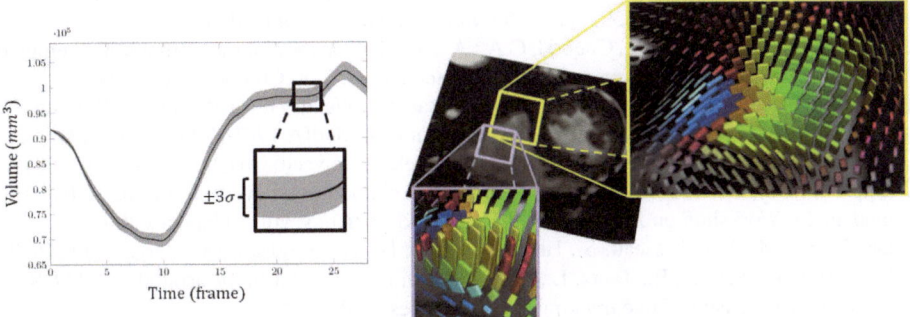

Fig. 4. (Left) LV volume with its associated confidence interval, estimated on the cine-MR data of volunteer V9. (Right) Spatial uncertainty visualized as a tensor map, with higher uncertainty in homogeneous regions and along contour lines.

edges and boundaries prove to be informative features to drive the registration. Lastly the uncertainty is higher in homogeneous regions, such as blood cavities.

Alternatively, for complete 3D+T sequences, displacement fields can be efficiently sampled at each time step t from the estimated posterior Gaussian distribution over $w_t \sim \mathcal{N}(\mu_t, \Sigma_t)$; such 3D+T samples can in turn be used to approximate the variance on integral quantities of relevance. Fig 4 (Left) illustrates such processing on the LV volume over the cycle. Note that while segmentation errors and mesh misalignment obviously accounts for a significant part of the uncertainty, our confidence bars only reflect uncertainty in the registration itself. Finally, all of our uncertainty estimates preserve the spatial covariance in the signal, unlike previous work [1] where concerns for computational tractability forced the approximation of Σ as a diagonal matrix.

5   Conclusion

We proposed a framework for registration that allows for the automatic determination of the relevant deformation model and of its hyperparameters, and demonstrated its performance on cardiac images of various modalities. Our work relies on statistical regression tools from the Sparse Bayes field, and extends them to handle multivalued output and any (quadratic) regularizing energy. As a generic machine learning tool, this work opens up many interesting perspectives for regression and classification problems. As a registration framework, its flexibility alleviates the need for manual supervision and makes the motion tracking process easier. As an added benefit, we have access to quantities that are directly interpretable in terms of uncertainty in the output.

Acknowledgments. This work was partly funded by the ERC Grant MedYMA.

References

1. Simpson, I.J., Schnabel, J.A., Groves, A.R., Andersson, J.L., Woolrich, M.W.: Probabilistic inference of regularisation in non-rigid registration. NeuroImage 59(3), 2438–2451 (2012)
2. Janoos, F., Risholm, P., Wells III, W.: Bayesian characterization of uncertainty in multi-modal image registration. In: Dawant, B.M., Christensen, G.E., Fitzpatrick, J.M., Rueckert, D. (eds.) WBIR 2012. LNCS, vol. 7359, pp. 50–59. Springer, Heidelberg (2012)
3. Richard, F.J., Samson, A.M., Cuénod, C.A.: A SAEM algorithm for the estimation of template and deformation parameters in medical image sequences. Stat. Comput. 19(4) (2009)
4. Shi, W., Jantsch, M., Aljabar, P., Pizarro, L., Bai, W., Wang, H., O'Regan, D., Zhuang, X., Rueckert, D.: Temporal sparse free-form deformations. MedIA 17(7), 779–789 (2013)
5. Tipping, M.E.: Sparse bayesian learning and the relevance vector machine. JMLR 1 (2001)
6. Tipping, M.E., Faul, A.C., et al.: Fast marginal likelihood maximisation for sparse bayesian models. In: Workshop on Artificial Intelligence and Statistics, vol. 1 (January 2003)
7. De Craene, M., Marchesseau, S., Heyde, B., Gao, H., Alessandrini, M., Bernard, O., Piella, G., Porras, A., Saloux, E., Tautz, L., et al.: 3d strain assessment in ultrasound (STRAUS): A synthetic comparison of five tracking methodologies. TMI (2013)
8. Tobon-Gomez, C., De Craene, M., McLeod, K., Tautz, L., Shi, W., Hennemuth, A., Prakosa, A., Wang, H., Carr-White, G., Kapetanakis, S., et al.: Benchmarking framework for myocardial tracking and deformation algorithms: An open access database. MedIA (2013)

Histology to μCT Data Matching Using Landmarks and a Density Biased RANSAC

Natalia Chicherova[1,2], Ketut Fundana[1], Bert Müller[2], and Philippe C. Cattin[1]

[1] Medical Image Analysis Center, University of Basel, Basel, Switzerland
[2] Biomaterials Science Center, University of Basel, Basel, Switzerland
natalia.chicherova@unibas.ch

Abstract. The fusion of information from different medical imaging techniques plays an important role in data analysis. Despite the many proposed registration algorithms the problem of registering 2D histological images to 3D CT or MR imaging data is still largely unsolved.

In this paper we propose a computationally efficient automatic approach to match 2D histological images to 3D micro Computed Tomography data. The landmark-based approach in combination with a density-driven RANSAC plane-fitting allows efficient localization of the histology images in the 3D data within less than four minutes (single-threaded MATLAB code) with an average accuracy of 0.25 mm for correct and 2.21 mm for mismatched slices. The approach managed to successfully localize 75% of the histology images in our database. The proposed algorithm is an important step towards solving the problem of registering 2D histology sections to 3D data fully automatically.

1 Introduction

Image registration is the art of automatically aligning or warping medical imaging data. Registered data allows a more in depth analysis of the probed tissues as different modalities often represent different physical properties important to better understand and interpret the data at hand. Many approaches have been proposed in the last decades for 2D-to-2D and 3D-to-3D registration of the same or even different modalities [11]. However, registering 2D histological images to 3D data is a largely unexplored problem.

The need for reasonable 2D histology to 3D data registration becomes more and more important with the availability of affordable micro Computed Tomography (μCT) devices with high spatial resolution and tissue contrast. Combining the functional information from histology with the structural imaging data of the μCT provides better insights in identifying anatomical features of hard and soft tissues.

Only few papers are insofar directly related to the research at hand as they describe the registration of histological sections to CT and MR data. Seise *et al.* [9] proposed an interactive registration of histological sections to CT in the context of radiofrequency ablation. However, this approach highly relied on manual intervention in the registration step as well as in segmentation. Sarve *et al.* [8]

P. Golland et al. (Eds.): MICCAI 2014, Part I, LNCS 8673, pp. 243–250, 2014.

registered histological images of bone implants with synchrotron radiation-based
μCT data. Their algorithm was based on segmentation of the implant by thresholding, which is not possible in our datasets, as the implant material is hardly
visible and highly assimilated in the jaw bone. Other approaches deal with the
registration of histological sections with soft tissue such as in the prostate [7] or
the human brain [6] where MRI is more useful than CT. An additional factor is
that the acquired μCT or μMR imaging data is generally of large size, amount-
ing up to several hundred megabytes of data. However, only very little research
has been devoted to efficiently register these type of datasets [5].

Using images of histological cross sections poses additional challenges to the
already ill-posed problem of image registration. First, the histology images are
susceptible to uneven lighting (vignetting artifact) and different contrasts from
staining. Second, the histological sections may suffer from severe non-rigid deformations originating from the cutting process. Moreover, the histological images
generally show different contrasts as compared to the μCT or μMR data that
must be handled appropriately. Lastly, the potentially non-uniform background
of the histological cuts may lead to erroneous results in the registration process.

In this paper we propose a novel approach for automatic registration of 2D
histological cross sections to 3D μCT scans. This fully automatic feature-based
registration approach makes use of the scale- and rotation-invariant feature detector SURF[2] and a modified density-driven RANSAC[3] plane-fitting. The
main advantage of our method is that it can detect corresponding slices under
different angulation that often appears in histological sectioning experiments.
Furthermore, the computation time of our algorithm is notably shorter than of
manual registration. The latter is estimated at 8 hours per slice. Finally, it does
not require insertion of any additional landmarks hence can be readily applied
to numerous biological data, where auxiliary inclusions are impossible.

2   Method

An illustration of the algorithmic pipeline is depicted in the Fig. 1. First, we
determine corresponding feature points between the histological image and each
image in the μCT volumetric data and extract their associated coordinates.
Then, based on these coordinates, we build a 3D point cloud, where the third
dimension corresponds to the slice number in the μCT data. As the distribution
of the matched points is higher in the plane that corresponds best to a given
histological slice (see Fig. 1(middle)) the remaining step reduces to a robust
plane fitting in a noisy point cloud.

2.1   Data Acquisition

The sample data used for this work [10] originates from a jaw bone volume
augmentation after tooth extraction study. In total ten clinical patients were
included in this study. Biopsies of the jaw bones were taken from 4 to 11 months
after implantation. The inner diameter of the specimen tubes was around 3 mm

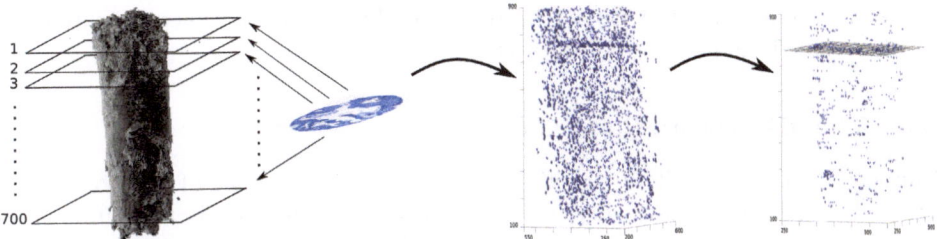

Fig. 1. Pipeline of the algorithm: (left) Feature matching of μCT data and histological image, (middle) 3D point cloud of matched points, (right) optimized RANSAC plane fitting

and the length was around 12 mm. The μCT of the whole specimen was acquired. Then five to nine histological cross-sections through the horizontal plane of the specimen were taken. Each histological slice (thickness 300 μm) resulted in an RGB image of size 2592 $\times$ 1944 pixels. The μCT data were 8 bit gray-scale 3D matrices with a range of data size 764 $\times$ 764 $\times$ (416 $\div$ 1939) pixels, where the vertical axis corresponds to the third dimension. The corresponding resolution along vertical axis differed from 0.03 mm to 0.006 mm per slice.

2.2 Feature Detection and Matching

Let $I(x, y)$ and $V(x, y, z)$ denote the histological image and the μCT data volume accordingly, where z is associated with a slice number in the μCT dataset. Hence, $I : \Omega_I \subset R^2 \to R$ and $V : \Omega_V \subset R^3 \to R$. The rigid registration problem between these two modalities can be formulated as finding coefficients of the plane section in the μCT space that corresponds best to the histological image. In a first step we match each of the histological images to all axial μCT slices using a landmark-based approach. As a feature detection algorithm we rely on the scale- and rotation-invariant feature detector and descriptor SURF [2]. The choice of this detector is based on performed comparative analysis with SIFT[4]. We have found that SURF was more accurate and computationally efficient for our application. For a Matlab implementation of the SURF algorithm we used the opensource code by D. Kroon of Sep 2010[1], saving the default parameters. The number of octaves was set to 5, threshold to 0.0002. The main principal of this detector is based on scale-space extrema detection and stable feature localization. Applying the feature detector to an image, *e.g.* histological image I, we obtain a small subset of distinctive feature points $P(x, y) \subset I$. The descriptor vectors are then used for matching the feature points between the μCT and histological images. As the matching algorithm, we use the second-nearest-neighbor-criteria [4,1] that calculates the Euclidean distance between the descriptor vectors. A match is only accepted when the smallest Euclidean distance is less than 0.8

---

[1] http://www.mathworks.ch/matlabcentral/fileexchange/
  28300-opensurf--including-image-warp-

times the second smallest Euclidean distance. This process is then repeated for all the axial slices in the μCT dataset.

2.3   The 3D Feature Point Cloud

Suppose that the result of the above matching step is a set of feature points $P_z \subset V_z$ with coordinates (x_i, y_i), where $i = 1...\kappa_j$ and κ_j is the number of found matching feature points in a slice z. Having matched features for each of the N slices in the μCT volume will subsequently allow us to plot them as a point cloud, *i.e.* the 3D set of the keypoints $C = \{(x_{ij}, y_{ij}, z_j)\}$ $(j = 1...N)$ with the third dimension z representing the slice number in the μCT data, see Fig. 1(middle). Here, the total number of feature points for the whole μCT data is determined as $M = \sum_{j=1}^{N} \kappa_j$.

As one would expect, the resulting point cloud shows an increased density of found matches at the correct location of the histology section. This holds true even for histological images that are tilted with respect to the z-axis of the μCT dataset. This plane - well visible in the point cloud of Fig. 1(middle) - corresponds to the best position for the histological slice. In order to efficiently extract the plane parameters, we define a binary matrix $B(x, y, z) : \Omega_V \subset R^3 \rightarrow R$ as

$$B(x, y, z) = \begin{cases} 1 & \text{if } (x, y, z) \in C \\ 0 & \text{otherwise,} \end{cases}$$

which is then convolved with a 3D Gaussian as $B_\sigma = G_\sigma * B$. Thus, in each point we obtain a new intensity value that is influenced by the neighboring keypoint distribution across the μCT space and thus reflects the local density of matched points.

2.4   Density-Driven RANSAC for Robust Plane Fitting

One of the most widely used robust algorithms for extracting shapes from a data set with outliers is RANSAC [3]. The algorithm randomly selects a minimum number of points that uniquely defines a fitting shape. Then the corresponding primitive is constructed. In our problem, the model of interest is a plane $Ax + By + Cz + D = 0$ and the minimum number of points is 3. Therefore, the output parameter of the algorithm is a four dimensional normal vector $n = [A\,B\,C\,D]^T$. RANSAC then counts the number of points within the distance threshold t to the obtained candidate model (inliers). If the number of inliers for one model is larger than in the previous iteration, the new model parameters are retained. Otherwise, another subset is randomly selected. Depending on the ratio of inliers over outliers, this process has to be repeated multiple times to assure with a high probability that a solution is found when present. The large amount of outliers in our data would result in a large number of iterations.

In this work we thus propose to bias the random sampling of the RANSAC plane fitting process towards points with high density *i.e.* points that are close to the plane of interest. To optimize the plane detection algorithm, the dataset

B_σ is further reduced to $\rho < M$ points by retaining features with the largest density values. However, the new dataset $B_\rho \subset B_\sigma$ still contains some outliers due to high similarities within a specimen along the vertical axis.

To further reduce the number of required sampling iterations, we bias the random sampling code towards preferring points with a higher local density. Thus points with a high local density have a higher probability of being selected. Suppose that each density value of the dataset B_ρ is assigned to the weighting vector $\mathbf{w} = \{w_l\}$, where $l = 1...\rho$. Therefore, instead of using the unbiased classical sampling of the original RANSAC, the probability of picking an element $b_m \in B_\rho$ is then defined as $p_m = w_m / \sum_{l=1}^{\rho} w_i$.

A further optimization is associated with the angle α between the z-axis and the plane formed by the currently randomly sampled points from the dataset. Based on our observations we restrict this angle to lie between $-\alpha_{hist} < \alpha < \alpha_{hist}$. In other words, for every iteration, the 3D coordinates of the sampled points $\{b_1, b_2, b_3\} \in B_\rho$ are used to calculate the normal of the plane that goes through these points $\boldsymbol{n} = (b_2 - b_1) \times (b_3 - b_1)$. We then find the angle $\alpha = \arccos(n_z \, / \|\boldsymbol{n}\|)$, subject to $-\alpha_{hist} < \alpha < \alpha_{hist}$. Therefore, only planes that satisfy this constraint are considered for further procession in RANSAC. These two modifications allow to robustly fit a plane to the selected points and to obtain its parameters. An example of the point cloud with corresponding plane fit is shown in the Fig. 1.

Finally, we make a cut through the μCT data matrix along the fitted plane. The image in this cut is the result of our algorithm and should be maximally similar to the histological image.

Algorithm 1. 2D-3D matching

Input: Histological image I and μCT 3D dataset V, RANSAC threshold $t=10$, $\rho=1000$, $\alpha_{hist} = \frac{\pi}{8}$

Output: Plane parameters $\boldsymbol{n}$

   Convert I to gray scale

   for all V_j, $(j = 1...N)$ **do** $\triangleright$ Detect coordinates of matching points

      $(x_i, y_i) = SURF(I, V_j)$

      Build 3D set of coordinates $C = \{(x_{ij}, y_{ij}, z_j)\}$

   end for

   Create a binary 3D matrix $B(x, y, z)$

   for $(x, y, z) \in B$ **do**

      if $(x, y, z) \in C$ **then**

         set $B(x, y, z)$ to 1

      end if

   end for

   Convolve with Gaussian: $B_\sigma = G_\sigma * B$

   Find ρ highest values in B_σ

   Define $B_\rho \subset B_\sigma$, *i.e.* keep ρ points with the highest values

   $\boldsymbol{n}=$RANSAC$(B_\rho, t, \alpha_{hist}, \mathbf{w})$ $\triangleright$ Fit a plane into B_ρ using its values as weights $\mathbf{w}$

   return $\boldsymbol{n}$

---

3   Results

Our framework was validated on ten μCT datasets with overall 60 histological cross section images. For each histological slice we obtained a four dimensional vector which uniquely describes a plane in a 3D space. To compare the automatically found results with manually found locations we estimated the z-coordinate along the μCT volume and the angle between z-axis and the normal to the plane which represents a cut of the specimen. The z-coordinate was calculated as a center point of the obtained plane. All manually found matching parameters were obtained from VG studio which provides a four-dimensional vector of the searching plane and automatically computes the center point of the plane, *i.e.*, z-coordinate. We also performed a visual assessment of the automatically found images. In Fig. 2, we showed two examples of a matched slice found automatically ((a) and (d)) in comparison with manually found ((b) and (e)) and histological image ((c) and (f)). The complete result of the visual estimation with corresponding comparison with the ground truth values is summarized in Table 1. In nine out of ten datasets our approach has allocated at least half of the histological slices with an average difference of 0.25 mm. For the datasets 4, 5 and 10 the algorithm showed poor performance. The average distance for mismatched slices averaged around 286 slices and an overall accuracy for mismatched slices reached 2.21 mm. This might be due to high intensity variations within the μCT dataset and the inhomogeneous dying of the histological slices (see Fig. 3(a)). The extrema detector was very sensitive to intensity changes and dirt spots on the histological slices. This caused wrong feature responses and consequently incorrectly matched images.

The comparison of the angles with the ground truth is shown in Table 2. For intuitive reasons, we provided negative angles instead of angles around 360° to stress small alternation of the cutting section slopes. For small angles (around 5°) our approach showed high efficiency, whereas, for the angles of more than 10°, which corresponded to 0.53 mm of the specimen, it often found only a close approximation to the desired section of the μCT volume. For example, for the dataset 10, it has found a very close slice number, but determined a wrong angulation.

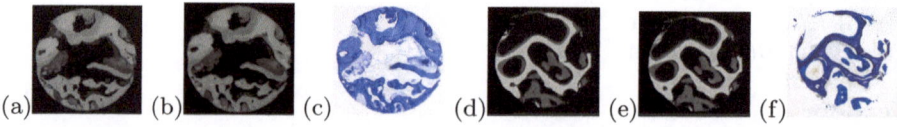

(a)   (b)   (c)   (d)   (e)   (f)

Fig. 2. (a),(d) Automatically found image. (b),(e) Manually found image. (c),(f) Histological image.

Table 1. Number of matched and mismatched images with corresponding average differences between automatically and manually found slices

Data set	1	2	3	4	5	6	7	8	9	10
Number of Matched slices	6	9	6	1	3	5	5	3	3	3
Average distance [mm]	0.06	0.04	0.9	0.17	0.05	0.59	0.24	0.07	0.16	0.13
Average difference [slices]	10	3	8	6	3	63	10	4	10	9
Number of Mismatched slices	0	0	1	4	3	1	1	1	2	3
Average distance [mm]	-	-	0.17	2.71	4.56	2.96	1.07	0.67	0.76	1.37
Average distance [slices]	-	-	15	94	286	314	45	40	47	91

*Note that number of slices per 1 mm is different for different samples.

Table 2. Comparison of average automatically found angles for matched slices with manually found angles

Data set	1	2	3	4	5	6	7	8	9	10
Average automatic angle [°]	1	1	1	-23	4	-1	-4	5	5	19
Manual angles [°]	-2	-5	5	-22	4	-19	-7	19	-8	-13

4 Discussion

Our novel algorithm for automatic 2D-3D registration showed a very high efficiency and small computational complexity and can be readily applied to the matching problem.

However, it has certain limitations regarding the feature detection step. Despite the good feature matching performance of SURF for most images it can not be considered a multi-modal approach but rather one that is robust against lightning changes. This also explains its poor performance when matching histological sections with non-uniform intensity variations. Moreover, additional complication arose from the histological slices that were compiled from disintegrated pieces (see Fig. 3(b)) and could not be readily matched with the same specimen. To overcome these limitations we want, firstly, to focus on developing a feature detector and descriptor that better will account for these specific characteristics and will efficiently work for multi-modal 2D-3D registration. Secondly, we want to include a non-rigid deformation estimation once the initial plane has been found. Lastly, we plan on further speeding up the calculation time by parallelization and GPU implementations. With a computation time of less than four minutes on a single-threaded MATLAB implementation, the algorithm still leaves room for further optimization and parallelization. This is irrespective of any angulation between the histology sections with respect to the μCT data.

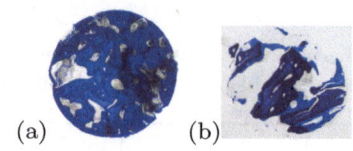

(a)   (b)

Fig. 3.   (a) Inhomogeneous dying of the histological slice from the 5th dataset.
(b) Compiled from pieces histological slice from the 8th dataset.

Acknowledgements. We would like to thank members of Biomaterials Science
Center (University of Basel): Anja Stalder for the manually found slices and
Simone Hieber for the help with the project. The work is funded by SNSF
(project 150164).

References

1. Baumberg, A.: Reliable feature matching across widely separated views. In: IEEE
   Conference on Computer Vision and Pattern Recognition, vol. 1, pp. 774–781
   (2000)
2. Bay, H., Ess, A., Tuytelaars, T., Van Gool, L.: Speeded-up robust features (SURF).
   Computer Vision and Image Understanding 110, 346–359 (2008)
3. Fischler, M.A., Bolles, R.C.: Random sample consensus: a paradigm for model
   fitting with applications to image analysis and automated cartography. Communications of the ACM 24, 381–395 (1981)
4. Lowe, D.G.: Distinctive image features from scale-invariant keypoints. International
   Journal of Computer Vision 60, 91–110 (2004)
5. Mosaliganti, K., Pan, T., Sharp, R., Ridgway, R., Iyengar, S., Gulacy, A., Wenzel,
   P., de Bruin, A., Machiraju, R., Huang, K., et al.: Registration and 3D visualization
   of large microscopy images. In: SPIE Medical Imaging, vol. 6144 (2006)
6. Osechinskiy, S., Kruggel, F.: Slice-to-volume nonrigid registration of histological
   sections to MR images of the human brain. Anatomy Research International (2010)
7. Ou, Y., Shen, D., Feldman, M., Tomaszewski, J., Davatzikos, C.: Non-rigid registration between histological and MR images of the prostate: A joint segmentation
   and registration framework. In: IEEE Computer Vision and Pattern Recognition
   Workshops, pp. 125–132 (2009)
8. Sarve, H., Lindblad, J., Johansson, C.B.: Registration of 2D histological images of
   bone implants with 3D SRμCT volumes. In: Advances in Visual Computing, pp.
   1071–1080 (2008)
9. Seise, M., Alhonnoro, T., Kolesnik, M.: Interactive registration of 2D histology
   and 3D CT data for assessment of radiofrequency ablation treatment. Journal of
   Pathology Informatics 2, 72 (2011)
10. Stalder, A.K., Ilgenstein, B., Chicherova, N., Deyhle, H., Beckmann, F., Müller,
    B., Hieber, S.E.: Combined use of micro computed tomography and histology to
    evaluate the regenerative capacity of bone grafting materials. International Journal
    of Materials Research (2014)
11. Zitova, B., Flusser, J.: Image registration methods: a survey. Image and Vision
    Computing 21, 977–1000 (2003)

Robust Registration of Longitudinal Spine CT

Ben Glocker[1], Darko Zikic[2], and David R. Haynor[3]

[1] Biomedical Image Analysis Group, Imperial College London, UK
[2] Microsoft Research, Cambridge, UK
[3] University of Washington, Seattle, WA, USA

Abstract. Accurate and reliable registration of longitudinal spine images is essential for assessment of disease progression and surgical outcome. Implementing a fully automatic and robust registration for clinical use, however, is challenging since standard registration techniques often fail due to poor initial alignment. The main causes of registration failure are the small overlap between scans which focus on different parts of the spine and/or substantial change in shape (e.g. after correction of abnormal curvature) and appearance (e.g. due to surgical implants). To overcome these issues we propose a registration approach which incorporates estimates of vertebrae locations obtained from a learning-based classification method. These location priors are used to initialize the registration and to provide semantic information within the optimization process. Quantitative evaluation on a database of 93 patients with a total of 276 registrations on longitudinal spine CT demonstrate that our registration method significantly reduces the number of failure cases.

1 Introduction

Assessment of disease progression and surgical outcome in the context of spinal pathologies is commonly performed using longitudinal imaging [1]. Clinical applications include but are not limited to correction of abnormal curvature, spinal fusion, treatment of fractures, vertebra disc replacement, and quantification of loss of bone mineral density. In order to detect, analyze and quantify changes between structures imaged at different time points it is essential to establish accurate anatomical correspondences which can be obtained by image registration. In the context of spinal imaging, longitudinal data such as pre- and post-operative scans can differ significantly which poses a major challenge to automatic registration methods. Relatively small overlap between pre- and post-operative data is particularly common in trauma cases. While whole-spine images are often acquired for diagnostic purposes when a patient is admitted to the hospital, more restricted scans with focus on the pathological region (e.g. fractures in the cervical part of the spine) are acquired after treatment. The overlap sometimes covers only a few vertebrae that are visible in both images. But even if the overlap of the visible anatomy is comparable, there are often large variations in spinal shape, for example after treatment of scoliosis, and change in appearance due to surgical implants such as metal screws, rods, and cages. These issues are the main cause of registration failure, which we aim to overcome with this work.

P. Golland et al. (Eds.): MICCAI 2014, Part I, LNCS 8673, pp. 251–258, 2014.
© Springer International Publishing Switzerland 2014

Our main contribution is a robust registration method which significantly reduces the number of failure cases in the context of the difficulties mentioned above. Robustness in the registration procedure is achieved by incorporating prior information about approximate locations of vertebrae. This semantic information is automatically extracted from the images by employing a vertebrae classification method. Our experiments demonstrate that the proposed approach yields accurate registrations in challenging cases where alternative methods fail.

The general idea of incorporating additional information into intensity-based registration is not new. Hybrid registration techniques [2], for example, which combine intensity information with automatically detected landmarks are based on such an approach. Also, registration methods which incorporate segmentation priors [3] or other semantic information such as bounding boxes of anatomical structures [4] fall into the same category. The key in such approaches is the integration of effective, application-specific components which can extract useful information from the images prior to registration. However, we are not aware of works that use such additional information to address the robustness in the context of volumetric spine registration. For 2D-3D spine registration robustness is achieved by using fiducial markers [5] which is not applicable in our scenario. Previous works on volumetric spine registration mainly focus on transformation models such as piecewise multi-rigid approaches [6,7] or aim at improving registration accuracy by highlighting spine specific image features [8] and anatomical structures [9]. However, these methods require good initialization which we aim to provide with the proposed registration approach.

2   Robust Registration Using Vertebrae Location Priors

Registration methods commonly rely on iterative optimization procedures which tolerate only a limited amount of initial misalignment. Reasonably accurate pre-alignment is therefore required in order to allow the registration to converge to an optimal solution. Often, application-specific heuristics can be employed in which initial transformations are automatically determined. For example, aligning the centers of intensity masses works often quite well for inter and intra-subject brain registration.

In the context of longitudinal spine registration, such heuristics are more difficult to find. We will later demonstrate that both center of mass alignment and exhaustive search along the main body axis often fail to provide good initialization. The problem of initialization seems particularly challenging for clinical spine data due to the issues discussed earlier such as small overlap, varying field of view and substantial change in shape and appearance. In addition, the presence of repetitive structures such as vertebrae bodies and ribs adds to the difficulty and imposes many local minima for the optimization. In this context, it should be beneficial to incorporate semantic information extracted from the images prior to registration. Recently, significant progress has been made towards automatic labeling and identification of individual vertebrae [10,11,12] and inter-vertebral discs [13,14]. Using such techniques within a registration approach seems a promising direction which can potentially overcome the issues of initialization. Following this idea, we introduce a registration approach which integrates a recently proposed learning-based vertebrae classification method [12]. This method has been shown to work reasonably well on pathological data which is essential for our purposes. The classification enables us to estimate prior information on approximate locations of vertebrae. Please note that the prior information does not need to be perfect as long as it can be used to start registration within the tolerance regime of the employed method.

2.1   Vertebrae Classification

Vertebrae localization in [12] is posed as a dense classification problem. A voxel-wise classifier based on randomized decision trees is learned using an annotated database of training images. Annotations in this approach are vertebrae centroids, from which dense label maps are generated and used for training.

At test time, the classifier produces probabilistic estimates for each image point. The estimates correspond to the likelihood of a point being part of a particular vertebra. Formally, the output of the classifier is the posterior distribution $p(v|f(x))$ where $v \in \mathcal{V}$ is a vertebra id and $f(x)$ is a feature vector extracted at image point $x \in \Omega_I$ in a test image I. A post-processing step based on mean shift and an outlier removal strategy [12] preserves the confident vertebrae centroid predictions while reducing the number of false positives.

Our approach does not require perfectly accurate prior information, since registration also relies on the rich intensity information. The uncertainty implicitly encoded in the probabilistic estimates will guide the optimization process to rely on the most confident information. The probability estimates generated by the classification approach can be directly integrated into the registration process, both for initialization as well as to guide the subsequent optimization process. To this end, we evaluate the posterior distribution in the spatial domain of the test image in order produce dense multi-channel probability maps $P_I(v, x) = p(v|f(x))$ with one channel per vertebra v. In Fig. 1, the thresholded maximum-a-posteriori output of the classifier is shown for two images of the same patient. Even though the output is noisy it contains sufficient semantic information for successful registration.

2.2   Registration with Location Priors

The probabilistic vertebrae priors obtained from the classifier are beneficial for two purposes. First, the inferred approximate locations of vertebrae can be used to determine an initial translational offset that is applied to the moving image prior to the actual registration. This offset is determined as the least squares solution which minimizes the distances between the estimated centroids of vertebrae which are detected in both images. Using this as an initialization works well even for image pairs with very small overlap and different field of views. The initial alignment is thus purely based on semantic information extracted from the images, without the need for any additional application-specific heuristics. Initialization results for one example are shown in Fig. 2.

The second purpose of the location priors is to drive the registration towards accurate alignment. This is achieved by augmenting the intensity-based objective function with a matching criterion defined on the probability maps P. The intensity information is suitable for precise alignment of structure boundaries, but only once those structures sufficiently overlap. The prior probabilities on the other hand help to avoid local minima by solving ambiguities between neighboring structures with locally similar appearance. The combination of intensity information and location priors obtained from a classifier makes the registration process very robust. We cast the registration of two images as the following optimization problem

$$\hat{T} = \arg\max_{T} \psi(I, J, P_I, P_J, T) \ , \tag{1}$$

where $T : \mathbb{R}^3 \mapsto \mathbb{R}^3$ is the transformation which aligns the moving image I with the fixed image J. The matching criterion ψ has the following form

$$\psi(I, J, P_I, P_J, T) = \rho(T(I), J) + \frac{1}{|\mathcal{V}_{IJ}|} \sum_{v \in \mathcal{V}_{IJ}} \phi(T(P_I(v, \cdot)), P_J(v, \cdot)) \ , \tag{2}$$

where P_I and P_J are the probability maps for the moving and fixed image, and $\mathcal{V}_{IJ}$ is the set of vertebrae that have been detected in both images. The criterion ψ is thus simply the sum of an intensity-based matching criterion ρ and another criterion ϕ evaluated on the probability maps. In the simplest case, the two criteria can be defined using one of the popular similarity measures. In this work, we use correlation coefficient both on the intensity information and on the prior probability maps and both terms equally contribute to the objective function. It could be beneficial to introduce a weighting factor that balances the two terms, in particular if other similarity measures are considered.

The actual registration procedure with the objective defined in Eq. (2) follows a common hierarchical setup. We first establish linear alignment with six degrees of freedom defining a rigid-body transformation. Subsequently, we run a non-rigid refinement using free-form deformations with three levels using 80, 40, and 20mm control grid spacing. Both the linear and the non-linear components make use of gradient-free optimization methods. For the linear registration we employ the Downhill-simplex optimizer, and the non-rigid part is optimized using discrete optimization [15]. This has the advantage that the objective function in Eq. (2) can be easily integrated into the existing registration code.

3   Experiments

The data used for experimental evaluation is a subset of our publicly available spine CT database[1]. Within this database we identified 93 patients for which at least two longitudinal scans are available. In some cases up to five follow-up scans are present. For each patient, we perform registration between all possible pairs of

---

[1] http://research.microsoft.com/spine/

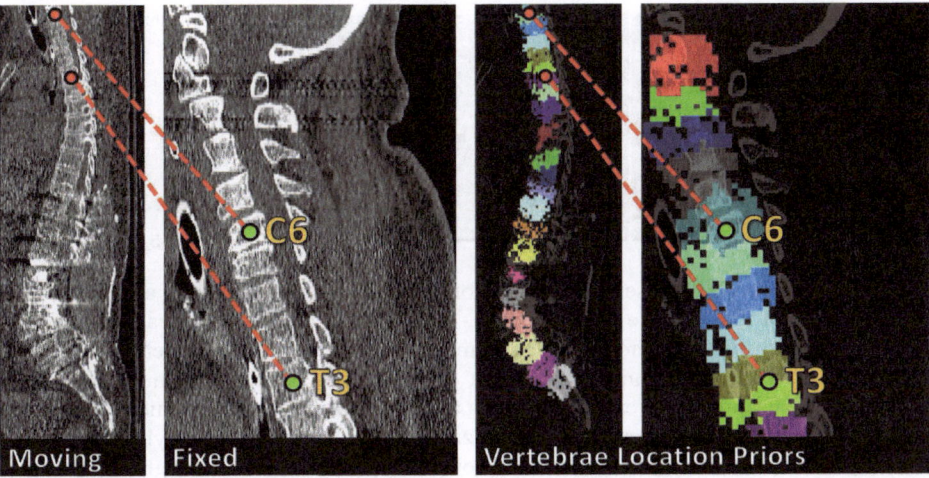

Fig. 1. Example of a challenging case of longitudinal spine registration where the source and the target image focus on different parts of the spine with only a few common vertebrae. After running our classification algorithm, location priors are obtained which be used to solve the initialization problem. The shown colored labelmaps correspond to the maximum-a-posteriori labels at each image point where each color corresponds to a particular vertebrae

scans if there is at least one common vertebra visible in both images. This results in a total of 276 intra-subject longitudinal registrations. Each dataset comes with manual annotations of vertebrae centroids which allows us to quantify the target registration. To this end we apply the resulting transformations to the manually annotated centroids of the moving image and determine the Euclidean mean distances to the centroids in the fixed image. The vertebrae classifier that is employed in our registration was trained on the remaining data from the original database, for which follow-up scans are not available.

3.1   Pre-processing

All evaluated registration methods operate on clamped intensity images. During initial experiments with different intensity-based methods we found that this yields best registration results when the aim is to establish correspondences between bony structures of the spine. We only consider intensities within an HU range of $[100, 1500]$. Setting an upper limit has also the effect of suppressing surgical implants and other artifacts caused by metal. This is particularly helpful when registering pre- and post-operative data.

3.2   Baselines

We compare our prior-augmented registration approach to three baselines. Each baseline employs a different strategy for obtaining an initial alignment, followed

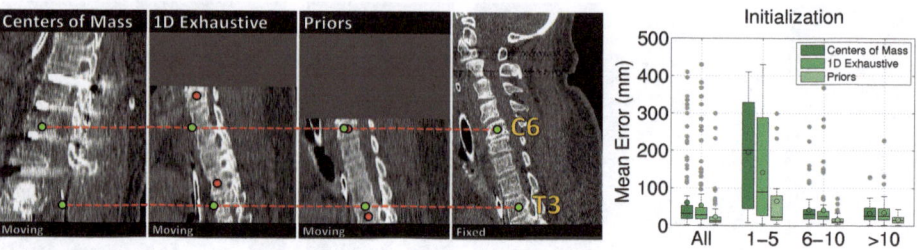

Fig. 2. The left image presents initialization results for three different approaches for the moving and fixed image shown in Fig. 1. Green circles are vertebrae centroids of C6 and T3 mapped from the fixed to the moving image space. Red circles are ground truth centroids. Initialization via alignment of 'Centers of Mass' fails completely in this case. The '1D Exhaustive' search converges to a local minimum from which subsequent registration fails (not shown). The initialization via location 'Priors' yields sufficient pre-alignment for successful registration (not shown). The plot on the right summarizes the alignment errors after initialization for all 276 image pairs grouped with respect to the amount of image overlap, expressed by number of vertebrae contained in both scans. Our prior-based alignment is particuarly beneficial when the overlap is small

by a standard registration driven by intensity information only. The first baseline 'Centers of Mass' uses the common heuristic of pre-aligning the centers of intensity masses. The second baseline '1D Exhaustive' uses a one-dimensional exhaustive search along the main anatomical axis with a small step size (around 2mm). The idea of this baseline is that it can potentially find reasonable alignments for images with very different a field of view. The third baseline 'Init with Priors' uses the proposed location prior-based initialization, but an intensity-only registration subsequently. This allows us to evaluate the impact of using priors for both initialization and within the objective function as it is done in our method. All baselines use exactly the same intensity-based registration components as our method. By using the identical setup for the transformation models and optimization procedures for our method and the baselines, we can isolate the effect of the location priors on the accuracy of the final registration result.

3.3 Results

Fig. 3 summarizes the main quantitative results in terms of error statistics, categorized by the number of overlapping vertebrae. We observe significantly better registration performance for our method compared to the three baselines on all cases. In particular, the difference in performance for the small overlap cases is remarkable. The overall mean registration error after non-rigid refinement on all 276 registration is 12.3mm for our method, 39.8mm for 'Centers of Mass', 35.5mm for '1D Exhaustive', and 14.0mm for 'Init with Priors'. With increasing overlap the registration errors decrease substantially. However, even if more than 10 vertebrae are visible in both images our registration method still outperforms the baselines, including the one that uses prior information for initialization.

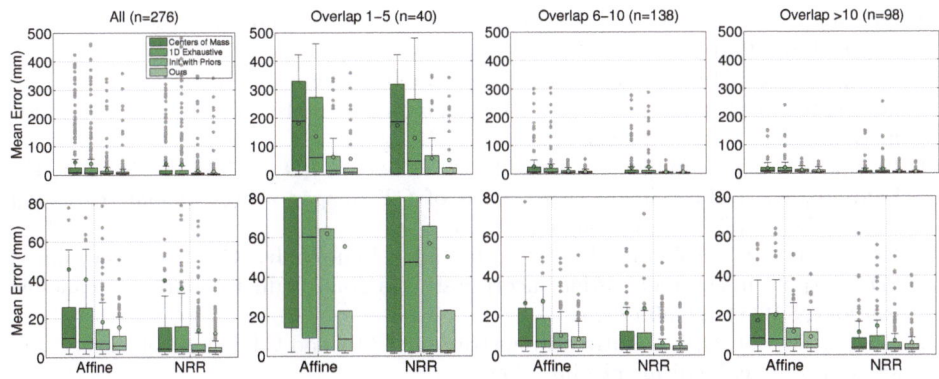

Fig. 3. Statistics of registration errors for two intensity-only baselines, a third baseline that uses prior maps for initialization only, and our registration which uses priors for both initialization and within the objective function. The errors are categorized by the number of overlapping vertebrae. The top row shows the full error range including extreme outliers. The bottom row is a zoom-in on a smaller error range. We observe that our method has significantly lower failure cases, and mean, median and standard deviations of registration errors are consistently lower in particular for the cases with small overlap

This indicates the importance of integrating the location priors also in the objective function. In terms of computational performance, our method is very efficient. Evaluating the classifier to obtain the probability maps takes less than one minute per image. The running time of the registration depends on the size of the images and takes about 2 minutes on average.

4   Conclusion

We demonstrated how volumetric spine registration can benefit from prior information about vertebrae locations yielding a fully automatic, robust registration tool that could be used in clinical routine on challenging data. Our approach immediately benefits from future improvements on learning-based vertebrae classification which could further reduce the number of failure cases. Establishing correspondences between longitudinal data for a large cohort of patients allows disease-specific modeling and a better understanding of underlying pathophysiological processes. Statistical analysis on such data could potentially be used to predict surgical outcome, which seems an interesting direction of research for future work.

References

1. Jarvik, J.J., Hollingworth, W., Heagerty, P., Haynor, D.R., Deyo, R.A.: The longitudinal assessment of imaging and disability of the back (LAIDBack) study: baseline data. Spine 26(10), 1158–1166 (2001)

2. Johnson, H.J., Christensen, G.E.: Consistent landmark and intensity-based image registration. TMI 21(5), 450–461 (2002)
3. Studholme, C., Hill, D., Hawkes, D.: Incorporating connected region labelling into automated image registration using mutual information. In: Mathematical Methods in Biomedical Image Analysis, pp. 23–31 (1996)
4. Konukoglu, E., Criminisi, A., Pathak, S., Robertson, D., White, S., Haynor, D., Siddiqui, K.: Robust linear registration of CT images using random regression forests. In: SPIE Medical Imaging (2011)
5. Russakoff, D.B., Rohlfing, T., Adler Jr., J.R., Maurer Jr., C.R.: Intensity-based 2D-3D spine image registration incorporating a single fiducial marker. Academic Radiology 12(1), 37–50 (2005)
6. Hu, Y., Haynor, D.R.: Multirigid registration of MR and CT images of the cervical spine. In: SPIE Medical Imaging (2004)
7. Cech, P., Andronache, A., Wang, L., Szekely, G., Cattin, P.: Piecewise rigid multi-modal spine registration. In: Handels, H., Ehrhardt, J., Horsch, A., Meinzer, H.P., Tolxdorff, T. (eds.) Bildverarbeitung fuer die Medizin 2006, pp. 211–215. Springer, Heidelberg (2006)
8. Li, W., Sode, M., Saeed, I., Lang, T.: Automated registration of hip and spine for longitudinal QCT studies: integration with 3D densitometric and structural analysis. Bone 38(2), 273–279 (2006)
9. Steger, S., Wesarg, S.: Automated Skeleton Based Multi-modal Deformable Registration of Head&Neck Datasets. In: Ayache, N., Delingette, H., Golland, P., Mori, K. (eds.) MICCAI 2012, Part II. LNCS, vol. 7511, pp. 66–73. Springer, Heidelberg (2012)
10. Klinder, T., Ostermann, J., Ehm, M., Franz, A., Kneser, R., Lorenz, C.: Automated model-based vertebra detection, identification, and segmentation in CT images. MedIA 13(3), 471–482 (2009)
11. Huang, S.H., Chu, Y.H., Lai, S.H., Novak, C.L.: Learning-based vertebra detection and iterative normalized-cut segmentation for spinal MRI. TMI 28(10), 1595–1605 (2009)
12. Glocker, B., Zikic, D., Konukoglu, E., Haynor, D., Criminisi, A.: Vertebrae Localization in Pathological Spine CT via Dense Classification from Sparse Annotations. In: Mori, K., Sakuma, I., Sato, Y., Barillot, C., Navab, N. (eds.) MICCAI 2013, Part II. LNCS, vol. 8150, pp. 262–270. Springer, Heidelberg (2013)
13. Schmidt, S., Kappes, J., Bergtholdt, M., Pekar, V., Dries, S., Bystrov, D., Schnörr, C.: Spine detection and labeling using a parts-based graphical model. In: Karssemeijer, N., Lelieveldt, B. (eds.) IPMI 2007. LNCS, vol. 4584, pp. 122–133. Springer, Heidelberg (2007)
14. Oktay, A., Akgul, Y.: Localization of the Lumbar discs using machine learning and exact probabilistic inference. In: Fichtinger, G., Martel, A., Peters, T. (eds.) MICCAI 2011, Part III. LNCS, vol. 6893, pp. 158–165. Springer, Heidelberg (2011)
15. Glocker, B., Komodakis, N., Tziritas, G., Navab, N., Paragios, N.: Dense image registration through MRFs and efficient linear programming. MedIA 12(6), 731–741 (2008)

Geometric-Feature-Based Spectral Graph Matching in Pharyngeal Surface Registration

Qingyu Zhao[1], Stephen Pizer[1], Marc Niethammer[1], and Julian Rosenman[2]

[1] Computer Science, UNC Chapel Hill, NC, United States
[2] Radiation Oncology, UNC Chapel Hill, NC, United States

Abstract. Fusion between an endoscopic movie and a CT can aid specifying the tumor target volume for radiotherapy. That requires a deformable pharyngeal surface registration between a 3D endoscope reconstruction and a CT segmentation. In this paper, we propose to use local geometric features for deriving a set of initial correspondences between two surfaces, with which an association graph can be constructed for registration by spectral graph matching. We also define a new similarity measurement to provide a meaningful way for computing inter-surface affinities in the association graph. Our registration method can deal with large non-rigid anatomical deformation, as well as missing data and topology change. We tested the robustness of our method with synthetic deformations and showed registration results on real data.

1 Introduction

The goal of surface registration is to find a dense set of corresponding points between two surfaces. Usually this is challenging because the surface may undergo large deformations, and sometimes there might be missing data, such as unexpected holes and different boundary locations, in the surface.

For example, in our application of the fusion between an endoscope movie and a CT image for head and neck cancer, one can acquire an endoscopic video clip of the pharyngeal region at radiation treatment planning time, from which a 3D reconstruction of the pharyngeal surface is derived. On the other hand, we can also segment a 3D pharyngeal surface from a head and neck CT image of the same patient. A registration between these two surfaces will permit fusion of the endoscopically available information about the tumor extent on the pharyngeal surface with the tumor information seen in the CT, thereby improving the radiation plan. As shown in Figs. 5a, 5b, a large deformation between the two surfaces is caused by the swallowing process and posture change of a patient. Due to the limitation of endoscope procedure, a part of the pharyngeal anatomy is visually inaccessible by the camera. Therefore, the reconstruction surface is only a partial surface with respect to the CT surface. The reconstruction artifacts will also create many holes in the surface. The fusion between endoscope and CT has been tried in other anatomies, but they consider only rigid or small deformations between the modalities and thus cannot be applied to the pharyngeal region.

P. Golland et al. (Eds.): MICCAI 2014, Part I, LNCS 8673, pp. 259–266, 2014.

For non-rigid surface registration some approaches directly solve for the deformation parameters [1–3] by minimizing the closeness of two surfaces in the original 3D domain, but they usually involve a non-convex optimization. Conformal mappings [4] and Möbius transformations [5] have also been proposed to map the surfaces onto a canonical domain conformally, and seek the matching in that space. Other methods [6, 7] for matching isometric shapes embed the surfaces into a Euclidean space to obtain isometry-invariant representations. Among those, spectral graph theory offers a nice mathematical framework for matching shapes in the spectral domain. Many registration methods adopt the idea of feature matching. To that end, spin images [8] and Heat Kernel Signature (HKS) [9] are the two most widely used surface features. However, spin images are variant to large deformations, and HKS can not handle missing data in the surface because of different boundary conditions.

Lombaert [10] found that by combining the two surfaces into one graph with some initial links, spectral decomposition could yield consistent eigenvectors, which he used for surface matching. In his application of cortical surface matching, he chose to use a conventional spectral matching to provide initial links. Expectedly, that method has been shown in our results not to be suitable for finding initial correspondences when facing large deformations and different topology.

We made the following contributions in our paper. First, we design a novel geometry-based feature descriptor that can be applied on any surface with notable geometric structures. Second, we define a correspondence confidence score based on feature comparison, with which an effective initial correspondence set can be derived to work with Lombaert's new form of spectral method. Third, we discuss the advantage of our method in the context of partial surface matching, which has not been studied before in any spectral matching framework.

2   Geometric Feature Extraction and Use

2.1   Feature Descriptor

In our application, a surface is represented by a triangulated mesh with a set of vertices $\{V\}$ and a set of edges $\{E\}$. We compute geometric feature descriptors at each vertex, on which vertex correspondences are based.

We design a special feature descriptor $f(v)$ to create a signature for each vertex. In order to describe the local shape around a vertex, we collect geometric information on both the vertex itself and a number of surrounding vertices. As shown in Fig. 1a, for each vertex v, we find 8 surrounding vertices $\{v_i | i = 1...8\}$ by going along 8 equally angularly spaced geodesic directions $\{g_i | i = 1...8\}$ from v by a certain distance d. We choose the nearest vertices at the end points of the 8 paths as the surrounding vertices. g_1 and g_3 overlap with the two principal directions p_1, p_2. Since the local shape can be captured by curvatures measured at different scales, the descriptor is defined as $f(v) = \{\mathbf{C}, \mathbf{S}, \Delta \mathbf{N}, \Delta \mathbf{F}, \Delta \mathbf{N}_{1,5}, \Delta \mathbf{N}_{3,7}\}$.

Koenderink's [11] informative curvature measures c, s derivable from the two principal curvatures k_1, k_2, are computed at the center vertex and 8 surrounding vertices to describe local curvatures by the tuple $\mathbf{C}, \mathbf{S}$. Larger scale measures of curvature between each of the surrounding vertices and the center vertex are computed as the normal direction difference magnitudes ΔN, as well as by the local coordinate frame rotation quaternions ΔF. The local coordinate frame is constructed as the two principal directions plus the normal direction. Also, normal direction differences between two extreme endpoint pairs (v_1, v_5) and (v_3, v_7) are computed to describe the general shape structure.

We used LMNN (Large Margin Nearest Neighbor) to learn the weights for different features using a set of ground truth corresponding vertices with their features and deleted features with near-zero weights, but we found the algorithm performed noticeably better when all features are used.

2.2 Computing Correspondence Confidence

We propose a similarity measurement between vertices from two different surfaces. This measurement is defined by a confidence score $\Delta_{i,j}$, indicating how likely $v_i \in S_1$ and $v_j \in S_2$ are corresponding. Define the two surfaces to be S_1, S_2 with N, M vertices respectively and v_i to be the ith vertex in a surface. Under the assumption that S_1 and S_2 are rigidly aligned first, the feature distance between $v_i \in S_1$ and $v_j \in S_2$ is defined as

$$\delta(i, j) = ||f(v_i) - f(v_j)||^2 + \alpha(1 + e^{-(||x_i - x_j|| - \tau)})^{-1} \tag{1}$$

where the second part is a sigmoid function penalizing a too large Euclidean distance between two corresponding vertices. Based on this feature distance function, we propose an efficient method to compute the confidence score $\Delta_{i,j}$.

A confidence score considers both-way corresponding likelihoods, namely v_i being the closest vertex to v_j and v_j being the closest vertex to v_i. $\kappa^1_{i,j}$ is defined as the likelihood of $v_j \in S_2$ being the closest vertex of $v_i \in S_1$, compared to all other vertices in S_2. It is computed by normalizing $\delta(i, j)$ to $[0, 1]$ using $\{\delta(i, k)|k = 1...M\}$ (Eq. 2). $\kappa^2_{i,j}$ is defined and computed vice versa (Eq. 3):

$$\kappa^1_{i,j} = 1 - (\delta(i, j) - \min_k \delta(i, k))/(\max_k \delta(i, k) - \min_k \delta(i, k)) \tag{2}$$

$$\kappa^2_{i,j} = 1 - (\delta(i, j) - \min_k \delta(k, j))/(\max_k \delta(k, j) - \min_k \delta(k, j)) \tag{3}$$

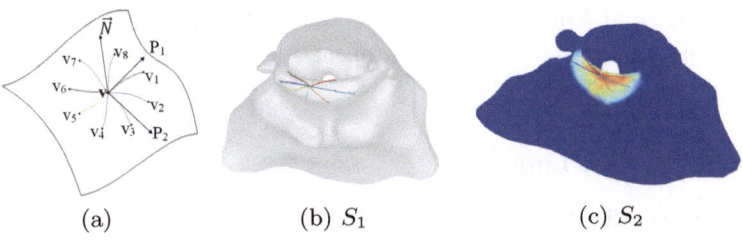

(a)   (b) S_1 (c) S_2

Fig. 1. (a) Local geometry from which $f(v)$ is computed. (b) A vertex is selected in S_1, indicated as the cross point. (c) The value of Δ's ith row (red indicates large value).

Because the two likelihoods are now at the same scale, the confidence score $\Delta_{i,j}$ is computed by taking the sum of $\kappa_{i,j}^1$ and $\kappa_{i,j}^2$. All the confidence scores will form a $N \times M$ confidence score matrix Δ. As shown in Figs. 1b, 1c, for a vertex $v_i \in S_1$, Δ's ith row is color-coded in S_2. The vertex with the largest value is selected as the corresponding point. The overall dense correspondences based on this strategy are color-coded as shown in Fig. 2b.

3   Spectral Graph Matching

3.1   Spectral Graph Matching on an Association Graph

We build two graphs $G_1 = \{V_1, E_1\}$ and $G_2 = \{V_2, E_2\}$ from the two surfaces S_1 and S_2 with the vertices and edges of the triangulated surface meshes. An association graph $G = \{V, E\}$ is built by connecting G_1 and G_2 with a set of initial links. Lombaert in his work defined the $|N + M| \times |N + M|$ affinity matrix W by the Euclidean distance between two vertices in the original 3D space for both intra-surface links and inter-surface links, i.e., $w_{i,j} = ||x_i - x_j||^{-2}$ if $\exists$ $e_{i,j} \in E$. The graph Laplacian operator L is defined as $L = D - W$, where D is a diagonal matrix with $d_i = \sum_j w_{i,j}$.

The spectral decomposition of L provides an orthogonal set of eigenvectors $[u^1, u^2, ..., u^{|N+M|}]$ with the corresponding non-*decreasing* eigenvalues, the first of which is zero for appropriate boundary conditions. Each of the eigenvectors u^i can be separated into two functions: u_1^i, the first N values of u^i, representing the ith vibration mode of G_1, and u_2^i, the last M values of u^i, representing the ith vibration mode of G_2. The inter-surface links ensure that they represent a consistent vibration mode. Moreover, the spectral embedding of the graph into a k-dimensional Euclidean space, also known as the spectral domain, is given by $[u^2, u^3, ..., u^{k+1}]$. In other words, we define $F = [f_1, f_2, ..., f_k]$ as an $n \times k$ matrix, and the first k eigenmodes with non-zero eigenvalues provide the solution to the problem:

$$\arg \min_{f_1, f_2, ..., f_k} \sum_{i,j=1}^{n} w_{i,j} \parallel f^{(i)} - f^{(j)} \parallel^2, \text{ with } F^T F = I \tag{4}$$

where $f^{(i)}$ is the ith row of F, representing the embedded Euclidean coordiantes of the ith vertex. Intuitively, the k eigenmodes define an embedding into a k-dimensional Euclidean space that tries to respect the edge lengths of the graph. The final matching is accomplished by a nearest-neighbor search in the k-dimensional spectral domain.

3.2   Finding Initial Links

The inter-surface affinity in the Lombaert paper was defined according to the Euclidean distance between two corresponding vertices, which is conceptually unnatural, because in most large deformation situations, two corresponding vertices might have a large Euclidean distance, ending up with a small affinity,

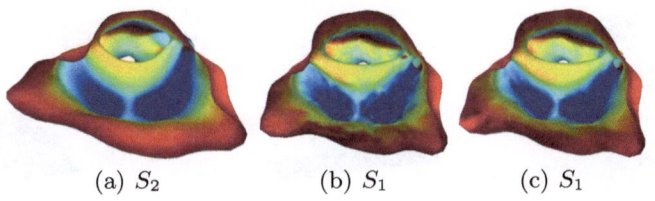

(a) S_2 (b) S_1 (c) S_1

Fig. 2. (a)S_2 is uniformly colored. The overall correspondences are indicated by the corresponding color in S_1. (b) Correspondences derived from the confidence scores. (c) Correspondences derived from spectral graph matching.

even though there is a clear evidence showing the correspondence is correct and should have a high affinity. Therefore, we propose to compute the inter-surface affinity based on the confidence score of the initial correspondences.

We use an iterative max-row-column approach described in [5] to construct a set of t initial correspondences based on the confidence score matrix Δ. In each iteration, we select the largest non-zero element $\Delta_{i,j}$ and add (v_i, v_j) to the initial correspondence set. To avert non-one-to-one correspondences, we zero out the ith row and jth column of Δ. We repeat this procedure t times to select t most credible correspondences. The affinity matrix W is now defined as

$$
w_{i,j} = \begin{cases} ||x_i - x_j||^{-2} & \text{if } v_i, v_j \text{ are in same the surface,} \\ \Delta_{i,j} & \text{if } (v_i, v_j) \text{ is in the initial correspondence set,} \\ 0 & \text{otherwise.} \end{cases} \tag{5}
$$

The final matching result is shown in Fig. 2c. As we can see, the correspondences are smoother than from the confidence scores directly.

4   Different Intrinsic Geometry

In our application, we have to register two surfaces with different intrinsic geometry, such as different boundary locations and holes (Fig. 5). Conventional separated spectral decompositions [12] in this situation will yield two totally different sets of eigenmodes. Just think of the simplest partial surface problem in Fig. 3a, in which one surface is a half of the other one. The first eigenmodes have distinct patterns, because surfaces with different sizes have different vibration modes. However, if we randomly assign only 5% initial correspondences between the two surfaces, as shown in Fig. 3b, the first eigenmodes become consistent with each other. Intuitively, we can achieve a joint vibration by patching the partial surface onto the other one using the initial links, so that the partial surface is forced to vibrate together with the other. Moreover, we can see this happening from the objective function (Eq. 4), because the energy is minimized when both intra-surface and inter-surface affinities are preserved in the spectral domain, which means corresponding vertices have similar embedded coordinates, as well as vibration properties.

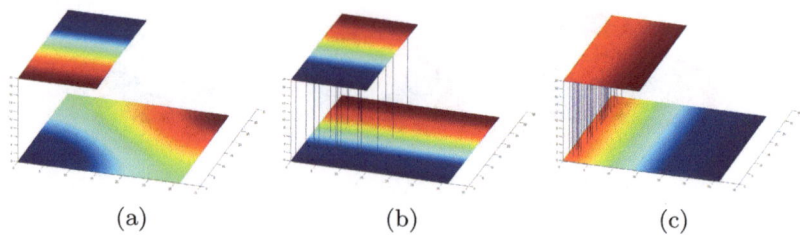

(a)   (b)   (c)

Fig. 3. The first eigenmodes derived from (a) separated spectral decompositions. (b) a spectral decomposition on an association graph. (c) a spectral decomposition on an association graph with initial links only on one side.

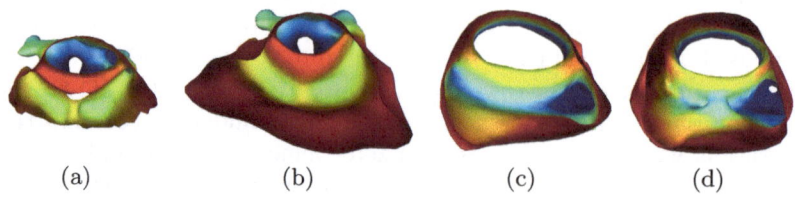

(a)   (b)   (c)   (d)

Fig. 4. The color-coded correspondences (a,b) between a complete surface and a partial surface with a hole and truncation. (c,d) between surfaces with a bridge.

We find that the initial links have to be scattered all over the surface, but not necessarily dense. For example, the first vibration modes are shown in Fig. 3c, if the initial links are only on one side of the surface. Intuitively, two pieces of paper won't be stuck together if there is only one piece glued together.

Therefore, it is essential to find a credible set of initial links. As shown before, conventional spectral matching is not able to provide correct correspondences. However, our geometric feature descriptor has the advantage of providing robust initial links regardless of whether the overall surface being partial or not, because the correspondences are derived only using local geometric features. For the same reason, in most situations where the partial surface has holes in it, the joint vibration can still be achieved. Figs. 4a, 4b show the final matching result for a partial surface with a hole and a truncated boundary.

Our method can also handle some other simple topology changes. However, in many cases, regions with complicated topology changes usually yield inconsistent geometric features, which makes the initial correspondences there unstable. For example, as shown in Figs. 4c, 4d, there is a bridge connecting the epiglottis and the pharyngeal wall, and the correspondence there is not reasonable.

5   Results

We tested our method on 12 surface pairs created from 6 patients. The pharyngeal surface from the pharynx down to the vocal cord was automatically segmented for the patient's CT. Each surface has 2K-6K vertices, with an approximately 2cm×3cm elliptical cross section. We manually applied synthetic deformations to the surfaces with the help of a medical physicist, ending up with 12 surface pairs, two for each patient. The synthetic deformation includes the distortion and contraction of the pharyngeal wall and the closing and opening of the laryngeal region and of the epiglottis. We measured the registration error of each vertex as the Euclidean distance between the resulting corresponding vertex and the ground truth. The registration error for each surface pair is defined as the average registration error over all vertices.

We studied the optimal choice of different parameters. 15 eigenmodes were used to perform the final matching. The size of the initial correspondence set was chosen as half the number of vertices. We set the geodesic path distance d to 4mm and the Euclidean distance threshold τ to 1cm. All the parameters were chosen according to a different set of surface pairs.

The average registration error for the 12 surface pairs using initial links derived by different options is provided in Table 1. In the first option, we used conventional spectral matching to compute a dense set of initial correspondences. In the second option, we used our method except that the inter-surface affinity was computed by Euclidean distance between two corresponding vertices in the original 3D space. The third option was exactly our method. We tested all options in both scenarios: complete surface matching and partial surface matching. In the partial surface matching context, we picked one surface from each pair and manually created holes in large deformation regions, such as the epiglottis, and truncated the surface in a different location. The registration error was only measured for boundary vertices for partial surface matching. We also ran the algorithm on several real data cases with large topology change. One of the results is shown in Figs. 5c, 5d.

Table 1. Registration error for complete surface and partial surface matching

	Complete Surface (mm)	Partial Surface (mm)
Initial Error	3.09±1.73	3.48±1.79
1. Conventional Spectral Matching	1.83± 2.37	3.26±6.71
2. Feature + Euclidean Distance	1.38±2.55	1.90±2.15
3. Feature + Confidence Score	0.67±0.96	1.15±1.36

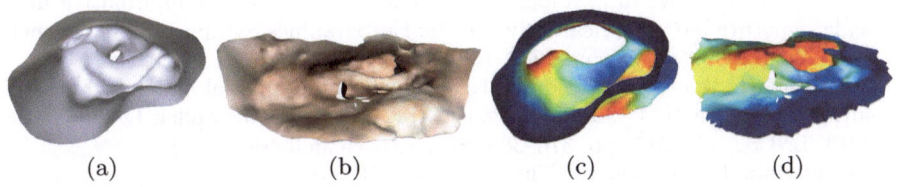

(a)   (b)   (c)   (d)

Fig. 5. The pharynx. (a) A CT segmentation. (b) An endoscopic video reconstruction. (c,d) Color-coded correspondences between a CT surface and a real reconstruction.

6   Conclusion

We have presented a non-rigid surface registration method based on spectral graph matching with the application of registering pharyngeal surfaces in CT/Endoscope fusion. We proposed an efficient approach for extracting initial correspondences using our novel geometric feature descriptor. The association graph based on this kind of initial correspondences produces better registrations. We showed the method's potential to handle partial surface matching and discussed its disadvantages when dealing with complicated topology change. Our results suggest that this approach might be applicable to other surface registrations with large deformations, holes and different boundary locations.

Acknowledgements. This work was supported by NIH grant R01 CA158925. The authors would like to thank Dr. Ron Alterovitz, Dr. Jan-Michael Frahm, Dr. Bisham Chera, Hina Shah and Federico Menozzi for the meaningful discussion and the preprocessing and 3D reconstruction work.

References

1. Allen, B., Curless, B., Popovic, Z.: The space of human body shapes: reconstruction and parameterization from range scans. In: ACM SIGGRAPH, vol. 22, pp. 587–594 (2003)
2. Li, H., Luo, L., Vlasic, D., Peers, P., Popovic, J., Pauly, M., Rusinkiewicz, S.: Temporally coherent completion of dynamic shapes. ACM Transactions on Graphics 31(2) (2012)
3. Huang, Q., Adams, B., Wicke, M., Guibas, L.: Non-rigid registration under isometric deformations. In: Symposium on Geometry Processing, pp. 1449–1457 (2008)
4. Zeng, W., Gu, X.D.: Registration for 3d surfaces with large deformations using quasi-conformal curvature flow. In: Computer Vision and Pattern Recognition, pp. 2457–2464 (2011)
5. Lipman, Y., Funkhouser, T.: Möbius voting for surface correspondence. ACM Transactions on Graphics 28(72) (2009)
6. Zigelman, G., Kimmel, R., Kiryati, N.: On bending invariant signatures for surfaces. IEEE Trans. Vis. Comput. Graph. 8(2), 198–207 (2002)
7. Sharma, A., Horaud, R.: Shape matching based on diffusion embedding and on mutual isometric consistency. In: IEEE CVPRW, pp. 29–36 (2010)
8. Johnson, A.E., Hebert, M.: Using spin images for efficient object recognition in cluttered 3d scenes. IEEE Transactions on PAMI 21(5), 433–449 (1999)
9. Sun, J., Ovsjanikov, M., Guibas, L.: A concise and provably informative multi-scale signature based on heat diffusion. In: Eurographics Symposium on Geometry Processing 2009, vol. 28, pp. 1383–1392 (2009)
10. Lombaert, H., Sporring, J., Siddiqi, K.: Diffeomorphic spectral matching of cortical surfaces. In: Gee, J.C., Joshi, S., Pohl, K.M., Wells, W.M., Zöllei, L. (eds.) IPMI 2013. LNCS, vol. 7917, pp. 376–389. Springer, Heidelberg (2013)
11. Koenderink, J.: Solid Shape. The MIT Press (1990)
12. Lombaert, H., Grady, L., Polimeni, J., Cheriet, F.: Fast brain matching with spectral correspondence. In: Székely, G., Hahn, H.K. (eds.) IPMI 2011. LNCS, vol. 6801, pp. 660–673. Springer, Heidelberg (2011)

Gaussian Process Interpolation for Uncertainty Estimation in Image Registration

Christian Wachinger[1,2], Polina Golland[1],
Martin Reuter[1,2], and William Wells[1,3]

[1] Computer Science and Artificial Intelligence Lab, MIT
[2] Massachusetts General Hospital, Harvard Medical School
[3] Brigham and Women's Hospital, Harvard Medical School

Abstract. Intensity-based image registration requires resampling images on a common grid to evaluate the similarity function. The uncertainty of interpolation varies across the image, depending on the location of resampled points relative to the base grid. We propose to perform Bayesian inference with Gaussian processes, where the covariance matrix of the Gaussian process posterior distribution estimates the uncertainty in interpolation. The Gaussian process replaces a single image with a distribution over images that we integrate into a generative model for registration. Marginalization over resampled images leads to a new similarity measure that includes the uncertainty of the interpolation. We demonstrate that our approach increases the registration accuracy and propose an efficient approximation scheme that enables seamless integration with existing registration methods.

1 Introduction

Registration is a fundamental tool in medical imaging for image alignment. Intensity-based registration commonly finds the transformation between images by an iterative procedure that resamples images on a common grid to evaluate their similarity. An inherent problem is the variation of the interpolation uncertainty across the image. Fig. 1 illustrates two images and an overlay of the corresponding grids. Intensity values on the moving grid (blue) are used to interpolate values on the fixed grid (red) to enable the comparison of both images. We point out two locations on the fixed grid that have very different distances to neighboring points on the moving grid. This difference causes variations in the interpolation uncertainty. Both locations contribute equally to the calculation of the similarity measure, although the interpolation from observations that are far away may not be very trustworthy.

To address this problem, we formulate the interpolation as Bayesian regression. The intensity values on the transformed grid serve as observations and the prediction yields samples on the fixed grid. We employ a Gaussian process (GP) prior over images and assume Gaussian noise on the observations. The inferred predictive distribution is Gaussian with mean and covariance functions serving as an interpolator and a confidence estimate. Depending on the design of the

P. Golland et al. (Eds.): MICCAI 2014, Part I, LNCS 8673, pp. 267–274, 2014.

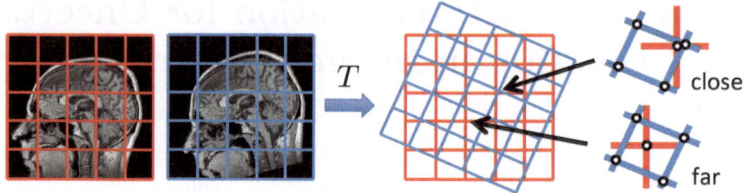

Fig. 1. Fixed (red) and moving (blue) images and the overlay of both grids after transformation (middle). The interpolation uncertainty varies across the resampled image due to different distances to neighboring points on the moving grid. Arrows point to two exemplary locations on the fixed grid where neighbors from the moving grid are close and far, respectively (right).

covariance matrix of the GP prior and the magnitude of the presumed noise in the images, we can account for smoothing and noise reduction in the prediction. This makes Gaussian processes a versatile framework for modeling image processing steps in registration.

The application of Gaussian processes introduces a new paradigm for the use of image interpolation in registration. Instead of only comparing the resampled intensity values, the similarity measure now takes into account the quality of the interpolation, which can vary dramatically across the image. To enable this change, we present a generative model for image registration with Gaussian processes. The inferred similarity measure emphasizes locations where samples are close to the original grid and deprecates locations that are equidistant from grid points. This is especially beneficial for anisotropically sampled data, frequently acquired in the clinical practice.

Related Work. The most common methods for interpolation are nearest neighbor, linear, cubic, and spline interpolation. The application of cubic B-splines for interpolation was proposed in [5]. Several excellent surveys of image interpolation exist [7,14]. Image interpolation in the context of registration is discussed in [4]. Further studies have been conducted to investigate the generation of interpolation artifacts and their influence on image registration, see for instance [1] and references therein. Gaussian processes have been applied in several fields of machine learning [11], *e.g.*, image denoising [8], interpolation [13] and segmentation [15]. Gaussian processes were also used to model flow fields [6] and deformation fields in hybrid registration [9]. Gaussian processes have not yet been used for image resampling in registration.

2   Method

Given two images I and J defined on discrete grids Ω_I and Ω_J, we calculate the transformation T that aligns the two images. We transform the grid Ω_J of the moving image J, yielding the transformed grid $T(\Omega_J) = \{T(\mathbf{x}), \mathbf{x} \in \Omega_J\}$.

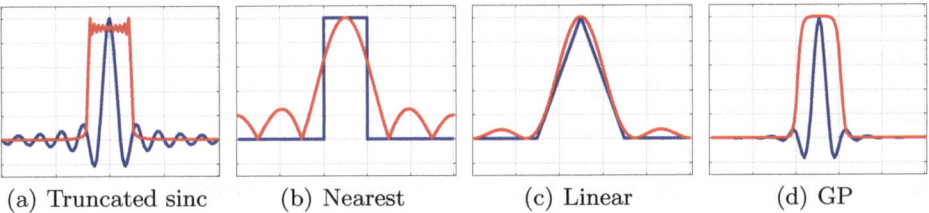

(a) Truncated sinc   (b) Nearest   (c) Linear   (d) GP

Fig. 2. Comparison of interpolation functions in spatial (blue) and frequency (red) domains. The optimal frequency response would correspond to a box function.

Except for axis-aligned transformations, we have to resample the transformed image from the grid $T(\Omega_J)$ to the grid of the fixed image Ω_I to compare the two images. For the resampling, a continuous version of the discrete input image is constructed with interpolation [10]. Fig 2 characterizes common image interpolation methods by showing their responses in spatial and frequency domains.

2.1   Image Interpolation with Gaussian Process Regression

In this section, we formulate image interpolation as Gaussian process regression to obtain the interpolator and uncertainty estimates. A Gaussian process is a stochastic process consisting of an infinite collection of random variables, where any finite subset has a multivariate Gaussian distribution [11]. A Gaussian process $\mathcal{GP}(m(\mathbf{x}), k(\mathbf{x}, \mathbf{x}'))$, is entirely characterized by the mean $m(\mathbf{x})$ and covariance $k(\mathbf{x}, \mathbf{x}')$ functions. The mean and covariance functions specify a distribution over functions, corresponding to a distribution over images in our case. We make the common assumption of a zero mean function [11].

Given moving image J on the transformed grid $X = T(\Omega_J)$, we predict the resampled image J^* on the fixed image grid $X^* = \Omega_I$. We employ a Gaussian process prior on the resampled image, $J^* \sim \mathcal{GP}(\mathbf{0}, k)$. Considering Gaussian noise $\varepsilon \sim \mathcal{N}(0, \sigma_J)$, the observations are distributed according to $p(J|J^*, X, X^*) = \mathcal{N}(\mathbf{0}|k(X, X) + \sigma_J^2 \mathbf{I})$, where $\mathbf{I}$ is the identity matrix. Under these assumptions, the posterior distribution for predicting the transformed image is

$$p(J^* \mid J; X^*, X) = \mathcal{N}(\boldsymbol{\mu}_J, \Sigma_J), \tag{1}$$

with mean and covariance

$$\boldsymbol{\mu}_J = k(X^*, X) \cdot [k(X, X) + \sigma_J^2 \mathbf{I}]^{-1} \cdot J, \tag{2}$$

$$\Sigma_J = k(X^*, X^*) - k(X^*, X) \cdot [k(X, X) + \sigma_J^2 \mathbf{I}]^{-1} \cdot k(X, X^*). \tag{3}$$

The covariance or kernel function k characterizes the properties of images. It captures the relation between the random variables, which correspond to the voxels in the image. We work with the squared exponential covariance function with length-scale l, $k(\mathbf{x}, \mathbf{x}') = \exp\left(-\|\mathbf{x} - \mathbf{x}'\|^2/(2 \cdot l^2)\right)$. The equivalent kernel characterizes the behavior of GP interpolation and is shown in Fig. 2 for the squared exponential function. Theoretical connections to sinc interpolation exist for specific settings of the kernel [12]. The squared exponential kernel corresponds to a Bayesian linear regression model with an infinite number of Gaussian-shaped basis functions [11].

2.2 Generative Model for Gaussian Process Registration

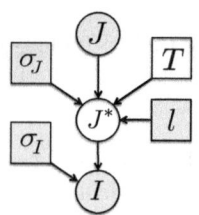

We derive the registration method with uncertainty estimates by integrating the Gaussian process in a new generative model for registration (see graphical model on the right). We treat input images I and J as observed random variables affected by image noise $\varepsilon_I \sim \mathcal{N}(0, \sigma_I^2)$ and $\varepsilon_J \sim \mathcal{N}(0, \sigma_J^2)$, respectively. The resampled image J^* is a latent random variable. The amount of smoothing in the image J^* is controlled by the length-scale l of the kernel. Following the graphical model, the joint distribution of images I, J, J^* factorizes

$$p(I, J, J^*; T, \sigma_J, \sigma_I, l) = p(J^*|J; T, \sigma_J, l) \cdot p(I|J^*; \sigma_I). \tag{4}$$

The probability $p(J^*|J; T, \sigma_J, l)$ is the predictive distribution of the Gaussian process. From the previous section on Gaussian process interpolation we have $p(J^*|J; T, \sigma_J, l) \sim \mathcal{N}(\boldsymbol{\mu}_J, \Sigma_J)$. The likelihood $p(I|J^*; \sigma_I)$ accounts for noise in the fixed image I with respect to the prediction J^*. Under the assumption of i.i.d. Gaussian noise, this leads to the multivariate Gaussian distribution $p(I|J^*; \sigma_I) \sim \mathcal{N}(J^*, \sigma_I^2 \mathbf{I})$. For calculating the optimal transformation $\hat{T}$, we perform maximum likelihood estimation on the joint distribution of images I and J

$$\hat{T} = \arg\max_T p(I, J; T, \sigma_J, \sigma_I, l). \tag{5}$$

For Bayesian inference, we marginalize over the latent random variable J^*

$$p(I, J; T, \sigma_I, \sigma_J, l) = \int p(I, J, J^*; T, \sigma_I, \sigma_J, l) \, \mathrm{d}J^* \tag{6}$$

$$= \int p(J^*|J; T, \sigma_J, l) \cdot p(I|J^*; \sigma_I) \, \mathrm{d}J^* \tag{7}$$

$$= \int \mathcal{N}(J^*; \boldsymbol{\mu}_J, \Sigma_J) \cdot \mathcal{N}(I; J^*, \sigma_I^2 \mathbf{I}) \, \mathrm{d}J^* \tag{8}$$

$$= \mathcal{N}(I; \boldsymbol{\mu}_J, \Sigma_J + \sigma_I^2 \mathbf{I}), \tag{9}$$

where we applied the factorization from the graphical model and product properties of multivariate Gaussian distributions [11]. The log-likelihood function is

$$\log p(I, J; T, \sigma_I, \sigma_J, l) = \log \left((2\pi)^{-\frac{k}{2}} |\Sigma|^{-\frac{1}{2}} \right) - \frac{1}{2}(I - \boldsymbol{\mu}_J)^\top \Sigma^{-1}(I - \boldsymbol{\mu}_J), \tag{10}$$

with $\Sigma = \Sigma_J + \sigma_I^2 \mathbf{I}$. This is the new similarity measure that we use for registration, where the covariance matrix Σ contains the uncertainty estimates. The presented approach models forward mapping in registration, where we obtain backward mapping by setting $X = \Omega_J$ and $X^* = T^{-1}(\Omega_I)$.

2.3   Practical Considerations

The computational cost of $\mathcal{O}(|\Omega_J|^3)$ for the matrix inversion $[k(X,X)+\sigma_J^2\mathbf{I}]^{-1}$ is challenging for large images. In order to reduce the computational cost, we split the volume into blocks. We perform the prediction for each block separately, where we identify the spatially closest observations. This comes at almost no additional cost, because the distances need to be calculated for constructing the kernel. Visual inspection has not shown boundary effects. With this approach, we do not construct the full covariance matrix Σ anymore, so that we cannot apply the similarity measure in Eq. (10). We consider only the diagonal entries of the covariance matrix Σ_{xx} and neglect the first term in Eq. (10), yielding

$$\log p(I, J; T, \sigma_I, \sigma_J, l) \approx - \sum_{x \in \Omega_I} \frac{(I(x) - \boldsymbol{\mu}_J(x))^2}{2 \cdot \Sigma_{xx}}. \tag{11}$$

We use this similarity measure in combination with block-wise estimation. For constant variances Σ_{xx}, this corresponds to the common sum of squared differences (SSD).

To make the concept of uncertainty estimation in interpolation easy to integrate in existing applications, we propose an approximation for the variance values Σ_{xx} without performing GP regression. In this case, we use classic interpolation methods to construct the resampled image. Considering the covariance matrix in Eq. (3), we see that it only depends on the *locations* of the observations and predictions, but not on the observed values. We use the interpolation weights, as defined in linear interpolation, to approximate the elementwise variance values Σ_{xx}. We consider the prediction for a point $\mathbf{x}^*$ on the regular grid with spacing $\mathbf{s}$ and let $\mathbf{d} = \mathbf{x}^* - \mathbf{x}$ be the difference vector to the closest point on the base grid $\mathbf{x}$. We approximate the variance at location x^* with

$$v(\mathbf{x}^*) = \sum_{i=1}^{D} |d_i| \cdot (s_i - |d_i|), \tag{12}$$

where D is the dimensionality of the image. $v(\mathbf{x}^*)$ is the highest for locations that are equidistant from the base grid nodes, and zero when $\mathbf{x}^*$ lies on the base grid. We illustrate the variances for the approximation and the Gaussian process in 1D and 2D in the supplementary material, which shows that the approximation closely follows the true estimates from the Gaussian process.

There are two important parameters that affect the interpolation; the noise variance σ_J^2 and the length-scale l of the kernel. If we set $\sigma_J^2 = 0$, the interpolator passes exactly through the observations. For $\sigma_J^2 > 0$, the method accepts noise in the observations so that the images can deviate from the observations. The length-scale determines the region of influence of each observation. For shorter length-scale, the prediction is only dependent on a few observations, causing more sensitive results. For larger length-scale, we obtain smoother results. Noise reduction and smoothing are common pre-processing steps for image registration and they can be naturally modeled within the proposed Gaussian process framework. Finally, the interpolation on irregular grids does not pose problems because the method depends on pairwise distances between points only.

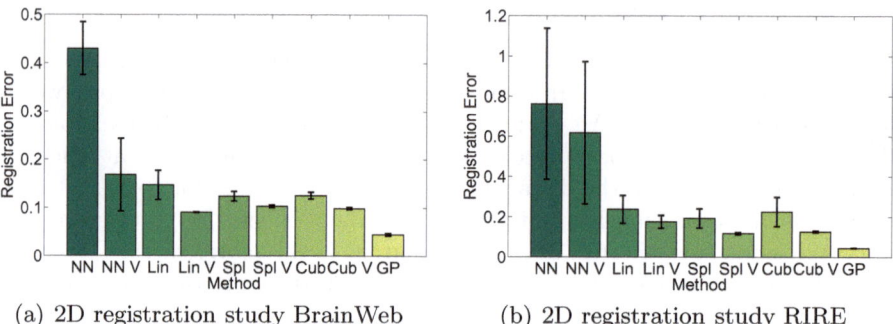

(a) 2D registration study BrainWeb   (b) 2D registration study RIRE

Fig. 3. Bars indicate mean registration error; error bars show standard error. Nearest neighbor (NN), Linear (Lin), Spline (Spl), Cubic (Cub), and Gaussian Process (GP) interpolation is reported. The use of the variance approximation is indicated with 'V'.

3   Results

In our registration experiments, we focus on a rigid transformation model. This choice allows us to better isolate the effects of image interpolation in registration, which is the contribution of this work. Moreover, rigid registration enables exact computation of registration errors with respect to ground truth transformations on real data, which is challenging for transformation models with more degrees of freedom. We perform the first set of registration experiments on the publicly available BrainWeb [2] and RIRE [3] datasets. We set $\sigma_I^2 = \sigma_J^2 = 0.1$ in all experiments. First, we select axial slices and perform 2D registration. We downsample the images in one direction by a factor of 5 to simulate anisotropic data. Such anisotropy is commonly present in clinical practice. We transform the grid and create the fixed image by downsampling the original image. For this 2D registration experiment, we can calculate the GP interpolation ($l = 2.5$) without splitting the image into blocks. Consequently, we use the similarity measure in Eq. (10) with the full covariance matrix. For comparison, we perform nearest neighbor, linear, cubic, and spline interpolation with SSD as a similarity measure. Moreover, we compute the approximated variance in Eq. (12) and use it in the similarity measures in Eq. (11), indicated with 'V' in the plots. The mean image μ_J from the Gaussian process regression is replaced by the nearest neighbor, linear, cubic, or spline interpolator in this case. Fig. 3 shows results over 50 runs from random initial transformations.

In a second experiment, we perform 3D experiments on the BrainWeb and RIRE datasets. Again we downsample the images in one direction by a factor of 5, to create anisotropic volumes. For the Gaussian process interpolation ($l = 2.5$), we split the image into $8 \times 8 \times 8$ cubes to limit the computational costs. Since we do not construct the entire covariance matrix Σ_J in this case, we work with a diagonal covariance matrix in the similarity measure in Eq. (10). The evaluation of the baseline methods with SSD and the variance approximation is analogous to the 2D experiment. Fig. 4 reports the mean RMS errors and standard errors.

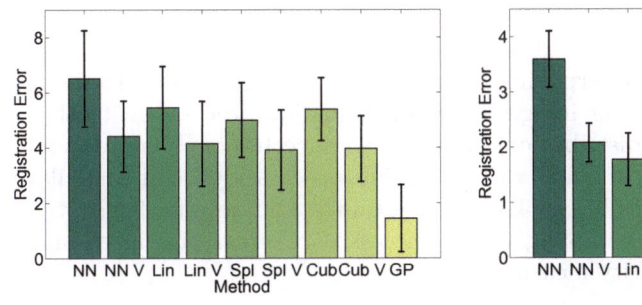

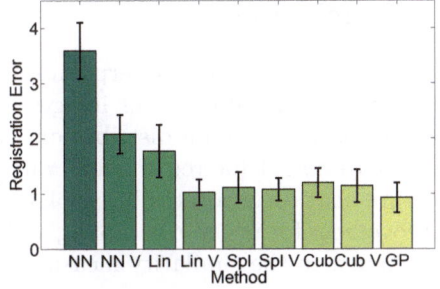

(a) 3D registration study BrainWeb   (b) 3D registration study RIRE

Fig. 4. Bars indicate mean registration error; error bars show standard error. Nearest neighbor (NN), Linear (Lin), Spline (Spl), Cubic (Cub), and Gaussian Process (GP) interpolation is reported. The use of the variance approximation is indicated with 'V'.

The final datatset consists of two MR images of the head that were acquired on two different grids in the MR scanner with a resolution of $3 \times 3 \times 3.6\text{mm}^3$. The primary slice direction is sagittal for the first image and axial for the second scan. We can access the transformation of each image with respect to the scanner coordinate system. Conse-

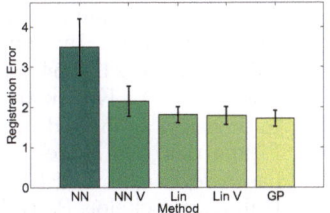

quently, the ground truth transformation in our rigid registration experiments that relates both volumes is available. The registration is repeated 50 times for each configuration. The mean RMS errors and standard errors are plotted in the figure on the right. We compare to the nearest neighbor and linear interpolation. For the Gaussian process interpolation ($l = 2.5$), we divide the image into $8 \times 8 \times 8$ cubes to limit the computational costs. Again, we only use the variance model and not the full covariance matrix Σ_J.

Our results show a large decrease in registration error for more complex interpolation techniques than nearest neighbor interpolation. The decrease from linear interpolation to cubic or spline interpolation is less pronounced. Spline interpolation leads to the best registration results among the classical interpolation schemes. In all experiments, using uncertainty estimates in the similarity measure leads to more accurate registration results. The improvement is largest for nearest neighbor interpolation, where the interpolation quality decreases the most when moving further away from the grid points. This finding is interesting for the registration of categorical or label data, where more complex interpolation methods cannot be applied. For the other interpolation schemes, we also notice a substantial improvement for the uncertainty estimate, especially for linear interpolation. Registration with Gaussian processes achieved the best performance in all experiments. This supports the use of the mean function as high quality interpolator and the covariance matrix as uncertainty estimate for registration.

4   Conclusion

We proposed to integrate interpolation uncertainty into registration. To this end, we defined distributions over images based on Gaussian processes with the covariance of the posterior distribution serving as an uncertainty estimate. A novel generative model for registration with Gaussian processes yielded a similarity measure that incorporates interpolation uncertainty. Our results demonstrated improvement for image resampling and the necessity of integrating interpolation uncertainty in the similarity measure.

Acknowledgements. This work was supported in part by the Humboldt foundation, the National Alliance for Medical Image Computing (U54-EB005149), the NeuroImaging Analysis Center (P41-EB015902) and the National Center for Image-Guided Therapy (P41-EB015898).

References

1. Aljabar, P., Hajnal, J., Boyes, R., Rueckert, D.: Interpolation artefacts in non-rigid registration. In: Duncan, J.S., Gerig, G. (eds.) MICCAI 2005, Part II. LNCS, vol. 3750, pp. 247–254. Springer, Heidelberg (2005)
2. Cocosco, C.A., Kollokian, V., Kwan, R.S., Evans, A.C.: Brainweb: Online interface to a 3d mri simulated brain database. NeuroImage 5(4) (May 1997)
3. Fitzpatrick, J.M., West, J.B., Maurer, C.R.: Predicting error in rigid-body point-based registration. IEEE Transactions on Medical Imaging 17(5), 694–702 (1998)
4. Hill, D., Batchelor, P., Holden, M., Hawkes, D.: Medical image registration. Physics in Medicine and Biology 46(3) (2001)
5. Hou, H., Andrews, H.: Cubic splines for image interpolation and digital filtering. IEEE Trans. on Acoustics, Speech and Signal Processing 26(6), 508–517 (1978)
6. Kim, K., Lee, D., Essa, I.: Gaussian process regression flow for analysis of motion trajectories. In: Int. Conference on Computer Vision, pp. 1164–1171 (2011)
7. Lehmann, T., Gonner, C., Spitzer, K.: Survey: Interpolation methods in medical image processing. IEEE Transactions on Medical Imaging 18(11), 1049–1075 (1999)
8. Liu, P.: Using Gaussian Process Regression to Denoise Images and Remove Artefacts from Microarray Data. Ph.D. thesis, University of Toronto (2007)
9. Lüthi, M., Jud, C., Vetter, T.: Using landmarks as a deformation prior for hybrid image registration. In: Mester, R., Felsberg, M. (eds.) DAGM 2011. LNCS, vol. 6835, pp. 196–205. Springer, Heidelberg (2011)
10. Parker, J., Kenyon, R., Troxel, D.: Comparison of interpolating methods for image resampling. IEEE Transactions on Medical Imaging 2(1), 31–39 (1983)
11. Rasmussen, C., Williams, C.: Gaussian processes for machine learning. MIT Press (2006)
12. Sollich, P., Williams, C.K.I.: Using the equivalent kernel to understand gaussian process regression. In: Neural Inform. Processing Systems, pp. 1313–1320 (2005)
13. Stytz, M.R., Parrott, R.W.: Using kriging for 3d medical imaging. Computerized Medical Imaging and Graphics 17(6), 421–442 (1993)
14. Thévenaz, P., Blu, T., Unser, M.: Image interpolation and resampling. In: Handbook of Medical Imaging, Processing and Analysis, pp. 393–420 (2000)
15. Wachinger, C., Sharp, G.C., Golland, P.: Contour-driven regression for label inference in atlas-based segmentation. In: Mori, K., Sakuma, I., Sato, Y., Barillot, C., Navab, N. (eds.) MICCAI 2013, Part III. LNCS, vol. 8151, pp. 211–218. Springer, Heidelberg (2013)

Hough Space Parametrization: Ensuring Global Consistency in Intensity-Based Registration

Mehmet Yigitsoy, Javad Fotouhi, and Nassir Navab

Computer Aided Medical Procedures (CAMP), TUM,
Munich, Germany
{yigitsoy,fotouhi,navab}@cs.tum.edu

Abstract. Intensity based registration is a challenge when images to be registered have insufficient amount of information in their overlapping region. Especially, in the absence of dominant structures such as strong edges in this region, obtaining a solution that satisfies global structural consistency becomes difficult. In this work, we propose to exploit the vast amount of available information beyond the overlapping region to support the registration process. To this end, a novel global regularization term using Generalized Hough Transform is designed that ensures the global consistency when the local information in the overlap region is insufficient to drive the registration. Using prior data, we learn a parametrization of the target anatomy in Hough space. This parametrization is then used as a regularization for registering the observed partial images without using any prior data. Experiments on synthetic as well as on sample real medical images demonstrate the good performance and potential use of the proposed concept.

1 Introduction

Intensity based image registration is often challenging when images to be registered have insufficient amount of information in their overlapping region. Classical registration approaches are bounded to use only the overlapping region since they use intensity correspondences or statistical relationships. Especially, in the absence of relevant structures such as strong edges in this region, assessing the local image similarity alone becomes inadequate, leading to an ill-posed registration problem. It is often the case in ultrasound (US) imaging that the acoustic window of the transducer is limited; therefore, to capture a large field of view, several acquisitions are needed where partial images have to be then stitched together [13]. However, due to the typical imaging artifacts inherent to US, the information in the overlapping region is often not salient enough for an image based compounding.

Figs. 1(a)-1(b) show a case where two US images of the liver with little overlap need to be registered. Obviously, most intensity-based registration methods would fail here due to the limited information in the overlap to drive the registration process. On the other hand, there is a rich amount of information beyond the overlap which can support the registration.

P. Golland et al. (Eds.): MICCAI 2014, Part I, LNCS 8673, pp. 275–282, 2014.

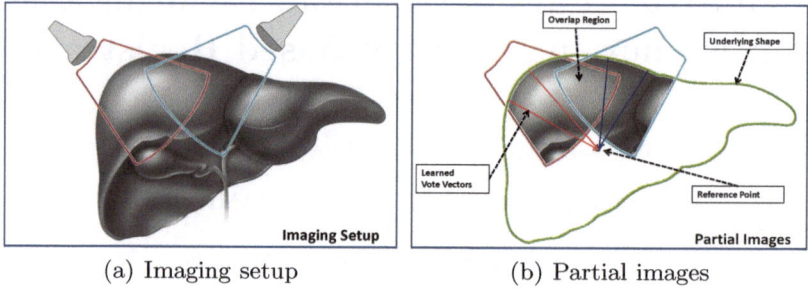

(a) Imaging setup   (b) Partial images

Fig. 1. (a) An illustration of the possible imaging setup where partial images may have limited overlap. (b) Given that the shape is known, dominant structures from non-overlapping regions can be utilized for regularization.

To alleviate this issue, acquisitions can be done such that there are large overlaps between partial images as done in [8] which obviously needs more time and effort. Similarly, methods based on matching extracted features [9] as well as patch-based voting schemes [7] require sufficient amount of overlap between images. Another typical approach is to augment the registration using previous data such as computed tomography (CT) scans [5] where each partial image is registered to the prior as well as to other partial images. For this approach to work, however, a previous scan of the same patient has to be readily available, which is often not the case. In the absence of previous scans, other prior data such as anatomical atlases are used for registration. Although it is possible to have good registration results using atlases, an explicit use of the intensity distribution of an atlas biases registration towards the chosen reference, making it inflexible and necessitating additional regularization. Recently, a method seeking for a consistent alignment of structures beyond overlapping region was proposed in [14]. The method, however, provides only local smoothness; thus, it cannot be generalized as a global regularization constraint.

All the previously mentioned approaches will have difficulties when the overlap size is small, non-salient or no prior data is given, therefore, they cannot ensure global consistency. In this work, we propose not to use prior data explicitly, but we learn a global parametrization $\mathcal{P}$ of the anatomy in question. To this end, we use Generalized Hough Transform (GHT) [1] to learn $\mathcal{P}_H$ of the target anatomy in the Hough space. GHT has the favorable property of being robust to partial occlusions and noise which we exploit here to enable global regularization for intensity based registration. Coupled with local similarity, $\mathcal{P}_H$ will serve as a regularization to ensure global consistency while registering partially overlapping images.

2   Methods

Generalized Hough Transform: Hough Transform was originally proposed for lines and edges, but later it was extended to other analytical shapes. Finally,

GHT was introduced as an extension where any arbitrary shape can be used as the prior for object detection [1]. GHT parametrizes a shape with the offsets of each shape element from a reference point. This parametrization is stored in a look-up table, so-called R-Table. This table is later used for detection where elements in a target image vote for the hypotheses that might have generated them. The peaks in the Hough space created by accumulating such votes correspond to parameters (such as the chosen reference point) of possible target object.

There is an ever increasing number of applications of GHT and its voting scheme in computer vision including object classification [6], detection [2] and tracking [3] to name a few. However, it has fewer applications in intensity based image registration where there is a large potential of usage. In [12], GHT was used to estimate the initial pose of intraoperative images where possible poses of target object are learned a priori. [10] addresses the initialization of intensity based rigid registration by using standard Hough Transform on gradient fields. To the best of our knowledge, GHT has not been used for global regularization of intensity based registration.

Global Consistency Measure: A Hough space parametrization $\mathcal{P}_H$ is learned from prior data such as previous scans, statistical shape models or atlases. Following the traditional Hough-like voting framework, using $\mathcal{P}_H$, the voting elements[1] in partial images vote for the hypotheses in a Hough space. Finally, a global consistency measure (GCM) is inferred from the resulting distribution. Various types of voting elements can be used ranging from edge pixels to more complex features such as keypoints or image patches [2]. Here, for the proof of concept, only edge pixels are considered as voting elements which can be extracted via standard edge detection methods such as Canny.

Let $\mathbf{I} = \left\{ I_i : \Omega_i \rightarrow \mathbb{R}, \Omega_i \subset \mathbb{N}^N \right\}_{i=1}^n$ be n partial images to be registered, N being the image dimension. Furthermore, let Ω_c be the common spatial domain of partial images and $\mathbf{T} = \left\{ T_i : \mathbf{x}_c \mapsto \mathbf{x}_i, |\mathbf{x}_i, \mathbf{x}_c \in \mathbb{R}^N \right\}_{i=1}^n$ be the corresponding transformations parametrized by $\mathbf{p} = \{p_i\}_{i=1}^n$, which, when optimal, will bring partial images into spatial alignment. Finally, we define Hough images $\mathbf{H} = \left\{ H_i(\mathbf{x}|I_i, p_i, \mathcal{P}_H) : \Omega_h \rightarrow \mathbb{R}, \Omega_h \subset \mathbb{N}^M \right\}_{i=1}^n$ where M is the dimensionality of Hough space.

In this work, the sum of pairwise distances between the maxima in Hough images is considered as the GCM. Using the same Hough space size for each partial image, the goal is to bring the strongest hypotheses into a cluster. We define GCM on the joint Hough space as

$$GCM(\mathbf{I}, \mathbf{p}, \mathcal{P}_H) = \frac{2}{n(n-1)} \sum_{i=1}^n \sum_{j=i+1}^n \left\| \arg\max_{\mathbf{h}_i} H_i(\mathbf{h}_i) - \arg\max_{\mathbf{h}_j} H_j(\mathbf{h}_j) \right\| \quad (1)$$

where $H_k(\mathbf{h}_k) = H_k(\mathbf{h}_k|I_k, p_k, \mathcal{P}_H)$, $\mathbf{h}$ is a hypothesis and $\arg\max$ locates the strongest hypothesis in the Hough image. The goal here is then to minimize the

---

[1] The elements do not have to be necessarily in the overlapping region which is one of the key idea behind this work.

GCM by clustering the peaks. This measure will be then coupled with a local intensity-based similarity term.

Registration: We define the local similarity measure (LSM) in terms of intensities as

$$LSM(\mathbf{I}, \mathbf{p}) = \frac{2}{n(n-1)} \sum_{k=1}^{|\Omega_c|} \sum_{i=1}^{n} \sum_{j=i+1}^{n} \xi(I_i(T_{p_i}^{-1}(\mathbf{x}_k)), I_j(T_{p_j}^{-1}(\mathbf{x}_k))) \qquad (2)$$

with T_{p_i} being the parametrization of T_i by p_i. Finally, we pose the alignment of all partial images as an optimization problem such that optimal transformations $\mathbf{T}$ optimizes an energy $\mathcal{E}$. Optimal parameters $\mathbf{p}$ then can be estimated via the following equation

$$\hat{\mathbf{p}} = \arg\min_{\mathbf{p}} \mathcal{E}(\mathbf{p}|\mathbf{I}, \mathcal{P}_H) \quad \text{with} \quad \mathcal{E}(\mathbf{p}|\mathbf{I}, \mathcal{P}_H) = LSM(\mathbf{I}, \mathbf{p}) + e^{GCM(\mathbf{I}, \mathbf{p}, \mathcal{P}_H) - \rho}.$$

$$(3)$$

LSM serves as a data fidelity term evaluated in the overlapping region, whereas the exponential term is a global regularization evaluated in the Hough space. ρ is a constant controlling the amount of regularization based on the uncertainty in GCM. The choice of ρ depends on the resolution of the Hough space as well as on the image content. For large Hough images, there is more uncertainty regarding the maxima in the Hough space, therefore, inconsistent local alignments should be penalized less. Similarly, object deformations cause dispersion in Hough space, thus, leading to an increased uncertainty.

The data term $\xi(\cdot)$ can be chosen according to the modalities being registered. In this paper, we use Normalized Cross Correlation (NCC). We also assume that the optimal transformations $\mathbf{T}$ are only rigid, leading to 3D Hough images. For the optimization of Eq. 3, Nelder-Mead Simplex algorithm as part of the NLopt package [4] is used.

3   Experimental Validation and Results

We have conducted experiments on synthetic and real images. For all experiments, we used 500 iterations for the optimizer and set ρ to 10 and 50 for synthetic and real experiments respectively. Through the synthetic experiments, we analyzed the robustness of our approach to the size of overlap and to the varying degrees of imaging noise. For this purpose, a binary image with 400x190 pixels size containing a shape was used as a template to learn the object. Two partially overlapping images are extracted from the same shape as the observed images (cf. Fig. 2(a)). Note that if the shape information is not utilized, a registration method will be insensitive to the horizontal translations in the overlapping region to a certain extent. Therefore, this synthetic experiment will also show the need for regularization when there is no global optimum in terms of intensity correspondences. The goal in this experiment is to reconstruct the same geometry starting from a randomly chosen initial relative positioning of partial images within a specified range.

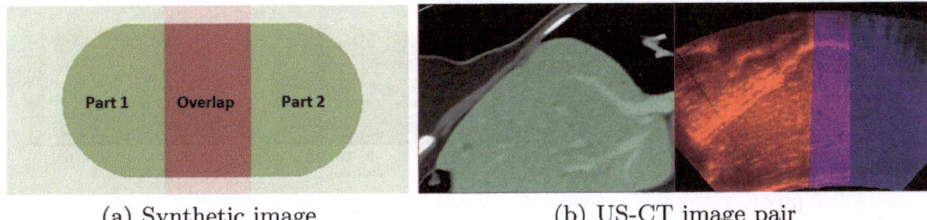

(a) Synthetic image   (b) US-CT image pair

Fig. 2. (a) An arbitrary shape and sample selection of partial images for experiments. (b) Used US-CT pair with CT segmentation overlayed on CT (left) and registered partially overlapping US images (right) where the overlapping region is highlighted.

Starting from a full overlap of objects in the partial images, we varied the overlap size by increments of 10% of the image width till we get a -60% overlap, which is a gap of size 60% of the image width. For each overlap size, we added uniform noise by varying its maximum relative to the the image dynamic range. For each overlap size and noise level, we applied 20 combinations of initial rigid transformations with translations and rotations chosen from $[-200, 200]$ pixels and $[-50, 50]$ degrees respectively. For evaluation, we warped the original partial images before adding noise using the optimal transformations and compared to the corresponding part of the original full image using Dice score. For comparison, we have conducted the same experiment without using the GCM. Results using GCM shown in Figs. 3(a)-(b) compared to Figs. 3(c)-(d) without GCM indicate the robustness of the method to varying degrees of noise as well as its good performance even in the presence of a gap. It is clear that usage of GCM improves the capture range of cost function and avoids undesired local optima.

In order to demonstrate the performance on real images, we performed an experiment where we took a pair of slices, each having 512x384 resolution with a pixel spacing 0.45mm, from a co-registered US-CT pair corresponding to the liver area. Then, we used the segmented CT for learning the parametrization $\mathcal{P}_H$ and cut the US image into two partially overlapping sub-images as shown in Fig. 2(b) which were used to reconstruct the original US image. The size of the overlap was about 15% of the original image size. We applied random initial rigid transformations in a range around the optimum where 50 combinations of translations and rotations were randomly sampled from $[-100, 100]$ pixels relative to the optimum and $[-30, 30]$ degrees respectively. For the evaluation of each case, we warped the segmentations of partial images and compared with the segmentation of the uncut US image using Dice score. Mean, median and STD values with and without using GCM were recorded as 0.95, 0.99, 0.07 and 0.48, 0.45, 0.34, respectively. Results shown in Fig. 4(a) support our previous observations in terms of robustness. Moreover, we calculated the scores with respect to changing uncertainty parameter ρ in Eq. 3 by varying it from 0 to 100. Fig. 4(b) shows that large values of uncertainty lead to a degradation of performance which is expected due to the reduced amount of regularization. This is also valid for small values resulting in a very strict regularization, thus, making it sensitive to the errors in detecting strongest hypotheses.

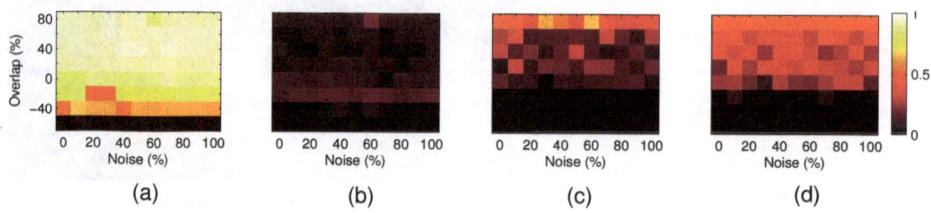

Fig. 3. Performance evaluation against noise and the amount of overlap using synthetic images. (a)-(b) Dice score and its standard deviation (STD) using GCM. (c)-(d) Dice score and STD without using GCM. A negative overlap value indicates a gap between images. It is clear from (a) that the method is robust to noise and can tolerate even gaps between the images. Whereas, without GCM, Dice score is very low with a high STD even when the overlap is sufficient and it is not possible to register with a gap.

For further evaluation in terms of Target Registration Error (TRE), we used 16 pairs of landmarks manually extracted from the overlapping region. The same experiments were repeated by using US and CT segmentations as well as their slightly deformed versions respectively for learning $\mathcal{P}_H$. As seen from Fig. 4(c), the best median TRE (8.46 pixels) was obtained by using CT for learning followed by using US (13.38 pixels). There were small degradations in each case when their deformed versions were used for learning, indicating the tolerance of the method to small deformations. A median error of 127.88 pixels was obtained when GCM was not employed. Obviously, most of the registrations without using GCM failed due to the small size of the overlap and the sensitivity to the initial parameters indicating a very limited capture range of the cost function. The slightly worse performance when using US compared to CT is due to the speckle and shadows in US images leading to false edges, thus, more uncertainty.

4   Discussion

The proposed concept differs from model based segmentation and registration methods in that we do not make any explicit use of prior data. We only learn a parametrization to employ it later for registering partial images which differentiates it also from the model-to-image alignment methods [11]. Therefore, once the parametrization is learned, the full intensity distribution of the prior image is not required for registration.

GCM term does not depend on the modality at hand as long as features required for the GHT can be extracted from the images. This makes the proposed framework suitable also for multi-modal applications. Theoretically, as prior data, it is possible to use 1) a different modality, 2) an image of the slightly deformed target anatomy, 3) a statistical shape model for learning the parametrization. This is one of the key features of the proposed concept allowing flexibility in model based reconstruction. Note that we are not making any comparison to the atlas based registration techniques. Here, we propose an alternative concept with its own advantages.

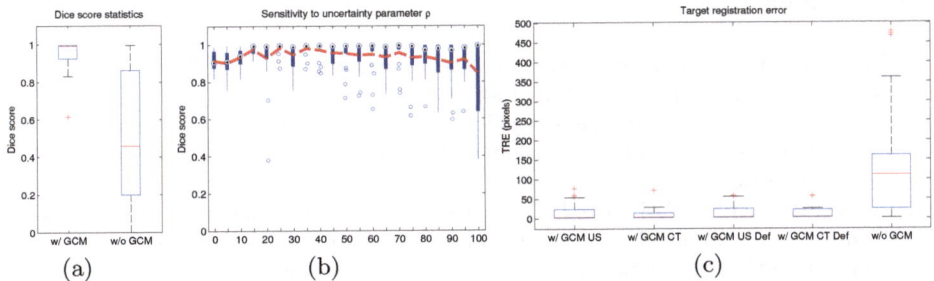

Fig. 4. Evaluation on US images. (a) Dice scores with and without using GCM. (b) Sensitivity analysis with respect to the changing uncertainty parameter (x-axis) in Eq. 3. Dashed line represents the mean value. (c) TREs when US(w/ GCM US), CT(w/ GCM CT), deformed US (w/ GCM US Def) and CT (w/ GCM CT Def) are used for learning. The last one is when GCM is not used at all.

We did not employ any sophisticated techniques for finding modes in the Hough space, emphasizing the simplicity of the proposed concept. Nevertheless, it is possible to augment the proposed Hough space parametrization approach by using advanced voting and mode finding techniques such as the ones used in computer vision applications. Here, a minimal implementation of the concept and its key features are presented through a proof-of-concept study.

The classical GHT is invariant to rotations and isotropic scaling of the object and tolerates small deformations which was confirmed by our experiments using slightly deformed segmentations for learning. However, it still cannot handle large deformations. This limitation, however, can be relaxed by employing large training datasets in the learning phase in a decision trees framework [3]. As future work, we will extend the proposed method by posing it as a regression problem and by solving it in a random forest framework. This will allow us to employ higher order features as voting elements [2]. Finally, using higher order transformations such as affine and deformable as well as mosaicing in 3D will be the immediate extensions of the proposed concept.

5   Conclusion

In this work, we have proposed a novel global regularization term using Generalized Hough Transform (GHT). It is used as a Global Consistency Measure (GCM) in intensity-based registration when the local information in the overlap of partial images is insufficient or corrupted. A Hough space parametrization of the target anatomy is learned from prior data such as previous scan, atlas or statistical shape model. This parametrization enables a global consistency voting through local information. The proposed concept is fully parallelizable and suited for reconstructing sparsely sampled scenes. Through experiments on synthetic and real images, it was shown that using GCM improves the registration quality when the partial images have less in common in their overlap.

References

1. Ballard, D.H.: Generalizing the hough transform to detect arbitrary shapes. Pattern Recognition 13(2), 111–122 (1981)
2. Gall, J., Lempitsky, V.: Class-specific hough forests for object detection. In: Decision Forests for Computer Vision and Medical Image Analysis, pp. 143–157. Springer (2013)
3. Godec, M., Roth, P.M., Bischof, H.: Hough-based tracking of non-rigid objects. Computer Vision and Image Understanding 117(10), 1245–1256 (2013)
4. Johnson, S.G.: The nlopt nonlinear-optimization package,
http://ab-initio.mit.edu/wiki/index.php/NLopt
(accessed February 21, 2014)
5. Kutter, O., Wein, W., Navab, N.: Multi-modal registration based ultrasound mosaicing. In: Yang, G.-Z., Hawkes, D., Rueckert, D., Noble, A., Taylor, C. (eds.) MICCAI 2009, Part I. LNCS, vol. 5761, pp. 763–770. Springer, Heidelberg (2009)
6. Leibe, B., Leonardis, A., Schiele, B.: Combined object categorization and segmentation with an implicit shape model. In: Workshop on Statistical Learning in Computer Vision (ECCV) (May 2004)
7. Ourselin, S., Roche, A., Prima, S., Ayache, N.: Block matching: A general framework to improve robustness of rigid registration of medical images. In: Delp, S.L., DiGoia, A.M., Jaramaz, B. (eds.) MICCAI 2000. LNCS, vol. 1935, pp. 557–566. Springer, Heidelberg (2000)
8. Øye, O., Wein, W., Ulvang, D., Matre, K., Viola, I.: Real time image-based tracking of 4d ultrasound data. In: Ayache, N., Delingette, H., Golland, P., Mori, K. (eds.) MICCAI 2012, Part I. LNCS, vol. 7510, pp. 447–454. Springer, Heidelberg (2012)
9. Schneider, R.J., Perrin, D.P., Vasilyev, N.V., Marx, G.R., del Nido, P.J., Howe, R.D.: Real-time image-based rigid registration of three-dimensional ultrasound. Medical Image Analysis 16(2), 402–414 (2012)
10. Shams, R., Barnes, N., Hartley, R.: Image registration in hough space using gradient of images. In: 9th Biennial Conference of the Australian Pattern Recognition Society on Digital Image Computing Techniques and Applications, pp. 226–232. IEEE (2007)
11. Toews, M., Wells III, W.M.: Efficient and robust model-to-image alignment using 3d scale-invariant features. Medical Image Analysis 17(3), 271–282 (2013)
12. Varnavas, A., Carrell, T., Penney, G.: Fully automated initialisation of 2D-3D image registration. In: 2013 IEEE 10th International Symposium on Biomedical Imaging (ISBI), pp. 568–571. IEEE (2013)
13. Wachinger, C., Wein, W., Navab, N.: Three-dimensional ultrasound mosaicing. In: Ayache, N., Ourselin, S., Maeder, A. (eds.) MICCAI 2007, Part II. LNCS, vol. 4792, pp. 327–335. Springer, Heidelberg (2007)
14. Yigitsoy, M., Navab, N.: Structure propagation for image registration. IEEE Transactions on Medical Imaging 32(9), 1657–1670 (2013)

2D/3D Registration of TEE Probe from Two Non-orthogonal C-Arm Directions

Markus Kaiser[1,2,3], Matthias John[3], Tobias Heimann[4], Alexander Brost[4],
Thomas Neumuth[1], and Georg Rose[2]

[1] Innovation Center Computer Assisted Surgery (ICCAS), Leipzig, Germany
[2] Otto von Guericke University, Magdeburg, Germany
[3] Siemens AG, Healthcare Sector, Forchheim, Germany
[4] Siemens AG, Corporate Technology, Imaging and Computer Vision,
Erlangen, Germany

Abstract. 2D/3D registration is a well known technique in medical imaging for combining pre-operative volume data with live fluoroscopy. A common issue of this type of algorithms is that out-of-plane parameters are hard to determine. One solution to overcome this issue is the use of X-ray images from two angulations. However, performing in-plane transformation in one image destroys the registration in the other image, particularly if the angulations are smaller than 90 degrees apart. Our main contribution is the automation of a novel registration approach. It handles translation and rotation of a volume in a way that in-plane parameters are kept invariant and independent of the angle offset between both projections in a double-oblique setting. Our approach yields more robust and partially faster registration results, compared to conventional methods, especially in case of object movement. It was successfully tested on clinical data for fusion of transesophageal ultrasound and X-ray.

Keywords: 2D/3D registration, X-ray & Ultrasound fusion.

1 Introduction

2D/3D registration is a key technology for image-guided medical interventions [1]. The ability to combine pre-operative clinical volume data sets and live fluoroscopy from a C-arm supports physicians during interventions and paves the way for novel procedures and workflows [2]. Usually, a CT or MRI volume is registered to C-arm X-ray images to provide additional anatomical information. Recently, different 2D/3D registration based systems were introduced, e.g. the registration of a transesophageal echocardiogram (TEE) ultrasound probe to X-ray images to track the device and to use it as indirect registration for the other live imaging modality [3]. Our presented registration framework targets the same clinical application. We adapted the approach of [3], combined it with a new method for parameter estimation and a new TEE probe prototype (Siemens AG, Healthcare Sector, Mountain View, CA, USA), shown in Fig.1.

In general, 2D/3D registration is an iterative process, where the six spatial parameters S of a 3D volume (translations (t_x, t_y, t_z) and rotations yaw, pitch

P. Golland et al. (Eds.): MICCAI 2014, Part I, LNCS 8673, pp. 283–290, 2014.
© Springer International Publishing Switzerland 2014

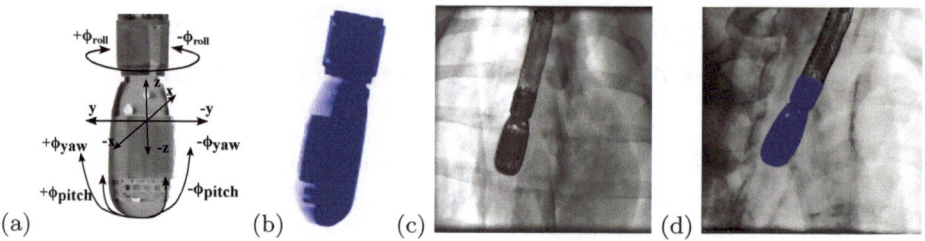

Fig. 1. (a) CT volume of the TEE probe prototype with object axes. (b) DRR of the TEE probe volume. (c) TEE probe under fluoroscopic X-ray. (d) Registered TEE probe with overlayed DRR from another C-arm angle.

and roll (ϕ_y, ϕ_p, ϕ_r)) are estimated by an optimizer until the projection of the 3D data is correctly aligned with the current image. A digitial reconstructed radiograph (DRR) is generated after each adaptation of the parameter set. This DRR is compared with the X-ray image by a similarity measure. Due to the projective characteristic of a C-arm system, S can be separated into in-plane and out-of-plane parameters. In-plane parameter transformation (t_x, t_z, ϕ_y) is parallel to the detector plane (i.e. the projected image). Therefore, a change in such a parameter can cause a significant image change and is easier to estimate. Changes in out-of-plane parameters like depth (t_y) or pitch (ϕ_p) and roll (ϕ_r) cause an object shift perpendicular to the image plane, which is more difficult to identify. Typically, there are two ways of registering multi-plane images.

1. Full 3D: all six spatial parameters are registered simultaneously along the object axes like in [3]. The optimizer will not distinguish between in-plane and out-of-plane parameters.
2. Subdivided in-plane: The decoupling of in- and out-of-plane parameters can be of major importance, particularly when registering on multi-plane system. The objects' in-plane parameters are registered alternately between both imaging planes. One can dramatically increase accuracy and capture range while registering only the in-plane parameters for each plane [4][5].

In a common biplane setup, the detector planes have a rotational offset of 90 degrees. Therefore, in-plane parameters of the first image become out-of-plane parameters in the second image and vice versa. Only one rotational parameter will always remain out-of-plane. In this work, we do not necessarily refer to a biplane C-arm system, but use images from a monoplane system from two angulations acquired consecutively. Since the TEE probe is in a fixed position for longer periods, performing imaging from a second angulation is a reasonable workflow, in particular for small angle offsets. Due to space constraints in hybrid operating rooms and catheter labs, orthogonal multi-plane imaging can be difficult to achieve. This leads to projection angle differences smaller than 90 degrees. The position of a C-arm system is defined by two angles, one for left-anterior-oblique and right-anterior-oblique given as α, and the second one for cranial-caudal as γ. The indices $_A$ and $_B$ are used to indicate the two

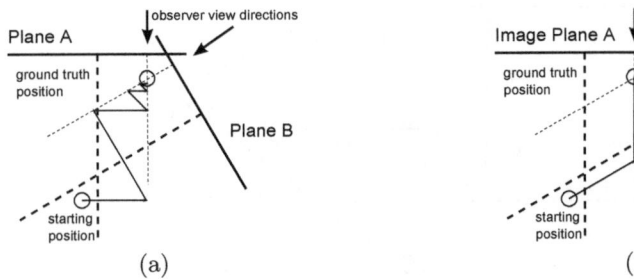

Fig. 2. (a) illustrates the in-plane approach and (b) the planar approach

different C-arm angles. If only one angle is changed between two images, this refers to a mono-oblique, otherwise to a double-oblique setting. In this work, we are considering the setup given by

$$\forall \alpha, \gamma : |\alpha_A - \alpha_B| \leq 90° \wedge |\gamma_A - \gamma_B| \leq 90°. \tag{1}$$

The drawback of a non-orthogonal setting is that the in-plane registration strategy results in an iterative process like in Fig. 2(a). Depending on the projection angles, this can have a significant influence on registration accuracy and runtime.

To resolve this issue, we improved the in-plane strategy to a planar approach. This approach keeps in-plane parameters invariant to the registration on the other image plane and establishes a one-step movement like illustrated in Fig. 2(b). The main idea is to transform the 3D object without disrupting previous in-plane registration results. For each view, only in-plane parameters t_x, t_z, ϕ_y are changed, while out-of-plane information is used from the other plane.

We employed the method in an automatic multi-plane image-based 2D/3D registration system for fusion of TEE ultrasound and X-ray. Our approach, which was basically introduced for manual registration in [6], is not limited to this application and could be used for various purposes.

2   Methods

Our approach is object-centerline-driven which initially lies in the cranial-caudal direction. Therefore, the rotation ϕ_r around the centerline c remains out-of-plane from both views. Aligning the other parameters correctly along the centerline will reduce the search space for ϕ_r.

In our setup, we have two image planes I_A and I_B, which are the detector planes of the C-arm in two different views. All object translations and rotations in one image are bound to the spanning plane of the other image. See Fig. 3 for an illustration. Considering I_A for example, every transformation is restricted by the plane P_B spanned by the focus eye_B and the centerline c. P_B is defined by its normal vector n_B as

$$n_B = (eye_B - m_{p_B}) \times (eye_B - c_{p_B}). \tag{2}$$

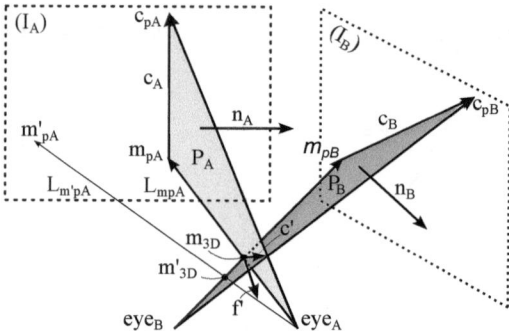

Fig. 3. Schema for multi-plane transformation

If the object is moved on I_A from image coordinate m_{pA} to a new one m'_{pA}, the new 3D position m'_{3D} of the object is determined by plane-line-intersection of plane P_B and line $L_{m'_{pA}}$. This ensures that the position of the object is changed for I_A, but is not influencing the independent translational in-plane parameters in I_B.

The vectors c_A and c_B that determine the in-plane yaw are obtained directly in the 2D image plane when projecting the centerline vector c of the object onto the image plane. Every yaw rotation ϕ_y is carried out in 2D by calculating the vector between the projected object center point m_p and the projected object point in center line direction c_p as

$$c_p = m_p + [sin(\phi_y), 0, cos(\phi_y)]. \tag{3}$$

The center line vector c' is thus defined by the intersection of planes P_A and P_B, which ensures that the yaw in I_B stays fixed even when the yaw in I_A is changed. The angle ϕ_p is not changed by the optimizer, but determined via n_B from I_B. The plane normal n_A determines the objects' 3D yaw rotation. The new rotation matrix R of the object is now built with the base vectors n_A, f', c' which are given as

$$c' = n_B \times n_A \tag{4}$$
$$f' = c' \times n_A. \tag{5}$$

The rotations ϕ_y and ϕ_p are covered by the matrix $R_{\phi_y \phi_p}$ which is given by

$$R_{\phi_y \phi_p} = \begin{pmatrix} n_{A_x} & f'_x & c'_x & 0 \\ n_{A_y} & f'_y & c'_y & 0 \\ n_{A_z} & f'_z & c'_z & 0 \\ 0 & 0 & 0 & 1 \end{pmatrix}. \tag{6}$$

Finally, the rotation ϕ_r around the centerline c' is given by the rotation matrix R_{ϕ_r}, which is build with the common Euler angle representation. The overall rotation matrix is then given by

$$R = R_{\phi_y \phi_p} \cdot R_{\phi_r}. \tag{7}$$

2.1   2D/3D Registration Framework

We employed our approach within a 2D/3D registration system for TEE probe registration. We use a Powell-Brent minimizer as optimizer. This algorithm is well understood and produces good results for non-linear optimization. It was also successfully employed in similar registration problems [3].

The optimization is multi-scale/multi-resolution driven. We use the regularized normalized gradient fields (NGF) [7] as similarity measure, which is based on gradient directions and magnitudes. We use it in the following configuration

$$NGF(I_1, I_2) = \frac{1}{2} \sum_{x \in I} \langle n_\epsilon(I_1, x), n_\epsilon(I_2, x) \rangle^2, \tag{8}$$

which evaluates the dot product between all gradients in the X-ray image (I_1) and the DRR image (I_2). Each pixel gradient n_ϵ is calculated as

$$n_\epsilon(I, x) = \frac{\Delta I(x)}{\sqrt{||\Delta I(x)|| + \epsilon^2}}, \tag{9}$$

where ϵ is the regularization condition to suppress gradients coming from image noise. For the X-ray image, we set ϵ to the mean value over all image gradients and $\epsilon = 0$ for the DRR, because there is no noise in the DRR.

2.2   In Case of Object Motion

The presented approach can also be used to overcome the influences of slight object movement caused by breathing or heart motion. This can result in wrong offsets between objects in the consecutively acquired X-ray images. Also uncalibrated C-arm projection matrices can cause differences between two views. It follows that one could not achieve a 3D position that correctly matches both 2D positions in the projection images. To solve that issue, we decouple the translation of both views. Therefore, in-plane translation parameters t_x, t_z of A and B are registered independently. The depth t_y is still obtained from the intersection point m'_{3D}. For our data, we recognized that the object motion causes a translational shift but only insignificant errors for rotation. Therefore, the rotation is still combined on both images.

3   Experiments and Results

We evaluated our approach on various multi-plane X-ray sequences acquired during a porcine study and compared it to the two conventional strategies. We

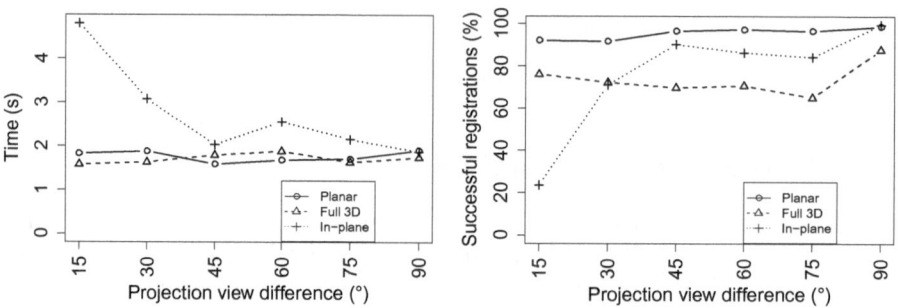

Fig. 4. Detailed registration performances on a mono-oblique system

acquired X-ray images within a wide range of projection angles to achieve different views to the TEE probe. The C-arm angles were in the range of $\alpha \in [-75, 90]$ and $\gamma \in [15, -30]$ degree. This range was limited by environmental constraints of the angiography lab. The probe was fixed to collect data without movement as well. The registration accuracy was evaluated while registering the TEE probe to different multi-plane X-ray image pairs. A ground truth registration was generated manually by careful visual inspection and automatic registration on different views. We tested the registration for a mono- and double-oblique setup, for data with and without movement. In total, we compared a various selection of image pairs from a set of 41 different X-ray scenes, similar to Fig. 1(c)(d).

We evaluated the registration error in terms of target registration error (TRE) [8], which can be seen as the overall 3D error of the registration process. We measured the mean error (mTRE) of 8 corner points of a bounding box around the TEE probe volume which are 5 cm away from the volume center and determined the capture range of the algorithm for each X-ray image pair. For each pair, we initialized 300 uniformly distributed random start positions of the TEE probe within an interval of $[-10, +10]$ mm and $[-10, +10]$ degree. If the final mTRE is below 2.5 mm, the registration is assumed to be successful.

The registration results for mono-oblique data is shown in Fig. 4. The evaluated scenes are merged over the difference between the projection angles. One can see on the left diagram that our approach is close to constant runtime, independent of the projection angle difference. In contrast to the conventional in-plane approach, particularly on small differences. The runtime of the planar and the full 3D approach is comparable, but has a lower success rate. The conventional in-plane method mostly fails on very low angle differences, while it adapts the planar results with increasing angle differences. The results are summarized in Tab. 1. As it can be seen in Tab. 2, the double-oblique views have a negative

Table 1. Results for mono-oblique setup

	Planar	In-plane	Full 3D
success [%]	**95.43**	75.83	73.57
time [s]	1.76	2.74	**1.70**

Table 2. Results for double-oblique setup

	Planar	In-plane	Full 3D
Success [%]	**85.92**	75.45	59.22
time [s]	2.29	1.67	**1.70**

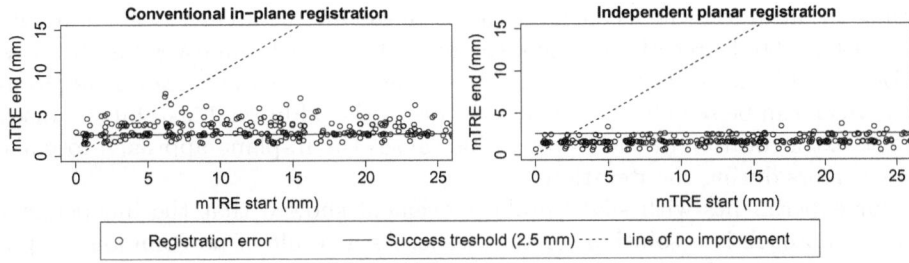

Fig. 5. Example result for registration on data with probe movement

influence on the overall registration accuracy while the planar approach is still more robust than the other. However, an increasing runtime can be observed.

In addition, we tested our approach on data, where we encountered a slight movement of the probe. Usually, the registration algorithm fails because of the varying 2D information. An example is given in Fig. 5. Compared to the independent approach, the conventional in-plane method has a low accuracy and a high variance in the final results. The summarized results in Tab. 3 show that, contrary to the independent approach, both conventional methods have poor results in accuracy. With 14.22 seconds, the runtime for in-plane is very high.

4   Discussion and Conclusion

In general, the planar approach shows about 25% higher accuracy than the compared methods. The accuracy and runtime of the conventional in-plane approach is limited by its iterative behaviour, Fig. 2(a). This effect can be observed especially for small angle differences. The smaller the angle, the more iterations are needed for convergence. For angles smaller than 15 degree, the error between the iterations is to large and the algorithm tends to converge to a local minimum. Because of the invariant in-plane parameters, the planar algorithm avoids additional iterations. Planar and in-plane methods have the identical behaviour for 90 degrees difference. The invariance of the in-plane parameters provides a better starting position on the respective other plane during optimization and increases the probability to find the correct minimum.

The full 3D strategy success rate is mostly lower. A reason is that the 3D position of the object is changed along the axes of the object which are not necessarily aligned with the image axes. In our implementation, the object is aligned to the in-plane directions of image A which is obviously not true for image B. Therefore, out- and in-plane parameters are mixed and are not separated

Table 3. Mean success and timing results for data with probe movement

	Planar independent	In-plane	Full 3D
Success [%]	**81.4**	38.3	30.1
time [s]	3.44	14.22	**1.59**

during optimization which can cause the optimizer ending up in a local minimum. Except for a 90 degree offset, where the full 3D approach improves significantly.

Double-oblique projection angles have an even bigger influence on the accuracy which can be seen in Tab. 2. This is due to the additional instability caused by the extra rotation of the C-arm. This causes the in-plane approach to make major errors during the iterations.

Our experiments with slight probe movement showed that the independent planar approach is a solution for that issue. As a result of no common 3D position, the conventional approaches try to find a compromise between both 2D image positions, respectively decide for one of the two possible positions. Decoupling the translation fixes this issue. Because of the iterative optimization, the in-plane approach tends to bounce between both positions which results in the increased runtime.

Our novel approach clearly achieves better results for non-perpendicular settings and with its constant runtime facilitates a seamless integration into clinical workflows. The presented approach is specialized on objects that have a "natural" centerline which represents the roll axis. Most technical objects in medical interventions (e.g. catheters, endoscopes) have a distinct centerline as well as anatomical structures like an aorta, vessels or head. That means, our presented approach can be potentially adopted to a various range of registration problems.

Disclaimer: The outlined concepts are not commercially available. Due to regulatory reasons its future availability cannot be guaranteed.

References

1. Markelj, P., Tomaževič, D., Likar, B., Pernuš, F.: A review of 3d/2d registration methods for image-guided interventions. Med. Image Anal. 16(3), 642–661 (2012)
2. Liao, R., Zhang, L., Sun, Y., Miao, S., Chefd'Hotel, C.: A Review of Recent Advances in Registration Techniques Applied to Minimally Invasive Therapy. IEEE Trans. on Multimedia 15(5), 983–1000 (2013)
3. Gao, G., Penney, G., Ma, Y., Gogin, N., Cathier, P., Arujuna, A., Morton, G., Caulfield, D., Gill, J., Aldo Rinaldi, C., et al.: Registration of 3D trans-esophageal echocardiography to X-ray fluoroscopy using image-based probe tracking. Med. Image Anal. 16(1), 38–49 (2012)
4. Brost, A., Wimmer, A., Liao, R., Bourier, F., Koch, M., Strobel, N., Kurzidim, K., Hornegger, J.: Constrained Registration for Motion Compensation in Atrial Fibrillation Ablation Procedures. IEEE Trans. on Med. Imag. 31(4), 870–881 (2012)
5. Miao, S., Liao, R., Pfister, M.: Toward smart utilization of two X-ray images for 2-D/3-D registration applied to abdominal aortic aneurysm interventions. Computers & Electrical Engineering 39(5), 1485–1498 (2013)
6. Kaiser, M., John, M., Heimann, T., Neumuth, T., Rose, G.: Improvement of Manual 2D/3D Registration by Decoupling the Visual Influence of the Six Degrees of Freedom. In: IEEE ISBI, pp. 766–769 (2014)
7. Haber, E., Modersitzki, J.: Intensity Gradient Based Registration and Fusion of Multi-modal Images. In: Larsen, R., Nielsen, M., Sporring, J. (eds.) MICCAI 2006. LNCS, vol. 4191, pp. 726–733. Springer, Heidelberg (2006)
8. van de Kraats, E., Penney, G., Tomazevic, D., van Walsum, T., Niessen, W.: Standardized evaluation methodology for 2-D-3-D registration. IEEE Trans. on Med. Imaging 24(9), 1177–1189 (2005)

Reduced-Dose Patient to Baseline CT Rigid Registration in 3D Radon Space

Guy Medan, Achia Kronman, and Leo Joskowicz

The Rachel and Selim Benin School of Computer Science and Engineering
The Hebrew University of Jerusalem, Israel
{gmedan,leo.josko}@mail.huji.ac.il

Abstract. We present a new method for rigid registration of CT scans in Radon space. The inputs are the two 3D Radon transforms of the CT scans, one densely sampled and the other sparsely sampled. The output is the rigid transformation that best matches them. The algorithm starts by finding the best matching between each direction vector in the sparse transform and the corresponding direction vector in the dense transform. It then solves the system of linear equations derived from the direction vector pairs. Our method can be used to register two CT scans and to register a baseline scan to the patient with reduced-dose scanning without compromising registration accuracy. Our preliminary simulation results on the Shepp-Logan head phantom dataset and a pair of clinical head CT scans indicates that our 3D Radon space rigid registration method performs significantly better than image-based registration for very few scan angles and comparably for densely-sampled scans.

1 Introduction

Rigid registration of CT scans acquired at different times plays a key role in numerous medical applications, including diagnosis, follow-ups, surgery planning and simulations. Rigid registration methods, including intensity, fiducial, and frequency-based methods are nowadays in routine clinical use.

Rigid registration plays an increasingly important role in image-guided interventional CT (ICT) procedures. ICT procedures include biopsies, catheter insertion, hematoma evacuation, and many more. Often times, a high-quality CT scan of the patient is available before the procedure. Since the diagnosis and procedure planning is usually performed on this CT scan, it is desirable to use it for guidance during the intervention. To monitor the progress of the surgery, evaluate anatomical changes, and determine the surgical tools location, repeated CT scanning is often performed. This results in the exposure of the patient to ionizing radiation, which has been shown to have risks for the patient [1,2]. It is thus highly desirable to develop methods that reduce the radiation dose required for intraoperative CT registration.

Two main approaches have been developed for rigid registration of CT scans: 1) image-based, and 2) Radon-based. Image-based methods, by far the most popular, perform the registration by comparing the intensity values of both

P. Golland et al. (Eds.): MICCAI 2014, Part I, LNCS 8673, pp. 291–298, 2014.

scans. To yield adequate results, they require both CT scans to be of high quality and free of image reconstruction artifacts. Radon-space methods use the CT scan's Radon transform representation (sinograms) for the registration. They are not subject to image reconstruction artifacts and have the potential to yield robust and accurate results with reduced-dose scanning.

Previous research addresses rigid registration in Radon space with a variety of methods. Freiman et al. [3] describe a method for 2D/3D registration of X-Ray to CT images. Their method uses invariant features in Fourier space to find the rigid parameters with out-of-plane coarse registration followed by in-plane fine registration. Mao et al. [4] describe a slice-by slice registration method in 2D Radon space and its extension to 3D/3D registration for small angles or with implanted fiducials. Mooser et al. [5] use an iterative optimization process to find the registration parameters in 3D Radon space. You et al. [6] investigate the mathematical relation between rigid movement in image space and Radon space and its invariants. Following this work, Lu et al. [7] use the Fourier phase matching technique applied to this relation to recover the rigid registration parameters of translation and rotation using the small angle approximation. The parameters are extracted in a stage-by-stage manner that employs the result of the previous stage in the evaluation of the next parameters, by decomposing the 3D problem into a series of 2D in-plane registrations.

In this paper we describe a new method for rigid registration of CT scans in 3D Radon space. The inputs are the two 3D Radon transforms of the CT scans, one densely sampled and the other sparsely sampled. The output is the rigid transformation that best matches the 3D Radon transforms. The algorithm first finds for each direction vector in the sparse 3D Radon transform the best matching direction vector in the dense 3D Radon transform. It then constructs and solves a system of linear equations from the direction vector pairs. The advantages of our method are: 1) it can be used both to register two CT scans and to register a baseline scan to the patient with reduced-dose scanning without compromising registration accuracy; 2) it supports fast on-line patient to baseline CT scan registration; 3) it is robust to noise, small anatomical differences, and has a wide convergence range because it relies on a closed-form solution of a set of linear equations instead of an iterative process. Our preliminary simulation results on the Shepp-Logan head phantom dataset and a pair of clinical head CT scans indicate that our Radon space method performs significantly better than image-based registration for very few scan angles.

2   Method

We first present the mathematical background of the Radon transform and its application to CT scan rigid registration. We then describe our new 3D Radon space method and algorithm details.

Mathematical Background. We follow the definitions and notations in [6] for parallel-beam scanning. Let $f : \Re^k \to \Re$ be an image function that maps

k-dimensional location vectors to intensity values. Let $H(\boldsymbol{n}, s)$ be the hyperplane defined by normal direction vector $\boldsymbol{n}$ and distance s from the origin in k-dimensional space. The Radon transform R of image function f is a function $Rf : S^{k-1} \times \Re \to \Re$ defined on unit sphere S^{k-1} of normal direction vector $\boldsymbol{n}$ and distance s:

$$Rf(\boldsymbol{n}, s) = \int_{H(\boldsymbol{n},s)} f(X)d\mu \tag{1}$$

where X is an k-dimensional vector and $d\mu$ is the standard measure on $H(\boldsymbol{n}, s)$. Let f, g be two image functions such that g is a similarity transformation of f:

$$g(X) = f(\rho A_{\boldsymbol{r},\theta} X + X_0) \tag{2}$$

where $\rho > 0$ is the scaling constant, $X_0 \in \Re^k$ is the constant offset vector, and $A_{\boldsymbol{r},\theta}$ is a unitary $k \times k$ matrix in which rotations are represented by an axis vector $\boldsymbol{r}$ and an angle θ of rotation about $\boldsymbol{r}$. A well-known relation between the Radon transforms Rf, Rg of image functions f, g is:

$$Rg(\boldsymbol{n}, s) = \rho^{n-1} Rf(\boldsymbol{n}', \rho^{-1}(s + \boldsymbol{n} \cdot X_0)) \tag{3}$$

where $\boldsymbol{n}$ and $\boldsymbol{n}'$ are normal unit direction vectors satisfying:

$$\boldsymbol{n}' = A_{\boldsymbol{r},\theta}^{-1} \boldsymbol{n} \tag{4}$$

This relation can be interpreted as follows. For a given normal unit direction vector $\boldsymbol{n}$, the Radon transforms of f and g, $Rf(\boldsymbol{n}, s)$ and $Rg(\boldsymbol{n}, s)$ are one-dimensional (1D) intensity signals of the distance s, which we denote by $F_{\boldsymbol{n}}(s) = Rf(\boldsymbol{n}, s)$ and $G_{\boldsymbol{n}}(s) = Rg(\boldsymbol{n}, s)$. Without offset and scaling, i.e. when $X_0 = \boldsymbol{0}$ and $\rho = 1$, Eq. 3 reduces to $Rg(\boldsymbol{n}, s) = Rf(\boldsymbol{n}', s)$, which means that the 1D signals $F_{\boldsymbol{n}'}(s)$ and $G_{\boldsymbol{n}}(s)$ are identical for direction vectors $\boldsymbol{n}$ and $\boldsymbol{n}'$. That is, the projection in the direction $\boldsymbol{n}'$ **before** the image f is rigidly rotated about the axis $\boldsymbol{r}$ is **identical** to the projection in a different direction $\boldsymbol{n}$ **after** the rotation, where the direction vectors $\boldsymbol{n}, \boldsymbol{n}'$ are related by the same rotation $A_{\boldsymbol{r},\theta}$. Furthermore, when the offset is not zero, that is $X_0 \neq \boldsymbol{0}$, we have:

$$G_{\boldsymbol{n}}(s) = F_{\boldsymbol{n}'}(s - \boldsymbol{n} \cdot X_0) \tag{5}$$

which means that $F_{\boldsymbol{n}'}(s)$ remains the same and is shifted by $\Delta = \boldsymbol{n} \cdot X_0$ for direction vectors $\boldsymbol{n}$ and $\boldsymbol{n}'$.

In physical space, the image functions f, g are volumetric images; their Radon transform, $R_{3D}f, R_{3D}g$ are 3D, and the direction vectors are points on the unit sphere S^2 (Fig. 1). The spatial rigid transformation that relates f and g can be described by a translational offset X_0, a rotation axis vector $\boldsymbol{r}$, and a rotation angle about it, θ. The goal of the rigid registration is to find the parameters $(\boldsymbol{r}, \theta, X_0)$ for which Eq. 2 holds.

The rigid transformation that aligns images f and g can be computed by matching their 3D Radon transforms, $R_{3D}f, R_{3D}g$, instead of matching the images themselves. This is called rigid registration in 3D Radon space. Furthermore,

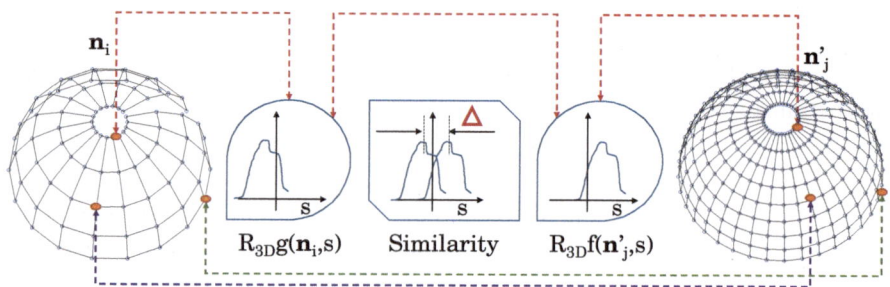

Fig. 1. Illustration of the matching procedure of 3D Radon transforms. n_i, n_j' are direction vectors represented as points on the unit sphere. Each direction vector corresponds to a 1D projection signal $R_{3D}g(n_i, s)$ or $R_{3D}f(n_j', s)$.

since Eq. 2 reduces to Eq. 5 without scaling, we can match $F_{n_j'}(s)$ and $G_{n_i}(s)$ where n_j' and n_i are the direction vectors of the 3D Radon transforms. When these Radon transforms are equal, that is when $G_{n_i}(s) = F_{n_j'}(s - \Delta_i)$ for offset Δ_i and direction vectors n_i, n_j', then, from Eqs. 4 and 5 we get:

$$\Delta_i = n_i \cdot X_0 \tag{6}$$
$$n_j' = A_{r,\theta}^{-1} n_i \tag{7}$$

which is a set of linear equations. The desired rigid transformation parameters (r, θ, X_0) can thus be computed by finding the pairs of direction vectors n_i, n_j' that satisfy Eqs. 6 and 7. Three pairs of independent direction vectors suffice to fully determine the resulting linear system of equations.

In general, the similarity between $F_{n_j'}$ and G_{n_i} does not imply Eqs. 6 and 7. Indeed, two identical 1D signals from two different direction vectors need not correspond to the same region of the images f and g: this similarity may be coincidental. However, such coincidental signal matches are unlikely in CT scans of human anatomy, which is rich in complexity and detail, and is radially asymmetric. For most direction vector pairs, the matchings correspond to the same image region after rigid transformation. In addition, not all direction vector pairs yield rigid transformations within the expected range.

3D Radon Rigid Registration Method. Based on these observation, we propose the following method for 3D Radon rigid registration of image g to image f. The inputs are the 3D Radon transforms of g and f defined by direction vectors $\{n_i\}_{i=1}^{K}$ and $\{n_j'\}_{j=1}^{L}$. The goal is to build a set of matching projection pairs with relative displacements (Fig. 1).

For each direction vector n_i we find the matching direction vector n_j' and relative displacement Δ_i for which the corresponding 1D signals G_{n_i} and $F_{n_j'}$ are most similar. The result is a set of matching pairs of projections, along with their relative displacements $\left\{ (F_{n_j'}, G_{n_i}, \Delta_i) \right\}_{i=1}^{K}$.

Substituting each direction vector pair in Eqs. 6 and 7 yields an overdetermined set of linear equations. We compute the desired rigid transformation parameters (r, θ, X_0) by least-squares minimization. Offset X_0 is estimated as $\hat{X}_0 = (N^T N)^{-1} N^T \Delta$ where $N = [n_1 \ ... \ n_K]^T$ and $\Delta = [\Delta_1 \ ... \ \Delta_K]^T$. This solution minimizes the term $\sum_{i=1}^{K} (\Delta_i - n_i \cdot X_0)^2$.

To estimate the rotation matrix $A_{r,\theta}$, we define the 3×3 matrix $M = \sum_{i=1}^{K} n'_i n_i^T$ and compute its Singular Value Decomposition $M = U^T \Sigma V$. From the values of U, V we obtain the estimate $\hat{A}_{r,\theta} = UV^T$. This solution minimizes the term $\sum_{i=1}^{K} (n_i - A_{r,\theta} n'_i)^2$.

A key property of this method is that it does not require a dense set of direction vectors of the 3D Radon transform of image g. Since the set of linear equations from which the transformation parameters are computed is of dimension 3, the set is overconstrained with more than three direction parings. Using more direction pairs that are not outliers usually increases robustness and improves accuracy. This is akin to point-based rigid registration, in which more than three point pairs are used. The method is therefore suitable for finding the rigid registration between sparsely and densely sampled set of direction vectors for $R_{3D}g$ and $R_{3D}f$. This is the situation of ICT procedures that require registering the patient with his/her earlier CT scan.

3D Radon Rigid Registration Algorithm. We now describe a new 3D Radon rigid registration algorithm based on the method described above. The inputs are the two Radon transforms $R_{3D}f$ and $R_{3D}g$ of images f and g. The output is the rigid transformation (r, θ, X_0). The algorithm consists of two steps. First, for each direction vector in the sparse $R_{3D}g$ transform, we find the matching direction vector in the dense $R_{3D}f$ transform. Then, we construct and solve the set of linear equations obtained by substituting each direction vector pair in Eqs. 6 and 7. We describe each step in detail next.

1. Direction vectors pairing. We evaluate the similarity of the two 1D signals from two direction vectors with Normalized Cross Correlation (NCC); the NCC value is the direction vectors pair score. For each direction vector n_i, we select the direction vector n_j' with the highest NCC score and compute its relative displacement Δ_i. We define an index function $match(i) = argmax_j \{NCC(R_{3D}g(n_i, s), R_{3D}f(n'_j, s)\}$ that pairs the direction vectors. In order to avoid searching all possible direction vectors n_j', we restrict the search to a neighbourhood of n_i defined by $\Phi(n_i) = \{n'_j : \cos^{-1}(n_i \cdot n'_j) < \varphi\}$ where φ is the largest expected relative orientation offset between the images.

2. Transformation computation. We construct and solve the set of linear equations obtained by substituting each direction vector pair in Eqs. 6 and 7 as described above. We use RANSAC to eliminate outliers. Since the resulting set of equations is 3-dimensional, we obtain high-quality results with a large number of RANSAC iterations in a short time. We set the RANSAC inliers threshold ψ for the relative angle $\cos^{-1}(n_i^T \hat{A}_{r,\theta} \ n'_j)$ to be half the angular resolution of the densely-sampled set $R_{3D}f$.

Computation of 3D Radon Transforms from 2D Sinograms. The 3D Radon transform $R_{3D}g$ of the baseline image f can be efficiently computed from the 2D sinograms of the slices as described in [5]. Our algorithm achieves the desired rigid registration with a sparse sampling of $R_{3D}g$, which takes place in the CT scanner. The reduced number of direction vectors required thus leads to a significant reduction of the radiation dose without compromising accuracy and without having to reconstruct the image g.

3   Experimental Results

To evaluate our method, we conducted the following simulation experiments in Matlab. We use the Shepp-Logan head phantom dataset whose size is $256 \times 256 \times 256$ voxels with intensity values in $[0, 1]$. To simulate data acquisition noise, we add $N(0, 0.05)$ Gaussian noise to the dataset to obtain the baseline image f. We then apply to f a series of rigid transformation including both rotations and translations to generate a new set of images h (Table 1). For each image h, we generate its sinograms by projection and create a set of new sparsely-sampled images $\{g_l\}$. Each image g_l is created by filtered back projection from 2 to 18 projection directions instead of the usual 180 required for full-resolution reconstruction. The resulting images include significant reconstruction artifacts.

We then perform two sets of rigid registrations: one in image space using Matlab's `imregtform` and the other one in Radon space with our method. In image space, we compute the rigid transformation parameters between the original phantom image f and the reconstructed and transformed phantom images g_l. In Radon space we applied our registration method on the 3D Radon transforms of f and g_l. The 3D Radon transform of f was computed at an angular resolution of $1°$ for 180 2D projection directions per slice, for a total of 32,400 direction vectors. The resulting rigid transformations of the image-based and Radon-based registration were then applied to the original image f. The resulting images were compared to the ground-truth rigid transformations of f by computing the RMS error between 3D voxel coordinates. The experiment was repeated between 3 to 10 times for each rigid transformations and sparse sampling settings. Fig. 2 shows the results. Note that our Radon space method performs significantly better than image-based registration for very few scan angles (< 12). Note also that our algorithm handles well rotation offsets $> 10°$, which are therefore unsuitable for small-angle approximation.

Table 1. Parameters and settings for the ground-truth transformations. A total of 18 rigid transformations (all $3 \times 3 \times 2$ combinations) were used.

Parameter Setting	Axis vector $\hat{r}$ not normalized	Angle θ degrees	Translation X_0 pixels
1	$(1, 2, 100)$	1.0	$(2, 0, -1)$
2	$(34, 45, 39)$	-7.7	$(14, 15.2, -18.5)$
3	$(23, -12, 1)$	13.2	

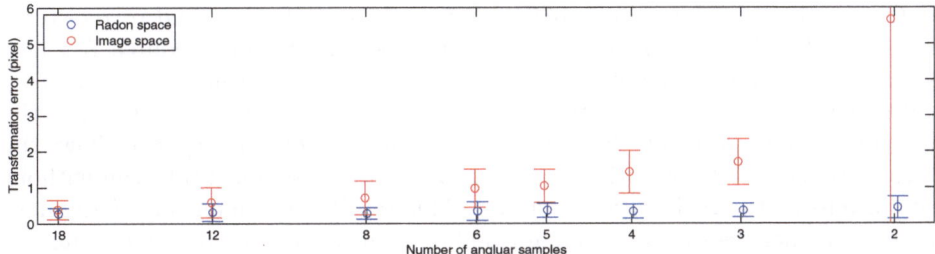

Fig. 2. Plot of the image-based (red) and 3D Radon (blue) rigid transformation error with respect to the ground-truth transformation (vertical axis) as a function of the number of scan angles (horizontal axis), 18 to 2

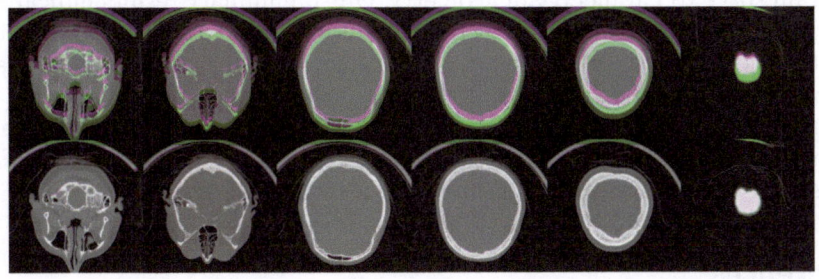

Fig. 3. Overlay of six representative slices from two head CT scans of the same patient: before registration (top row), after 3D Radon space registration (bottom row)

In a second experiment, we test our method on a pair of CT scans from a patient head taken at two different times. The voxel sizes are $0.42 \times 0.42 \times 0.67$ mm^3. Prior to registration, we removed the scanning bed from both images, as it is not rigidly attached to the patient and introduces errors in the Radon space signals. In practice, this can be done automatically, since the Radon transform of the bed without the patient is always the same and can be precomputed and subtracted from the patient scan. We then computed the image-based registration of the full-resolution scans and our Radon space registration with the second image from 18 angles using our method and compared the results (Fig. 3). The RMSE between the image space registration and our method is 0.64mm. This indicates that our method yields results comparable to full-resolution image-space registration with about 10% of the radiation dose of the second scan.

4 Conclusions

We have presented a new 3D Radon space rigid registration method for CT scans registration. Our method is the first which does not require in-plane decompositions in 2D Radon space [6], or small-angle approximations [4], [5], [7].

Our method can be used to register two existing CT scans and to register a baseline CT scan to the patient for interventional CT (ICT) procedures. It is also suitable for adaptive incremental scanning registration during the intervention without producing an image, thus allowing very sparse scanning well below the imaging Nyquist rate. The key characteristic of our method is that it allows the registration of a full-resolution CT scan to a sparsely-sampled CT scan without compromising the registration accuracy. This results in a significant X-ray dose reduction when registering a diagnostic CT scan to the patient prior to image-guided ICT procedures. Another advantage of our method is that it supports fast on-line patient to baseline CT scan registration, as most of the 3D Radon space computation on the baseline image can be performed prior to the intervention. Note that our method can also handle the common fan-beam and cone-beam scanning geometries used in commercial CT scanners by re-sampling the acquired sinogram space to parallel beam geometry. Our preliminary results indicate that a very small number of scan directions are sufficient to obtain voxel size accuracy, that the method has a wide convergence range, and that it is robust to small anatomical differences.

Future work includes extending our formulation to cone-beam and spiral CT acquisition without re-sampling, conducting more extensive simulation experiments, and conducting studies with actual CT sinograms.

References

1. Chodick, G., Ronckers, C.M., Shalev, V., Ron, E., et al.: Excess lifetime cancer mortality risk attributable to radiation exposure from computed tomography examinations in children. IMAJ-RAMAT GAN 9(8), 584 (2007)
2. Mettler Jr., F.A., Wiest, P.W., Locken, J.A., Kelsey, C.A.: CT scanning: patterns of use and dose. Journal of Radiological Protection 20(4), 353 (2000)
3. Freiman, M., Pele, O., Hurvitz, A., Werman, M., Joskowicz, L.: Spectral-based 2d/3d X-ray to CT image rigid registration. In: SPIE Medical Imaging, International Society for Optics and Photonics, pp. 79641B–79641B (2011)
4. Mao, W., Li, T., Wink, N., Xing, L.: CT image registration in sinogram space. Medical Physics 34(9), 3596–3602 (2007)
5. Mooser, R., Forsberg, F., Hack, E., Székely, G., Sennhauser, U.: Estimation of affine transformations directly from tomographic projections in two and three dimensions. Machine Vision and Applications 24(2), 419–434 (2013)
6. You, J., Lu, W., Li, J., Gindi, G., Liang, Z.: Image matching for translation, rotation and uniform scaling by the radon transform. In: Proceedings of the 1998 International Conference on Image Processing, ICIP 1998, vol. 1, pp. 847–851. IEEE (1998)
7. Lu, W., Fitchard, E.E., Olivera, G.H., You, J., Ruchala, K.J., Aldridge, J.S., Mackie, T.R.: Image/patient registration from (partial) projection data by the fourier phase matching method. Physics in Medicine and Biology 44(8), 2029 (1999)

Hierarchical Label Fusion with Multiscale Feature Representation and Label-Specific Patch Partition

Guorong Wu and Dinggang Shen

BRIC and Department of Radiology, University of North Carolina at Chapel Hill, USA
{grwu,dgshen}@med.unc.edu

Abstract. Recently, patch-based label fusion methods have achieved many successes in medical imaging area. After registering atlas images to the target image, the label at each target image point can be subsequently determined by checking the patchwise similarities between the underlying target image patch and all atlas image patches. Apparently, the definition of patchwise similarity is critical in label fusion. However, current methods often simply use entire image patch with fixed patch size throughout the entire label fusion procedure, which could be insufficient to distinguish complex shape/appearance patterns of anatomical structures in medical imaging scenario. In this paper, we address the above limitations at three folds. *First*, we assign each image patch with multiscale feature representations such that both local and semi-local image information can be encoded to increase robustness of measuring patchwise similarity in label fusion. *Second*, since multiple *variable* neighboring structures could present in one image patch, simply computing patchwise similarity based on the entire image patch is not specific to the particular structure of interest under labeling and can be easily misled by the surrounding *variable* structures in the same image patch. Thus, we partition each atlas patch into a set of new label-specific atlas patches according to the existing label information in the atlas images. Then, the new label-specific atlas patches can be more specific and flexible for label fusion than using the entire image patch, since the complex image patch has now been semantically divided into several distinct patterns. *Finally*, in order to correct the possible mis-labeling, we hierarchically improve the label fusion result in a coarse-to-fine manner by iteratively repeating the label fusion procedure with the gradually-reduced patch size. More accurate label fusion results have been achieved by our hierarchical label fusion method with multiscale feature presentations upon label-specific atlas patches.

1   Introduction

Many medical imaging based studies demand accurate segmentation of anatomical structures, in order to quantitatively measure structure differences across individuals or between two groups. To this end, automatic ROI (Region of Interest) labeling has been a hot topic in medical image processing areas, as evidenced by hundreds of labeling and label fusion methods that have been developed to improve both segmentation accuracy and robustness.

P. Golland et al. (Eds.): MICCAI 2014, Part I, LNCS 8673, pp. 299–306, 2014.

In order to deal with high structural variations in the population, multiple atlases with delineated labels are commonly used for labeling the latent ROIs of the target image [1]. The basic assumption behind multi-atlas based segmentation is that the target image should bear the same label as the atlas image if both of them present similar shape/appearance. Thus, all atlas images are required to be registered to the target image before label fusion. To alleviate the possible mis-registration, patch-based label fusion technique [1, 2] is also advocated by measuring the patchwise similarity at each point. Intuitively, the higher the similarity between target image and a particular atlas image is, the more confidence we assign the label on that atlas to the target image.

It is apparent that the patchwise similarity is the key in patch-based label fusion methods. Most of the current state-of-the-art methods only use the fixed patch size throughout entire label fusion procedure. For example, $7 \times 7 \times 7$ or $9 \times 9 \times 9$ cubic patches are usually used in the literature. In order to make the label fusion robust to noise, image patches are required to be large enough in order to capture sufficient image content. However, large image patch could raise a critical issue in labeling small anatomical structures, since the patchwise similarity could be dominated by the surrounding large structures in the image patch. The main reason for such dilemma is that the simple use of whole image patch lacks high-level knowledge to distinguish complex appearance patterns in medical imaging data.

Many efforts have been made to improve the discrimination power of image patches. For instance, sparse dictionary learning technique is used in [3] to find the best feature representations in label fusion. However, the dictionary is still confined in using the whole image patch with fixed size. In this paper, we address the above limitations in a new perspective of developing hierarchical and high-level feature representations for image patch. In general, our contribution has three folds.

First, we propose to adaptively treat each image point within the image patch by designing the image patch with multi-scale feature representations. We argue that image points close to the patch center should use fine-scale features to characterize the details of patch center, while the level of image features could gradually turn from fine to coarse as the distance toward the patch center increases. To this end, we assign the conventional image patch with the *layerwise* multi-scale feature representation by adaptively capturing image features in each layer with different scale.

Second, it is very common that the to-be-segmented ROI, e.g., hippocampus, is surrounded by other complex structures. Those surrounding *variable* structures may mislead the patchwise similarity measurement. In computer vision area, recognizing object could be much easier if the foreground pattern can be separated from the background clutters [4]. In light of this, we present a new concept of label-specific patch partition to enhance the discriminative power of each atlas patch in label fusion. Specifically, since each atlas patch bears the well-determined labels, such information can provide the valuable heuristic about anatomical structures and thus can be used to guide the splitting of each atlas patch into a set of new complementary label-specific (or structure-specific) image patches. It is worth noting that each label-specific image patch carries only the image information at selected locations with same label. Therefore, our label-specific partition *not only* enriches the representations for each atlas patch *but also* encapsulates the high-level label information. To the best of our knowledge, such important label information is poorly used in the current label fusion methods. Afterwards, sparsity constraint is further used in our proposed label fusion method to deal with the increased number of label-specific image patches.

Third, current label fusion methods fix the patch size throughout the entire label fusion procedure. Here, we go one step further, e.g., propose to iteratively refine the labeling results by gradually reducing the patch size with the progress of label fusion. Specifically, we use the large image patches in the beginning, in order to make the label fusion robust. Sparsity constraint is used to allow only a small number of atlas patches for joining the label fusion. Then, for those selected atlas patches, we can reduce their patch size and repeat the label fusion procedure to refine their respective weights in the final label fusion.

We comprehensively evaluate the performance of our new label fusion method both in segmenting hippocampus in ADNI dataset and labeling 54 ROIs in LPBA40 dataset. More accurate labeling results are achieved, compared with the state-of-the-art label fusion methods.

2   Methods

Given the target image T, the goal of label fusion is to automatically determine a label map L_T for the target image T. To achieve it, we need to first register all atlas images as well as their labeled maps to the target image space. Here, we use $I = \{I_s | s = 1, ..., N\}$ and $L = \{L_s | s = 1, ..., N\}$ to denote N registered atlases and label maps, respectively. For each target image point x ($x \in T$), all the atlas patches[1] within a certain search neighborhood $n(x)$, denoted as $\vec{\beta}_{s,y}$ ($\vec{\beta}_{s,y} \subset I_s$, $y \in n(x)$), are used to compute the patchwise similarities w.r.t. the target image patch $\vec{\alpha}_{T,x}$ ($\vec{\alpha}_{T,x} \subset T$). It is worth noting that we arrange each patch, $\vec{\beta}_{s,y}$ and $\vec{\alpha}_{T,x}$, into a column vector.

Next, label fusion strategies, e.g., non-local averaging, can be used to calculate the weighting vector $\vec{w} = [w_{s,y}]_{s=1,...,N, y \in n(x)}$ for each atlas patch $\vec{\beta}_{s,y}$. As we will explain in Section 2.2, we adopt the sparsity constraint in our method by regarding the label fusion procedure as the problem of finding optimal combination among a set of atlas patches $\{\vec{\beta}_{s,y}\}$ for the target image patch $\vec{\alpha}_{T,x}$ [5, 6]:

$$\widehat{\vec{w}} = \arg\min_{\vec{w}} \left\| \vec{\alpha}_{T,x} - B\vec{w} \right\|^2 + \lambda \|\vec{w}\|_1, \text{ s.t. } \vec{w} > 0 \qquad (1)$$

where the scalar λ controls the strength of sparsity constraint and B is the matrix by assembling all column vectors $\{\vec{\beta}_{s,y}\}$ in a columnwise way. Assuming that we have M possible labels $\{l_1, ..., l_m, ..., l_M\}$ in the atlases, then the label on target image point x can be efficiently determined by:

$$\hat{L}_T(x) = \arg\max_{m=1,...,M} \sum_{s=1}^{N} \sum_{y \in n(x)} [w_{s,y} \cdot \delta(L_s(y), l_m)] \qquad (2)$$

---

[1] Some label fusion methods use patch pre-selection to discard the less similar patches.

where Dirac function $\delta(L_s(y), l_m)$ is always zero except for the case when $L_s(y)$ bears the label l_m. In that case, $\delta(L_s(y), l_m)$ equals to 1.

It is clear that image intensities in the entire image patch are used in label fusion (Eq. 1). Since one image patch may contain more than one anatomical structures and the to-be-segmented ROI may have very complex shape/appearance pattern, current patch-based label fusion methods have high risk of being misled by the current definition of patchwise similarities that are computed based on the entire image patch. In the following, we propose three ways to improve the label fusion accuracy: **(1)** substantially upgrading the feature discrimination power by using multi-scale feature representations (Section 2.1); **(2)** adaptively building label-specific atlas patches by using the existing label information in the atlases (Section 2.2); and **(3)** hierarchically improving label fusion accuracy in a coarse-to-fine manner by gradually reducing the patch size (Section 2.3).

2.1   Multi-scale Feature Representations

In current patch-based label fusion methods, every point in the image patch uses its own intensity value and equally contributes in computing the patchwise similarity. Here, we allow each point to use adaptive scale for capturing local appearance characteristics. Specifically, we first partition the whole image patch into several nested non-overlapping *layers*, spreading from the center point to the bound of image patch. Next, we use small scale to capture the fine-scale features for the layer closest to the patch center. Gradually, we use larger and larger scale to capture the coarse-scale information as the distance to the patch center increases. Although advanced pyramid image technique can be applied for multiscale feature representation, we choose a more efficient way by replacing the intensity value with the average intensity in a certain neighborhood, due to the consideration of computational time. For example, for the points in the first layer that is the closest to the patch center (including the patch center and its 6 immediate neighboring points), we still keep using their original intensities. For each point in the second layer, we replace its intensity value with the average intensity value in its $3 \times 3 \times 3$ neighborhood. Similarly, we use intensity average in a larger neighborhood as the feature representation for the image points beyond the second layer. In this way, the image patch is now equipped with the multi-scale feature representation. Hereafter, $\vec{\alpha}_{T,x}$ and $\vec{\beta}_{s,y}$ denote the image patches after replacing the original intensities with the multi-scale feature representations.

2.2   Label-Specific Atlas Patch Partition

Since atlas image patches have label information, we can partition each atlas patch into a set of new label-specific atlas patches for encoding the label information. Given the atlas patch $\vec{\beta}_{s,y}$, we use $\vec{\gamma}_{s,y}$ to denote its associated labels. Suppose there are M kinds of labels in $\vec{\gamma}_{s,y}$. Then, the proposed label-specific atlas patch set $\boldsymbol{P}_{s,y}$ consists of M label-specific atlas patches, i.e., $\boldsymbol{P}_{s,y} = \{\vec{p}_{s,y}^m | m = 1, \ldots, M\}$, where $\vec{p}_{s,y}^m$ is the column vector. Each element u in $\vec{p}_{s,y}^m$ keeps the intensity value $\vec{\beta}_{s,y}(u)$ if and only if $\vec{\gamma}_{s,y}(u)$ has label l_m; otherwise, $\vec{p}_{s,y}^m(u) = 0$. Mathematically, we have $\vec{p}_{s,y}^m(u) = \vec{\beta}_{s,y}(u) \cdot \delta(\vec{\gamma}_{s,y}(u), l_m)$, where $\delta(.,.)$ is the same Dirac function as used in Eq. 2.

Note that the number of image patches increases significantly after we partition each atlas patch into the label-specific atlas patch set. Thus, we propose to use the sparsity constraint again in label fusion, in order to select only a small number of label-specific atlas patch $\vec{p}_{s,y}^m$ to represent the target image patch $\vec{a}_{T,x}$. By replacing each conventional atlas patch with label-specific atlas patches, the matrix of atlas patches B in Eq. 1 now expands to $P = [P_{s,y}]_{s=1,...,N,y\in n(x)}$. Then, the new energy function for label fusion can be reformulated as:

$$\vec{\xi} = \arg\min_{\vec{\xi}}\|\vec{a}_{T,x} - P\vec{\xi}\|^2 + \lambda\|\vec{\xi}\|_1, \text{ s.t. } \vec{\xi} > 0, \tag{3}$$

where $\vec{\xi} = [\xi_{s,y}^m]$ is the weighting vector for each label-specific atlas patch $\vec{p}_{s,y}^m$. Since each $\vec{p}_{s,y}^m$ is only related with a particular label l_m, each element $\xi_{s,y}^m$ in $\vec{\xi}$ represents the probability of labeling the center point x of the target image patch $\vec{a}_{T,x}$ by label l_m. Therefore, the labeling result on the target image point x can be obtained by:

$$\hat{L}_T(x) = \arg\max_{m=1,...,M} \sum_{s=1}^N \sum_{y\in n(x)} \xi_{s,y}^m \tag{4}$$

Fig. 1 demonstrates the construction of label-specific atlas patch set P for the case with only two labels, i.e., $M = 2$. As displayed in Fig. 1(a), each atlas patch $\vec{\beta}_{s,y}$ is split into two label-specific atlas patches $\vec{p}_{s,y}^1$ and $\vec{p}_{s,y}^2$, where we use the black to denote the zero elements. For example, the zero elements in $\vec{p}_{s,y}^1$ have their label as l_2, instead of l_1. The objective function in Eq. 1 is to minimize the appearance difference between $\vec{a}_{T,x}$ and $B\vec{w}$. In our method, we first divide each whole atlas patch into several label-specific patches and then recognize the structural patterns in $\vec{a}_{T,x}$ in a label-by-label manner. In this way, our method makes the representation of $\vec{a}_{T,x}$ more selective and flexible.

The advantage of using label-specific atlas patches is demonstrated by the toy example in Fig. 1(b), where we use red and blue to denote two different labels and numbers represent the intensity values. To be simple, only two atlas patches are used in this example. Apparently, the first atlas patch (first column in B) and $\vec{a}_{T,x}$ belongs to the same structure since their intensity values are both in the ascending order. If we estimate the weighting vector $\vec{w}$ based on the entire atlas patch by Eq. 1 ($\lambda = 0.01$), the weights for the first and second atlas patches are 0.43 and 0.49, respectively. According to Eq. 2, we have to assign the target point with the blue (incorrect) label. In our method, we first extend the matrix B to label-specific atlas patch set P, as shown in the bottom of Fig. 1(b) and then solve the new weighing vector $\vec{\xi}$ by Eq. 3. As suggested by $\vec{\xi}$, the overall weights for red and blue labels are 0.885 (0.88+0.005) and 0.800 (0.69+0.11), respectively. Therefore, we can correctly assign the target point with red label. This example demonstrates the power of our method.

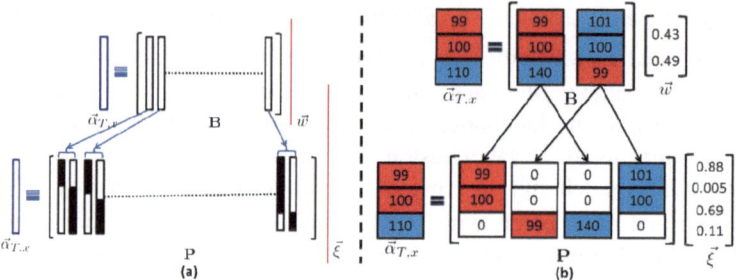

Fig. 1. (a) Construction of label-specific atlas patch set and (b) the advantage in label fusion

2.3 Hierarchical Patch-Based Label Fusion

In the beginning of patch-based label fusion, we often use a large patch size in order to obtain global image information. Since we use the sparsity constraint in solving the weighing vector $\vec{\xi}$, only a small number of image patches are selected to represent the target image patch $\vec{\alpha}_{T,x}$, as many weights in $\vec{\xi}$ are zero or almost zero. After discarding those non-selected atlas patches, we are more confident to reduce the patch size of those selected atlas patches and then repeat the whole label fusion procedure as described in Section 2.1 and 2.2 by using more detailed local features. In this way, our label fusion method can iteratively improve the labeling results in a hierarchical way.

3   Experiments

In the following experiments, we compare our label fusion method (by Eq. 3 and Eq. 4) with the sparse patch-based label fusion method (by Eq. 1 and Eq. 2). To label the target image, we first use FLIRT in FSL package to linearly register all atlas images onto the target image and then use diffeomorphic Demons [7] to compute the remaining local deformations[2]. After optimization, λ is set to 0.1 for both the label fusion methods. The patch size is $5 \times 5 \times 5$ for the sparse patch-based label fusion method. In our method, the patch size is initialized with $11 \times 11 \times 11$ in the first iteration and reduced to $5 \times 5 \times 5$ in the second iteration. Here, we use Dice ratio on each ROI to measure the labeling accuracy.

3.1   Evaluation on Hippocampus Labeling

In this experiment, we randomly select 66 elderly brains from ADNI dataset[3], where hippocampus has been manually labeled for each brain. Besides comparing with the

---

[2] The main parameters for running diffeomorphic Demons are: 15, 10, and 5 iterations in low, middle, and high resolution, respectively. The smoothing kernel size is 2.0.
[3] www.adni-info.org

baseline sparse patch-based label fusion method (*Sparse PBL*), to evaluate the contribution of each component in our label fusion method, we further compare our method with the three degraded versions of our method, (1) Degraded_1: our method using only the multi-scale feature representation (with patch size $11 \times 11 \times 11$), (2) Degraded_2: our method using only the label-specific atlas patches (with patch size $11 \times 11 \times 11$), and (3) Degraded_3: our method using only the hierarchical labeling mechanism.

We evaluate each of the above five label fusion methods with a leave-one-out cross-validation. From all 66 leave-one-out cases, the mean and standard deviation of Dice ratios in hippocampus and the surface distance are calculated and provided in Table 1. It is clear that: (1) Our full method achieves the highest Dice ratio and lowest surface distance over other four comparison methods, where we obtain almost 1.2% improvement over the baseline *Sparse PBL* method; (2) Each component in our label fusion method has contribution in improving the labeling accuracy, as evidenced by 0.6%, 0.9%, and 0.3% Dice ratio increases over the baseline *Sparse PBL* by Degraded_1, Degraded_2, and Degraded_3, respectively. Also, we find all degraded methods have significant improvement over the baseline method in paired *t*-test.

Table 1. The statistics of Dice ratios in hippocampus labeling by 5 different methods

	Sparse PBL	Degraded_1	Degraded_2	Degraded_3	Our method
Dice Ratio	87.3±3.4	87.9±3.0	88.2±2.5	87.6±2.9	**88.5±2.2**
Surf. Dist	0.38mm	0.35mm	0.34mm	0.35mm	**0.33mm**

3.2   Evaluation on LPBA40 Dataset

LPBA 40 dataset[4] consists of 40 MR brain images, each with 54 manually labeled ROIs. We randomly select 20 images as atlases and another 20 as the target images. The statistics of overall Dice ratio across 54 ROIs are given in Table 2, where our full method achieves 1.5% improvement over the baseline *Sparse PBL* method. Apparently, each component in our proposed label fusion method has its contribution in enhancing the label fusion results. Fig. 2 shows the Dice ratio in each left-and-right-combined ROI by *Sparse PBL* (in blue) and our full method (in red), from which we can observe significant improvements in 12 out of 27 ROIs ('*' denoting the significant improvement confirmed by paired *t*-test ($p < 0.05$)).

Table 2. The statistics of Dice ratios in labeling 54 ROIs on LPBA40 dataset by 5 diffent methods

	Sparse PBL	Degraded_1	Degraded_2	Degraded_3	Our method
Dice Ratio	80.3±3.2	81.1±2.5	81.5±2.4	80.6±3.0	**81.8±2.1**

---

[4] http://www.loni.usc.edu/atlases/Atlas_Detail.php?atlas_id=12

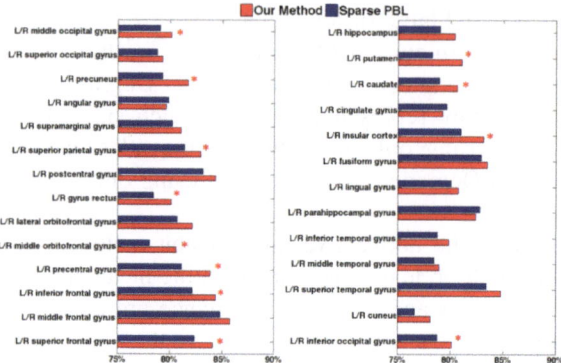

Fig. 2. The Dice ratios of 27 ROIs (left and right combined) in LPBA 40 dataset by *Sparse PBL* (in blue) and our method (in red)

4   Conclusion

In this paper, we explore a new perspective to substantially enhance the discriminative power of the conventional, widely used, image patch in label fusion. Specifically, we assign each atlas patch with multi-scale feature representation, and further develop label-specific atlas patches according to the existing label information in the atlases for making each atlas patch more flexible during label fusion. Moreover, we present a hierarchical label fusion mechanism to iteratively improve the labeling results by gradually reducing the patch size. Promising labeling results have been obtained on ADNI and LPBA40 dataset, by comparing with state-of-the-art methods.

References

1. Coupe, P., Manjoh, J., Fonov, V., Pruessner, J., Robles, M., Collins, L.: Patch-based segmentation using expert priors: Application to hippocampus and ventricle segmentation. NeuroImage 54(2), 940–954 (2011)
2. Rousseau, F., Habas, P.A., Studholme, C.: A Supervised Patch-Based Approach for Human Brain Labeling. IEEE Trans. Medical Imaging 30(10), 1852–1862 (2011)
3. Tong, T., Wolz, R., Coupe, P., Hajnal, J., Rueckert, D.: Segmentation of MR images via discriminative dictionary learning and sparse coding: application to hippocampus labeling. NeuroImage 76, 11–23 (2013)
4. Li, L., Su, H., Xing, E., Li, F.: Object Bank: A High-Level Image Representation for Scene Classification and Semantic Feature Sparsification. In: Proceedings of the Neural Information Processing System (NIPS) (2010)
5. Tong, T., et al.: Segmentation of Brain Images via Sparse Patch Representaion. In: MICCAI Workshop on Sparsity Techniques in Medical Imaging, Nice, France (2012)
6. Zhang, D., Guo, Q., Wu, G., Shen, D.: Sparse patch-based label fusion for multi-atlas segmentation. In: Yap, P.-T., Liu, T., Shen, D., Westin, C.-F., Shen, L. (eds.) MBIA 2012. LNCS, vol. 7509, pp. 94–102. Springer, Heidelberg (2012)
7. Vercauteren, T., Pennec, X., Perchant, A., Ayache, N.: Diffeomorphic demons: efficient non-parametric image registration. NeuroImage 45(suppl. 1), S61–S72 (2009)

Simultaneous Segmentation and Anatomical Labeling of the Cerebral Vasculature

David Robben[1,*], Engin Türetken[2], Stefan Sunaert[3], Vincent Thijs[4], Guy Wilms[3], Pascal Fua[2], Frederik Maes[1], and Paul Suetens[1]

[1] iMinds - Medical Image Computing (ESAT/PSI), KU Leuven, Belgium
[2] CVLab, EPFL, Lausanne, Switzerland
[3] Department of Radiology, University Hospitals Leuven, KU Leuven, Belgium
[4] Department of Neurology, University Hospitals Leuven, KU Leuven, Belgium
david.robben@esat.kuleuven.be

Abstract. We present a novel algorithm for the simultaneous segmentation and anatomical labeling of the cerebral vasculature. The method first constructs an overcomplete graph capturing the vasculature. It then selects and labels the subset of edges that most likely represents the true vasculature. Unlike existing approaches that first attempt to obtain a good segmentation and then perform labeling, we jointly optimize for both by simultaneously taking into account the image evidence and the prior knowledge about the geometry and connectivity of the vasculature. This results in an Integer Program (IP), which we solve optimally using a branch-and-cut algorithm. We evaluate our approach on a public dataset of 50 cerebral MRA images, and demonstrate that it compares favorably against state-of-the-art methods.

Keywords: Cerebral Vasculature, Segmentation, Reconstruction, Anatomical Labeling, Circle of Willis, Integer Programming.

1   Introduction

Automated segmentation and anatomical labeling of blood vessels is an important problem with many practical applications. In clinical settings, it can give an interventional radiologist extra guidance when navigating through a patient's vasculature, or it can allow automatic quantification of specific vessel segments. In a research context, it can be used to detect patterns in the vasculature that may be correlated to the incidence of vascular pathologies.

In this work, we focus on the cerebral vasculature and more specifically on the Circle of Willis (CoW) as well as its adjacent vessels. The CoW is a circle of arteries in the skull base that connects the left and right side of the anterior cerebral circulation with the posterior cerebral circulation (Fig. 1). It is supplied with blood via three large arteries, namely the left and right ICA and VBA. Although the CoW has a very characteristic morphology, it is highly variable:

---

* David Robben is supported by a Ph.D. fellowship of the Research Foundation - Flanders (FWO).

P. Golland et al. (Eds.): MICCAI 2014, Part I, LNCS 8673, pp. 307–314, 2014.

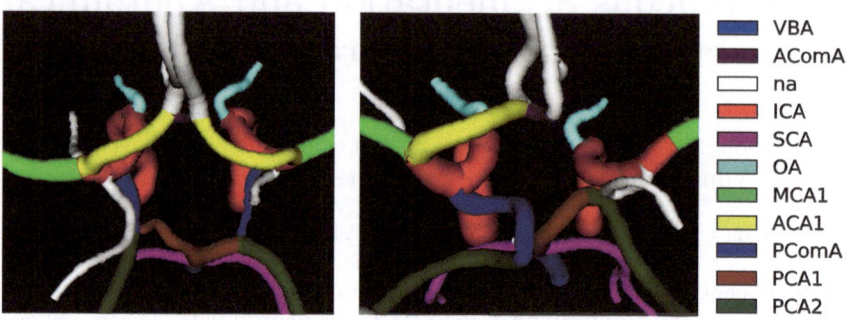

Fig. 1. Configuration of the Circle of Willis for two different subjects as segmented from MRA. The colors indicate the anatomical names of the vessel segments. The left CoW is complete, while the right misses several segments.

less than half of the population has a complete circle, while in the majority of cases, one or more arteries are missing.

Most existing approaches to anatomical labeling of the vasculature pose the problem in a graph-based setting, in which the vertices represent furcations and the edges the branches of the segmented vasculature. For example, Robben et al. [6] label the CoW by matching bifurcations in this graph to a probabilistic atlas, taking into account both unary potentials of the bifurcations and also pairwise potentials between them. Bogunović et al. [1] also label the CoW by matching bifurcations to an atlas. They use the bifurcation properties and have several reference graphs to model the topology of the bifurcations. The method is evaluated on ground truth segmentations as it requires topologically correct segmentations. Mori et al. [5] label the bronchial branches, which are tree-like with no loops, in an edge matching approach. A trained classifier gives a probability to each possible pair of branch and label. The solution is the global optimal assignment of labels taking into account several topological constraints. All these approaches rely on a pre-existing segmentation in terms of a graph of potential blood vessels. They account for the fact that vasculature is not a random set of tubular structures but an organ with specific connectivity patterns. However they fail to exploit this knowledge to improve the segmentations. Finally, Lu et al. [4] segment and label three non-branching coronary arteries by generating many possible segmentations and selecting – based solely on geometry – for each label the most likely.

By contrast, in this paper, we propose to perform the segmentation and labeling jointly. To the best of our knowledge, we are the first to propose such a simultaneous model-based approach for vascular structures. Not only does this approach yield better results than state-of-the-art methods [7] but it is also very generic and could equally well be applied to other curvilinear structures.

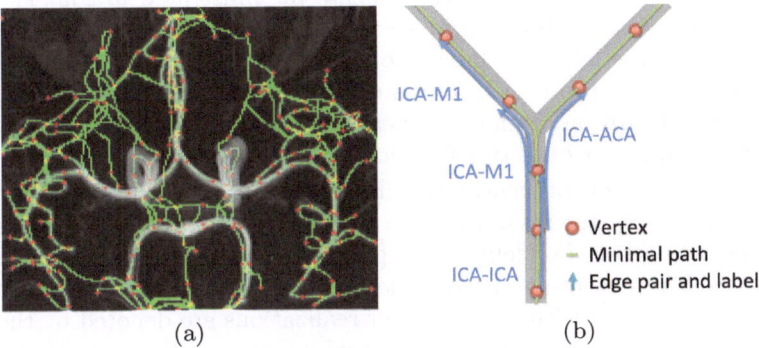

(a)   (b)

Fig. 2. (a) Maximum intensity projection of the overcomplete graph capturing the cerebral vasculature overlaid on the MRA image. (b) Illustration of the edge and edge pair labels.

2   Methodology

Following of Türetken et al. [7], we first compute a 4D scale-space *tubularity* volume, in which the last dimension stands for the vessel radius, or scale. The values represent the likelihood that there is a vessel of that radius centered at the voxel in the image. We sample local maxima of this volume at regular intervals (5 mm) and treat the samples as vertices V_I in a directed graph $G_I = (V_I, E_I)$, which contains the vasculature (Fig. 2a). The edges E_I represent tubular paths and are obtained by connecting pairs of samples that are within a certain distance from each other, using the Fast Marching Algorithm [3] in the scale space. We assume that G_I is overcomplete such that its edges cover all the vessels in the image, but it also contains spurious branches that are not part of the vasculature.

We then select a subgraph in G_I and anatomically label its edges such that it most likely represents the true vasculature. This is done jointly by optimizing a global objective function that captures both the image evidence and the prior knowledge about the geometry and connectivity of the labeled arteries.

In contrast to earlier approaches that attempt to sample their vertices from the true furcations of the vasculature, which are very hard to obtain accurately, the vertices in our graphs do not need to coincide with the furcations. As a consequence, an edge can belong to multiple anatomical segments as illustrated in Fig. 2b. However, we infer the position of the furcations once the optimal solution is obtained by merging its overlapping edges that occupy the same 3D space.

Notation. Given an image I, let $G = (V, E)$ be the directed graph obtained by adding a virtual vertex v_v to G_I such that $V = \{v_i\} = V_I \cup \{v_v\}$ and $E = \{e_{ij} = (v_i, v_j)\} = E_I \cup \{(v_v, v_i) | v_i \in V_I\}$. Let also $S = \{s_i\}$ be the set of the anatomical labels for distinct segments of the vasculature extended with a void label (na) for unnamed vessel segments (as illustrated in Fig. 1). This is necessary since we are interested in segmenting the whole cerebral vasculature rather than only the labeled segments of the CoW.

We formulate our problem in terms of consecutive edge pairs in G, since it allows us to capture more global appearance and geometry information, and it gives rise to a linear objective function and constraints [7]. Let $F = \{e_{ijk} = (e_{ij}, e_{jk})\}$ be the set of consecutive directed edge pairs and and $\hat{L} = \{(s_1, .., s_n)|1 \leq n \leq 4, \forall i : s_i \in S\}$, the set of the edge pair labels, where an edge pair label is a tuple of segment labels. We define $\boldsymbol{X} = \{X_{ijk}^l\}$ to be the vector of binary random variables, each representing the (non-)existence of a vessel segment along the directed edge pair e_{ijk} with label l. Their realizations are denoted by the vector of binary variables $\boldsymbol{x} = \{x_{ijk}^l\}$. In the following, we pose the joint segmentation and labeling problem as an integer program (IP) over $\boldsymbol{x}$ subject to a set of constraints. We solve the resulting IPs to provable optimality (with a solution gap of $1e^{-4}$) using the branch-and-cut procedure of the Gurobi Optimizer[1]. The optimization took on average 20 mins. per image on a single core.

Objective Function. We formulate the problem as a maximum likelihood (ML) inference over the binary variables $\boldsymbol{x}$:

$$\boldsymbol{x}^* = \arg\max_{\boldsymbol{x} \in \mathcal{X}} P(I, G|\boldsymbol{X} = \boldsymbol{x}) \tag{1}$$

where $\mathcal{X}$ denotes the set of feasible solutions that satisfy the constraints described later in this section. We decompose $\boldsymbol{X} = \{X_{ijk}^l\}$ into two sets of random variables $\boldsymbol{T} = \{T_{ijk}\}$ and $\boldsymbol{L} = \{L_{ijk}\}$, with the binary variable T_{ijk} representing whether the edge pair e_{ijk} belongs to the underlying vasculature and L_{ijk} representing the label $l \in \hat{L}$ of the edge pair. We write:

$$P(I, G|\boldsymbol{X} = \boldsymbol{x}) \propto P(\boldsymbol{T} = t|I, G)\frac{P(\boldsymbol{L} = l|\boldsymbol{T} = t, I, G)}{P(\boldsymbol{T} = t, \boldsymbol{L} = l)}. \tag{2}$$

We omit here the derivation of the first term $P(\boldsymbol{T} = t|I, G)$ as it is given in [7]. To derive the second term, we assume conditional independence of the image evidence given X_{ijk}^l, a uniform distribution $P(L_{ijk}|T_{ijk} = 0)$ – if the edge is not part of the solution, the choice of label is arbitrary – and a uniform prior distribution over $\boldsymbol{T}$. As we show in the supplementary material[2] , this yields:

$$\frac{P(\boldsymbol{L} = l|\boldsymbol{T} = t, I, G)}{P(\boldsymbol{T} = t, \boldsymbol{L} = l)} \propto \prod_{e_{jk} \in E} \prod_{e_{ij} \in E} \prod_{l \in \hat{L}} \left[\frac{P(L_{ijk} = l|I, G, T_{ijk} = 1)}{P(L_{ijk} = l|T_{ijk} = 1)}\right]^{x_{ijk}^l}. \tag{3}$$

Taking the logarithm of Eq. 2 results in an objective function that is linear in the x_{ijk}^l variables:

$$\sum_{e_{ijk} \in F} \sum_{l \in \hat{L}} \left[\log \frac{P(T_{ijk} = 1|I, G)}{1 - P(T_{ijk} = 1|I, G)} + \log \frac{P(L_{ijk} = l|I, G, T_{ijk} = 1)}{P(L_{ijk} = l|T_{ijk} = 1)}\right] x_{ijk}^l. \tag{4}$$

---

[1] http://www.gurobi.com
[2] http://www.medicalimagingcenter.be/public/MIC/publications/DR201405/

Table 1. Comparison of the labeling performance on the ground truth centerlines

Bifurcation	Proposed			Bogunović et al.[1]		
	accuracy	precision	recall	accuracy	precision	recall
ICA-OA	99	100	99	-	-	-
ICA-M1	99	99	100	99	100	99
ICA-PComA	93	94	96	97	98	98
ACA1-AComA	92	93	97	98	97	100
M1-M2	89	89	100	82	82	100
VBA-SCA	95	98	97	-	-	-
VBA-PCA1	94	100	93	96	96	100
PCA1-PComA	96	100	94	98	97	100
PCA2-PCA3	89	92	93	-	-	-

The probabilities $P(T_{ijk} = 1|I, G)$ are obtained using the path classifier introduced in [7], and $P(L_{ijk} = l|I, G, T_{ijk} = 1)$ is obtained from a random forest classifier using geometrical features such as the mean position, direction and radius of the edge pair e_{ijk}.

Constraints. Not every x gives rise to a biologically plausible and feasible solution. For example, we force the active edge pairs in the final solution to be connected to the virtual vertex v_v as in [7], and every edge e_{jk} to have at most one incoming edge pair e_{ijk} as illustrated in Fig. 2b. Furthermore, our algorithm learns from the annotated training data which edge pair labels – and more importantly – configurations of labels are possible in the final solution: labels of overlapping edge pairs should be compatible, some labels can occur only in a furcation, etc. All these constraints are expressed by the linear inequality $Wx <= b$, where $W_{ij} \in \{-1, 0, 1\}$ and b is a binary vector. A more detailed description is given in the supplementary material.

3   Evaluation

In this section, we first evaluate the labeling and segmentation performance of our algorithm separately, each against the state-of-the-art approach for the respective task and then report our combined performance. All experiments are done with a leave-one-image-out cross-validation, using 50 MRA images of the cerebral vasculature from a public dataset [2] together with their ground truth segmentations (as used in and provided by [1]) and anatomical labels manually annotated by an expert. The images are rigidly aligned and cropped to the region that covers the segmentations [1].

Anatomical Labeling on the Ground Truth Centerlines. Instead of using an overcomplete graph constructed from the image, we create a graph from the ground truth centerlines. This graph is unlabeled, but contains only valid edges.

Table 2. Results of the simultaneous segmentation and labeling. (a) Comparison of the segmentation performance. Reported numbers are the mean and standard deviation (in parenthesis) over the images. (b) Labeling performance.

(a)

Metric	Proposed	Türetken [7]
Prec. overlap	83(5)	84(6)
Recall overlap	76(5)	77(5)
Prec. topology	61(39)	44(44)
Recall topology	70(43)	65(42)

(b)

Bifurcation	acc.	prec.	recall
ICA-OA	60	79	69
ICA-M1	91	95	95
ICA-PComA	68	73	79
ACA1-AComA	55	52	98
M1-M2	59	59	98
VBA-SCA	82	95	85
VBA-PCA1	83	90	90
PCA1-PComA	42	28	52
PCA2-PCA3	71	73	88

By setting $P(T_{ijk} = 1|I, G) = 1$, we can use our algorithm to only perform labeling. The result is an edge labeled graph, from which we can infer the positon of several named bifurcations. The positions are compared with those in the ground truth annotation. If the Euclidean distance is smaller than 2mm, it is considered a true positive. Since we use the same dataset as [1], we can directly compare the performance. Results are given in table 1.

On average, the accuracy is about the same, but on individual PoI, there is quite some difference, especially on the furcation formed by M1-M2. This furcation has many variations and to infer its position, medical experts look at the end positions of its daughter branches. This is done implicitly by our edge labeling algorithm. Finally, it should be noted that the method of Bogunović et al. [1] requires topologically correct segmentations, and uses reference graphs explicitly stating PoI connectivity and order for the entire vasculature. Extending it to a larger number of bifurcations requires a steep increase in the number of reference graphs. For example, inclusion of the left and right VBA-SCA, which can lie either before or after VBA-PCA1 and not necessarily next to each other, would already triple the number of reference graphs from 8 to 24 in their approach.

Simultaneous Segmentation and Labeling. We compare the segmentation quality of our method with the method of Türetken et al. [7], which can be thought of as our algorithm without the labeling step. The comparison is performed based on two criteria: overlap and topology of the solutions. The former is computed by measuring the distance between the centerline points of the ground truth and the solution. We consider a point in the solution to be a true (false) positive if its distance to the closest ground truth point is less (more) than half the ground truth's radius at that point.

The topology criterion, on the other hand, is a more global measure since it captures connectivity of the vasculature. We compute it by first finding all the paths that extend between the start points of the VBA or ICAs segments in

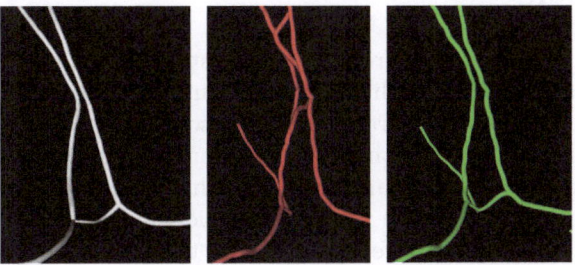

Fig. 3. The centerlines of the ACA1 and AComA according to the ground truth (left), the method of Türetken et al. (middle), which contains spurious branches, and the proposed method (right).

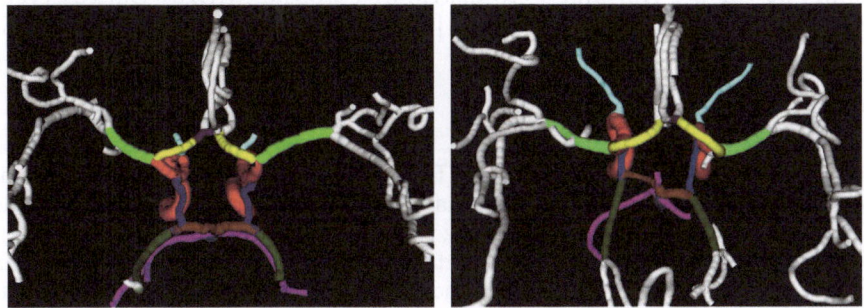

Fig. 4. Two automatically segmented and labeled vasculatures. As in Fig. 1, the colors indicate the anatomical labels of the vessel segments.

the ground truth. Note that such a path visits multiple anatomical segments in the CoW. We only compute the paths between the VBA and ICAs segments because they are the brain supplying arteries, and therefore, the origin of the blood supply to the entire vasculature. We then enumerate all the paths between these three segments in the obtained solution and find their corresponding paths in the ground truth if they exist. We consider a path in the solution to be a true positive if the overlap precision and recall of its centerline points (as described earlier in this section) are both above 0.7.

Table 2a gives the precision and recall values over the evaluated images for the two measures. The overlap values of the two methods are relatively similar but still significantly better than thresholding and thinning, as used in [6] (precision: 73(7), recall 64(6)). In terms of the topology criterion, our approach clearly outperforms that of [7], which is also illustrated in the close-ups of Fig. 3.

The labeling results are given in Table 2b, which are calculated as described in Section 3. The results show that the additional difficulty of segmenting the image causes the labeling accuracy to drop. Finally, Fig. 4 shows automated segmentation and labeling results of our algorithm for two complete vasculatures.

4   Conclusion

To the best our knowledge, we presented the first algorithm for simultaneous segmentation and anatomical labeling of the vasculature. Our probabilistic formulation results in an integer program, which we solved optimally on the evaluated dataset of 50 images. We demonstrated that our approach compares favorably against specialized state-of-the-art algorithms that address the segmentation and labeling problems separately. In future work, we will evaluate the segmentation quality more extensively on different structure types and imaging modalities.

Acknowledgement. This work was supported in part by the EU ERC project MicroNano. The MR brain images from healthy volunteers used in this paper were collected and made available by the CASILab at The University of North Carolina at Chapel Hill and were distributed by the MIDAS Data Server at Kitware Inc. We thank the authors of [1] for sharing their centerline delineations.

References

1. Bogunovic, H., Pozo, J.M., Cardenes, R., Roman, L.S., Frangi, A.F.: Anatomical labeling of the Circle of Willis using maximum a posteriori probability estimation. IEEE Transactions on Medical Imaging 32(9), 1587–1599 (2013)
2. Bullitt, E., Zeng, D., Gerig, G., Aylward, S., Joshi, S., Smith, J.K., Lin, W., Ewend, M.G.: Vessel tortuosity and brain tumor malignancy: A blinded study. Academic Radiology 12(10), 1232–1240 (2005)
3. Li, H., Yezzi, A.: Vessels as 4-D curves: global minimal 4-D paths to extract 3-D tubular surfaces and centerlines. IEEE Transactions on Medical Imaging 26(9), 1213–1223 (2007)
4. Lu, L., Bi, J., Yu, S., Peng, Z., Krishnan, A., Zhou, X.S.: Hierarchical Learning for Tubular Structure Parsing in Medical Imaging: A Study on Coronary Arteries Using 3D CT Angiography. In: ICCV, pp. 2021–2028 (2009)
5. Mori, K., Ota, S., Deguchi, D., Kitasaka, T., Suenaga, Y., Iwano, S., Hasegawa, Y., Takabatake, H., Mori, M., Natori, H.: Automated anatomical labeling of bronchial branches extracted from CT datasets based on machine learning and combination optimization and its application to bronchoscope guidance. In: Yang, G.-Z., Hawkes, D., Rueckert, D., Noble, A., Taylor, C. (eds.) MICCAI 2009, Part II. LNCS, vol. 5762, pp. 707–714. Springer, Heidelberg (2009)
6. Robben, D., Sunaert, S., Thijs, V., Wilms, G., Maes, F., Suetens, P.: Anatomical labeling of the Circle of Willis using maximum a posteriori graph matching. In: Mori, K., Sakuma, I., Sato, Y., Barillot, C., Navab, N. (eds.) MICCAI 2013, Part I. LNCS, vol. 8149, pp. 566–573. Springer, Heidelberg (2013)
7. Turetken, E., Benmansour, F., Andres, B., Pfister, H., Fua, P.: Reconstructing loopy curvilinear structures using integer programming. In: CVPR, pp. 1822–1829 (2013)

Atlas-Based Under-Segmentation

Christian Wachinger[1,2] and Polina Golland[1]

[1] Computer Science and Artificial Intelligence Lab, MIT
[2] Massachusetts General Hospital, Harvard Medical School

Abstract. We study the widespread, but rarely discussed, tendency of atlas-based segmentation to under-segment the organs of interest. Commonly used error measures do not distinguish between under- and over-segmentation, contributing to the problem. We explicitly quantify over- and under-segmentation in several typical examples and present a new hypothesis for the cause. We provide evidence that segmenting only one organ of interest and merging all surrounding structures into one label creates bias towards background in the label estimates suggested by the atlas. We propose a generative model that corrects for this effect by learning the background structures from the data. Inference in the model separates the background into distinct structures and consequently improves the segmentation accuracy. Our experiments demonstrate a clear improvement in several applications.

1 Introduction

Atlas-based segmentation exploits knowledge from previously labeled training images to segment the target image. In this paper, we focus on multi-atlas segmentation methods that map all labeled images onto the target image, which helps to reduce segmentation errors [6,8,11]. Label fusion combines the transferred labels into the final segmentation [9]. A common tendency of atlas-based segmentation to under-segment has largely been ignored in the field. We conjecture that one of the reasons that this phenomenon has not received more attention is that common error metrics do not capture the under-segmentation effect. For instance, the Dice volume overlap [3] and the Hausdorff distance [4] do not indicate if the segmentation is too large or too small. We are only aware of one recent article that addresses the spatial bias in atlas-based segmentation [12]. In that work, the bias is approximated by spatial convolution with an isotropic Gaussian kernel, modeling the distribution of residual registration errors. This model implies under-segmentation of convex shapes and over-segmentation of concave shapes. To reduce the spatial bias, a deconvolution is applied to the label maps. Results were reported for the segmentation of the hippocampus [12].

We present an alternative hypothesis for the bias in segmentation and propose a strategy to correct for such bias. First, we quantify the under-segmentation in atlas-based segmentation with new volume overlap measures. Our hypothesis ties the under-segmentation to the asymmetry of most segmentation setups where we seek to identify a single organ and merge all surrounding structures

P. Golland et al. (eds.): MICCAI 2014, Part I, LNCS 8673, pp. 315–322, 2014.
© Springer International Publishing Switzerland 2014

into one large background class. We show that this foreground-background segmentation strategy exhibits stronger bias than multi-organ segmentation. We propose a generative model of the background to correct under-segmentation even if the segmentation labels for multiple organs are not available. The posterior probability distribution of the Dirichlet process mixture model yields the splitting of the background into several components. Our experiments illustrate that this refined voting scheme improves the segmentation accuracy.

2   Under-Segmentation in Multi-atlas Segmentation

In multi-atlas segmentation, the training set includes images $\mathcal{I} = \{I_1, \ldots, I_n\}$ with the corresponding manual segmentations $\mathcal{S} = \{S_1, \ldots, S_n\}$ and $S_i(x) \in \{1, \ldots, \eta\}$, where η is the number of labels. The objective is to infer segmentation S for a new input image I. Probabilistic label maps $\mathcal{L} = \{L^1, \ldots, L^\eta\}$ specify the likelihood of each label $l \in \{1, \ldots, \eta\}$ at location $x \in \Omega$ in the new image

$$L^l(x) = \sum_{i=1}^{n} p(S(x) = l|S_i) \cdot p(I(x)|I_i). \tag{1}$$

The label maps satisfy $\sum_l L^l(x) = 1$ and $0 \leq L^l(x) \leq 1$. For obtaining label likelihood, we register all training images $\mathcal{I}$ to the test image I, yielding deformation fields $\{\phi_1, \ldots, \phi_n\}$, and define

$$p(S(x) = l|S_i) = \begin{cases} 1 & \text{if } S_i(\phi_i(x)) = l, \\ 0 & \text{otherwise.} \end{cases} \tag{2}$$

Alternatively, probabilistic segmentations S_i can be included in the label likelihood, with the rest of the analysis unchanged. For majority voting (MV) [6,8], the image likelihood is constant, $p(I(x)|I_i) \propto 1$. For intensity-weighted (IW) voting [9], also referred to as locally-weighted voting, the likelihood depends on image intensities

$$p(I(x)|I_i) \propto \exp\left(-(I(x) - I_i(\phi_i(x)))^2/2\sigma^2\right), \tag{3}$$

where σ^2 is the variance of the image noise. We obtain the final segmentation $\hat{S}(x)$ by choosing the most likely label

$$\hat{S}(x) = \arg\max_l L^l(x). \tag{4}$$

For one structure (η=2), we directly compare foreground and background likelihoods to obtain the segmentation by identifying image locations x for which $L^f(x) > L^b(x)$, or equivalently $L^f(x) > 0.5$.

2.1   Quantifying Under-Segmentation

Since the Dice volume overlap [3] and the Hausdorff distance [4] do not capture the type of segmentation error, we introduce two measures that explicitly

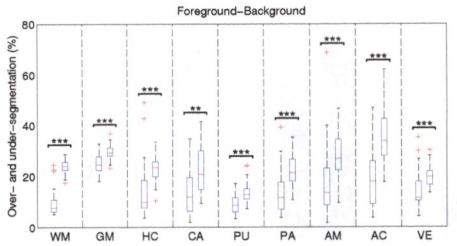
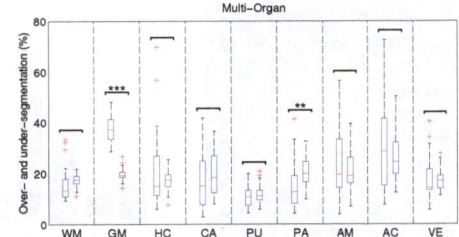

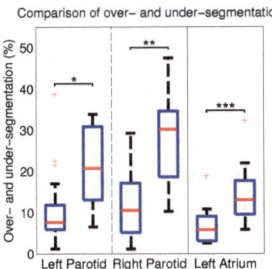

Fig. 1. Statistical analysis of over-segmentation O (left bar) and under-segmentation U (right bar). Top: Segmentation of brain structures with foreground-background (left panel) and multi-organ (right panel) scheme. Left: Segmentation statistics for foreground-background segmentation of parotid glands and left atrium. Red line indicates the median, the boxes extend to the 25th and 75th percentiles, and the whiskers reach to the most extreme values not considered outliers (red crosses). *, **, and *** indicate statistical significance levels at 0.05, 0.01, and 0.001, respectively.

quantify the over- and under-segmentation. Given the manual segmentation $\bar{S}$ and the automatic segmentation $\hat{S}$, we define

$$O(\hat{S}, \bar{S}) = \frac{|\hat{S} \setminus \bar{S}|}{|\bar{S}|} \qquad \text{and} \qquad U(\hat{S}, \bar{S}) = \frac{|\bar{S} \setminus \hat{S}|}{|\bar{S}|} \qquad (5)$$

to quantify over- and under-segmentation, respectively. To examine the problem of under-segmentation, we compute and report statistics in three different segmentation applications using intensity-weighted voting in Fig. 1. The applications target the segmentation of (i) nine brain structures in magnetic resonance (MR) images, (ii) left and right parotid glands in CT images, and (iii) the left atrium of the heart in magnetic resonance angiography (MRA) images. For the brain, we perform foreground-background segmentation by segmenting each brain structure separately and merging all other structures into a background label. The structures we segment are white matter (WM), gray matter (GM), hippocampus (HC), caudate (CA), putamen (PU), pallidum (PA), amygdala (AM), accumbens (AC), ventricles (VE). Under-segmentation errors are significantly higher than over-segmentation errors in all three applications, suggesting a bias towards under-segmentation in atlas-based segmentation.

2.2 Foreground-Background Segmentation Causes Spatial Bias

Our hypothesis for the cause of under-segmentation is the asymmetry in how the foreground and background labels are treated by binary classification methods. Merging all surrounding structures into background causes this new meta-label to dominate in the voting process even if the evidence for the foreground label

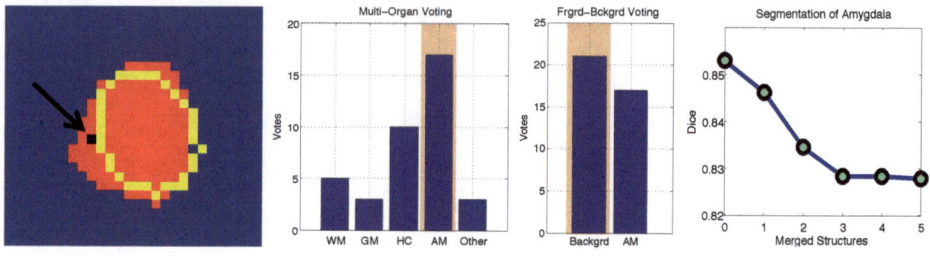

Fig. 2. Left: Manual segmentation of amygdala is shown in red, the outline of the automatic segmentation with foreground-background scheme is shown in yellow. Two middle panels: Distribution of votes for the location marked in black in the image on the left. Multi-organ segmentation correctly assigns the AM label. The foreground-background segmentation assigns the background label, which is an error. Right: Dice volume overlap as a function of the number of merged neighboring structures.

is stronger than that for any of the surrounding structures. We illustrate this phenomenon on the example of the amygdala in Fig. 2. The atlas-based segmentation with the foreground-background scheme yields an under-segmentation (yellow outline). Investigating the votes for one location (black voxel in the left image), we observe that labels from several structures are present. Amygdala is assigned the highest number of votes and would win the voting in a multi-organ scheme. However, merging all other structures into a background label causes the background to win, leading to a segmentation error. To further illustrate the impact of merging neighboring structures, we examine the drop in the Dice volume overlap as we accumulate more and more structures into the background label (Fig. 2, right panel).

To further quantify the difference between foreground-background and multi-organ segmentation, we report the under- and over-segmentation statistics for the brain segmentation in Fig. 1. In comparison to the foreground-background segmentation, the under-segmentation is reduced and most of the significant differences between over- and under-segmentation are reduced or eliminated when we use multiple labels. Interestingly, the gray matter segmentation changes from under- to over-segmentation, which may be attributed to its complex shape. While it is possible for the brain segmentation algorithms to use multi-organ schemes because many structures have been delineated in training data, it is not possible for many other applications (*e.g.*, left atrium or parotid glands), where no multi-label training data exists.

3   Latent Multi-label Model of the Background

We introduce a generative model that estimates latent labels for the background structures from the available images. We emphasize that the method does not require multi-label training segmentations. We use image intensities of the training data to perform unsupervised separation of the background into K components while simultaneously estimating the number of components K. Estimated components serve as labels in the voting procedure. We assume that image patches $P_{ix} = I_i(\mathcal{M}(x))$, with patch neighborhood $\mathcal{M}$, are sampled from a Gaussian mixture model (GMM). Since we do not know the number of components a priori, we employ a Dirichlet process Gaussian mixture model (DP-GMM) [5,10] to account for the potentially infinite number of components. In practice, the number of components is determined as part of the inference procedure. Formally, our generative model and the corresponding graphical model are as follows

$$
\begin{aligned}
P_{ix}|z_{ix} &\sim \mathcal{N}(\mu_{z_{ix}}, \Sigma_{z_{ix}}), \\
z_{ix} &\sim \mathrm{Cat}(\pi), \\
\pi &\sim \mathrm{GEM}(\alpha), \\
(\mu_k, \Sigma_k) &\sim H(\lambda),
\end{aligned}
$$

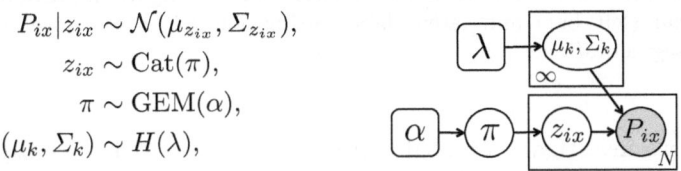

where (μ_k, Σ_k) are the mean and covariance of the normal distribution. We choose the conjugate Normal-Wishart distribution H with hyperparameter λ as a prior on the parameters (μ_k, Σ_k) [5]. Mixture weights π follow a stick-breaking process GEM with parameter α [10]. Setting $\Sigma_u = \sigma I$, the asymptotic case of $\sigma \to 0$ yields the DP-means algorithm [7], which is an extension of the k-means algorithm that assumes a variable number of clusters during the estimation procedure. We compare the performance of k-means, DP-means, GMM, and DP-GMM in our experiments. For k-means and DP-means, we use k-means++ seeding for initialization [1].

Once the inference yields a model with K components, the index $z_{ix} \in \{1, \ldots, K\}$ specifies the component that generates the patch P_{ix}. Since we only consider background patches, we replace the background label $S_i(x) = b$ with the component index $S_i(x) = z_{ix}$ in the voting procedure. The labels for the foreground-background segmentation therefore change from $\{f, b\}$ to $\{f, 1, \ldots, K\}$. Voting on this updated label set as defined in Eq. (4) yields the segmentation.

3.1   Model Inference

The increased model complexity of DP mixture models makes the posterior inference difficult. Variational inference algorithms that approximate the result lack convergence guarantees. Instead, we use a recently proposed inference scheme based on efficient Markov chain Monte Carlo sampling, which shows improved convergence properties [2]. The method combines non-ergodic, restricted Gibbs iteration with split-merge moves yielding an ergodic Markov chain.

It is not necessary to perform the inference on the entire background region, as it will affect the voting only in voxels close to the organ boundary. We restrict the inference to the atlas-induced region $\Gamma = \{x \in \Omega : 0.1 < L^f(x) < 0.5\}$, since our procedure does not change the vote of foreground locations. Within

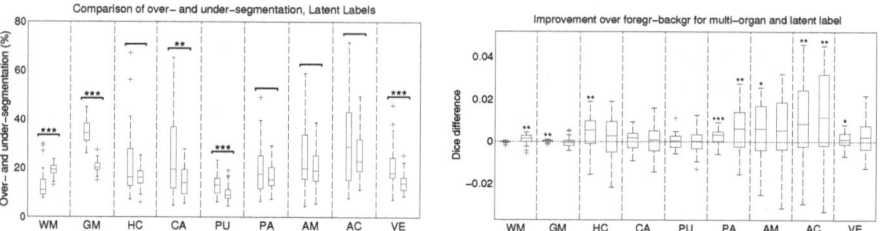

Fig. 3. Segmentation statistics for brain data. Left: Over- and under-segmentation for each brain structure after inference of latent labels. Right: Improvement offered by multi-organ (left bar) and latent label estimation (right bar) over foreground-background segmentation.

this region, we investigate a global and a local approach. The global approach considers background patches in the region Γ for all training images, $\mathcal{P} = \{P_{ix} : x \in \Gamma, S_i(x) = b\}$. The local approach selects patches in a small region R around a current location $\mathcal{P}(x) = \{P_{iy} : y \in R(x), S_i(y) = b\}$. Considering patches in a small region is necessary to have more relevant samples for learning the parameters. For the local approach, we perform separate inferences for each location on $\mathcal{P}(x)$, instead of one global inference on $\mathcal{P}$.

4   Results

We evaluate our approach on three datasets. The first set contains 39 brain MR T1 scans with 1mm isotropic resolution and dimensions $256 \times 256 \times 256$ that were used to construct the FreeSurfer atlas. The second dataset includes 18 CT scans from patients with head and neck cancer [11], containing between 80 and 200 axial slices with a slice thickness of 2.5mm. The in-plane resolution is 0.9mm, the slice size is 512×512 pixels. The third dataset contains 16 heart MRA images that are electro-cardiogram gated to counteract considerable volume changes of the left atrium and contrast-enhanced (0.2 mmol/kg, Gadolinium-DTPA, CIDA sequence, TR=4.3ms, TE=2.0ms). The in-plane resolution varies from 0.51mm to 0.68mm and slice thickness varies from 1.2mm to 1.7mm with an image resolution of $512 \times 512 \times 96$. We use intensity-weighted voting for creating baseline label maps that serve as input to our algorithm ($\sigma = 10$ for brain, $\sigma = 45$ for head and neck, $\sigma = 0.5$ for heart). We compare to the deconvolution with a generalized Gaussian [12], where we sweep kernel parameters for each application to determine the best setting. We quantify the segmentation accuracy with the Dice volume overlap between manual and automatic segmentation.

We set the patch size $\mathcal{M}$ to $(3, 3, 3)$ for brain and $(3, 3, 1)$ for the other two applications to account for anisotropy in the data. For the global approach, we evaluate k-means, DP-means, GMM, and DP-GMM. We set $\alpha = 0.1$ for DP-GMM and create a new cluster in DP-means if the distance to a cluster center exceeds 10 times the average distance within a cluster. For GMM and k-means,

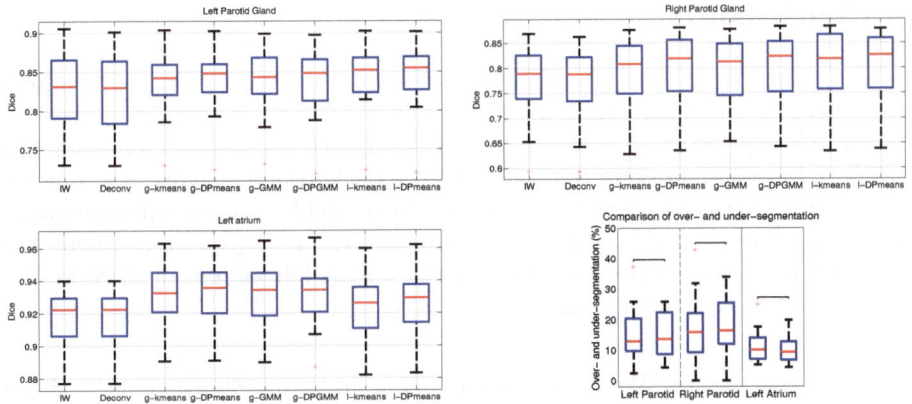

Fig. 4. Segmentation accuracy of parotid glands (top) and left atrium (bottom left). We compare global (g-) and local (l-) approaches with intensity-weighted voting (IW) [9] and the deconvolution approach (Deconv) [12] as baseline methods. The plot in the bottom right shows the over- and under-segmentation statistics after latent label estimation for all three structures.

we set the number of clusters to 5. For the local approach, we set the region R to $(3, 3, 3)$ and only consider k-means and DP-means because other methods become computationally prohibitive. The number of clusters is set to 3 for the local approach, as we expect fewer structures to be present at one location.

Fig. 3 reports segmentation results of brain structures with the inference of latent background labels using DP-GMM. The under-segmentation is reduced when compared to the foreground-background segmentation in Fig. 1. The latent label estimation offers improvements in accuracy that are comparable to those of the multi-organ scheme, without requiring the multiple organ segmentations for the training set. Fig. 4 illustrates segmentation results for the parotid glands and the left atrium, where we experiment with different inference methods and add the deconvolution approach to the comparison. We also quantify the under-segmentation for the proposed method. We observe that the differences between over- and under-segmentation are no longer significant.

Our results demonstrate the advantage of estimating latent background labels over foreground-background segmentation. The non-parametric methods based on the Dirichlet process yield a slight additional gain compared to their parametric counterparts. This is a consequence of the simultaneous estimation of component membership and number of components, which enables dynamic adaptation to the data. The comparison of global and local approaches indicates that the performance is application dependent. While local approaches perform better for parotid glands, they are slightly worse for the left atrium. Our experiments with majority voting are not included in the article but they confirm the presented results.

5 Conclusion

We demonstrated that a significant bias exists in atlas-based segmentation that leads to under-segmentation. We proposed the asymmetry in foreground-background segmentation as a new hypothesis for the cause of this phenomenon. To reduce the domination of the voting by the background, we introduced a generative model for the background based on the Dirichlet process mixture model. Inference of latent labels yielded partitioning of the background. Segmentation results for brain structures, parotid glands, and the left atrium illustrated clear improvement in the segmentation quality.

Acknowledgements. We thank Jason Chang and Greg Sharp. This work was supported in part by the National Alliance for Medical Image Computing (U54-EB005149) and the NeuroImaging Analysis Center (P41-EB015902).

References

1. Arthur, D., Vassilvitskii, S.: k-means++: the advantages of careful seeding. In: ACM-SIAM Symposium on Discrete Algorithms (SODA), pp. 1027–1035 (2007)
2. Chang, J., Fisher III, J.W.: Parallel sampling of dp mixture models using sub-clusters splits. In: Neural Information Processing Systems, pp. 620–628 (2013)
3. Dice, L.: Measures of the amount of ecologic association between species. Ecology 26(3), 297–302 (1945)
4. Dubuisson, M., Jain, A.: A modified hausdorff distance for object matching. In: International Conference on Pattern Recognition, vol. 1, pp. 566–568 (1994)
5. Görür, D., Rasmussen, C.E.: Dirichlet process gaussian mixture models: Choice of the base distribution. Computer Science and Technology 25(4), 653–664 (2010)
6. Heckemann, R., Hajnal, J., Aljabar, P., Rueckert, D., Hammers, A.: Automatic anatomical brain MRI segmentation combining label propagation and decision fusion. NeuroImage 33(1), 115–126 (2006)
7. Kulis, B., Jordan, M.I.: Revisiting k-means: New algorithms via bayesian nonparametrics. In: International Conference on Machine Learning, pp. 513–520 (2012)
8. Rohlfing, T., Brandt, R., Menzel, R., Maurer, C., et al.: Evaluation of atlas selection strategies for atlas-based image segmentation with application to confocal microscopy images of bee brains. NeuroImage 21(4), 1428–1442 (2004)
9. Sabuncu, M., Yeo, B., Van Leemput, K., Fischl, B., Golland, P.: A Generative Model for Image Segmentation Based on Label Fusion. IEEE Transactions on Medical Imaging 29 (2010)
10. Sudderth, E.B.: Graphical Models for Visual Object Recognition and Tracking. Ph.D. thesis, Massachusetts Institute of Technology (2006)
11. Wachinger, C., Sharp, G.C., Golland, P.: Contour-driven regression for label inference in atlas-based segmentation. In: Mori, K., Sakuma, I., Sato, Y., Barillot, C., Navab, N. (eds.) MICCAI 2013, Part III. LNCS, vol. 8151, pp. 211–218. Springer, Heidelberg (2013)
12. Wang, H., Yushkevich, P.A.: Spatial bias in multi-atlas based segmentation. In: Computer Vision and Pattern Recognition (CVPR), pp. 909–916 (2012)

Bayesian Model Selection for Pathological Data

Carole H. Sudre[1,2], Manuel Jorge Cardoso[1,2], Willem Bouvy[3],
Geert Jan Biessels[3], Josephine Barnes[2], and Sébastien Ourselin[1,2]

[1] Translational Imaging Group, CMIC, University College London, NW1 2HE, UK
[2] Dementia Research Centre, UCL Institute of Neurology, London, WC1N 3BG, UK
[3] Department of Neurology and Neurosurgery, UMC Utrecht, Netherlands

Abstract. The detection of abnormal intensities in brain images caused by the presence of pathologies is currently under great scrutiny. Selecting appropriate models for pathological data is of critical importance for an unbiased and biologically plausible model fit, which in itself enables a better understanding of the underlying data and biological processes. Besides, it impacts on one's ability to extract pathologically meaningful imaging biomarkers. With this aim in mind, this work proposes a fully unsupervised hierarchical model selection framework for neuroimaging data which permits the stratification of different types of abnormal image patterns without prior knowledge about the subject's pathological status.

1 Introduction

Measures of pathological load visible on MRI and comparison with healthy tissues can be used to ascertain clinical correlations and infer disease progression [6]. As the presence of pathology leads to unexpected observations (i.e. outlier intensities), from a modelling perspective, two main problems arise: first, bias is introduced in the model parameters' estimation by the pathological outliers when segmenting non-pathological tissues [3], [12]; second, there is a need for prior knowledge in order to design better pathology-specific segmentation algorithms. Due to pathology specific tuning and the reliance on knowledge-based heuristic rules [14], [7], these methods are not easily transposed from one pathology to another [1]. Furthermore, multiple types of outliers might be present [16].

Using a finite weighted sum of Gaussian components, also known as a Gaussian mixture model (GMM), is probably the most widespread way of modelling the distribution of observed intensities in neuroimaging data [2]. Optimising the model parameters is usually performed through the Expectation-Maximisation algorithm (EM) introduced in [4]. Due to the presence of pathology, an *a priori* fixed number of Gaussian components might not be appropriate to tackle the problems related to the presence of pathology-linked intensities [5]. Moreover, as underlined in [10] and [15], natural appearing features such as the cerebrospinal fluid (CSF) are not well explained by a single Gaussian component due to the high variability of their contents.

This work proposes a Bayesian inference criterion (BIC) regularised adaptive hierarchical Gaussian mixture model selection framework, enabling an automated selection of the number of components necessary to model both the

P. Golland et al. (Eds.): MICCAI 2014, Part I, LNCS 8673, pp. 323–330, 2014.

outlier (pathologies such as lesions, tumours or vasculature) and the inlier part (normal anatomical tissues such as white matter (WM), grey matter (GM), CSF or non-brain (NB)) of the observed data. The model selection framework exploits a split-and-merge strategy (SM) [9] for model search, which combined with the BIC, ensures a balance between computational burden, model fit and model complexity. Additional spatial knowledge is introduced through the use of probabilistic tissue atlases and a Markov Random Field (MRF) [14]. After describing the data generative model and the model selection and inference strategies, we present results illustrating the generality of the proposed method both on simulated and clinical data.

2   Methods

2.1   General Modelling and EM Algorithm

The proposed framework models the intensity observations as a hierarchical mixture of Gaussian and uniform components. In the following, $\mathcal{Y}$ denotes the set of N log-transformed intensity vectors of dimension d, $\{\mathbf{y}_1, \cdots, \mathbf{y}_n, \cdots \mathbf{y}_N\}$, where N and d are respectively the number of voxels and the number of available modalities (T1w, T2w, PD, etc). The data likelihood for model $\mathbf{K}$ is defined as $F(\mathcal{Y}|\boldsymbol{\Theta}_{\mathbf{K}})$, where $\boldsymbol{\Theta}_{\mathbf{K}}$ represents the model parameters. More specifically, we propose a three level hierarchical model: a first level (l) characterising if an observation is an outlier or an inlier, a second level (j) characterising its tissue class (i.e. if an inlier/outlier voxel belongs to WM, GM, CSF or NB) and a third level (k) characterising the multiple intensity clusters/distributions of each inlier or outlier tissue class. In order to robustly model the data, one can separate the first level of the model into two density functions I and O, that correspond respectively to the inlier part, modelling the healthy tissues, and to the outlier part, related to the unexpected tissues, such that $F(\mathbf{y}_n|\boldsymbol{\Theta}_{\mathbf{K}}) = b_I \cdot I(\mathbf{y}_n|\boldsymbol{\Theta}_{\mathbf{K}}) + b_O \cdot O(\mathbf{y}_n|\boldsymbol{\Theta}_{\mathbf{K}})$ with $b_I + b_O = 1$. In this scenario, previously proposed models have classically assumed a uniform distribution for O [17]. At the second level of the hierarchical model, the distribution is $F(\mathbf{y}_n|\boldsymbol{\Theta}_{\mathbf{K}}) = \sum_{l \in I,O} b_l \sum_{j=1}^{J} a_{l_j} \Phi(\mathbf{y}_n|\boldsymbol{\Theta}_{l_j})$ where b_l, a_{l_j} and $\Phi(\mathbf{y}_n|\boldsymbol{\Theta}_{l_j})$ are respectively the mixing weight for l, the class weight for l_j and the likelihood of the data at voxel n for the tissue class l_j. In the third level of this multi-layered model, indexed by k, each anatomical class density distribution is finally modelled by a mixture of Gaussian and/or uniform components such that $\Phi(\mathbf{y}_n|\boldsymbol{\Theta}_{l_j}) = \sum_{k=1}^{K_{l_j}} w_{l_{j_k}} \mathcal{G}(\mathbf{y}_n|\theta_{l_{j_k}}) + w_{l_{j_{unif}}} \mathcal{U}_{l_j}$ where K_{l_j} is the number of Gaussian components in class l_j, $w_{l_{j_k}}$ is the mixing proportion of class l_{j_k}, $\mathcal{G}$ is a Gaussian density distribution and $\mathcal{U}$ is a uniform distribution. The parameters of the Gaussian distribution are $\theta_{l_{j_k}} = \left\{\boldsymbol{\mu}_{l_{j_k}}, \Lambda_{l_{j_k}}\right\}$, where $\boldsymbol{\mu}$ and Λ are respectively the multivariate mean and covariance matrix. Assuming iid observations, the multi-layered mixture model can finally be written as follows:

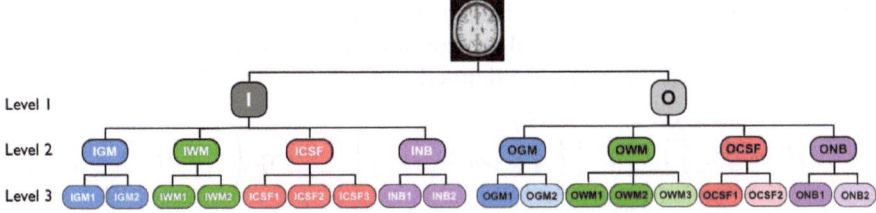

Fig. 1. Example of hierarchical model with 4 main tissue classes (GM, WM, CSF and NB). The lighter colored components follow a uniform distribution.

$$F\left(\mathcal{Y}|\boldsymbol{\Theta}_{\mathbf{K}}\right) = \prod_{i=1}^{N} \sum_{l \in I, O} \sum_{j=1}^{J} \left[\sum_{k=1}^{K_{l_j}} b_l a_{l_j} w_{l_{j_k}} \mathcal{G}\left(\mathbf{y}_n \Big| \theta_{l_{j_k}}\right) + b_l a_{l_j} w_{l_{j_{\text{unif}}}} \right].$$

The final model structure is depicted in Figure 1 where both the inlier and outlier versions of the GM, WM, CSF and NB classes are separated into their sub-clusters. The EM algorithm is used within this setting to optimise the model parameters. Introducing the labelling configuration set $\mathcal{Z} = \{\mathbf{z}_1, \cdots, \mathbf{z}_n, \cdots, \mathbf{z}_N\}$, where $\mathbf{z}_n$ is a unity vector of dimension $\sum_l \sum_j K_{l_j}$, with one component being equal to 1 and all the others to 0, the EM algorithm alternates between the expectation of the complete data log-likelihood $\mathbb{E}_{\boldsymbol{\Theta}_{\mathbf{K}}^{(t)}}\left[\log\left(F\left(\mathcal{Y}|\mathcal{Z}, \boldsymbol{\Theta}_{\mathbf{K}}, \boldsymbol{\pi}\right) F\left(\mathcal{Z}|\boldsymbol{\pi}\right)\right)\right]$ at iteration t, also known as the E-step, and the maximisation of this function with respect to the different parameters, also known as the M-step, where $\boldsymbol{\pi} = \{\mathcal{B}, \mathcal{A}, \mathcal{W}\}$ are the sets of weights attributed to the different components of the mixture levels. At this point, three main types of parameters have to be optimised: first, the parameters of each Gaussian distribution $\theta_{l_{j_k}}$; second, the contribution $w_{l_{j_k}}$ of each distribution to the overall observation model; and third and most importantly, the number of Gaussian components K_{l_j} necessary to describe the underlying distribution of tissue class l_j.

2.2 Spatial and Smoothness Priors

Probabilistic tissue atlases are used to introduce knowledge in the generative model about the location of each tissue class l_j. As b_l is initialised to a global value, $\boldsymbol{\pi}$ has to be normalised to $\boldsymbol{\pi} = \{\tilde{\mathcal{B}}, \tilde{\mathcal{A}}, \mathcal{W}\}$, so that $\forall n, \sum_{j=1}^{J} \tilde{a}_{nj} = 1$ and $\sum_{l \in \{I,O\}} \tilde{b}_{nl} = \sum_{l \in \{I,O\}} \tilde{b}_l = 1$. The priors $\tilde{\mathcal{B}}$ and $\tilde{\mathcal{A}}$ follow a Dirichlet distribution as in [11].

In addition, a MRF is used to spatially regularise the labelling l_{j_k} as in [11,14]. This work defines a symmetric MRF energy matrix H of size $K_{l_j} \times K_{l_j}$ containing the neighborhood clique energies, such that

$$H(l'_{j'_{k'}}, l_{j_k}) = H(l_{j_k}, l'_{j'_{k'}}) = \begin{cases} 0 & \text{if } j = j' \\ 0.2 & \text{if } (j, j') = (\text{WM}, \text{CSF}) \text{ or } (\text{G/WM,NB}) \\ 0.1 & \text{otherwise} \end{cases}$$

Let $\mathbf{p}_m$ be the set of responsibilities for voxel m, updated with Bayes' Rule during the E-step. Under a mean field approximation, with $\mathcal{N}_n$ the set of neighbours of voxel n, the labelling $\mathcal{Z}$ can be defined as:

$$F\left(\mathcal{Z}|H,\boldsymbol{\pi}\right) \propto \prod_{n=1}^{N} \prod_{l\in I,O} \prod_{j=1}^{J} \prod_{k=1}^{K_{l_j}} \left[\tilde{b}_{nl}\tilde{a}_{nl_j}w_{l_{j_k}}\right]^{z_{nl_{j_k}}} \exp\left(-\mathbf{z}_n^t H \sum_{m\in\mathcal{N}_n} \mathbf{p}_m\right).$$

2.3   Model Selection

The flexibility of the proposed model lies in the automatic selection of the appropriate number of components K_{l_j} needed to model each l_j class. Ideally, this parameter could be optimised using a Markov Chain Monte Carlo algorithm. However, due to the computational complexity of such an approach, here, a split-and-merge (SM) algorithm is used for model selection [9,13]. In this framework, a merge operation consists of transforming two close enough Gaussian distributions of the same l_j class, $l_{j_{k_1}}$ and $l_{j_{k_2}}$, into a single component l_{j_k}. A split operation is the transformation of a single distribution, Gaussian or Uniform, into two subcomponents. The symmetric Kullback-Leibler Divergence (KLD) is used to define which component(s) should be split (largest KLD compared to the observations) or merged (smallest KLD between the components' distributions). The SM algorithm alternates between a split and a merge operation given the current model estimates. Parameters' initialisation when splitting or merging Gaussian distribution(s) follows the strategy used in [9]. As no closed-form solution exists when splitting a uniform distribution, a 2-class k-means algorithm is used to estimate the 2 sub-clusters of the samples $\mathcal{U}_{l_j}$. The mean and covariance of the cluster with the smallest variance is used to initialise a new Gaussian class. Finally, the proposed method is optimised using an iterative conditional modes (ICM) approach, where it switches between the optimisation of the model parameters and the model selection. In order to provide a bias-variance trade-off between accuracy and complexity of the model, the Bayesian inference criterion for model $\boldsymbol{K}$, expressed as $\mathrm{BIC}(\boldsymbol{K}) = \kappa\log\left(F\left(\mathcal{Y}|\boldsymbol{\Theta_K}\right)\right) - C(\boldsymbol{K})$ is used as an objective function. It penalises the log-likelihood of the model according to the cost function $C(\boldsymbol{K}) = \left[\sum_l \sum_j K_{l_j}\left(\frac{(d+1)d}{2}+1\right) - j\right] \cdot \log(N\cdot\kappa)$ that depends on the number of free parameters to optimise. Here, κ is a correction factor accounting for the proportion of voxels considered as independent [8]. For each ICM iteration, the model evolves given the most probable model. If the selected model fails to increase the objective function $\mathrm{BIC}(\boldsymbol{K})$ after convergence of the EM, the next most probable model is tested. The SM search stops when all models have been tested.

Implementation Details. In this implementation, the weight for the inlier uniform class is set to 0, as inlier classes are expected to follow a GMM. Also, in order to avoid instability in the inference strategy, the Dirichlet priors are only updated when the initial model converges. The code and further implementation details will be made publicly available.

Table 1. DSC and KLD when using EMS and BaMoS for different modality combinations and lesion loads on the Brainweb MS model

	Modalities	Mild		Moderate		Severe	
		EMS	BaMoS	EMS	BaMoS	EMS	BaMoS
DSC (%)	T1T2PD	4.13	53.31	28.77	54.8	53.78	65.45
	T1T2	2.43	50.94	16.57	52.08	35.28	63.82
	T1PD	13.93	24.63	50.44	59.67	69.24	78.77
	T2PD	3.74	11.58	27.42	39.50	53.43	64.42
KLD($\times 10$)	T1T2PD	6.10	4.21	6.16	4.12	6.13	4.08
	T1T2	0.95	0.29	0.95	0.28	0.93	0.28
	T1PD	1.98	0.46	1.99	0.46	1.99	0.45
	T2PD	3.03	1.01	3.05	1.00	3.05	0.99

3   Validation

3.1   Simulated Images - Brainweb

The simulated multiple sclerosis (MS) lesion model provided by Brainweb http://brainweb.bic.mni.mcgill.ca, with ground truth lesion segmentations, was used to evaluate the performance of the proposed model, here denoted as BaMoS (Bayesian Model Selection). All combinations of the 3 available modalities (T1w, T2w, PD) on the 3 lesion loads (mild, moderate, severe), at 3% of noise and without magnetic field inhomogeneity were assessed. In this experiment, the parameter b_O was initialised to 0.01. The proposed method was compared with the classical lesion segmentation method by van Leemput *et al.* [14], here denoted as EMS, with the parameter 3 for the Mahalanobis distance threshold and MRF parameters as defined in Sec 2.2. The outlier components O_{j_k} of the proposed model with $\mu_{O_{j_k}} > \mu_{I_{WM}}$ and $j = $ WM, for the T2 and PD modalities, were automatically selected as lesion-related intensity clusters. These MS lesion clusters are then added together to form the total lesion segmentation. The Dice similarity coefficient (DSC) and the KLD between the modelled distribution and the observations, here used to compare respectively the binary lesion segmentation overlap and the quality of the model fit, are gathered in Table 1, showing the general improvement brought by BaMoS. Figure 2 depicts the different intensity clusters associated with MS lesions. Note that each lesion component is related to the lesion density in the ground truth.

3.2   Clinical Data - Type 2 Diabetes

Type 2 Diabetes (T2DB) patients typically present white matter hyperintensities (WMH) that correlate with cognitive decline. Segmentation of such variable outliers is needed to study their evolution and their clinical correlates. The behavior of BaMoS on clinical data with multiple types of outliers was evaluated using data with WMH from the MICCAI MRBrainS2013 challenge. For this study, brain images from T2DB patients and controls (age > 50) were acquired on a

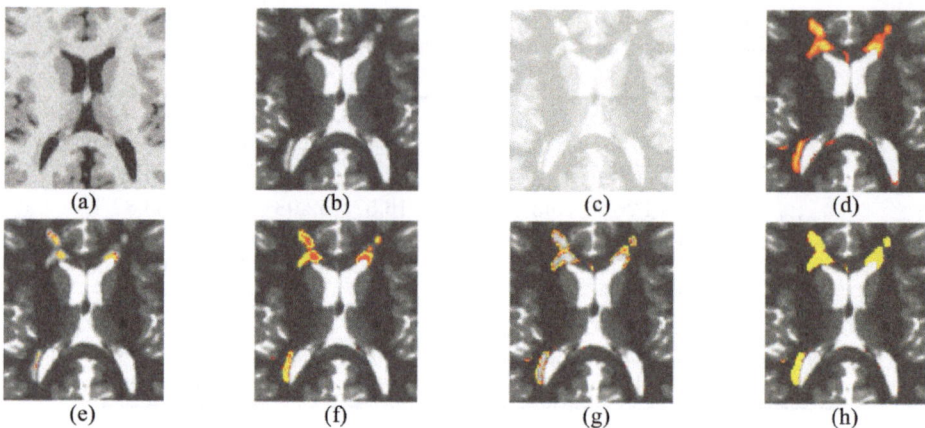

Fig. 2. Top) A zoomed-in section of the T1w (a), T2w (b) and PD (c) simulated Brainweb images with severe MS lesion load followed by the ground truth lesion segmentation (d). Bottom) The three automatically extracted probabilistic lesion maps (e-g), followed by their sum (h) overlayed on the T2 image.

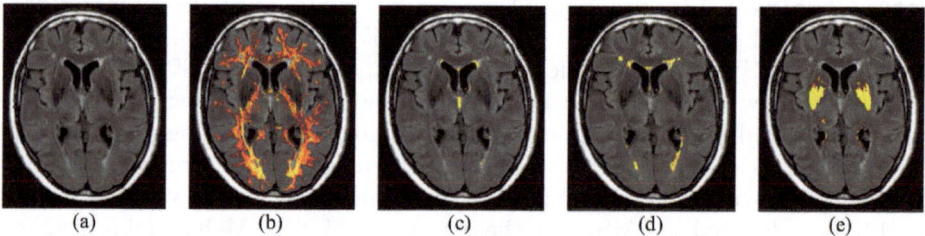

Fig. 3. Components of interest obtained using BaMoS. From left to right) FLAIR image (a), inlier component of WM related to penumbra (b), lesion-related WM outliers (c - d) and WM outlier component localising cysteine-iron complex deposition in the globus pallidus (e).

3T Philips scanner. Multi-slice T2-FLAIR images ($0.958 \times 0.958 \times 3$ mm) and T1w 3D registered images were used. Further details about the acquisition and preprocessing can be found at `http://mrbrains13.isi.uu.nl`. Manual WMH segmentation was performed on 16 FLAIR images. BaMoS was run using the parameters detailed in Sec. 3.1 after extraction of the brain tissues and registration of the statistical atlases to the T1w image. The results obtained for BaMoS and EMS are gathered in Table 2. A 1-tailed t-test showed a significant improvement in terms of both model fit (p-value<0.01) and DSC (p-value<0.05) for BaMoS compared to EMS. The R^2 measure of correlation with the manually segmented WMH's volumes was improved with BaMoS (0.938) compared to EMS (0.887). Figure 3 presents an example of different components of interest separated by BaMoS. BaMoS automatically found separate clusters for both

Table 2. DSC and KLD when comparing EMS and BaMoS performance on WMH segmentation for the studied T2DB and control cases

Case	1	2	4	5	6	7	8	9	10	11	13	15	17	18	19	20
DSC (%)																
EMS	24.2	5.4	40.9	47.4	69.2	5.9	45.7	7.3	20.0	55.5	33.3	24.7	41.7	52.9	3.7	9.3
BaMoS	57.6	8.0	67.8	64.2	80.3	0	69.1	4.0	19.4	49.1	32.0	0	56.4	75.3	4.3	15.3
KLD ($\times$10)																
EMS	1.23	1.06	1.59	1.36	1.22	1.34	1.17	1.08	1.57	1.30	1.11	1.27	1.23	1.39	1.38	1.25
BaMoS	0.67	0.84	0.69	0.86	0.73	0.71	0.88	0.65	0.76	0.72	0.69	0.84	0.83	2.21	0.76	0.74

WM lesion-related hyperintensities and WM hypointensities, strengthening the generalisability argument of the proposed method. The lesion-penumbra related subclass of the WM inlier class might be of interest to study WMH evolution and apparition. In low performance cases, corresponding to milder hyperintensities, the information in the data and model complexity constraints did not support the existence of an extra outlier lesion-related subclass. Finally, we noted the stability in the number of components for each inlier class of the selected model across all subjects.

4 Discussion and Conclusion

This work presents an automated model selection strategy that differentiates between different types of outliers. The main interest of the developed outliers modelling strategy resides in its generality. Indeed, its performance in terms of detection of specific types of outliers, such as MS lesions or white matter hyperintensities, is comparable to other methods specifically tuned towards this goal. However, the proposed method can also simultaneously model other types of outliers (e.g. vessels, iron deposition, etc). This property is of major interest in neurodegenerative disease studies, since different pathological changes might be present concomitantly. Furthermore, the ability to distinguish different lesion densities and their spatial location might be of further interest to help characterise the underlying pathophysiological process. Further work will investigate the balance between the different model parameters, their relationship with the image characteristics and the contribution of the different used modalities.

Acknowledgements. This work was supported by the Wolfson Foundation, the Faculty of Engineering Science UCL, EPSRC (EP/W046410/1, EP/H046410/1, EP/J020990/1, EP/K005278), the MRC (MR/J01107X/1), the EU-FP7 project VPH-DARE@ IT (FP7-ICT-2011-9-601055), NIHR Queen Square Dementia Biomedical Research UK, the NIHR UCLH/UCL Biomedical Research Centre (High Impact Initiative) and Alzheimer's Research UK (ARUK). The Dementia Research Centre is supported by ARUK, Brain Research Trust and the Wolfson

Foundation. The authors would like to thank the staff and patients of the Vascular Cognitive Impairment Group at UMC Utrecht without whom collection and generation of the diabetes-related data would not be possible.

References

1. Admiraal-Behloul, F., van den Heuvel, D., Olofsen, H., van Osch, M., van der Grond, J., van Buchem, M., Reiber, J.: Fully automatic segmentation of white matter hyperintensities in MR images of the elderly. NeuroImage 28 (2005)
2. Balafar, M.A.: Gaussian mixture model based segmentation methods for brain MRI images. Artificial Intelligence Review (2012)
3. Battaglini, M., Jenkinson, M., De Stefano, N.: Evaluating and reducing the impact of white matter lesions on brain volume measurements. HBM 33, 2062–2071 (2012)
4. Dempster, A.P., Laird, N.M., Rubin, D.B.: Maximum likelihood from incomplete data via the EM Algorithm. J. R. Stat. Soc. B 39(1), 1–38 (1977)
5. Fraley, C., Raftery, A.E.: Model-based clustering, discriminant analysis, and density estimation. J. Am. Statist. Assoc. 97(458), 611–631 (2002)
6. García-Lorenzo, D., Francis, S., Narayanan, S., Arnold, D.L., Collins, D.L.: Review of automatic segmentation methods of multiple sclerosis white matter lesions on conventional magnetic resonance imaging. Medical Image Analysis 17, 1–18 (2013)
7. García-Lorenzo, D., Prima, S., Douglas, A.L., Collins, D.L., Barillot, C.: Trimmed-likelihood estimation for focal lesions and tissue segmentation in multisequence mri for multiple sclerosis. IEEE TMI 30(8), 1455–1467 (2011)
8. Groves, A.R., Beckmann, C.F., Smith, S.M., Woolrich, M.W.: Linked independent component analysis for multimodal data fusion. NeuroImage 54(3) (2011)
9. Li, Y., Li, L.: A split and merge EM algorithm for color image segmentation. In: IEEE ICIS 2009, vol. 4, pp. 395–399 (2009)
10. Sajja, B.R., Datta, S., He, R., Mehta, M., Gupta, R.K., Wolinsky, J.S., Narayana, P.A.: Unified approach for multiple sclerosis lesion segmentation on brain MRI. Ann. Biomed. Eng. 34(1), 142–151 (2006)
11. Shiee, N., Bazin, P.-L., Cuzzocreo, J., Blitz, A., Pham, D.L.: Segmentation of brain images using adaptive atlases with application to ventriculomegaly. In: Székely, G., Hahn, H.K. (eds.) IPMI 2011. LNCS, vol. 6801, pp. 1–12. Springer, Heidelberg (2011)
12. Shroeter, P., Vesin, J.M., Langenberger, T., Meuli, R.: Robust parameter estimation of intensity distributions for brain magnetic resonance images. IEEE TMI 17(2), 172–186 (1998)
13. Ueda, N., Nakano, R., Ghahramani, Z., Hinton, G.E.: SMEM Algorithm for Mixture Models. Neural Comput. 12(9), 2109–2128 (2000)
14. Van Leemput, K., Maes, F., Vandermeulen, D., Colchester, A., Suetens, P.: Automated segmentation of multiple sclerosis lesions by model outlier detection. IEEE TMI 20(8), 677–688 (2001)
15. Wolff, Y., Miron, S., Achiron, A., Greespan, H.: Improved CSF classification and lesion detection in MR brain images with multiple sclerosis. In: SPIE, vol. 6512 (2007)
16. Wu, Y., Warfield, S.K., Tan, I.L., Wells III, W.M., Meier, D.S., van Schijndel, R.A., Barkhof, F., Guttmann, C.R.: Automated segmentation of multiple sclerosis lesion subtypes with multichannel MRI. NeuroImage 32, 1205–1215 (2006)
17. Zhuang, X., Huang, Y., Palaniappan, K., Zhao, Y.: Gaussian mixture density modeling, decomposition, and applications. IEEE TIP 5(9), 1293–1302 (1996)

Automatic Localization of Cochlear Implant Electrodes in CT

Yiyuan Zhao[1], Benoit M. Dawant[1], Robert F. Labadie[2], and Jack H. Noble[1]

[1] Dept. of Elect. Eng. and Comp. Sci., Vanderbilt University, Nashville, TN, USA
[2] Dept. of Otolaryngology – Head & Neck Surg., Vanderbilt University, Nashville, TN, USA

Abstract. Cochlear Implants (CI) are surgically implanted neural prosthetic devices used to treat severe-to-profound hearing loss. Recent studies have suggested that hearing outcomes with CIs are correlated with the location where individual electrodes in the implanted electrode array are placed, but techniques proposed for determining electrode location have been too coarse and labor intensive to permit detailed analysis on large numbers of datasets. In this paper, we present a fully automatic snake-based method for accurately localizing CI electrodes in clinical post-implantation CTs. Our results show that average electrode localization errors with the method are 0.21 millimeters. These results indicate that our method could be used in future large scale studies to analyze the relationship between electrode position and hearing outcome, which potentially could lead to technological advances that improve hearing outcomes with CIs.

Keywords: cochlear implant, electrode array, snake, segmentation.

1 Introduction

Cochlear Implants (CI) are surgically implanted neural prosthetic devices used to treat severe-to-profound hearing loss. In CI surgery, an electrode array is threaded into the cochlea. After surgery, a processor worn behind the ear sends signals to the implanted electrodes, which activate auditory nerve pathways inducing the sensation of hearing. Although CIs have been remarkably successful, a significant number of CI recipients experience marginal hearing restoration. Recent research has suggested that hearing outcomes with CIs are correlated with the location where the electrodes are placed [1-5]. However, without post-implantation imaging, the position of the electrodes is generally unknown since the array is blindly threaded into a small opening of the cochlea during surgery, with its insertion path guided only by the walls of the spiral-shaped intra-cochlear cavities.

In efforts to analyze the relationship between electrode location and outcome, several groups have proposed coarse electrode position measurements that can be visually assessed in CT images, e.g., whether all electrodes are within one of the two principal intra-cochlear cavities, depth of insertion of the first and last electrode, etc. [1-5]. Studies using these techniques have indicated that placement and outcome are indeed correlated, but it has not been possible to determine specific factors that affect outcome because dataset size was limited and because the electrode positions were never precisely quantified with these techniques. One factor that has limited the size

P. Golland et al. (Eds.): MICCAI 2014, Part I, LNCS 8673, pp. 331–338, 2014.
© Springer International Publishing Switzerland 2014

of the datasets in the studies is the amount of manual effort that must be undertaken to analyze the images. Our group has shown that knowledge of electrode location can be used to select better CI processor settings to significantly improve hearing outcomes compared to standard clinical results [6]. In the current work, we propose a fully automatic approach for localizing CI electrodes in CT images. An electrode localization approach that is automatic and accurate would be significant as it could facilitate precise quantification of electrode position on large numbers of datasets to better analyze the relationship between electrode position and outcome, which may lead to advances in implant design or surgical techniques. It could also automate the electrode localization process in systems designed to determine patient-customized CI settings such as the one proposed in [6], reducing the technical expertise required to use such technologies and facilitating transition to large scale clinical use.

Figure 1 shows an example of an electrode array in a CT slice. Localizing the electrodes in CT images is difficult because (a), as seen in the figure, the beam hardening artifacts caused by the metallic electrodes distort intensities in the region around the electrode array, leading to incorrect assignment of very high intensities during image reconstruction to nearby voxels that are not occupied by metal, thus making it difficult to segment electrodes via thresholding; and (b) the individual electrodes are so close that there is no contrast between them in standard CT images, even when acquired at very fine slice thickness and resolution. Our solution is to identify the centerline of the voxels occupied by the CI electrodes using a snake-based localization approach [7] and then to fit a 3D model of the electrode array to the extracted centerline. This is a similar approach to that which we proposed in [8]. However, the technique we presented in that paper leads to inaccurate results around the first and last electrodes due to curve shrinkage. This shrinking phenomenon is caused by the use of an intensity-based attraction function since the image intensity decreases mildly at the array endpoints relative to the rest of the array. Further, we found that the "forward energy," an external energy term designed to counteract endpoint shrinking errors by expanding the curve, became unstable and led to failures when applying the technique on clinical image datasets. As will be described in the following section, in this work, we propose a new technique to counteract the shrinking effect by localizing and fixing the endpoints prior to snake optimization. Our results, presented and discussed in Sections 3 and 4, will show that this fully automatic approach can reliably be applied to clinical images.

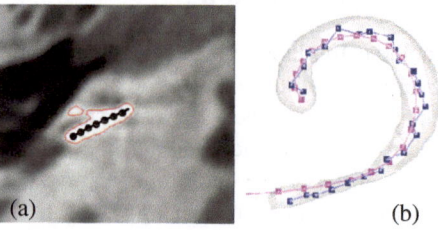

(a)   (b)

Fig. 1. Panel (a) shows a portion of an electrode array in an axial slice of a CT. Black dots indicate locations of individual electrodes. An isocontour around high intensity voxels is shown in red. Panel (b) shows a 3D isosurface of an electrode array with a manually determined centerline in purple. The blue curve is the coarse approximation to the centerline determined using our automatic initialization process discussed in Section 2.2.

2   Methods

The automatic segmentation method we propose is outlined in Figure 2. As can be seen in the figure, the first step (1) involves coarsely estimating the location of the region of interest (ROI), which is a local region ~1 cm^3 around the cochlea. This is done through registration with a known volume. The subsequent processing steps are then performed solely within the ROI. The next step (2) is to initialize our electrode array centerline localization. This is done by segmenting via thresholding the region of the image that contains the metallic electrodes and then computing the initialized centerline as the medial axis of the result. The thresholding step will produce a segmentation that includes electrode voxels as well as those that appear bright due to partial volume or beam hardening artifacts, but the medial axis extraction step is able to reliably and coarsely approximate the centerline of the electrode array. After initialization, the next steps (3-4) are to refine the centerline using a snake-based optimization approach [7]. In the third step, the curve endpoints are first localized within the neighborhood of their initialized positions using an endpoint detection filter we have designed. In the fourth step, the endpoints are fixed and the points in the rest of the curve are optimized. This is done using a snake with its external energy defined using the output of a vesselness filter that is applied to the original image to enhance the centerline of the electrode array [9]. By detecting and fixing the endpoints prior to snake optimization, curve shrinking effects discussed in the previous section are eliminated. The final step (5) is a straightforward resampling of the extracted centerline to determine individual electrode locations using *a priori* knowledge about the distance between neighboring electrodes. The following subsections detail this approach.

2.1   Data

The images in our dataset include images from 15 subjects acquired with a Xoran xCAT$^®$. The images have voxel size 0.4 x 0.4 x 0.4 mm^3. As a pre-processing step, an ROI bounding the region around the electrode array in each target image is automatically localized by using a mutual information-based affine registration computed between the target image and a known reference image [10]. The ROI is then automatically cropped from the original target image and all subsequent steps are performed on the cropped image. Each cropped image includes approximately 30 × 30 × 30 mm^3. Each subject in this study was implanted with a Cochlear™ Contour Advance®. Thus, the methods presented are focused on segmenting this type of electrode array but could prove in future studies to be applicable to other implant models.

2.2   Centerline Initialization

The centerline is initialized by thresholding the region of the image that includes the electrode array and computing the medial axis of the result. We determine the threshold dynamically using a maximum likelihood estimation-based (MLE) threshold selection approach [11] since the best threshold can vary across subjects due to the relatively low signal-to-noise ratio (SNR) achieved using the low-dose acquisition

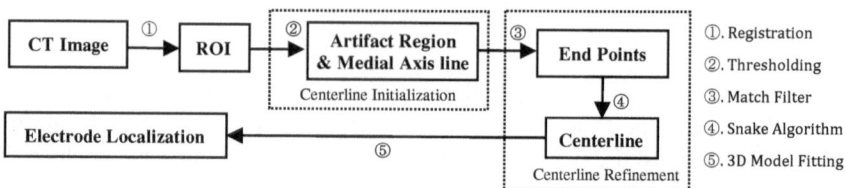

Fig. 2. Flow chart of the electrode array centerline localization process

protocols on a flat panel scanner. We would also expect that a dynamic threshold would account for differences between scanners, but this was not tested in this study. The MLE approach we have designed is to fit a model, defined as the sum of two Gaussian distributions, to the ROI image histogram and compute a threshold based on this result. One distribution $G(\mu_1, \sigma_1)$ corresponds to soft tissue and another $G(\mu_2, \sigma_2)$ corresponds to bony tissue. While air and metal are present in the ROI image, their relatively small volumes contribute little to the shape of the histogram, and thus these intensity classes are ignored in the histogram fitting. Once the distributions are estimated, the threshold is selected based on the upper tail of the Gaussian that models the intensity distribution of bone to be $\mu_2 + 5\sigma_2$, which was empirically determined to lead to good results. We chose to use this MLE-based approach, rather than a simpler percentile-based approach, because this approach is not sensitive to differences in ROI volume or differences in volume of metal present in the ROI, which can vary across subjects. After a threshold is determined, the medial axis of the resulting thresholded volume is computed using the medial axis extraction techniques presented by Bouix et al. [12]. The resulting curve provides a close but coarse approximation to the centerline of the electrode array. An example result of this process is shown in blue in Figure 1b.

2.3   Centerline Refinement

After the curve is initialized, we refine its position using a snake-based algorithm. The traditional snake algorithm localizes a contour by minimizing the energy equation

$$E = \int_0^1 \rho_1 \|x'(s)\|^2 + \rho_2 \|x''(s)\|^2 + E_{ext}(x(s)) \, ds, \tag{1}$$

where $x(s)$ is the position of the parameterized curve at s, ρ_1 and ρ_2 are the tension and rigidity weighting terms, and E_{ext} is the external energy term. In our experiments, we set $\rho_1 = 0.03$ and $\rho_2 = 0.08$ as these values were empirically determined to lead to good results, and we define E_{ext} to be the output of a vesselness response filter applied to the ROI image [9]. We apply the filter at scales $\sigma = \{0.08, 0.16, ..., 0.8\}$ mm and set the other internal parameters to be $\alpha = 0.5$, $\beta = 0.5$, and $\gamma = 500$. Vesselness response, rather than, for example, a direct function of image intensity is used as an external energy because the high intensity voxels in the region around the electrode array can be noisy, and voxels with intensity that is locally maximal often do not fall on the centerline of the homogeneous bright region in the image (see Figure 1). Since the electrode array has the appearance of a tubular structure, a vesselness response filter is a natural choice to enhance the centerline of the electrode array.

The robustness of the vesselness filter in detecting the centerline of the electrode array is high along the length of the array but diminishes at the endpoints. Thus, with no additional information, optimizing the snake would result in a shrinking of the curve at the endpoints. To address this, we determine the endpoint positions using an endpoint detection filter and fix them during the snake optimization. The endpoint detection filter we have constructed, $M_{\hat{p}}(\boldsymbol{\omega})$, is a match filter. For the sake of simplicity, we define $M_{\hat{p}}(\boldsymbol{\omega})$ such that $\boldsymbol{\omega} = \mathbf{0}$ lies at the center of the filter (see Figure 3a). We also orient the filter using $\hat{v}$, which represents the orientation of the centerline of the electrode array at the endpoint. To define $M_{\hat{p}}(\boldsymbol{\omega})$, we first define $M'_{\hat{p}}(\boldsymbol{\omega})$ as

$$M'_{\hat{p}}(\boldsymbol{\omega}) = \begin{cases} r^2 - \|\boldsymbol{\omega}\|^2 & \boldsymbol{\omega} \cdot \hat{v} \geq 0 \\ r^2 - \|\boldsymbol{\omega} - (\boldsymbol{\omega} \cdot \hat{v})\hat{v}\|^2 & \boldsymbol{\omega} \cdot \hat{v} < 0 \end{cases}. \qquad (2)$$

This equation defines $M'_{\hat{p}}(\boldsymbol{\omega})$ such that when $\boldsymbol{\omega} \cdot \hat{v} \geq 0$, i.e., in the $\hat{v}$ direction from the origin as seen in Figure 3a, $M'_{\hat{p}}(\boldsymbol{\omega})$ matches a semispherical structure, whereas in the opposite direction where $\boldsymbol{\omega} \cdot \hat{v} < 0$, the filter matches a tubular structure. The radius, r, of the sphere and tube are set to be 0.3 mm, which is approximately the radius of the electrode arrays in our images. The final form of the filter is defined as $M_{\hat{p}}(\boldsymbol{\omega}) = M'_{\hat{p}}(\boldsymbol{\omega})\left(\rho_3 H\left(M'_{\hat{p}}(\boldsymbol{\omega})\right) + (1-\rho_3)H\left(-M'_{\hat{p}}(\boldsymbol{\omega})\right)\right)$, where $H(\cdot)$ is the Heaviside function and $\rho_3 = 0.97$ is a parameter we chose empirically to optimize results and tunes the weighting between the fore- and background regions of the filter.

To find each endpoint using this filter, we set $\hat{v}$ to be the orientation of the central axis of the electrode array as estimated by the vesselness response at x_e^i, the location that the endpoint was initialized using the methods described in Section 2.2, and then compute the endpoint location x_e as

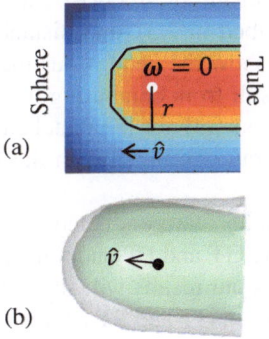

(a)

(b)

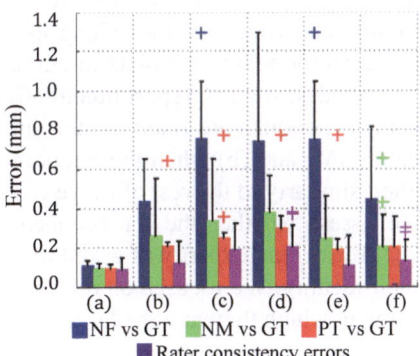

Fig. 3. (a) shows a slice of $M'_{\hat{p}}(\boldsymbol{\omega})$ with $M'_{\hat{p}}(\boldsymbol{\omega}) = 0$ isocontour in black and $\boldsymbol{\omega} = \mathbf{0}$ shown as white dot. (b) shows the 3D isosurface of $M'_{\hat{p}}(\boldsymbol{\omega})$ (white) aligned with the tip of an electrode array (green).

Fig. 4. Barplots of mean (a) and max (c) curve distances; mean (b) and max (d) electrode distances; and tip (e) and base (f) endpoint distances.

$$\boldsymbol{x}_e = \text{argmax}_{\boldsymbol{x} \in N(\boldsymbol{x}_e^i)} \sum_{\boldsymbol{y} \in L(\boldsymbol{x})} I(\boldsymbol{y}) M_{\hat{v}}(\boldsymbol{y} - \boldsymbol{x}). \qquad (3)$$

$N(\boldsymbol{x}_e^i)$ is a neighborhood function that we define as the set of 16 x 16 x 16 points uniformly sampled in a 1.2 x 1.2 x 1.2 mm^3 box surrounding $\boldsymbol{x}_e^i$, I is the ROI image, and $L(\boldsymbol{x})$ is a neighborhood function defined as the set of 21 x 21 x 21 points uniformly sampled in a 1.2 x 1.2 x 1.2 mm^3 box oriented in the $\hat{v}$ direction surrounding $\boldsymbol{x}$. In summary, Eqn. (3) selects the endpoint as the point in a local region around the initial endpoint that maximizes the response of the endpoint enhancement filter, and the filter response should be maximized when it is aligned with and centered on the tip of the electrode array.

After the endpoints are determined, they are fixed and the positions of the remaining points in our curve are optimized by iterating the standard snake update equations [7] until convergence or until reaching 100 iterations. Once the final curve is localized it is straightforward to resample the curve to identify the location of individual electrodes based on *a priori* knowledge of the distance between electrodes in the array.

2.4   Validation

We quantified the accuracy of our automatic electrode array extraction technique in a dataset of fifteen head CT images by comparing centerlines computed automatically using the proposed technique (PT) to ground truth (GT) curves, which were created by averaging of three sets of curves independently defined by an expert. Metrics used to characterize distance between two curves include mean and max curve distance (mean and max of the distances computed from each point on curve 1 to the closest point on curve 2 and vice versa), mean and max electrode distance (distance between each electrode location in curve 1 to the corresponding electrode in curve 2 after determining electrode locations along the curves as described in 2.3), and distance between corresponding endpoints in curves 1 and 2. To show the benefit our matched filter provides, we also report quantitative errors that result from computing the curve when (a) endpoints are fixed at their initialization position without the matched filter update (NM) and (b) when the endpoints are not fixed but optimized with the snake method similarly to the rest of curve (NF).

To assess whether the PT produces acceptable results, we conducted a second study in which an expert was asked to select between the GT and PT endpoints, blind to their identity. We focused on the endpoints because, as our results will show, this is the area in which there are the largest discrepancies between GT and PT curves.

3   Results

The quantitative comparisons between the GT and PT centerlines for all the datasets are shown in Figure 4 in red, and Figure 5 shows visualizations of two cases. In Figure 4, for each barplot, the height of the bars, crosses, and black whiskers denote the mean, outlier data, and maximum non-outlier value. Data are considered outliers if they fall above $q_3 + 1.5(q_3 - q_1)$, where q_3 and q_1 are the 25th and 75th percentiles

of the dataset. As can be
seen in the figure, our
proposed method results
in mean curve errors of
0.09 mm (0.13 of a voxel
diagonal) and average
maximum curve errors of
0.25 mm (0.36 of a voxel
diagonal) with an overall
maximum of 0.80 mm.
Our method extracts a
much more accurate cen-

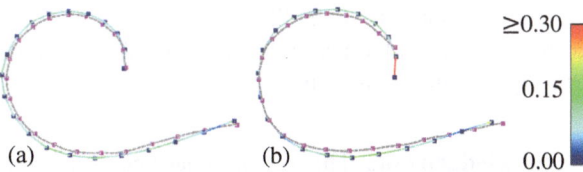

Fig. 5. 3D renderings of GT (colormapped with curve distance in mm) and PT (shown in transparent black) curves for our best (a) and worst (b) case errors. Points indicate electrode locations along curves determined by distance priors

terline compared to prior work in which we achieved mean curve errors of 0.2 millimeters [8]. Further, the mean electrode localization error with our currently proposed method is only 0.21 mm. The utility of fixing the endpoints and optimizing them with our matched filter is also apparent in Figure 4 as NF and NM lead to much larger electrode and endpoint localization errors. This difference is not as pronounced in mean curve errors since curve distances along the length of the curve are not sensitive to errors at the endpoints. The mean tip and base endpoint errors with PT are 0.19 mm and 0.2 mm. These quantities are slightly higher for NM and substantially higher for NF. The outlier values for PT that fall above 0.6 mm all correspond to the case shown in Figure 5b, where the tip of the array was localized incorrectly due to lower than normal SNR in the image. We also show in purple in Figure 4 rater consistency errors computed among the three sets of curves manually delineated by an expert. We find mean and overall maximum consistency curve errors of 0.09 and 0.35 mm, suggesting that except for the outlier case, errors in our PT are close to the level of rater repeatability.

In the expert endpoint selection test, among the 30 endpoints in the 15 cases, 8 PT endpoints were judged to be equally accurate to GT, and 29 of 30 PT endpoints were judged to be acceptable. The lone exception was the tip endpoint shown in Figure 5b.

4   Conclusions

In this work, we have designed an automatic cochlear implant electrode array centerline extraction method. Our experiments show that our method is highly accurate, even when applied to clinical images. Compared to our prior method reported in [8], the method we propose here achieves results with errors that are half as large on average. This improvement is due in large part to the use of our matched filter, which leads to better endpoint localization. Our approach requires approximately 3 minutes of computation time on a standard PC.

Our method did result in unacceptably large errors for one of fifteen images. Future studies will involve developing techniques to detect and handle such errors. Additionally, we plan to test our method with images acquired with different scanners and of subjects with different implant models. We also plan to apply our method to large numbers of datasets to facilitate studying how the location of individual electrodes correlates with outcomes with the goal of developing technologies that can improve hearing outcomes with CIs.

Acknowledgements. This research has been supported by NIH grants R01DC014037, R01DC008408, and R21DC012620. The content is solely the responsibility of the authors and does not necessarily represent the official views of this institute.

References

1. Verbist, B.M., Frijns, J.H.M., Geleijns, J., van Buchem, M.A.: Multisection CT as a Valuable Tool in the Postoperative Assessment of Cochlear Implant Patients. Am. J. Neuroradiol. 26, 424–429 (2005)
2. Aschendorff, A., Kubalek, R., Turowski, B., Zanella, F., Hochmuth, A., Schumacher, M., Klenzner, T., Laszig, R.: Quality control after cochlear implant surgery by means of rotational tomography. Otol Neurotol 26, 34–37 (2005)
3. Skinner, M.W., Holden, T.A., Whiting, B.R., Voie, A.H., Brundsen, B., Neely, G.J., Saxon, E.A., Hullar, T.E., Finley, C.C.: In vivo estimates of the position of advanced bionics electrode arrays in the human cochlea. Annals of Otology, Rhinology and Laryngology Supplement 197, 2–24 (2007)
4. Wanna, G.B., Noble, J.H., McRacken, T.R., Dawant, B.M., Dietrich, M.S., Watkins, L.D., Schuman, T.A., Labadie, R.F.: Assessment of electrode placement and audiologic outcomes in bilateral cochlear implantation. Otol Neurotol 32, 428–432 (2011)
5. Wanna, G.B., Noble, J.H., Carlson, M.L., Gifford, R.H., Dietrich, M.S., Haynes, D.S., Dawant, B.M., Labadie, R.F.: Impact of electrode design and surgical approach on scalar location and cochlear implant outcomes. Laryngoscope (in press, 2014)
6. Noble, J.H., Labadie, R.F., Gifford, R.H., Dawant, B.M.: Image-guidance enables new methods for customizing cochlear implant stimulation strategies. IEEE Trans. on Neural Systems and Rehabilitiation Engineering 21(5), 820–829 (2013)
7. Kass, M., Witkin, A., Terzopoulos, D.: Snakes: Active Contour Models. Int'l Jour. of Computer Vision, 321–331 (1988)
8. Noble, J.H., Schuman, T.A., Wright, C.G., Labadie, R.F., Dawant, B.M.: Automatic Identifi-cation of Cochlear Implant Electrode Arrays for Post-Operative Assessment. In: Dawant, B.M., Haynor, D.R. (eds.) Medical Imaging 2011: Image Processing, Proc. of the SPIE Conf. on Med. Imag., vol. 7962, p. 796217 (2011)
9. Frangi, A.F., Niessen, W.J., Vincken, K.L., Viergever, M.A.: Multiscale vessel enhancement filtering. In: Wells, W.M., Colchester, A., Delp, S. (eds.) MICCAI 1998. LNCS, vol. 1496, pp. 130–137. Springer, Heidelberg (1998)
10. Maes, F., Collignon, A., Vandermeulen, D., Marchal, G., Suetens, P.: Multimodality image registration by maximization of mutual information. IEEE Trans. Med. Imag. 16, 187–198 (1997)
11. Duda, R.O., Hart, P.E.: Pattern Classification and Scene Analysis. A Wiley-Interscience Publication, pp. 192–202. Wiley, New York (1973)
12. Bouix, S., Siddiqi, K., Tannenbaum, A.: Flux driven automatic centerline extraction. Medical Image Analysis 9, 209–221 (2005)

Coronary Lumen and Plaque Segmentation from CTA Using Higher-Order Shape Prior

Yoshiro Kitamura[1,2], Yuanzhong Li[1], Wataru Ito[1], and Hiroshi Ishikawa[2]

[1] Imaging Technology Center, Fujifilm Corporation, Tokyo, Japan
[2] Department of Computer Science and Engineering, Waseda University, Tokyo, Japan

Abstract. We propose a novel segmentation method based on multi-label graph cuts utilizing higher-order potentials to impose shape priors. Each higher-order potential is defined with respect to a candidate shape, and takes a low value if and only if most of the voxels inside the shape are foreground and most of those outside are background. We apply this technique to coronary lumen and plaque segmentation in CT angiography, exploiting the prior knowledge that the vessel walls tend to be tubular, whereas calcified plaques are more likely globular. We use the Hessian analysis to detect the candidate shapes and introduce corresponding higher-order terms into the energy. Since each higher-order term has any effect only when its highly specific condition is met, we can add many of them at possible locations and sizes without severe side effects. We show the effectiveness of the method by testing it on the standardized evaluation framework presented at MICCAI segmentation challenge 2012. The method achieved values comparable to the best in each of the sensitivity and positive predictive value, placing it at the top in average rank.

Keywords: Shape prior, Graph cuts, Multiple labels, Higher order function, Coronary stenosis.

1   Introduction

Cardiovascular disease is one of the largest causes of death in developed countries. Thanks to the recent progress of multi-detector CT techniques, 3D CT angiography has become a standard examination for the disease. Since coronary artery disease (stenosis) is caused by a narrowing of the arteries, accurate lumen segmentation is an important step toward determination of the degree of stenosis. Despite the great amount of past studies, computer aided detection and quantification of coronary stenosis remains a challenging task. A comprehensive analysis and categorization of vessel segmentation techniques can be found in [1] and a quantitative comparison of different algorithms in [2]. Coronary stenosis detection algorithms are classified into two types: classification-based and segmentation-based. Classification-based methods directly detect a plaque (or a stenosis) using extracted features [3], while most of segmentation-based methods aim at accurate lumen segmentation by estimation of healthy vessel diameter to detect stenosis [4,10,12]. On the other hand, early accumulation of plaques in coronary arteries is associated with compensatory enlargement of

P. Golland et al. (Eds.): MICCAI 2014, Part I, LNCS 8673, pp. 339–347, 2014.
© Springer International Publishing Switzerland 2014

vessel walls (positive remodeling). Therefore, segmenting vessel walls as well as lumen is a key to accurate assessment of stenosis grade. For this purpose, several methods such as the model-guided level-sets [5] have been proposed.

In this paper, we present a novel segmentation method based on the Conditional Random Field (CRF) framework. As the plaque tissue and surrounding tissues have nearly the same intensities, typical graph-cut methods utilizing first-order potentials tend to fail in distinguishing them. To overcome this challenge, we utilize higher-order functions that can model more complex structures than mere continuity. Kohli et al. [7] presented a framework utilizing higher-order functions that can combine multiple segmentations generated using unsupervised segmentation algorithms. Recently, Kadoury et al. [8] presented a segmentation approach in which higher-order potentials ensure regional consistency. In contrast, we take advantage of the prior knowledge regarding the shape of the vessel walls and calcified plaques.

Even when arteries are narrowed with (calcified or soft) plaques, their walls tend to be tubular, while calcified plaques are more likely globular. We use the Hessian analysis to detect such candidate shapes and introduce higher-order terms to encourage segmentation along them. Such a higher-order term takes a low value if and *only if* most of the voxels on the border stick together inside or outside. Since each higher-order term has an effect only when its highly specific condition is met, we can add many of them at possible locations and sizes without worrying about side effects.

We show the effectiveness of the method by testing it on the standardized evaluation framework presented at MICCAI segmentation challenge workshop in 2012.

2   Method

In this paper, we address the problem of segmentation of coronary lumen and plaques in order to quantify the stenosis grades of the coronary arteries. We assume that the centerlines of coronary arteries have been extracted and a stacked volume has been reconstructed from each centerline by generating multi-planar reconstructed (MPR) images perpendicular to the direction along the centerline. Our goal is to detect the double boundaries of vessel wall and lumen from the stacked volume (Fig. 1). Since a lumen boundary is always inside the vessel wall, we solve this as an ordered three-class labeling problem, where the three classes are {1: *Background*, 2: *Plaque*, 3: *Lumen*}. In the following, we first describe the general multi-label CRF energy setup. Then we explain the higher-order potentials in more specifics. Finally, we describe the unary and pairwise potentials as well as our stenosis detection algorithm.

2.1   Multi-label CRFs with Higher Order Potentials

First, we describe the multi-label Conditional Random Field (CRF) with higher-order potentials. We consider minimizing a function of the form:

$$E(\mathbf{y}) = \sum_{a \in V} \theta_a(y_a) + \sum_{a \in V, b \in N_a} \theta_{ab}(y_a, y_b) + \sum_{c \in C} \theta_c(\mathbf{y}_c), \tag{1}$$

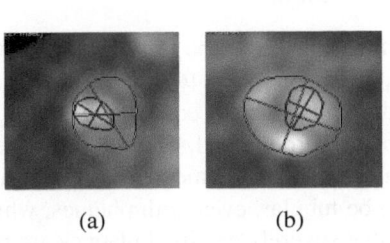

Fig. 1. The sectional images of the vessel with (a) soft plaque, and (b) calcified plaque. The cyan and magenta lines represent the vessel-wall and the lumen boundaries, respectively.

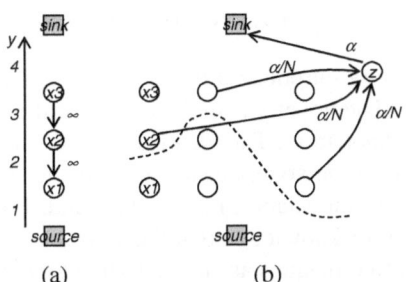

Fig. 2. (a) Encoding of a multi label to binary variables. (b) The graph construction for higher order multi-label function. z is an auxiliary variable. This construction penalizes any labeling above the dashed line.

where $\mathbf{y}$ is the vector of variables y_i indexed by the set V of voxels taking values in a label set $L = \{1, 2, \ldots, l\}$ with a linear order and N_a is the set of a's neighbors. The functions θ_a and θ_{ab} are the potentials for the label y_a and the label pair (y_a, y_b), respectively, while the higher order potential $\theta_c(\mathbf{y}_c)$ depends on the variables y_i for voxels in its *clique* $c \subset V$. According to [6], the multi-label variables y_i can be encoded by $l-1$ binary variables $\{x_1, \ldots, x_{l-1}\}$. For instance, $\{1, 2, 3\}$ can be mapped to the labelings of two binary labels $x_1 x_2 = \{11, 01, 00\}$. In order to ensure a bijective encoding, very high costs are assigned to the unused labelings such as $x_1 x_2 = \{10\}$ (see Fig. 2 (a)). Next, multi-label higher-order functions with the form:

$$\theta_c(\mathbf{y}_c) = \begin{cases} \alpha & \text{if } \exists i \in c : y_i < l_i, \\ 0 & \text{otherwise} \end{cases} \tag{2}$$

can be converted to submodular quadratic pseudo Boolean functions, where α is a positive weight and the threshold label l_i can vary from voxel to voxel. This potential encourages every variable y_i in the clique to take the value equal to or more than l_i. Similarly, there is a family of functions that encourage the variables y_i to take the label less than l_i. Although eq. (2) is a "hard" function that takes two values depending on whether or not *all* the variables satisfy the condition, we can introduce the idea of the "robust P^n Potts model" [7] into this and let the function to take gradually larger value as the number of voxels that violate the condition increases. With a positive integer N, such a potential is formulated as:

$$\theta_c(\mathbf{y}_c) = \min\left\{\alpha, \sum_{i \in c : y_i < l_i} \frac{\alpha}{N}\right\}, \tag{3}$$

which gives an increasing penalty as more voxels violate the condition, until it saturates at N violating voxels. The graph construction in this case is shown in Fig. 2 (b).

2.2   Shape Constraints Using Higher Order Potentials

We now introduce a novel use of higher-order functions as shape prior in segmentation. The novelty is in the choice of the voxels in the clique c for $\theta_c(\mathbf{y}_c)$, which we call the shape term. The idea is to add the higher-order terms such as eq. (3) to encourage: a) all of the voxels inside a candidate shape to be foreground and, b) all of the voxels outside the shape to be background. For lumen and plaque segmentation, we utilize the prior knowledge that the vessel walls tend to be tubular, even with plaques, while calcified plaques are liable to be globular. Note that severely calcified plaques are not always globular. However, they tend to be brighter than other structures, enough to be distinguished based on the intensities (i.e. by the unary term).

Since the vessel wall is represented as the summed regions of *Lumen* and *Plaque* (labels 2 and 3, respectively), we encourage the segmentation to be tubular by setting the "soft" constraint $y_i < 2$ for voxels inside the tube, and $y_i \geq 2$ for voxels outside. Similarly, we encourage $y_i < 2$ and $y_i \geq 3$ for voxels inside the globular shape. Of course, we do not know the position and the size of the candidate shapes in advance. So we place the shape term cliques at various positions and scales, choosing the candidates using the Optimally Oriented Flux (OOF) [9]. The OOF computes the Hessian matrices at the boundaries of spherical regions. As is well known, their eigenvalues can be used to estimate the shape of the object, such as tubular or globular, and the eigenvector corresponding to the smallest eigenvalue indicates the orientation of the tubular object. Since the computation of the OOF is localized at the spherical surface, we can estimate the boundaries of the vessel walls accurately (Fig. 3). In our experiments, we computed the OOF at multiple kernel radii from 0.5 to 4.0mm in steps of scale 1.26. We create a clique out of the voxels just inside the circle regions on the plane orthogonal to the main axis, and create another clique from the voxels just outside the circle. This way, several to hundreds of voxels were selected in a clique, when the resolution of the reconstructed MPR image was 0.25mm.

The advantage of our higher-order terms is that, because each shape term does not affect the energy unless the voxels in its clique satisfy the specific condition, there is not severe side effect by including as many of them as desired, except for the computational cost. If instead we tried to influence the energy using pairwise terms by, for instance, placing many of them along the boundary, each term would independently affect the outcome in a way difficult to control. Also, by using the robust P^n Potts model, we can encourage not only the exact candidate shape but also similar shapes, without increasing auxiliary variables.

2.3   Learning Weights of Higher Order Potentials

Next, we describe how to set the weight α for the shape term. We learn the weight from the reference segmentation data that was manually prepared. Computing the OOF in the reference image, we obtain the objective label y_i at each $i \in c$ and the feature vector at each position and scale. Since the responses of the Hessian filters cannot discriminate complicated structures, to improve the prediction accuracy the feature vector consists of twelve eigenvalues sampled at the same position but at different scales. We set the shape constraint using the robust P^n Potts model by setting the N in eq. (3) to 20% of the total number of voxels in the clique; thus the potential allows up to 20% of the voxels violating the assumed shape. For each of the two cases whether 80% of the labels are less than the certain label or not, we generate the histograms for the feature values and learn the log likelihood ratio of their probabilities:

$$-\log\left(\Pr_{c \in C}\left(\#\{i \in c \mid y_i < l_i\} \geq N\right)/\Pr_{c \in C}\left(\#\{i \in c \mid y_i < l_i\} < N\right)\right). \tag{4}$$

As a result, we confirmed that the shape terms regarding the vessel walls and calcified plaques were significantly predicted when the feature vectors represented tubular patterns or spherical patterns. The likelihood value corresponding to the feature value for given data is directly used as the weight of the shape term. Note that the weight α of the energy must be positive in order to keep the potential submodular. Then the shape terms are set at where the candidate shapes were detected. Fig. 4 is a visualization of the shape terms and the resulting segmentation.

2.4   Unary and Pairwise Potentials

The unary and pairwise potentials in eq. (1) are set as follows. First, we estimate the intensity distributions of lumen and two types of plaques (soft-plaque and calcified-plaque). The mean and the standard deviation of lumen (I_z^{lumen} and σ_z^{lumen}) and soft-plaque (I_z^{soft} and σ_z^{soft}) at the slice position z along the stacked volume are calculated from the upper sides and lower sides of the histogram of the regions determined by the initial centerline and radii (R_z). The mean value of calcified plaque is given by shifting the center to higher level: $I_z^{\text{calcified}} = I_z^{\text{lumen}} + 3\sigma_z^{\text{lumen}}$. Finally, $I_z^{\text{background}}$ is the mean of low intensity regions around the initial centerline.

Unary potentials: The unary potentials are given by

$$\theta_a(y_i = Lumen) \propto 1 - \exp\left(-\frac{(I_i - I_z^{\text{lumen}})^2}{2(\sigma_z^{\text{lumen}})^2}\right) \cdot h(D_i), \tag{5}$$

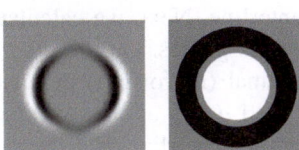

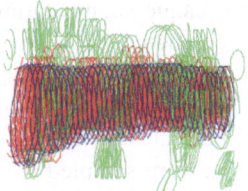

Fig. 3. (LEFT) A sectional plane of OOF filter kernel. (RIGHT) The higher-order potentials set according to the filter response. The voxels in the white and black regions are encouraged to be foreground and background, respectively.

Fig. 4. The visualization of the shape terms. The red circles represent the active terms, i.e., most voxels inside them were labeled as plaque or lumen in the optimization. The green circles represent inactive terms. The blue lines correspond to the vessel-wall boundaries after optimiza-

where I_i is the intensity at voxel y_i, D_i is the distance of the voxel from the centerline, and $h(D_i)$ is 0 if $D_i < R_z$ and 1 otherwise. Similarly, the likelihood of the *Plaque*, $\theta_a(y_i = Plaque)$ takes a small value when I_i is close to I_z^{soft} or $I_z^{\text{calcified}}$. Finally, $\theta_a(y_i = Background)$ is set to take a small number at voxels with $D_i \gg R_z$.

Pairwise Potentials: The pairwise potentials are defined as functions of the image gradient and the absolute intensity at each pair of 18-neighboring voxels:

$$\theta_{ij}(y_i, y_j) \propto \begin{cases} N(I_i - I_j, \sigma_g^2) \cdot (1 - N(I_i - (I_z^{\text{plaque}} + I_z^{\text{lumen}})/2), \sigma_z^2)/D_i & \text{, if } y_i < 3 \text{ and } y_j = 3 \\ N(I_i - I_j, \sigma_g^2) \cdot (1 - N(I_i - (I_z^{\text{background}} + I_z^{\text{plaque}})/2), \sigma_z^2)/D_i & \text{, if } y_i < 2 \text{ and } y_j \geq 2 \\ 0 & \text{, otherwise.} \end{cases} \quad (6)$$

I_z^{plaque} is I_z^{soft} if $I_i < I_z^{\text{lumen}}$ and $I_z^{\text{calcified}}$ otherwise. These potentials encourage label changes at voxels with strong image gradient or intensity close to the middle of the estimated distributions of each class. The weights between unary, pairwise and higher order potentials in eq. (1) were determined heuristically.

2.5   Stenosis Detection and Quantification Algorithm

We implemented automatic stenosis detection and quantification algorithm for verification with the standardized evaluation framework presented at MICCAI segmentation challenge workshop in 2012 [2]. The evaluation is done in three categories: 1) Stenosis detection, 2) Stenosis quantification, and 3) Lumen segmentation. For categories 1 and 2, participants are required to report 3D positions of detected stenoses and their stenosis grades that represent the diameter reduction between 0% (healthy) to 100% (occluded). Category 1 evaluates the sensitivity and positive predictive value (PPV) of the algorithm only for severe stenoses with diameter reductions more than 50%. Category 2 evaluates the differences of the estimated stenosis grades and the reference, which have been prepared for Quantitative coronary angiography (QCA) and CT angiography (CTA) by three observers.

We reported these measures in the following steps. We used extraction results obtained by the method in [11] as the initial input of coronary centerlines. After the lumen and plaque segmentation, short axis lengths of lumen (d_{lumen}) and vessel wall (d_{wall}) are computed at every position z along the centerline. Next, we calculated the ratio of the two measures: $d_{\text{lumen}} / d_{\text{wall}}$ for CTA stenosis grades. On the other hand, QCA stenosis grades are defined as the ratio of minimal (narrowing) diameter and estimated normal lumen diameter (d_{normal}). We estimated d_{normal} as the average value of d_{lumen} that were sampled from 50 mm length along the centerline. For the category 3, the boundaries of lumen obtained by the proposed method were evaluated.

To reduce false detections, the following rules were considered in the stenosis detection. 1) The segments in the coronary tree were labeled according to the model matching method in [11]. Then, clinically relevant 18 segments defined by the Society of Cardiovascular Computed Tomography (SCCT) were evaluated. 2) Only z positions along the centerline from the ostia till 100mm length point were evaluated, excluding around branching points.

3   Results and Discussion

The summary of the three evaluation categories, comparing our method with other top participants for each metric as of May 2014 are shown in Table 1, 2 and 3, respectively. The processing time was at most 10 seconds per a centerline, depending on its length, on a quad-core 3.4GHz PC. As can be seen in Table 1, the method achieved a sensitivity of 51.1% and a PPV of 33.3% compared to CTA reference, which are almost equal to the best ones for each measure. And it achieved the best quantification performance compared to the CTA reference with kappa value: 0.32. Fig. 5 shows an example of the segmentation result compared to the reference. The boundaries obtained by the proposed method are close to observer's one. On the other hand, the quantification performance compared to the QCA was not very good. Our method underestimated the QCA stenosis grades because the normal lumen diameter calculated as an average value of local lumen diameters did not show significant decrease in some cases. As is discussed in [2], robust regression may improve the accuracy of QCA-based stenosis quantification.

An advantage of our method in stenosis detection is accurate detection of the vessel wall boundaries. Fig. 6 shows a comparison of segmentation results obtained with and without the shape terms. It can be seen that the shape terms improve the segmentation accuracy of vessel wall boundary, and successfully segment calcified regions. The method can improve stenosis quantification accuracy by avoiding the difficulty of estimating the normal diameter, and can also assess the positive remodeling effect accurately. A limitation of the method derives from the Hessian-based features, which cannot distinguish very wide variety of structures. For example, the shape constraints do not work well around branching points. The method also tends to over or under-segment where surrounding structures form a tubular pattern.

Table 1. Stenosis detection results compared to other top participants for each metric

Method	QCA Sensitivity		QCA PPV		CTA Sensitivity		CTA PPV		Avg. rank
	%	rank	%	rank	%	rank	%	rank	
Proposed method	35.7	12	32.3	6	51.1	6	**33.3**	**5**	**7.2**
Lugauer et al. [12]	60.7	6	24.6	7	46.8	9	25.0	10	8.0
Cetin et al. [3]	53.6	9	19.2	10	**53.2**	**5**	26.0	8	8.0
Wang. et al. [5]	25.0	14	**50.0**	**3**	10.6	17	**33.3**	**5**	9.8
Eslami et al. [10]	**67.9**	**4**	9.4	16	51.1	6	4	16	10.5

Table 2. Stenosis quantification results compared to other top participants for each metric

Method	QCA Avg. Abs. diff.		QCA R.M.S. diff.		CTA Weighted Kappa		Avg. rank
	%	rank	%	rank	K	rank	
Proposed method	30.8	5	36.6	5	**0.32**	**5**	**5.0**
Wang et al. [5]	**28.8**	**1**	**33.7**	**1**	0.18	10	5.5
Lugauer et al. [12]	49.0	11	55.1	12	0.30	6	8.8

Table 3. Lumen segmentation results compared to other top participants for each metric

Method	DICE diseased		DICE healthy		MSD diseased		MSD healthy		MAXSD diseased		MAXSD healthy		Avg. rank
	%	rank	%	rank	%	rank	%	Rank	%	rank	%	rank	
Lugauer et al. [12]	**0.74**	**3.6**	0.73	**4.3**	**0.35**	**3.9**	0.55	**4.6**	2.99	4.2	3.73	4.2	**4.2**
Mohr et al. [4]	0.70	4.9	0.73	4.5	0.40	5.5	**0.39**	4.7	**2.68**	**3.6**	**2.75**	**2.7**	**4.2**
Proposed method	0.71	5.2	**0.75**	4.6	0.42	6.2	0.41	5.4	3.17	5.4	3.69	4.3	5.1

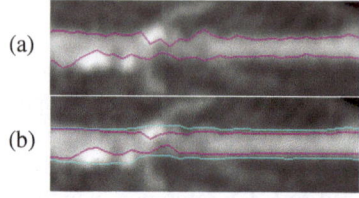

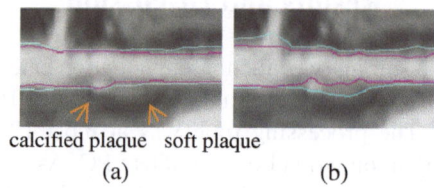

calcified plaque   soft plaque
(a)   (b)

Fig. 5. The results in segment LAD7 in training dataset #08. (a) manually annotated reference of observer #1, (b) the result obtained by the proposed method.

Fig. 6. Segmentation results for the stenosed artery obtained (a) without the shape terms, and (b) with the shape terms. The cyan and magenta lines represent the vessel-wall and the lumen boundaries, respectively.

4   Conclusion

We proposed a novel segmentation method for coronary lumen and vessel wall segmentation from CT angiography images. Our contribution is presenting effective use of higher-order potentials that enable us to introduce shape priors to a CRF energy. The verification tests for stenosis detection and quantification showed the state of the art performance. The method could be applied for general vessel segmentation. Extending its utility would be an interesting future work.

Acknowledgment. In the course of this work, H. Ishikawa was partially supported by the JSPS Grant-in-Aid for Scientific Research (B) #24300075 and the JSPS Grant-in-Aid for Challenging Exploratory Research #25540075.

References

1. Lesage, D., Angelini, E., Bloch, I., Funka-Lea, G.: A review of 3D vessel lumen segmentation techniques: Models, features and extraction schemes. Medical Image Analysis 13(6), 819–845 (2009)
2. Kirişli, H.A., Schaap, M., Metz, C., et al.: Standardized evaluation framework for evaluating coronary artery stenosis detection, stenosis quantification and lumen segmentation algorithms in computed tomography angiography. Medical Image Analysis 17(8), 859–876 (2013)
3. Cetin, S., Unal, G.: Automatic detection of coronary artery stenosis in CTA based on vessel intensity and geometric features. In: Proc. of MICCAI 2012 Workshop 3D Cardiovascular Imaging: A MICCAI Segmentation Challenge (2012)
4. Mohr, B., Masood, S., Plakas, C.: Accurate stenosis detection and quantification in coronary CTA. In: Proc. of MICCAI 2012 Workshop 3D Cardiovascular Imaging: A MICCAI Segmentation Challenge (2012)
5. Wang, C., Moreno, R., Smedby, Ö.: Vessel segmentation using implicit model-guided level sets. In: Proc. of MICCAI 2012 Workshop 3D Cardiovascular Imaging: A MICCAI Segmentation Challenge (2012)

6. Ramalingam, S., Kohli, P., Alahari, K., Torr, P.H.S.: Exact inference in multi-label CRFs with higher order cliques. In: Proc. of CVPR (2008)
7. Kohli, P., Ladicky, L., Torr, P.H.S.: Robust higher order potentials for enforcing label consistency. In: Proc. of CVPR (2008)
8. Kadoury, S., Abi-Jaoudeh, N., Valdes, P.A.: Higher-Order CRF Tumor Segmentation with Discriminant Manifold Potentials. In: Mori, K., Sakuma, I., Sato, Y., Barillot, C., Navab, N. (eds.) MICCAI 2013, Part I. LNCS, vol. 8149, pp. 719–726. Springer, Heidelberg (2013)
9. Law, M.W.K., Chung, A.C.S.: Three Dimensional Curvilinear Structure Detection Using Optimally Oriented Flux. In: Forsyth, D., Torr, P., Zisserman, A. (eds.) ECCV 2008, Part IV. LNCS, vol. 5305, pp. 368–382. Springer, Heidelberg (2008)
10. Eslami, A., Aboee, A., Hodaei, Z., Moghaddam, M.J., Carlier, S., Katouzian, A., Navab, N.: Quantification of coronary arterial stenosis by inflating tubes in CTA images. In: Proc. of MICCAI 2012 Workshop 3D Cardiovascular Imaging: A MICCAI Segmentation Challenge (2012)
11. Kitamura, Y., Li, Y., Ito, W.: Automatic coronary extraction by supervised detection and shape matching. In: Proc. of ISBI, pp. 234–237 (2012)
12. Lugauer, F., Zhang, J., Zheng, Y., Hornegger, J., Kelm, M.: Improving Accuracy in Coronary Lumen Segmentation via Explicit Calcium Exclusion, Learning-based Ray Detection and Surface Optimization. In: Proc. of SPIE MI, 90343U (2014)

Multi-atlas Spectral PatchMatch: Application to Cardiac Image Segmentation

Wenzhe Shi[1], Herve Lombaert[3], Wenjia Bai[1], Christian Ledig[1],
Xiahai Zhuang[2], Antonio Marvao[1], Timothy Dawes[1],
Declan O'Regan[1], and Daniel Rueckert[1]

[1] Biomedical Image Analysis Group, Imperial College London, UK
[2] Shanghai Advanced Research Institute, Chinese Academy of Sciences, China
[3] INRIA, Asclepios Project-Team, Sophia-Antipolis, France

Abstract. The automatic segmentation of cardiac magnetic resonance images poses many challenges arising from the large variation between different anatomies, scanners and acquisition protocols. In this paper, we address these challenges with a global graph search method and a novel spectral embedding of the images. Firstly, we propose the use of an approximate graph search approach to initialize patch correspondences between the image to be segmented and a database of labelled atlases. Then, we propose an innovative spectral embedding using a multi-layered graph of the images in order to capture global shape properties. Finally, we estimate the patch correspondences based on a joint spectral representation of the image and atlases. We evaluated the proposed approach using 155 images from the recent MICCAI SATA segmentation challenge and demonstrated that the proposed algorithm significantly outperforms current state-of-the-art methods on both training and test sets.

1 Introduction

An important step in the analysis of cardiac magnetic resonance (MR) images is the segmentation of the image into different anatomical structures or regions. One of the most popular segmentation approaches is based on multi-atlas label fusion [1,2,3]. The main components of these methods are atlas selection, atlas propagation and label fusion.

In the atlas propagation step, affine or non-rigid registration methods are commonly used, such as the free-form deformation (FFD) [4] registration or the Demons [5] algorithm. The registration is commonly based on intensity similarities and constrained to ensure one-to-one correspondences between the target image and the atlas. This restriction ensures a realistic deformation that preserves the topology of the atlas structures in the target image. However, it also limits the ability of the registration to capture large or local variations in shape.

To relax the method's dependence on accurate registrations, recent research has focused on patch-based label fusion methods [6,7,8,9,10] including their application to cardiac MR images [7,11]. These approaches compensate registration error by searching for correspondences between the target image and atlas within a limited search window. However, intensity based features, which are

P. Golland et al. (Eds.): MICCAI 2014, Part I, LNCS 8673, pp. 348–355, 2014.
© Springer International Publishing Switzerland 2014

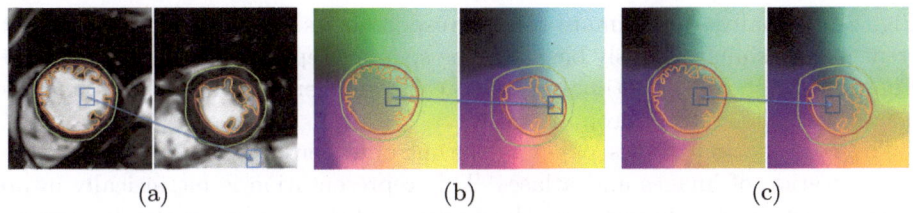

(a)   (b)   (c)

Fig. 1. This figure shows the most similar patches under different representations of the images. Red, green, and orange contours are the manual segmentation of endocardial, epicardial boundaries and trabeculae/papillary muscles respectively. For spectral representations, RGB color represents the first three eigenmodes. (a) shows the intensity images and the correspondence; (b) shows the independent spectral representations and the correspondence; (c) shows the joint spectral representation and the correspondence.

often used as patch selection criteria, can have ambiguous matches especially for larger search windows as shown in Fig. 1a.

PatchMatch [12] is a popular search method to find global patch correspondences between two images based on an approximate graph search. This approach is appealing due to its unique ability to capture large variations while remaining computationally feasible. However, there is no intrinsic regularization and corresponding patches do not necessarily preserve the topology of anatomical structures as shown in Fig. 3d.

In this paper, we aim to search for patch correspondences between the target image and warped atlases without any restriction of the search window size for the purpose of label fusion. There are two challenges, as discussed above: Firstly, cardiac MR images exhibit significant variability in terms of anatomy. This renders the application of conventional registration methods difficult. Secondly, the optimal matching patches, in terms of intensity features, may come from different anatomical regions around the heart. This limits the usefulness of patch selection methods like label fusion or the PatchMatch algorithm [12].

In this paper, we propose a novel method called multi-atlas spectral Patch-Match (MASP) to overcome these limitations. Here we combine spectral matching [13] with multi-atlas PatchMatch (MAPM) [14]. Recent advances in spectral matching [13], based on spectral graph theory [15], allow global correspondences to be established between two graphs by linking them together. By modelling images as graphs, this method can be applied to image registration [16]. However, any alteration in the images will inherently change the graph representation and result in perturbations in shape isometry. These alterations include variation of the objects, changes of the regions of interest, and different views of the scene. This will lead to the change in the spectral representation as shown in Fig.2d and Fig. 1b, thus, affect the performance of matching.

In order to build a consistent spectral embedding of the images, we first represent the images as graphs [16]. However, different from [16], we construct a multi-layered graphical representation of the image and atlases by using the patch correspondence stemming from the PatchMatch (Fig. 2a). We then learn the joint spectral representation of the graph using the principles from [13]

(Fig. 2b). Finally, we estimate the correspondences using MAPM across different images simultaneously based on the spectral representation of the patches (Fig. 2c). Based on the estimated patch correspondences, we then segment the images with the method proposed in [6].

The contribution of this paper is the introduction of a novel joint spectral representation of images and atlases. This representation is intrinsically aware of the image content, in our case, the anatomy of the cardiac region. In contrast to the application of [16], we capture shape properties among all images simultaneously. By using this new representation, we enable a multi-layered graph search strategy and recover unambiguous global patch correspondences between the unseen image and atlases. Our results demonstrate that the proposed algorithm significantly outperforms state-of-art algorithms. We confirm our results through a blinded and external online evaluation.

2   Method

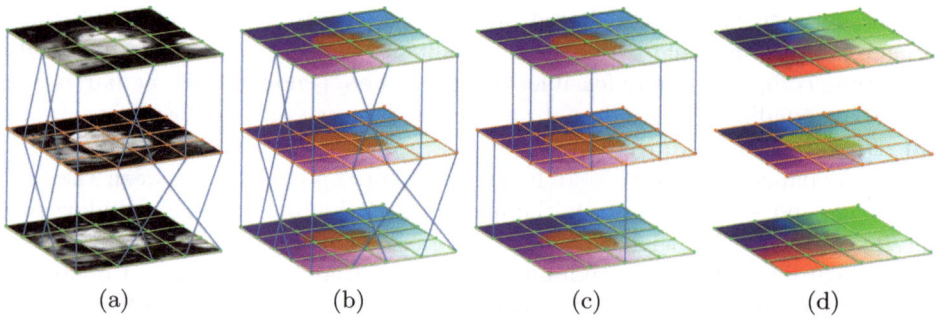

(a)   (b)   (c)   (d)

Fig. 2. Algorithm overview – intermediate steps for segmenting an unseen image and two atlases. The number of atlases, vertices and edges has been simplified for better illustration. The unseen image is overlaid with an orange grid and atlases are overlaid with a green grid. (a) shows the image-atlas graph as initialized by PatchMatch; (b) shows the spectral representation of the image-atlas graph; (c) shows the final estimation of the correspondences using the spectral representation and MAPM; (d) shows the spectral representation of individual images.

2.1   Image-Atlas Graph Initialization

The PatchMatch algorithm proposed by Barnes et al. [12] finds corresponding patches between two images or regions without any restriction of the search space. It is based on the assumption that given a good match of one patch, it is very likely that the neighbouring patches share the same or similar correspondences [12]. The first step of our segmentation method is to construct a multi-layered image-atlas graph from the unseen image and atlases using the correspondences estimated with PatchMatch.

Given an unseen image $\mathbf{U}$ and an warped atlas database $\mathbf{A}$ (individual atlases are denoted as $\mathbf{A_k}, K = |\mathbf{A}|$), we find for each point $\mathbf{p} = (x, y, z)$ in image $\mathbf{U}$

a correspondence in each atlas $\mathbf{A_k}$, $\mathbf{C_k(p)} = (\mathbf{q}, k)$ where $\mathbf{q} = (x', y', z')$ is the closest match in atlas $\mathbf{A_k}$ for a given distance function $D(\mathbf{p}, \mathbf{q})$ between patches $\mathbf{P}$ and $\mathbf{Q}$ centered at $\mathbf{p}$ and $\mathbf{q}$. Here, the distance is the Euclidean distance of the feature vectors. For each patch $\mathbf{P}$, the feature vector consists of the intensity, the intensity gradients in all three directions, and the spatial location x, y, z of each point $\mathbf{x} \in \mathbf{P}$. This is equivalent to embedding each patch of the unseen image and the K atlases in a M dimensional space, where $M = 7|\mathbf{P}|$ is the number of features in the feature vector. The choice of the Euclidean distance ensures the triangle inequality so that the multi-layered image-atlas graph introduced in the next section is embedded in a metric space.

2.2   Image-Atlas Graph Construction

Using the estimated correspondence fields $\mathbf{C_1}, ..., \mathbf{C_K}$, we can construct a single multi-layered undirected graph $\mathbf{G} = (\mathbf{V}, \mathbf{E})$ from image $\mathbf{U}$ and atlases $\mathbf{A}$ as shown in Fig.2a. The graph is constructed with the vertices $\mathbf{V} = \mathbf{V_U} \cup \mathbf{V_A}$ representing voxels of image $\mathbf{U}$ and atlases $\mathbf{A}$ and the edges $\mathbf{E}$ consisting of the union of $\mathbf{E_U}$, $\mathbf{E_{A_1}}, ..., \mathbf{E_{A_K}}$ and $\mathbf{E_{C_1}}, ..., \mathbf{E_{C_K}}$. Within the unseen image $\mathbf{U}$ and atlases $\mathbf{A}$, we define $\mathbf{E_U}$, $\mathbf{E_{A_1}}, ..., \mathbf{E_{A_K}}$ such that each voxel is connected to its immediate spatial neighbours within the same image. Between the unseen image and atlases, the edges $\mathbf{E_{C_1}}, ..., \mathbf{E_{C_K}}$ are given by the corresponding fields $\mathbf{C_1}, ..., \mathbf{C_K}$. The distance $D(\mathbf{p}, \mathbf{q})$ between the vertices is defined as in Sec.2.1.

For the multi-layered graph $\mathbf{G}$ the $|\mathbf{V_U} \cup \mathbf{V_A}| \times |\mathbf{V_U} \cup \mathbf{V_A}|$ weighted adjacency matrix has the form:

$$\mathbf{W} = \begin{bmatrix} \mathbf{W_U} & \mathbf{W_{C_1}} & ... & \mathbf{W_{C_K}} \\ \mathbf{W_{C_1}^T} & \mathbf{W_{A_1}} & 0 & 0 \\ ... & 0 & ... & 0 \\ \mathbf{W_{C_K}^T} & 0 & 0 & \mathbf{W_{A_K}} \end{bmatrix}, \quad (1)$$

where $\mathbf{W_U}$ and $\mathbf{W_{A_k}}$ are the adjacency matrices of intra-image edges of the unseen image and atlas $\mathbf{A_k}$. $\mathbf{W_{C_k}}$ are the weighted adjacency matrices of inter image-atlas edges defined by the correspondence field $\mathbf{C_k}$. For each $w_{\mathbf{p},\mathbf{q}}$ where $\mathbf{p}$ and $\mathbf{q}$ are two voxels of the unseen image and/or atlases, we define $w_{\mathbf{p},\mathbf{q}} = \exp(-D(\mathbf{p}, \mathbf{q})^2/2\sigma^2)$ if $\exists e_{\mathbf{p},\mathbf{q}} \in \mathbf{E}$ or 0 otherwise. The parameter σ is set to the standard deviation of $D(\mathbf{p}, \mathbf{q})$ $\forall e_{\mathbf{p},\mathbf{q}} \in \mathbf{E}$. The resulting graph is simplified and illustrated in Fig. 2a. Examples are presented in the supplementary material.

2.3   Spectral Feature Extraction

Inspired by [13], we use the image-atlas graph $\mathbf{G}$ to exploit the joint spectral representation of the unseen image and atlases. In this paper, we use the symmetric normalized Laplacian [15] for the spectral embedding. The Laplacian is defined as $\mathbf{L^{norm}} = \mathbf{D^{-1/2}(D - W)D^{-1/2}}$ where $\mathbf{D}$ is the diagonal degree matrix [15]. The spectral decomposition of the graph Laplacian $\mathbf{L^{norm}} = \mathbf{S \Lambda S^{-1}}$ provides eigenvalues $\mathbf{\Lambda}$ and associated eigenvectors $\mathbf{S} = (s_{.,0}, s_{.,1}, ..., s_{.,|\Lambda|})$, where $s_{.,i}$ is the ith

column of S. We denote the spectral representation, $\mathbf{S^N} = (s_{\cdot,0}, s_{\cdot,1}, ..., s_{\cdot,N})$, a N-dimensional embedding of the images. Each voxel $\mathbf{x}$ of images in $\mathbf{U}$ and $\mathbf{A}$ has the spectral feature defined as $s^{norm}_{\mathbf{x},(1,...,N)}$, which is a row of $\mathbf{S^N}$ normalized to the intensity range of the unseen image.

2.4   Multi-atlas Spectral PatchMatch

MAPM was proposed to find the corresponding patches between one unseen image and multiple atlases in [14]. Different from PatchMatch as described in Sec.2.1, it finds only one correspondence for each point $\mathbf{p} = (x, y, z)$ in image $\mathbf{U}$ $\mathbf{C}(\mathbf{p}) = (\mathbf{q}, k)$, so that $\mathbf{A_k}(\mathbf{q})$ is the closest match in all atlases $\mathbf{A}$. The MAPM algorithm [14] consists of three different steps which we briefly describe as follows: The correspondence $\mathbf{C}(\mathbf{x}) = (\mathbf{x}, R(K))$ is initialised by a uniform random selection $R(K)$ that selects between $\mathbf{A_1}$ to $\mathbf{A_K}$. After initialization, the correspondence $\mathbf{C}$ is improved by iterating between propagating good matches to its neighbours and searching for better matches across different atlases simultaneously. This process is performed until the sum of all distances between each patch in the unseen image and its correspondence converges.

The advantage of MAPM is that it can find global patch correspondences between an unseen image and multiple atlases simultaneously. The complexity of the algorithm does not increase with the number of atlases [14]. However, using intensity features, the match can be ambiguous and may connect different anatomical structures. In this paper, we propose adding the spectral feature s^{norm} into MAPM. We redefine the distance function as follows,

$$D_s(\mathbf{p}, \mathbf{q}) := D(\mathbf{p}, \mathbf{q}) + \sqrt{\sum_{\mathbf{p'} \in \mathbf{P}} \sum_{i=1}^{N} (s^{norm}_{\mathbf{p'},i} - s^{norm}_{\mathbf{q'},i})^2}, \qquad (2)$$

where $\mathbf{q'}$ are corresponding points to $\mathbf{p'}$ in the atlas patch $\mathbf{Q}$. Using this approach, the shape context contained in the spectral features can be used to support MAPM to identify differences between different anatomical structures as shown in Fig. 1. Compared to Spectral Demons [16], this is the first attempt to build a joint spectral representation of multiple images. If we build the image graph independently, large perturbations of the graph will cause fundamental differences in the spectral representations which are difficult to recover [13]. The final label probability $P_L(\mathbf{x})$ at each voxel $\mathbf{x}$ is estimated with the method proposed in [6]. We use a weighting function identical to the one in Sec. 2.2.

3   Application to Cardiac MR Image Segmentation

The proposed framework was applied to cardiac cine MR images. The images used were from healthy and clinical cohorts of the cardiac atlas project [17] and demonstrated a wide range of shape variations. This data set was also used in the MICCAI-SATA 2013 segmentation challenge [18]. A standard acquisition was performed, including an axial stack of cine b-SSFP MR images in the left ventricular short axis plane. The image dimensions are 192 x 192 x 16 x 30 and the voxel sizes are 1.5 x 1.5 x 6 mm. Ground truth segmentations of the myocardium were provided throughout the cardiac cycle for the training set of 83 subjects. In addition, a test set of 72 subjects were provided without ground truth segmentations.

MASP was applied between slices of the unseen image and the atlases to deal with the respiratory motion and large slice thickness. Before label fusion, the atlases were aligned to the unseen image followed by intensity normalization [19]. The initial alignment was obtained using five manual landmarks similar to [11]. In the experiments, the patch size was set to 3 x 3 voxels [11]. To initialize the image-atlas graph, each pixel was connected to its four neighbouring pixels within the same image and one inter image-atlas neighbour from the unseen image to each atlas using PatchMatch [12]. The dimension of spectral features was $N = 3$ [16].

3.1   Results

We performed a leave-one-out cross-validation using the end diastolic (ED) frame of the training set. We compared the Dice metric between the segmentation result and the ground truth using different segmentation techniques including the majority voting, patch-based fusion [7], joint label fusion [9], MAPM [14] and MASP. To ensure fair comparison, all methods were based on the same

Table 1. The mean and standard deviation of Dice metric for different methods. The first, second and third rows show the results using affine registration, the result using FFD registration and the differences between the FFD and affine registration respectively. Paired sample t-test shows a significant difference between the proposed method and the other approaches (p-value < 0.01 indicated by *)

	Majority	Patch based [7]	Joint label [9]	MAPM [12]	MASP
Affine	0.673 (0.098)*	0.736 (0.090)*	0.729 (0.068)*	0.720 (0.050)*	0.800 (0.054)
FFD	0.737 (0.086)*	0.762 (0.083)*	0.761 (0.060)*	0.728 (0.050)*	0.801 (0.048)
Differences	0.065 (0.029)*	0.026 (0.021)*	0.035 (0.022)*	0.008 (0.013)*	0.001 (0.015)

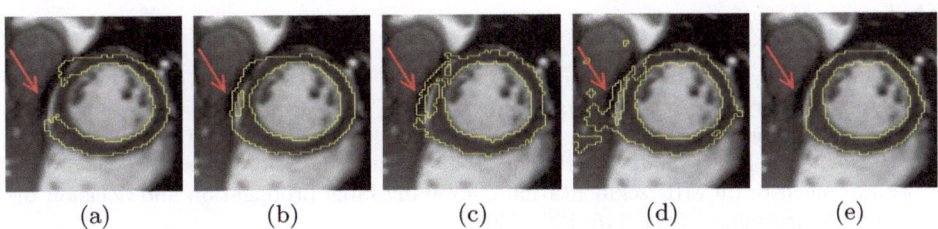

(a)   (b)   (c)   (d)   (e)

Fig. 3. This figure illustrates the segmentation results of different methods using FFD. (a) shows majority voting; (b) shows patch-based segmentation [7]; (c) shows joint label fusion [9]; (d) shows the MAPM [14]; (e) shows the proposed MASP.

affine registration and refined by FFD registration. To estimate the sensitivity of the methods against different registrations approaches, we presented results based on both affine and FFD registration. For each unseen image, 20 atlases were selected from a pool of 82 images after affine registration as in [3].

The results are summarized in Tab. 1. MASP yields a significant improvement in the segmentation accuracy. MASP is also significantly less sensitive to the initial registration as shown in the third row. In addition, the difference when using MASP with different initialisation methods (affine, FFD) was not significant. The intensity based methods have difficulties in distinguishing the difference between liver and myocardium (Fig.3b,Fig.3c and Fig.3d). In particular, MAPM did not preserve the topology of the myocardium. In contrast, MASP can recover large variation in shape while preserving the topology (Fig.3e). This is due to the fact that MASP uses a global search strategy which is, due to spectral features, aware of the anatomical context.

We also submitted our result based on affine registration on the test set to the SATA segmentation challenge. To label the myocardium consistently across temporal frames, we used graph cuts [21] with the label probability $P_L(\mathbf{x})$ as the data term and linked between neighboring frames as the smoothness term. The results are summarized in the leader board[1] under the entry name MASP_AREG_GC with a mean Dice metric of 0.807 and a mean Hausdorff distance of 1.287mm.

4   Conclusion

In this paper we developed MASP: a segmentation method for, but not limited to, cardiac MR images. By creating a multi-layered image-atlas graph, we used spectral embedding to estimate spectral features of the unseen image and multiple atlases simultaneously. Compared to the intensity features, the spectral features contain shape context and facilitate the estimation of an unambiguous correspondence field. We have shown that our method is less sensitive to the initial registration and robust to the presence of large shape variations.

Acknowledgement. This research was supported by British Heart Foundation grant PG/12/27/29489.

References

1. Rohlfing, T., Brandt, R., Menzel, R., Maurer, C.: Evaluation of atlas selection strategies for atlas-based image segmentation with application to confocal microscopy images of bee brains. NeuroImage 21(4), 1428–1442 (2004)
2. Heckemann, R., Hajnal, J., Aljabar, P., Rueckert, D., Hammers, A.: Automatic anatomical brain MRI segmentation combining label propagation and decision fusion. NeuroImage 33(1), 115–126 (2006)
3. Aljabar, P., Heckemann, R., Hammers, A., Hajnal, J., Rueckert, D.: Multi-atlas based segmentation of brain images: Atlas selection and its effect on accuracy. Neuroimage 46(3), 726–738 (2009)

---

[1] http://masi.vuse.vanderbilt.edu/submission/leaderboard.html

4. Rueckert, D., Sonoda, L., Hayes, C., Hill, D., Leach, M., Hawkes, D.: Nonrigid registration using free-form deformations: application to breast MR images. IEEE Transactions on Medical Imaging 18(8), 712–721 (1999)
5. Thirion, J.: Image matching as a diffusion process: an analogy with maxwell's demons. Medical Image Analysis 2(3), 243–260 (1998)
6. Rousseau, F., Habas, P.A., Studholme, C.: A supervised patch-based approach for human brain labeling. IEEE Transactions on Medical Imaging 30(10), 1852–1862 (2011)
7. Coupé, P., Manjón, J., Fonov, V., Pruessner, J., Robles, M., Collins, D.: Patch-based segmentation using expert priors: Application to hippocampus and ventricle segmentation. Neuroimage 54(2), 940–954 (2011)
8. Asman, A.J., Landman, B.A.: Non-local statistical label fusion for multi-atlas segmentation. Medical Image Analysis 17(2), 194–208 (2013)
9. Wang, H., Suh, J., Das, S., Pluta, J., Craige, C., Yushkevich, P.: Multi-atlas segmentation with joint label fusion. IEEE Transactions on Pattern Analysis and Machine Intelligence 35(3), 611–623 (2013)
10. Liao, S., Gao, Y., Lian, J., Shen, D.: Sparse patch-based label propagation for accurate prostate localization in CT images. IEEE Transactions on Medical Imaging 32(2), 419–434 (2013)
11. Bai, W., Shi, W., O'Regan, D.P., Tong, T., Wang, H., Jamil-Copley, S., Peters, N.S., Rueckert, D.: A probabilistic patch-based label fusion model for multi-atlas segmentation with registration refinement: Application to cardiac MR images. IEEE Transactions on Medical Imaging 32(7), 1302–1315 (2013)
12. Barnes, C., Shechtman, E., Goldman, D.B., Finkelstein, A.: The generalized patchMatch correspondence algorithm. In: Daniilidis, K., Maragos, P., Paragios, N. (eds.) ECCV 2010, Part III. LNCS, vol. 6313, pp. 29–43. Springer, Heidelberg (2010)
13. Lombaert, H., Sporring, J., Siddiqi, K.: Diffeomorphic spectral matching of cortical surfaces. In: Gee, J.C., Joshi, S., Pohl, K.M., Wells, W.M., Zöllei, L. (eds.) IPMI 2013. LNCS, vol. 7917, pp. 376–389. Springer, Heidelberg (2013)
14. Shi, W., et al.: Cardiac image super-resolution with global correspondence using multi-atlas patchMatch. In: Mori, K., Sakuma, I., Sato, Y., Barillot, C., Navab, N. (eds.) MICCAI 2013, Part III. LNCS, vol. 8151, pp. 9–16. Springer, Heidelberg (2013)
15. Chung, F.R.: Spectral graph theory, vol. 92. AMS Bookstore (1997)
16. Lombaert, H., Grady, L., Pennec, X., Ayache, N., Cheriet, F.: Spectral log-demons: Diffeomorphic image registration with very large deformations. International Journal of Computer Vision (2013)
17. Fonseca, C., Backhaus, M., Bluemke, D., Britten, R., Do Chung, J., Cowan, B., Dinov, I., Finn, J., Hunter, P., Kadish, A., et al.: The cardiac atlas project: an imaging database for computational modeling and statistical atlases of the heart. Bioinformatics 27(16), 2288–2295 (2011)
18. Andrew, A., Alireza, A.A., Hongzhi, W., Brian, A., Simon, K.W., Bennett, L.: MICCAI 2013 segmentation algorithms, theory and applications (SATA) challenge results summary (2013)
19. Nyúl, L., Udupa, J., et al.: On standardizing the MR image intensity scale. Magnetic Resonance in Medicine 42(6), 1072 (1999)
20. Lin, X., Cowan, B.R., Young, A.A.: Automated detection of left ventricle in 4D MR images: Experience from a large study. In: Larsen, R., Nielsen, M., Sporring, J. (eds.) MICCAI 2006. LNCS, vol. 4190, pp. 728–735. Springer, Heidelberg (2006)
21. Boykov, Y., Veksler, O., Zabih, R.: Fast approximate energy minimization via graph cuts. IEEE Transactions on Pattern Analysis and Machine Intelligence 23(11), 1222–1239 (2001)

Robust Bone Detection in Ultrasound Using Combined Strain Imaging and Envelope Signal Power Detection

Mohammad Arafat Hussain[1], Antony Hodgson[2], and Rafeef Abugharbieh[1]

[1] Department of Electrical and Computer Engineering
[2] Department of Mechanical Engineering, The University of British Columbia,
Vancouver, BC, Canada
{arafat,rafeef}@ece.ubc.ca, ahodgson@mech.ubc.ca

Abstract. Bone localization in ultrasound (US) remains challenging despite encouraging advances. Current methods, e.g. local image phase-based feature analysis, showed promising results but remain reliant on delicate parameter selection processes and prone to errors at confounding soft tissue interfaces of similar appearance to bone interfaces. We propose a different approach combining US strain imaging and envelope power detection at each radio-frequency (RF) sample. After initial estimation of strain and envelope power maps, we modify their dynamic ranges into a modified strain map (MSM) and a modified envelope map (MEM) that we subsequently fuse into a single combined map that we show corresponds robustly to actual bone boundaries. Our quantitative results demonstrate a marked reduction in false positive responses at soft tissue interfaces and an increase in bone delineation accuracy. Comparisons to the state-of-the-art on a finite-element-modelling (FEM) phantom and fiducial-based experimental phantom show an average improvement in mean absolute error (MAE) between actual and estimated bone boundaries of 32% and 14%, respectively. We also demonstrate an average reduction in false bone responses of 87% and 56%, respectively. Finally, we qualitatively validate on clinical in vivo data of the human radius and ulna bones, and demonstrate similar improvements to those observed on phantoms.

Keywords: Ultrasound, bone, strain imaging, segmentation.

1 Introduction

Fluoroscopy remains the primary intraoperative imaging modality for bone boundary visualization in computer assisted orthopaedic surgery systems. The associated radiation exposure posing risks to both patients and surgical teams gave rise to recent interest in safer non-ionizing real-time intraoperative imaging alternatives such as US [1].

In US guided surgical intervention, bone localization in US images is essential for visualization and guidance, e.g. during fragment positioning in fracture reduction surgeries [1]. Despite recent advancement in US intensity-based automatic

P. Golland et al. (Eds.): MICCAI 2014, Part I, LNCS 8673, pp. 356–363, 2014.

bone segmentation, results remain unpredictable due to the high levels of speckle noise, reverberation, and signal drop out [1]. Recent work by Hacihaliloglu et. al. [2] on local image phase feature-based bone segmentation addressed some of these limitations however remains prone to false positive bone responses at soft tissue interfaces that commonly exhibit similar intensity profiles as bone interfaces.

Elastography is an emerging medical diagnostic tool for capturing the mechanical properties (e.g. stiffness) of biological tissue [3]. Elastography has shown promise in the detection of breast and prostate tumors, liver cirrhosis, vascular plaques [3], and ligament-bone insertion. However, in the bone imaging literature, US elastography has been very limited. In [4], bone detection using US elastography was investigated. The reported strain images, however, showed low contrast between the hard bone and soft tissue regions. In addition, problems arose from signal windowing as window-based elastography (WBE) methods have limitations associated with the size of the window segments. A significant amount of noise in the strain image can be easily introduced with the choice of smaller window size and/or large overlap between successive windows [3].

In this paper, we propose a novel method for robust bone boundary localization based on combined US strain imaging and envelope power signal detection. Our method uses real-time strain imaging based on analytic minimization (AM) of regularized cost functions [5]. The AM method estimates strain for each of the RF samples, so the resulting strain image has better spatial resolution than that of the WBE methods, and does not suffer from window-related artifacts. Furthermore, WBE methods often produce distorted strain estimates due to the amplitude modulation effect even if there is no displacement estimation error [6]. In contrast, the cost functions used in the AM method incorporate a measure of the similarity of RF data intensity as well as displacement continuity, which makes the method robust to echo de-correlations present throughout the image; in turn, this produces smoother transitions across bone/soft tissue interfaces. To better delineate the bone boundary, we combine the envelope power map with the strain image. We use the envelope power map rather than an envelope or log-compressed envelope map (i.e. B-mode) as it possesses a higher dynamic range. As elastography estimates tissue stiffness, we achieve a marked reduction of false positive bone responses at the soft tissue interfaces.

2 Methods

Our method is divided into three parts. In Sect. 2.1, we discuss the strain map estimation and subsequent processing of it. Then, in Sect. 2.2, we discuss the estimation of the envelope power map and its further processing. Finally, in Sect. 2.3, we discuss our integration procedure of the strain and envelope power maps.

2.1 Estimation of Modified Strain Map (MSM)

The AM-based strain estimation method has been described in detail elsewhere [5]. However, in brief, the AM method estimates tissue displacement from the pre- and post-compression RF echo frames using a regularized cost function that incorporates three regularizing parameters and representations of the estimated axial and lateral displacements. The cost function is partial-differentiated with respect to the displacements and set to zero. Assumptions related to the depth dependence of US attenuation, the size of lateral displacements and the displacement at the transducer face are introduced to simplify the solution of the problem, and a Kalman filter-based method is adopted to estimate the final strain $\mathbf{S}$ from the estimated displacement map [5]. Finally, to produce a strain map with a dynamic range roughly equivalent to that of the envelope power map, we estimate the MSM $= \hat{\mathbf{S}}/\hat{\mathbf{S}}_M$, where $\hat{\mathbf{S}} = \mid (-\mathbf{S})+ \mid median(-\mathbf{S}) \mid \mid$, $\hat{\mathbf{S}}_M$ is the maximum of $\hat{\mathbf{S}}$, and *median* is the median operator.

2.2   Estimation of Modified Envelope Map (MEM)

As the strain is mapped with respect to the pre-compression RF frame, we use the same pre-compression RF frame to generate the MEM so that it can be spatially matched to the MSM. The envelope of a RF scan-line at column j is calculated as $\mathbf{E}_j(i) = \mid H[I_{1,j}(i)] \mid$ [7], where H denotes the Hilbert transform. Finally, we estimate MEM $= \hat{\mathbf{E}}/\hat{\mathbf{E}}_M$, where $\hat{\mathbf{E}} = \mathbf{E}^2$ and $\hat{\mathbf{E}}_M$ is the maximum of $\hat{\mathbf{E}}$.

2.3   Fused Map (FM) Estimation and Bone Boundary Localization

Our final step involves fusing the MSM and MEM into a single FM measure as

$$FM = \lambda \times MSM + (1 - \lambda) \times MEM, \tag{1}$$

where λ is the weight. To choose a suitable value of λ, we analyse the effect of this choice on the accuracy of the bone boundary localization in an FEM-based simulation of a noisy environment (i.e. 10dB SNR). Fig. 1(h) shows the MAE as a function of different values of λ ranging from 0.3 to 0.7. From this figure we see that the mean MAE is minimized for $\lambda = 0.5$. While this value for λ may not be optimal under all possible imaging situations, the results seem to be relatively insensitive to this choice, so we opted to set $\lambda = 0.5$ for this study. However, after estimating the FM, the maximum intensity point along each scan-line of the FM is detected and the final bone boundary is estimated using a local linear-fit with a length of 3mm over the detected intensity points.

3   Validation Setup

Simulated Phantom. We built a 40mm×40mm FEM phantom using the ANSYS analysis software (ANSYS, Inc., Canonsburg, PA) and then generated an ultrasound simulation of the model using Field II [8]. Our phantom mimicked an US scan of the human distal radius bone with a total number of nodes of 55,180. The stiffness of the homogeneous soft tissue and bone region were set to

10kPa and 10GPa, respectively as previously reported in the literature [9]. Our phantom was compressed from the top using a larger-width planar compressor in free-hand fashion. An ultrasonic transducer of center frequency, $f_0 = 5$MHz and band-width = 50% was used to simulate the phantom scan from the top. The total number of scan lines was set to 128. We set an applied pressure level that corresponds to 1% average strain. In addition, we did not model out-of-plane motion.

Experimental Physical Phantom. We constructed an experimental phantom using a radio-opaque Sawbones hemi-pelvis (Sawbones, Pacific Research Laboratories, Inc., Vashon Island, WA), model number 1297-22. A portion of the pelvis was suspended in a PVC gel and placed in an acrylic tube. A high resolution peripheral quantitative computed tomography (CT) machine, model HR pQCT Xtreme CT (Scanco USA, Inc., Wayne, PA) was used to acquire a single $482 \times 482 \times 402$ (lateral×axial×elevational) voxel volume with a resolution of 0.25mm^2. In addition, US was acquired using a SonixRP (Ultrasonix Medical Corporation, Richmond, BC) scanner integrated with a L14-5W/60 probe operating at 10MHz.

Real In Vivo Data. We acquired three sets of in vivo US data with free-hand compression from three volunteers (volunteer-I: 25-year old male; volunteer-II: 26-year old male; volunteer-III: 24-year old male) after proper prior consent was obtained. US was acquired using a SonixRP (Ultrasonix Medical Corporation, Richmond, BC) scanner integrated with a L14-5W/60 probe operating at 10MHz. The study was approved by our institutional review board (IRB).

4 Results and Discussion

We provide comparative results of our proposed method with the automatic adaptive parameterization in local phase feature-based bone segmentation in US (APS) [2] method using the FEM phantom, experimental phantom and in vivo data. The initial parameters in the APS method are chosen according to [2] such that the best possible bone map is generated. We calculate MAE that is defined as MAE $= \frac{1}{N} \sum_{k=1}^{N} \mid A(k) - G(k) \mid$, where N is the approximated number of columns on which the bone boundary spans, A is the matrix containing the actual bone boundary points (ground truth), and G is the matrix containing the estimated bone boundary points. As ground truth, we use the estimated bone boundaries from the ideal elastogram and CT image for the FEM and experimental phantom, respectively. We also estimate mean signed distance (MSD) [2] for quantitative evaluation of the false positive responses produced by the proposed and APS method using the FEM and experimental phantom data. Signed distance of a bone response in any scan-line is estimated with respect to the actual bone position along that particular scan-line. Note that to estimate MSD for the proposed method, we use the bone boundary points before applying the regression.

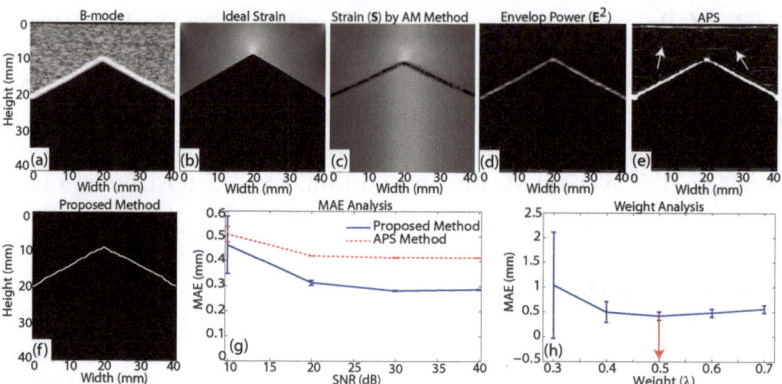

Fig. 1. Illustration of bone boundary detection using the FEM phantom. (a) B-mode image, (b) ideal strain image, (c) strain image **S** generated by the AM method, (d) envelop power map **Ê**, (e) estimated bone boundary by the APS method, (f) estimated bone boundary by the proposed method, (g) MAE analysis of the proposed and APS methods at different SNRs, and (h) weight analysis at 10dB SNR (weight at minimum error is shown with red arrow).

FEM Results. We provide comparative qualitative and quantitative results of our proposed and APS method using the FEM data. In Figs. 1(a), (b), (c) and (d), we show the B-mode, ideal strain, estimated strain **S**, and envelop power **Ê** images, respectively. Note that we are dealing with anatomy that includes bone, hence, the RF intensities fall sharply (compared to soft tissue) beneath the bone surface. In such a situation, the regularization terms in the cost equation become larger than the signal part in the region beneath the bone surface and over-smoothing tends to occur [5]. In Figs. 1(e) and (f), we show the bone boundaries detected by the APS and proposed methods, respectively. The figures demonstrate that the APS method produces several false positive bone responses (indicated by white arrows) due to the presence of ridge-like features in the B-mode image. In contrast, the bone boundary produced by our method (Fig. 1(f)) is apparently free of such artifacts. Note that if the false positive responses produced by the APS method could be ignored, then a local fitting over the actual bone responses similar to the proposed method could produce better bone boundary. We also compare the quantitative performance of the proposed and APS methods in terms of MAE in Fig. 1(g) with four different signal-to-noise ratio (SNR) simulations (40, 30, 20, and 10dB) with 100 realizations each. As can be seen in this figure, up to 20dB SNR, the APS method produces greater mean MAE than that of the proposed method, though the mean MAE of both the methods are almost flat and standard deviations (SD) are close to zero. In addition, the mean MAE of the APS method at 10dB SNR is higher though the SD of the proposed method in this case somewhat higher. Moreover, the estimated MSDs are found to be 0.68 ± 2.5mm and 5.47 ± 6.20mm for the proposed and APS methods, respectively. Therefore, we can say that the proposed method shows better performance in terms of reduced false positive bone responses than that of the APS method.

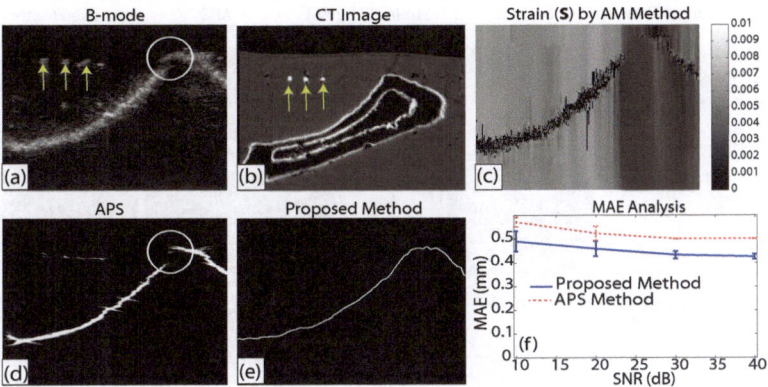

Fig. 2. Illustration of the bone boundary detection using the experimental phantom. (a) B-mode image, (b) a CT projection along which US scanning is performed, (c) strain image **S**, (d) estimated bone boundary by the APS method, (e) estimated bone boundary by the proposed method, and (f) MAE analysis of the proposed and APS methods at different SNRs.

Experimental Phantom Results. Figure 2 demonstrates the qualitative and quantitative performance comparison of the proposed and APS methods using the experimental phantom. In Fig. 2(a), we show the B-mode image. Figure 2(b) shows the CT projection slice along which the US scanning is performed and fiducials in Fig. 2(a) corresponds to fiducials in Fig. 2(b) (shown with yellow arrows) in the same order. The estimated strain image is shown in Fig. 2(c). We show the detected bone boundaries by the APS and proposed methods in Figs. 2(d) and (e), respectively. We can see from Fig. 2(d) that the bone boundary image estimated by the APS method produces false positive responses in soft tissue regions and fails to estimate bone boundary where US back-scatter response is very weak (shown with white circles in Figs. 2(a) and (d)). In contrast, the bone boundary estimated by the proposed method has no discontinuity as well as produces no noticeable false positive response. We also show the quantitative performance of both the methods in Fig. 2(f). Here too, we use four different SNRs (40, 30, 20, and 10dB) with 100 realizations for each of them to analyze the MAE. Since the quality of the ultrasound machine-acquired RF data is dependent on user-defined parameters, the signals may have different signal to noise ratios in different situations. Therefore, we have used a range of SNRs to evaluate the robustness of our proposed scheme. We can see from this figure that the mean MAE values of the proposed method are lower than that of the APS method at all SNRs though the SDs of the proposed method are slightly higher. In addition, the estimated MSDs are found to be 0.66 ± 0.64mm and 1.51 ± 3.34mm for the proposed and APS methods, respectively. Therefore, from here too, we can say that the proposed method shows better performance in terms of reduced false positive bone responses than that of the APS method.

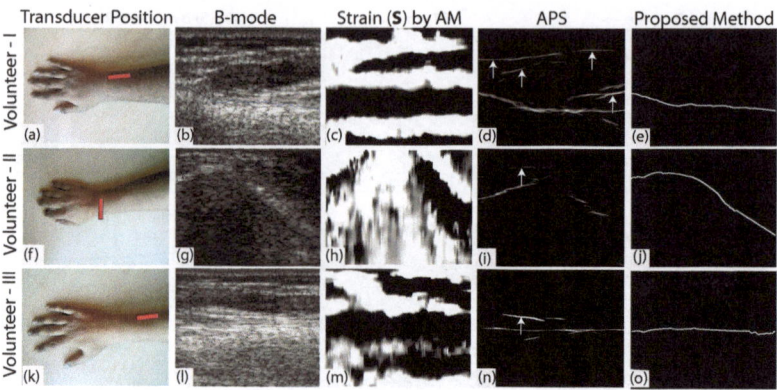

Fig. 3. Illustration of the bone boundary detection using the in vivo data. (a), (f) and (k) show the transducer face positions on each volunteer's hand (with red rectangles), (b), (g) and (l) are the B-mode images, (c), (h) and (m) are strain images **S**, (d), (i) and (n) show the detected bone boundaries by the APS method, and (e), (j) and (o) are the detected bone boundaries by the proposed method.

In Vivo Results. We compared the bone boundary detection performance of our proposed and APS methods using the in vivo data. The transducer positions on the anatomies as well as the B-mode images of volunteer-I, II and III are shown in Figs. 3(a) and (b), (f) and (g), and (k) and (l), respectively. Note that for volunteer-II, only half of the total scan-lines are considered for both methods since almost half of the transducer face laterally was in the air. We can see from Figs. 3(d), (i) and (n) that the APS method produced false positive response for bone in the soft tissue interfaces (shown with white arrows). In addition, in Fig. 3(i), the APS method fails to show the bone boundary. In contrast, in all three cases, the bone boundaries estimated by our proposed method better match the shapes visible in the corresponding B-mode images. (see Figs. 3(e), (j) and (o)). In addition, our method did not produce false positives at soft tissue interfaces.

5   Conclusions

We proposed a novel method for robust bone boundary localization based on the fusion of strain imaging and envelope signal power detection. We combined real-time strain imaging based on analytic minimization of regularized cost functions with an envelope power map of the pre-compression RF frame. Our results demonstrated reduced bone localization error through better elastogram resolution, adoption of envelope power map of higher dynamic range, addressing the false positive bone response, and exploiting the smoothing feature of the AM method to better delineate the bone boundary in strain image. We demonstrated our improved performance on a wide range of validation data including a simulated FEM phantom, a physical experimental phantom, and in vivo data of the human with reported improvements of approximately 32% and 14% in terms of MAE, and 87% and 56% in terms of MSD in the FEM and experimental phantom tests, respectively, when compared with current state-of-the-art. We plan to follow up this promising initial study with a more extensive range of clinical test cases to better identify situations in which our method does not produce accurate results. We anticipate that it will be more problematic in situations where the bone boundary lies relatively far below the skin surface due to signal dropout and inhomogeneous tissue deformation near the bone boundary. However, preliminary indications are that the technique is quite robust when the bone boundary lies close to the skin surface.

References

1. Hacihaliloglu, I., Abugharbieh, R., Hodgson, A.J., Rohling, R.N.: Bone Segmentation and Fracture Detection in Ultrasound Using 3D Local Phase Features. In: Metaxas, D., Axel, L., Fichtinger, G., Székely, G. (eds.) MICCAI 2008, Part I. LNCS, vol. 5241, pp. 287–295. Springer, Heidelberg (2008)
2. Hacihaliloglu, I., Abugharbieh, R., Hodgson, A.J., Rohling, R.N.: Automatic Adaptive Parameterization in Local Phase Feature-based Bone Segmentation in Ultrasound. Ultrasound in Med. and Biol. 37(10), 1689–1703 (2011)
3. Hussain, M.A., Anas, E.M.A., Alam, S.K., Lee, S.Y., Hasan, M.K.: Direct and Gradient Based Average Strain Estimation by Using Weighted Nearest Neighbor Cross-correlation Peaks. IEEE Trans. Ultra. Ferro. Freq. Cont. 59(8), 1713–1728 (2012)
4. Wen, X., Salcudean, S.E.: Enhancement of Bone Surface Visualization Using Ultrasound Radio-frequency Signals. In: IEEE Ultra. Symp., vol. 1051, pp. 2535–2538 (2007)
5. Rivaz, H., Boctor, E.M., Choti, M.A., Hager, G.D.: Real-time Regularized Ultrasound Elastography. IEEE Trans. Med. Imag. 30(4), 928–945 (2011)
6. Lindop, J.E., Treece, G.M., Gee, A.H., Prager, R.W.: Estimation of Displacement Location for Enhanced Strain Imaging. IEEE Trans. Ultra. Ferro. Freq. Cont. 54(9), 1751–1771 (2007)
7. Hussain, M.A., Alam, S.K., Lee, S.Y., Hasan, M.K.: A Robust Strain Estimation Algorithm Using Combined Radio-frequency and Envelope Cross-correlation with Diffusion Filtering. Ultrason. Imag. 34(2), 93–109 (2012)
8. Jensen, J.A.: Field: A Program for Simulating Ultrasound Systems. In: 10th Nordicbaltic Conf. on Biomed. Imag. Part I, vol. 4(1), pp. 351–353 (1996)
9. Pistoia, W., Rietbergen, B.V., Lochmüller, E., Lill, C.A., Eckstein, F., Rüegsegger, P.: Estimation of Distal Radius Failure Load With Micro-Finite Element Analysis Models Based on Three-dimensional Peripheral Quantitative Computed Tomography Images. Bone 30(6), 842–848 (2002)

SIMPLE Is a Good Idea
(and Better with Context Learning)

Zhoubing Xu[1], Andrew J. Asman[1],
Peter L. Shanahan[2], Richard G. Abramson[2], and Bennett A. Landman[1,2]

[1] Electrical Engineering, Vanderbilt University, Nashville, TN, USA 37235
{zhoubing.xu,andrew.j.asman,bennett.landman}@vanderbilt.edu
[2] Radiology and Radiological Science, Vanderbilt University, Nashville, TN, USA 37235
{peter.l.shanahan,richard.abramson}@vanderbilt.edu

Abstract. Selective and iterative method for performance level estimation (SIMPLE) is a multi-atlas segmentation technique that integrates atlas selection and label fusion that has proven effective for radiotherapy planning. Herein, we revisit atlas selection and fusion techniques in the context of segmenting the spleen in metastatic liver cancer patients with possible splenomegaly using clinically acquired computed tomography (CT). We re-derive the SIMPLE algorithm in the context of the statistical literature, and show that the atlas selection criteria rest on newly presented principled likelihood models. We show that SIMPLE performance can be improved by accounting for exogenous information through Bayesian priors (so called context learning). These innovations are integrated with the joint label fusion approach to reduce the impact of correlated errors among selected atlases. In a study of 65 subjects, the spleen was segmented with median Dice similarity coefficient of 0.93 and a mean surface distance error of 2.2 mm.

Keywords: Selective and Iterative Method for Performance Level Estimation (SIMPLE), Context Learning, Multi-Atlas Segmentation, Abdomen.

1 Introduction

Multi-atlas segmentation is a technique for transferring information from canonical atlases to target images via registration. While this family of techniques has proven effective in neuroimaging [2], the importance of atlas selection has become increasingly clear for variable anatomical targets (e.g., the prostate [3]).

Here, we revisit atlas selection and fusion techniques in the context of segmenting the spleen in metastatic liver cancer patients with possible splenomegaly using clinically acquired computed tomography (CT). Abdominal anatomy is variable both between individuals (e.g., weight, stature, age, disease status) and within individuals (e.g., pose, respiratory cycle, clothing). Splenomegaly exacerbates inter-individual spleen variability (and can result in a ≈10 fold increase in spleen volume over normal individuals) and complicates inter-subject registration (Figure 1). Note that in this situation a majority of atlases tend to be poorly registered, but a subset (shown for

P. Golland et al. (Eds.): MICCAI 2014, Part I, LNCS 8673, pp. 364–371, 2014.
© Springer International Publishing Switzerland 2014

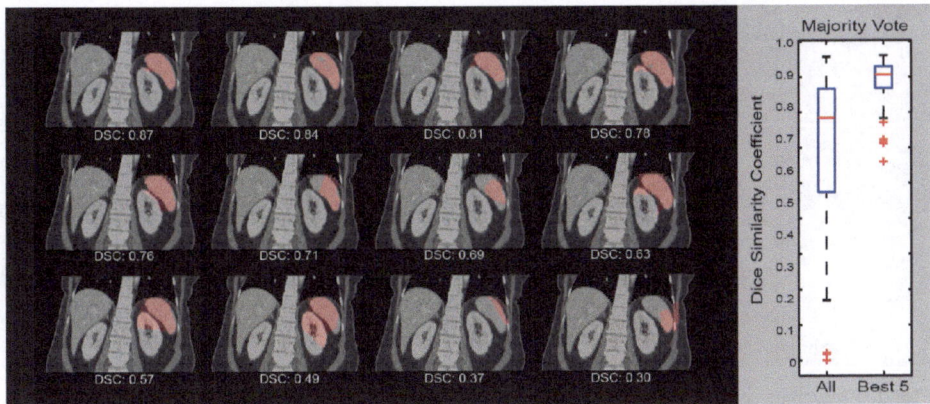

Fig. 1. (left) 12 registered (using [1]) spleen labels are overlaid on a slice of a target image. DSC values are computed on a volumetric basis as examples. (right) Using leave-one-out validation, multi-atlas segmentation is tested on 65 subjects for spleen segmentation. For each subject, majority vote is used to fuse either all registered atlases or the best five atlases in terms of DSC.

five best matches) could result in excellent segmentation *if* they could be identified without using the true labels to compute Dice similarity coefficient (DSC) [4] (as in the Figure 1 illustration).

Two broad families of techniques have emerged to address these issues: voting (well synthesized in [2]) and statistical fusion (largely following [5, 6]). The selective and iterative method for performance level estimation (SIMPLE) [3] algorithm identifies and combines a set of registered images by selecting self-consistent sets of atlases based on DSC. SIMPLE addressed extensive variation in prostate anatomy and was presented from the perspective of voting using sensible, but *ad hoc,* criteria to reduce the impact of outlier atlases. Recently, joint label fusion (JLF) [7] has provided a technique to reduce the impact of correlated errors among atlases. SIMPLE and JLF effectively address different aspects of the fusion problem: atlas selection and label determination. Hitherto, they have not been combined into a common framework.

The primary contributions of this manuscript are as follows (Figure 2). (1) We present SIMPLE in the context of the statistical literature and show that "simple" atlas selection criteria rest on principled likelihood models. (2) We generalized the SIMPLE theoretical framework to account for exogenous information (e.g., from separate models of tissue likelihood) – referred to as *context learning*. (3) We integrate context learning and SIMPLE with JLF. (4) Finally, we combine these contributions to segment the spleen on metastatic liver cancer patients.

2   Theory

First, we consider SIMPLE from the perspective of Expectation-Maximization (EM) while focusing on the atlas selection step. Consider the hidden true segmentation as a vector, $T \in L^{N \times 1}$, where $L = \{0, ..., L - 1\}$ is the set of possible label types.

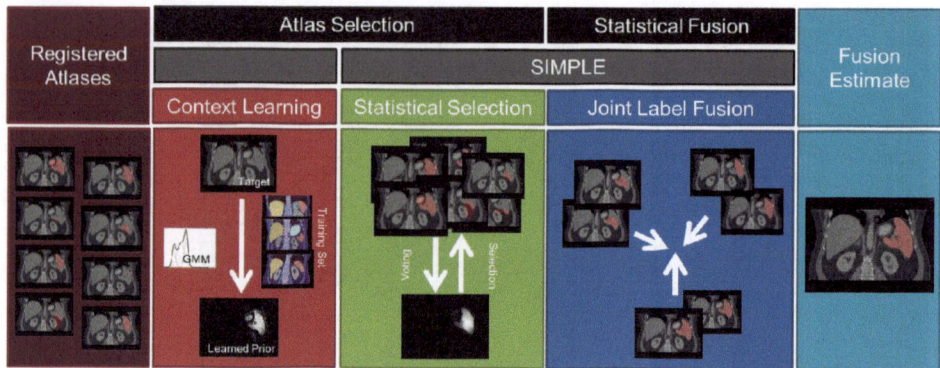

Fig. 2. Flowchart of the proposed method. Given registered atlases with variable qualities, atlas selection and statistical fusion are considered as two necessary steps to obtain a reasonable fusion estimate of the target segmentation. The SIMPLE algorithm implicitly combines these two steps to fusion selected atlases; however, more information can be incorporated to improve the atlas segmentation, and a more advanced fusion technique can be used after the atlases are selected. We propose to (1) extract a probabilistic prior of the target segmentation by context learning to regularize the atlas selection in SIMPLE and (2) use Joint Label Fusion to obtain the final segmentation while characterizing the correlated errors from among atlases.

Consider a collection of R registered atlases with label decisions, $\boldsymbol{D} \in \boldsymbol{L}^{N \times R}$. Let $\boldsymbol{c} \in \boldsymbol{S}^R$ represent the atlas selection decisions, where $\boldsymbol{S} = \{0,1\}$ indicates that the associated atlas is ignored or selected, respectively. We propose a non-linear rater model, $\theta \in \mathbb{R}^{R \times 2 \times L \times L}$, where each elemen $\theta_{jns's}$ represents the probability that the registered atlas j observes label s' given the true label is s and the atlas selection decision is n. Let the ignored atlases be no better than random chance, and the selected atlases be slightly inaccurate with error factors $\boldsymbol{\epsilon} \in \boldsymbol{E}^{R \times 1}$, where $\boldsymbol{E} \in (0, \frac{L-1}{L})$. Thus

$$\theta_{j0s's} = \frac{1}{L}, \quad \forall s' ; \; \theta_{j1s's} = \begin{cases} 1 - \epsilon_j, & s' = s \\ \dfrac{\epsilon_j}{L-1}, & s' \neq s \end{cases} \tag{1}$$

For a registered atlas j at each voxel i, the generative model is

$$f(D_{ij} = s' | T_i = s, c_j = n, \epsilon_j) \equiv \theta_{jns's} \tag{2}$$

Following [5, 6], let $\boldsymbol{W} \in \mathbb{R}^{L \times N}$, where W_{si} represents the probability that the true label associated with voxel i is label s. Using Bayesian expansion and conditional independence between the atlases, the kth iteration of $\boldsymbol{W}$ is

$$W_{si}^{(k)} = \frac{f(T_i = s) \prod_j f(D_{ij} | T_i = s, c_j^{(k)} = n, \epsilon_j^{(k)})}{\sum_{s'} f(T_i = s') \prod_j f\left(D_{ij} | T_i = s', c_j^{(k)} = n, \epsilon_j^{(k)}\right)} \tag{3}$$

where $f(T_i = s)$ is a voxel-wise *a priori* distribution of the underlying segmentation. Note that the ignored atlases do not affect $\boldsymbol{W}$, and the selected atlases contribute to $\boldsymbol{W}$ in a similar way as majority vote (MV) given the symmetric form of $\theta_{1s's}$.

The estimate of the parameters (M-Step) is obtained by maximizing the expected value of the conditional log likelihood function found in Eq. 3. For the error factor,

$$\epsilon_j^{(k+1)} = \arg\max_{\epsilon_j} \sum_i E\left[\ln f\left(D_{ij}|T_i, c_j^{(k)}, \epsilon_j\right)|\boldsymbol{D}, c_j^{(k)}, \epsilon_j^{(k)}\right]$$

$$= \arg\max_{\epsilon_j} \sum_{s'} \sum_{i:D_{ij}=s'} \sum_s W_{si}^{(k)} \ln \theta_{jc_j^{(k)}s's} \equiv L_{\epsilon_j} \tag{4}$$

Consider the binary segmentation for simplicity, let $M_{TP} = \sum_{i:D_{ij}=1} W_{1i}^{(k)}$, $M_{FP} = \sum_{i:D_{ij}=1} W_{0i}^{(k)}$, $M_{FN} = \sum_{i:D_{ij}=0} W_{1i}^{(k)}$, $M_{TN} = \sum_{i:D_{ij}=0} W_{0i}^{(k)}$, and $M_T = M_{TP} + M_{TN}$, $M_F = M_{FP} + M_{FN}$. After taking partial derivative of L_{ϵ_j},

$$\epsilon_j^{(k+1)} = \frac{M_F}{M_T + M_F}, i.e., 1 - \epsilon_j^{(k+1)} = \frac{M_T}{M_T + M_F} \tag{5}$$

Then for the atlas selection decision

$$c_j^{(k+1)} = \arg\max_{c_j} \sum_i E\left[\ln f\left(D_{ij}|T_i, c_j, \epsilon_j^{(k+1)}\right)|\boldsymbol{D}, c_j^{(k)}, \epsilon_j^{(k+1)}\right]$$

$$= \arg\max_{c_j} \sum_{s'} \sum_{i:D_{ij}=s'} \sum_s W_{si}^{(k)} \ln \theta_{jc_js's}. \tag{6}$$

In general, this is a combinatoric problem; however, assuming known true labels, it can be maximized separately for each 0/1 atlas selection decision. Noting the behavior of selecting/ignoring atlases in Eq. 6 is parameterized with the error factor ϵ_j, and thus, as in Eq. 5, affected by the four summed values of True Positive (TP), False Positive (FP), False Negative (FN), and True Negative (TN).

In SIMPLE, atlases are selected based on DSC with the previous majority vote estimate. Above, Eq. 3 reduces to a majority vote of atlases with $c_j^{(k)} = 1$ and the relative weight of atlases is scaled by Eq. 5, which differs from DSC in that DSC does not factor the impacts of TN. Typical practice for a fusion approach might use the prior probability, $f(T_i = s)$, to weight by expected volume of structure. With outlier atlases, one could reasonably expect a much larger region of confusion (i.e., non "consensus"[8]) than true anatomical volume. Hence, an informed prior would greatly deemphasize the TN and yield a metric similar to DSC. Therefore, we argue that SIMPLE is legitimately viewed as a statistical fusion algorithm that is approximately optimal for the non-linear rater model proposed in Eq. 1.

2.1   Context Learning (CL)

Different classes of tissues in CT images can be characterized with multi-dimensional Gaussian mixture models using intensity and spatial "context" features. On a voxel-wise basis, let $v \in \mathbb{R}^{d \times 1}$ represent a d dimensional feature vector, $m \in \boldsymbol{M}$ indicate the tissue membership, where $\boldsymbol{M} = \{1, ..., M\}$ is the set of possible tissues. The probability of the observed features given the tissue is m can be represented with the mixture of N_G Gaussian distributions,

$$f(v|m = t) = \sum_{k=1}^{N_G} \frac{\alpha_{kt}}{(2\pi)^{\frac{d}{2}}|C_{kt}|^{\frac{1}{2}}} exp\left[-\frac{1}{2}(v - \mu_{kt})^T C_{kt}^{-1}(v - \mu_{kt})\right] \qquad (7)$$

where $\alpha_{kt} \in \mathbb{R}^{1\times1}$, $\mu_{kt} \in \mathbb{R}^{d\times1}$, and $C_{kt} \in \mathbb{R}^{d\times d}$ are the unknown mixture probability, mean, and covariance matrix to estimate for each Gaussian mixture component k of each tissue type t by the EM algorithm following [9].

The context model can be learned from datasets with known tissue separations, and then the tissue likelihoods on unknown dataset can be inferred by Bayesian expansion and flat tissue membership probability from extracted feature vectors.

$$f(m = t|v) = \frac{f(v|m = t)f(m = t)}{\sum_{t'} f(v|m = t')f(m = t')} = \frac{f(v|m = t)}{\sum_{t'} f(v|m = t')} \qquad (8)$$

3   Methods and Results

Under an Institutional Review Board (IRB) waiver, the first-session CT abdomen scans of 65 metastatic liver cancer patients were randomly selected from an ongoing colorectal cancer chemotherapy trial. Images are with variable field of views (approx. 300 x 300 x 400 mm ~ 500 x 500 x 700 mm) and resolutions (approx. 0.5 x 0.5 x 1.5 mm ~ 1.0 x 1.0 x 7.0 mm). Spleens were manually labeled by an experienced graduate student on a volumetric basis using the MIPAV software (NIH, Bethesda, MD [10]). All images and labels are cropped along the cranio-caudal axis with a tight border without excluding liver, spleen, and kidneys before any processing (following [1]).

We used 12 of the 65 subjects as training datasets for learning context models for eight tissue types, including five manually traced organs (i.e., spleen, liver, kidneys, pancreas, and stomach) and three automatically retrieved tissues (i.e., muscle, fat, and other) using intensity clustering and excluding the traced organ regions. These 12 datasets were not considered for quantitative evaluation in the leave-one-out analyses. Six context features were extracted, including intensity, gradient, and local variance, and three spatial coordinates with respect to a single landmark, which was loosely identified as the mid-frontal point of the lung at the plane with the largest cross-sectional lung area. We specified the number of components of Gaussian mixture model, $N_G = 3$. The spleen and non-spleen likelihoods on each target image were inferred, and used as a two-fold spatial prior to regularize the SIMPLE atlas selection, referred as CL+SIMPLE. We constrained the number of selected atlases as no less than five and no larger than ten. When using JLF, we specified the local search radii as $3 \times 3 \times 3$, the local patch radii as $2 \times 2 \times 2$, and set the intensity difference mapping parameter (β), and the regularization term (α) as 2 and 0.1, respectively (i.e., default parameters). We appended Markov Random Field (MRF) for smoothing the Gaussian filtered ($\sigma_G = 1$) result of CL+SIMPLE+JLF with the smoothness parameter as 0.2, and the incompatibility parameter as -5.

3.1   Motivating Simulation

To demonstrate and motivate the benefits of the CL+SIMPLE approach, a simulation was constructed using a single CT slice from a representative subject with the spleen manually labeled (see Figure 3). Eighty simulated observations were estimated by

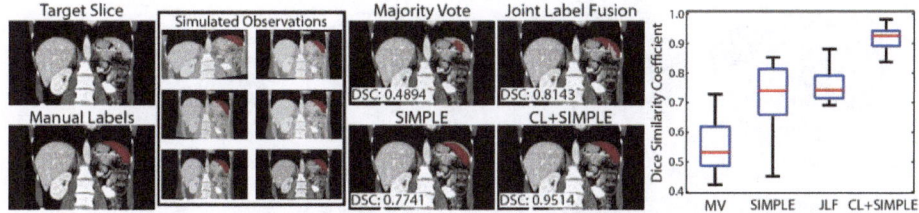

Fig. 3. The results of the motivating simulation demonstrate the benefits of the CL+SIMPLE approach. Using a model in which simulations are drawn from a randomly generated affine transformation, CL+SIMPLE more accurately estimates the location, size, and orientation of the spleen, and significantly outperforms the considered benchmarks.

applying a random five degree-of-freedom affine transformation to the target slice. Each transformation consisted of a rotational component as well as two translational and two scaling components, with the effect of each component drawn from a zero-mean Gaussian distribution with standard deviations of 2 degrees for the rotational component, 1 mm for the translational components and 0.1 mm for the scaling components. A representative fusion result is shown for MV, JLF, SIMPLE, and CL-SIMPLE, with CL+SIMPLE resulting in an estimate that substantially more accurately represents the shape, location, and orientation of the spleen. With 20 Monte Carlo iterations, the spread of DSC values demonstrate significant improvement exhibited by CL+SIMPLE, with a median DSC improvement of approximately 0.15 over SIMPLE and JLF, and approximately 0.4 over majority vote.

3.2   Volumetric Spleen Multi-atlas Segmentation

We performed leave-one-out cross validation for the multi-atlas spleen segmentation for 53 scans (excluding the 12 subjects used for context learning). For each scan, all other scans (including the training dataset) were considered as atlases (hence, 64 atlases), and aligned to the target with a multi-stage registration, in the order of rigid, affine and a multi-level non-rigid registration using free-form deformations with B-spline control point spacings of 20, 10, and 5mm [11]. We tested on seven label fusion methods (as listed in Table 1). The performances of the methods were evaluated on DSC, symmetric mean surface distance (Sym. MSD), and symmetric Hausdorff distance (Sym. HD).

Combined with CL, CL+SIMPLE and CL+SIMPLE+JLF improved mean DSC by at least 0.03 over SIMPLE and SIMPLE+JLF, respectively, while the direct integration of SIMPLE with JLF does not provide higher accuracy over JLF. CL+SIMPLE+JLF outperforms the other methods with the higher median DSC, narrower range of DSC, and lower MSD. An extra MRF step effectively removes outlier speckled structures in the segmentation (Figure 4), and thus further reduces the surface distance errors (Table 1).

4   Discussion

We reformulated SIMPLE as a statistical fusion algorithm that is approximately optimal for a newly presented non-linear rater model tailored for heterogeneous atlases. Revealed in the generalized SIMPLE theoretical framework, we find

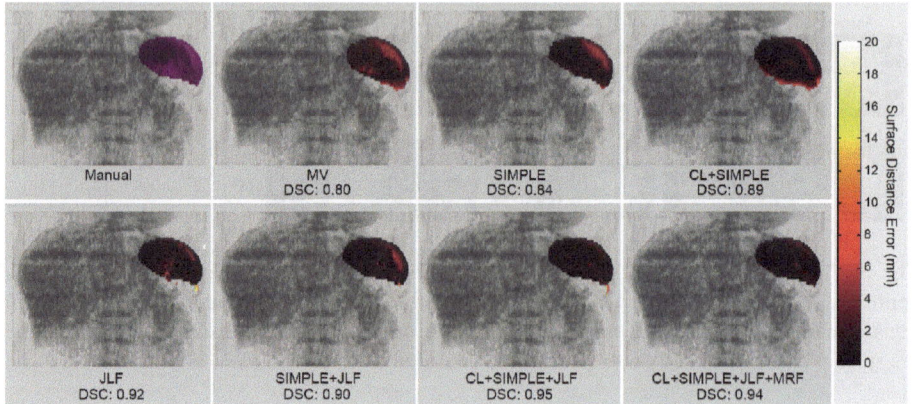

Fig. 4. Representative qualitative results. The subject above was selected to fall within 30th and 70th percentile in terms of DSC for each tested method. The 3D rendered segmentation of each method is colored in terms of the voxel-wise surface distance from the estimated segmentation to the manual segmentation.

Table 1. Quantitative metrics for tested methods on 53 of 65 subjects

Methods \ Metrics	Dice Similarity Coefficient		Surface Distance (mm)	
	Median [Min, Max]	Mean ± Std	Sym. MSD	Sym. HD
MV	0.74 [0, 0.94]	0.65 ± 0.25	6.28 ± 4.81	25.89 ± 11.95
SIMPLE	*0.84 [0.24, 0.95]	0.78 ± 0.16	*4.27 ± 3.87	*21.71 ± 11.03
CL+SIMPLE	*0.87 [0.44, 0.95]	0.83 ± 0.11	*3.35 ± 2.78	*19.91 ± 9.96
JLF	*0.9 [0.4, 0.98]	0.86 ± 0.13	4.45 ± 7.67	*67.07 ± 41.75
SIMPLE+JLF	0.91 [0.33, 0.97]	0.85 ± 0.14	*4.04 ± 7.85	*28.17 ± 26.4
CL+SIMPLE+JLF	***0.93 [0.54, 0.97]**	**0.89 ± 0.1**	***2.2 ± 2.27**	**22.16 ± 9.73**
CL+SIMPLE+JLF+MRF	***0.93 [0.54, 0.97]**	**0.88 ± 0.1**	**2.17 ± 2.33**	***18.46 ± 9.85**

* indicates that the DSC, Sym. MSD, or Sym. HD values are statistically different than the corresponding value in the row immediately above (e.g, SIMPLE vs. MV) as determined by a Wilcoxon signed rank test (p<0.05).

adaptation of the spatial priors to be critical for contexts with large numbers outliers. Using exogenous information, these can be estimated separately with the proposed context learning. In a study of 65 liver cancer patients with potential splenomegaly using clinically acquired CT, we combined context learning and SIMPLE with JLF to address the problems of atlas selection and label determination in multi-atlas segmentation, achieving a mean DSC of 0.89 with a range of 0.54 to 0.97 (evaluated on the 53 that were not used for context learning). In a study of 150 gastric / cholecystitis / colorectal cancer patients, Wolz *et al.* applied multi-scale non-rigid registration followed by non-local fusion and graph-cut post processing to achieve a mean DSC of 0.92 with a range of 0.26 to 0.98 [1]. The body shape variations of their patient population (acquired in Japan) is expected to be relatively smaller comparing to ours (acquired in U.S.), while all their scans were acquired in portal venous phase as opposed to ours with variable phases. With larger variations on our clinically data, our method yields a slightly lower DSC, but substantially narrower range. The performance of the Wolz approach using our dataset was disappointing (mean DSC of

0.73); however, we considered the direct comparison unfair since our atlas structure, i.e., single organ on 65 datasets, did not support some innovative aspects of the Wolz approach (re-weighting atlases based on different organs). Lastly, we note that proposed generative model naturally leads to an iterative atlas selection, which differs from the STEPS approach [12] that first locally ranks atlases, and uses the top local atlases for statistical fusion. In the further study, a systematic integration between CL+SIMPLE and JLF theories could yield atlas selection and label determination.

Acknowledgements. This research was supported by NIH 1R03EB012461, NIH 2R01EB006136, NIH R01EB006193, ViSE/VICTR VR3029, NIH UL1 RR024975-01, and NIH UL1 TR000445-06. The content is solely the responsibility of the authors and does not necessarily represent the official views of the NIH.

References

1. Wolz, R., Chu, C., Misawa, K., Fujiwara, M., Mori, K., Rueckert, D.: Automated abdominal multi-organ segmentation with subject-specific atlas generation. IEEE Transactions on Medical Imaging 32, 1723–1730 (2013)
2. Sabuncu, M.R., Yeo, B.T., Van Leemput, K., Fischl, B., Golland, P.: A generative model for image segmentation based on label fusion. IEEE Transactions on Medical Imaging 29, 1714–1729 (2010)
3. Langerak, T.R., van der Heide, U.A., Kotte, A.N., Viergever, M.A., van Vulpen, M., Pluim, J.P.: Label fusion in atlas-based segmentation using a selective and iterative method for performance level estimation (SIMPLE). IEEE Transactions on Medical Imaging 29, 2000–2008 (2010)
4. Dice, L.R.: Measures of the amount of ecologic association between species. Ecology 26, 297–302 (1945)
5. Warfield, S.K., Zou, K.H., Wells, W.M.: Simultaneous truth and performance level estimation (STAPLE): an algorithm for the validation of image segmentation. IEEE Transactions on Medical Imaging 23, 903–921 (2004)
6. Rohlfing, T., Brandt, R., Menzel, R., Maurer Jr., C.R.: Evaluation of atlas selection strategies for atlas-based image segmentation with application to confocal microscopy images of bee brains. NeuroImage 21, 1428–1442 (2004)
7. Wang, H., Suh, J.W., Das, S.R., Pluta, J., Craige, C., Yushkevich, P.A.: Multi-Atlas Segmentation with Joint Label Fusion. IEEE Transactions on Pattern Analysis and Machine Intelligence (2012)
8. Asman, A.J., Landman, B.A.: Robust statistical label fusion through COnsensus Level, Labeler Accuracy, and Truth Estimation (COLLATE). IEEE Transactions on Medical Imaging 30, 1779–1794 (2011)
9. Van Leemput, K., Maes, F., Vandermeulen, D., Suetens, P.: Automated model-based bias field correction of MR images of the brain. IEEE Trans. Med. Imaging 18, 885–896 (1999)
10. McAuliffe, M.J., Lalonde, F.M., McGarry, D., Gandler, W., Csaky, K., Trus, B.L.: Medical image processing, analysis and visualization in clinical research. In: Proceedings of the 14th IEEE Symposium on Computer-Based Medical Systems, pp. 381–386. IEEE (2001)
11. Rueckert, D., Sonoda, L.I., Hayes, C., Hill, D.L.G., Leach, M.O., Hawkes, D.J.: Nonrigid registration using free-form deformations: Application to breast MR images. IEEE Trans. Med. Imaging 18, 712–721 (1999)
12. Jorge Cardoso, M., Leung, K., Modat, M., Keihaninejad, S., Cash, D., Barnes, J., Fox, N.C., Ourselin, S.: STEPS: Similarity and Truth Estimation for Propagated Segmentations and its application to hippocampal segmentation and brain parcelation. Med. Image Anal. 17, 671–684 (2013)

Segmentation of Multiple Knee Bones from CT for Orthopedic Knee Surgery Planning

Dijia Wu, Michal Sofka, Neil Birkbeck, and S. Kevin Zhou*

Imaging & Computer Vision, Siemens Corporate Technology, Princeton, NJ, USA

Abstract. Patient-specific orthopedic knee surgery planning requires precisely segmenting from 3D CT images multiple knee bones, namely femur, tibia, fibula, and patella, around the knee joint with severe pathologies. In this work, we propose a fully automated, highly precise, and computationally efficient segmentation approach for multiple bones. First, each bone is initially segmented using a model-based marginal space learning framework for pose estimation followed by non-rigid boundary deformation. To recover shape details, we then refine the bone segmentation using graph cut that incorporates the shape priors derived from the initial segmentation. Finally we remove overlap between neighboring bones using multi-layer graph partition. In experiments, we achieve simultaneous segmentation of femur, tibia, patella, and fibula with an overall accuracy of less than 1mm surface-to-surface error in less than 90s on hundreds of 3D CT scans with pathological knee joints.

1 Introduction

American Academy of Orthopedic Surgeons reports that over 500,000 patients have their degenerative knees replaced each year in United States. In recent years, the knee replacement procedure has advanced with personalized surgery designed specifically for each patient. The procedure starts with a CT scan of patient's knee joint from which a 3D knee anatomy model of this patient is extracted. This model is then used for subsequent knee surgery planning. To streamline workflow and reduce cost, fully automatic and highly accurate segmentation of knee bones from 3D CT images is critical in clinical practices.

Most of previous studies on automatic knee bone segmentation focused on MR data, including the voxel based [1] or block-wise classification [2] with texture features and intensity distribution. However, all these methods are ineffective in dealing with the strong intensity and texture inhomogeneities between cortical and cancellous bone in CT and MR images. To improve the segmentation robustness, statistical shape models [3] are often used as prior knowledge to guide the segmentation [4–6]. In these methods, fast and accurate model initialization and adaptation remains a challenge. Graph-based algorithms [7] have been extensively used to solve different vision problems, including bone segmentation

---

* Zhou is corresponding author. Wu is with Microsoft, Sofka with Cisco and Birkbeck with Google. All work was done while they were with Siemens.

P. Golland et al. (Eds.): MICCAI 2014, Part I, LNCS 8673, pp. 372–380, 2014.

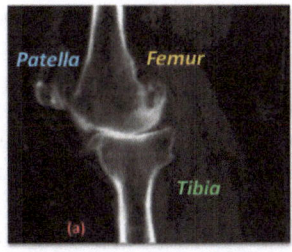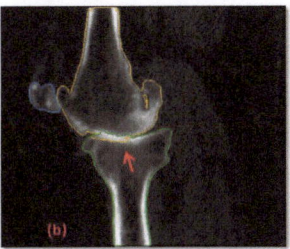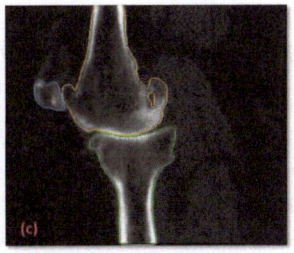

Fig. 1. (a) Example CT image of femur and tibia where two bones touch each other. (b) Segmentation result where overlap occurs. (c) Joint segmentation results.

[2, 4, 8–10] as well; but the accuracy of such algorithms usually depend on seed points often manually provided. Also the bones are segmented individually instead of jointly, which often leads to sub-optimal segmentation results that even overlap with each other particularly in regions where bones are too close or touch each other. This happens more often in the osteoarthritis patients with degenerative cartilage as shown in Fig.1(a). To handle the bone overlap, Li *et al.* [11] proposed a novel column graph-based algorithm to solve coupled surface segmentation problems, which was later used for simultaneous bone and cartilage segmentation in the knee [12]. It exploits the geometric constraints between multiple terrain-like and cylindrical surfaces; but unfolding the structures like femur with two condyles to terrain-like surfaces is nontrivial. Kainmueller *et al.* [13] proposed coupled deformable model for multiple-object segmentation, which does not completely prohibit but discourages the overlap.

Here we present an approach for segmenting multiple knee bones that makes two key contributions. The first contribution is its novel combination of three state-of-the-art methods for *precise* segmentation of multiple knee bones of diseased knees: (i) Marginal space learning(MSL) [14]. Each bone is first detected using MSL and then deformed with a statistical shape model [3]. (ii) Graph cut [7]. The adapted model is then used as a shape prior in a graph cut formulation for refined segmentation. (iii) Multi-layer graph cut [18]. Because each bone is separately segmented, their results possibly overlap. We utilize multi-layer graph cut to remove such overlap error. The second contribution is its full automation and computational efficiency because it needs no image unwrapping and the joint segmentation can be performed in a small local region where the overlap occurs. This efficiency is *clinically significant* for reduced cost and streamlined workflow. Currently our approach is already deployed in Siemens image-to-implant system.

2   Learning-Based Bone Detection and Model Fitting

2.1   Pose Estimation

For a given volume I, each bone is first individually detected from the volume by searching for the optimal similarity transformation parameters or pose parameters including translation $\mathbf{t} = (t_x, t_y, t_z)$, orientation $\mathbf{r} = (r_x, r_y, r_z)$ and anisotropic scaling $\mathbf{s} = (s_x, s_y, s_z)$. The pose estimation task can be formulated by maximizing the posterior probability as follows:

$$(\hat{\mathbf{t}}, \hat{\mathbf{r}}, \hat{\mathbf{s}}) = \arg\max_{\mathbf{t},\mathbf{s},\mathbf{r}} P(\mathbf{t}, \mathbf{s}, \mathbf{r}|I). \tag{1}$$

Solving equation (1) involves the search in a nine dimensional parameter space, which can be computationally expensive in practice. Here we adopt an efficient inference scheme, MSL[14], to decompose the whole search space into marginal space inference. The object localization is split into three steps: position estimation, position-orientation estimation, and full similarity transformation estimation.

$$(\hat{\mathbf{t}}, \hat{\mathbf{r}}, \hat{\mathbf{s}}) \approx (\arg\max_{\mathbf{t}} P(\mathbf{t}|I), \arg\max_{\mathbf{r}} P(\mathbf{r}|I, \hat{\mathbf{t}}), \arg\max_{\mathbf{s}} P(\mathbf{s}|I, \hat{\mathbf{t}}, \hat{\mathbf{r}})). \tag{2}$$

After each step only a limited number of best candidates is kept to reduce the search space and speed up the inference. To learn the marginal posterior probabilities in Eq.(2), discriminative classifiers such as the probabilistic boosting tree (PBT) [15] or the probabilistic boosting network [16] can be used. Moreover, 3D Haar features are used for location detection and steerable features are used for orientation and scale inferences [14]. Fig.2(a) shows an example of the pose estimation result, where the pose parameters are represented as a bounding box.

2.2   Model Initialization and Boundary Deformation

After pose estimation, the shape of the target object is initialized using the statistical shape model (SSM) as follows:

$$\mathbf{x} = f(\mu; \hat{\mathbf{t}}, \hat{\mathbf{r}}, \hat{\mathbf{s}}), \tag{3}$$

where $\mathbf{x}$ denotes the initialized shape, f is the rigid transformation with the pose parameters $(\hat{\mathbf{t}}, \hat{\mathbf{r}}, \hat{\mathbf{s}})$ estimated by MSL, μ represents the mean of the statistical shape model obtained from the training annotations.

The initialized shape is then deformed with the boundary detectors. Here, boundary detection is again formulated as a classification problem: whether there is a boundary passing point at (X, Y, Z) with orientation (O_x, O_y, O_z). The boundary detectors are used to move the mesh points on the current estimated shape surface along its normal direction to the optimal position, where the classification score is the highest. After adjustment, the deformed shape is projected to the SSM subspace to smooth out and constrain the surface. In our experiments, the dimension of the SSM subspace is selected to capture 98% of the shape variations from the training annotations. The process is repeated a few iterations until convergence. As an example shown in Fig.2(b), the derived shape after boundary deformation fits the image well, but is still subject to noticeable errors due to the loss of shape details by the statistical shape model, as well as possible boundary detection errors.

3   Bone Refinement with Shape Prior in Graph Cut

To further improve the accuracy, we formulate the following graph-based energy function with the previous segmentation result used as the shape prior:

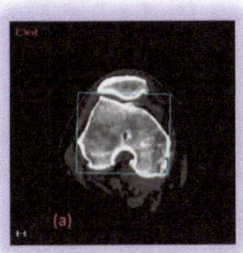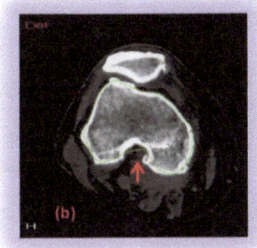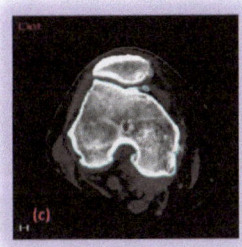

Fig. 2. The example result of (a) MSL pose estimation, (b) boundary detector based deformation, and (c) graph cut based refinement

$$E(L) = \sum_{p \in \mathcal{P}} D_p(L_p) + \sum_{(p,q) \in \mathcal{N}} V_{p,q}(L_p, L_q), \tag{4}$$

where $L = \{L_p \mid p \in \mathcal{P}\}$ is the binary labeling ($L_p \in \{0, 1\}$) of volume $\mathcal{P}$, $D_p(L_p)$ is the unary data term which is defined as below:

$$D_p(L_p) = L_p(1 - g(\mathbb{M}(p))) + (1 - L_p)g(\mathbb{M}(p)). \tag{5}$$

Here, $\mathbb{M}(p)$ measures the signed shortest distance of voxel p to the boundary of the prior segmentation. $\mathbb{M}(p) > 0$ when p lies inside the segmentation (foreground), $\mathbb{M}(p) < 0$ if p is outside (background), and $\mathbb{M}(p) = 0$ if p locates on the boundary. Therefore, $\mathbb{M}$ can also be viewed as a confidence map of the prior segmentation. The larger (smaller) $\mathbb{M}(p)$ is, the more likely voxel p should be classified as the foreground (background). When voxel p approaches the boundary ($\mathbb{M}(p) \approx 0$), label L_p becomes more uncertain and therefore more likely to be updated by the graph cut refinement. $\mathbb{M}(p)$ can be efficiently computed in linear time using the convolution method [17]. The sigmoid function $g(.)$ is defined as $g(x) = \frac{1}{1 + e^{-x/\tau}}$, where τ is the parameter that controls the range of uncertainty of the previous segmentation result. In Eq.(4), $\mathcal{N}$ is the set of all pairs of neighboring voxels and $V_{p,q}$ is the pairwise interaction term:

$$V_{p,q} = \lambda e^{-\frac{(I_p - I_q)^2}{2\sigma^2}} \delta(L_p \neq L_q), \tag{6}$$

where $\delta(.)$ is the Kronecker delta function $\delta(L_p \neq L_q) = 1$ if $L_p \neq L_q$ and equal to 0 otherwise, λ and σ are the regularization parameter and contrast coefficient, respectively, and I_p and I_q denote the intensity of voxels p and q. The pairwise term encourages the neighboring voxels with similar intensities to be assigned the same label.

The segmentation is refined by minimizing the energy in Eq.(4) using the max-flow/min-cut algorithm. Fig.2(c) shows the improved result after graph based refinement.

4   Joint Bone Segmentation

Because each bone is separately initialized and refined in the previous steps, the overlap error can not be prevented when two bones touch each other, as one

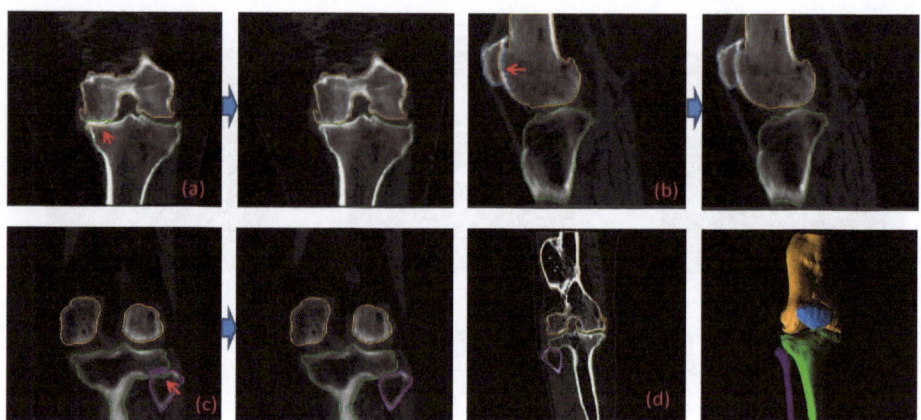

Fig. 3. The example of overlap error removed by joint segmentation. (a) pair of femur and tibia (b) pair of patella and femur (c) pair of tibia and fibula (d) pathological example with osteoporosis and 3D rendering of the segmentation.

example shown in Fig.1(b). To remedy this, we present a joint re-segmentation method to co-segment the pair of bones that overlap in the initial segmentation. With specific spatial exclusion constraint introduced [18], the joint segmentation can guarantee a complete removal of erroneously overlapping boundaries.

Without loss of generality, we denote the pair of bones as A and B. L_A and L_B stand for the labeling of bone A and B, respectively. It means that voxel p is inside bone A if $L_{A(p)} = 1$ and otherwise if $L_{A(p)} = 0$, likewise for bone B. The energy function Eq.(4) can thus be extended to the case of two bones as follows:

$$
E(L_A, L_B) = E(L_A) + E(L_B) = \sum_{p \in \mathcal{P}} D_{A(p)}(L_{A(p)}) + \sum_{(p,q) \in \mathcal{N}} V_{A(p,q)}(L_{A(p)}, L_{A(q)})
$$
$$
+ \sum_{p \in \mathcal{P}} D_{B(p)}(L_{B(p)}) + \sum_{(p,q) \in \mathcal{N}} V_{B(p,q)}(L_{B(p)}, L_{B(q)}), \tag{7}
$$

where all the symbols follow exactly the same meaning as in Eq.(4) except that $\mathbb{M}$ is now based on the segmentation result after refinement as described in Section 3. As shown in Eq.(7), the minimization of $E(L_A, L_B)$ can be decomposed to the minimization of $E(L_A)$ and $E(L_B)$ separately because no interaction terms between L_A and L_B exist in the energy function Eq.(7). Therefore bone A and B are essentially segmented separately.

There is, however, a spatial exclusion constraint between L_A and L_B because bone A and B can not overlap in the space. It means that if $L_{A(p)} = 1$, $L_{B(p)}$ must $= 0$, and vice versa. This spatial constraint can be easily incorporated into the energy function Eq.(7) by adding the pairwise terms as follows:

$$
\tilde{E}(L_A, L_B) = E(L_A, L_B) + \sum_{p \in \mathcal{P}} W(L_{A(p)}, L_{B(p)}), \tag{8}
$$

Table 1. The statistics of symmetric surface segmentation errors. All units are in mm.

sym. surface error (mm)	mean	std. dev.	min	median	80 percentile
Femur (boundary deformation)	1.20	3.22	0.38	0.85	1.22
Femur (graph cut refinement)	0.83	3.35	0.43	0.55	0.67
Femur (joint segmentation)	0.82	3.33	0.43	0.55	0.67
Tibia (boundary deformation)	1.07	1.39	0.42	0.79	1.13
Tibia (graph cut refinement)	0.70	1.28	0.42	0.55	0.63
Tibia (joint segmentation)	0.69	1.25	0.42	0.55	0.63
Fibula (boundary deformation)	1.26	4.57	0.31	0.47	0.65
Fibula (graph cut refinement)	0.98	4.31	0.38	0.53	0.59
Fibula (joint segmentation)	0.96	4.29	0.38	0.53	0.59
Patella (boundary deformation)	0.72	2.07	0.35	0.62	0.67
Patella (graph cut refinement)	0.68	2.05	0.33	0.55	0.62
Patella (joint segmentation)	0.68	2.06	0.33	0.54	0.61

where

$$W(L_{A(p)}, L_{B(p)}) = \begin{cases} +\infty & \text{if } L_{A(p)} = L_B(p) = 1 \\ 0 & \text{otherwise} \end{cases}$$

Therefore the optimal solution that minimizes the energy function $\tilde{E}(L_A, L_B)$ guarantees that $L_{A(p)}$ and $L_{B(p)}$ can not be both 1 at the same time ($\forall p \in \mathcal{P}$). However, the introduced pairwise term $W_{A(p),B(p)}(L_{A(p)}, L_{B(p)})$ is supermodular because $W(0,1) + W(1,0) < W(0,0) + W(1,1)$, hence it can not be directly optimized via min-cut/max-flow algorithm [19]. To address this problem, we flip the binary meaning of label $\bar{L}_B = 1 - L_B$, then the new energy function $\tilde{E}(L_A, \bar{L}_B)$ becomes submodular everywhere and min-cut/max-flow can be used to find the optimal labeling of L_A and L_B jointly.

The major advantage of the multi-layer graph cut is its 'simplicity'. The existing methods [10, 12, 13] based on the multi-column graph segmentation [11] all require point correspondence on adjacent surfaces for coupled deformation. Thus they are limited to terrain-like or cylindrical surfaces. Otherwise, complex methods are required to find so called shared profiles [13] or electric lines of force [10] which connect corresponding points on two surfaces and constitute the non-intersecting columns of the graph. By contrast, multi-layer graph cut makes no assumption of the shape of interactive surfaces, and does not need any such preprocessing. Hence it is easy to implement and also runs fast, taking less than 1s to remove all the segmentation overlaps in our implementation.

5   Experiments

In the experiment, we collect 465 CT volumes around the knee with an average size of $200 \times 200 \times 150$ voxels and $1 \times 1 \times 1 mm$ voxel spacing, as shown in Fig.1. The annotations are obtained by experts based on visual assessment and consensus review. We randomly select 217 volumes for training the learning pipeline in Section 2, and use the remaining 248 volumes for testing. First, we compare the

Table 2. The size (mm^3) of the overlap area between femur segmentation and tibia ground truth also between tibia segmentation and femur ground truth

femur segmentation	1	2	3	4	5	6	7	8	9	10
before joint segmentation	3493	2075	1165	912	802	237	228	213	146	137
after joint segmentation	161	40	27	4	3	86	18	1	0	0
reduction %	95.4	98.1	97.7	99.6	99.6	63.7	92.1	99.5	100	100
tibia segmentation	1	2	3	4	5	6	7	8	9	10
before joint segmentation	3791	2729	1745	1562	896	522	491	448	312	286
after joint segmentation	1198	257	142	838	602	515	62	324	302	302
reduction %	68.4	90.6	91.9	46.4	32.8	1.3	87.4	27.7	3.2	-12.9

segmentation result after each step in the proposed method. As error measure we first computed the shortest Euclidean distances between each result mesh and its corresponding annotated mesh at every vertex of the former as well as every vertex of the latter, and then averaged all such distances. As shown in Table 1, the proposed method achieves quality segmentation with average symmetric surface error lower than $1mm$ for all four bones, and that is less than the 1mm voxel resolution. The graph cut refinement with shape prior decreases the mean error about $5 \sim 35\%$. Still we have failed cases (albeit very few) that contribute to the large variance in the surface error.

The overlaps after initial segmentation could happen when two bones almost touch each other (cartilages severely worn out). Those volumes are about 5% to 10% in our database. But this overlap usually occurs only around touching surfaces of neighboring bones, a very small region compared to the whole bone surface, so the numerical improvement by joint segmentation is not that obvious in Table 1. We use a different measurement to evaluate the effectiveness of the joint segmentation step to remove the overlap error. As shown in Table 2, we compare the size of the overlap area between *femur* result and *tibia* ground truth, as well as between *tibia* result and *femur* ground truth. For brevity, we only listed the 10 worst volumes with the largest overlap errors generated from previous individual segmentation step. The results show that the proposed joint segmentation can significantly reduce the overlap up to 100% in most of the cases, especially for the femur segmentation. Consistent improvements (except one case[1]) can be observed for the pair of patella and femur and the pair of tibia and fibula too. The joint segmentation result also depends on initial segmentation result of each bone. Fig. 3 shows examples of the overlap error eliminated by joint segmentation with a pathological example.

For each bone, the individual segmentation as described in Section 2 and 3 takes about 20 seconds to complete (Intel®Core™CPU @ 2.29 GHz and 3.23GB RAM). Because the joint re-segmentation in Section 4 is only applied to the local overlap region, it can be computed efficiently and only takes about 1

---

[1] If initial femur segmentation leaks into tibia too much, it will affect the final tibia result adversely. That is why joint Tibia #10 is worse, although very rare.

second on the average. If the the initial segmentation does not overlap, the joint re-segmentation can be skipped with little extra computational cost.

6   Conclusion

In this work, we present a fully automated method and system for segmenting multiple knee bones from 3D CT images. Our novel combination of marginal space learning, graph cut with shape-prior, and joint multi-layer graph cut for overlap removal achieves sub-mm segmentation accuracy needed for orthopedic surgery planning with a running speed of less than 90s for reduced cost and streamlined planning workflow in clinical practices, while guaranteeing no overlap in the segmentation results between knee bones. In future, we plan to apply it for segmentation of other objects such as organs from other imaging modalities.

References

1. Bourgeat, P., et al.: MR image segmentation of the knee bone using phase information. Med. Image Anal. 11, 325–335 (2007)
2. Ababneh, S.Y., et al.: Automatic graph-cut based segmentation of bones from knee magnetic resonance images for osteoarthritis research. Med. Image Anal. 15 (2011)
3. Cootes, T.F., et al.: Active Shape Models - Their Training and Application. Comput. Vis. Image Und. 61(1), 38–59 (1995)
4. Seim, H., et al.: Model-based auto-segmentation of knee bones and cartilage in MRI data. In: Medical Image Analysis for the Clinic: A Grand Challenge, Beijing (2010)
5. Schmid, J., Magnenat-Thalmann, N.: MRI Bone Segmentation Using Deformable Models and Shape Priors. In: Metaxas, D., Axel, L., Fichtinger, G., Székely, G. (eds.) MICCAI 2008, Part I. LNCS, vol. 5241, pp. 119–126. Springer, Heidelberg (2008)
6. Fripp, J., et al.: Automatic segmentation of the bone and extraction of the bone-cartilage interface from magnetic resonance images of the knee. Phys. Med. Biol. 52(6), 1617–1631 (2007)
7. Boykov, Y.: Graph cuts and efficient N–D image segmentation. Int. J. Comput. Vision 70(2), 109–131 (2006)
8. Liu, L., Raber, D., Nopachai, D., Commean, P., Sinacore, D., Prior, F., Pless, R., Ju, T.: Interactive separation of segmented bones in CT volumes using graph cut. In: Metaxas, D., Axel, L., Fichtinger, G., Székely, G. (eds.) MICCAI 2008, Part I. LNCS, vol. 5241, pp. 296–304. Springer, Heidelberg (2008)
9. Freedman, D., Zhang, T.: Interactive Graph Cut Based Segmentation With Shape Priors. In: Proc. CVPR (2005)
10. Shim, H., et al.: Knee cartilage: efficient and reproducible segmentation on high-spatial-resolution MR images with the semiautomated graph-cut algorithm method. Radiology 251(2), 548–556 (2009)
11. Li, K., et al.: Optimal surface segmentation in volumetric images-a graph-theoretic approach. IEEE Trans. Pattern Anal. Mach. Intell. 28(1), 119–134 (2006)
12. Yin, Y., et al.: LOGISMOS–layered optimal graph image segmentation of multiple objects and surfaces: Cartilage segmentation in the knee joint. IEEE Trans. Med. Imag. 29(12), 2023–2037 (2010)

13. Kainmueller, D., et al.: Multi-Object Segmentation with Coupled Deformable Models. In: Annals of BMVA (2009)
14. Zheng, Y., et al.: Four-Chamber Heart Modeling and Automatic Segmentation for 3-D Cardiac CT Volumes Using Marginal Space Learning and Steerable Features. IEEE Trans. Med. Imag. 27(11), 1668–1681 (2008)
15. Tu, Z.: Probabilistic Boosting-Tree: Learning Discriminative Models for Classification, Recognition, and Clustering. In: Proc. ICCV, vol. 2, pp. 1589–1596 (2005)
16. Zhang, J., et al.: Joint Real-Time Object Detection and Pose Estimation Using Probabilistic Boosting Network. In: Proc. CVPR (2007)
17. Felzenszwalb, P., Huttenlocher, D.: Distance Transforms of Sampled Functions Cornell Computing and Information Science (2004)
18. Delong, A., Boykov, Y.: Globally Optimal Segmentation of Multi-Region Objects. In: Proc. ICCV (2009)
19. Kolmogorov, V., Zabin, R.: What Energy Functions Can Be Minimized Via Graph Cuts? IEEE Trans. Pattern Anal. Mach. Intell. 26(2), 147–159 (2004)

TRIC: Trust Region for Invariant Compactness and Its Application to Abdominal Aorta Segmentation

Ismail Ben Ayed[1], Michael Wang[2], Brandon Miles[3], and Gregory J. Garvin[4]

[1] GE Healthcare, London, ON, Canada
[2] McGill University, Montreal, QC, Canada
[3] Simon Fraser University, Burnaby, BC, Canada
[4] St. Joseph's Health Care Hospital, London, ON, Canada

Abstract. This study investigates segmentation with a novel invariant compactness constraint. The proposed prior is a high-order *fractional* term, which is not directly amenable to powerful optimizers. We derive first-order *Gateâux* derivative approximations of our compactness term and adopt an iterative trust region paradigm by splitting our problem into constrained sub-problems, each solving the approximation globally via a Lagrangian formulation and a graph cut. We apply our algorithm to the challenging task of abdominal aorta segmentation in 3D MRI volumes, and report quantitative evaluations over 30 subjects, which demonstrate that the results correlate well with independent manual segmentations. We further show the use of our method in several other medical applications and demonstrate that, in comparison to a standard level-set optimization, our algorithm is one order of magnitude faster.

1   Introduction

Embedding shape priors in medical image segmentation is necessary in numerous applications [13,11,10,14], more so when the target segment has an intensity profile very similar to other parts in the image. Based on standard techniques such as statistical shape models [14] and probabilistic atlases [10], most of the existing medical image segmentation algorithms require (i) an intensive learning from a large, manually-segmented training set; and (ii) registration or pose optimization procedures (i.e., w.r.t rotation, translation, and scaling). Although they can yield excellent results in some applications, training-based algorithms may have difficulty in capturing the substantial variations that occur in a clinical context, with the results often being dependent on the choice of a specific training set. This is due to the fact that they enforce a strict *pixelwise* consistency between the solution and the template shapes in a training set.

Recently, there has been an ongoing research effort towards embedding *global* shape constraints in segmentation [13,12,11,2,5,16]. These include constraints on segment convexity [16], axial symmetry [13], area [12] and compactness [5], as well as geometric inter-segment relationships [2]. Several recent studies have

P. Golland et al. (Eds.): MICCAI 2014, Part I, LNCS 8673, pp. 381–388, 2014.
© Springer International Publishing Switzerland 2014

shown that such global shape constraints can lead to excellent performances in various medical applications [13,12,11,2], while removing the need for intensive training and pose estimation. Unfortunately, such constraints are high-order functionals, which result in difficult optimization problems that are not directly amenable to standard powerful optimizers, e.g., graph cuts or convex-relaxation techniques. The following summarizes the contributions of this study.

Contributions in the General-Purpose Context: We propose a novel global shape constraint, which measures segment compactness w.r.t a point set. Our compactness constraint can be invariant w.r.t scale, rotation and translation, unlike the shape compactness in [5] (which is pose dependent). Unfortunately, our prior is a high-order *fractional* functional, which is not directly amenable to powerful optimizers. We derive first-order *Gateâux* derivative approximations of our compactness term and adopt an iterative trust region paradigm [7] by splitting our problem into constrained sub-problems, each solving the approximation globally via a Lagrangian formulation and a graph cut. We show the use of our method in several medical applications and demonstrate that, in comparison to a standard level-set optimization, our algorithm is one order of magnitude faster.

Contributions in the Application Context: Abdominal aorta segmentation is an essential step towards accurate assessments of abdominal aortic aneurysms (AAA) [6,4]. Most of the existing works addressed the problem in CTA, except the recent interactive-segmentation study in [6] (which also considered MRI). In MRI, the task is seriously challenged by the intensity similarities and very weak edges between the aorta and its neighboring structures. Furthermore, this tubular structure may have sudden/unpredictable changes in the scale (size) of the 2D aorta cross-sections (e.g., due to aneurysms). With the scale-invariance property, our method can handle such unpredictable changes in scale. We report comprehensive evaluations over a set of 30 MRI volumes acquired from 30 subjects, which show a Dice metric of 0.91 ± 0.03, an excellent agreement with independent manual segmentations.

2   Formulation

Proposed Functional: Let $I(\mathbf{p}) : \Omega \subset \mathbb{R}^2 \to \mathbb{R}$ be an image function defined over a domain Ω. Our objective is to find an optimal region in Ω, so that the region is compact with respect to a point set and follows some appearance and boundary priors. We optimize a functional containing three terms:

$$\min_{u \in \{0,1\}} E(u) = \alpha \mathcal{A}(u) + \beta \mathcal{S}(u) + \gamma \mathcal{C}(u) \tag{1}$$

The following details each of the variables and terms that appear in (1):

- $u : \Omega \to \{0,1\}$ is binary function, which defines a variable segmentation of Ω: $\{\mathbf{p} \in \Omega / u(\mathbf{p}) = 1\}$, corresponding to the target segment, and $\{\mathbf{p} \in \Omega / u(\mathbf{p}) = 0\}$, corresponding to the complement of the target segment in Ω.

– We introduce the following invariant compactness prior:

$$\mathcal{C}(u) = \frac{\int_\Omega u(\mathbf{p})\mathcal{D}^2\left(\mathbf{p}, \mathcal{Q}\right)d\mathbf{p}}{\left(\int_\Omega u(\mathbf{p})d\mathbf{p}\right)^2} \tag{2}$$

where $\mathcal{D}\left(\mathbf{p}, \mathcal{Q}\right)$ is the shortest-path distance between each point $\mathbf{p} \in \Omega$ and a set of reference points $\mathcal{Q}$: $\mathcal{D}\left(\mathbf{p}, \mathcal{Q}\right) = \min_{\mathbf{q} \in \mathcal{Q}} \|\mathbf{p} - \mathbf{q}\|$, with $\|.\|$ denoting the L_2 norm. Depending on the application, point set $\mathcal{Q}$ can be either a variable, which depends on the segmentation (i.e., on function u), or fixed (e.g., obtained from user inputs). To understand the meaning of the proposed compactness prior, let us first consider the particular case of a single reference point, which depends on u and corresponds to the centroid of the target segment, i.e., $\mathcal{Q}$ is a singleton containing $\frac{\int_\Omega \mathbf{p}d\mathbf{p}}{\int_\Omega u(\mathbf{p})d\mathbf{p}}$. In this case, $\mathcal{C}(u)$ becomes one of the well known *Hu moment invariants* (invariant to translation, rotation and scaling). The recent study in [17] has shown that this invariant can be effectively used to measure shape circularity (i.e., the deviation of a given shape from the most compact a shape–a circle). The lower the value of this invariant, the closer the shape to a circle. Our extension of this compactness measure to multiple reference points can accommodate a more general class of shapes that deviate significantly from a circle (See the liver example in Fig. 2, where reference points are obtained from a user scribble). It is worth noting that, in applications where point set $\mathcal{Q}$ is fixed (e.g., obtained from user inputs), $\mathcal{C}(u)$ loose its invariance w.r.t translation but remains invariant w.r.t scaling and rotation.

– $\mathcal{A}$ is a log-likelihood appearance term [3]: $\mathcal{A}(u) = \int_\Omega u(\mathbf{p}) \log \frac{M_t(I(\mathbf{p}))}{M_c(I(\mathbf{p}))} d\mathbf{p}$, where M_t and M_c are fixed (learned *a priori*) model distributions of intensity within the target segment and its complement in Ω, respectively.

– $\mathcal{S}(u)$ is a pairwise term, which regularizes the segmentation boundary and biases it towards strong edges [3]: $\mathcal{S}(u) = \sum_{\{\mathbf{p},\mathbf{q}\} \in \mathcal{N}} \frac{exp(-\sigma\|I(\mathbf{p})-I(\mathbf{q})\|^2)}{\|\mathbf{p}-\mathbf{q}\|} \delta_{u(\mathbf{p}) \neq u(\mathbf{q})}$, with $\delta_{x \neq y}$ equal to 1 if $x \neq y$ and 0 otherwise. $\mathcal{N}$ is a 16-neighborhood system containing all unordered pairs $\{\mathbf{p}, \mathbf{q}\}$ of neighboring elements of Ω.

– α, β, γ and σ are positive constants, which have to be fixed empirically.

Trust Region Optimization: Our prior is a *fractional* term, which is not directly amenable to powerful optimizers, e.g., graph cuts [3]. We derive first-order *Gateâux* derivative approximations of the compactness term and adopt an iterative trust region paradigm [7]: We split our problem into a sequence of easier sub-steps, each approximating the functional within a trust region around the current solution (i.e., a region where the approximation can be trusted).

Constrained sub-problems: At each iteration k, we solve the following constrained sub-problem via a Lagrangian formulation and a graph cut:

$$\min_{u:\Omega \to [0;1]} \widetilde{E}_k(u) \quad \text{s.t.} \quad \|u - u_k\| < d_k, \quad \text{For } k = 0, 1, 2, \dots$$

$$\text{with } \widetilde{E}_k(u) = \alpha\mathcal{A}(u) + \beta\mathcal{S}(u) + \gamma\widetilde{\mathcal{C}}_k(u) \tag{3}$$

where u is relaxed in $[0; 1]$ and $\widetilde{\mathcal{C}}_k(u)$ is the first-order *Gateâux* derivative approximation of the compactness term near current solution u_k. d_k defines the size of the trust region, which is adjusted automatically at previous iteration k (see Algorithm 1, line 7). We derive the approximation in the case $\mathcal{Q}$ is fixed (scale and rotation invariant case):

$$\widetilde{\mathcal{C}}_k(u) = K_1 + \frac{\int_\Omega u(\mathbf{p})d\mathbf{p}}{\left(\int_\Omega u_k(\mathbf{p})d\mathbf{p}\right)^2} - \frac{2\int_\Omega u_k(\mathbf{p})\mathcal{D}^2(\mathbf{p}, \mathcal{Q})\,d\mathbf{p}}{\left(\int_\Omega u_k(\mathbf{p})d\mathbf{p}\right)^3}\int_\Omega u(\mathbf{p})\mathcal{D}^2(\mathbf{p}, \mathcal{Q})\,d\mathbf{p} \quad (4)$$

where K_1 a constant independent of u.

Lagrangian formulation of the sub-problems: We state each sub-problem in (3) as an unconstrained optimization: $\min_{u:\Omega\to[0;1]} \widetilde{E}_k(u) + \lambda\|u - u_k\|$. For binary functions u and u_k in $\{0, 1\}$, $\|u - u_k\|$ can be approximated with a unary potential [7]: $\|u - u_k\| \approx \int_\Omega \phi_k(p)(u(\mathbf{p}) - u_k(\mathbf{p}))d\mathbf{p}$, where ϕ_k is the signed distance function corresponding to the boundary defined by u_k, i.e., $\{\mathbf{p} \in \Omega | \nabla u_k \neq 0\}$.

Algorithm: A summary of the procedure is given in *Algorithm 1*. Each sub-problem in line 3 can be solved globally with a graph cut [3]. Note that the use of graph cuts is an option, among others, to solve the trust-region sub-problems. One can use other global optimization techniques, e.g., those based on convex relaxation [11]. Once candidate solution u^* is computed, the merit of the approximation is evaluated by the ratio between the actual and approximate reduction in the functional. Based on this ratio, the solution is updated in line 6 and the trust region is adjusted in line 7. We set parameter τ_2 in line 7 to 0.25.

Algorithm 1: TRUST REGION FOR INVARIANT COMPACTNESS (TRIC)

---

1 **Repeat**

2   //**Solve trust region sub-problem**

3     $u^* \longleftarrow \min_{u:\Omega\to\{0,1\}} \widetilde{E}_k(u) + \lambda\int_\Omega \phi_k(p)(u(\mathbf{p}) - u_k(\mathbf{p}))d\mathbf{p}$

4     $\widetilde{\mathcal{R}} = \widetilde{E}_k(u_k) - \widetilde{E}_k(u^*)$ //Approximate functional reduction

5     $\mathcal{R} = E(u_k) - E(u^*)$ //Actual functional reduction

6   //**Update current solution:** $u_{k+1} \longleftarrow \begin{cases} u^* \text{ if } \frac{\mathcal{R}}{\widetilde{\mathcal{R}}} > 0 \\ u_k \text{ otherwise} \end{cases}$

7   //**Adjust the trust region** $d_{k+1} \longleftarrow \begin{cases} d_k \cdot \gamma \text{ if } \frac{\mathcal{R}}{\widetilde{\mathcal{R}}} > \tau_2 \\ d_k/\gamma \text{ otherwise} \end{cases}$

8 **Until Convergence**

---

3   Experiments

We report several sets of experiments to demonstrate the benefit of the proposed prior, including: (i) Quantitative evaluations of supervised abdominal aorta segmentations over a set of 30 MRI volumes acquired from 30 subjects; (ii) Additional examples, which show the use of our method in other applications,

Table 1. Quantitative evaluations of abdominal aorta segmentations over 30 subjects

Dice metric (with compactness)	Dice metric (without compactness) [3]
0.91 ± 0.03	0.33 ± 0.05

e.g., liver segmentation in CT and delineations of cardiac structures (the cavity and myocardium) in MRI; and (iii) Comparisons in regard to speed/optimality with a standard level-set optimization applied to the same compactness functional, which show that our method is one order of magnitude faster and is less likely to get trapped into weak local minima (See the plot in Fig. 3).

Abdominal Aorta Segmentation

Typical examples: Fig. 1 depicts aorta segmentations in 3D T2-weighted MRI volumes. The problem is challenging due to the intensity similarities and very weak edges between the aorta and its neighboring structures, as well as the sudden/unpredictable changes in the sizes of the 2D aorta cross-sections. The first row of Fig. 1 depicts the cross-sectional results for one subject at different slices, along with the ground truth and the segmentations obtained *without* compactness (this corresponds to the well known method in [3]). The solution of [3] leaked into several parts of the background, whereas our method yielded segmentations that are very close to the ground truth. The second row of Fig. 1 depicts 3D results obtained for another subject. The scale invariance of our method handled well the sudden/unpredictable changes in the size of the 2D aorta cross-sections. For this application, we assume that the centroid of the aorta cross-section within each 2D slice is given. Such a reference point is used to define the shortest-path distance and build the appearance models. The method belongs to the class of tubular/vascular structure segmentation techniques that use the centerline of the structure as input, e.g., [15]; See [8] for a complete categorization of prior works. Standard semi-automated centerline extraction techniques [8], which use minimum user inputs (e.g., one or two seed points for the whole volume), can further automate the process. The parameters were fixed as follows: $\alpha = 5 \times 10^{-3}$, $\beta = 10^{-2}$ and $\gamma = 10^{8}$. The appearance models are learned from inside/outside a disc centered at the reference point, with a radius equal to 10 pixels.

Quantitative evaluations: The evaluation was carried out over a data set of 30 T2-weighted MRI volumes acquired from 30 subjects. We segmented a total of 1968 cross-sectional 2D slices. The results were compared to independent manual segmentations performed by an expert using the well known Dice metric (DM) measure. DM evaluates the similarity (overlap) between the automatically detected and ground-truth segments: $DM = \frac{2S_{am}}{S_a + S_m}$, with S_a, S_m, and S_{am} corresponding respectively to the sizes of the segmented aorta volume, the corresponding hand-labeled volume, and the intersection between them. The parameters were fixed for all subjects, and were similar to those used in the

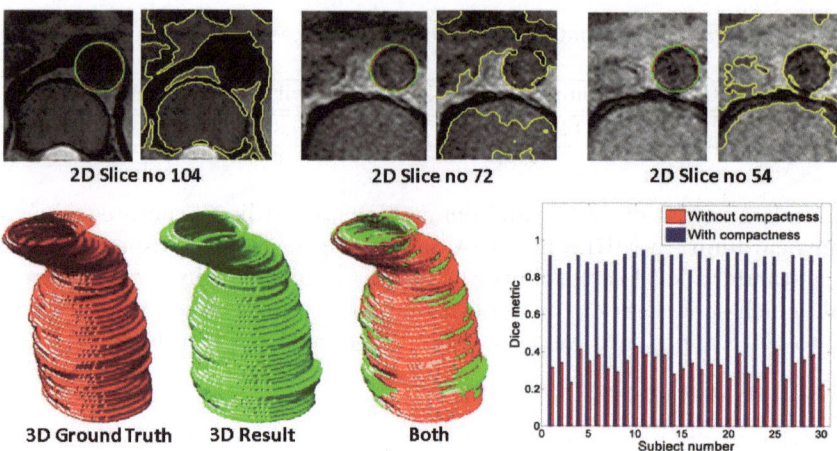

Fig. 1. Abdominal aorta segmentation in 3D MRI volumes. The first row depicts cross-sectional results for one subject at different slice levels, with the red curve showing the ground truth, the green curve showing the result with our compactness prior and the yellow curve showing the result without compactness (i.e., using [3]). Second row, left: 3D result obtained for another subject. Second row, right: the Dice metrics obtained for 30 subjects *with* and *without* compactness.

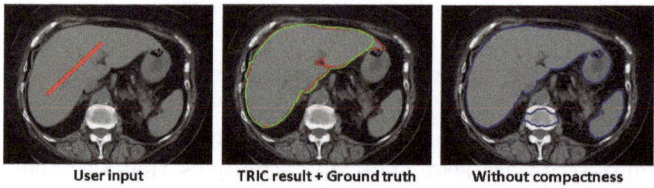

Fig. 2. Interactive liver segmentation in CT. $\alpha = 5 \times 10^{-3}$, $\beta = 10^{-1}$ and $\gamma = 5 \times 10^{8}$.

examples above. Table 1 reports the DM mean and standard deviation *with* and *without* compactness (i.e., using the method in [3]). The plot in Fig. 1 (bottom-right) depicts the Dice metrics obtained for the 30 subjects. The results confirm that the compactness term brings a substantial improvement in accuracy.

Liver Segmentation in CT: Fig. 2 illustrates the application of our compactness term to interactive liver segmentation in CT. This example shows how our compactness term can accommodate a more general class of shapes that deviate significantly from a circle. Here, the shortest-path distance is defined w.r.t multiple reference points (a segment), which were obtained from a simple two-point user input (Fig. 2, first column). The second column depicts the obtained result (green curve) along with the ground truth (red curve). The last column depicts the result obtained without compactness (i.e., with [3]).

Cardiac Segmentation in MRI: Fig. 3 shows delineations of the cavity/myocardium boundaries in MRI, a well-known problem in cardiac image analysis

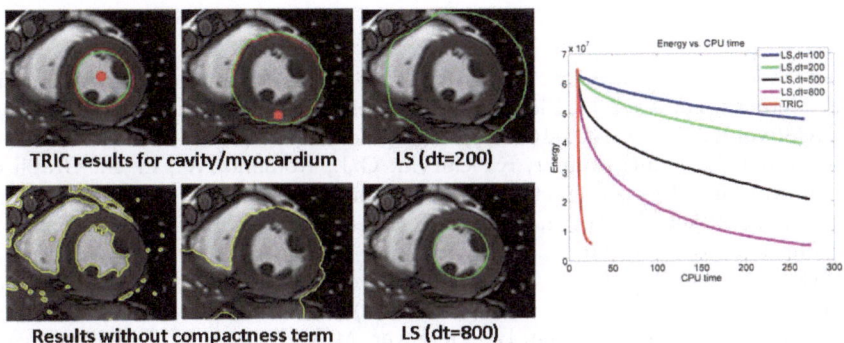

Fig. 3. Delineation of the cavity/myocardium boundaries in cardiac MRI. First column: delineation of the cavity boundary; Second column: delineation of the external boundary of the myocardium; Third column: results obtained with a level set optimization [9] for two different time steps (dt). Last column: Plots of the evolution of the cavity-segmentation functional w.r.t CPU time for TRIC and level-set optimization (LS) with different time steps.

[1]. The first column depicts cavity segmentation starting from a single-point user input, which serves as a reference to define the shortest-path distance and build the appearance models. The upper figure depicts the user input (red point), obtained result (green curve) and ground truth (red curve), whereas the lower one depicts the result without compactness. The parameters were fixed as follows: $\alpha = 5 \times 10^{-3}$; $\beta = 0$; $\gamma = 5 \times 10^{8}$; the appearance models are learned from inside/outside a disc centered at the reference point, with a radius of 10 pixels. The second column depicts epicardium delineation using an additional user-specified point to learn myocardium appearance. The upper figure shows the obtained result (green curve) along with the ground truth (red curve) and the additional user input (red point). The lower figure depicts segmentation without compactness. In this example, we added a hard constraint [3] to ensure that the solution includes the cavity segment (which was computed at the previous step), and fixed the parameters as follows: $\alpha = 5 \times 10^{-3}$; $\beta = 10^{-1}$; $\gamma = 10^{8}$.

Comparisons with Level Sets in Regard to Speed/Optimality: For the cavity segmentation example, we plotted the evolution of our functional w.r.t CPU time for TRIC and level-set gradient-descent optimization (LS), implemented via the well known scheme in [9] (See the right-hand side of Fig. 3). For the LS method, we varied the artificial time step (dt) in interval [100; 800] so as to ensure that the curve evolution is stable[1]. The plot shows that, in the case of our compactness prior, the LS method is highly sensitive to the gradient-descent time step and is one order of magnitude slower that our method.

---

[1] In comparison to level set implementations based on re-initialization procedures, the scheme in [9] allows much larger time steps (and therefore faster curve evolution). However, the value of dt still have to be fixed carefully; a very large value would cause instability in curve evolution.

References

1. Ben Ayed, I., Lu, Y., Li, S., Ross, I.: Left ventricle tracking using overlap priors. In: Metaxas, D., Axel, L., Fichtinger, G., Székely, G. (eds.) MICCAI 2008, Part I. LNCS, vol. 5241, pp. 1025–1033. Springer, Heidelberg (2008)
2. Ben Ayed, I., Punithakumar, K., Garvin, G.J., Romano, W., Li, S.: Graph cuts with invariant object-interaction priors: Application to intervertebral disc segmentation. In: Székely, G., Hahn, H.K. (eds.) IPMI 2011. LNCS, vol. 6801, pp. 221–232. Springer, Heidelberg (2011)
3. Boykov, Y., Funka-Lea, G.: Graph cuts and efficient n-d image segmentation. International Journal of Computer Vision 70(2), 109–131 (2006)
4. de Bruijne, M., van Ginneken, B., Viergever, M.A., Niessen, W.J.: Interactive segmentation of abdominal aortic aneurysms in cta images. Medical Image Analysis 8(2), 127–138 (2004)
5. Das, P., Veksler, O., Zavadsky, V., Boykov, Y.: Semiautomatic segmentation with compact shape prior. Image and Vision Computing 27(1-2), 206–219 (2009)
6. Duquette, A.A., Jodoin, P.M., Bouchot, O., Lalande, A.: 3D segmentation of abdominal aorta from ct-scan and mr images. Computerized Medical Imaging and Graphics 36(4), 294–303 (2012)
7. Gorelick, L., Schmidt, F., Boykov, Y.: Fast trust region for segmentation. In: CVPR, pp. 1714–1721 (2013)
8. Lesage, D., Angelini, E.D., Bloch, I., Funka-Lea, G.: A review of 3d vessel lumen segmentation techniques: Models, features and extraction schemes. Medical Image Analysis 13(6), 819–845 (2009)
9. Li, C., Xu, C., Gui, C., Fox, M.D.: Level set evolution without re-initialization: A new variational formulation. In: CVPR, pp. 430–436 (2005)
10. Linguraru, M.G., Pura, J.A., Pamulapati, V., Summers, R.M.: Statistical 4D graphs for multi-organ abdominal segmentation from multiphase CT. Medical Image Analysis 16(4), 904–914 (2012)
11. Nambakhsh, C.M.S., Peters, T.M., Islam, A., Ben Ayed, I.: Right ventricle segmentation with probability product kernel constraints. In: Mori, K., Sakuma, I., Sato, Y., Barillot, C., Navab, N. (eds.) MICCAI 2013, Part I. LNCS, vol. 8149, pp. 509–517. Springer, Heidelberg (2013)
12. Niethammer, M., Zach, C.: Segmentation with area constraints. Medical Image Analysis 17(1), 101–112 (2013)
13. Qiu, W., Yuan, J., Ukwatta, E., Sun, Y., Rajchl, M., Fenster, A.: Fast globally optimal segmentation of 3d prostate mri with axial symmetry prior. In: Mori, K., Sakuma, I., Sato, Y., Barillot, C., Navab, N. (eds.) MICCAI 2013, Part II. LNCS, vol. 8150, pp. 198–205. Springer, Heidelberg (2013)
14. Rousson, M., Cremers, D.: Efficient kernel density estimation of shape and intensity priors for level set segmentation. In: Duncan, J.S., Gerig, G. (eds.) MICCAI 2005, Part II. LNCS, vol. 3750, pp. 757–764. Springer, Heidelberg (2005)
15. Schaap, M., et al.: Coronary lumen segmentation using graph cuts and robust kernel regression. In: Prince, J.L., Pham, D.L., Myers, K.J. (eds.) IPMI 2009. LNCS, vol. 5636, pp. 528–539. Springer, Heidelberg (2009)
16. Veksler, O.: Star shape prior for graph-cut image segmentation. In: Forsyth, D., Torr, P., Zisserman, A. (eds.) ECCV 2008, Part III. LNCS, vol. 5304, pp. 454–467. Springer, Heidelberg (2008)
17. Zunic, J.D., Hirota, K., Rosin, P.L.: A Hu moment invariant as a shape circularity measure. Pattern Recognition 43(1), 47–57 (2010)

Small Sample Learning of Superpixel Classifiers for EM Segmentation

Toufiq Parag, Stephen Plaza, and Louis Scheffer

Janelia Farm Research Campus- HHMI, Ashburn, VA, USA
paragt@janelia.hhmi.org

Abstract. Pixel and superpixel classifiers have become essential tools for EM segmentation algorithms. Training these classifiers remains a major bottleneck primarily due to the requirement of completely annotating the dataset which is tedious, error-prone and costly. In this paper, we propose an interactive learning scheme for the superpixel classifier for EM segmentation. Our algorithm is 'active semi-supervised' because it requests the labels of a small number of examples from user and applies label propagation technique to generate these queries. Using only a small set ($< 20\%$) of all datapoints, the proposed algorithm consistently generates a classifier almost as accurate as that estimated from a complete groundtruth. We provide segmentation results on multiple datasets to show the strength of these classifiers.

1 Introduction

Connectomics is an emerging field in neuroscience where the goal is to discern neural connectivity in an organism. Recent advances of Electron Microscopy (EM) techniques have enabled us to image neurons and their components in an unprecedented level of details. The sizes of such datasets suggest that (semi-)automated region labeling or segmentation is the most viable strategy to conduct subsequent biological analysis. The outputs of such automated algorithms require manual correction afterwards [1].

Motivated by the advances in natural image segmentation techniques (see [2] and references therein), there have been many fruitful attempts to segment neural regions recently [3][4][5] [6][7][8][9]. Most of these studies initially apply a pixel (2D or 3D)-wise classifier [10] to compute the boundary confidence at any location and produce an initial (over-)segmentation comprising superpixels through methods such as Watershed [11]. Different approaches use different methods to refine, as well as register in anisotropic problem, the initial region labeling in order to generate the final segmentation. We adopt an Agglomerative or Hierarchical clustering scheme [6][7] due to its advantages e.g., low space, time complexity and flexibility to tune for over/under segmentation.

Identifying a potential merge between two superpixels (either in 2D or 3D) through classification is a crucial step for almost all successful EM segmentation algorithms [3][4][5][7][8][9]. This classifier may act as a region boundary predictor; given two adjacent superpixels, it classifies the separating boundary to be a true cell boundary or a false separation generated by the over-segmentation algorithm [9][7][12]. For anisotropic dataset, the classifier may also be trained to identify which superpixels on different

P. Golland et al. (Eds.): MICCAI 2014, Part I, LNCS 8673, pp. 389–397, 2014.

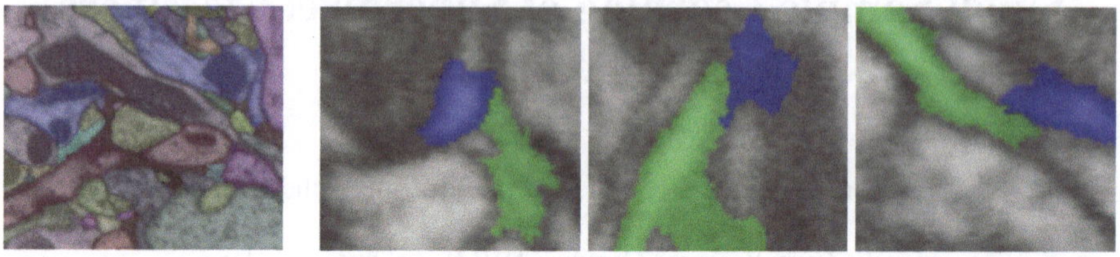

| (a) Exhaustive groundtruth | (b) example query 1 | (c) example query 2 | (d) example query 3 |

Fig. 1. Leftmost: complete groundtruth. Right 3 images: examples of queries generated by the proposed algorithm.

planes indeed belong to the same neural body [3][4][5]. This study investigates an interactive small sample learning method to generate a robust and accurate classifier to be used primarily for region boundary detection.

While it is critical to have highly accurate classifiers for accurate segmentation [8] [7], training such classifiers, both pixel and superpixelwise, is considered to be a major bottleneck in EM segmentation literature [13]. On one hand, training algorithms typically demand complete groundtruth labels, which assigns a label to each location of a volume or a set of images as displayed in Figure 1(a) where each color represents a label. Generating such labeling from either the actual grayscale images or a preliminary segmentation output is costly, tedious and entails the risk of human errors (e.g., due to loss of attention over time) and therefore could significantly stifle the performance of such predictors [13]. While dependence on complete groundtruth may sometimes be alleviated by using the interactive tool Ilastik [14] for pixel-wise detection [12], it can not be eliminated altogether due to the subsequent superpixel classifier training step. The work of [9] attempts to train the superpixel boundary predictor in an interactive fashion similar to Ilastik, but it has not been shown to be comparable, in terms of accuracy, to the one learned from a complete labeling.

On the other hand, the frameworks that require multiple training phases [7][12] are less amenable to have a small sample variant. Since a single class, such as cytoplasm, may comprise several sub-classes possessing widely varying characteristics, it seems to be crucial for these algorithms to recursively refine the hypotheses and accumulate training sets for satisfactory performance. In contrast, a context-aware approach [15], which processes different components (sub-structures) of the same class separately, was demonstrated to attain improved segmentation performance with predictors trained from fewer examples than those in [7][12]. The context-aware approach of [15] motivated us to pursue a training method for a superpixel boundary classifier with even fewer numbers of examples while retaining the accuracy of that learned on complete groundtruth.

This paper proposes an active semi-supervised algorithm for training a superpixel face detector utilizing a significantly small subset ($< 20\%$) of all such faces. In the proposed framework, the user is repeatedly asked to assign binary class labels (true/false) to a few of all region boundaries, such as the ones shown in Figure 1(b), (c), (d), generated by an over-segmentation algorithm[1]. Provided these labels, the algorithm updates the classifier learned so far and generates a new set of queries for the next round.

Active learning algorithm are known to suffer from inconsistent performance and low noise tolerance [16]. Experimentally, the incorporation of a semi-supervised method has been shown to achieve a greater degree of robustness for 'actively' trained predictors [17] [18]. Similar to [17], our proposed interactive learning employs a semi-supervised method along with a classifier to identify the most useful examples to be queried next. *The boundary predictors produced by the proposed method are shown to consistently achieve (almost) the same performance as that learned with full groundtruth* and to be more robust than those trained using several standard active learning techniques.

Our framework has a substantial implication on the overall EM reconstruction process. Together with an interactive pixel boundary detector (e.g., Ilastik), the proposed method paves the way for EM segmentation without exhaustive annotation. This enables us to learn and apply segmentation quickly and is advantageous for large volume reconstruction (e.g., whole animal brain) where one may anticipate to learn different predictors for different areas to improve accuracy. A quick segmentation output on preliminary images, generated with different sample preparations, could also assist the imaging expert to decide the optimal preparation during EM imaging.

2   Interactive Learning of Region Boundary Predictor

Let us suppose the initial over-segmentation process generated N superpixels $\mathcal{S} = \{S_1, S_2, \ldots, S_N\}$ on an EM dataset with M neurites (neuronal regions) where $N \gg M$. Let $L(S)$ be the neurite region that S actually belongs to. Our goal is to iteratively merge these N superpixels such that each $S_i, i = 1, 2, \ldots, N$ is merged into its corresponding $L(S_i)$.

We denote a boundary between two oversegmented regions by a pair of regions $e \triangleq \{S_i, S_j\}$ and the set of all such boundaries by E. In a graph representation, each of the regions S_i is considered to be a node and the boundary or face between two regions is regarded as an edge – a notation we will be using throughout the paper. Also, let the binary boundary label map $B : \mathcal{S} \times \mathcal{S} \to \{-1, 1\}$ assign a 1 to a boundary that actually separates one neurite region from another and a -1 to the boundary incorrectly generated due to over-segmentation. In agglomerative clustering methods, a real-valued superpixel boundary confidence function $h : \mathcal{S} \times \mathcal{S} \to \mathbb{R}$ approximates $B(e)$. In this paper, we describe how this predictor h can be estimated from a small subset rather than all boundaries of E.

2.1   Active Semi-supervised Learning

The primary challenge of an active learning algorithm is to fit a classifier with few examples respecting the actual class boundaries in the feature distribution of the whole

---

[1] Access to an over-segmented volume computed by an interactive (or other limited sample) pixel-wise classifier and an appropriate region growing algorithm is assumed in this study.

dataset. Without any additional information, any classifier will concentrate on separating the members of different classes within the small sample set at hand. It is, however, possible to extrapolate the labels of other datapoints, through the most similar ones to the small set, by a semi-supervised algorithm called the label propagation technique [19][17]. A datapoint is more informative for classification if it is classified differently than the examples 'nearby' (or the ones it is strongly connected to based on the affinities among them) – in other words, the samples for which the generative label propagation estimate disagrees with the discriminative prediction.

The proposed algorithm starts with a small subset $E_l \subset E$ which is initially fully labeled. A (Random Forest [20]) classifier is trained on this initial dataset E_l and the confidences of all the remaining edges $E_u = E \setminus E_l$ are computed. In addition, another set of confidences for E_u is computed by a generative model. The disagreement among these two types of estimates are quantified in a ranking formula. The first k examples in descending order of disagreement measure are presented to the user as queries. The set E_l is augmented by this new queries and the whole process is repeated until some stopping criterion is satisfied.

Generative View: The generative view for our approach consists of a graph based label propagation technique of semi-supervised learning [19][17]. Let us denote $\mathbf{x}$ to be the feature representation of a boundary sample e. Given a set E of examples, this algorithm computes a pairwise affinity matrix $W = \exp\{-\frac{1}{2}(\mathbf{x}_i - \mathbf{x}_j)^T \Sigma^{-1}(\mathbf{x}_i - \mathbf{x}_j)\}$ where $e_i, e_j \in E$ and its corresponding degree D and Laplacian matrix $L = D - W$. The smoothness on the labels $\mathbf{y}$, given the pairwise affinities, can be enforced by requiring the quantity $\frac{1}{2}\sum_{i \sim j} W_{ij}(y_i - y_j)^2 = \mathbf{y}^T W \mathbf{y}$ to be minimized. This energy term is minimized at $(D - W)\mathbf{y} = 0$.

Provided a set of known labels $\mathbf{y}_l$ for $e \in E_l$, the factorization of the labels and weight matrix enables us to compute the unknown labels $\mathbf{y}_u$ for the remaining set E_u as follows.

$$\mathbf{y} = \begin{bmatrix} \mathbf{y}_l \\ \mathbf{y}_u \end{bmatrix}, \quad W = \begin{bmatrix} W_{ll} & W_{lu} \\ W_{ul} & W_{uu} \end{bmatrix}, \quad L_{uu}\,\mathbf{y}_u = W_{ul}\,\mathbf{y}_l, \tag{1}$$

where L_{uu} is the corresponding graph Laplacian of W_{uu}. Relaxing the values of $\mathbf{y}_u$ to real values, this system of linear equations can be solved efficiently by existing algorithms.

Ranking: Given the real valued confidences $h_c(e)$, $e \in E_u$ from the current classifier (discriminative view) and the estimates $\mathbf{y}_u$ of the label propagation method, we use the following formula to compute disagreement between them.

$$R(e) = 1 - h_c(e)\, y_u(e). \tag{2}$$

The k boundaries with largest $R(e)$ constitute the set E_q of queries. The sets of edges are updated as follows: $E_l = E_l \cup E_q, E_u = E_u \setminus E_q$.

3   Implementation Details

An efficient solver for the linear system in Equation 1 is essential for the implementation of an interactive learner. Notice that, the Laplacian matrix L_{uu} is a symmetric diagonally dominant one. Fortunately, it has been shown that such systems can be solved in nearly linear time in terms of the number of edges on the graph [21][22]. In our implementation, we employed an efficient Algebraic Multigrid solver freely available at [23].

Similarly, we need a classifier for the discriminative view to be trained quickly. One of the reasons for our choice of Random Forest classifier [20] is that the decision trees within the forest can be trained in parallel and therefore can be computed efficiently on multi-core machines.

To reduce redundancy, the initial labeled set E_l was populated by the k centers of the output of a clustering algorithm (in our case k-means). Another alternative is to select the k datapoints with the largest degrees (w.r.t W) which are not neighbors to one another. The latter approach is deterministic and faster than clustering algorithms, but performs with same degree of accuracy in our dataset.

4   Experiments and Results

The interactive training method has been tested for 3D FIBSEM volumes as well as 2D ssTEM images (without alignment across planes). We generate the over-segmentation from the output of a multi-class (e.g., cell boundary, cytoplasm, mitochondria, mito-chondria boundary) *pixel classifier trained on only few pixels selected from the volume/images* using Ilastik [14] for both data modalities. Following [9][15], the boundary predictor h_c is trained only on cytoplasm superpixel boundaries with the superpixel features similar to [15][8]. To compute the affinities of W, a diagonal Σ was used where $\Sigma(a, a)$ is the variance of a-th feature.

This paper reports the segmentation performance of a context-aware agglomeration strategy [15] given the predictor h_c trained by the proposed method. In this agglomeration scheme, the cytoplasm superpixels are first clustered using the predictor h_c and then the mitochondria are merged based on their boundary ratios. The performances were measured using split-VI and split-RI values as described in [15]. The extended version of this paper (the arXiv version) contains the segmentation performance of the Global method [9] with h_c learned by our method.

4.1   FIBSEM Data

Initial over-segmentation on two training volumes (Tr set1, TrSet2, each of size 250^3) generated roughly 30,000 edges each, the proposed algorithm utilized 3% of all edges to populate the initial E_l. At each iteration, 10 new samples were queried until the total number of samples reaches 5000 (roughly 17%) at which point the algorithm terminates. We also trained the following standard active learning techniques and compared the performances on two different 520^3 volumes(Test vol 1, Test vol 2) : 1) Bootstrap variant of Importance Weighted Active Learning [16]. 2) Active version of Co-training method [24] where the initial set of E_l is divided and two different Random Forest classifiers were learned. Each example, on which the predictions of these two classifiers differ, is queried and inserted on the training set of the one that misclassified it. 3)Uncertain queries: train a Random forest from small set of samples and query all samples

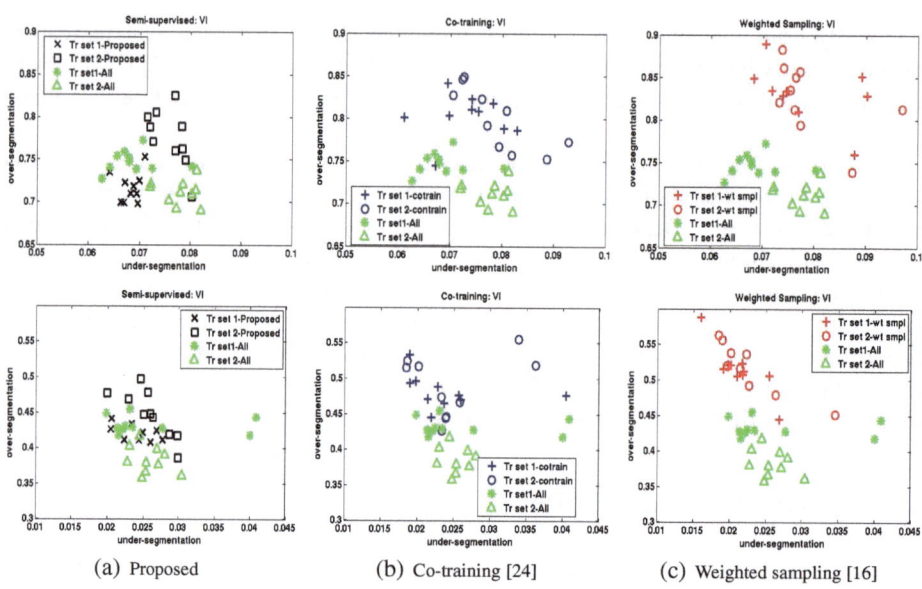

Fig. 2. Segmentation error (split-VI) on FIBSEM volume . Test volume 1 and 2 in top and bottom rows respectively.

with prediction in range $[-0.3, 0.3]$. 4) Random queries. Unless otherwise specified, all the parameters for these methods were kept the same as those of the proposed method. In order to evaluate robustness, the training algorithms are executed 10 times on two training volumes (Tr set 1 and Tr set 2) and the corresponding segmentation errors, in terms of split-VI[2], are displayed on Figure 2 (top: Test vol 1, bottom: Test vol 2). The threshold δ_c, which remains fixed for the multiple trials, was chosen such that the under-segmentation error of any particular actively trained predictor remains close to that produced by the one learned from full groundtruth agglomerated upto $\delta_c = 0.2$. Each plot compares the errors of the two predictors estimated by a certain active learning scheme (e.g., proposed in black + and square on Figure 2(a)) with those of boundary predictors learned with full groundtruth (Green * and triangle). *For both the test volumes (row 1 and 2 of Figure 2), the over and under-segmentation errors of proposed method are the closest to those of full groundtruth training model* (see arXiv version for mean and std dev of the errors).

For practical reasons, we are constrained to use far less samples than what is required by the importance weighted sampling method (Figure 2 Column (c)) to achieve an accuracy similar to the full groundtruth classifier as suggested by the results in [16]. The co-training algorithm (Figure 2 Column (b)) is apparently less capable than the proposed strategy in reinforcing the performances of the two hypotheses – this is not surprising since each of these hypotheses is trained on half of the training set. The random and uncertain query models both manifests inconsistent results (see arXiv version) over multiple trials – such outcome from these models is known in the active learning community [16].

---

[2] Plots showing split-RI are provided in the arXiv version.

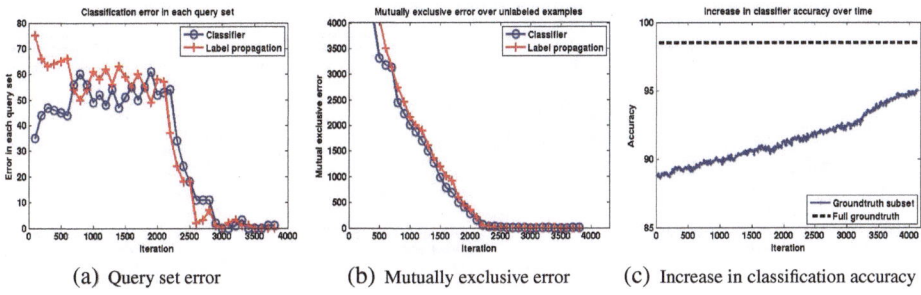

(a) Query set error   (b) Mutually exclusive error   (c) Increase in classification accuracy

Fig. 3. Analyzing errors of discriminative and generative views

The discriminative and generative views of the dataset utilized in the proposed method attempts to rectify each others mistakes through the queries presented. In Figure 3(a), we show the number of misclassified examples in each 100 queries generated by the RF classifier (blue) and the label propagation method (red) generated during one of the trials of the proposed method. Figure 3(b) displays the number of mutually exclusive errors (label propagation correct but RF incorrect and vice versa) on all the unlabeled examples (E_u) against the number of iterations. As these plots show, both the classifier and the label propagation techniques initially produce mutually exclusive errors. Over time, these errors are corrected and their respective models are updated accordingly. The steady increase in predictor accuracy (on all the unlabeled examples) plotted in Figure 3(c) suggests that this interaction also reduces the common errors made by these two views.

As Figure 3(a) indicates, both the generative and discriminative views appear to correctly classify the query samples once sufficient number of queries have been presented. Continuing the query process further would generate ambiguous or uncertain samples with confidences near 0. Intuitively, these samples would improve the margins of the interactive learner. We utilize this empirical observation to devise a **stopping criterion** for the proposed algorithm: the interactive process is repeated until the query set error reaches zero and then is continued for approximately 500 more examples before terminating.

4.2   ssTEM Data

The proposed algorithm has also been tested on 2D ssTEM images. We have trained the superpixel boundary predictor on 15 500 × 500 images following the same procedure as used in FIBSEM data and applied on 15 1000 × 1000 pixel images to segment the images (in 2D) in a context-aware fashion. The total number of queries used was 6000 out of approximately 41000 samples ($< 15\%$). The split-VI errors produced by the predictors learned using the proposed method, random queries and co-training method in 10 trials are shown in Figure 4; other algorithms performed too poorly on this data to be practically useful (see arXiv version). In this dataset too, the proposed method estimated a predictor producing the same segmentation errors as those resulted by the ones learned on full groundtruth.

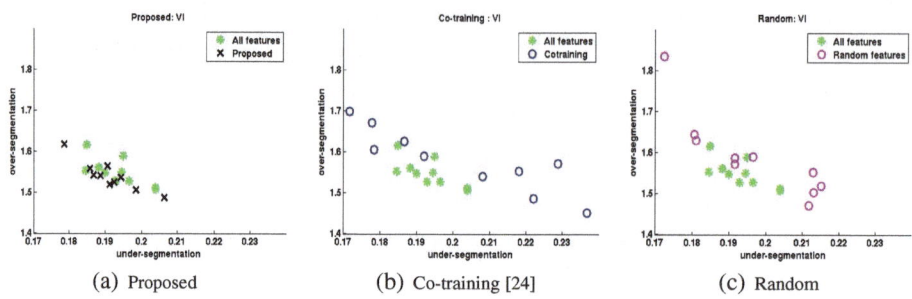

(a) Proposed   (b) Co-training [24]   (c) Random

Fig. 4. Segmentation error (split-VI) on TEM data

5   Conclusion

This paper presents an algorithm to train a superpixel boundary predictor from a few of all training examples. The predictors estimated by the the proposed method are shown to be as robust and accurate as those learned from complete groundtruth for segmentation purposes. Such a training algorithm will expedite learning tools for EM segmentation considerably and pave the way for practical semi-automatic segmentation systems for large volumes with diverse region characteristics.

Acknowledgement. The authors are grateful to Stuart Berg of Janelia Farm Research for his support in software development.

References

1. Takemura, S.Y., et al.: A visual motion detection circuit suggested by Drosophila connectomics. Nature 500(7461), 175–181 (2013)
2. Arbelaez, P., Maire, M., Fowlkes, C., Malik, J.: Contour detection and hierarchical image segmentation. IEEE Transactions on PAMI 33(5), 898–916 (2011)
3. Funke, J., Andres, B., Hamprecht, F., Cardona, A., Cook, M.: Efficient automatic 3D-reconstruction of branching neurons from EM data. In: CVPR (2012)
4. Kaynig, V., Fuchs, T., Buhmann, J.: Neuron geometry extraction by perceptual grouping in sstem images. In: CVPR (2010)
5. Vitaladevuni, S., Basri, R.: Co-clustering of image segments using convex optimization applied to em neuronal reconstruction. In: CVPR (2010)
6. Chklovskii, D.B., Vitaladevuni, S., Scheffer, L.K.: Semi-automated reconstruction of neural circuits using electron microscopy. Current Opinion in Neurobiology 20(5), 667–675 (2010)
7. Jain, V., Turaga, S.C., Briggman, K., Helmstaedter, M.N., Denk, W., Seung, H.S.: Learning to agglomerate superpixel hierarchies. In: NIPS, vol. 24, pp. 648–656 (2011)
8. Andres, B., Köthe, U., Helmstaedter, M., Denk, W., Hamprecht, F.: Segmentation of SBFSEM Volume Data of Neural Tissue by Hierarchical Classification. Pattern Recognition 5096(15), 142–152 (2008)
9. Andres, B., Kroeger, T., Briggman, K.L., Denk, W., Korogod, N., Knott, G., Koethe, U., Hamprecht, F.A.: Globally optimal closed-surface segmentation for connectomics. In: Fitzgibbon, A., Lazebnik, S., Perona, P., Sato, Y., Schmid, C. (eds.) ECCV 2012, Part III. LNCS, vol. 7574, pp. 778–791. Springer, Heidelberg (2012)

10. Jain, V., Bollmann, B., Richardson, M., Berger, D., Helmstaedter, M., Briggman, K., Denk, W., Bowden, J., Mendenhall, J., Abraham, W., Harris, K., Kasthuri, N., Hayworth, K., Schalek, R., Tapia, J., Lichtman, J., Seung, H.: Boundary learning by optimization with topological constraints. In: CVPR (2010)
11. Beucher, S., Meyer, F.: The Morphological Approach to Segmentation: The Watershed Transformation. In: Mathematical Morphology in Image Processing, pp. 433–481 (1993)
12. Nunez-Iglesias, J., Kennedy, R., Parag, T., Shi, J., Chklovskii, D.B.: Machine learning of hierarchical clustering to segment 2D and 3D images. PLoS ONE 8(8) (August 2013)
13. Helmstaedter, M.: Cellular-resolution connectomics: challenges of dense neural circuit reconstruction. Nat. Methods 10(6), 501–507 (2013)
14. Sommer, C., Straehle, C., Koethe, U., Hamprecht, F.A.: Ilastik: Interactive learning and segmentation toolkit. In: ISBI (2011)
15. Parag, T., Chakraborty, A., Plaza, S.: A context-aware delayed agglomeration framework for EM segmentation. arXiv 1406:1476 (2014)
16. Beygelzimer, A., Dasgupta, S., Langford, J.: Importance weighted active learning. In: ICML 2009 (2009)
17. Zhu, X., Lafferty, J., Ghahramani, Z.: Combining Active Learning and Semi-Supervised Learning Using Gaussian Fields and Harmonic Functions. In: ICML 2003 Workshop on The Continuum from Labeled to Unlabeled Data in Machine Learning and Data Mining (2003)
18. Muslea, I., Minton, S., Knoblock, C.A.: Active + semi-supervised learning = robust multi-view learning. In: ICML (2002)
19. Chapelle, O., Schölkopf, B., Zien, A. (eds.): Semi-Supervised Learning. MIT Press, Cambridge (2006)
20. Breiman, L.: Random forests. Machine Learning 45(1), 5–32 (2001)
21. Spielman, D.A., Teng, S.H.: A local clustering algorithm for massive graphs and its application to nearly-linear time graph partitioning. CoRR abs/0809.3232 (2008)
22. Koutis, I., Miller, G., Peng, R.: A nearly-m log n time solver for sdd linear systems. In: Foundations of Computer Science (FOCS), pp. 590–598 (2011)
23. Demidov, D.: Algebraic multigrid solver, https://github.com/ddemidov/amgcl
24. Zhu, X., Goldberg, A.B., Brachman, R., Dietterich, T.: Introduction to Semi-Supervised Learning. Morgan and Claypool Publishers (2009)

A Cautionary Analysis of STAPLE
Using Direct Inference of Segmentation Truth

Koen Van Leemput[1,2] and Mert R. Sabuncu[1]

[1] A.A. Martinos Center for Biomedical Imaging, MGH, Harvard Medical School, USA
[2] Technical University of Denmark, Denmark

Abstract. In this paper we analyze the properties of the well-known segmentation fusion algorithm STAPLE, using a novel inference technique that analytically marginalizes out all model parameters. We demonstrate both theoretically and empirically that when the number of raters is large, or when consensus regions are included in the model, STAPLE devolves into thresholding the average of the input segmentations. We further show that when the number of raters is small, the STAPLE result may not be the optimal segmentation truth estimate, and its model parameter estimates might not reflect the individual raters' actual segmentation performance. Our experiments indicate that these intrinsic weaknesses are frequently exacerbated by the presence of undesirable global optima and convergence issues. Together these results cast doubt on the soundness and usefulness of typical STAPLE outcomes.

1 Introduction

Since its introduction a decade ago, the Simultaneous Truth and Performance Level Estimation (STAPLE) algorithm [1] has become an established technique for estimating the true underlying segmentation of a structure from multiple imperfect segmentations. Its applications range from combining manual delineations by different human expert raters, to fusing registration-based automatic segmentations in multi-atlas label fusion methods. The algorithm is based on an explicit probabilistic model of how an (unknown) true segmentation degrades into (observed) imperfect segmentations, allowing for different frequencies of segmentation errors by different raters. Starting from its basic formulation, it has since been extended in several directions, including accounting for spatially-varying rater performance [2,3], putting "error bars" on estimated rater performance measures [4], and modeling missing or repeat segmentations [5].

A detailed theoretical understanding of the results produced by STAPLE and its variants is hampered by the fact that the algorithm depends on a numerical optimization procedure for the parameters of its model. Here, we show that this optimization procedure can actually be avoided, since the parameters can be marginalized out analytically. This allows us to theoretically predict the behavior of STAPLE and its variants in several often-used scenarios – which we empirically verify – revealing several undesirable properties.

P. Golland et al. (Eds.): MICCAI 2014, Part I, LNCS 8673, pp. 398–406, 2014.

To the best of our knowledge, this is the first detailed analysis of the theoretical properties of STAPLE, although it has been criticized before in empirical studies (e.g., [6]).

2   Theoretical Analysis

2.1   The STAPLE Model

Let $\mathbf{d}^j = (d_1^j, \ldots, d_I^j)^T$ denote the segmentation of a structure by rater j, where $d_i^j \in \{0, 1\}$ is the one of two possible labels assigned to voxel i, and I is the total number of voxels. Given J raters, the collection of all segmentations is given by $\mathbf{D} = (\mathbf{d}^1 \ldots \mathbf{d}^J)$. Letting $\mathbf{t} = (t_1, \ldots, t_I)^T$ with $t_i \in \{0, 1\}$ denote the true underlying structure, the STAPLE algorithm is based on the following generative model for the observed segmentations:

$$p(\mathbf{t}|\boldsymbol{\pi}) = \prod_i \pi_{t_i} \quad \text{and} \quad p(\mathbf{D}|\mathbf{t}, \boldsymbol{\theta}) = \prod_j p(\mathbf{d}^j|\mathbf{t}, \boldsymbol{\theta}^j), \quad p(\mathbf{d}^j|\mathbf{t}, \boldsymbol{\theta}^j) = \prod_i \theta_{d_i^j, t_i}^j.$$

Here the vector $\boldsymbol{\pi} = (\pi_0, \pi_1)^T$, with $0 \leq \pi_t \leq 1$ and $\sum_t \pi_t = 1$, contains the expected frequencies of occurrence for each label t. Furthermore, $\theta_{d,t}^j$ denotes the probability that rater j assigns label d to a voxel if the true label is t, so that $\sum_d \theta_{d,t}^j = 1$. Finally, the vector $\boldsymbol{\theta}^j = (\boldsymbol{\theta}_0^{j^T}, \boldsymbol{\theta}_1^{j^T})^T$ with $\boldsymbol{\theta}_t^j = (\theta_{0,t}^j, \theta_{1,t}^j)^T$ collects the segmentation performance parameters of rater j, and the vector $\boldsymbol{\theta} = (\boldsymbol{\theta}^{1^T}, \ldots, \boldsymbol{\theta}^{J^T})^T$ collects all performance parameters of all raters.

Letting the vector $\boldsymbol{\omega} = (\boldsymbol{\theta}^T, \boldsymbol{\pi}^T)^T$ denote all the parameters of the model, a prior of the form

$$p(\boldsymbol{\omega}) = p(\boldsymbol{\pi})p(\boldsymbol{\theta}), \quad p(\boldsymbol{\pi}) \propto \pi_0^{\alpha_0} \pi_1^{\alpha_1}, \quad p(\boldsymbol{\theta}) \propto \prod_j \prod_t (\theta_{0,t}^j)^{\alpha_{0,t}} (\theta_{1,t}^j)^{\alpha_{1,t}}$$

is often used, where $\{\alpha_t, \alpha_{d,t}\}$ are hyperparameters whose values are assumed given. By selecting hyperparameter values $\alpha_{d,t} = 0, \forall d, t$ (implying that all values of $\theta_{d,t}^j$ are equally likely) and $\alpha_t = \rho \sum_j \sum_i [d_i^j = t], \rho \to \infty$ (effectively clamping the values of π_t to the average frequency of occurrence in the raters' segmentations), the original STAPLE model [1] is obtained. Alternatively, $\alpha_{d,t}$ can be set to specific positive values to encode an expectation of better-than-random segmentation performance [2,5]; and by setting $\alpha_t = 0, \forall t$ the expected frequencies of occurrence π_t can automatically be inferred from the data [5].

2.2   STAPLE Inference

Given the collection of available segmentations $\mathbf{D}$, the STAPLE algorithm first seeks the maximum a posteriori (MAP) estimate *of the model parameters*:

$$\widehat{\boldsymbol{\omega}} = \arg\max_{\boldsymbol{\omega}} p(\boldsymbol{\omega}|\mathbf{D}) = \arg\max_{\boldsymbol{\theta}, \boldsymbol{\pi}} \prod_i \left(\sum_{t_i} (\prod_j \theta_{d_i^j, t_i}^j) \pi_{t_i} \right) p(\boldsymbol{\theta})p(\boldsymbol{\pi}), \quad (1)$$

using a dedicated expectation-maximization (EM) optimizer that exploits the specific structure of Eq. (1). Once a MAP parameter estimate $\widehat{\boldsymbol{\omega}}$ is found, it is then used to infer the segmentation truth as: $\hat{\mathbf{t}}_{STAPLE} = \arg\max_{\mathbf{t}} p(\mathbf{t}|\mathbf{D}, \widehat{\boldsymbol{\omega}})$, which involves only voxel-wise binary decisions [1]. In some cases one is also interested in the performance parameters $\boldsymbol{\theta}_t^j$ of individual raters. In that scenario, the corresponding component $\hat{\boldsymbol{\theta}}_t^j$ is simply extracted from the high-dimensional parameter vector $\widehat{\boldsymbol{\omega}}$ and inspected [1]. In addition, "error bounds" around these values are sometimes computed by locally approximating the posterior $p(\boldsymbol{\omega}|\mathbf{D})$ using a Gaussian distribution and estimating its covariance structure [4].

2.3   STAPLE Inference as an Approximation

Given the raters' segmentations $\mathbf{D}$, the MAP estimate *of the segmentation truth* is given by $\hat{\mathbf{t}} = \arg\max_{\mathbf{t}} p(\mathbf{t}|\mathbf{D})$, which will generally be different from the STAPLE result $\hat{\mathbf{t}}_{STAPLE}$ obtained by maximizing $p(\mathbf{t}|\mathbf{D}, \widehat{\boldsymbol{\omega}})$. Furthermore, the distribution $p(\boldsymbol{\theta}_t^j|\mathbf{D})$ is a low-dimensional projection of a higher dimensional distribution $p(\boldsymbol{\omega}|\mathbf{D})$; its properties – including its maximum – cannot generally be inferred by simply ignoring all other components in $\boldsymbol{\omega}$.

The crux of this paper is that the STAPLE inference of both the segmentation truth and performance parameters will only be a good approximation when the distribution $p(\mathbf{t}|\mathbf{D})$ is strongly peaked around its optimal value $\hat{\mathbf{t}}$. To understand this, it is instructive to write out the parameter posterior as:

$$p(\boldsymbol{\omega}|\mathbf{D}) = \sum_{\mathbf{t}} p(\boldsymbol{\omega}|\mathbf{t}, \mathbf{D})p(\mathbf{t}|\mathbf{D}) \tag{2}$$

with

$$p(\boldsymbol{\omega}|\mathbf{t}, \mathbf{D}) = \frac{p(\mathbf{t}, \mathbf{D}|\boldsymbol{\omega})p(\boldsymbol{\omega})}{p(\mathbf{t}, \mathbf{D})} = p(\boldsymbol{\pi}|\mathbf{t})\prod_{j}\prod_{t} p(\boldsymbol{\theta}_t^j|\mathbf{t}, \mathbf{D}), \tag{3}$$

where $p(\boldsymbol{\pi}|\mathbf{t})$ and $p(\boldsymbol{\theta}_t^j|\mathbf{t}, \mathbf{D})$ are beta distributions. The last step in Eq. (3) is based on the fact that the normalizer

$$p(\mathbf{t}, \mathbf{D}) = \int_{\boldsymbol{\omega}} p(\mathbf{t}, \mathbf{D}|\boldsymbol{\omega})p(\boldsymbol{\omega})\mathrm{d}\boldsymbol{\omega} = \int_{\boldsymbol{\theta}} p(\mathbf{D}|\mathbf{t}, \boldsymbol{\theta})p(\boldsymbol{\theta})\mathrm{d}\boldsymbol{\theta} \int_{\boldsymbol{\pi}} p(\mathbf{t}|\boldsymbol{\pi})p(\boldsymbol{\pi})\mathrm{d}\boldsymbol{\pi} \propto$$

$$\mathrm{B}(N_0 + \alpha_0 + 1, N_1 + \alpha_1 + 1)\left(\prod_{j}\prod_{t} \mathrm{B}\left(N_{0,t}^j + \alpha_{0,t} + 1, N_{1,t}^j + \alpha_{1,t} + 1\right)\right) \tag{4}$$

involves a marginalization over the model parameters that is given in analytical form. Here $\mathrm{B}(\cdot, \cdot)$ denotes the beta function, $N_{d,t}^j$ the number of voxels assigned to label d by rater j when the truth label in $\mathbf{t}$ is t, and N_t the total number of voxels where the truth label is t.

Referring to Eq. (2), the posterior $p(\boldsymbol{\omega}|\mathbf{D})$ is obtained by summing conditional posteriors $p(\boldsymbol{\omega}|\mathbf{t}, \mathbf{D})$, one for each possible $\mathbf{t}$ and weighed according to how probable that $\mathbf{t}$ is. When $p(\mathbf{t}|\mathbf{D})$ is strongly peaked around $\hat{\mathbf{t}}$, the resulting summation will be dominated by the contribution of $\hat{\mathbf{t}}$ only: $p(\boldsymbol{\omega}|\mathbf{D}) \simeq p(\boldsymbol{\omega}|\hat{\mathbf{t}}, \mathbf{D})$. As Eq. (3) shows, this distribution factorizes across the individual parameter components, so that the location of the maximum of $p(\boldsymbol{\theta}_t^j|\mathbf{D})$ can indeed be obtained by extracting the corresponding component from the joint maximum location $\widehat{\boldsymbol{\omega}}$. Furthermore, since the individual factors are (narrow) beta distributions, their product will be strongly peaked around $\widehat{\boldsymbol{\omega}}$, so that in turn $p(\mathbf{t}|\mathbf{D}) = \int_{\boldsymbol{\omega}} p(\mathbf{t}|\mathbf{D}, \boldsymbol{\omega})p(\boldsymbol{\omega}|\mathbf{D})\mathrm{d}\boldsymbol{\omega} \simeq p(\mathbf{t}|\mathbf{D}, \widehat{\boldsymbol{\omega}})$ and therefore $\hat{\mathbf{t}}_{STAPLE} \simeq \hat{\mathbf{t}}$.

2.4   Two Cases Where STAPLE Inference Will Be Accurate

There are two common scenarios, analyzed below, where $p(\mathbf{t}|\mathbf{D})$ is sharply peaked around $\hat{\mathbf{t}}$ and where STAPLE therefore provides accurate inference. However, as we shall see, both scenarios will also render the STAPLE results akin to simply thresholding the average segmentation map $\bar{\mathbf{d}} = \sum_j \mathbf{d}^j / J$ – similar to majority voting which thresholds $\bar{\mathbf{d}}$ at level 0.5.

We start by writing the conditional posterior distribution of the segmentation truth label in a single voxel. Because of Eq. (4), we have that

$$p(t_i|\mathbf{D}, \mathbf{t}_{\setminus i}) \propto \left(\prod_j \frac{N^j_{d^j_i, t_{i \setminus i}} + \alpha_{d^j_i, t_i} + 1}{\sum_d (N^j_{d, t_{i \setminus i}} + \alpha_{d, t_i} + 1)} \right) (N_{t_{i \setminus i}} + \alpha_t + 1), \qquad (5)$$

where $\mathbf{t}_{\setminus i}$ denotes the truth labels in all voxels except voxel i, and $N^j_{d, t_{\setminus i}}$ and $N_{t_{\setminus i}}$ are the corresponding voxel counts.

Many Raters: When the number of raters is very large ($J \gg 0$), we have that, around the optimum $\hat{\mathbf{t}}$, the log of the ratio of conditional posterior probabilities in a voxel i behaves approximately as a simple linear function of the fraction of raters that assigned voxel i to foreground, denoted by $f_i = \sum_j d^j_i / J$:

$$\log \left(\frac{p(t_i = 1|\mathbf{D}, \hat{\mathbf{t}}_{\setminus i})}{p(t_i = 0|\mathbf{D}, \hat{\mathbf{t}}_{\setminus i})} \right) \simeq s_{\hat{\mathbf{t}}} \cdot f_i + o_{\hat{\mathbf{t}}}, \qquad (6)$$

with slope $s_{\hat{\mathbf{t}}} = J(\bar{c}_{0,0} + \bar{c}_{1,1} - \bar{c}_{1,0} - \bar{c}_{0,1})$ and offset $o_{\hat{\mathbf{t}}} = J(\bar{c}_{0,1} - \bar{c}_{0,0}) + (c_1 - c_0)$, where $\bar{c}_{d,t} = \frac{\sum_j c^j_{d,t}}{J}$, $c^j_{d,t} = \log \left(\frac{\hat{N}^j_{d,t} + \alpha_{d,t} + 1}{\sum_d (\hat{N}^j_{d,t} + \alpha_{d,t} + 1)} \right)$, and $c_t = \log \left(\hat{N}_t + \alpha_t + 1 \right)$. This is because of the large number of summations involved when $J \gg 0$ (law of large numbers), and because $\hat{N}^j_{d, t_{\setminus i}} \simeq \hat{N}^j_{d, t}$ and $\hat{N}_{t_{\setminus i}} \simeq \hat{N}_t$. When the foreground fraction f_i exceeds a certain threshold, the "log odds" of Eq. (6) becomes positive and the voxel is assigned to label $t_i = 1$, *independent of which raters exactly labeled the voxel as fore- or background*. Furthermore, the same threshold applies to all voxels, since the slope $s_{\hat{\mathbf{t}}}$ and offset $o_{\hat{\mathbf{t}}}$ are independent of i. Note that the slope $s_{\hat{\mathbf{t}}}$ depends directly on J, so that the joint posterior $p(\mathbf{t}|\mathbf{D})$ will be strongly peaked when $J \gg 0$ – therefore $\hat{\mathbf{t}}_{STAPLE}$ can be expected to correspond to a thresholded average segmentation map $\bar{\mathbf{d}}$ (although not necessarily at the threshold level 0.5 used by majority voting).

Large Consensus Regions: Even if the number of raters J is small, Eq. (6) will still be a good approximation when large values for the hyperparameters $\alpha_{d,t}$ are used, as these effectively make the different $c^j_{d,t}$ similar across all raters. This will happen when large "consensus regions" are included in the analysis, i.e., image regions where all raters agree on the same label, since the net effect of such voxels will be to act as large hyperparameters $\alpha_{0,0} \gg 0$ (for background areas) and $\alpha_{1,1} \gg 0$ (for foreground areas) on the remaining, non-consensus voxels. In that specific scenario, $c_{0,1}$ and $c_{1,0}$ will attain large negative values, yielding a large slope $s_{\hat{\mathbf{t}}}$ indicative of a sharply peaked $p(\mathbf{t}|\mathbf{D})$, so that again $\hat{\mathbf{t}}_{STAPLE}$ can be expected to be a thresholded map $\bar{\mathbf{d}}$ in this case as well.

2.5   Direct Inference of Segmentation Truth

In addition to providing theoretical insight, Eq. (5) also suggests a new way of *directly* inferring the segmentation truth using discrete optimization – without estimating continuous model parameters first. In particular, starting from some initial labeling, the MAP segmentation truth $\hat{\mathbf{t}} = \arg\max_{\mathbf{t}} p(\mathbf{t}|\mathbf{D})$ can be estimated by visiting each voxel in turn, assigning it to the label that maximizes Eq. (5), and repeating this procedure until no voxels change labels. A similar procedure can also be used to generate Monte Carlo samples from $p(\mathbf{t}|\mathbf{D})$: by repeatedly visiting each voxel, in random order, and assigning label t_i with probability $p(t_i|\mathbf{D}, \mathbf{t}_{\setminus i})$, a large number S of samples $\{\mathbf{t}^{(s)}\}_{s=1}^{S}$ of the segmentation truth can be obtained (so-called Gibbs sampling). Such samples can then be used to assess the full posterior distribution of specific (combinations of) performance parameters, e.g., $p(\boldsymbol{\theta}_t^j|\mathbf{D}) = \sum_{\mathbf{t}} p(\boldsymbol{\theta}_t^j|\mathbf{t}, \mathbf{D}) p(\mathbf{t}|\mathbf{D}) \simeq \frac{1}{S} \sum_{s=1}^{S} p(\boldsymbol{\theta}_t^j|\mathbf{t}^{(s)}, \mathbf{D})$.

3   Experiments

In order to verify our theoretical analysis, we performed experiments in the context of multi-atlas label fusion, in which a manually annotated brain MR scan of each of 39 subjects was non-linearly warped to the remaining 38 subjects as described in [7]. These warps were applied to the manual segmentations of 10 brain structures (cerebral white matter, cerebral cortex, lateral ventricle, thalamus, caudate, putamen, pallidum, hippocampus, and amygdala in the left hemisphere, as well as brain stem), which were subsequently used as input to a binary STAPLE set-up (treating each structure in turn as foreground and the remaining voxels as background).

We studied three variations of STAPLE. In the original "Basic" variant [1], all voxels in the image are considered; a flat prior on the segmentation performance parameters is used (i.e., $\alpha_{d,t} = 0$); and a pre-computed spatial prior $\boldsymbol{\pi}$ is clamped to the average relative size of the foreground/background in the input segmentations. The "Restricted" variant is identical except that all voxels in which all raters agreed on the same label ("consensus areas") are excluded from the analysis [8]. Finally, the "Advanced" variant also discards all consensus areas, but encourages better-than-random segmentation performance by setting $\alpha_{0,0} = \alpha_{1,1} = 2$ and $\alpha_{0,1} = \alpha_{1,0} = 0$ [5,2]; in addition $\alpha_0 = \alpha_1 = 0$ so that the spatial prior $\boldsymbol{\pi}$ is automatically estimated from the data [5].

As is common in the literature, each variant was initialized with high sensitivity and specificity parameters (we used $\theta_{0,0}^j = \theta_{1,1}^j = 0.99$); for the "Advanced" variant π_1 was initialized as 0.5. To reduce the number of experiments, we only studied a random subset of 20 subjects from the available 39. We ran experiments in 2D, selecting, for each experiment, the coronal slice in which the structure being studied was the largest in the co-registered 3D volumes. To quantify the influence of the number of raters, each experiment was run with the segmentations restricted to the first 5, 15, and 37 of the available 38 ones.

4   Results

Since our analysis predicts thresholding behavior in certain scenarios but not the applicable threshold level (which itself depends on the found solution), we conducted the following experiment. For each STAPLE result, we thresholded $\bar{\mathbf{d}}$ at varying levels $(l - 1/2)/J, l = 1, \ldots, J$ and recorded the level yielding the highest Dice score with $\hat{\mathbf{t}}_{STAPLE}$. The resulting threshold levels and corresponding Dice scores, averaged across all 20 subjects and all 10 structures, are shown in the table below (standard deviations are in parentheses):

ra-ters	Basic		Restricted		Advanced	
	threshold	Dice	threshold	Dice	threshold	Dice
5	0.30 (±0.00)	1.00 (±0.01)	0.41 (±0.04)	0.89 (±0.09)	0.45 (±0.05)	0.91 (±0.08)
15	0.17 (±0.03)	0.99 (±0.01)	0.46 (±0.05)	0.98 (±0.02)	0.46 (±0.06)	0.98 (±0.01)
37	0.14 (±0.06)	1.00 (±0.01)	0.44 (±0.14)	0.99 (±0.01)	0.43 (±0.15)	0.99 (±0.01)

For the Basic variant, which includes large consensus regions, the thresholding behavior of STAPLE is apparent for all number of raters. The threshold level, which corresponds to the point of zero-crossing $-o_{\hat{\mathbf{t}}}/s_{\hat{\mathbf{t}}}$ of the line of Eq. (6), is clearly below the majority voting 0.5 level because the size of the background is very large, which through $c_{1,0}$ increases $s_{\hat{\mathbf{t}}}$ but not $o_{\hat{\mathbf{t}}}$. The threshold level also decreases as more raters are added – thereby gradually yielding the *union* of all segmentations – because the fixed spatial prior favors background, making $c_1 < c_0$ and therefore rendering $-o_{\hat{\mathbf{t}}}/s_{\hat{\mathbf{t}}}$ dependent on J.

Both the Restricted and Advanced variants, which only consider non-consensus voxels, clearly exhibit the predicted thresholding behavior for $J \gg 0$, with Dice scores around 0.99 for both methods when $J = 37$, and around 0.98 when $J = 15$. However, for the Restricted case these numbers mask a more complex underlying phenomenon: As can be seen from Eq. (1), when $p(\boldsymbol{\pi})$ clamps $\boldsymbol{\pi}$ to $(0.5, 0.5)^T$ and $p(\boldsymbol{\theta}) \propto 1, p(\boldsymbol{\omega}|\mathbf{D})$ is invariant to swaps of the type $\theta_{d,0}^j \leftrightarrow \theta_{d,1}^j$, which corresponds to interchanging the role of the background and foreground label. Since the spatial prior was very close to 0.5 across all experiments (mean value 0.46, standard deviation 0.06), the posteriors $p(\boldsymbol{\omega}|\mathbf{D})$ were typically bimodal (cf. Fig (1)). In this variant a spatial prior different from 0.5 is the only factor discerning between the two modes, but in more than 20% of the cases for 15 and 37 raters, finding the global optimum would have yielded a solution similar to thresholding $\bar{\mathbf{d}}$ *and subsequently inverting the labels*. The fact that this is not apparent from the table above is because STAPLE got trapped in the wrong solution in all these cases (cf. Fig. (1)). When the number of raters was 5, STAPLE failed to locate the global maximum in 55% of the cases; the spatial prior encouraged the wrong solution in 46% of the cases.

The Advanced variant discerns between the two modes by encouraging performance parameters that are better-than-random, and the resulting models were found to always identify the correct solution. For all 15 and 37 rater cases, for which $p(\boldsymbol{\omega}|\mathbf{D})$ is strongly peaked, STAPLE also successfully located this solution. When initializing the proposed discrete optimizer at $\hat{\mathbf{t}}_{STAPLE}$ to see if further improvements in $\log p(\mathbf{t}|\mathbf{D})$ could be achieved, only modest improvements were obtained (0.150 and 1.225 on average for 37 and 15 raters, respectively,

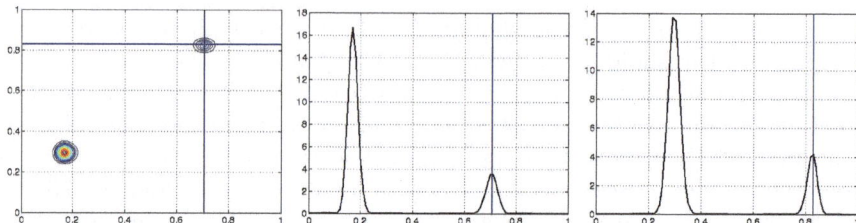

Fig. 1. Example of the bimodal parameter posterior often seen with the Restricted variant (37 raters, left lateral ventricle). The left shows a contour plot of $p(\theta_{1,1}^j, \theta_{0,0}^j|\mathbf{D})$ for one rater j, computed using the proposed Gibbs sampler; the two other plots show $p(\theta_{1,1}^j|\mathbf{D})$ and $p(\theta_{0,0}^j|\mathbf{D})$. The blue lines indicate the location of the (suboptimal) STAPLE parameter estimate – the global optimum would swap the fore- and background.

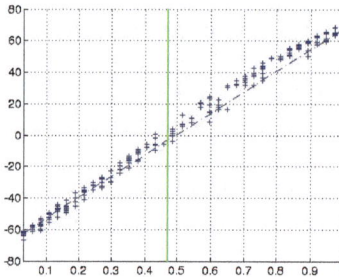

Fig. 2. Plot of the linear behavior of the "log odds": each cross corresponds to a voxel plotted against its foreground fraction (Advanced variant, 37 raters, left hippocampus). Voxels above the 0 level are assigned to foreground; a very similar result (Dice overlap 0.989) can be obtained by thresholding $\bar{\mathbf{d}}$ at level 0.472 (indicated by the thick green line).

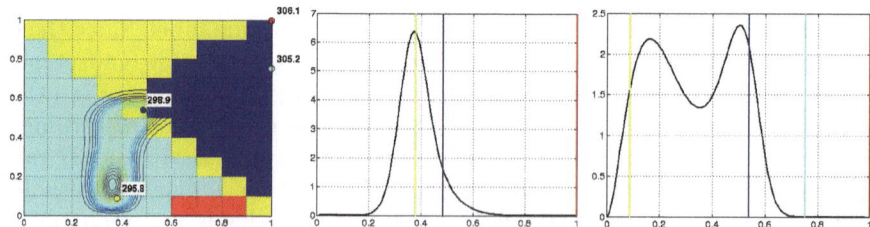

Fig. 3. Example of the broad, complex parameter posteriors often seen when only 5 raters are used (Advanced variant, left hippocampus). The plots are similar to those shown in Fig. 1, except that local optima arrived at when re-initializing STAPLE differently are shown in different colors. Tiles with the same color in the left plot indicate initializations in a 10×10 grid that arrive at the same optimum (indicated with a color-filled circle with the value of $-\log p(\mathbf{D}|\mathbf{t})p(\mathbf{t})$ indicated). Note that the (presumably global) yellow optimum is not found by STAPLE (shown in blue), and that the local optima in the high-dimensional parameter space do not generally correspond to local optima in the lower-dimensional marginal distributions.

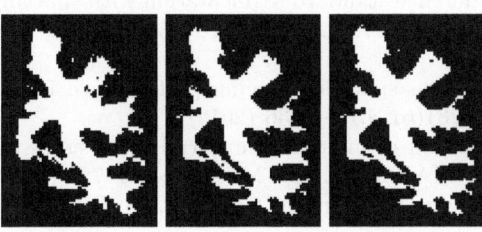

Fig. 4. When the number of raters is small, STAPLE may not yield the optimal segmentation truth estimate, even when it finds globally optimal parameters (as is the case in this example). From left to right: majority voting, STAPLE, and proposed discrete optimizer (Advanced variant, 5 raters, left cerebral white matter).

corresponding to 1.162 and 3.404 ratios in probabilities), which is in line with our theoretical predictions. Fig. (2) shows the "log odds" for each voxel under consideration for a 37-rater case, plotted vs. its foreground fraction f_i; the match with the predicted line of Eq. (6) is clear. When only 5 raters were used, much larger improvements in $\log p(\mathbf{t}|\mathbf{D})$ could be obtained with the discrete optimizer: 11.850 on average, which corresponds to solutions that are over $100,000$ times more likely. Some of this is attributable to the fact that $p(\boldsymbol{\omega}|\mathbf{D})$ is often a complex distribution that makes STAPLE susceptible to getting trapped in local optima: For each case we repeatedly re-ran STAPLE using a 10×10 parameter grid for initialization of $(\theta_{1,1}^j, \theta_{0,0}^j)$ (cf. Fig. (3)), and found that in 23% a better optimum could be located this way. However, even when the correct parameter estimate $\hat{\boldsymbol{\omega}}$ was found, the broad distribution $p(\boldsymbol{\omega}|\mathbf{D})$ typically makes the STAPLE solution $\hat{\mathbf{t}}_{STAPLE}$ amendable to further improvement (Fig. (4)). Note in Fig. (3) also the difficulty in interpreting the value of individual components of $\hat{\boldsymbol{\omega}}$ in these cases.

5 Discussion

In this paper we have analyzed the theoretical properties of the STAPLE algorithm, revealing several fundamental shortcomings that cast doubt on the soundness and usefulness of results obtained with this method. We note that, although we only considered the binary STAPLE case here, the obtained results readily translate to cases with more than two labels.

Acknowledgments. This research was supported by NIH NCRR (P41-RR14075), NIBIB (R01EB013565, K25EB013649), and a BrightFocus grant (AHAF-A2012333).

References

1. Warfield, S.K., et al.: Simultaneous truth and performance level estimation (STAPLE): an algorithm for the validation of image segmentation. IEEE TMI 23(7), 903–921 (2004)

2. Commowick, O., et al.: Estimating a reference standard segmentation with spatially varying performance parameters: Local MAP STAPLE. IEEE TMI 31(8), 1593–1606 (2012)
3. Asman, A.J., Landman, B.A.: Formulating spatially varying performance in the statistical fusion framework. IEEE TMI 31(6), 1326–1336 (2012)
4. Commowick, O., Warfield, S.K.: Estimation of inferential uncertainty in assessing expert segmentation performance from STAPLE. IEEE TMI 29(3), 771–780 (2010)
5. Landman, B., et al.: Robust statistical fusion of image labels. IEEE TMI 31(2), 512–522 (2012)
6. Langerak, T.R., et al.: Label fusion in atlas-based segmentation using a selective and iterative method for performance level estimation (SIMPLE). IEEE TMI 29(12), 2000–2008 (2010)
7. Sabuncu, M.R., et al.: A generative model for image segmentation based on label fusion. IEEE TMI 29(10), 1714–1729 (2010)
8. Rohlfing, T., Russakoff, D.B., Maurer, C.R.: Expectation maximization strategies for multi-atlas multi-label segmentation. In: Taylor, C.J., Noble, J.A. (eds.) IPMI 2003. LNCS, vol. 2732, pp. 210–221. Springer, Heidelberg (2003)

Auto Localization and Segmentation of Occluded Vessels in Robot-Assisted Partial Nephrectomy

Alborz Amir-Khalili[1], Jean-Marc Peyrat[2], Julien Abinahed[2], Osama Al-Alao[3], Abdulla Al-Ansari[2,3], Ghassan Hamarneh[4], and Rafeef Abugharbieh[1]

[1] BiSICL, University of British Columbia, Vancouver, Canada
[2] Qatar Robotic Surgery Centre, Qatar Science & Technology Park, Doha, Qatar
[3] Urology Department, Hamad General Hospital, Hamad Medical Corporation, Qatar
[4] Medical Image Analysis Lab, Simon Fraser University, Burnaby, Canada

Abstract. Hilar dissection is an important and delicate stage in partial nephrectomy during which surgeons remove connective tissue surrounding renal vasculature. Potentially serious complications arise when vessels occluded by fat are missed in the endoscopic view and are not appropriately clamped. To aid in vessel discovery, we propose an automatic method to localize and label occluded vasculature. Our segmentation technique is adapted from phase-based video magnification, in which we measure subtle motion from periodic changes in local phase information albeit for labeling rather than magnification. We measure local phase through spatial decomposition of each frame of the endoscopic video using complex wavelet pairs. We then assign segmentation labels based on identifying responses of regions exhibiting temporal local phase changes matching the heart rate frequency. Our method is evaluated with a retrospective study of eight real robot-assisted partial nephrectomies demonstrating utility for surgical guidance that could potentially reduce operation times and complication rates.

1 Introduction

Approximately 30,000 new cases of kidney cancer, generally renal cell carcinoma, are detected each year in the U.S. alone. Kidney resection, also known as a nephrectomy, is the only known effective treatment for this type of localized cancer [1]. Robot-assisted partial nephrectomy (RAPN) refers to nephron-sparing techniques performed with surgical robots in which only the cancerous cells are excised while the kidney is reconstructed to retain functionality.

The intraoperative aspect of RAPN procedures can be organized into five stages [2]: 1) Bowel mobilization; 2) Hilar dissection and control; 3) Identification and demarcation of tumor margins; 4) Resection of tumor; and 5) Reconstruction of the kidney (renorrhaphy). Hilar dissection stands out as a daunting stage that requires significant expertise since improper clamping due to overlooked accessory renal vessels can cause significant bleeding during resection [3].

Hilar dissection is a delicate procedure during which the surgeon dissects through the Gerota's fascia and removes the connective tissue that surrounds

P. Golland et al. (Eds.): MICCAI 2014, Part I, LNCS 8673, pp. 407–414, 2014.
© Springer International Publishing Switzerland 2014

the renal artery (RA) and vein (RV). This task is complex due to the variability in patient vasculature and the amount of perinephric fat which surrounds the kidney. Access to the hilum grants the surgeon control over the flow of blood into and out of the kidney, which is very important as warm ischemia is required during the excision of the tumor to minimize internal hemorrhaging.

In some cases, accessory vessels that branch off from the RA or the abdominal aorta are accidentally missed as they lie hidden behind a thick layer of perinephric fat. In one study of 200 laparoscopic partial nephrectomy cases by world leading surgeons, seven incidents of intraoperative bleeding were reported as a result of inadequate hilar control, two of which were directly caused by missed accessory vessels [4]. Although the number of incidents is low, other studies have observed the existence of accessory vessels in up to 35% of patients [5,6]. If the surgeon's level of experience is limited, the incidence of bleeding may be much higher. The implications are many, aside from obvious complications that would arise from internal hemorrhaging, bleeding may also jeopardize the surgical outcome by occluding the surgeon's view as the tumor is being resected.

Surgeons often make use of preoperative medical images in identifying troublesome accessory vessels [7]. Even with a detailed scan and segmented pre-op plan, surgeons are still burdened with the task of mentally transferring this abstraction onto the surgical site during the operation. Reducing the difficulty of navigation has been attempted by state-of-the-art approaches that used multimodal registration to align the preoperative surgical map of the vessels onto the surgeon's endoscopic view [8]. Such techniques have to date not been extensively validated in clinical practice, possibly because they require very delicate selection of parameters, use of invasive fiducials, or are computationally complex to the extent that the algorithms cannot perform in real-time. Recent methods favor the use of hardware solutions such as near infrared flourescence imaging [9] or algorithmic methods that only use color intensity information from the endoscope for enhancing RAPN by highlighting vasculature based on perfusion models [10]. Hardware solutions are not widely accessible as they are cost restrictive and both methods fail to identify vessels that are hidden under a layer of fat.

Our work is motivated by the need for an automated guidance system that can work in parallel to the techniques mentioned above to reduce the complications and the time required to perform hilar dissection by assisting the surgeon in localizing hidden accessory vessels. Our proposed system aims at highlighting occluded vessels by analyzing the complementary temporal motion characteristics of the scene as acquired by the endoscope. Our method is inspired by video magnification techniques developed for natural scenes [11,12], where an Eulerian approach to analyzing flow within a video sequence can be used to magnify periodic motions that are nearly invisible to the human eye. An extension of [11] was very recently implemented in the context of robot-assisted surgery [13]. In our case, we adapted the phased-based video magnification [12] to detect and label subtle motion patterns instead of magnifying them. Our method is evaluated with a retrospective study of eight RAPN cases to show its potential utility for surgeons.

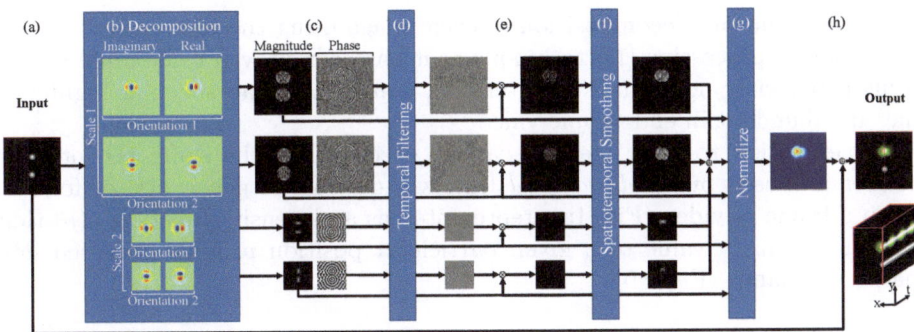

Fig. 1. Overview of our proposed method: (a) First frame of a synthetic input video composed of one circle that pulsates (top) and another that remains stationary (bottom). (b) Steerable filter bank with illustrated impulse responses are used to decompose the information inside each frame into (c) magnitude and local phase at different scales and orientations. (d) The phase information of all frames of the video is temporally filtered using an ideal bandpass filter centered on the frequency of the pulsating circle. (f) A spatiotemporal median filter is applied to (e) the magnitude weighted response of the filtered phases to remove phase noise. (g) The filtered results are then combined and (h) added back to the input as an overlay. A spatiotemporal cross section of the video illustrates four pulsations across 30 frames of the synthetic video.

2   Methods

The goal is to highlight occluded vasculature near the renal hilum. These regions in the video exhibit periodic pulsatile motion within a narrow temporal passband centered around the heart rate. This sub-pixel motion is faintly visible on the surface of the occluding adipose tissue. We can relate the position p of such a region at time t to its original position P, at time $t = 0$, with the displacement vector $u(P,t)$ such that $p = u(P,t) + P$. By analyzing the vector u with respect to time, for a dense set of regions starting at every pixels in the first frame of acquisition, we can label regions that exhibit the desired behaviour.

Dense tracking of pixels in an image through time is computationally expensive, more so when the motions occur at the subpixel level [14]. To overcome this limitation, our proposed segmentation method (Fig. 1) relies on Eulerian motion processing techniques to label regions that pulsate like a vessel.

The Eulerian motion magnification work [11] relies on the first-order approximation of changes in intensities to estimate motion. Analysis in [11], demonstrated that this approximation is susceptible to noise at high spatial frequencies, especially at spatial locations where the curvature of change in intensity is high. A recent study demonstrated that a second order approximation of the change in intensity using the Hessian matrix is less susceptible to errors and provides a metric for attenuating noise locally [13]. Even with a second order approximation, these gradient based methods are prone to error in salient regions. We have chosen to estimate this local motion from the change in instantaneous phase of complex sinusoid decomposition of each image using the more recent phase-based motion processing [12] technique as it has been proven to be more robust to high frequency noise and, by extension, non-Lambertian specular highlights that are abundant in endoscopic video.

Our extension to their method can be described in the same 1D intuitive manner proposed by *Wadhwa et al* [12], without loss of generality, as follows. Given a frame of video (Fig. 1a), represented as an intensity function $f(p)$ that maps an intensity value to a given particle at position p, is decomposed into spatial sub-bands (Fig. 1b)

$$f(p) = f(P + u(P,t)) = \sum_{\omega=-\infty}^{\infty} A_\omega e^{i\omega(P+u(P,t))} \tag{1}$$

with each sub-band representing a complex sinusoid $S_\omega(p,t) = A_\omega e^{i\omega(P+u(P,t))}$ at spatial frequency ω, the local phase (Fig. 1c) is defined as $\omega(P + u(P,t))$.

The motion vectors $u(P,t)$ can be extracted from a temporal sequence of local phase measurements using a DC balanced bandpass filter (Fig. 1d); the filter response of the temporal bandpass filter is denoted by B_ω. If the passband is wide enough, we can compute the displacement vector entirely at each sub-band such that $B_\omega(p,t) = \omega u(P,t)$. If the passband of the filter is tuned to the typical heart rate of a patient, we can isolate components of the local motion that are synchronous with the heart rate and vascular pulsation.

We adapt our method to generate fuzzy segmentation labels from the computed local motion. Local phase changes, B_ω, are first attenuated in regions where the magnitude response A_ω of the spatial sub-band is weak by computing the product between the bandpassed phases and the normalized magnitude of the spatial filter response vectors to obtain $Q_\omega = \hat{A}_\omega B_\omega$ (Fig. 1e). Local phase measurements are wrapped between the interval $(-\pi, \pi]$ so Q_ω will contain impulse noise. We remove noise from the product Q_ω using a spatiotemporal median filter (Fig. 1f). This denoised product $\tilde{Q}_\omega$ is finally incorporated into a voting scheme (Fig. 1g) using magnitude weighted averaging to obtain fuzzy labels

$$H(p,t) = \frac{\sum_{\omega=-\infty}^{\infty} \lfloor \frac{A_\omega \tilde{Q}_\omega}{2\pi\omega} - T \rfloor}{\sum_{\omega=-\infty}^{\infty} A_\omega + \epsilon}, \tag{2}$$

where T is an optional noise compensation term representing the maximum response that can be generated from noise alone and ϵ is a small number to avoid division by zero. The resulting sequence of fuzzy labels H may be displayed as an overlay or separately to highlight this pulsatile motion (Fig. 1h).

3   Results

Video sequences from eight real RAPN interventions were used for validation. All endoscopic video data were acquired by a da Vinci Si surgical system (Intuitive Surgical, California, USA). HD (1080i) videos were resized to 480×270 pixels.

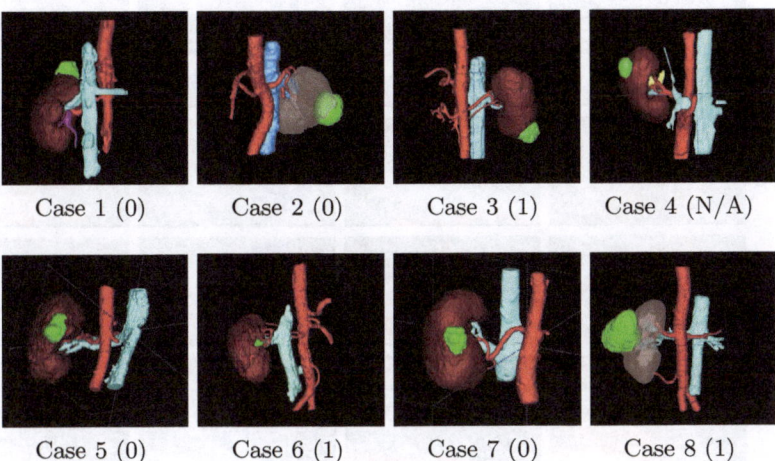

Case 1 (0)   Case 2 (0)   Case 3 (1)   Case 4 (N/A)

Case 5 (0)   Case 6 (1)   Case 7 (0)   Case 8 (1)

Fig. 2. Manual segmentation of each RAPN case, number of accessory vessels in paren-thesis, showing kidney (brown), tumor/cyst (green), veins (cyan), and arteries (red)

Sixteen complex steerable filter pairs were used (four orientations at four scales) with one filter per octave using publicly available code [15]. The passband of the temporal filter was set between 60 to 120 beats per minute and the noise threshold T was set to zero. Average runtime of our unoptimized MATLAB code to process a four second clip (120 frames) was 65 seconds.

In order to provide a framework for validation, we compare the segmentations obtained through our guidance system against manually localized vasculature. To achieve this, we segmented the kidney, tumor/cyst, inferior vena cava, ab-dominal aorta, RA, RV, and accessory vessels (Fig. 2) using a semi-automatic segmentation algorithm [16]. The resulting meshes were manually aligned onto the first frame of each endoscopic scene (Fig. 3a) using a rigid transformation. Anatomical landmarks such as the contour of the kidney or visible parts of the vessels were used to guide the registration process. Our best estimate of the ground truth is presented in Fig. 3b. Small observable discrepancies between the aligned model and the endoscopic view are attributed to non-rigid deforma-tions of the organs and vasculature caused by deformation during insufflation, retraction, or the mobilization of organs during the dissection.

In our experiments, it was observed that although venous and arterial struc-tures pulsate at the same frequency, their pulsations are not in-phase. The mo-tion of the inferior vena cava and RV typically succeeds that of the RA and abdominal aorta by an average of six frames. The results in Fig. 3 illustrate this phenomenon in two frames of the segmented video. Compared to the reference in Fig. 3b, the motions highlighted in Fig. 3c correspond to the cyan structures (venous) and Fig. 3d corresponds to the red structures (arterial).

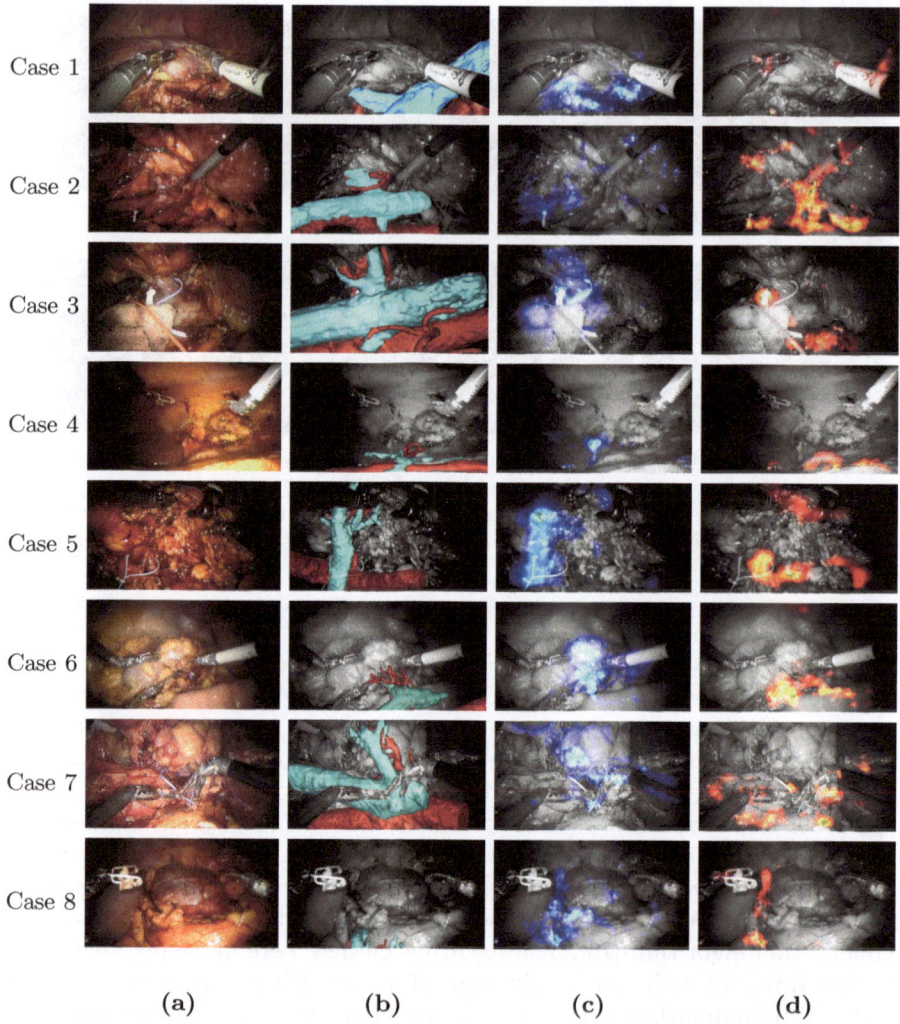

(a)   (b)   (c)   (d)

Fig. 3. Exemplar video frames with the proposed automatic localization of veins and arteries in the scene. (a) The first frame of the sequence, (b) manually localized venous (cyan) and arterial (red) structures, and segmentation of (c) veins and (d) arteries.

From the results we can further observe that, in Case 1, the small RA is correctly identified at the hilum. The mislabeling of the RA in Case 2 is attributed to retraction by the surgical instrument. The small accessory RA to the left of RV is also identified in Case 3. In Case 4, the suprarenal vein is misaligned due to mobilization of the spleen. Case 5 illustrates that retraction has shifted the abdominal aorta up. Branching of RA is detected on both sides of RV in Case 6 and the pulsation of heavy vascular region has casued the tumor to pulsate in the centre of the frame. False positives are observed in Case 7 due to the motion

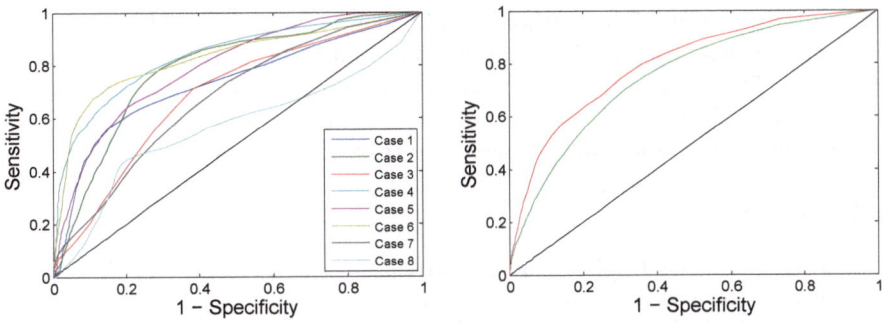

Fig. 4. Left: ROC of all cases. Right: median (red) and mean (green) of all ROC. Mean area under all ROC is 0.76 with a standard deviation of 0.08.

of the tools in the scene. Ideally, surgical instruments should remain motionless during the acquisition of the video. The last case posed a big challenge as the vasculature is heavily occluded by the bowel and many false positives are detected in fluid filled cavities to the left of the cyst.

To validate our labels quantitatively, the segmentations were binarized (at a fixed threshold throughout the sequence) and combined across the frames of the video. This resulting binarized image was then compared to the binarized version of the reference manual segmentation in Fig. 3b, combining all vasculature into a single mask. Fig. 4 illustrates the segmentation performance of all cases, at different threshold values, via their receiver operating characteristics (ROC).

4   Conclusion

We have described a novel method for localizing and labelling regions in endoscopic video that contain occluded vessels. Our method extends Eulerian phase-based video motion processing techniques to detect and label small motions that are barely visible on the surface of the perinephric fat. To the best of our knowledge, we are the first to attempt the challenging task of localizing occluded vasculature in endoscopic video without the use of additional hardware or preoretative scans. We validated our novel method qualitatively in a retrospective *in vivo* study to verify its application in a clinical setting. Conservative quantitative validation of our method demonstrates that it is suitable for integration alongside existing techniques (as an additional cue) that use other visible features such as color, shape and texture. In the future, we plan to extend this method by developing an adaptive estimation for noise and optimizing the code to operate in real-time. We are actively exploring the use of obtained segmentations as an additional data term for guiding automatic non-rigid registration of preoperative surgical models with endoscopic video in the context of RAPN. Finally, we aim to assess its applicability to other surgical interventions.

Acknowledgement. The authors would like to thank Mr. Masoud Nosrati, Mr. Jeremy Kawahara, and Mr. Ivan Figueroa for their assistance with the data acquisition. This publication was made possible by NPRP Grant #4-161-2-056 from the Qatar National Research Fund (a member of the Qatar Foundation). The statements made herein are solely the responsibility of the authors.

References

1. Drucker, B.J.: Renal cell carcinoma: current status and future prospects. Cancer Treatment Reviews 31(7), 536–545 (2005)
2. Gill, I.S., et al.: Laparoscopic partial nephrectomy for renal tumor: Duplicating open surgical techniques. The Journal of Urology 167(2, Part 1), 469–476 (2002)
3. Singh, I.: Robot-assisted laparoscopic partial nephrectomy: Current review of the technique and literature. Journal of Minimal Access Surgery 5(4), 87 (2009)
4. Ramani, A.P., Desai, M.M., Steinberg, A.P., Ng, C.S., Abreu, S.C., Kaouk, J.H., Finelli, A., Novick, A.C., Gill, I.S.: Complications of laparoscopic partial nephrectomy in 200 cases. The Journal of Urology 173(1), 42–47 (2005)
5. Urban, B.A., Ratner, L.E., Fishman, E.K.: Three-dimensional volume-rendered CT angiography of the renal arteries and veins: Normal anatomy, variants, and clinical applications. RadioGraphics 21(2), 373–386 (2001)
6. Sampaio, F., Passos, M.: Renal arteries: anatomic study for surgical and radiological practice. Surgical and Radiologic Anatomy 14(2), 113–117 (1992)
7. Mottrie, A., De Naeyer, G., Schatteman, P., et al.: Impact of the learning curve on perioperative outcomes in patients who underwent robotic partial nephrectomy for parenchymal renal tumours. European Urology 58(1), 127–133 (2010)
8. Teber, D., Guven, S., Simpfendörfer, T., Baumhauer, M., Güven, E.O., Yencilek, F., Gözen, A.S., Rassweiler, J.: Augmented reality: a new tool to improve surgical accuracy during laparoscopic partial nephrectomy? Preliminary in vitro and in vivo results. European Urology 56(2), 332–338 (2009)
9. Tobis, S., Knopf, J., Silvers, C., Yao, J., et al.: Near infrared fluorescence imaging with robotic assisted laparoscopic partial nephrectomy: initial clinical experience for renal cortical tumors. The Journal of Urology 186(1), 47–52 (2011)
10. Crane, N.J., Gillern, S.M., Tajkarimi, K., Levin, I.W., Pinto, P.A., et al.: Visual enhancement of laparoscopic partial nephrectomy with 3-charge coupled device camera: assessing intraoperative tissue perfusion and vascular anatomy by visible hemoglobin spectral response. The Journal of Urology 184(4), 1279–1285 (2010)
11. Wu, H.Y., Rubinstein, M., Shih, E., Guttag, J., Durand, F., Freeman, W.T.: Eulerian video magnification for revealing subtle changes in the world. ACM Transactions on Graphics 31(4), 65 (2012)
12. Wadhwa, N., Rubinstein, M., Durand, F., Freeman, W.T.: Phase-based video motion processing. ACM Transactions on Graphics 32(4), 80 (2013)
13. McLeod, A.J., Baxter, J.S., de Ribaupierre, S., Peters, T.M.: Motion magnification for endoscopic surgery. In: SPIE: Medical Imaging, vol. 9036, pp. 9036–9011 (2014)
14. Liu, C.: Beyond pixels: exploring new representations and applications for motion analysis. PhD thesis, Massachusetts Institute of Technology (2009)
15. Portilla, J., Simoncelli, E.P.: A parametric texture model based on joint statistics of complex wavelet coefficients. IJCV 40(1), 49–70 (2000)
16. Yushkevich, P.A., Piven, J., Cody Hazlett, H., Gimpel Smith, R., Ho, S., Gee, J.C., Gerig, G.: User-guided 3D active contour segmentation of anatomical structures. Neuroimage 31(3), 1116–1128 (2006)

3D Global Estimation and Augmented Reality Visualization of Intra-operative X-ray Dose

Nicolas Loy Rodas and Nicolas Padoy

ICube, University of Strasbourg, CNRS, IHU Strasbourg, France
{nloyrodas,npadoy}@unistra.fr

Abstract. The growing use of image-guided minimally-invasive surgical procedures is confronting clinicians and surgical staff with new radiation exposure risks from X-ray imaging devices. The accurate estimation of intra-operative radiation exposure can increase staff awareness of radiation exposure risks and enable the implementation of well-adapted safety measures. The current surgical practice of wearing a single dosimeter at chest level to measure radiation exposure does not provide a sufficiently accurate estimation of radiation absorption throughout the body. In this paper, we propose an approach that combines data from wireless dosimeters with the simulation of radiation propagation in order to provide a global radiation risk map in the area near the X-ray device. We use a multi-camera RGBD system to obtain a 3D point cloud reconstruction of the room. The positions of the table, C-arm and clinician are then used 1) to simulate the propagation of radiation in a real-world setup and 2) to overlay the resulting 3D risk-map onto the scene in an augmented reality manner. By using real-time wireless dosimeters in our system, we can both calibrate the simulation and validate its accuracy at specific locations in real-time. We demonstrate our system in an operating room equipped with a robotised X-ray imaging device and validate the radiation simulation on several X-ray acquisition setups.

Keywords: Surgical workflow analysis, hybrid surgery, radiation monitoring, augmented reality, RGBD cameras.

1 Introduction

The increasing use of intra-operative X-ray imaging in minimally invasive surgical procedures is increasing the exposure of clinical staff to radiation. Although the use of radioprotective equipment such as lead vests and aprons can minimize exposure, an accurate real-time estimation of the amount of radiation absorbed by clinicians during such procedures is important to improve OR safety, increase clinical staff awareness of radiation risk, and influence their behavior in high-radiation environments. For instance, such estimates can be used to generate warnings in cases of potential radiation overdose, allow surgeons to understand which steps of the surgery put them at greater risk of radiation exposure and enable the design of a safer OR layout. Large-scale efforts are being made to

P. Golland et al. (Eds.): MICCAI 2014, Part I, LNCS 8673, pp. 415–422, 2014.
© Springer International Publishing Switzerland 2014

measure radiation exposure during surgery, understand the parameters that affect it, and devise recommendations to reduce the exposure of clinical staff. The ORAMED project [1,2] comprehensively measured the dose absorbed by operators at different body locations during several interventional procedures, and highlighted the need to increase clinicians' awareness of the behavior of scattered radiation. In [2], Monte Carlo based studies were performed for selected interventional radiology scenarios, varying X-ray tube parameters, and varying operator and protective equipment positions to understand the relationship between these factors and radiation exposure. Doses were also measured in the different body parts of anthropomorphic phantoms placed near a radiation source, and several configurations that reduce extremity and eye lens exposure were proposed.

Current practice requires surgeons to wear a single dosimeter at chest level under the lead vest to measure their dose exposure. Whereas traditional thermoluminescent dosimeters (TLDs) provide the dose accumulated over time, semiconductor dosimeters provide real-time measurements. The recent development of wireless dosimeters [3] further enables the real-time display of radiation dose absorption on a screen, and has been received with strong interest by clinicians. However, the use of a single dosimeter does not provide the complete picture of radiation exposure as it only measures exposure at a single location in the body. Indeed, the ORAMED study [1] demonstrated that radiation exposure differs at different body parts. Since it would be impractical for the staff to wear a multitude of dosimeters on a regular basis, especially on their head and arms, there exists a need to complement these devices with a global radiation awareness system. In this paper, we propose a system that generates a 3D radiation risk map, validated by real-measurements, and overlays it onto a reconstructed model of the OR.

Previous work has addressed the problem of radiation monitoring. [4] propose a method to simulate the propagation of radiation and to display the risk on a 3D mesh tracking the clinician's body. However, that study was a proof of concept that was demonstrated in a simple lab setup, using an invalid simulation that did not take into account real parameters and conditions. Furthermore, the application of body mesh tracking of clinicians in a real work environment is challenging due to the presence of numerous obstructions and is yet to be successfully demonstrated. In [5], a training tool was proposed that shows the propagation of radiation in a virtual setup. While such a system can be used to improve clinicians' understanding of radiation scattering, an intra-operative system that provides real-time feedback will permit better *in situ* awareness of radiation exposure risk among physicians and can improve overall OR safety.

Our contributions are therefore threefold: 1) we propose to *combine* the simulation with data from real-time wireless dosimeters in order to calibrate and validate the simulation *in situ*; 2) we propose to use a computer vision system based on multiple RGBD cameras in order to display the augmented reality risk map in a real OR setup thus providing intuitive awareness about the distribution of intra-operative scattered radiation; 3) we provide experimental results using a real X-ray device to demonstrate the proposed system.

2 Methods

We propose a system that combines real-time dose measurements with simulations of intra-operative radiation propagation for providing information about the behavior of scattered radiation in an augmented reality manner. A multi-camera RGBD system is used to capture real-time data and generate a 3D model of the room, which includes the configuration of the robotized C-arm and the clinicians. Then a Monte Carlo based simulation, built from the recorded layout of the room and calibrated with the dose values measured at certain points of the scene, is used to estimate the propagation of scattered radiation in the room. Wireless dosimeters placed at key locations are also used to estimate the accuracy of the simulation. Finally, visualization is provided by overlaying a color-coded radiation risk map onto a 3D point cloud representation of the scene.

2.1 System Setup

Three RGBD cameras are mounted on the ceiling of the OR using articulated arms in order to obtain images of different views of the room. These are then fused to generate a 3D point cloud representation of the scene. In the calibration step, a checkerboard is placed over the left corner of the OR table for computing the transformation of each camera frame with respect to this point. This procedure is done once per setup since the position of the motorized table can be re-obtained from the robotized C-arm.

Eight wireless Raysafe dosimeters [3] are placed at different locations in the room in order to measure the dose of scattered radiation. These sensors provide real-time dose measurements calibrated in $H_p(10)$, namely the personal dose equivalent in soft tissue at a 10 mm depth below the position where it is worn. Two of them are used for calibrating the simulation framework while the other six for providing a real-time measure of the accuracy of the simulation results. The calibration sensors are placed over the table, to the left and to the right of the isocenter of the C-arm thus receiving high scattered radiation doses, while the evaluation dosimeters are distributed in key locations of the room.

2.2 Simulation of Intra-operative Scattered Radiation

The GEANT4 [7] toolkit was used to simulate the behavior of intra-operative scattered radiation. GEANT4 applies Monte Carlo methods for simulating the passage of particles through matter by iteratively calculating the trajectories and interactions between photons and atoms from the materials present in the scene. The 3D point cloud is used to obtain the position and orientation of dosimeters and clinicians with respect to the room reference frame while the source configuration and its pose with respect to the operating table is obtained from the robotized C-arm system.

The simulation model (shown in Fig. 1a) was built by defining detector geometries having the same physical characteristics, namely shape, material and position with reference to the world reference frame, as in the real-world setup.

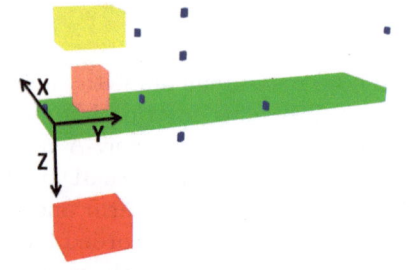
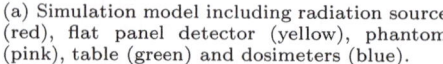
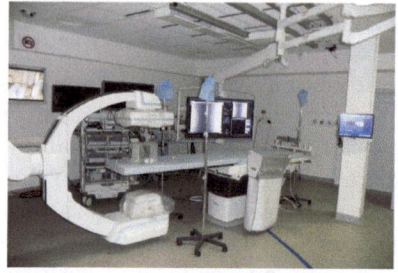

(a) Simulation model including radiation source (red), flat panel detector (yellow), phantom (pink), table (green) and dosimeters (blue).

(b) Experimental setup: Robotic C-arm (at 0° rotation), three RGBD cameras fixed on the ceiling and eight dosimeters placed at key locations.

Fig. 1. Simulation model and experimental setup for validating the system using an Artis Zeego [6] and its motorized operating table, a multi-camera RGBD system, RaySafe i2 dosimeters [3] and a water-filled slab phantom.

As in [5], the interventional room was represented by a volume filled with the material "air" and centered at the origin of the room reference frame obtained in 2.1. Inside, iron volumes were added to represent the image intensifier and radiation source. Their position and orientation were adapted according to the simulated C-arm configuration. In the same way, a carbon fiber parallelepiped was added for the OR table and a cubic volume filled with water and plexiglas walls for the phantom. For modeling the personal dosimeters, a $45 \times 45 \times 20$ mm volume of ICRU [8] soft tissue equivalent material (density 1 $g.cm^{-3}$ and mass composition: 76.2% oxygen, 11.1% carbon, 10.1% hydrogen and 2.6% nitrogen) was placed in the same position with respect to the radiation source as in the real-world setup. The $H_p(10)$ dose was evaluated by defining small sensitive cells of $45 \times 45 \times 0.5$ mm inside those volumes located at 10 mm depth from the outer surface. These sensitive detectors collect information about the particle interactions that occur on the volume during a run; the total energy deposited divided by the mass, obtained from the material definition, is used to represent the personal dose equivalent. In order to compute the propagation of scattered radiation all over the room, the world volume was divided into cubic voxels forming a 3D grid. Each of these voxels was defined as a sensitive volume so that at the end of each run it is possible to obtain the accumulated dose at any given location of the room by checking the corresponding voxel. A primary generator that produces a user defined number of photons was used to model the X-ray beam. The particles' energies were sampled from simulated X-ray spectra generated for selected peak tube voltages, filtrations and Air Kerma values using the X-ray Toolbox from Siemens [9]. Their moment direction was randomly sampled inside a cone of the same diameter as the considered X-ray field of view. The physics models leading to the production of scattered radiation, namely Compton Scattering, Rayleigh Scattering and the Photoelectric Effect were also modeled.

Simulations were performed for a large number of particles n. The computed doses were normalized by n, thus the number of histories only has an impact on the statistical error. A correction factor defined as the mean ratio between the measured and the simulated dose obtained from the calibration dosimeters is computed and applied to all simulation results.

2.3 Scattered Radiation Visualization

The proposed system provides three different approaches for visualizing the propagation of scattered radiation in an augmented reality manner. After a simulation run for given C-arm parameters and room layout, dose values inside every voxel element from the world volume are known. First, a color-coded radiation risk map can be overlaid onto the 3D model by coloring points according to the dose measured in the voxel that they belong to. This can help clinicians identify regions of high risk, enabling them to choose the safest position during the radiograph generation process. Second, scattered radiation isosurfaces can be generated and displayed over the model using volume rendering. This feature, besides showing the highly irradiated areas of the scene, can also be applied as an intuitive assistance tool to teach about the diffusion effects for given C-arm configurations. Third, by tracking the positions of the clinicians in the 3D point cloud, color-coded dose values in different parts of their bodies can be shown according to the simulated measures obtained in the corresponding voxels. This provides a complete picture of radiation exposure in the whole body thus complementing the information from the usual dosimeter worn at chest-level. The proposed global radiation awareness system is thereby able to make visible what is not perceived by any human sense.

3   Experiments

The system was validated with a set of experiments performed in a real operating room using an Artis Zeego X-ray robotized imaging device [6] and using the setup described in section 2.1. A 20×20×24 cm slab phantom with 10 mm thick plexiglas walls filled with water was placed over the operating table in the center of the primary beam in order to model the patient and generate scattered radiation during the imaging process. The two calibration dosimeters were placed over the bed at a distance of 30 cm on either side of the phantom. Nobody was irradiated during our tests, instead five test dosimeters were taped on drip rods installed around the operating table for reproducing the position of clinicians during a procedure. Three dosimeters were placed at different heights on the first drip rod in order to measure the radiation a clinician would receive in legs, chest and head. Two other drip rods with dosimeters taped at chest level were added to the scene: one close to the radiation source (opposite from the first) and the other at the end of the table, next to the bed control panel hence simulating the operator's position. Furthermore, an eighth dosimeter was taped on the corner of a lead panel, installed at mid distance between the radiation source and the bed control panel. Thus for each irradiation test performed we measured $H_p(10)$ values over eight sparse locations in the operating room, which

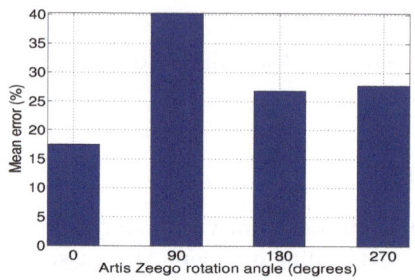
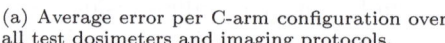
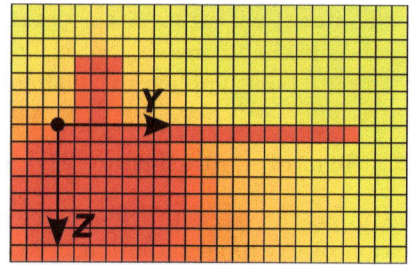

(a) Average error per C-arm configuration over all test dosimeters and imaging protocols.

(b) Radiation map summed along the x axis, illustrating radiation backscattering.

Fig. 2. (a) Average simulation error and (b) 2D radiation risk map, where the C-arm is vertical, the source is under the phantom and red indicates higher dose.

were later used for calibrating and/or testing our system. The complete setup is shown in figure 1b. Five fluoroscopy protocols were carried out, three Digital Radiography (DS) and two Digital Subtraction Angiography (DSA) protocols, with default peak tube voltages and Air Kerma values, using the inherent 0.4 mm Al filtration proper to the Artis Zeego, for a 20-second exposure time and for four different C-arm configurations: 0°, 90°, 180° and 270° rotation. The dose values measured by each dosimeter were recorded for each of the 20 experiments.

3.1   Validation of the Simulation Framework

The positions of the C-arm, operating table, phantom and dosimeters with reference to the room frame were obtained from the 3D point cloud or from the devices and used to initialize the radiation simulation framework. Five runs with n equal to 500 million particles were performed for each tested C-arm configuration and fluoroscopy protocol parameter; the dose values measured on each sensitive cell were normalized per particle and the results were averaged over all runs. The results were compared to the dose measured by the test dosimeters after applying the correction factor obtained during the calibration of the simulation with the remaining two dosimeters. A 30% average error over all test dosimeters, all radiograph protocols and C-arm rotations was obtained. This error can be explained by the approximations made in the simulation model, in particular in the geometry and parameters, as well as in the angular limitations of the semiconductor dosimeters. While it is superior to the 10% accuracy measured in [2] using TLD dosimeters, it should be noted that the TLDs used in [2] are located 10 cm from the phantom, while we span a much larger space. Fig. 2a shows the average error for each of the four C-arm configurations. In Fig. 2b a 2D radiation risk map obtained for a C-arm in vertical position with source under the phantom (0° rotation) is provided. It is obtained by summing the 3D risk map along the x axis using the coordinate system shown in Fig. 2b. One can clearly observe the expected backscattering of the radiation under the table in this particular configuration.

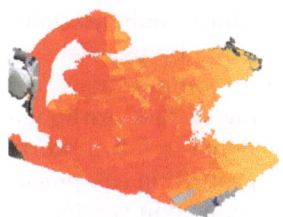 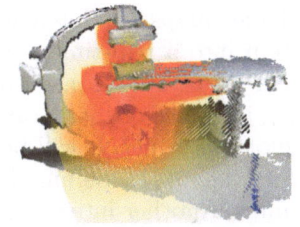 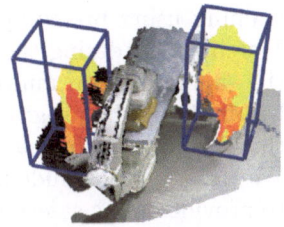

(a) Color-coded radiation risk map overlaid onto the 3D point cloud of the room.

(b) Volume rendered radiation isosurface illustrating the backscattering effect in 3D.

(c) Body-part dose vizualisation: risk map shown in the clinician's bounding box.

Fig. 3. Augmented reality visualization of scattered radiation propagation by overlaying radiation risk maps over the scene's 3D point cloud representations. Red indicates higher dose.

3.2 Visualization of Scattered Radiation Results

The pre-computed dose maps are used to visualize the propagation of scattered radiation over the room's 3D point cloud reconstruction. A 3D radiation risk map is overlaid by coloring the points according to the dose estimated at their location in the simulation (Fig. 3a). Also, the radiation volume can be displayed using volume rendering to provide an intuitive visualization of 3D radiation propagation and risk isosurfaces (Fig. 3b). The clinician's 3D position is tracked by applying a background subtraction approach on the depth maps. Body-part dose can thus be shown by displaying the risk map inside the clinicians' bounding boxes only, as illustrated in Fig. 3c.

The images of Fig. 3 demonstrate how our radiation simulation and augmented reality framework can be useful to visualize the 3D propagation of scattered radiation for safety purposes. Such information is particularly useful because the radiation field depends on multiple and simultaneously interacting parameters. This field can change drastically when the OR configuration is modified.

4   Discussion and Conclusion

In this paper, we have proposed a system for visualizing the propagation of scattered radiation during intra-operative X-ray procedures. By combining the simulation with data obtained from a multi-RGBD camera system, we are able to show the radiation exposure risk intuitively by overlaying the risk map onto a point cloud, either to show the exposure of the entire room or solely of the tracked clinician. The strength of the proposed system is the combination of the simulation with data from wireless real-time dosimeters, not only to calibrate the simulation, but also to validate its accuracy online so as to provide confidence in the presented risk map. Currently, our system is not real-time because of the long computational time required for the simulation and also because the positions of the robotic C-arm and table are read manually on the devices. The system can however be used in a real-environment for augmented reality training using pre-computed risk maps validated for standard configurations. Moreover, rendering the system into a real-time one is feasible by parallelising the simulations on multiple GPUs to obtain quasi-real time computations and by obtaining the programming interface of the X-ray imaging system. Although this was not within the scope of this paper, it will be considered in future work. We also plan to include the tracking and modeling of radio protection equipment to provide online safety warnings. Another interesting but challenging extension of this system would be to use a body part tracking system in the OR instead of the clinician box tracking that we currently use: this would allow us to compute the accumulation of radiation doses per body part over time, providing very useful information in the long term to clinicians and radio protection officers.

Acknowledgements. This work was supported by French state funds managed by the ANR within the Investissements d'Avenir program under references ANR-11-LABX-0004 (Labex CAMI), ANR-10-IDEX-0002-02 (IdEx Unistra) and ANR-10-IAHU-02 (IHU Strasbourg). The authors would like to thank Siemens and RaySafe for their help with the devices as well as Nicolas Clauss and Ziad El Bitar for interesting discussions.

References

1. Krim, S., Brodecki, M., Carinou, E., Donadille, L., Jankowski, J., Koukorava, C., Dominiek, J., Nikodemova, D., Ruiz-Lopez, N., Sans-Merce, M., Struelens, L., Vanhavere, F.: Extremity doses of medical staff involved in interventional radiology and cardiology: Correlations and annual doses (hands and legs). Radiation Measurements 46(11), 1223–1227 (2011)
2. Koukorava, C., Carinou, E., Ferrari, P., Krim, S., Struelens, L.: Study of the parameters affecting operator doses in interventional radiology using monte carlo simulations. Radiation Measurements 46(11), 1216–1222 (2011)
3. RaySafe: Raysafe i2 active dosimetry system,
   http://www.raysafe.com/en/Products/Staff/RaySafe%20i2
4. Ladikos, A., Cagniart, C., Ghotbi, R., Reiser, M., Navab, N.: Estimating radiation exposure in interventional environments. In: Jiang, T., Navab, N., Pluim, J.P.W., Viergever, M.A. (eds.) MICCAI 2010, Part III. LNCS, vol. 6363, pp. 237–244. Springer, Heidelberg (2010)
5. Bott, O.J., Wagner, M., Duwenkamp, C., Hellrung, N., Dresing, K.: Improving education on C-arm operation and radiation protection with a computer-based training and simulation system. Int. J. Computer Assisted Radiology and Surgery 4(4), 399–407 (2009)
6. Siemens: Artis zeego robotised x-ray imaging system,
   http://www.healthcare.siemens.com/medical-imaging/angio/artis-zee
7. GEANT4, http://geant4.cern.ch/
8. ICRU: Report. Number n 33 in 1956-1964: National Bureau of Standards handbook. International Commission on Radiation Units and Measurements (1980)
9. Siemens: X-ray toolbox,
   https://w9.siemens.com/cms/oemproducts/Home/X-rayToolbox

An Augmented Reality Framework for Soft Tissue Surgery

Peter Mountney[1], Johannes Fallert[2], Stephane Nicolau[3],
Luc Soler[3,4], and Philip W. Mewes[5]

[1] Imaging and Computer Vision, Siemens Corporate Technology, Princeton, NJ, USA
[2] Imaging Technologies Research, Karl Storz, Tuttlingen, Germany
[3] Institut de Recherche contre les Cancers de l'Appareil Digestif (IRCAD),
Strasbourg, France
[4] Institut Hospitalo-Universitaire de Strasbourg (IHU Strasbourg),
Strasbourg, France
[5] Angiography & Interventional X-Ray Systems, Siemens Healthcare, Germany

Abstract. Augmented reality for soft tissue laparoscopic surgery is a growing topic of interest in the medical community and has potential application in intra-operative planning and image guidance. Delivery of such systems to the operating room remains complex with theoretical challenges related to tissue deformation and the practical limitations of imaging equipment. Current research in this area generally only solves part of the registration pipeline or relies on fiducials, manual model alignment or assumes that tissue is static. This paper proposes a novel augmented reality framework for intra-operative planning: the approach co-registers pre-operative CT with stereo laparoscopic images using cone beam CT and fluoroscopy as bridging modalities. It does not require fiducials or manual alignment and compensates for tissue deformation from insufflation and respiration while allowing the laparoscope to be navigated. The paper's theoretical and practical contributions are validated using simulated, phantom, *ex vivo*, *in vivo* and non medical data.

1 Introduction

Interest in augmented reality (AR) for soft tissue surgery, such as liver resection and partial nephrectomy, has grown steadily within the medical community. The role of AR in this context is procedure- and workflow-dependent. It can be used at the beginning of the surgical procedure for intra-operative planning to rapidly identify target anatomy and critical sub surface vessels, or it can facilitate image guidance to display tumor resection margins and improve dissection accuracy [1].

A number of theoretical and practical challenges remain for the translation of such systems into the operating room. The core challenge is registration of the pre-operative image (CT/MRI) with the intra-operative laparoscopic image. This in itself is challenging due to the lack of cross modality landmarks and the laparoscopic camera's small viewing field. Furthermore, surgical procedures require insufflation of the abdomen causing an initial organ shift and tissue deformation, which must be reconciled. The registration problem is further

P. Golland et al. (Eds.): MICCAI 2014, Part I, LNCS 8673, pp. 423–431, 2014.

complicated during the procedure itself due to continuous tissue deformation caused by respiration and tool-tissue interaction.

Due to the complex registration pipeline required to deliver AR to the operating room, current research tends to focus on individual components of the process and do not provide complete solutions. For example, notable work exists in deformable tissue modeling [2,3], dense reconstruction [4,3], non-rigid registration of CT to cone beam CT (CBCT) [5], tissue tracking [6], surface registration [7] and laparoscopic camera pose estimation [8,9].

A handful of end-to-end systems have been proposed for the operating room that rely on additional fiducials, manual registration, or the baseline assumption that tissue is static. Challenges persist in each scenario. Fiducials act as cross modality landmarks and have been attached externally on the patient's skin [10] and to the organ itself [11]. Their use however, can be disruptive to the clinical workflow. Manual registration, on the other hand, requires experts to visually align a 3D model to the laparoscopic image [12]. Accuracy is user dependent even when alignment is constrained with a single cross modality landmark [13]. Finally, as per the static environment assumption, a comprehensive system has been proposed for skull surgery [8], but deformation compromises its accuracy.

This paper proposes an AR framework for intra-operative planning in liver surgery[1]. The novel system registers pre-operative CT and stereo laparoscopic images to a common coordinate system using CBCT and fluoroscopy as bridging modalities. It does not require fiducials or manual model alignment. Tissue deformation caused by insufflation, organ shift and respiration are accounted for along with laparoscopic camera motion. The framework is evaluated on simulated, phantom, *ex vivo*, *in vivo* and non medical data.

2   Method

A key component of the AR system is the introduction of CBCT into the operating room. CBCT machines capture 3D CT-like images and 2D fluoroscopy —in the same coordinate system —while the patient is on the operating table. CBCT and fluoroscopy are used as bridging modalities to co-register pre-operative CT and laparoscopic images. The framework consists of three registration phases: 1) a registration of CT to CBCT (Fig. 1), which takes into account tissue deformation resulting from insufflation 2) a registration of the laparoscope to CT via CBCT coordinate system (Fig. 2), accounting for tissue deformation caused by respiration and 3) a temporal registration of laparoscopic images (Fig. 3), which deals with camera motion and tissue deformation caused by respiration.

2.1   Non Rigid Registration of CT to CBCT

Pre-operative CT and organ segmentation are performed in the days or weeks prior to the operation. With the patient in the supine position, two CT images are captured using a contrast injection at the arterial and venous phases. The images

---

[1] Not currently commercially available.

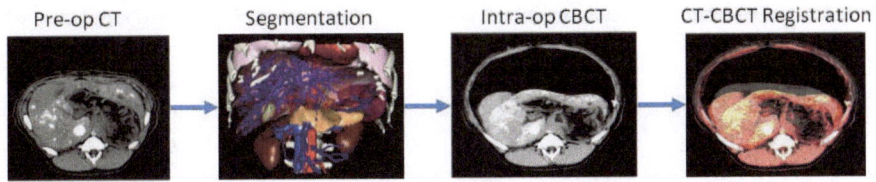

Fig. 1. Registration of pre-operative CT to intra-operative CBCT

are registered together and segmented[2] into 3D anatomical models including the liver, tumor, vessels and abdomen wall as shown in Fig. 1.

During the procedure, the patient is positioned for easy of access (e.g. reverse Trendelenburg) and the abdomen is insufflated with CO_2 causing organ shift and deformation. The tools and laparoscope are removed or positioned safely and a CBCT is acquired during an inhale breath hold. Fig. 1, shows the significant difference between the CT and CBCT images. The CT is registered to the CBCT using a non-rigid biomechanically driven registration technique [5]. This registration approach consists of three steps: 1) rigid alignment of the spine, 2) biomechanical insufflation modeling, and 3) diffeomorphic non-rigid registration. The final deformation field can be applied to the pre-operative planning data and models, thus bringing this information into the CBCT coordinate system.

2.2   Registration of the Laparoscope to CBCT Coordinate System

With the CT to CBCT registration complete, the next task is registering the laparoscope to the CBCT coordinate system. This is challenging due to the lack of cross modality landmarks and the camera's small field of view. A two step registration is proposed- an initial position estimation and local refinement.

The initial position of the laparoscope in the CBCT coordinate system is estimated using fluoroscopic images. A mechanical device holds the laparoscope in position and two mono fluoroscopic images are acquired, each $90°$ apart. A semi-automated method is used to select two points along the shaft which are triangulated to estimate the laparoscope's position and pose with 5 degrees of freedom. The rotation around the laparoscope's optical imaging axis is not estimated due to its symmetrical appearance in the fluoroscopic images. Furthermore, the physical position of the camera center along the shaft is not known, and this introduces additional errors.

A local registration refinement is performed directly between the laparoscopic images and the 3D surface model of the organ in the CBCT coordinate system. At this point in the surgical workflow the patient is not at breath hold. Their breathing is periodic and controlled by a ventilator. This respiration causes the abdominal tissue to deform periodically. The first challenge, therefore, lies in the registration of the laparoscopic images to a 3D model representing the tissue at an inhale breath hold. Registering to any other point in the respiration cycle would introduce error into the system.

---

[2] `www.visiblepatient.com`

Detect Scope in Fluoro   Detect Respiration Phase   Stereo Reconstruction   CT-Scope Registration

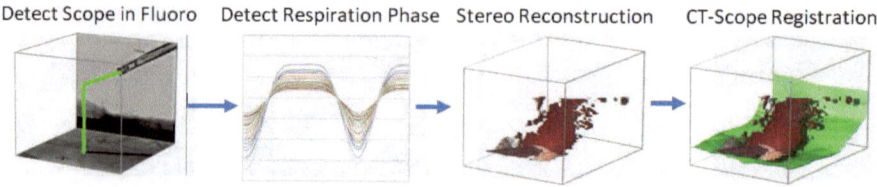

Fig. 2. Registration of laparoscope to CBCT coordinate system

The temporal motion of the tissue in the laparoscopic images is used to estimate the current point in the respiration cycle. Features are detected on the tissue surface and matched in the left and right stereo laparoscope images to estimate their 3D position relative to the camera. The 3D features are transformed into CBCT space using the initial laparoscope alignment and features which are not position near the liver are removed. The features are tracked from frame to frame and their 3D position is computed. Principal Component Analysis (PCA) is applied to extract a 1D respiration signal from the 3D motion of the features [9]. The first component corresponds to respiration, this data is smoothed using a moving average filter to obtain a 1D respiration signal for each feature.

The maximum inhalation position is estimated by fitting a respiration model

$$z(t) = z_0 - bcos^{2n}(\frac{\Pi t}{\tau} - \phi) \tag{1}$$

where z_0 is the position of the liver at the exhale, b is the amplitude, τ is the respiration frequency, ϕ is the phase and n describes the gradient of the model and is empirically set to 4. The parameters of Eq. 1 are estimated using Levenberg-Marquardt minimization algorithm. Before the model is fit, outliers are removed by applying RANSAC to the orientation of the PCA transformation and thresholding the periodicity of the respiration signal which corresponds to τ and ϕ. The remaining inliers are averaged and the model parameters are estimated to identify the point in the respiration cycle corresponding to maximum inhale.

Given the initial estimate of the laparoscope's position and the point in the respiration cycle, the final step remains to perform the direct registration between stereo images and the 3D model. A 3D-3D registration aligns a stereo reconstruction [4] to a point set extracted from the 3D model surface. This point set is extracted using the initial estimate of the laparoscope's position from the previous step, the camera's intrinsic parameters, and z-buffering.

The accurate registration of the 3D model point set and the stereo reconstruction is challenging. At a macro level the point sets represent the same shape, however at a local level they are structurally different because of the way the point sets are generated. The 3D model is continuous, smooth and isotropic. The stereo reconstruction is discretized, contains steps due to pixel level disparity estimates, is anisotropic and may not be a complete surface representation. As a result, even after correct alignment it is impossible to get an exact match for

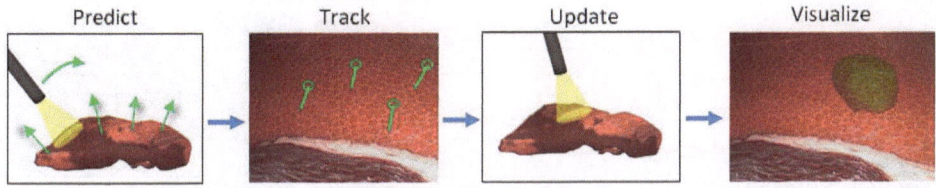

Fig. 3. Temporal registration of laparoscope and tissue

each point. This can cause point-to-point algorithms such as Iterative Closest Point (ICP) to converge a sub-optimal solution as shown in [7].

A probabilistic approach is used [14] that models noise in both the target and source point sets. It makes use of the underlying surface structure while remaining computationally efficient by combines point-to-point and point-to-plane ICP in a single framework. The goal is to align two point sets $A = \{a_i\}_{i=1,\ldots,n}$ and $B = \{b_i\}_{i=1,\ldots,n'}$. The proposed approach replaces the traditional ICP minimization step $\mathbf{T} \leftarrow \mathrm{argmin}_{\mathbf{T}} \sum_i \{\mathbf{T}b_i - m_i\|^2\}$ which finds the optimal transformation $\mathbf{T}$ between point b_i and m_i (the closest corresponding point in A) with

$$\mathbf{T} = \underset{\mathbf{T}}{\mathrm{argmin}} \sum_i \left\{ d_i^{(\mathbf{T})^\top} (C_i^B + \mathbf{T} C_i^A \mathbf{T}^\top)^{-1} d_i^{\mathbf{T}} \right\} \tag{2}$$

where $d_i^{\mathbf{T}} = b_i - \mathbf{T}a_i$ and C_i^A and C_i^B are the covariance matrices used to model noise in the system. By setting high covariance along the local plane and a low covariance along the surface normal, the registration algorithm is guided to use the surface information in both the 3D model point set and the stereo reconstruction point set. The stereo point set is a subset of the 3D model point set. A maximum correspondence distance is empirically set to account for the fact that some points do not have matches.

2.3   Temporal Alignment

Section 2.2 outlined an approach for registering the laparoscope to the CBCT system where the laparoscope is static and the tissue is temporally static, i.e. at maximum inhale. However, during abdominal surgery, tissue and organs are continuously deforming and the surgeon is free to move the laparoscopic camera.

The position of the laparoscopic camera and tissue deformation are jointly estimated using a modified Simultaneous Localization and Mapping (SLAM) technique [9]. This approach models the position and orientation of the camera in conjunction with a dynamic 3D tissue model which is driven by a respiration model. Within an Extended Kalman Filter (EKF) framework the state vector $\hat{x}$ is comprised of the camera position r^W, its orientation R^{RW}, translational velocity v^W and angular velocity w^R and the respiration model parameters estimated in section 2.2 $\{z_0, b, \tau, \phi\}$. In addition, for each feature, the state contains $\hat{y}_i = (\bar{y}, eig)$ where $\bar{y}$ is the average 3D position of the feature and eig is the PCA

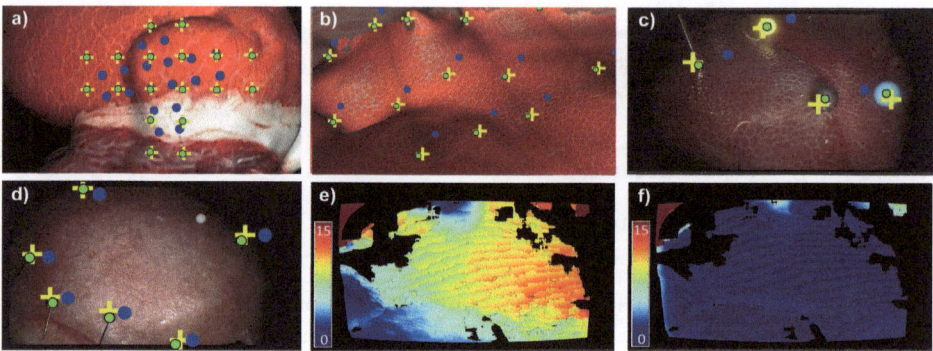

Fig. 4. Laparoscope to CBCT registration: Fiducials shown in green (ground truth), blue (before registration), yellow (after registration). a) non medical, b) sim, c) *ex vivo*, d) phantom. *In vivo* SRE (mm) e) before and f) after registration.

transformation. As shown in Fig. 3, the system iterates between prediction and update steps to estimate the camera's position and tissue deformation. Further details can be found in [9].

The SLAM algorithm initalization follows the registration in section 2.2. As a result, the 3D SLAM features are co-registered to the CBCT coordinate system. In the subsequent image frames, computing the transformation, using singular value decomposition, between the feature positions at time t and time 0 yeilds the estimated 3D model position.

3   Experiments and Results

A range of experiments were performed to validate the proposed framework on simulated, phantom, *ex vivo*, *in vivo* and non medical data. The phases of the pipeline are evaluated separately here, both for clarity and because not all data contain temporal deformation. CT to CBCT obtains accuracy of <1mm on liver, due to space constraints the reader is directed to [5] for evaluation. A description of the datasets follows. **Simulated**: a mesh generated form a CT and textured with laparoscopic images. **Phantom**: a visually realistic silicon liver phantom with surface fiducials for ground truth. **Ex vivo**: porcine with fiducials for ground truth. **In vivo**: two porcine without fiducials. **Non Medical**: meshes from Stanford dataset[3] textured with laparoscopic images.

Registration of laparoscopic camera to CBCT. 50 datasets with ground truth were available- simulated (20), phantom (10), *ex vivo* (10) and non medical (10). Random noise (Up to ±20mm) was added to the initial position of the laparoscope in the CBCT system to quantitatively evaluate the registration. 10 noisy datasets were created for each ground truth dataset, making a total of 500 datasets. 11 *in vivo* datasets were evaluated without ground truth fiducials. The results are shown in Table 1 and illustrated in Fig. 4.

---

[3] http://graphics.stanford.edu/data/3Dscanrep#bunny

Table 1. Quantitative validation: Registration of laparoscope to CBCT

Dataset	SRE Before	SRE After	TRE Before	TRE After
Sim	5.3mm	0.8mm	10.4mm, 289.9 px	1.69mm, 56.8 px
Phantom	5.7mm	1.1mm	10.2mm, 90.5 px	4.1mm, 29.9 px
Ex vivo	4.7mm	1.3mm	10.28mm, 136.5 px	3.4mm, 48.7 px
In vivo	5.4mm	0.9mm	N/A	N/A
Non Medical	5.5mm	0.9mm	10.2mm, 321.2 px	0.3mm, 10.6 px

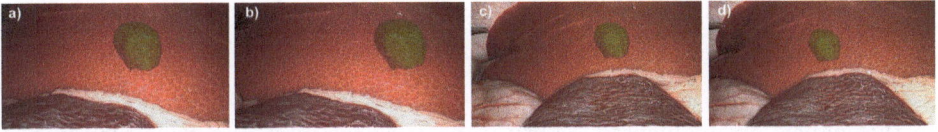

Fig. 5. Augmented reality overlay of a virtual tumor for intra-operative planning

The metrics Surface Registration Error **(SRE)** $= \frac{1}{n}\sum_{i=0}^{n}\{\sqrt{(a_i - m_i)^2}\}$ and Target Registration Error **(TRE)** $= RMSError(Fiducials1 - Fiducials2)$ are used for evaluation. The registration refinement process reduces the TRE for all datasets converging to results of between 0.3-4.1mm. The phantom data has the largest error which is attributed to its homogenous shape. Additional errors may be introduced by manual fiducial annotation. The 2D TRE is dependent on the proximity of the fiducials to the camera and image size. The *in vivo* and *ex vivo* image size is 1280x720 and all others are 1920x1080. The 2D TRE is visualized in Fig. 4. Fig. 4a) shows a successful registration where the added noise is 10° around the optical axis and 10mm along the optical axis. The registration reduces the SRE for all datasets. Fig. 4 e-f) show the SRE for *in vivo* data before and after registration with Fig. 4 f) demonstrates a converged registration. Stereo reconstruction takes 5.1s and registration takes 7.2s however, the proposed surgical workflow does not requrie these step to be real-time.

Temporal registration was quantitatively evaluated on 20 simulated and five *in vivo* datasets. Simulated data was generated by applying a realistic

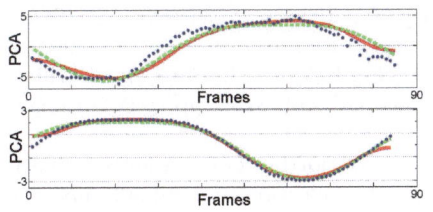

Fig. 6. Respiration model. *in vivo* (top), sim (bot). 1D respiration signal (b), smoothed data (r), model(g).

Table 2. Quantitative evaluation of temporal registration of laparoscopic images

Dataset	TRE Error 3D	Camera Position 3D
Sim	3.6mm	1.9 mm
In vivo	n/a	4.1 mm

biomechanical deformation to the organ model and moving the camera. Evaluation with respect to TRE and camera position are shown in Table 2. For *in vivo* data ground truth was obtained by annotating the position of the scope in fluoro images at the start and end of each sequence. The annotation contains absolute positional errors in the CBCT coordinate system but it can be considered accurate relative to the camera coordinate system. The results are shown in Table 2. Qualitative validation is provided for *in vivo* data in Fig. 5 where a segmented virtual tumor is augmented. This illustrates the accurate estimation of the camera's position and the point in the respiration cycle. The respiration models are visualized in Fig 6. Temporal registration runs at 15fps.

4   Conclusion

In this paper, an augmented reality framework for intra-operative planning is proposed which co-registering pre-operative CT to laparoscope images. It does not require fiducials, manual model alignment and accounts for camera motion and tissue deformation. The framework has been validated on simulated, phantom, *ex vivo* (porcine), *in vivo* (porcine) and non medical data. Future work will focus on improving computational efficiency and more complex tissue modelling.

References

1. Hughes-Hallett, A., Mayer, E.K., Marcus, H.J., Cundy, T.P., Pratt, P.J., Darzi, A.W., Vale, J.A.: Augmented reality partial nephrectomy: Examining the current status and future perspectives. Urology, 266–273 (2013)
2. Allard, J., Cotin, S., Faure, F., Bensoussan, P.J., Poyer, F., Duriez, C., Delingette, H., Grisoni, L.: Sofa-open framework for medical simulation. In: MMVR (2007)
3. Collins, T., Bartoli, A.: Towards live monocular 3d laparoscopy using shading and specularity information. In: Abolmaesumi, P., Joskowicz, L., Navab, N., Jannin, P. (eds.) IPCAI 2012. LNCS, vol. 7330, pp. 11–21. Springer, Heidelberg (2012)
4. Stoyanov, D., Scarzanella, M.V., Pratt, P., Yang, G.-Z.: Real-time stereo reconstruction in robotically assisted minimally invasive surgery. In: Jiang, T., Navab, N., Pluim, J.P.W., Viergever, M.A. (eds.) MICCAI 2010, Part I. LNCS, vol. 6361, pp. 275–282. Springer, Heidelberg (2010)
5. Oktay, O., Zhang, L., Mansi, T., Mountney, P., Mewes, P., Nicolau, S., Soler, L., Chefd'hotel, C.: Biomechanically driven registration of pre- to intra-operative 3D images for laparoscopic surgery. In: Mori, K., Sakuma, I., Sato, Y., Barillot, C., Navab, N. (eds.) MICCAI 2013, Part II. LNCS, vol. 8150, pp. 1–9. Springer, Heidelberg (2013)
6. Puerto Souza, G.A., Adibi, M., Cadeddu, J.A., Mariottini, G.L.: Adaptive multi-affine (AMA) feature-matching algorithm and its application to minimally-invasive surgery images. In: IROS, pp. 2371–2376 (2011)
7. Maier-Hein, L., Franz, A., dos Santos, T., Schmidt, M., Fangerau, M., Meinzer, H., Fitzpatrick, J.: Convergent iterative closest-point algorithm to accomodate anisotropic and inhomogenous localization error. PAMI 34(8), 1520–1532 (2012)

8. Mirota, D., Uneri, A., Schafer, S., Nithiananthan, S., Reh, D., Ishii, M., Gallia, G., Taylor, R., Hager, G., Siewerdsen, J.: Evaluation of a system for high-accuracy 3D image-based registration of endoscopic video to c-arm cone-beam CT for image-guided skull base surgery. Transactions on Medical Imaging 32, 1215–1226 (2013)

9. Mountney, P., Yang, G.Z.: Motion compensated slam for image guided surgery. In: Jiang, T., Navab, N., Pluim, J.P.W., Viergever, M.A. (eds.) MICCAI 2010, Part II. LNCS, vol. 6362, pp. 496–504. Springer, Heidelberg (2010)

10. Nicolau, S.A., Pennec, X., Soler, L., Buy, X., Gangi, A., Ayache, N., Marescaux, J.: An augmented reality system for liver thermal ablation: Design and evaluation on clinical cases. Medical Image Analysis 13(3), 494–506 (2009)

11. Teber, D., Guven, S., Simpfendrfer, T., Baumhauer, M., Gven, E.O., Yencilek, F., Gzen, A.S., Rassweiler, J.: Augmented reality: a new tool to improve surgical accuracy during laparoscopic partial nephrectomy? preliminary in vitro and in vivo results. European Urology 56(2), 332–338 (2009)

12. Su, L.M., Vagvolgyi, B.P., Agarwal, R., Reiley, C.E., Taylor, R.H., Hager, G.D.: Augmented reality during robot-assisted laparoscopic partial nephrectomy: toward real-time 3D-CT to stereoscopic video registration. Urology 73(4), 896–900 (2009)

13. Pratt, P., Mayer, E., Vale, J., Cohen, D., Edwards, E., Darzi, A., Yang, G.Z.: An effective visualisation and registration system for image-guided robotic partial nephrectomy. Journal of Robotic Surgery 6(1), 23–31 (2012)

14. Segal, A., Haehnel, D., Thrun, S.: Generalized-ICP. In: RSS, p. 4 (2009)

Pico Lantern: A Pick-up Projector for Augmented Reality in Laparoscopic Surgery

Philip Edgcumbe[1], Philip Pratt[2], Guang-Zhong Yang[2],
Chris Nguan[3], and Rob Rohling[1,4]

[1] Department of Electrical and Computer Engineering,
University of British Columbia, Vancouver, BC, Canada
{edgcumbe,rohling}@ece.ubc.ca
[2] Hamlyn Centre for Robotic Surgery
Imperial College of Science, Technology and Medicine, London, UK
{p.pratt,g.z.yang}@imperial.ac.uk
[3] Department of Urologic Sciences
University of British Columbia, Vancouver, BC, Canada
chris.nguan@ubcurology.com
[4] Mechanical Engineering, University of British Columbia, Vancouver, BC, Canada

Abstract. The Pico Lantern is proposed as a new tool for guidance in laparoscopic surgery. Its miniaturized design allows it to be picked up by a laparoscopic tool during surgery and tracked directly by the endoscope. By using laser projection, different patterns and annotations can be projected onto the tissue surface. The first explored application is surface reconstruction. The absolute error for surface reconstruction using stereo endoscopy and untracked Pico Lantern for a plane, cylinder and *ex vivo* kidney is 2.0 mm, 3.0 mm and 5.6 mm respectively. The absolute error using a mono endoscope and a tracked Pico Lantern for the same plane, cylinder and kidney is 0.8mm, 0.3mm and 1.5mm respectively. The results show the benefit of the wider baseline produced by tracking the Pico Lantern. Pulsatile motion of a human carotid artery is also detected *in vivo*. Future work will be done on the integration into standard and robot-assisted laparoscopic surgery.

Keywords: pico projector, laparoscopic surgery, augmented reality.

1 Introduction

Laparoscopic surgery is minimally invasive and has several advantages over open surgery. However, one disadvantage is the reduced visibility through the endoscope. In particular, monocular endoscopy reduces the ability to perceive the depth of the tissue surface and spatial relationships. Several companies market stereo endoscopy cameras as a way to improve visual perception, but they are not widely used. Two examples are the Viking 3DHD Vision System (Viking Systems, Westborough, MA, USA) and the Endoeye Flex 3D (Olympus, Shinjuku, Tokyo, Japan).

The da Vinci robotic system for minimally invasive surgery (Intuitive Surgical, Sunnyvale, CA) offers stereo vision and dexterous tele-manipulation of the surgical tools and camera. Because of these advantages it has become the predominant system

P. Golland et al. (Eds.): MICCAI 2014, Part I, LNCS 8673, pp. 432–439, 2014.
© Springer International Publishing Switzerland 2014

for several types of surgery in the United States, such as radical prostatectomy (RP). RP is a common treatment for prostate cancer, the second leading cause of cancer-related deaths for men in the United States. During RPs, preservation of the neurovascular bundle near the prostate helps maintain potency and continence. In this and other applications, there is a clear need for accurate guidance tools in both standard and robotic surgery to see subsurface anatomy such as blood vessels and nerves.

There is a wealth of research on a wide range of guidance tools for minimally invasive surgery. One research area is augmented reality (AR). An early example of AR in laparoscopic surgery used a combination of a camera, projector and helmet-mounted display of computer-generated subsurface anatomy structures [1]. Ongoing challenges include the accurate registration and alignment of the structures with the possibly deformed tissue [2, 3], the transformation of the structures into the endoscope view, and the natural depiction and spatial perception of structures [4].

A common requirement in many surgical guidance tools is the ability to reconstruct the 3D surface of the tissue accurately and quickly. A recent survey paper on this topic [5] provides a highly detailed review of the state of the art. The five main approaches are stereo endoscopy (requiring a stereo endoscope), monocular shape-from-X, SLAM (Simultaneous Localization and Mapping from a moving camera), time-of-flight from a specialized illumination unit, and structured light. All methods have advantages and disadvantages. We are particularly interested in structured light because of its advantages in speed, accuracy, and ability to map even smooth featureless organ surfaces. One approach is a sophisticated multi-spectral fiber-based structured light probe [6]. It has a diameter of 1.7 mm and it can fit in the biopsy channel of an endoscope. It projects 127 differently colored spots which are uniquely identified in the endoscope images. The spot colors are fixed so it cannot project AR.

This paper describes a new low cost (<$500US) source of structured light and AR that leverages recent advances in laser-based pico projectors. It uses the laser diodes and a micro electro mechanical system (MEMS) from the Microvision ShowWX+ projector (Redmond, WA, USA). The proposed system is called a "Pico Lantern" because it is designed to be dropped into the abdominal cavity, then picked up and moved around the cavity to illuminate a region of interest. We have three Pico Lantern prototypes with nearly identical hardware components. The first is the calibrated ShowWX+ projector used for the experiments in this paper. The second separates the integrated photonics module (IPM) and electronics platform module (EPM) of the ShowWX+ projector via a new housing and cabling so that the EPM is kept outside of the patient (Fig. 1). It has the same 3-color functionality as the ShowWX+ projector, a diameter of 28 mm and it can be placed through the skin incision with the cable beside the trocar. It has the same grasp as in Schneider *et al.* [7] so it is compatible with the da Vinci robot. The third prototype (Fig. 1) has a diameter of 12mm and it can be placed through a trocar. In the third prototype two of the three laser diodes have been removed and the one blue laser is in a new location. This prototype is still under development.

As mentioned above, the use of projectors in surgery has a long history [1]. What is new here is leveraging the miniaturization of projectors for consumer electronics to create a pick-up projector for laparoscopic surgery. The Pico Lantern image is always in focus because it has a raster scanning laser pico projector (MEMS scanner mirror: 2.9×2.2×1 mm) and a single-pixel beam expansion that matches the rate of expansion of the projected image size. It can project on any surface, including irregular surfaces, with a higher sharpness, contrast, and color space than non-laser projectors [8].

The Pico Lantern can project different patterns and annotations from a range of positions in the cavity. Thus, augmented reality can be implemented by directly projecting computer-generated structures on the tissue surface using the same coordinate system transformations used to calculate the 3D tissue surface. There are challenges of projecting on curved non-white surfaces, but solutions to these problems have been proposed [9]. It is possible to modify the projected pattern on the curved surface so that it appears undistorted in the endoscope view [10]. Like a real lantern, several other uses for the Pico Lantern could be envisioned in addition to the delivery of structured light. For example, the Pico Lantern could be simply used as a supplementary light source that can cast shadows of small surface features when lit from a shallow angle. It could also reduce undesired bright specular reflections from a constant light source by reducing the illumination of only those reflecting regions (seen in the camera and converted to Pico Lantern coordinates). The da Vinci surgical system is ideal for testing the Pico Lantern because it can hold the Pico Lantern steady in different poses. It also has a stereo endoscope to help reconstruct the 3D tissue surface.

In summary, tests on phantoms and animal tissue demonstrate the feasibility and accuracy of 3D tissue surface reconstruction using the Pico Lantern with a stereo endoscope and mono endoscope. Novel aspects include the explicit tracking of the Pico Lantern, the detection with the Pico Lantern of tiny tissue movement from the pulsatile motion of an underlying blood vessel and showing how the image projected by the Pico Lantern for AR could enhance the appearance of that motion.

2   Methods and Materials

2.1   Materials

A 1280×960 pixel Flea2 camera (Point Grey Research, Richmond, Canada) is used for the laser calibration. All tests are done using a da Vinci Si Surgical System with images of 1280×1024 pixels. The Pico Lantern has an HDMI input, a frame rate of 60 Hz, projection resolution of 848×480 pixels, and a brightness of 15 lumens.

A checkerboard with 3.175 mm squares is affixed onto a flat surface of the Pico Lantern prototypes. The inner 2x6 checks and associated saddle points (suitable for the 12mm prototype) are used for tracking. The checkerboard is made of surgical identification tape (Key Surgical Inc., MN, USA) that is designed to be semi-permanently attached to surgical instruments through repeated sterilization cycles, and it is approved for use in humans [11].

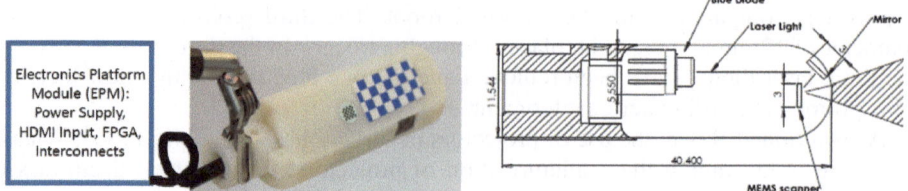

Fig. 1. Picture of Pico Lantern prototype #2 with tether to external electronics platform module (left), and schematic of the Pico Lantern prototype # 3 with units of mm (right)

2.2   3D Surface Reconstruction

Two methods are proposed for 3D surface reconstruction in the two sections below:

2.2.1   Method 1 - Stereo Endoscope and Untracked Pico Lantern

In method 1, the Pico Lantern projects a checkerboard pattern onto the surface for stereo-correspondence determination between left and right cameras to calculate the 3D position of the checkerboard saddle points [12].

2.2.2   Method 2 - Mono endoscope and Tracked Pico Lantern

Method 2 is suitable for either a mono or stereo endoscope; mono vision is used here. The location of the Pico Lantern, in the coordinate system of the endoscope/camera, is determined by visually tracking the checkerboard that is affixed to the Pico Lantern. This enables surface reconstruction using *wide baseline* triangulation with the camera and Pico Lantern at two of the vertices of the triangle.   The 3D position of each projected checkerboard saddle point is at the third vertex of the triangle and is at the intersection of the ray *V* (from P to a saddle point in I, converted using ^IT_P) of the Pico Lantern and the corresponding ray *R* (from C to saddle point in I, converted using ^IT_C) in the camera images (Eqn. 1) [12].

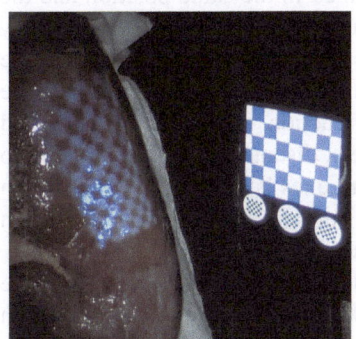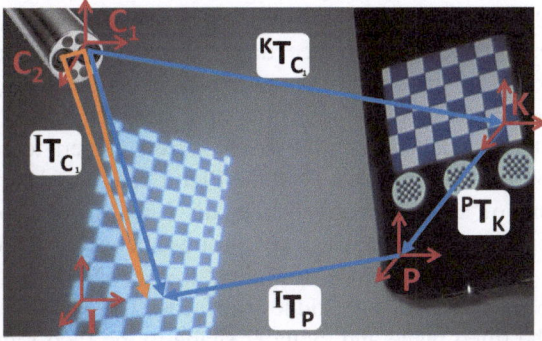

Fig. 2. Projection of blue checkerboard onto an *ex vivo* kidney with medium intensity lighting (40/100) from the da Vinci Si light source (left). Overview of the two methods used for surface reconstruction (right). The orange lines show the narrow-triangle geometry of method 1 and the blue lines show the wider geometry of method 2.

The Caltech Camera Calibration stereo triangulation toolbox [13] is used to solve the scalar parameters S and u to determine the coordinates of the saddle points on the object.§

$$^C\begin{bmatrix} sR_x & sR_y & sR_z & s \end{bmatrix}' = {}^CT_P * {}^P\begin{bmatrix} uV_x & uV_y & uV_z & u \end{bmatrix}' \tag{1}$$

The transformation from the projector to camera coordinate system, ^CT_P, is equal to $^CT_K * {}^KT_P$ where ^CT_K is the transformation from the Key Surgical checkerboard (K) on the Pico Lantern to the camera (C) that is calculated in each camera frame (C), and ^KT_P is the fixed transformation from the Pico Lantern keyhole aperture (P) to the Key Surgical checkerboard (K). ^KT_P is calibrated offline using corresponding points between the known location of projected checkerboard saddle points onto a plane in the Pico Lantern (P) and Key Surgical checkerboard (K) coordinates [14]. Twelve images from the Flea2 camera with 98 points each are used for this calibration. The method uses the Bouguet's Camera Calibration Toolbox [13] which is based on Zhang's algorithm [15]. The key is to model the projector as a camera in reverse. The endoscope cameras are also calibrated for intrinsic and extrinsic parameters [13].

2.2.3   Saddle Point Selection

For method 1 and method 2, regions with saddle points are selected manually, and the saddle point detection algorithm [13] is then used to determine the checkerboard corner locations with sub-pixel accuracy. In the future, an automatic tracking algorithm will be implemented that has been successfully used on porcine [16] and human [17] surgical subjects, hence the extra circular targets in Fig. 2.

2.3   Validation of 3D Surface Reconstruction

The objects for 3D surface reconstruction are a white plane, cylinder (52.63±0.05 mm diameter) and an *ex vivo* porcine kidney for a more realistic appearance of a tissue surface. For each object, the camera and object remained in the same position and the Pico Lantern is moved to 5 different poses within the field of view of the stationary endoscope. The surface data from the 5 poses are then combined together. The identical images and poses are used for evaluating the accuracy of both 3D surface reconstruction methods. For all the surface reconstruction tests, the average and standard deviation of the distance from camera to object, distance from Pico Lantern to object, and angle between the Pico Lantern and camera axes is 166±7 mm, 49±11 mm and 61°±12° respectively. The da Vinci Si endoscope surgical light is set to a medium brightness (40/100) as a compromise between ambient lighting and projected contrast.

For all tests, a Certus optical tracker (NDI, Waterloo, Canada) stylus measured the plane, cylinder and kidney surfaces. The *relative error* is the average distance from the fitted plane and cylinder shape to the Pico Lantern measured surface points. The *absolute error* is the average distance from the Certus measured surfaces of the plane/cylinder/kidney to the Pico Lantern measured surface points. To minimize tissue deformation from the stylus, the kidney is frozen and only the surface is defrosted.

2.4   Augmented Reality Display of Tissue Movement

The Pico Lantern can be used to both *measure* pulsatile motion of a subsurface artery using the above method, and *depict* its motion/location. There are challenges for depicting computer-generated features such as vessels, and suitable visual cues have been proposed by others [4]. Here we propose to simply display dots that are sized in proportion to the surface motion in the frequency domain of 0.82–1.1 Hz over a 10 second period. By combining the checkerboard and dots, measurement and depiction can be simultaneous. The projector and endoscope is pointed towards the carotid artery of the volunteer, and method 2 is used to track the 3D surface map of the region.

3   Results

The 3D surface reconstruction relative error for method 1 was 1.6 ± 1.6 mm for the plane and 2.4 ± 2.1 mm for the cylinder. The relative error for method 2 was 0.8 ± 0.7 mm for the plane, and 0.3 ± 0.3 mm for the cylinder. The absolute error for method 1 was 2.0 ± 1.7 mm for the plane, 3.0 ± 2.9 mm for the cylinder and 5.6 ± 4.9 mm for the kidney. The absolute error for method 2 was 1.4 ± 1.1 mm for the plane, 1.5 ± 0.6 mm for the cylinder and 1.5 ± 0.6 mm for the kidney. During data collection, the range of covered by the Pico Lantern, in the camera coordinate system, was 27×21×49 mm for the plane, 14×53×36 mm for the cylinder and 20×28×29 mm for the kidney. The extent of the *ex vivo* kidney surface included in the surface reconstruction is shown in Fig. 3.

The results of the *in vivo* human test of the pulsatile motion of the neck near the carotid artery is shown in the right of Fig. 3. The dot size corresponds to the magnitude of the pulsatile motion in the frequency range of 0.82–1.1 Hz. The larger dots denotes the carotid artery path that runs vertically through the image on the right side of the checkerboard. The carotid artery path was determined by typical anatomical landmarks and the pulsation sensed by palpation. The top graph in Fig. 3 shows the periodic pulsatile displacement of a saddle point which has a maximum 3D vector magnitude of 0.9mm. The lower graph shows a point that is about 10mm away from the carotid artery and has a maximum displacement of 0.3mm and is not as periodic.

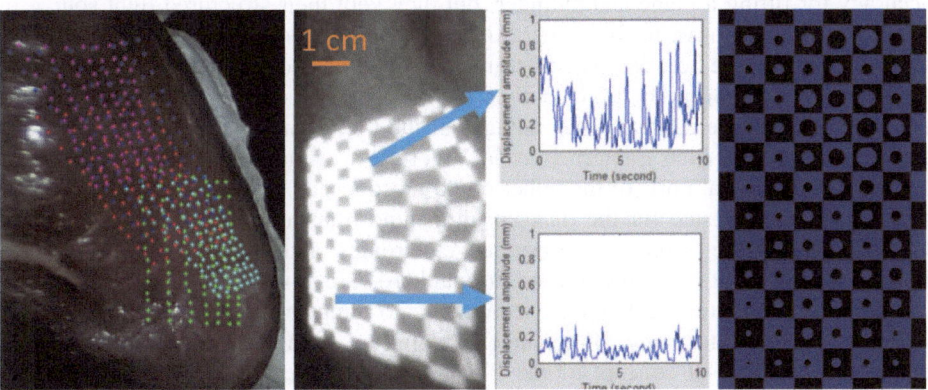

Fig. 3. Endoscope view of the combined surface measurements of the *ex vivo* kidney with the Pico Lantern projector in five different locations (left). Endoscope view while measuring motion of the human neck *in vivo* with graphs showing 10 secs of displacement of the saddle points indicated by the arrows (middle). Depiction of the motion of the carotid artery using dot size: large dots correspond to large motion (right).

4   Discussion and Conclusion

In this paper we have proposed the Pico Lantern, a pick-up laser projector for minimally invasive surgical guidance that is based on low-cost, fast, commercially available technology. We test the surface reconstruction accuracy that can be achieved using the Pico Lantern and show it can stitch multiple views of the surface together.   Method 1 uses a stereo endoscope with an untracked Pico Lantern method and achieves an accuracy comparable to other stereo endoscope results for the plane and cylinder [18]. However, it is sensitive to the detection of the saddle point, so the accuracy decreases for the kidney because a simple correspondence method is used, the surface of the kidney causes the projected image to become blurrier and the stereo endoscope has a small baseline of 5mm. Method 2, the mono endoscope with tracked Pico Lantern, was more accurate and consistent. This is because method 2 has a wide baseline between the camera/endoscope and Pico Lantern and the high-contrast checkerboard on the Pico Lantern make it easy to accurately track. Other potential advantages of method 2 include: easier identification of the structured light features in the endoscope view since the Pico Lantern rays can be calculated in camera coordinates; mono-vision endoscopy to be used in 3D surface reconstruction; particular effectiveness compared to other technique on tissues with a low density of natural and unique surface features; it can cover a wide region of interest by stitching reconstructed surfaces together; the surgeon can move the Pico Lantern as close as necessary to achieve desired accuracy/field-of-view tradeoff; an effective way to add AR which only requires the laparoscopic video feed and does not require any change to the laparoscopic hardware.   The sub-millimeter level relative accuracy of the method 2 mono endoscope approach compares very favorably to surface reconstruction techniques in which a single mono endoscope is used with no additional components.   As mentioned previously, Clancy *et al.* used a mono-endoscope and multi-spectral illumination and reported sub-millimeter relative accuracy for fitting a plane and cylinder, but they kept their structured light source in a fixed position relative to the camera throughout the experiment and did not report the baseline distance between the structured light source and mono endoscope [6].

A disadvantage of method 2 is that the Pico Lantern must be in the field of view of the endoscope. More general disadvantages of the Pico Lantern are: the need to grasp and manipulate the Pico Lantern (the da Vinci 3rd arm may be a solution); a tether through an additional port (or the tether could be squeezed between an existing trocar and tissue, as suggested for the pick-up ultrasound transducer [7]); the brightness is limited (this is the same for consumer electronics and luminance continues to improve); the Pico Lantern requires additional hardware, unlike stereo endoscopy.

As pico projector technology continues to improve, we will see further improvements in accuracy, luminance, resolution, miniaturization and cost. In conclusion, a proof-of-concept of the Pico Lantern suggests sub-millimeter surface reconstruction is possible and could be used for detecting and displaying subsurface pulsatile vessel motion. The next steps include sterilization and clinical validation.

Acknowledgements. This work was funded by CIHR and NSERC and proudly funded by Prostate Cancer Canada – Grant # GS2014-05. Thanks to Caitlin Schneider and Tim Salcudean for advice, help and equipment.

References

1. Fuchs, H., et al.: Augmented Reality Visualization for Laparoscopic Surgery. In: Wells, W.M., Colchester, A.C.F., Delp, S.L. (eds.) MICCAI 1998. LNCS, vol. 1496, pp. 934–943. Springer, Heidelberg (1998)

2. Pratt, P., Stoyanov, D., Visentini-Scarzanella, M., Yang, G.-Z.: Dynamic Guidance for Robotic Surgery Using Image-Constrained Biomechanical Models. In: Jiang, T., Navab, N., Pluim, J.P.W., Viergever, M.A. (eds.) MICCAI 2010, Part I. LNCS, vol. 6361, pp. 77–85. Springer, Heidelberg (2010)

3. Benincasa, A.B., Clements, L.W., Duke Herrell, S., Galloway, R.L.: Feasibility study for image-guided kidney surgery: Assessment of required intraoperative surface for accurate physical to image space registrations. Med. Phys. 35(9), 4251–4261 (2008)

4. Hansen, C., Wieferich, J., Ritter, F., Rieder, C., Peitgen, H.-O.: Illustrative Visualization of 3D Planning Models for Augmented Reality in Liver Surgery. IJCARS 5, 133–141 (2010)

5. Maier-Hein, L., Mountney, P., Bartoli, A., Elhawary, H., Elson, D., Groch, A., Kolb, A., Rodrigues, M., Sorger, J., Speidel, S., Stoyanov, D.: Optical Techniques for 3D Surface Reconstruction in Computer-Assisted Laparoscopic Surgery. Med. Img. 17, 974–996 (2013)

6. Clancy, N.T., Stoyanov, D., Maier-Hein, L., Groch, A., Yang, G.-Z., Elson, D.S.: Spectrally Encoded Fiber-Based Structured Lighting Probe for Intraoperative 3D Imaging. Biomedical Optics Express 2(11), 3119–3128 (2011)

7. Schneider, C., Guerrero, J., Nguan, C., Rohling, R., Salcudean, S.: Intra-operative "Pick-Up" Ultrasound for Robot Assisted Surgery with Vessel Extraction and Registration: A Feasibility Study. In: Taylor, R.H., Yang, G.-Z. (eds.) IPCAI 2011. LNCS, vol. 6689, pp. 122–132. Springer, Heidelberg (2011)

8. Lincoln, J.: March of the Pico Projectors. IEEE Spectrum 47, 40–45 (2010)

9. Park, H., Lee, M.-H., Kim, S.-J., Park, J.-I.: Surface-Independent Direct-Projected Augmented Reality. In: Narayanan, P.J., Nayar, S.K., Shum, H.-Y. (eds.) ACCV 2006. LNCS, vol. 3852, pp. 892–901. Springer, Heidelberg (2006)

10. Tardif, J.P., Roy, S., Meunier, J.: IEEE: Projector-based augmented reality in surgery without calibration. In: IEEE EMBS, pp. 548–551. IEEE Press, New York (2003)

11. Edgcumbe, P., Nguan, C., Rohling, R.: Calibration and Stereo Tracking of a Laparoscopic Ultrasound Transducer for Augmented Reality in Surgery. In: Liao, H., Linte, C.A., Masamune, K., Peters, T.M., Zheng, G. (eds.) MIAR 2013 and AE-CAI 2013. LNCS, vol. 8090, pp. 258–267. Springer, Heidelberg (2013)

12. Geng, J.: Structured-Light 3D Surface Imaging: a Tutorial. Advances in Optics and Photonics 3, 128–160 (2011)

13. Bouguet, J.-Y.: Visual Methods for Three-dimensional Modeling, Phd Thesis (1999)

14. Falcao, G., Hurtos, N., Massich, J., Fofi, D.: Projector-Camera Calibration Toolbox. Erasumus Mundus Masters in Vision and Robotics (2009)

15. Zhang, Z.: A Flexible New Technique for Camera Calibration. IEEE T PAMI 22, 1330–1334 (2000)

16. Pratt, P., Di Marco, A., Payne, C., Darzi, A., Yang, G.-Z.: Intraoperative ultrasound guidance for transanal endoscopic microsurgery. In: Ayache, N., Delingette, H., Golland, P., Mori, K. (eds.) MICCAI 2012, Part I. LNCS, vol. 7510, pp. 463–470. Springer, Heidelberg (2012)

17. Hughes-Hallett, A., Pratt, P., Mayer, E., Di Marco, A., Yang, G.-Z., Vale, J., Darzi, A.: Intraoperative Ultrasound Overlay in Robot-assisted Partial Nephrectomy: First Clinical Experience. Eur. Urol. 65(3), 671–672 (2014)

18. Röhl, S., Bodenstedt, S., Suwelack, S., Dillmann, R., Speidel, S., Kenngott, H., Müller-Stich, B.P.: Dense GPU-Enhanced Surface Reconstruction From Stereo Endoscopic Images for Intraoperative Registration. Med. Phys. 39, 1632–1645 (2012)

Efficient Stereo Image Geometrical Reconstruction at Arbitrary Camera Settings from a Single Calibration

Songbai Ji[1,2], Xiaoyao Fan[1], David W. Roberts[2,3], and Keith D. Paulsen[1,2,3]

[1] Thayer School of Engineering, Dartmouth College, Hanover, NH 03755, USA
[2] Geisel School of Medicine, Dartmouth College, Hanover, NH 03755, USA
[3] Dartmouth Hitchcock Medical Center, Lebanon, NH 03756, USA
{songbai.ji,xiaoyao.fan,david.w.roberts,
keith.d.paulsen}@dartmouth.edu

Abstract. Camera calibration is central to obtaining a quantitative image-to-physical-space mapping from stereo images acquired in the operating room (OR). A practical challenge for cameras mounted to the operating microscope is maintenance of image calibration as the surgeon's field-of-view is repeatedly changed (in terms of zoom and focal settings) throughout a procedure. Here, we present an efficient method for sustaining a quantitative image-to-physical space relationship for arbitrary image acquisition settings (S) without the need for camera re-calibration. Essentially, we warp images acquired at S into the equivalent data acquired at a reference setting, S_0, using deformation fields obtained with optical flow by successively imaging a simple phantom. Closed-form expressions for the distortions were derived from which 3D surface reconstruction was performed based on the single calibration at S_0. The accuracy of the reconstructed surface was 1.05 mm and 0.59 mm along and perpendicular to the optical axis of the operating microscope on average, respectively, for six phantom image pairs, and was 1.26 mm and 0.71 mm for images acquired with a total of 47 arbitrary settings during three clinical cases. The technique is presented in the context of stereovision; however, it may also be applicable to other types of video image acquisitions (e.g., endoscope) because it does not rely on any *a priori* knowledge about the camera system itself, suggesting the method is likely of considerable significance.

1   Introduction

Camera images provide texture intensity from the surface of objects in the scene, and are an increasingly popular form of data in image-guided procedures such as neurosurgery [1]. Calibration is central to obtaining quantitative geometrical information from the camera system to project 2D image pixels into their 3D coordinates in physical space in the case of stereovision. Techniques for calibrating a camera system at fixed zoom and focal settings are well studied [2]. However, many cameras offer a wide range of zoom factors and focal lengths that can be arbitrarily varied to obtain an optimal view [3]; thus, maintenance of camera calibration becomes a practical challenge. Because these images depend on acquisition settings, recovering the camera calibration parameters efficiently and for an arbitrary setting is

P. Golland et al. (Eds.): MICCAI 2014, Part I, LNCS 8673, pp. 440–447, 2014.

essential for applications like stereovision in the operating room (OR) where the surgeon is repeatedly altering the field-of-view through the operating microscope.

Existing techniques for camera calibration at an arbitrary setting either actively re-calibrate at a given setting on-demand [3] or interpolate camera parameters via bivariate fitting by explicitly modeling each as a polynomial function of zoom and focal length based on data from a dense set of pre-calibrations [4, 5]. Although calibration at a given setting can be fully automated with an on-demand approach [2], repeatedly imaging an instrumented calibration target [3] is inconvenient and cumbersome in the OR. While interpolation of pre-determined camera parameters minimizes disruption of surgical workflow, a dense combination of zoom and focal length settings have to be calibrated (and re-calibrated for quality assurance and/or when camera extrinsic parameters are changed, e.g., from repositioning) which too adds to pre-operative activity and personnel time requirements. Consequently, suggestions of a fixed zoom and focus have been made to ensure optimal accuracy [5], but such restrictions significantly limit the effective OR use of camera systems.

In this study, we present a method to recover geometry from stereo images at arbitrary camera settings using a single calibration at a fixed (reference) zoom and focal setting. The approach is especially appealing for OR applications because it does not disrupt surgical workflow nor does it require tedious calibration at numerous zoom-focus combinations. The performance of the technique is evaluated on a physical phantom and in three clinical cases involving open cranial surgery with a microscope-mounted stereovision system. However, the general strategy appears to be applicable to other types of stereo/video images (e.g., endoscope).

2 Material and Methods

A custom-designed stereovision system consisting of two C-mount cameras (Flea2 model FL2G-50S5C-C, Point Grey Research Inc., Richmond, BC, Canada) was rigidly mounted to a Zeiss surgical microscope (OPMI® Pentero™, Carl Zeiss, Inc., Oberkochen, Germany) through a binocular port [6]. The position and orientation of the microscope was available from a StealthStation® navigation system via StealthLink (Medtronic, Inc., Louisville, CO) through a rigidly-attached tracker. In addition, the microscope zoom, m, and focal length, f, are also directly available from StealthLink, which eliminates the need to manually record the acquisition settings.

The technical details of stereovision calibration at a single acquisition setting and subsequent surface reconstruction have been well studied [2]. Both the left (I_L) and right (I_R) camera images depend on image acquisition settings such as m and f. Conceptually, the following functional forms define the images acquired:

$$I_L = G_L(m, f), \text{ and } I_R = G_R(m, f) . \tag{1}$$

For notational simplicity, we drop the subscripts throughout the rest of the paper when an image is not specifically associated with either the left (L) or right (R) camera. We also denote the image acquired at a set of reference settings, S_0, as $I_0 = G(m_0, f_0)$, which represents the lowest magnification (m_0) and shortest focal length (f_0) that the microscope offers. The choice of S_0 is selected for convenience because of the ease with which the microscope can be returned to these settings;

however, a different set of reference settings or multiple settings could be utilized (see Discussion). An image obtained at an arbitrary setting, S, is referred to as a "deformed" image ($I = G(m, f)$). The "deformation field" relating the deformed image to the reference or "undeformed" image is found via optical flow (OF) motion-tracking, which has been well studied [7] and successfully employed in image-guided procedures [1] including stereovision in neurosurgery [6]. Essentially, our technique for stereovision reconstruction at S warps the deformed images into the reference image as if the data were acquired at S_0 using deformation/distortion fields obtained from a series of phantom images. Because stereo images at S_0 have been calibrated, the warped stereo images acquired at S can then be reconstructed with the same single calibration once the warping is complete.

2.1   Image Deformation due to the Change in Acquisition Settings

To determine image deformation due to the change in image acquisition settings, m and f, a phantom was created by printing squares in random positions and intensities on paper. The phantom was first imaged at the reference setting, S_0, and then a series of images was acquired by successively changing either m or f (while maintaining the partnered parameter at its respective reference value). Image acquisitions at multiple m values at each f settings were unnecessary because the resulting 2D image deformation induced by a change in m was independent of f settings, at least for the Zeiss Pentero surgical microscope based on setting values from StealthLink.

Because the OF algorithm is designed to detect small displacements, deformation fields between images obtained from two adjacent m or f values (instead of relative to the reference values) were computed. The resulting displacement vectors were found to vary radially relative to the focal point along the optical axis (Fig. 1). Thus, a local cylindrical coordinate system was established with its origin at the focal point in order to fit the deformation field as a function of radial distance, r. Because the OF algorithm can produce artifacts especially in image corners with poor lighting conditions, regions near the boundary (<100 pixels) were excluded from the processing. A least-squares linear fitting was found to be sufficient to represent the deformation field (difference between the measured and recovered values was 0.06 pixels on average with a maximum value of 0.2 in the region used for fitting). This procedure yielded an analytical expression for the magnitude of radial displacement

$$F_m^{i \to (i-1)}(r) = k_m^{i \to (i-1)} r \text{ , and } F_f^{i \to (i-1)}(r) = k_f^{i \to (i-1)} r \text{ ,} \tag{2}$$

where $k_m^{i \to (i-1)}$ and $k_f^{i \to (i-1)}$ are linear scaling factors independently determined from fitting the deformation fields obtained from image pairs acquired at the ith and $(i-1)^{st}$ setting of m and f, respectively (Fig. 1).

The following pseudo-algorithm summarizes the process of generating and fitting image deformation fields resulting from changes in m and f:

1.   Set $f = f_0$, successively increase m from m_0 in small steps to acquire images at each setting. Compute deformation field between images obtained from two adjacent m values, and determine the corresponding scaling factor, $k_m^{i \to (i-1)}$;

2. Set $m = m_0$, successively increase f from f_0 in small steps to acquire images at each setting. Compute deformation field between images obtained from two adjacent f values, and determine the corresponding scaling factor, $k_f^{i\to(i-1)}$.

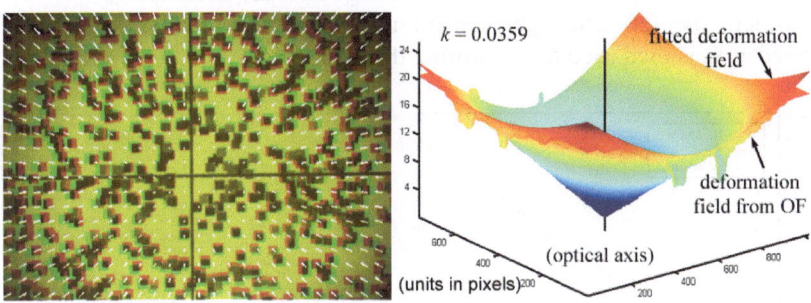

Fig. 1. Typical deformation field for $F_m^{i\to(i-1)}(r)$ (analogous for $F_f^{i\to(i-1)}(r)$, not shown). Left: overlays of undeformed (red) and deformed (green) images and the resulting displacement field (reduced lighting condition is evident in the corners). Right: magnitudes of radial displacements (measured and fitted) expressed in a cylindrical coordinate system with the optical axis focal point as the origin (unit in pixels). The corresponding linear scaling factor is also shown.

2.2   Image Warping into Reference Setting

Because the deformation scaling factors were obtained between two adjacent m and f values, tracking the position of each individual pixel in the current image (acquired at m or f; in the local cylindrical coordinate system) through the chain of image deformations is required to warp it into the equivalent position acquired at m_0 or f_0. For example, the corresponding position of a specific pixel in the image acquired at setting m^i, can readily be obtained in the image acquired at m^{i-1} as $r \times (1 + k_m^{i\to(i-1)})$. Following the chain of deformation scaling, the corresponding pixel location at m_0, and analogously, at f_0, is obtained with the closed-form equation

$$P_m^{i\to0}(r) = r\prod(1 + k_m^{i\to(i-1)}), \text{ and } P_f^{i\to0}(r) = r\prod(1 + k_f^{i\to(i-1)}). \tag{3}$$

The resulting ratios define the "pixel cumulative radial scaling (PCRS)" in the local cylindrical coordinate system with respect to m and f. Based on the set of m and f values at which phantom images were acquired, the corresponding characteristic curves can be found that define the image deformation behavior of the stereovision system (Fig. 2). These curves were further fit to a polynomial form in order to warp images acquired at arbitrary m or f values (ratios were constrained to 1.0 at the reference settings). A third-order polynomial was sufficient to produce differences with respect to the measured data that were less than 5×10^{-5} for both m and f. The same measurement and data-fitting schemes were applied to both the left and right camera images of the stereovision system. We found that the characteristic curves were virtually identical in the two cases (difference $<10^{-3}$).

The following pseudo-algorithm summarizes the procedure to warp an image acquired at an arbitrary setting, S, into the reference setting, S_0:

1. Use the fitted data, $P_m^{i \to 0}(r)$, to interpolate the PCRS for the given m;
2. Re-position pixels and interpolate image as if acquired at (m_0, f);
3. Use the fitted data, $P_f^{i \to 0}(r)$, to interpolate the PCRS for the given f;
4. Re-position pixels and interpolate image as if acquired at (m_0, f_0).

After both the left and right camera images were warped into S_0, calibration performed at S_0 is then used to reconstruct the 3D surface.

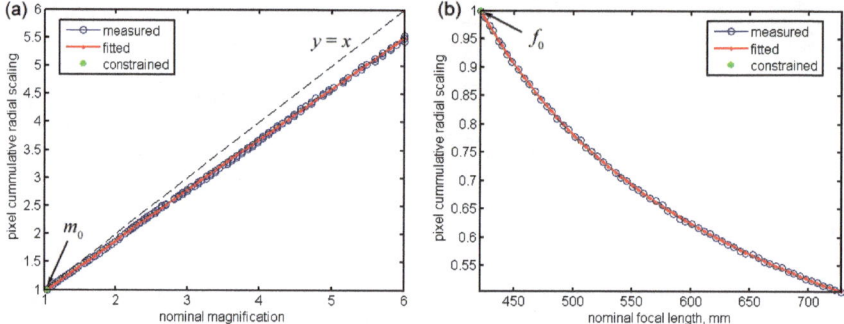

Fig. 2. Characteristic PCRS curves with respect to (a) magnification, m, and (b) microscope focal length, f, for the left camera. The characteristic curves for the right camera (not shown) were virtually identical (difference $< 10^{-3}$). The measured radial scaling ratios were fit to a third-order polynomial with ratios constrained to 1.0 at the reference points, m_0 and f_0.

2.3   Data Analysis

Six combinations of (m, f) were arbitrarily selected to evaluate the performance of our technique on a phantom skull with hand-drawn feature lines. Images acquired with 47 arbitrary zoom and focal settings, S, during 3 epilepsy surgeries were also considered. For each S, a pair of stereo images of the exposed surface was acquired, warped, and reconstructed into a 3D surface. The "ground-truth" surface was also reconstructed using image pairs acquired at S_0. For each object (phantom or cortical surface), the overlapping region of all reconstructed surfaces corresponded to the same physical surface, and allowed the reconstruction accuracy at S to be measured as the average surface nodal distances along (d_1) and perpendicular to (d_2) the optical axis of the microscope based on the triangulated surfaces. To compute the lateral distance (i.e., d_2), the two texture-encoded surfaces were projected onto the XY-plane in a local coordinate system (with the optical axis as the Z-axis), and an average displacement magnitude was obtained through OF motion tracking. Finally, the accuracy of the "ground-truth" surface reconstructed at S_0 was evaluated using independently sampled points acquired from a tracked stylus to report an average relative distance between two sets of homologous points (e.g., vessel intersections).

3   Results

Table 1 summarizes d_1 and d_2 for two arbitrary settings, S, from the phantom skull and from each of the 3 patient cases (m and f ranged 1.02–6.05 and 417.9–728.2 mm, respectively). Based on all settings tested, the average accuracies of d_1 and d_2 were 1.05 ± 0.33 mm (range 0.59–1.4 mm) and 0.59 ± 0.32 mm (range 0.15–0.79 mm) for the phantom, and 1.26 ± 0.31 mm (range 0.61–1.90 mm) and 0.71 ± 0.39 mm (range 0.08–1.56 mm) for the patient cases, respectively. The average accuracy in terms of point-to-point distances between homologous features on the surfaces reconstructed at S_0 using independently sampled probe tip data was 1.57 ± 0.27 mm (based on a total of 16 data points from 3 patient cases). Fig. 3 illustrates the reconstructed surfaces from the phantom skull and cortical surfaces from the 3 patient cases using camera calibration at S_0 and the corresponding surfaces formed from images acquired at a selected arbitrary setting, S, by the warping technique described in Section 2.2. For comparison of reconstruction accuracy, independently sampled probe points from a tracked stylus are also shown together with their homologous features on the cortical surfaces reconstructed at S_0.

Table 1. Summary of d_1 and d_2 (in mm) between surfaces reconstructed at S_0 and S at representative settings (m, f) for phantom and patient cases, as well as their average values ($\overline{d_1}$ and $\overline{d_2}$) from all settings tested (n is the number of settings tested for each case)

Parame ter	Phan- tom	Phan- tom	Patient 1	Patient 1	Patient 2	Patient 2	Patient 3	Patient 3
M	1.20	4.30	3.02	4.43	2.71	2.16	3.65	6.03
F	417.9	501.7	472.2	545.2	520.9	420.2	521.1	728.2
d_1	0.59	1.40	1.08	1.32	1.65	0.82	1.38	1.54
d_2	0.55	0.35	0.74	0.66	0.10	0.20	0.63	0.84
$\overline{d_1}$	1.05±0.33 (n=6)		1.13±0.24 (n=24)		1.34±0.39 (n=11)		1.44±0.24 (n=12)	
$\overline{d_2}$	0.59±0.32		0.90±0.33		0.51±0.44		0.48±0.28	

4   Discussion and Conclusion

Efficient image reconstruction at an arbitrary camera setting is critical for effective deployment of intraoperative stereovision especially when the data is presented in the operating room (OR). We have described a simple, yet effective strategy for maintaining quantitative correspondence of camera image data with physical OR coordinates despite intraoperative changes in camera zoom and focal length settings based on a one-time collection of images of a planar phantom from which the deformation field is derived to warp subsequent images acquired at arbitrary settings. The resulting sub-millimeter to millimeter accuracy of the reconstructed surfaces at arbitrary settings relative to "ground-truth" especially in the clinical cases (maximum d_1 and d_2 error of 1.90 mm and 1.56 mm, respectively) was excellent, particularly since the magnitude of cortical surface pulsation, itself, can be up to 1 mm [6]. Since our approach does not require (repeatedly) imaging a calibration target, it is especially appealing for applications in the OR because it does not interrupt surgical workflow. Similarly to fitting individual camera parameters into bivariate functions of m and f [4, 5], image acquisitions of a phantom are still necessary with our approach (in order to derive 2D image deformation fields). However, instead of requiring as many as $p \times q$ individual settings (p and q are the number of discrete m and f settings needed to calibrate, respectively; [4, 5]), the number of image acquisitions required with our method is limited to $p + q$ because the 2D image deformation induced by a change in m does not depend on f settings for the Zeiss Pentero surgical microscope. If such independence does not hold elsewhere, our method would similarly require $p \times q$ acquisitions. However, our strategy only needs to model 1D radial scaling (or 2D deformation at worst) instead of 11 camera parameters explicitly for every calibration. In addition, accurate interpolation of parameters (Fig. 2) can be obtained with sparse (m, f) pairs because of the smooth deformation field (Fig. 1). In contrast, conventional methods require dense (m, f) pairs because of the jagged/nonlinear parametric surfaces [4]. The simple radial scaling is sufficient to accurately characterize the induced image deformations, as expected from a pinhole camera model. The closed-form expressions for the PCRS curves (Eqn. 3) further simplify our approach because they allow image deformation to be easily interpolated and images to be efficiently warped to the reference setting for accurate 3D reconstruction. When a closed analytical form is otherwise not available (e.g., perhaps for a different camera system), a chain of *implicit* deformation fields can still be used to interpolate and warp the images, in which case the general concept of image warping to a reference setting for reconstruction would be applicable as well.

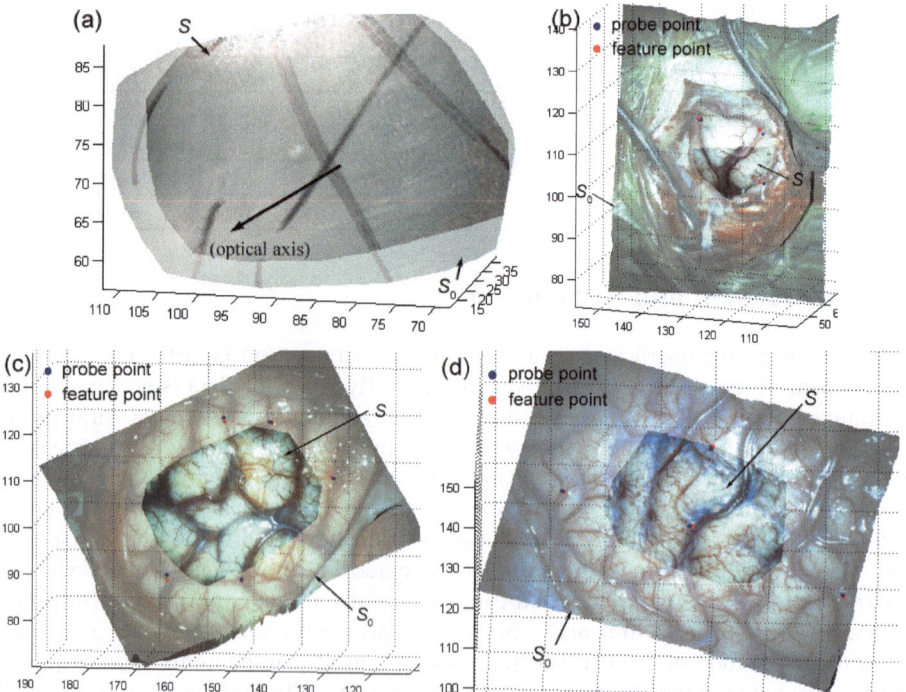

Fig. 3. Overlays of reconstructed surfaces using the reference setting S_0 and an arbitrary setting S for the phantom (a) and three patient cases (c–d) in MR image space (units in mm). Surfaces reconstructed at S (manually masked) through the warping technique virtually coincide with their counterparts reconstructed at S_0. Independently sampled probe points from a tracked stylus are shown together with their homologous feature locations on the cortical surfaces.

We chose the lowest m and f values as the reference setting in this study because of the ease with which the microscope can be manually returned to this state. Because image reconstruction was performed at a single calibration setting, some loss of resolution or reduction in the field of view occurs when images are acquired at a higher m or f, respectively. However, our technique can be extended by calibrating the camera system at a small number of discrete reference settings, e.g., at higher m and/or f values. For each new reference setting, the PCRS curves can be re-established using the same set of phantom planar images without re-collection.

Essentially, our reconstruction framework treats the calibration process as a transfer function by directly modeling the smooth (and hence, more accurate) relationship between input (changes in m, f) and output (image warping) instead of intermediate parameters that are often nonlinear and co-dependent in parametric space [4]. Therefore, we expect that our general image warping strategy will be advantageous and important for broad deployment of intraoperative stereovision and applicable to other types of stereo/video images as well (e.g., endoscope) because it does not rely on any *a priori* knowledge about the camera system itself other than the induced image deformation remaining constant and being reproducible. In addition, the general strategy does not dictate the specific techniques used for calibration at the reference setting or 3D surface reconstruction [1, 2], suggesting this methodological approach has potential to be of considerable clinical significance.

Acknowledgement. This work was supported in part by National Institutes of Health grant number R01 CA159324–01 and 1R21 NS078607.

References

1. Mirota, D.J., Ishii, M., Hager, G.D.: Vision-based navigation in image-guided interventions. Annual Review of Biomedical Engineering 13, 297–319 (2011)
2. Hemayed, E.E.: A survey of camera self-calibration. In: Proceedings of the IEEE Conference on Advanced Video and Signal Based Surveillance, pp. 351–357 (2003)
3. Figl, M., Ede, C., Hummel, J., Wanschitz, F., Ewers, R., Bergmann, H., Birkfellner, W.: A fully automated calibration method for an optical see-through head-mounted operating microscope with variable zoom and focus. IEEE Trans. Med. Imag. 24(11), 1492–1499 (2005)
4. Willson, R.: Modeling and Calibration of Automated Zoom Lenses, CMU-RI-TR-94-03, Robotics Institute, Carnegie Mellon University (1994)
5. Edwards, P.J., King, A.P., Maurer, C.R., de Cunha, D.A., Hawkes, D.J., Hill, D.L., Gaston, R.P., Fenlon, M.R., Jusczyzck, A., Strong, A.J., Chandler, C.L., Gleeson, M.J.: Design and evaluation of a system for microscope-assisted guided interventions (MAGI). IEEE Trans. Med. Imag. 19(11), 1082–1093 (2000)
6. Ji, S., Fan, X., Roberts, D.W., Paulsen, K.D.: Cortical surface strain estimation using stereovision. In: Fichtinger, G., Martel, A., Peters, T. (eds.) MICCAI 2011, Part I. LNCS, vol. 6891, pp. 412–419. Springer, Heidelberg (2011)
7. Liu, C.: Beyond Pixels: Exploring New Representations and Applications for Motion Analysis. Doctoral Thesis. Massachusetts Institute of Technology (May 2009)

A Compact Active Stereovision System with Dynamic Reconfiguration for Endoscopy or Colonoscopy Applications

Yingfan Hou[1], Erwan Dupont[1], Tanneguy Redarce[2], and Frederic Lamarque[1]

[1] Université de Technologie de Compiègne (UTC), Laboratory Roberval(UMR 7337),
1, rue du Dr Schweitzer 60200 Compiègne, France
yingfan.hou@utc.fr
[2] Institut National des Sciences Appliquées de Lyon (INSA-Lyon), Laboratoire
Ampère(UMR 5005), 20 av Albert Einstein 69100 Villeurbanne, France
tanneguy.redarce@insa-lyon.fr

Abstract. A new concept of endoscopic device based on a compact optical probe which can capture 3D shape of objects using an active stereovision method is presented. The distinctive feature of this probe is its capability to dynamically switch between two distinct points of view. If the first measurement angle of view does not give results with sufficient quality, the system can switch to a second mode which sets distinct angle of view within less than 25 milliseconds. This feature consequently allows selecting the angle that provides the more useful 3D information and enhances the quality of the captured result.

The instrumental setup of this measurement system and the reconstruction algorithms are presented in this paper. Then, the advantages of this new endoscopic probe are explained with an experimental 3D reconstruction of a coin's surface. Finally, first measurements on a phantom colon are provided. In future works, further miniaturization of the device and its integration into a real colonoscope will be implemented.

1 Introduction

Recent advances in the technology of medical devices have allowed for the surgeons to provide more precise and reliable diagnosis and for the patient a quicker recovery time and shorter hospital stays. Miniaturization is one of these advances with technologies such as swallowable wireless capsule endoscopy in [1], or more generally the various technologies employed in Minimally Invasive Surgery (MIS) [2]. Many researchers have presented great perspectives of endoscopy or colonoscopy in detecting small objects and minimizing invasiveness at the same time.

Using computer vision algorithm with enhanced endoscopy or colonoscopy devices offers a convenient way to obtain accurate 3D surface information. In [3], Schmalz et al. have proposed an endoscopic 3D scanner with single-shot-color-ring pattern structured light, which offers an axial resolution of less than $200 \mu m$ for the reconstructed surface. Maurice et al. [4] have presented a laparoscope

P. Golland et al. (Eds.): MICCAI 2014, Part I, LNCS 8673, pp. 448–455, 2014.

with real-time organs' surface reconstruction in MIS. These devices are both based on projection of one static pattern.

There is a great variety of methods to achieve 3D reconstruction in a medical environment, such as fringe projection [5], stereo matching [6], structure from shading [7], shape from motion [8] , time of flight [9] etc. Although all these methods have their own pros and cons, it is still a challenging problem to obtain accurate 3D results in gastrointestinal condition or in MIS.

Active stereovision is one of these methods. Its principle is to project patterns on the measured surface from a first angle of view and to capture the image of the patterns from a second angle of view. Through this triangulation, the 3D depth information of the object is obtained. A review of the active methods for stereovision is proposed in [5]. These active methods can been applied in endoscopic medical devices [10,11].

Although active stereovision methods can extract surface information with good quality, some factors such as surface occlusions, shadows, specular areas or absorptive materials can lead to loss of 3D information during the reconstruction process. One basic principle to overcome some of these difficulties is to capture more images of the object in different positions [12], with the drawback of time consumption.

Another possibility, proposed in this paper, is to dynamically generate two distinct measurement results by switching between projection and capture channels. Combining these two results can be an additional way to enrich the surface information obtained from the measurement.

In order to design a compact system, flexible image guides have been integrated in a compact optical probe. This probe is an improved model of the one presented in [13] and its size is fitted for colonoscopy. The view angle switch is achieved with two miniature digital electromagnetic actuators on witch mobile mirrors are mounted. This type of actuator is chosen because it provides a non-consuming holding force, which is obtained with magnetic interactions between permanent magnets, at its discrete states without the need of external electrical energy [14]. Another property of the proposed device is its ability to dynamically modify the projected patterns during the measurement to make them suitable for various reconstruction algorithms.

The structure of our system and its measurement principle are described in section 2. Section 3 presents the new designed compact optical probe. Some details on the algorithms are provided in section 4. Measurement results are shown in section 5 and the conclusion and perspectives of our work are finally discussed in section 6.

2   System Structure Description

In standard active stereovision systems, optical and mechanical configurations are generally static. In this section a dynamic system configuration obtained with the integration of miniature digital actuators is presented. This new configuration enhances the 3D reconstruction capability of the proposed system.

A schematic description of the proposed system is shown in two distinct configurations in Fig.1. As shown in Fig.1(a), a white light source illuminate the DMD (Digital Micro-mirror Device, a projecting device fabricated by Texas Instrument Inc). The patterns generated by DMD go through the lenses and image guide 1 (these image guides are fiber bundle composed of 60 000 optical fibers for a total diameter of $1.4mm$, FIGH-60-1200N, fabricated by Fujikura Inc) to enter the compact optical probe. These patterns are then projected onto the objects' surface and reflected back into the compact optical probe. Due to the stereoscopic angle between the two channels of the probe, the projected patterns are deformed and captured by the image guide 2. These deformed patterns are finally projected on a CCD sensor and depth analysis is performed on the captured images.

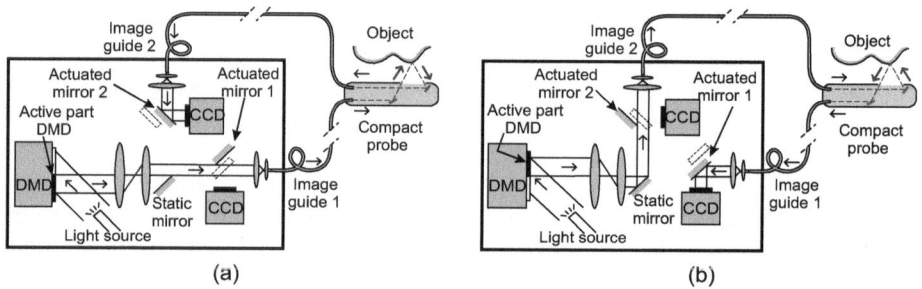

Fig. 1. Principle of the measurement modes.(a): active mode 1.(b): active mode 2.

In Fig.1(a), only half of the pattern generated by the DMD go through the system by image guide 1 because the other part of the DMD is used on the other mode (Fig.1(b)) to inject the image guide 2. Actuated mirror 1 and 2 are mounted on two digital electromagnetic miniature actuators(each of them have two discrete states) to switch between positive and negative positions. The first mode (Fig.1(a)) is obtained by setting actuated mirror 1 in negative position and by setting the actuated mirror 2 in positive position to reflect the patterns from image guide 2 to the CCD sensor.

The other active stereovision mode is obtained by switching the position of both actuated mirrors (Fig.1(b)). The other half of DMD is used to inject the patterns into image guide 2 after being reflected by static mirror 1. Another CCD sensor captures the patterns from image guide 1. In the following sections, the configuration of Fig.1(a) will be called "mode 1" and Fig.1(b) "mode 2".

Even though the object and the measure area are identical in mode 1 and mode 2, the captured images and the reconstruction results are different because the projection and view angles are exchanged between these two modes. It means that some sides of the measured object are more precisely captured with the first mode (i.e. the first view angle of mode 1) and other sides of the object are better measured with the second mode. In the final reconstruction the more precise measurements from each mode can be selected to optimize the quality of the result.

3   Structure of Compact Optical Probe

To fulfill requirements in gastrointestinal diagnosis, a new compact optical probe was designed. The structure of the probe is shown in Fig.2.

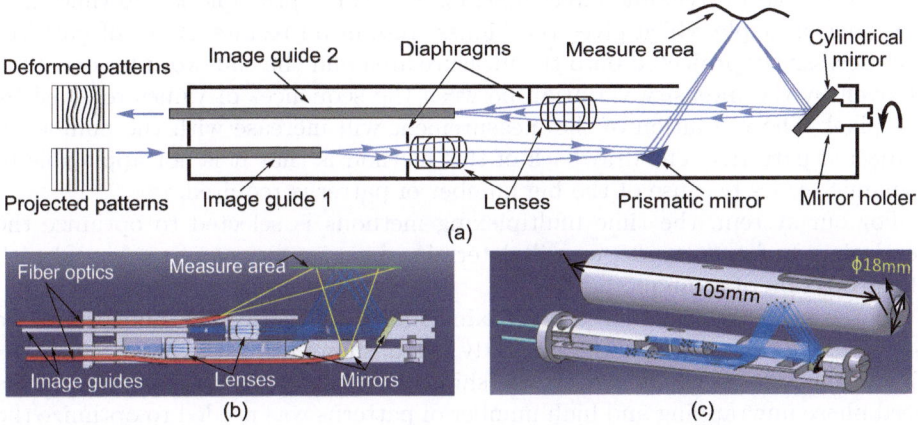

Fig. 2. Principle structure of compact optical probe.(a): Functional schematic for mode 1.(b): Schematic with two integrated fibers optics and two image guides. (c): Overall view of compact optical probe.

Two image guides are connected with two Steinheil Triplet Achromat Lenses of $6.5mm$ diameter and two diaphragms. Some mirrors are also used in the probe to reflect the patterns either from the image guides to the object or from the object to the image guides. As shown in Fig.2, the measurement area is at the side of the cylindrical probe. This is suitable for measurement in gastrointestinal diagnosis. In such a way, a 360° esophagus or intestine stripe can be measured by just rotating the probe during the operation. In this compact optical probe, two optical fibers can be added, as shown in Fig.2(c). Non-structured light can be projected directly on the surface of the objects by these optical fibers if the object must be seen without pattern projection. The circular mirror at the end of the probe can be rotated. This allows tuning the reflecting angle to make sure the two channels are capturing or projecting on the same area of the object. The probe size is about $\phi18 \times 105mm$ and the capture area is about $16mm^2$. In future works, this compact optical probe will be enhanced to capture a much larger area, which can be a necessity when the capture of large areas is needed. And the miniaturization will be tried for the size of this probe.

4   Reconstruction Algorithm

Structured light projection techniques are generally classified in three principles [5], [15]: the first one is the spatial neighborhood principle, where generally a unique pattern is projected onto the measure area. This method can be used in dynamic scenes but has difficulties to provide accurate results in presence of shadows or occlusions. The second principle is the direct codification strategy. Each pixel of the projected pattern has a specific color or grey level which is used to detect the corresponding projected pixel. This method is very sensitive to the scene noise and generally request to capture more than one image, which is not suitable in dynamic environments. The third principle is the time multiplexing principle which gives the highest resolution results. A set of patterns are successively projected onto the measure area and the codeword for one pixel is given by the intensity variation between the sequences of values received by the pixel. The resolution of the measurement will increase with the number of projected patterns. The drawback of this method is that it is not applicable to dynamic scenes because of the big number of patterns required.

For our system, the time multiplexing methods is selected to optimize the resolution. In future works, we will determine what quality can be achieved with the projection of a unique pattern.

In the scope of the time multiplexing methods, phase-shift and gray code methods are two possibilities. Our study in [13] showed that the best reconstruction results were obtained with phase shift algorithms, however these algorithms need phase unwrapping and high number of patterns was needed to optimize the axial resolution. Gray code is well suited for lower resolution results, but with fewer projected patterns.

In the following experimental section, phase-shift method is used for accurate measurement on a 10 cents euro coin because more objects' detail information is included in coin's surface, and Gray-code method is applied to do faster measurement on a colon phantom because only surface form information want to be detected.

5   Measurement Results

Some experimentations were carried out with the presented prototype and the two modes were tested. Firstly, a 10 cent euro coin has been measured to validate the properties of our proposed system (noted Test 1). Then measurements have been applied on a colon phantom to test the device in a medical environment (noted Test 2).

In test 1, the letter "N" of the "CENT" word has been measured on the euro coin, the results are presented in Fig.3. Phase-shift method was used to obtain a more precise reconstructed 3D model. Vertical line patterns were projected onto the object. In Fig.3(b) and (c), which are the two captured results of the two modes, the vertical line patterns are deformed because of the height of letter "N". Moreover, the orientation of patterns' deformation is opposite between these

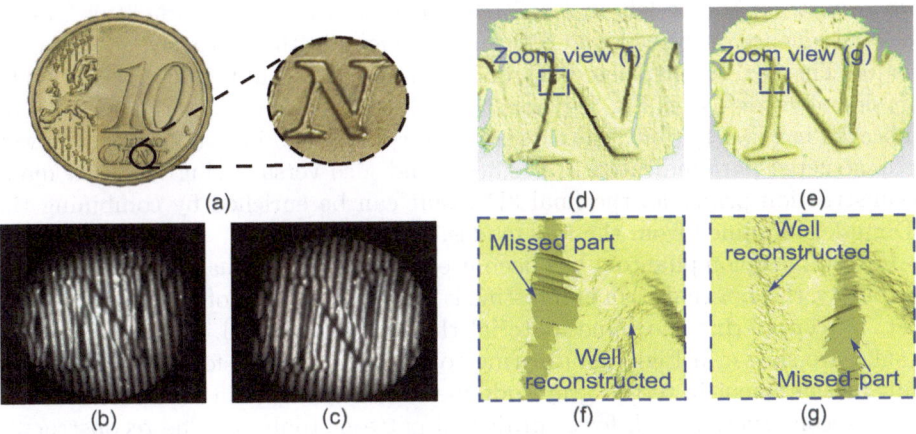

Fig. 3. Experimental measurement results for test 1.(a): measured letter N from a 10 cent of euro coin. (b) and (c): result of active mode 1 and 2. (d) and (e): reconstruction results of mode 1 and mode 2 with phase shift method. (f) and (g): zoom view of (d) and (e).

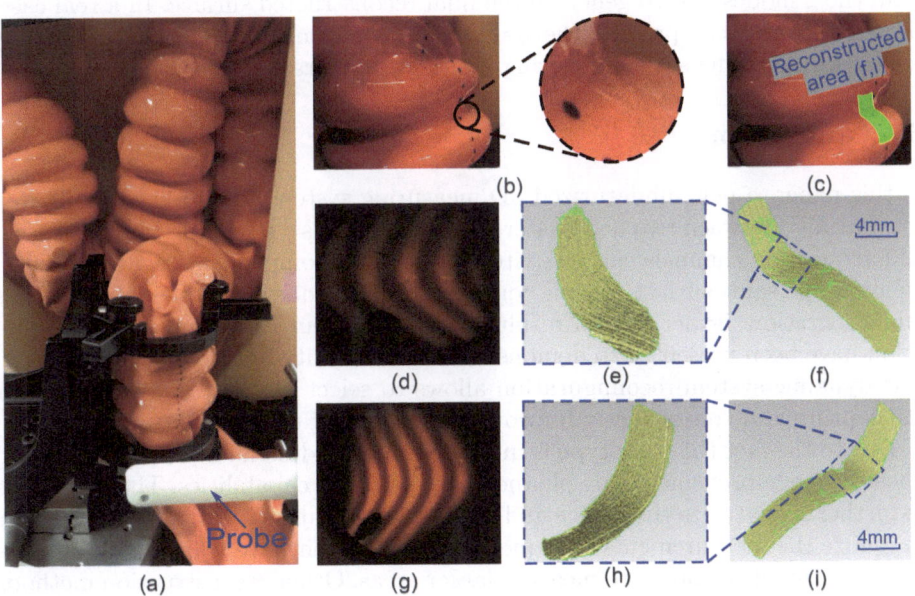

Fig. 4. Experimental measurement results for test 2.(a): setup for the test 2(the reference points are drawn onto the dummy intestine's surface to make sure series measurement position are in line). (b): external form of dummy intestine is measured in one measurement. (c): 15 measurements are taken to reconstruct a large zone of external form. (d) and (g): result of active mode 1 and 2. (e) and (h): reconstruction results of mode 1 and mode 2 with gray code method. (f) and (i): enlarged measurement area of mode 1 and mode 2.

two results: on to the left in Fig.3(b) and on to the right in Fig.3(c). This is the consequence of the two different angle of views in the two active stereovision modes. The final reconstructed 3D models are presented in Fig.3(d) and (e). The left side of letter "N" in Fig.3(d) was not well reconstructed (e.g. the missed part indicated in Fig.3(f)), but this side is well reconstructed in Fig.3(e)(e.g. the well reconstructed part indicated in Fig.3(g)) and vice versa. Using the dual mode reconstruction principle, the final 3D result can be enriched by combining the 3D models obtained from the two modes.

In test 2, a colon phantom has been used to measure its shape. For the sake of simplicity, the external form of intestine is measured instead of inside form in this test, by considering the same material they have possessed. The experimental results are shown in Fig.4. Comparing to 32 patterns used for a precise phase-shift measurement in test 1, gray code method was chosen in this test 2 to do a faster reconstruction with fewer projected patterns (only 8). The reconstructed surface (Fig.4(e) and (h)) shows a small part of the colon captured in these two measurement modes. The measurement area can be enlarged by moving the probe with small increments. 15 more positions were measured with the two modes, and the surface results are stitched in Fig.4(f) and Fig.4(i). The Geomagic Studio software was used to merge the captured point cloud data from the 2 modes and to generate the final reconstructed surface. In a real case, the view angle that provide the best quality of result could be automatically selected to help the surgeons during its surgical operation.

6   Conclusions

In this paper, a new miniaturized 3D measuring system able to be reconfigured dynamically between two active stereovision modes is presented. The projection and acquisition channels can be switched to obtain complementary 3D measurements of the same surface. A new compact optical probe was designed to achieve miniaturization. Experimental results on a 10 cent euro coin and on a phantom colon have been presented to demonstrate its feasibility in medical environment. The dynamic system reconfiguration allows to select the best angle of view for the capture and consequently improve the quality of the result.

Due to the fact the prototype is in its preliminary design and experimentation phase, some improvements are planned to enhance its capabilities. The first one is to further miniaturize the device and study its integration into a real colonoscope to realize the measurements on a medical environment. We will also modify the optical setup of the probe to measure larger areas. Other reconstruction methods will be studied to meet the real-time reconstruction condition with a unique pattern projection and consequently no time multiplexing.

References

1. Cavallotti, C., Piccigallo, M., Susilo, E., Valdastri, P., Menciassi, A., Dario, P.: An integrated vision system with autofocus for wireless capsular endoscopy. Sensors and Actuators A: Physical 156(1), 72–78 (2009)

2. Valdastri, P., Simi, M., Webster III, R.J.: Advanced technologies for gastrointestinal endoscopy. Annual Review of Biomedical Engineering 14, 397–429 (2012)
3. Schmalz, C., Forster, F., Schick, A., Angelopoulou, E.: An endoscopic 3d scanner based on structured light. Medical Image Analysis 16(5), 1063–1072 (2012)
4. Maurice, X., Albitar, C., Doignon, C., de Mathelin, M.: A structured light-based laparoscope with real-time organs' surface reconstruction for minimally invasive surgery. In: 2012 Annual International Conference of the IEEE Engineering in Medicine and Biology Society (EMBC), pp. 5769–5772. IEEE (2012)
5. Gorthi, S.S., Rastogi, P.: Fringe projection techniques: whither we are? Optics and Lasers in Engineering 48(2), 133–140 (2010)
6. Cui, H., Dai, N., Liao, W., Cheng, X.: Intraoral 3d optical measurement system for tooth restoration. Optik-International Journal for Light and Electron Optics 124(12), 1142–1147 (2013)
7. Wu, C., Narasimhan, S.G., Jaramaz, B.: A multi-image shape-from-shading framework for near-lighting perspective endoscopes. International Journal of Computer Vision 86(2-3), 211–228 (2010)
8. Collins, T., Compte, B., Bartoli, A.: Deformable shape-from-motion in laparoscopy using a rigid sliding window. In: Medical Image Understanding and Analysis Conference (2011)
9. Penne, J., et al.: Time-of-flight 3-d endoscopy. In: Yang, G.-Z., Hawkes, D., Rueckert, D., Noble, A., Taylor, C. (eds.) MICCAI 2009, Part I. LNCS, vol. 5761, pp. 467–474. Springer, Heidelberg (2009)
10. Wong, C., Chen, N., Sheppard, C.: Study on potential of structured illumination microscopy utilizing digital micromirror device for endoscopy purpose. In: International Symposium on Biophotonics, Nanophotonics and Metamaterials, Metamaterials 2006, pp. 218–221. IEEE (2006)
11. Dupont, E., Lamarque, F., Prelle, C., Redarce, T., et al.: Tri-dimensional optical inspection based on flexible image guide: first step toward 3D industrial endoscopy. In: Proc. of the 11th Biennial Conference on Engineering Systems Design and Analysis, vol. 19 (2012)
12. Cui, H., Liao, W., Dai, N., Cheng, X.: Registration and integration algorithm in structured light three-dimensional scanning based on scale-invariant feature matching of multi-source images. Chinese Optics Letters 10(9), 091001–091001 (2012)
13. Dupont, E., Hou, Y., Lamarque, F., Redarce, T.: Binary pattern codification strategies in an active stereoscopic system based on flexible image guides. In: SPIE MOEMS-MEMS, International Society for Optics and Photonics, pp. 86180H–86180H (2013)
14. Miao, X., Dai, X., Wang, P., Huang, Y., Ding, G., Zhao, X.: Electromagnetic bistable microactuator fabricated on a single wafer. Micro & Nano Letters, IET 7(2), 99–100 (2012)
15. Salvi, J., Pages, J., Batlle, J.: Pattern codification strategies in structured light systems. Pattern Recognition 37(4), 827–849 (2004)

Continuous Zoom Calibration by Tracking Salient Points in Endoscopic Video*

Miguel Lourenço[1], João P. Barreto[1,2], Fernando Fonseca[3], Hélder Ferreira[4],
Rui M. Duarte[4], and Jorge Correia-Pinto[4]

[1] Institute of Systems and Robotics, University of Coimbra, Coimbra, Portugal
[2] Perceive 3D, Coimbra, Portugal
[3] Coimbra Hospital and Universitary Centre, Faculty of Medicine, Coimbra, Portugal
[4] Life and Health Sciences Research Institute, University of Minho, Braga, Portugal

Abstract. Many image-based systems for aiding the surgeon during minimally invasive surgery require the endoscopic camera to be calibrated at all times. This article proposes a method for accomplishing this goal whenever the camera has optical zoom and the focal length changes during the procedure. Our solution for online calibration builds on recent developments in tracking salient points using differential image alignment, is well suited for continuous operation, and makes no assumptions about the camera motion or scene rigidity. Experimental validation using both a phantom model and *in vivo* data shows that the method enables accurate estimation of focal length when the zoom varies, avoiding the need to explicitly recalibrate during surgery. To the best of our knowledge this the first work proposing a practical solution for online zoom calibration in the operation room.

1 Introduction

Minimally Invasive Surgery has a number of well documented benefits for the patient, such as faster recovery time, and less trauma to surrounding tissues. However, since the surgeon has limited access to the anatomical cavity and the visualisation is carried indirectly through the video acquired by an endoscopic camera, the execution of MIS is more difficult than the (equivalent) open-surgery. In this context, systems for CAS that process the endoscopic video can be very helpful in assisting the doctor during the procedure, either by improving the visualisation [1], or by recovering the camera motion [2].

Most image-based CAS systems that use the endoscopic video as primary sensory input require the intrinsic camera calibration to be known at all times during the procedure [1,2]. Endoscopic camera calibration in the context of CAS is challenging for three reasons [1,3]: (i) since the optics are exchangeable and

---

* Miguel Lourenço and João Barreto want to thank *QREN-Mais Centro* by generous funding through *Novas Tecnologias para apoio à Saúde e Qualidade de Vida, Projecto A- Cirurgia e Diagnóstico Assistido por Computador Usando Imagem* and the Portuguese Science Foundation by funding through grant SFRH/BD/63118/2009.

P. Golland et al. (Eds.): MICCAI 2014, Part I, LNCS 8673, pp. 456–463, 2014.

the camera cannot be pre-calibrated, the calibration procedure must be carried in the operation room (OR) by a non-expert user [1], (ii) in the case of oblique-viewing endoscopes the surgeon often rotates the lens scope with respect to the camera head, which changes the calibration parameters [3], and (iii) high-end endoscopy systems provide optical zoom, which means that camera focal length changes during the intervention. Melo *et al.* [1] describe effective solutions for overcoming challenges (i) and (ii). They improve usability by proposing a fully automatic calibration method that uses as input a single image of a planar checkerboard pattern and, in the case of oblique viewing endoscopes, they show that it is possible to estimate the lens rotation and update the initial calibration by tracking the image boundary contour. This paper addresses challenge (iii) meaning that it is shown that under varying zoom the only parameter that changes significantly is the focal length, and that it is possible to update the initial calibration information without the need of re-calibrate the camera.

Zoom calibration is closely related to the problem of unknown/variable focal length estimation [4,5]. Stoyanov *et al.* [4] propose a solution for stereo endoscopy where the focal lengths are directly estimated from the fundamental matrix [6]. Given the offline extrinsic stereo calibration, the focal lengths can be determined using only two point matches across the stereo pair. Unfortunately, the solution only generalizes for monocular endoscopy if the camera motion is known. Stewenius *et al.* [5] propose a minimal solution for computing the relative camera pose and unknown focal length from 6 correspondences that is used within a sample consensus framework. The method assumes a rigid scene and requires in practice a considerable baseline between images, which makes its use problematic in continuous video. Related to this article is the work of Lee *et al.* [7] that does online estimation of focal length based on the image of the boundary contour of the endoscope. This approach has the disadvantage of requiring explicit camera calibration for multiple zoom positions and, more importantly, it does not work whenever the boundary contour is not visible in the image. This article reports a solution for efficient and accurate focal length estimation in endoscopic video. We built on recent advances in tracking image features between frames with radial distortion [8] to show that it is possible to recover the focal length variation in sequences with zoom variation. Since we built on tracking theory, our approach is well suited for processing continuous monocular endoscopic video, does not make assumptions about camera motion [4] or scene rigidity [5], and does not require the boundary contour of the lens to be visible [7]. Quantitative and qualitative validation in synthetic and *in vivo* scenarios show that the proposed method enables accurate, online estimation of the focal length when the camera zoom changes.

2   Methods

This section details the proposed method for online focal length calibration. We start by introducing the adopted camera model before moving to the method description.

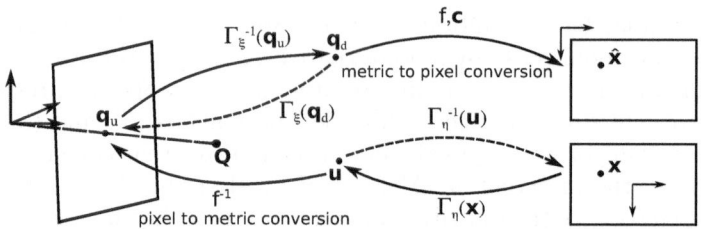

Fig. 1. Illustration of endoscopic camera modeling in the presence of radial distortion

2.1   Endoscopic Camera Modeling

We assume that the radial distortion present in endoscopic cameras can be conveniently described using the so-called division model [1,9]. Let $\mathbf{q}_d$ be a generic 2D point with distortion. This point can be mapped in its undistorted counterpart $\mathbf{q}_u$ by the function $\mathbf{\Gamma}_\xi(\cdot)$

$$\mathbf{q}_u = \mathbf{\Gamma}_\xi(\mathbf{q}_d) = \left(1 + \xi\mathbf{q}_d{}^\mathsf{T}\mathbf{q}_d\right)^{-1} \cdot \mathbf{q}_d, \tag{1}$$

with ξ quantifying the amount of distortion.

Direct Projection Model and Single Image Calibration: Let $\mathbf{q}_u$ be the perspective projection of a 3D point $\mathbf{Q}$ in the canonical projective plane (see Fig.1). In the presence of distortion, and assuming the camera to be skewless and having unitary aspect ratio, point $\mathbf{q}_u$ is mapped into the point $\hat{\mathbf{x}}$ in the image plane by

$$\hat{\mathbf{x}} = f\,\mathbf{\Gamma}_\xi^{-1}(\mathbf{q}_u) + \mathbf{c}, \tag{2}$$

with $\mathbf{\Gamma}^{-1}(\cdot)$ being the inverse of Eq. 1 that maps $\mathbf{q}_u$ in its distorted counterpart

$$\mathbf{q}_d = \mathbf{\Gamma}_\xi^{-1}(\mathbf{q}_u) = 2\left(1 + \sqrt{1 - 4\xi\mathbf{q}_u{}^\mathsf{T}\mathbf{q}_u}\right)^{-1} \cdot \mathbf{q}_u, \tag{3}$$

f is the camera focal length that converts metric units into pixel units, and $\mathbf{c} = (c_x, c_y)$ is the principal point in pixels. With the single image calibration of [1] we can easily estimate ξ, f and $\mathbf{c}$ at an initial reference zoom position. Remark that ξ is the amount of distortion in metric units that is a characteristic of the lens and therefore independent of the zoom variation.

Modeling Radial Distortion in the Image Plane: An alternative way of modelling the projection is to consider that the radial distortion acts in the image plane as opposed to act in the metric projective plane. From the inversion of Eq. 2 it comes in a straightforward manner that

$$\mathbf{q}_u = \mathbf{\Gamma}_\xi(f^{-1}(\hat{\mathbf{x}} - \mathbf{c})). \tag{4}$$

For simplicity, let's assume that $\mathbf{x} = \hat{\mathbf{x}} - \mathbf{c}$, which means that image points are expressed in a coordinate frame centred in the principal point. Replacing $\boldsymbol{\Gamma}_\xi$ by the expression of Eq. 1 it comes that

$$f \cdot \mathbf{q}_u = \left(1 + \frac{\xi}{f^2}\mathbf{x}^\mathsf{T}\mathbf{x}\right)^{-1} \cdot \mathbf{x}. \tag{5}$$

Let $\mathbf{u} = f \cdot \mathbf{q}_u$ be the undistorted image point in pixel units. From the equation above it follows that $\mathbf{u}$ is related with its distorted version $\mathbf{x}$ by $\mathbf{u} = \boldsymbol{\Gamma}_\eta(\mathbf{x})$ with

$$\eta = \xi \cdot f^{-2} \tag{6}$$

being the parameter that quantifies the distortion in pixel units. We conclude that, if the radial distortion is expressed in metric units, i.e. before the intrinsics, the corresponding parameter ξ does not depend of the camera focal length. However, if we quantify this same distortion in pixel units using η, then there is a dependence on the focal length which means that the distortion parameter varies with the zoom. We will use the relation of Eq. 6 for recovering the focal length f at each frame by combining offline calibration of the constant parameter ξ using [1] with online estimation of η using the tracking framework of [8].

2.2   Estimating Image Distortion at Every Frame Using uRD-KLT

Lourenço and Barreto show in [8] that it is possible to estimate the radial distortion in the image plane by tracking feature points between adjacent frames. Their uncalibrated KLT algorithm for images with radial distortion (uRD-KLT) starts by extracting reference templates $\mathsf{T}(\mathbf{x})$ around a set of salient points $\mathbf{x}$ that are detected based on image derivatives [8]. Given an incoming image $\mathsf{I}(\mathbf{x})$, the goal is to align the templates $\mathsf{T}(\mathbf{x})$ with the corresponding image regions subject to the squared intensity difference and under the assumption of a 2D deformation model $\mathbf{v}(\mathbf{x}; \mathbf{p})$, with parameters $\mathbf{p}$, that accounts for both the local motion $\mathbf{w}$ and the global effect of distortion. The deformation model is given by:

$$\mathbf{v}(\mathbf{x}; \mathbf{p}) = \left(\boldsymbol{\Gamma}^{-1} \circ \mathbf{w} \circ \boldsymbol{\Gamma}\right)(\mathbf{x}; \mathbf{p}), \tag{7}$$

with $\mathbf{p} = (\mathbf{m}, \eta)$ where $\mathbf{m}$ is the vector of motion parameters that describes the local deformation undergone by each image patch in the absence of distortion [10], and η is the global distortion parameter that is common to all image regions.

Given an initial estimate of $\mathbf{p}$ the goal is to iteratively compute the updates $\delta\mathbf{p}$ of the warp parameters by minimizing the following cost function

$$\epsilon = \sum_{\mathbf{x} \in \mathcal{N}} \left[\mathsf{I}(\mathbf{v}(\mathbf{x}; \mathbf{p})) - \mathsf{T}(\mathbf{v}(\mathbf{x}; \delta\mathbf{p}))\right]^2 \tag{8}$$

This error function can linearised with respect to $\mathbf{p}$ by computing the first order Taylor expansion, and the final updates $\delta\mathbf{p}$ can be computed in closed-form as:

$$\delta\mathbf{p} = \mathcal{H}^{-1} \sum_{\mathbf{x} \in \mathcal{N}} \left[\nabla\mathsf{T}\frac{\partial\mathbf{v}(\mathbf{x}; \mathbf{0})}{\partial\mathbf{p}}\right]^\mathsf{T} \left(\mathsf{I}(\mathbf{v}(\mathbf{x}; \mathbf{p})) - \mathsf{T}(\mathbf{x})\right), \tag{9}$$

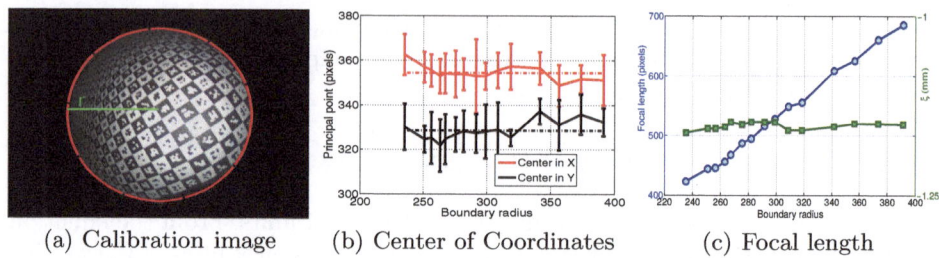

(a) Calibration image   (b) Center of Coordinates   (c) Focal length

Fig. 2. Intrinsic parameters for different zoom positions. Fig. 2(a) shows a calibration image where the radius of the boundary is used to index the current zoom position. Fig. 2(b) shows the variation of the center of coordinates and Fig. 2(c) shows the variation of the focal length (blue) and distortion in metric units (green) for increasing zoom. The experiment confirms that the focal length increases, while the principal point $\mathbf{c}$ and the distortion parameter ξ are virtually constant ($-\xi = 1.1515 \pm 0.007$).

with $\mathcal{H}$ being a 1st order approximation of the Hessian matrix, and $\partial\mathbf{v}(\mathbf{x};\mathbf{0})/\partial\mathbf{p}$ being the Jacobian of the warp evaluated at the identity warp [8,10]. Since the η is a global parameter common to every image point, the corresponding distortion updates are computed using all tracked features, while the feature local motion $\mathbf{m}$ is computed for each feature separately [8].

2.3 Calibrating Zoom by Image Alignment

So far, we have derived the relation between distortion parameters in metric and pixel units and showed that the distortion in pixels can be estimated at each time instant using the uRD-KLT. While in [8] it is assumed that the camera calibration is not known and that the principal point $\mathbf{c}$ is coincident with the image center, we use the single image calibration [1] at an initial zoom position to obtain the principal point $\mathbf{c}$ and the lens distortion ξ in metric units. The uRD-KLT is applied during operation to continuously estimate the image distortion parameter η and the focal length is estimated at each frame time instant using the relation of Eq. 6. The approach works as far as $\mathbf{c}$ and ξ remain constant.

3   Results

In this section we evaluate the proposed solution for recovering the focal length in continuous video. We start by conducting a set of experiments with ground truth to validate the assumptions made for the derivation of our solution. Afterwards, the method is validated in both a synthetic environment and in a *in vivo* sequence acquired in a porcine uterus.

3.1 Variation of Intrinsic Camera Parameters with Zoom Changes

In this experiment we used a Storz H3-Z endoscopy system with a Dyonics' arthroscopic lens with 4mm diameter. We placed the camera zoom in 15 distinct

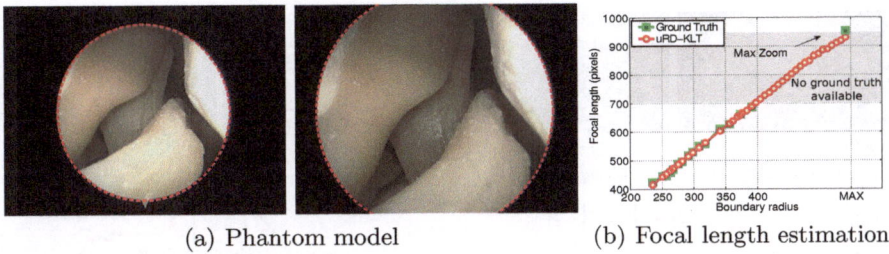

(a) Phantom model   (b) Focal length estimation

Fig. 3. Simulation experiment with a zoom only sequence. Fig. 3(a) shows the two phantom images with the corresponding boundary radius at different zoom positions. Fig. 3(b) shows that the focal length estimation of the uRD-KLT is accurate.

positions and, for each position, we collected 5 images of a checkerboard pattern that were used to obtain 5 independent intrinsic calibrations using the method described in [1]. Figure 2(b) shows the principal point estimation for successive zoom positions that are referenced using the radius of the boundary contour. Fig. 2(c) does the same for the focal length f and the lens distortion parameters ξ. The assumption that $\mathbf{c}$ and ξ are kept constant while the zoom varies holds in practice.

3.2   Validation with a Phantom Model

This experiment uses the camera setup of section 3.1 for acquiring a video sequence of a phantom model of the knee. The endoscope is kept stationary, while the zoom is increased. The focal length is estimated at each frame time instant by using the uRD-KLT to track 20 automatically detected points. The focal length estimates are related with the calibration results of section 3.1 using the radius of the boundary contour like in [7]. Figure 3 compares the on-line estimation results with the calibration ground truth. Please note that high-zoom values have no ground truth because the boundary contour is not visible and there is no manner of relating the f estimates with calibration results. Nevertheless, the estimation seems to be plausible and consistent with the calibration obtained for the end zoom position. The maximum relative estimation error was 2.5% for the maximum zoom position when the image distortion η reaches its minimum.

3.3   Validation in *in-vivo* Data

The data used in this experiment was recorded in a *in-vivo* porcine uterus during a robotic assisted procedure. The sequence of 1000 frames with resolution 1920 × 1080 was acquired at 30Hz with a Storz H3-Z camera system equipped with a laparoscopic lens of 10 mm from Dyonics. We used the procedure of section 3.1 to obtain calibration ground truth. The surgeon was asked to vary the zoom against the direction of motion of the endoscope in an attempt to keep the size of the image structures constant and evaluate the robustness to changes

462   M. Lourenço et al.

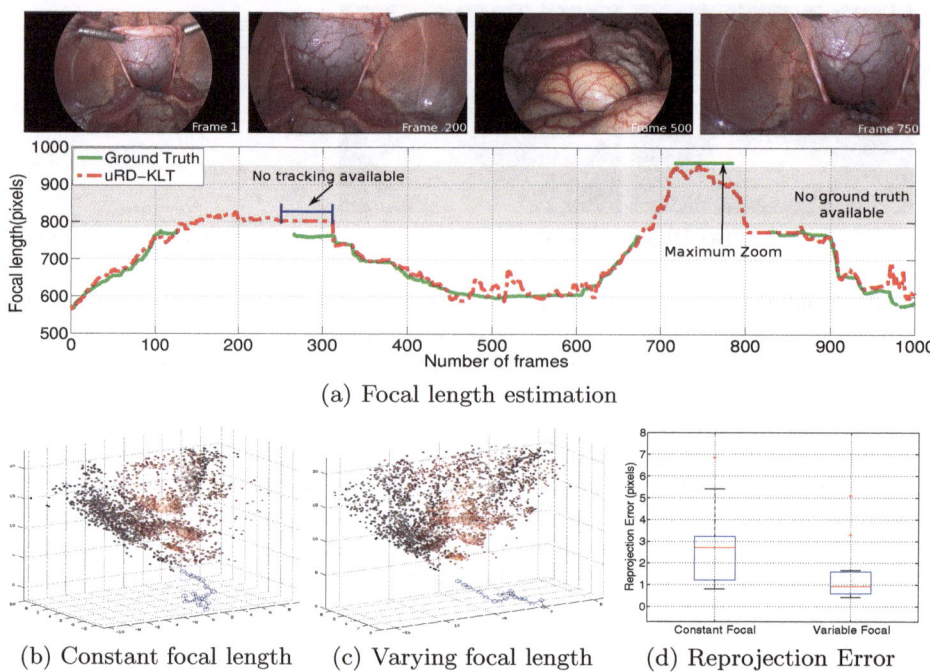

(a) Focal length estimation

(b) Constant focal length   (c) Varying focal length   (d) Reprojection Error

Fig. 4. Results in *in-vivo* data. (a) shows some sample video frames, and the focal length estimation. (b) and (c) show a visual odometry experiment without and with focal length compensation, respectively. Compensating the focal length bring clear benefits for visual odometry, as it can be seen in Fig. 4(d) where the reprojection error of the reconstructed 3D points decreases from ≈ 3 pixels to less than 1 pixel.

in scale. Figures 4(a) shows the online estimation results for the focal length by performing uRD-KLT tracking in the *in-vivo* sequence. These results were obtained with a straightforward Matlab implementation that ran at 2fps on a single core of an Intel i7-3630QM CPU @ 2.40GHz processor. It can be observed that the uRD-KLT-based estimation is quite accurate with an average relative error of $2.1927 \pm 2.3959\%$ when compared with the calibration ground truth. Please note that there are sequence segments for which there are no salient points (frames 250 to 300) or the accuracy of the estimation decreases due to temporary poor tracking (frames 475-525). However, and since the focal length measurement is carried in a frame-by-frame basis, these errors do not accumulate. Finally Fig. 4(b) to 4(d) show comparative visual odometry results for a sub-sequence of 17 frames where the camera moves forward while the zoom decreases. Since most of the scene is rigid the camera motion is computed by applying the five-point algorithm [11] using image correspondences obtained with sRD-SIFT [12]. Fig. 4(b) and 4(d) depict the motion estimation results when the focal length is kept constant and when the focal length is updated.

4   Discussion and Conclusion

This article presents a practical solution for keeping the camera calibrated when the camera zoom changes during operation. The method builds on recent developments in image alignment for tracking keypoints in video with radial distortion and, since there are no distortion free endoscopic cameras, it can be virtually used in any MIS. The approach was validated in both synthetic and *in-vivo* data, showing that is possible to keep the camera calibrated under zoom variations without the need to re-calibrate the camera during operation. To the best of our knowledge, this is the first work proposing an effective solution for the zoom calibration in continuous medical endoscopic video.

References

1. Melo, R., Barreto, J., Falcao, G.: A New Solution for Camera Calibration and Real-Time Image Distortion Correction in Medical Endoscopy-Initial Technical Evaluation. IEEE Transactions on Biomedical Engineering 59, 634–644 (2012)
2. Burschka, D., Li, M., Taylor, R., Hager, G.: Scale-Invariant Registratiou of Monocular Endoscopic Images to CT-Scans for Sinus Surgery. In: Barillot, C., Haynor, D.R., Hellier, P. (eds.) MICCAI 2004. LNCS, vol. 3217, pp. 413–421. Springer, Heidelberg (2004)
3. Yamaguchi, T., et al.: Camera Model and Calibration Procedure for Oblique-Viewing Endoscope. In: Ellis, R.E., Peters, T.M. (eds.) MICCAI 2003. LNCS, vol. 2879, pp. 373–381. Springer, Heidelberg (2003)
4. Stoyanov, D., Darzi, A., Yang, G.Z.: Laparoscope Self-calibration for Robotic Assisted Minimally Invasive Surgery. In: Duncan, J.S., Gerig, G. (eds.) MICCAI 2005. LNCS, vol. 3750, pp. 114–121. Springer, Heidelberg (2005)
5. Stewenius, H., Nister, D., Kahl, F., Schaffalitzky, F.: A minimal solution for relative pose with unknown focal length. In: IEEE Conference on Computer Vision and Pattern Recognition, vol. 2, pp. 789–794 (2005)
6. Hartley, R.I., Zisserman, A.: Multiple View Geometry in Computer Vision, 2nd edn. Cambridge University Press (2004) ISBN: 0521540518
7. Lee, T.Y., et al.: Automatic distortion correction of endoscopic images captured with wide-angle zoom lens. IEEE Transactions on Biomedical Engineering 60, 2603–2613 (2013)
8. Lourenço, M., Barreto, J.P.: Tracking Feature Points in Uncalibrated Images with Radial Distortion. In: Fitzgibbon, A., Lazebnik, S., Perona, P., Sato, Y., Schmid, C. (eds.) ECCV 2012, Part IV. LNCS, vol. 7575, pp. 1–14. Springer, Heidelberg (2012)
9. Fitzgibbon, A.: Simultaneous linear estimation of multiple view geometry and lens distortion. In: IEEE Conference on Computer Vision and Pattern Recognition, vol. 1, pp. 125–132 (2001)
10. Baker, S., Matthews, I.: Lucas-kanade 20 years on: A unifying framework. International Journal of Computer Vision 56, 221–255 (2004)
11. Nister, D.: An efficient solution to the five-point relative pose problem. IEEE Transactions on Pattern Analysis and Machine Intelligence 26, 756–770 (2004)
12. Lourenco, M., Barreto, J., Vasconcelos, F.: sRD-SIFT: Keypoint Detection and Matching in Images With Radial Distortion. IEEE Transactions on Robotics 28, 752–760 (2012)

Instrument Tracking via Online Learning in Retinal Microsurgery

Yeqing Li[1], Chen Chen[1], Xiaolei Huang[2], and Junzhou Huang[1]

[1] Department of Computer Science and Engineering,
University of Texas at Arlington, Arlington TX 76019, USA
[2] Computer Science and Engineering Department, Lehigh University,
Bethlehem, PA 18015, USA

Abstract. Robust visual tracking of instruments is an important task in retinal microsurgery. In this context, the instruments are subject to a large variety of appearance changes due to illumination and other changes during a procedure, which makes the task very challenging. Most existing methods require collecting a sufficient amount of labelled data and yet perform poorly in handling appearance changes that are unseen in training data. To address these problems, we propose a new approach for robust instrument tracking. Specifically, we adopt an online learning technique that collects appearance samples of instruments on the fly and gradually learns a target-specific detector. Online learning enables the detector to reinforce its model and become more robust over time. The performance of the proposed method has been evaluated on a fully annotated dataset of retinal instruments in in-vivo retinal microsurgery and on a laparoscopy image sequence. In all experimental results, our proposed tracking approach shows superior performance compared to several other state-of-the-art approaches.

1 Introduction

Retinal microsurgery (RM) is an important treatment for sight-threatening conditions. The procedure is performed by a surgeon using a microscope for visualization and manipulating a set of surgical instruments. The operating surgeon faces several difficulties such as indirect visualization of the surgical target, hand tremors and lack of tactile feedback. To overcome these difficulties, new techniques have been developed. Accurate visual tracking of surgical tools in microscopic images is an important technique to complement the previously developed smart tools. In this paper, we focus on the task of robust visual tracking of instruments in in-vivo RM monocular image sequences.

This task is challenging due to the great variability in the appearance of surgical tools because of illumination and other factors. Many existing methods focus on training the appearance model based on color features or the instrument geometry [1–4]. However, these methods often perform poorly under complex appearance changes due to their oversimplified appearance models. Sznitman et al. proposed an approach, namely Data-Driven Visual Tracking (DDVT) [5],

P. Golland et al. (Eds.): MICCAI 2014, Part I, LNCS 8673, pp. 464–471, 2014.

which integrates an instrument detector based on deformable features with a simple gradient-based tracker. DDVT is able to run in video frame rate and achieves state-of-the-art results on challenging human in-vivo surgery datasets. To our best knowledge, DDVT is by far the best visual tracking approach in RM. However, there are two drawbacks to DDVT. First, it needs manually labelled instrument positions in many video frames for training the offline detector. Second, it performs poorly in handling appearance changes that were not observed in the training sequences and could not be modelled by the trained offline detector.

Currently, it draws more and more attentions to integrate online learning techniques in visual tracking system [6, 7]. How to extract new reliable samples without corrupting the current model is a key problem to this kind of systems. Therefore, many techniques have been exploited to constrain the learning process [8, 9]. However, many existing models are not robust enough to apply on RM tracking problem due to the challenges discussed above.

To this end, we propose a new approach based on online learning—Instrument Tracker via Online Learning (ITOL). In this approach, we adopt the paradigm of combining tracking and detection in the same framework [10, 11]. ITOL uses a robust gradient-based tracker capable of failure detection as the basic tracker. Then, a cascade appearance classifier is used as the instrument detector. The appearance model of the detector is initialized by manually clicking the instrument position in the first frame. It is adaptively trained and updated on the fly. Samples for online updating are collected by a filtering process, which selects "unfamiliar" positive samples and "hard" negative samples. The obtained training set is used to augment the model of the detector and prevent the detector from making the similar mistakes. The performance of the proposed approach is evaluated in three human in-vivo retinal microsurgery videos and one laparoscopy image sequence. The experimental results demonstrate that our method significantly outperforms the state-of-the-art approaches.

The rest of this paper is organized as follows: Section 2 introduces the framework and each components of our approach. Then we present our experimental results in Section 3 and conclude the proposed approach in Section 4.

2   Method

In this section, we will detail our proposed method ITOL. Methods for visual tracking usually fall into two groups: tracking through local optimization and tracking by detection [2]. Tracking through local optimization is fast, accurate and able to handle appearance changes of the target. However, continuous template updating is needed in order to maintain accurate position tracking when there are significant changes in target appearance [5]. Tracking by detection has the advantage of being able to handle target disappearance, but the ability of detection is limited by the training data.

Instrument tracking is challenging due to often unexpected appearance changes and extreme deformations of the instrument. We use a multi-component tracking framework to address these problems. A flowchart diagram of the framework is shown in Fig. 1. First, a robust gradient-based **tracker** with the ability of failure detection is used to handle unexpected appearance changes. Then an instrument **detector** is adopted to compensate for tracking loss and it automatically re-initializes the tracker when the instrument reappears after disappearance or tracking loss. To provide more reliable tracking results, outputs of the tracker and the detector will be integrated into a unique target position by a component named **integrator**. Finally, a component named **sample expert** will be used to efficiently select image patches for online updating of appearance model of the detector. In the whole framework, we only need to manually click the position of the instrument in the first frame for training data. Then, the tracking system is fully automatic. Details of each component of the system will be discussed in the following sections.

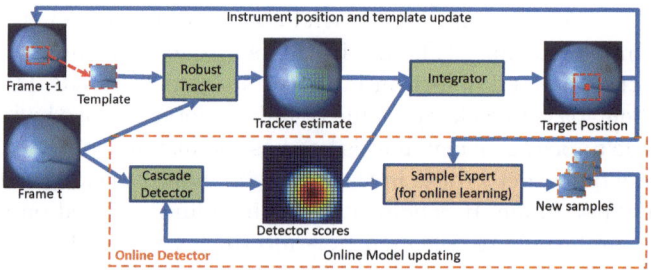

Fig. 1. Diagram of our ITOL framework

2.1   Robust Tracker

The tracker is used to handle instrument appearance changes and bring in new appearance samples. In many cases, although the appearance in the current frame is new to the current model of the detector, it is gradually adapted over time from seen samples. Since we use a gradient based tracker, which is only concerned with similarity between two consecutive frames, it can adaptively collect new appearance samples while tracking. The tracker is based on the Median Flow (MF) algorithm [12]. In the Median Flow tracker, the target is represented by a bounding box around it. For robustness, the bounding box is divided into a $k \times k$ grid ($k = 10$ in our experiments), where each cell of the grid is tracked by the pyramidal L-K algorithm [13]. The displacement of the target is voted by 50% of the most reliable cells. The reliability level of a cell is measured by normalized cross-correlation (NCC).MF also uses a quantity named Forward-Backward (FB) error for failure detection. The tracking is performed both forward and backward along the time axis and the FB error is computed based on the discrepancies between these two trajectories of the target [12]. Since the instrument sometimes move severely or is out of view, this failure detection ability is critical to prevent the tracker from importing false samples.

2.2 Cascade Detector

The gradient-based MF tracker assumes that the target is always in view and under continuous changes. In practice, instruments or tools during RM often undergo large appearance changes, which breaks the assumption. An online detector is developed to compensate for this shortcoming of the tracker and to re-initialize the tracker when an instrument reappears after loss. The detector scans the current frame by sliding window and decides whether the target is present in each window. A complex object detector often requires high computational cost, which makes it impossible for real-time surgical tracking. This problem is addressed by combining successively more complex classifiers in a cascade structure, which rejects most negative windows in the early stages of the cascade thus increasing the processing speed of the detector [14].

In our method, each frame is scanned by the detector at multiple scales using sliding window. All the candidate bounding boxes will be resized to the same size. Inspired by [11], we use a three-stage detector. The first stage is a variance filter that checks if the variance of the patch is under certain threshold related to the variance of trained positive samples. The variance filter can be evaluated efficiently by using integral images [14]. The second stage is random ferns (forest) [15] on patches for comparing the pixel values. Pixels in a patch are first divided into several groups. The probability is then computed for each group based on the number of times that the same feature combination appeared in previous frames as positive or negative examples. The final confidence score is computed by averaging the probabilities of each group. The third stage is a 1-Nearest-Neighbour (1NN) classifier using Normalized Correlation Coefficient (NCC) as the distance between the candidate patch and two sets of patches: positive patches and negative patches. Usually, the first two stages are able to reject more than 95% of the candidate windows, which makes the detector very efficient. In fact, this detector is able to run at nearly 30fps in our experiments.

2.3 Integrator

As discussed above, the detector and the tracker have their respective advantages and disadvantages. Therefore, we use the integrator to integrates their outputs to achieve an optimal estimation. The rules for this integration are: 1) If neither the tracker nor the detector output any positions, the target is declared as not visible; 2) Otherwise, all the outputs of the tracker and the detector are clustered into one by their scores. Suppose s_+ is the similarity between a candidate patch and its nearest neighbour in the positive sample set and s_- is the similarity between the patch and its nearest neighbour in the negative sample set, and $\rho = \frac{s_+}{s_-}$. Then the score of the patch is defined as $s = \frac{1}{1+\rho}$.

2.4 Online Updating of Detector's Model

The sample expert is designed to select new training samples for online model updating of the detector. Online updating make the detector capable of handling unexpected appearance changes and more robust to the noises. Given new samples, the updating process is straightforward. For random ferns, the probability of each branch is updated by adding the results of the pixel comparison. The 1NN classifier simply adds new samples to its sample sets.

The online learning method is detailed in the following. To prevent false positive samples, the sample expert use higher threshold than the detector. Then we consider these bounding boxes as potential positive samples. Starting from the output of the integrator, the sample expert will generate the new positive samples by choosing bounding boxes that are very close to the output one. Second, we filter them by our 1NN classifier and only accept the samples that are rejected by the 1NN classifier. The second step has two effects: 1) It rules out those "easy" samples to avoid redundancy; 2) The remaining samples are "new" enough so that the model will improve very rapidly. In order to accelerate the growth of the model, positive sample are rotated and blurred to generate more data. For negative examples, a common practice is focusing on "hard" samples. Therefore, only samples that have passed the first two stages of the detector and far away from the output are considered candidates of negative samples.

3   Experiment and Results

In this section, we conduct experiments to evaluate ITOL on two public datasets: **Retina Microsurgery Dataset** and **Laparoscopy Sequence** [5].

- **Retina Microsurgery Dataset** consists of 3 sequences of in-vivo vitreo-retinal surgery, which contains a total of 1171 images (640 × 480 pixels). See Fig. 2 for examples. These sequences are challenging due to variations in illumination type and quantity, light source position and the presence of blur and shadows.
- **Laparoscopy Sequence** consists of 1000 images with labelled locations of the tool tip. The original video is from Youtube. There are two instruments in each image, hence there are roughly 2000 instrument locations.

We compare our method **ITOL** with four baseline methods: **DDVT** [5], **SCV** [16], **MI** [4], **SSD** [17]. We also compare two components used in the proposed method: **Median-Flow (MF)** and **Detector-Tracker (DT)**. **MF** is the gradient-based tracker that we used. **DT** is MF plus the cascade detector without online model updating. For fair comparison, two measures are used by following the experimental setting of [5]: the accuracy on the thresholding distance to groundtruth and the number of the consecutive tracking frame. The accuracy is defined as the percentage of the detection within δ pixels of the groundtruth annotation. We vary δ from 15 to 40 in experiments (same as the setting in DDVT [5]).

The proposed method is implemented in Matlab. All experiments are conducted on a Desktop PC, 3.4GHz Intel Core i7-3770 and 12GB RAM. Our method runs at nearly 20fps and should run even faster implemented on parallel architecture (e.g. GPU or Mutlti-core).

3.1 Retina Microsurgery Dataset

The experimental results on the RM dataset are shown in Fig. 2. Results of each video sequence are shown in one row. In all the results, DDVT [5] outperforms the others except the proposed ITOL. ITOL also outperforms MF and DT, which validates the benefits of the online detector. Similar trends have been witness in all three videos where ITOL always achieves the best accuracy and unstableness. We accredit the advantages of the proposed ITOL to the online learning component that effectively updates the detector and makes it adapt to the appearance changes of instruments. One thing that is worth to note is DDVT uses the offline detector and therefore requires sufficient amount of training data before tracking (e.g. 500 manually labelled frames [5]), while our method bases on online learning techniques and only requires one labelled position in the first frame as training data before tracking.

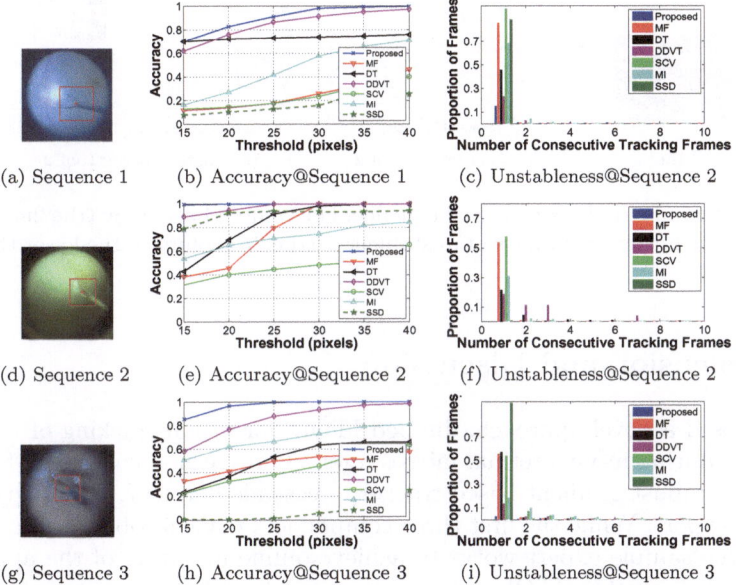

(a) Sequence 1   (b) Accuracy@Sequence 1   (c) Unstableness@Sequence 2

(d) Sequence 2   (e) Accuracy@Sequence 2   (f) Unstableness@Sequence 2

(g) Sequence 3   (h) Accuracy@Sequence 3   (i) Unstableness@Sequence 3

Fig. 2. The results on Retina Microsurgery Dataset. For values of accuracy (the 2nd column), the higher the better. For values of unstableness (the 3rd column), the lower the better.

3.2 Laparoscopy Sequence

Finally, we also evaluate our method on the laparoscopic instrument sequence. The sequence is provided by [5]. DDTV uses the first 500 images for training and the last 500 images for testing. For fair comparison, we follow the setting of [5] and use the last 500 images for testing. However, we only need one image frame for training before tracking because of the online learning technique.

There are two tools in this video. For better visualization, we separately present the experimental results of two instruments in Fig. 3, one in each row. In the sequence, the first tool is under big changes in terms of the instrument structure and movement. Our method significantly outperforms DDVT [5] and two component methods. The second tool is relatively stable in shapes and positions in the whole testing image sequence. The results of the proposed approach are similar to those of the DDVT.

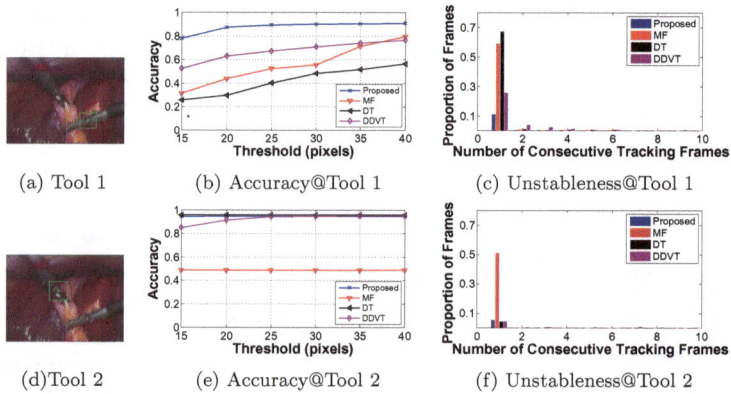

(a) Tool 1   (b) Accuracy@Tool 1   (c) Unstableness@Tool 1

(d)Tool 2   (e) Accuracy@Tool 2   (f) Unstableness@Tool 2

Fig. 3. The results on Laparoscopy Sequence. For values of accuracy (the 2nd column), the higher the better. For values of unstableness (the 3rd column), the lower the better.

4   Conlcusion and Discussion

We proposed a novel approach, dubbed ITOL, for visual tracking of retinal instruments during in-vivo retinal microsurgery. Our method consists of four components: a robust gradient-based tracker, a cascade detector, an integrator and a sample expert. While the first three components make a robust and automatic tracker, the sample expert works to achieve online updating of the appearance model of the detector. ITOL only needs manually labelled position in the first frame and all remaining steps are fully automated, which makes it an approach needing much less user input than other existing methods. ITOL can also automatically re-initialize the tracker after failure. Experimental results on two video datasets demonstrate that the proposed method outperforms the state-of-the-art approaches. Our method makes tracking in RM much more feasible than before.

References

1. Pezzementi, Z., Voros, S., Hager, G.D.: Articulated object tracking by rendering consistent appearance parts. In: IEEE International Conference on Robotics and Automation, ICRA 2009, pp. 3940–3947 (2009)

2. Sznitman, R., Basu, A., Richa, R., Handa, J., Gehlbach, P., Taylor, R.H., Jedynak, B., Hager, G.D.: Unified detection and tracking in retinal microsurgery. In: Fichtinger, G., Martel, A., Peters, T. (eds.) MICCAI 2011, Part I. LNCS, vol. 6891, pp. 1–8. Springer, Heidelberg (2011)
3. Burschka, D., Corso, J.J., Dewan, M., Lau, W., Li, M., Lin, H., Marayong, P., Ramey, N., Hager, G.D., Hoffman, B., et al.: Navigating inner space: 3-D assistance for minimally invasive surgery. Robotics and Autonomous Systems 52(1), 5–26 (2005)
4. Richa, R., Balicki, M., Meisner, E., Sznitman, R., Taylor, R., Hager, G.: Visual tracking of surgical tools for proximity detection in retinal surgery. In: Taylor, R.H., Yang, G.-Z. (eds.) IPCAI 2011. LNCS, vol. 6689, pp. 55–66. Springer, Heidelberg (2011)
5. Sznitman, R., Ali, K., Richa, R., Taylor, R.H., Hager, G.D., Fua, P.: Data-driven visual tracking in retinal microsurgery. In: Ayache, N., Delingette, H., Golland, P., Mori, K. (eds.) MICCAI 2012, Part II. LNCS, vol. 7511, pp. 568–575. Springer, Heidelberg (2012)
6. Grabner, H., Grabner, M., Bischof, H.: Real-time tracking via on-line boosting. In: BMVC, vol. 1, p. 6 (2006)
7. Babenko, B., Yang, M.H., Belongie, S.: Visual tracking with online multiple instance learning. In: IEEE Computer Vision and Pattern Recognition (CVPR), pp. 983–990 (2009)
8. Liu, B., Huang, J., Yang, L., Kulikowsk, C.: Robust tracking using local sparse appearance model and k-selection. In: IEEE Computer Vision and Pattern Recognition (CVPR), pp. 1313–1320 (2011)
9. Liu, B., Yang, L., Huang, J., Meer, P., Gong, L., Kulikowski, C.: Robust and fast collaborative tracking with two stage sparse optimization. In: Daniilidis, K., Maragos, P., Paragios, N. (eds.) ECCV 2010, Part IV. LNCS, vol. 6314, pp. 624–637. Springer, Heidelberg (2010)
10. Sznitman, R., Richa, R., Taylor, R.H., Jedynak, B., Hager, G.D.: Unified detection and tracking of instruments during retinal microsurgery. IEEE Transactions on Pattern Analysis and Machine Intelligence 35(5), 1263–1273 (2013)
11. Kalal, Z., Mikolajczyk, K., Matas, J.: Tracking-learning-detection. IEEE Transactions on Pattern Analysis and Machine Intelligence 34(7), 1409–1422 (2012)
12. Kalal, Z., Mikolajczyk, K., Matas, J.: Forward-backward error: Automatic detection of tracking failures. In: 20th International Conference on Pattern Recognition (ICPR), pp. 2756–2759 (2010)
13. Baker, S., Matthews, I.: Lucas-kanade 20 years on: A unifying framework. International Journal of Computer Vision 56(3), 221–255 (2004)
14. Viola, P., Jones, M.: Rapid object detection using a boosted cascade of simple features. In: Computer Vision and Pattern Recognition (CVPR), vol. 1, pp. I-511–I-518 (2001)
15. Ozuysal, M., Fua, P., Lepetit, V.: Fast keypoint recognition in ten lines of code. In: IEEE Computer Vision and Pattern Recognition (CVPR), pp. 1–8 (2007)
16. Pickering, M.R., Muhit, A.A., Scarvell, J.M., Smith, P.N.: A new multi-modal similarity measure for fast gradient-based 2d-3d image registration. In: IEEE Engineering in Medicine and Biology Society, EMBC 2009, pp. 5821–5824 (2009)
17. Benhimane, S., Malis, E.: Homography-based 2d visual tracking and servoing. The International Journal of Robotics Research 26(7), 661–676 (2007)

Estimating a Patient Surface Model for Optimizing the Medical Scanning Workflow

Vivek Singh[1], Yao-jen Chang[1], Kai Ma[1], Michael Wels[2],
Grzegorz Soza[2], and Terrence Chen[1]

[1] Imaging and Computer Vision
Siemens Corporation, Corporate Technology, Princeton, NJ, USA
[2] Siemens AG, Healthcare Sector
Forchheim, Germany

Abstract. In this paper, we present the idea of equipping a tomographic medical scanner with a range imaging device (e.g. a 3D camera) to improve the current scanning workflow. A novel technical approach is proposed to robustly estimate patient surface geometry by a single snapshot from the camera. Leveraging the information of the patient surface geometry can provide significant clinical benefits, including automation of the scan, motion compensation for better image quality, sanity check of patient movement, augmented reality for guidance, patient specific dose optimization, and more. Our approach overcomes the technical difficulties resulting from suboptimal camera placement due to practical considerations. Experimental results on more than 30 patients from a real CT scanner demonstrate the robustness of our approach.

1 Introduction

State-of-the-art medical imaging technologies such as CT, MR or PET provide high quality visual images of the inside of the patient body to the radiologists and physicians for better diagnosis. Nevertheless, the workflow of the existing scanning procedure depends heavily on the experience and subjective decisions of the technician, which often results in suboptimal image quality, large inter-technician variability, unnecessary radiation to the patient (in case of CT), and prolonged scanning time. In this paper, we propose to equip the scanner with visual capability and the knowledge about the patient surface geometry to improve scanning in all these aspects.

In order to provide the knowledge about the 3D patient surface, we propose a novel framework to obtain a detailed body surface model of the patient (on the table) using a range imaging device, which can ease scan planning in several ways. The estimated surface model includes a detailed body surface mesh as well as the location of various anatomical landmarks (such as the shoulders, thyroid, etc.) in the coordinate reference frame of the scanner. These surface landmarks provide a rough estimate of the organ positions which enables automatic table height adjustment. Furthermore, it can also be used to restrict the scan range to reduce unnecessary irradiation. Other potential clinical benefits include but are

P. Golland et al. (Eds.): MICCAI 2014, Part I, LNCS 8673, pp. 472–479, 2014.

not limited to motion compensation for better image quality, consistent imaging quality across technicians, automatic sanity check based on movement of patient during scan, optimized dose based on patient body size, breathing motion detection, and much more.

Besides the algorithm for surface estimation, appropriate placement of the range imaging device also plays an important role for the optimal surface estimation. Keeping track of key factors such as patient visibility in the camera's field of view, ease of the installation, cost and sensor noise characteristics, we mounted an ASUS Xtion (a structured light sensor that captures depth and color information) on top of the gantry as shown in Figure 1. The camera was positioned carefully to keep as much of the patient in the view as possible while avoiding occlusion by the gantry surface. Mounting the sensor on the gantry also simplifies the installation procedure and avoids structural modifications to the scanning room. Note that range imaging devices for patient positioning in a medical scanning setup have been discussed in the literature before, although primarily in the context of fractionated Radiation Therapy. For instance, [2] use a Microsoft Kinect sensor for coarse patient setup by aligning the range image data of the patient (on the table) with a previously obtained CT scan. [4] use the laser surface scanning system GALAXY to perform a similar task. In our work, we produce a 3D patient deformable mesh from one single camera shot without prior scan. The information can be used in real time for improving various aspects of subsequent scanning.

We validate the performance of our approach by data captured from 33 people with different body shapes, sizes, clothing and ethnicity. Our results demonstrate that the patient surface can be estimated with high accuracy and can potentially enable aforementioned applications.

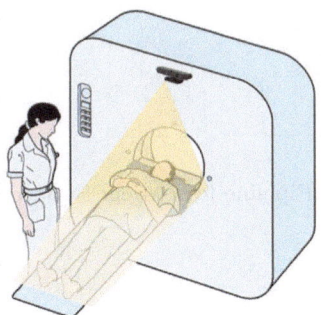

Fig. 1. Structured Light Depth Sensor mounted on top of a CT Scanner

2   Machine Learnt Patient Surface Model Estimation

In this section, we describe the approach to estimate the human body surface geometry from data captured from a single snapshot from a range imaging device such as ASUS Xtion mounted on top of the scanner gantry. While the problem of estimating human body pose and surface geometry in an unconstrained setting is very difficult, we systematically consider the constraints imposed in a medical scanning workflow to solve this problem to a high accuracy. For instance, the knowledge that the patient is lying down on the examination table significantly reduces the degree of articulation of the body pose as well as simplifies the problem of separating the patient region from the background scene information. Furthermore for medical scanning the patient is often required to be in one of the few poses depending on which body region needs to be scanned. For instance, when a head scan is requested, patient pose should be such that the head is close to the gantry and arms are either folded on the abdomen or on the side. While such constraints on body pose help reduce the search space, the system still has to deal with significant shape variations from patient clothing as well as body shape. Furthermore, the depth sensor on the gantry captures data at an angle (about 45 degrees) which can lead to occlusion when a knee rest is used. The approach must also deal with the noise in the data captured from the sensor such as noise due to stereo analysis as well as depth quantization.

In our approach, we systematically take the prior knowledge into account and use machine learning to estimate the patient surface geometry with a high accuracy, while being fast enough for a seamless integration in the patient scanning workflow. Our algorithm consists of 4 modules, as shown in Figure 2 - Patient Isolation (to extract patient region from the rest of the scene), Body Pose Classification (to classify the body pose as prone or supine and head first or feet first), Patient Surface Model Estimation (to fit a kinematic model of body landmarks) and finally, Dense Body Shape Estimation (to fit a deformable body mesh to the range data).

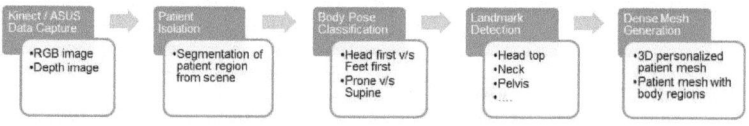

Fig. 2. Processing Pipeline for Patient Surface Model Estimation

2.1   Patient Isolation

Given the color and range data from the sensor (represented as a point cloud), we first localize the image region only containing the patient and the table. Note that the relative position of the range sensor w.r.t. the scanner is known (established during the calibration process) and the range of table movement is limited. We use this spatial prior to automatically crop the image region enclosed by the 3D volume containing the patient and the table. We then transform the cropped data such that the x-axis is aligned with the ground normal and z-axis is aligned with the table length. The transformed depth data (and associated color information) is then orthographically projected on the y-z plane to generate a color and depth image pair (referred as reprojected image), which is then used for subsequent processing. Next, to further refine the position and extent of the patient, we apply a full body detector on the reprojected image. For detection, we employ Probabilistic Boosting Tree (PBT) [8] with 2D HAAR features extracted over reprojected depth and surface normal data (computed using PCL [5]).

2.2 Body Pose Classification

Given the coarse patient position information, we then classify the patient pose in prone or supine, and head first or feet first. We again employ the Probabilistic Boosting Tree (PBT) [8] for this task; for better results, we extend the PBT framework to multiple channels by considering HAAR features extracted from reprojected depth image, surface normal data, saturation image as well as U and V channels from LUV space. In our experiments, we observed that use of multiple channels provides a significant improvement over only using the depth information.

Instead of training one multi-class classifier, we train multiple binary classifiers to systematically handle the variations in the data. We first apply a head first vs. feet first classifier by considering half of the patient region that is close to the sensor (this region covers the upper half of the body for the head first case and lower half for the feet first case). Based on whether pose is head first and feet first, we then apply a prone vs supine classifier. Note that we train separate prone classifiers based on whether the patient is head first or feet first. This is because when the patient is lying on the examination table the data statistics on the head in the head first case are significantly different compared to the feet first case; this is due to the large angle between the camera and body surface as well as the increase in data noise with increasing distance from the sensor.

2.3 Patient Surface Model Estimation

Given the patient pose information, we then fit a sparse body surface model with anatomical landmarks to the data. The body model is represented as a Directed Acyclic Graph (DAG) over the anatomical landmarks on the body surface, such as thyroid etc., where the graph captures the relative position of the landmarks w.r.t. each other. The patient surface is modeled using 10 body landmarks - head, groin, left and right landmarks for shoulders, waist, knees as well as ankles. For each landmark, we train a multi-channel PBT classifier with HAAR features over the same channels as used to train the pose classifier. Due to the camera and body surface angle as well as sensor noise, the image statistics vary significantly over the body surface. The data distribution over a landmark in the head first case is different from that in the feet first case. Thus, we train separate landmark detectors for both these cases. Note that during inference, since the pose category is already known at this stage, only one set of landmark detectors is applied. The relative position of the landmarks is modeled using a

Gaussian whose parameters are obtained from annotations over a training data set.

During inference, the landmark detectors are applied sequentially taking contextual constraints of the neighboring landmarks into account. For each landmark l_i, we obtain the position hypotheses based on the detector response as well as the position hypotheses for the parent landmarks in the DAG.

$$p(l_i|I, l_j) = \prod p(I|l_i)p(l_i|l_j) \quad where, \ l_j \in Parent(l_i) \quad (1)$$

Given the position information for the patient, first the groin landmark detection is applied in the center region. Next the knee detector is applied on the image region estimated based on the constraints from the pose information as well as relative position information from the hypotheses from the groin region. One by one the landmark hypotheses are obtained for each landmark by traversing the DAG. After all the landmark hypotheses are obtained a global reasoning is performed on these hypotheses, to obtain the set of the landmarks with highest joint likelihood based on detection as well as contextual information. Note that this sequential process also handles the size and scale variations across patients of different age, which may be difficult using body pose estimation approaches that first performs a pixel level body region labeling [6]. Furthermore, due to a large angle between camera and body surface, approaches based on body part detection [7] also may not work well due to significant foreshortening of part geometry.

Figure 3 shows landmark detection results on a few images with patients in different poses. For clarity, the figure also shows the body regions estimated by averaging appropriate landmark positions.

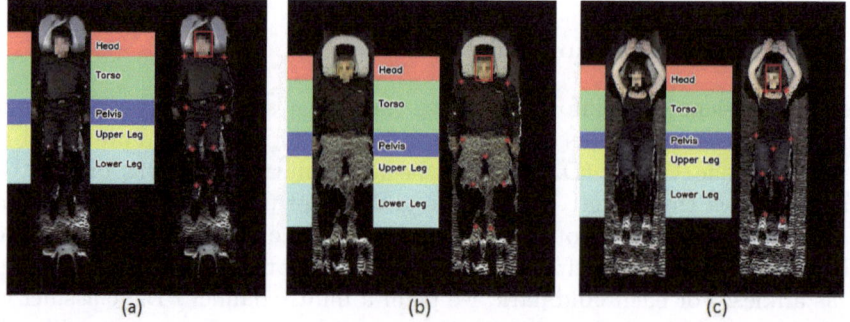

Fig. 3. Landmark detection results and estimated body regions for various poses. Results are rendered on the reprojected images generated by orthographic projection, based on the 3D range data (with associated color information) on the patient table.

2.4   Detailed Body Shape Estimation

Given the location of the landmarks, next we reconstruct the 3D dense patient body surface, represented as a polygon mesh. The reconstructed 3D model is obtained using a parametrized deformable mesh (SCAPE [1]) which can be efficiently perturbed to a target body pose and shape. To model the complex body shape perturbations in compact fashion, [1] decouples the pose and shape perturbation model and during inference, optimizes the pose and shape parameters in an iterative framework. The optimization function for fitting the deformable mesh is modeled as a weighted combination of the surface regularization term (that captures the consistency and smoothness between the neighboring triangles) and a data term (that penalizes for mismatch between the mesh and the input surface data).

In this work, we perform the mesh fitting in a coarse to fine manner for efficiency. We first fit the deformable mesh based on the estimated landmark positions on the patient surface (coarse fit). Next, we apply ICP-based [3] registration to create the correspondences between the deformed template mesh and the 3D surface data. Based on the registration, we optimize the mesh fitting (in an iterative framework) to get a more accurate reconstruction. In our experiments, 2 to 3 iterations were sufficient. Figure 4(a) shows an example of the deformable mesh before and after the optimization. Please observe that the optimized mesh fits the person shape more accurately. Furthermore, the detailed mesh fitting also makes the landmark estimation more precise (as in Figure 4(b)).

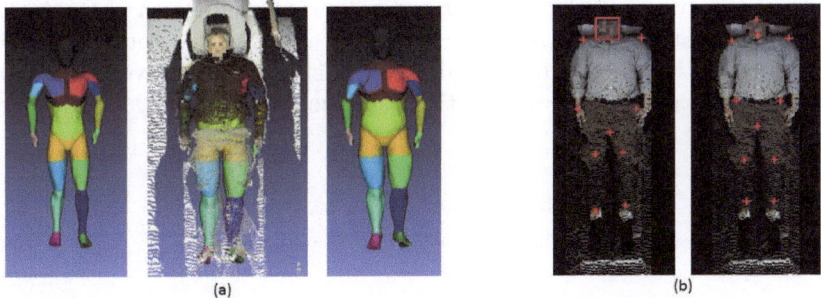

Fig. 4. Detailed Body Shape Estimation. (a) shows the improvement in the body shape estimate before and after the optimization. (b) shows the improvement in landmark precision

3   Experiments

To validate the performance of our approach, we collected data using an ASUS Xtion sensor mounted on the gantry of a Siemens' Somatom CT scanner. The sensor was calibrated w.r.t. the CT scanner by using standard calibration techniques for cameras with color and depth sensors. For our experiments, data was collected from over 33 people with different age, body shapes/sizes, clothing and ethnicity. For each person, about 40 images were obtained to capture data at different table height and for various body poses that are commonly used in the typical scanning workflow (head first vs feet first, prone vs supine and various hand positions). More than 1000 images were obtained for evaluation purpose.

Although the data was captured at the CT scanner, the people who volunteered for the study were not real patients; hence, we only have access to the color and depth data but not the medical data such as CT or MR. For the purpose of evaluation, we generated ground truth by manual annotation of the anatomical landmarks on the image and depth data. However accurately annotating such landmarks on images can be very difficult and ambiguous due to clothing. For this reason, during the data acquisition process, we captured 2 images for each pose of each patient - one with colored markers at the landmarks and one without any markers. The images with colored markers are only used to assist annotations but not included in the evaluation.

For experimental validation, we split the data into train and test sets of 17 and 16 patients respectively. The total processing time for an image was about 3.5 seconds. We report results for various modules in our processing pipeline. The body pose classification module achieved an accuracy of 0.994178 and 0.989811 for head-first vs feet-first and prone vs. supine, respectively.

To measure the landmark estimation accuracy, we report the error as the distance between the ground truth location and the estimated location along the z-axis. This measure is suitable to evaluate the accuracy of the landmarks to define the extent of various body regions (abdomen, pelvis etc) along the table length, which is relevant to typical medical scanning tasks. Figure 5 shows the error at various stages of the processing pipeline, averaged over the entire test dataset. Note that for depth sensors (based on structured light), the error in depth estimation increases quadratically with distance (red curve in the figure) and hence, the error in landmark estimation increases as well. However, even

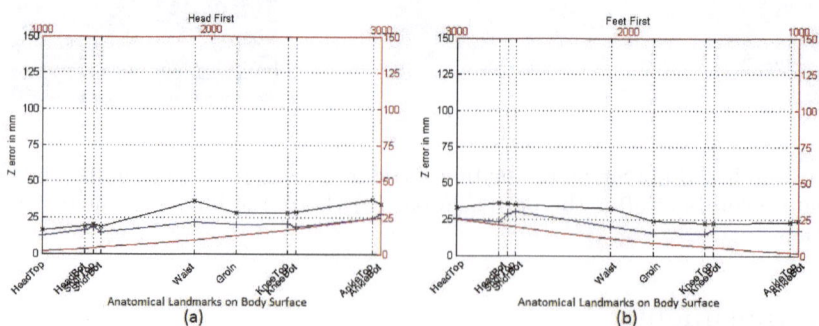

Fig. 5. Quantitative Results. (a) and (b) show the landmark estimation errors for head first and feet first poses respectively. The red curve indicates the error in mm in depth estimation from the depth sensor. Black and blue curves indicate the initial and optimized landmark detection results, respectively.

with the sensor noise, our algorithm still localizes the landmarks with less than 15 mm error for landmarks close to the gantry with error increasing only to 25 mm for the farthest landmarks.

4   Conclusion

A technical approach, which is able to obtain the 3D patient surface model from a single shot of a camera mounted on top of the scanner gantry is proposed. The technology is applicable to different types of medical scanner, such as CT, MR or PET. We validated the approach on real-world data and show robust and promising results. The proposed approach can potentially be used to provide several significant clinical benefits to existing scanning workflows, including time saving, radiation reduction, higher image quality, and real time guidance. Our future work includes capturing real patient camera data with their CT, MR, or PET data to further validate the performance for specific use cases as well as quantitatively evaluate the performance of the dense shape estimation, and to speed up the computation time to potentially update the model in real time.

References

1. Anguelov, D., Srinivasan, P., Koller, D., Thrun, S., Rodgers, J., Davis, J.: SCAPE: shape completion and animation of people. ACM Trans. Graph. 24, 408–416 (2005)
2. Bauer, S., Wasza, J., Haase, S., Marosi, N., Hornegger, J.: Multi-modal surface registration for markerless initial patient setup in radiation therapy using microsoft's kinect sensor. In: IEEE International Conference on Computer Vision Workshops (ICCV Workshops), pp. 1175–1181 (November 2011)
3. Chen, Y., Medioni, G.: Object modeling by registration of multiple range images. In: IEEE International Conference on Robotics and Automation, vol. 3, pp. 2724–2729 (1991)
4. Frenzel, T.: Patient setup using a 3d laser surface scanning system. In: Dossel, O., Schlegel, W.C. (eds.) World Congress on Medical Physics and Biomedical Engineering. IFMBE Proceedings, vol. 25/1, pp. 217–220. Springer, Heidelberg (2009)
5. Rusu, R.B., Cousins, S.: 3D is here: Point cloud library (pcl). In: International Conference on Robotics and Automation. Shanghai, China (2011)
6. Shotton, J., Fitzgibbon, A., Cook, M., Sharp, T., Finocchio, M., Moore, R., Kipman, A., Blake, A.: Real-time human pose recognition in parts from single depth images. In: Proceedings of the 2011 IEEE Conference on Computer Vision and Pattern Recognition, pp. 1297–1304 (2011)
7. Sigal, L., Isard, M., Haussecker, H., Black, M.: Loose-limbed people: Estimating 3d human pose and motion using non-parametric belief propagation. International Journal of Computer Vision 98(1), 15–48 (2012)
8. Tu, Z.: Probabilistic boosting-tree: Learning discriminative models for classification, recognition, and clustering. In: International Conference on Computer Vision (ICCV), vol. 2, pp. 1589–1596. IEEE (2005)

3D Steering of a Flexible Needle by Visual Servoing

Alexandre Krupa

Inria Rennes - Bretagne Atlantique and IRISA, F-35042 Rennes Cedex, France
Alexandre.Krupa@inria.fr
http://www.irisa.fr/lagadic/welcome-eng.html

Abstract. This paper presents a robotic control method for 3D steering of a beveled-tip flexible needle. The solution is based on a new duty-cycling control strategy that makes possible to control three degrees of freedom of the needle. A visual servoing control scheme using two orthogonal cameras observing a translucent phantom is then proposed to automatically steer a needle toward a 3D target point. Experimental results show a final positioning error of 0.4 mm and demonstrate the feasibility of this promising approach and its robustness to model errors.

Keywords: Flexible needle steering, visual servoing.

1 Introduction

The needle is a tool used in many medical procedures as for example aspiration biopsy for cancer diagnosis. However, steering a needle requires a lot of skills from the clinician in order to reach the target successfully. A new community of researchers are currently working to provide robotic assistance solutions and more particularly for steering bevel-tip flexible needles [1]. By applying a translation motion to this kind of needle, this later bends during the insertion due to asymmetric forces exerted by the soft tissue onto the beveled tip. As a consequence the needle follows an arc in a 2D plane as reported in [2,3]. This bending becomes an advantage for targeting anatomical elements that were not possible to reach with a standard rigid needle. Several research works have therefore been conducted to automatically steer a flexible needle actuated by a robot. In most approaches a path planning initial step based on inverse kinematics is required to predict the needle trajectory. A finite element mesh was also considered in [4] to predict soft tissue deformations and plan the path thanks to a numerical optimization. Probabilistic methods were also tested, like the Rapidly-Exploring-Random Tree (RRT) algorithm [5], or the Stochastic roadmap [6]. In [7] a kinematic model was proposed for bevel-tip needle steering by constantly spinning the needle during its insertion. This model allows proportional control of the needle curvature and was used in a control-loop that online adapts the evolution of the needle trajectory along an arc in a 2D plane [8]. Other approaches based on the RRT algorithm were proposed to take into account obstacles during the path planning. For example, a RRT algorithm with backchaining was

P. Golland et al. (Eds.): MICCAI 2014, Part I, LNCS 8673, pp. 480–487, 2014.

presented in [9] to steer the needle in 3D with obstacle avoidance. More recently, a combination of the RRT algorithm and duty-cycling control technique was proposed in [10] for needle steering in a 2D plane. In this paper, we propose a new approach to steer a needle in 3D that has several advantages. First, it does not require a trajectory planning that can be time consuming. Second, it does not constraint the needle to follow a succession of planar arcs but allows non planar 3D trajectories. Third, with the proposed method the direct control of the two lateral angular velocities and the insertion velocity of the needle extremity is possible. This last point is crucial since, in opposite to approaches based on path planning, it opens numerous control scheme possibilities as for example visual control using the classical framework of visual servoing [11]. The paper is organized as follows. Section 2 presents the kinematic model of the flexible needle and recalls the principle of the classic 2D duty-cycling control technique. We present in Section 3 our 3D duty-cycling strategy that allows to control the two lateral angular velocities and the insertion velocity of the needle. Section 4 presents the control scheme we propose for automatic soft tissue targeting using visual servoing. Finally, experimental results on the visual targeting task are reported and discussed in section 5.

2 Needle Kinematic Model and Duty-Cycling Technique

Let $\mathcal{F}_n$ and $\mathcal{F}_w$ be respectively a Cartesian frame attached to the needle tip and the world frame as shown in Figure 1a. We describe the 3D pose $\mathbf{p}$ (with $\mathbf{p} \in \mathrm{SE}(3)$) of the needle tip with respect to $\mathcal{F}_w$ by the homogeneous 4×4 transformation matrix :

$$^{w}\mathbf{M}_n = \begin{bmatrix} ^{w}\mathbf{R}_n & ^{w}\mathbf{T}_n \\ \mathbf{0}_{[1 \times 3]} & 1 \end{bmatrix} \tag{1}$$

where $^{w}\mathbf{R}_n$ is a 3×3 rotation matrix representing the orientation of $\mathcal{F}_n$ with respect to $\mathcal{F}_w$ and $^{w}\mathbf{T}_n$ is the 3×1 translation vector defining the origin of $\mathcal{F}_n$ in

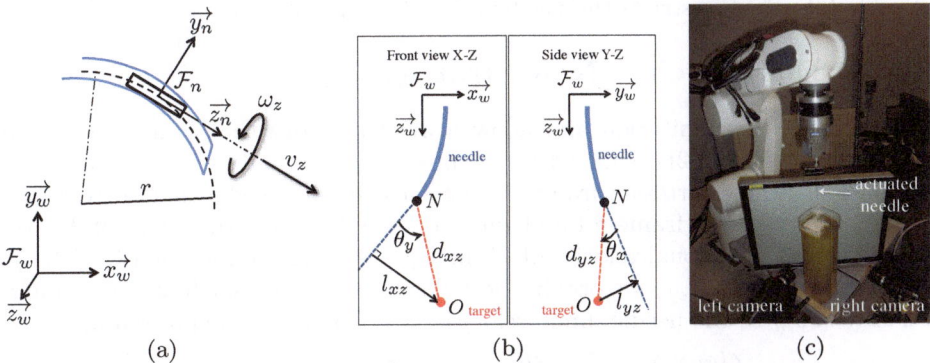

(a)   (b)   (c)

Fig. 1. (a) needle beveled tip modeled by an unicycle following an arc of radius r. (b) Geometry of selected visual features. (c) Experimental setup.

$\mathcal{F}_w$. We also denote the instantaneous screw velocity vector $^{(n)}\mathbf{v}_n$ of the needle frame $\mathcal{F}_n$ with respect to the world $\mathcal{F}_w$. It is composed by the translational velocities $^{(n)}v_x$, $^{(n)}v_y$, $^{(n)}v_z$ along each axis of $\mathcal{F}_n$ and the angular velocities $^{(n)}\omega_x$, $^{(n)}\omega_y$, $^{(n)}\omega_z$ around each axis. Note that the upper script $^{(n)}$ indicates that this velocity is expressed in the frame $\mathcal{F}_n$. If we apply a forward insertion motion to the needle, then this later can only move in the plane y-z of $\mathcal{F}_n$. Thus, the velocity components $^{(n)}v_x$, $^{(n)}v_y$, $^{(n)}\omega_y$ are constraint to be null and only the insertion velocity $^{(n)}v_z$, and angular spin velocity $^{(n)}\omega_z$ can be applied by the user to steer the needle. As experimentally demonstrated in [2], the bending effect due to the asymmetric beveled tip introduces a rotation velocity around the x axis of $\mathcal{F}_n$ that depends on the insertion velocity and natural curvature K of the needle such as $\omega_x = K\,^{(n)}v_z$. The screw velocity vector is therefore linked to the needle input velocities by the following kinematic relation that expresses the nonholonomic contraints:

$$^{(n)}\mathbf{v}_n = \begin{bmatrix} 0 & 0 & 1 & K & 0 & 0 \\ 0 & 0 & 0 & 0 & 0 & 1 \end{bmatrix}^T \begin{pmatrix} ^{(n)}v_z \\ ^{(n)}\omega_z \end{pmatrix} \tag{2}$$

The duty cycling method [7] was introduced to allow the proportional control of the curvature of a bevel-tip needle during insertion. It works by alternating between time period T_{trans} of pure insertion where the needle will follow an arc of maximum curvature K, with time period T_{rot} of both insertion and rotation, where the needle will follow a helical curve. This later becomes a straight line if the rotation velocity is highly superior than the insertion velocity. Those two phases compose a cycle of period $T = T_{rot} + T_{trans}$. Therefore, it is possible to obtain a desired effective needle curvature $K_{eff} = K(1 - DC)$ by controlling the duty-cycle ratio $DC = \frac{T_{rot}}{T}$. In [8,10] this method has been implemented by inserting during each cycle the needle on a constant fixed distance Δz, and by applying a constant rotational velocity $\omega_z = \omega_c$ such as:

$$T_{rot} = \frac{2\pi}{\omega_c}, T_{trans} = \frac{T_{rot}(1 - DC)}{DC}, v_z = \frac{\Delta z}{T} \tag{3}$$

However, this technique applies a complete rotation (2π rad) during each cycle of period T which restricts the needle to evolve only in a plane.

3 3D Duty-Cycling New Strategy

To overcome this limitation and allow a 3D trajectory that is not composed from a succession of 2D planar arcs, we propose a new duty-cycle strategy. Let us consider a new cartesian frame $\mathcal{F}_{\tilde{n}}$ attached to the needle that corresponds to the current needle frame rotated with an angle θ around the z axis of $\mathcal{F}_n$. By expressing the rotational velocity of $\mathcal{F}_{\tilde{n}}$ in $\mathcal{F}_n$ and using the relation (2) with the effective curvature K_{eff} we obtain the following relation that links the angular velocity of $\mathcal{F}_n$ to the needle input velocities $^{(\tilde{n})}v_z$ and $^{(\tilde{n})}\omega_z$ expressed in $\mathcal{F}_{\tilde{n}}$:

$$\begin{pmatrix} ^{(n)}\omega_x \\ ^{(n)}\omega_y \\ ^{(n)}\omega_z \end{pmatrix} = \begin{bmatrix} \cos(\theta) & -\sin(\theta) & 0 \\ \sin(\theta) & \cos(\theta) & 0 \\ 0 & 0 & 1 \end{bmatrix} \begin{pmatrix} K_{eff}\,^{(\tilde{n})}v_z \\ 0 \\ ^{(\tilde{n})}\omega_z \end{pmatrix} \tag{4}$$

As $\mathcal{F}_{\tilde{n}}$ and $\mathcal{F}_n$ have the same origin and their z-axis are aligned, we have $^{(n)}v_z = ^{(\tilde{n})}v_z$ that we replace in (4) to formulate the angular velocity of $\mathcal{F}_n$ by:

$$^{(n)}\omega_x = cos(\theta)K_{eff}\,^{(n)}v_z \text{ and } ^{(n)}\omega_y = sin(\theta)K_{eff}\,^{(n)}v_z \tag{5}$$

One can notice that it is therefore possible to control the velocities $^{(n)}\omega_x$ and $^{(n)}\omega_y$ at each cycle period T by applying an angle θ around its z-axis before inserting the needle and applying then the desired curvature such as:

$$\theta = atan(^{(n)}\omega_y/\,^{(n)}\omega_x) \text{ and } K_{eff} = (\sqrt{^{(n)}\omega_x^2 + ^{(n)}\omega_y^2})/^{(n)}v_z \tag{6}$$

Note that if $^{(n)}v_z$ is null we set $K_{eff} = 0$ since the needle is not moving in this case. In practice, our 3D duty-cycling approach is performed by the following successive steps:

1) measure the current absolute needle spin angle: θ_a
2) compute the desired absolute spin angle to achieve by accumulating 2π rad and the control angle input θ given by eq. (6) such as: $\theta_a = \theta_a + 2\pi + \theta$
3) compute the desired period T_{rot} and desired spin angular velocity profile $^{(n)}\omega_z$ needed to achieve θ_a based on a trapezoidal acceleration profile with a nominal needle spin velocity of ω_c
4) compute the desired insertion distance $\Delta z = ^{(n)}v_z\,T_{rot}$
5) perform the rotation and insertion thanks to the position-based robot low-level controller to reach the desired angle θ_a and translation Δ_z
6) measure the real period T_{rot} that was taken by the system
7) compute the desired duty-cycle ratio $DC = 1 - K_{eff}/K$ with K_{eff} given by (6), the desired pure translation period $T_{trans} = T_{rot}(1 - DC)/DC$ and the desired insertion distance $\Delta z = ^{(n)}v_z\,T_{trans}$
8) perform the insertion thanks to the position-based robot low-level controller to reach the desired relative translation Δ_z
9) go back to step 1) to start a new cycle.

4   Automatic Targeting by Visual Servoing

We consider that a 3D image containing the needle is available thanks for example to the use of a 3D ultrasound probe. It is therefore possible to extract the shape of the needle by performing some image processing. We will not detail any method to extract the needle but the reader can refer for example to the RANSAC-based approach proposed in [12]. By the use of such extraction algorithm it is therefore possible to obtain the current location of the needle tip point that we denoted N of coordinates $^w\mathbf{T}_n = (t_{nx}, t_{ny}, t_{nz})$ and its tip direction orientation $^w\mathbf{R}_n$ with respect to the world frame $\mathcal{F}_w$. As the target coordinates that we denote $^w\mathbf{T}_o = (t_{ox}, t_{oy}, t_{oz})$ are expressed in the world frame $\mathcal{F}_w$ and not directly in the needle frame $\mathcal{F}_n$, it is more suitable to express the needle lateral angular control velocities in the fixed world frame $\mathcal{F}_w$. The lateral angular velocities applied to the needle frame will then be obtained from the lateral control velocities $^{(w)}\omega_x$, $^{(w)}\omega_y$ expressed in $\mathcal{F}_w$ thanks to the following relation:

$$\begin{pmatrix} ^{(n)}\omega_x \\ ^{(n)}\omega_y \end{pmatrix} = {}^{w}\mathbf{R}_{n_{[2\times2]}}{}^{T} \begin{pmatrix} ^{(w)}\omega_x \\ ^{(w)}\omega_y \end{pmatrix} \qquad (7)$$

where $^{w}\mathbf{R}_{n_{[2\times2]}}{}^{T}$ is the transpose of the $[2 \times 2]$ upper-left part of $^{w}\mathbf{R}_n$.

To perform the targeting task we propose to apply a constant needle insertion velocity $^{(n)}v_z = v_c$ and online adapt the angular control velocities $^{(w)}\omega_x$, $^{(w)}\omega_y$ by visual servoing in such a way to orientate the needle z-axis toward the target. The set of visual features that we chose is $\mathbf{s} = (l_{xz}, l_{yz})$ where l_{xz} and l_{yz} are respectively the distances between the target point O and their orthogonal projections onto the needle line direction projected in the x-z plane and y-z plane of $\mathcal{F}_w$ as shown in Figure 1b. Let us denote d_{xz} and d_{yz} the distances of the projections of vector $\overrightarrow{NO}$ into the x-z plane and y-z plane of $\mathcal{F}_w$. We also define θ_x and θ_y as being respectively the angles around the world frame x and y axes that describe the relative orientation of the vector $\overrightarrow{NO}$ with respect to needle unitary orientation vector $^{w}\mathbf{u}$ (see Figure 1b). Note that all these geometrical features can be easily computed from the measured 3D positions of the needle and target. The visual features can therefore be obtained from: $l_{xz} = d_{xz} \sin(\theta_y)$ and $l_{yz} = -d_{yz} \sin(\theta_x)$. The visual servoing task consists then in aligning the needle line direction on the target by regulating $\mathbf{s}$ to the desired value $\mathbf{s}^* = (0,0)$. As we previously mentioned, one important advantage of our new 3D duty-cycling strategy is that we can apply the classical framework of visual servoing [11]. Therefore we first determine the image jacobian $\mathbf{J}$ that relates the variation $\dot{\mathbf{s}}$ of the selected visual features to the needle velocity inputs and obtain the following expression from basic angular kinematic relationships:

$$\dot{\mathbf{s}} = \begin{pmatrix} \dot{l}_{xz} \\ \dot{l}_{yz} \end{pmatrix} = \underbrace{\left[\mathbf{J}_{\omega_{xy}} \; \mathbf{J}_{v_z}\right]}_{=\mathbf{J}} \begin{pmatrix} ^{(w)}\omega_x \\ ^{(w)}\omega_y \\ ^{(n)}v_z \end{pmatrix} \quad \text{with } \mathbf{J}_{\omega_{xy}} = \begin{bmatrix} 0 & \cos(\theta_y)d_{xz} \\ -\cos(\theta_x)d_{yz} & 0 \end{bmatrix}$$

$$(8)$$

and $\mathbf{J}_{v_z} = \begin{bmatrix} 0 & 0 \end{bmatrix}^{T}$. Finally we applied the following classical control law that gives the control angular velocity inputs in such a way to obtain an exponential decrease of the visual error $\mathbf{e} = \mathbf{s} - \mathbf{s}^*$:

$$\begin{pmatrix} ^{(w)}\omega_x \\ ^{(w)}\omega_y \end{pmatrix} = -\lambda \mathbf{J}_{\omega_{xy}}^{-1} \mathbf{e} \text{ where } \lambda > 0 \text{ is a proportional gain.} \qquad (9)$$

5   Experimental Results

The experiment setup is presented in Figure 1c. It is composed of a 6-DOF anthropomorphic robot holding a 22 gauge bevel-tip flexible aspiration biopsy needle of 20 cm length (Angiotech Chiba MCN2208). A homemade translucent gelatin phantom built relatively less flexible than the needle (assuring the model non-holonomic assumption) is employed to simulate a piece of organic soft tissues and is observed by two orthogonal video cameras. The cameras are used to

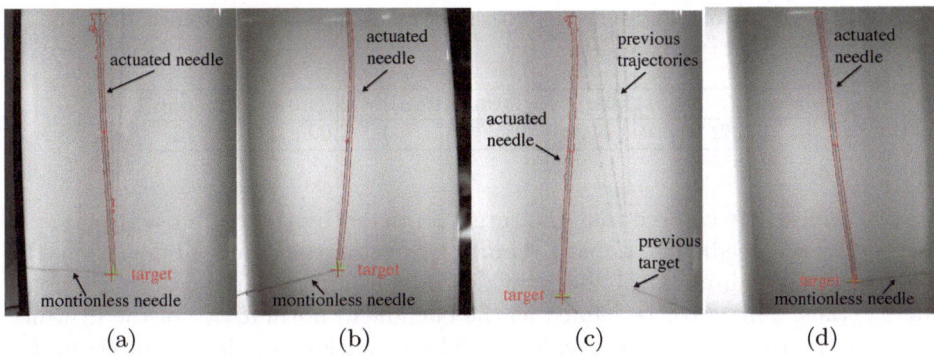

Fig. 2. (a) right camera (x-z plane) and (b) left camera (y-z plane) views of the needle trajectory obtained with the targeting task by visual servoing for one trial. (c) right and left (d) views obtained for another trial. The extracted shape of the actuated needle is displayed in red and the needle tip location is shown by the green cross. The red cross corresponds to the target that was defined by indicating in the images the location of the tip of a second motionless needle that was previously manually inserted. One can see the hole in the phantom performed by other previous trials which also successfully reached the target.

perform a 3D localization of the needle tip, but another image modality could be used as for example 3D ultrasound as we plan to consider in future work. The flat screen monitor positioned behind the phantom is used to illuminate the phantom. The image processing and robot motion control is implemented on a PC equiped with a Dual-core 2.4 Ghz Intel Pentium. The needle tip 3D location is measured by first thresholding the images and applying basic morphological operations (erosion, dilatation). Then an algorithm that extracts connected pixels is employed to retain only the pixels corresponding to the needle shape. The tip location and direction vector of the needle is then computed in each image and their 3D coordinates are obtained thanks to the intrinsic parameters of the two calibrated cameras. We coarsely fixed the natural curvature value of the needle that is used in the control to $K = 2$ m^{-1} (corresponding to a radius of 0.5 m). In all experiments we applied a constant insertion velocity of 1 mm/s and the control gain of the visual servoing was empirically set to $\lambda = 0.02$. In order to simulate a target point in the phantom we manually inserted another needle from an entry point realized on a lateral wall of the phantom as shown in the bottom of the camera views presented in Figure 2. This allows us to obtain the target 3D coordinates ground truth by clicking on the tip of this motionless needle in the two images. We performed 25 trials of our automatic targeting task by visual servoing with different target positions that were fixed in a 3D region that is reachable by the needle. For each experiment the entry point of the needle actuated by the robot was slightly shifted for avoiding insertion in a previous hole of the phantom. For all these trials the target was successfully reached. Figure 2 presents the needle trajectories observed in the left and right images

Table 1. Mean, standard deviation, maximum and minimum values of the final positioning error d_{error} of the needle tip with respect to the target obtained from the 25 automatic targeting trials

Mean (mm)	Standard deviation (mm)	Max (mm)	Min (mm)
0.432	0.262	1.023	0.113

for two trials. One can see that the target depicted by the red cross is perfectly reached by the needle tip. Table 1 reports the mean, the standard deviation, the maximum and minimum of the final positioning error that are obtained from the 25 trials. This error is defined as the euclidiean norm d_{error} of the distance between the target and the needle tip. The evolutions of the visual errors for the trial corresponding to the views of Figures 2a-2b are presented in Figures 3a-3b. They correspond as expected to exponential decreases toward zero. Figure 3c shows the evolution of the distance between the needle tip and target and Figures 3d-3e show the projection of the needle trajectory onto the x-z and y-z planes of $\mathcal{F}_w$. The evolution of the duty-cycling control ratio DC input applied to our 3D duty-cycling low-level controller is reported in Figure 3f. The results also experimentally demonstrate that the targeting task by visual servoing is robust to modelling errors since we do not consider the torsional effect of the needle in its kinematic model and we employ a coarse estimated constant value of its natural curvature.

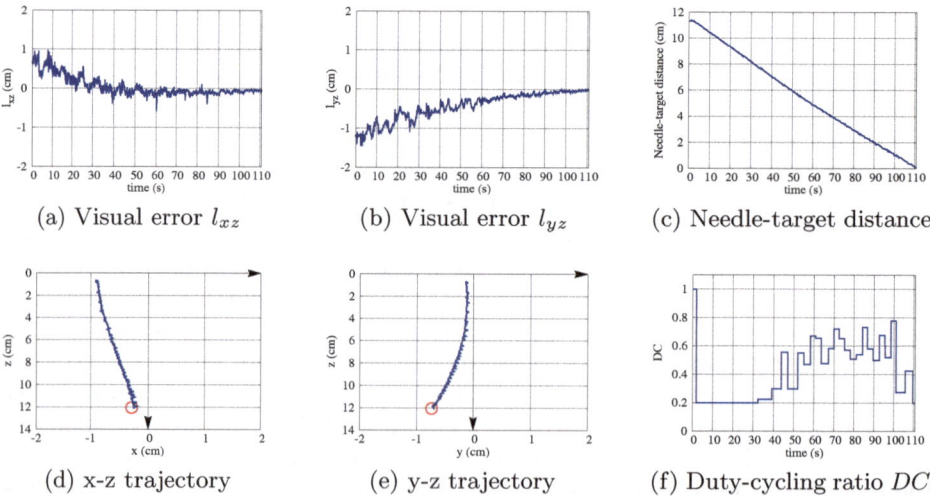

(a) Visual error l_{xz} (b) Visual error l_{yz} (c) Needle-target distance

(d) x-z trajectory   (e) y-z trajectory   (f) Duty-cycling ratio DC

Fig. 3. Results of one trial of the targeting task by visual servoing: (a)-(b) visual features errors. (c) distance between the needle and target. (d)-(e) obtained needle 3D trajectory projected in the x-z and y-z world frame planes. (f) applied duty-cycling ratio with a lower saturation of 0.2 to limit the period time of pure translation.

6   Conclusion

In this paper we presented a new duty-cycling strategy that allows to control the insertion velocity and the two lateral angular velocities of a bevel-tip flexible needle. Experimental results demonstrate the efficiency of our approach to steer the needle to reach a 3D target directly by visual servoing without relying like other methods on a computationally expensive path planning that generates a trajectory composed from successive planar arcs. We are currently implementing our approach to automatically steer a flexible needle by ultrasound visual servoing thanks to the use of a 3D ultrasound probe. We are also planning to design a hierarchical multi-task control law for obstacle avoidance.

References

1. Reed, K., Majewicz, A., Kallem, V., Alterovitz, R., Goldberg, K., Cowan, N., Okamura, A.: Robot-assisted needle steering. IEEE Robotics and Automation Magazine 18(4), 35–46 (2011)
2. Webster III, R., Kim, J., Cowan, N., Chirikjian, G., Okamura, A.M.: Nonholonomic modeling of needle steering. The International Journal of Robotics Research 25(5-6), 509–525 (2006)
3. Misra, S., Reed, K., Schafer, B., Ramesh, K., Okamura, A.: Mechanics of flexible needles robotically steered through soft tissue. The International Journal of Robotics Research 29(13), 1640–1660 (2010)
4. Alterovitz, R., Goldberg, K., Okamura, A.: Planning for steerable bevel-tip needle insertion through 2D soft tissue with obstacles. In: IEEE Int. Conf on Robotics and Automation, pp. 1640–1645 (2005)
5. LaValle, S., Kuffner, J.: Randomized kinodynamic planning. In: IEEE Int. Conf. on Robotics and Automation, vol. 1, pp. 473–479 (1999)
6. Alterovitz, R., Siméon, T., Goldberg, K.: The stochastic motion roadmap: A sampling framework for planning with markov motion uncertainty. In: Burgard, W., et al. (eds.) Robotics: Science and Systems III, pp. 233–241. MIT Press (2008)
7. Minhas, D., Engh, J., Fenske, M., Riviere, C.: Modeling of needle steering via duty-cycled spinning. In: IEEE Int. Conf. on Engineering in Medicine and Biology Society, pp. 2756–2759 (2007)
8. Wood, N., Shahrour, K., Ost, M., Riviere, C.: Needle steering system using duty-cycled rotation for percutaneous kidney access. In: IEEE Int. Conf on Engineering in Medicine and Biology Society (EMBS), pp. 5432–5435 (2010)
9. Xu, J., Duindam, V., Alterovitz, R., Goldberg, K.: Motion planning for steerable needles in 3D environments with obstacles using rapidly-exploring random trees and backchaining. In: IEEE Int. Conf on Automation Science and Engineering, pp. 41–46 (2008)
10. Bernardes, M., Adorno, B., Poignet, P., Borges, G.: Robot-assisted automatic insertion of steerable needles with closed-loop imaging feedback and intraoperative trajectory replanning. Mechatronics 23, 630–645 (2013)
11. Chaumette, F., Hutchinson, S.: Visual servo control, part i: Basic approaches. IEEE Robotics and Automation Magazine 13(4), 82–90 (2006)
12. Uhercik, M., Kybic, J., Liebgott, H., Cachard, C.: Model fitting using ransac for surgical tool localization in 3-D ultrasound images. IEEE Trans. on Biomedical Engineering 57(8), 1907–1916 (2010)

Improved Screw Placement for Slipped Capital Femoral Epiphysis (SCFE) Using Robotically-Assisted Drill Guidance

Bamshad Azizi Koutenaei[1,2], Ozgur Guler[1], Emmanuel Wilson[1],
Ramesh U. Thoranaghatte[3], Matthew Oetgen[1], Nassir Navab[2,4], and Kevin Cleary[1]

[1] Children's National Medical Center, Washington D.C, United States
{bazizi,oguler,ewilson,moetgen,kcleary}@cnmc.org
[2] Chair for Computer Aided Medical Procedures (CAMP), TUM, Munich, Germany
{bazizi,nassir}@cs.tum.edu
[3] NeoMedz Sarl, Switzerland
rameshtu@yahoo.com
[4] Computer Aided Medical Procedures, Johns Hopkins University, USA

Abstract. Slipped Capital Femoral Epiphysis (SCFE) is a common hip displacement condition in adolescents. In the standard treatment, the surgeon uses intra-operative fluoroscopic imaging to plan the screw placement and the drill trajectory. The accuracy, duration, and efficacy of this procedure are highly dependent on surgeon skill. Longer procedure times result in higher radiation dose, to both patient and surgeon. A robotic system to guide the drill trajectory might help to reduce screw placement errors and procedure time by reducing the number of passes and confirmatory fluoroscopic images needed to verify accurate positioning of the drill guide along a planned trajectory. Therefore, with the long-term goals of improving screw placement accuracy, reducing procedure time and intra-operative radiation dose, our group is developing an image-guided robotic surgical system to assist a surgeon with pre-operative path planning and intra-operative drill guide placement.

Keywords: Slipped Capital Femoral Epiphysis (SCFE), Robotically-assisted orthopedic surgery, Computer-aided intervention.

1 Introduction

Slipped capital femoral epiphysis (SCFE) is a common hip disorder in early adolescence that results in displacement of the proximal femoral epiphysis into a posterior and inferior position in relation to the proximal femoral metaphysis. Symptoms of SCFE include groin or knee pain, decreased hip range of motion, and a limp. Due to the risk of permanent injury to the hip joint with continued displacement, SCFE is considered an orthopedic emergency. Surgical treatment is aimed at stabilization of the proximal femoral epiphysis to prevent further displacement, and traditionally has been done by placing one or two screws from the proximal femoral metaphysis across

P. Golland et al. (Eds.): MICCAI 2014, Part I, LNCS 8673, pp. 488–495, 2014.

the physis into the femoral head (shown in fig. 1). The SCFE procedure is done in a minimally invasive manner using X-ray fluoroscopic imaging for visualization. Minimally invasive surgical techniques are advantageous to patients, as they are less disruptive to the soft tissues and often lead to faster functional patient recovery. Despite this benefit, the lack of direct field visualization while operating, as opposed to open surgery, makes these techniques much more technically challenging and requires the surgeon to have an extensive three-dimensional understanding of anatomy to perform the procedure safely. Minimally invasive techniques in orthopedic surgery are often aided by X-ray fluoroscopic imaging. However, concerns exist regarding radiation dose when using fluoroscopy, particularly in pediatrics.

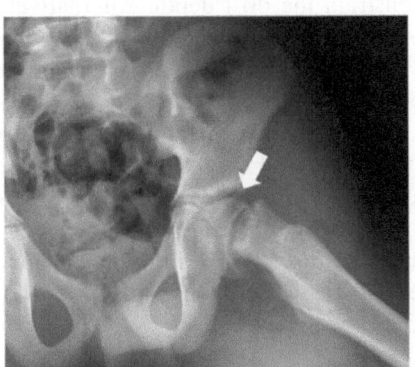 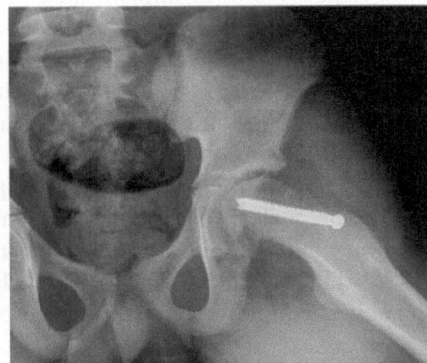

Fig. 1. (Left) Presenting radiograph of a child with slipped capital femoral epiphysis. The proximal epiphysis is displaced posteriorly on the femoral neck (arrow). (Right) Hip radiograph showing fixation of the slipped capital femoral epiphysis with a single screw into the hip.

In the current treatment of SCFE, the surgeon uses intra-operative fluoroscopic imaging to guide the placement of the screw guide pin, confirm the drill trajectory, and direct the final screw placement. Optimal placement of the screw requires precision, with the best position being perpendicular to the physis and deep and central in the femoral head. Improper screw placement, either off center or poorly angled in relation to the physis, leads to the possibility of significant complications from the implant including hip joint penetration, chondrolysis, femoral head vascular injury, proximal femoral avascular necrosis, and poor patient outcomes. The accuracy, duration, and efficacy of this procedure are dependent on surgeon skill and experience. Longer procedures involve higher radiation dose, to both the patient and surgeon.

Other researchers have investigated navigation techniques for orthopedic procedures. For distal locking of intramedullary implants, Suhm et al. showed that radiation exposure time could be decreased from 108 seconds to 7 seconds by using a computer aided surgery navigation system. While procedure time was increased slightly by the use of the navigation system, radiation dose was decreased significantly [1]. In another study of distal locking by Rohilla et al., the average number of fluoroscopy images used for the complete procedure was 48.27 [2], which results in significant radiation exposure. To improve visualization during minimally invasive procedures and reduce radiation exposure, many researchers have proposed augmented reality systems such as video see-through binocular systems [3], half-mirror display devices [4], systems that directly project images onto the patient's body [5], and single laser-beam pointers [6]. However, these systems have some other challenges such as complexity in surgical tool alignment in proper position and orientation.

In many orthopedic surgeries, navigating the surgical tool to the desired target position is crucial. In addition to image-guided navigation techniques, other methods have been investigated, either to augment the available visual information or to provide additional guidance to a conventional surgical approach. An infrared system was used to track the surgical tool position and provide depth guidance during drilling [7]. Simpler mechanical frames, in the form of a physical stopper, depth guide and depth guidance rings have been implemented to constrain the drill depth. Alternatively, a combination of image-guided and robot-assisted navigation would be a reliable method to provide all required information to perform an intervention in the most efficient and precise way. In regards to the placement of implants to treat SCFE, a navigated robotic system could help reduce both screw placement errors and procedure time by allowing more precise screw placement and decreasing the number of fluoroscopic images needed to accurately position the drill guide along the planned trajectory. The goal of this study was to improve screw placement accuracy, and reduce procedure time and intra-operative radiation dose, by developing an image-guided robotic surgical system to assist the orthopedic surgeon with pre-operative path planning and intra-operative drill guide placement.

2   Methodology

A conventional SCFE procedure relies on fluoroscopy to provide the visual feedback needed by the surgeon to accurately place the fixation screw. This exposes the surgeon to significant radiation exposure over their operating lifetime. In addition, the precision of screw placement is highly dependent on the surgeon's skill and ability to visualize the 3D trajectory of the screw from 2D X-ray images. A few millimeters of screw misplacement could potentially lead to major complications. It requires an experienced surgeon to determine the proper position and orientation of the screw and mentally transform the patient space to image space. All these reasons lead us to develop our robotic assist system for the SCFE procedure. The major contribution of this paper is developing and demonstrating an integrated platform for surgeons that assists in path planning by choosing the entry and target point easier and faster. In addition, we aim to increase the precision of screw placement and decrease the time of the SCFE procedure by navigating the robot to align the drill tip position and drill path along a planned trajectory. When the drill guide is at the planned target location, it provides a rigid and constrained trajectory for the drill to advance.

Pre-operative Planning: The surgical workstation uses preoperative CT data to provide a four-quadrant view of the surgical anatomy. The workstation was created using the open source software package the image-guided surgical toolkit (IGSTK)[8]. This four-quadrant view consists of axial, sagittal, coronal and 3D rendered volumetric views, which can be used by the surgeon to define skin entry and final target points for screw placement (as shown in fig. 2).

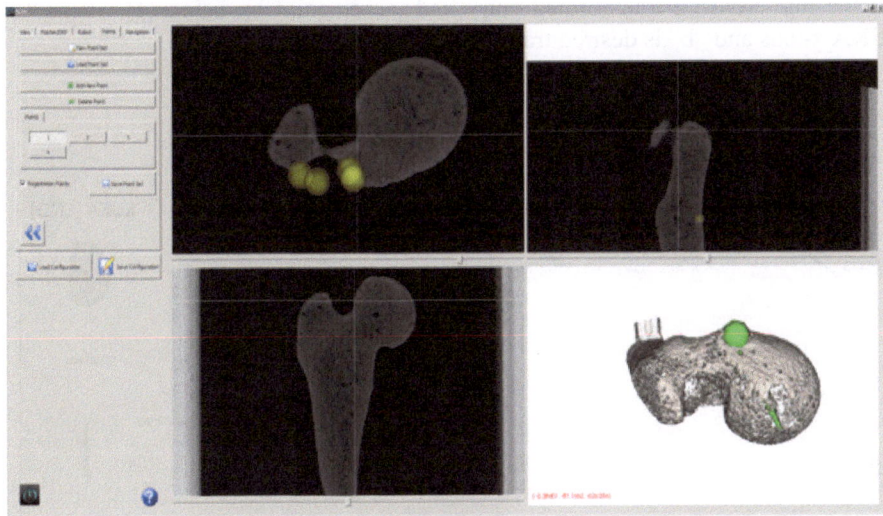

Fig. 2. Surgical navigation workstation showing axial, sagittal, coronal, and 3D views

Trajectory Planning and Calculation of Robot Transformation: The robotic arm used to position the drill guide is a 7 DOF KUKA Light Weight Robot (LWR) robot[1]. The KUKA Fast Research Interface (FRI) API is used to establish a communication between workstation PC and KUKA robot. The application and FRI communication run in parallel using multi-threading. FRI can transfer 20 packets per second which allows the system to update the current position and orientation of the robot in real-time. This update rate means any position change of patient, tracking system, or KUKA base will be compensated quickly via FRI. The surgical navigation component measures the current position of the patient and the robot end-effector and calculates the transformation needed to move the robot from its current position to the planned position. The transformation is then sent to the robot via FRI. A Polaris[TM] optical tracking system[2] is used to track the locations of the bone phantom and KUKA end-effector and provides a means of computing the transformations between patient and robotic workspace, shown in fig. 3 Two unique rigid body markers, one mounted to the KUKA drill guide tool and one mounted to the bone phantom, are used to track their locations in tracker camera coordinates. The surgical navigation component provides registration between the pre-operative CT dataset and tracker coordinates. This is done using paired-point registration [9] of identifiable phantom surface

---

[1] KUKA Robotics GMBH, Germany.
[2] Northern Digital Inc., Waterloo, Canada.

features. The transformation from CT to camera coordinates is then used to transform the skin entry and target points (selected by the surgeon within the surgical planning application) to robot coordinate space. Since the drill guide is aligned precisely to the X-axis of the KUKA, our application finds the angles between the X-axis of KUKA and the line crossing transformed entry and target point by using (1) where "a" is KUKA x-axis and "b" is desired trajectory.

$$\cos\theta = \frac{\bar{a}.\bar{b}}{|a|\times|b|} \qquad (1)$$

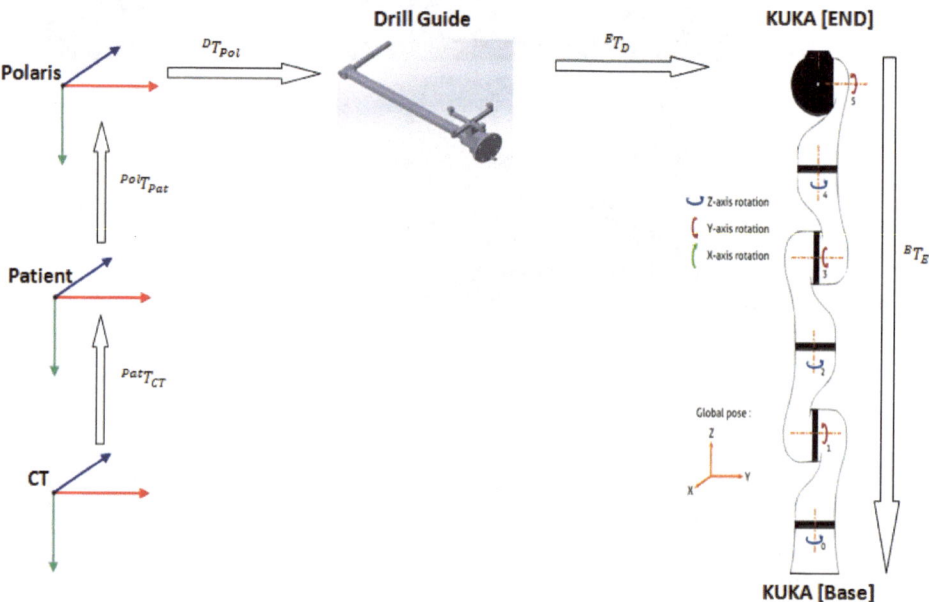

Fig. 3. Chain of transformation from patient coordinate system to KUKA[3] coordinate system

Intra-operative Robot Positioning: A drill guide was designed and fabricated through rapid prototyping[4] to affix to the KUKA end-effector, and securely align the drill along a planned trajectory. The drill guide was designed with a long offset to give the surgeon room to manipulate the drill through the guide. The desired robot end-effector path is converted to joint space using inverse kinematics and communicated to the KUKA controller via FRI. Once the drill guide has reached the commanded position, the KUKA thread inside the application software updates the KUKA coordinates 20 times in one second and calculates the average position and orientation. This helps to reduce the effects of noise in tracker measurements. The

---

[3] KUKA from http://www.openrobots.org/morse/doc/
latest/user/actuators/kuka_lwr.html
[4] Objet Connex500, Stratasys Ltd., USA.

robotic arm then maintains its position in a docked state and the surgeon can use the drill to create the pilot hole for screw placement. Several safety concerns have been addressed in this project. First, a virtual region in the KUKA controller has been set in addition to the internal safety features of the KUKA robot. Therefore, the KUKA robot will be turned off if it goes outside of this region. Second, there is a physical stop in the drill guide and a safety offset in the application to prevent the surgeon from drilling beyond a pre-specified depth.

Once the integrated software application was developed, we conducted preliminary tests to assess the contribution of errors from the different system components within the transformation chain. The first proof of concept test conducted in the lab used a CT dataset of a Lego model in the KUKA coordinate system and moved the robot to several predefined points in different orientations. After the lab test, we completed a study in the operating room to position all required devices for image-guided robotic system without any interference with other existing tools and devices. We used 10 pre-scanned sawbones in the operating room test and the surgeon selected entry and target points for screw placement on our interventional workstation. Then we navigated the KUKA to the proper position and the surgeon drilled the wire into the sawbones models.

3   Results

After the initial experiment described above, the overall procedural workflow was tested again and validated in a laboratory environment to get more precise results. First, we redesigned the drill guide to make it stiffer and position the optical tracking frame closer to the tip to minimize offset error. Second, we ran the KUKA robot iteratively to filter the tracking system noise by averaging. The KUKA can receive 20 message packets including new accessible positions and orientations in each second. After system accuracy optimization, additional tests were then conducted in the operating room. Left femur bone models with slipped capital epiphysis deformity were used to perform the drilling and screw placement tasks, as shown in fig. 4. The results from 10 robotic assisted trials performed by an orthopedic surgeon showed sufficient accuracy in comparison to 10 manual trials as detailed below. Of primary note is that all the procedures were done very quickly in these phantom studies, with average times of 4:49 (minutes:seconds). Secondarily, the accuracy results show an overall error that is sufficient for the clinical application [10]. The results are shown in Tables 1- 3.

Table 1. Average time of each step in robotic assisted SCFE surgery phantom experiment (minutes:seconds)

	Planning	Registration	Navigation	Drilling	Total
Average of 10	2:35	0:33	0:43	0:58	4:49

Table 2. Accuracy results (all results in mm). Average of Entry Error and Target error calculated based on distance of desired points and drilled points. Total Error is average of sum of robotic system error and surgeon path planning error for target points.

	Registration Error	Entry Error	Target Error	Total Error
Average of 10	0.588	1.95	2.36	7.04

Table 3. 10 manual trial result conducted by same surgeon. Total Error is measured just for target points based on distance of desired points and drilled points.

	Time	# of fluoroscopy images	Total Error (mm)
Average of 10	2:46	20.4	7.6

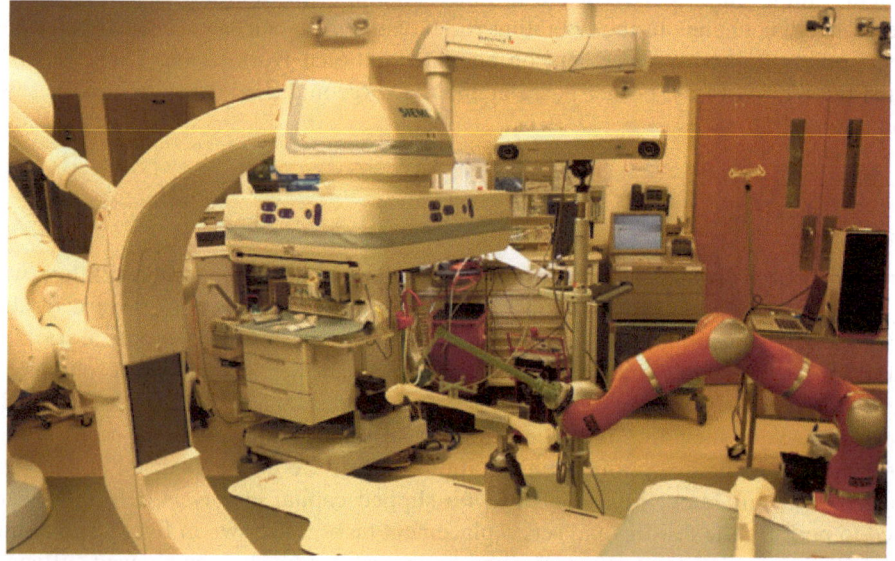

Fig. 4. Phantom study in interventional suite. It demonstrates orange KUKA robotic arm, 3D printed drill guide mounted to the KUKA, bone model and Polaris tracking system.

4   Conclusion and Future Work

Slipped capital femoral epiphysis is a relatively common orthopedic procedure where the accurate placement of the fixation screw is critical to the success of the operation. This paper introduces the system concept and overall architecture for robotically-assisted SCFE procedures. We also present our initial results using phantom models in the operating room. The long term goal is to pursue a clinical trial to determine if this approach could lead to an improved SCFE procedure for patients. For this purpose we also need to improve the workstation and obtain clinical approvals for the system.

Acknowledgment. This research was partially supported by an internal grant from the Sheikh Zayed Institute for Pediatric Surgical Innovation at Children's National Medical Center, which is funded by the government of Abu Dhabi. Partial support was also provided by a Board of Visitor's Grant from Children's and by NIH grant R01CA172244. We would also like to acknowledge the assistance of Radiology Technologists Moaaz Ali and William Powell.

References

1. Suhm, N., Messmer, P., Zuna, I., Jacob, L.A., Regazzoni, P.: Fluoroscopic guidance versus surgical navigation for distal locking of intramedullary implants. a prospective, controlled clinical study. Injury 35(6), 567–574 (2004)
2. Rohilla, R., Singh, R., Magu, N., Devgan, A., Siwach, R., Sangwan, S.: Simultaneous use of cannulated reamer and schanz screw for closed intramedullary femoral nailing. ISRN Surg. (2011) (published online)
3. Fuchs, H., State, A., Pisano, E.D., Garrett, W.F., Hirota, G., Livingston, M., Whitton, M.C., Pizer, S.M.: Towards Performing Ultrasound-Guided Needle Biopsies from within a Head-Mounted Display. In: Höhne, K.H., Kikinis, R. (eds.) VBC 1996. LNCS, vol. 1131, pp. 591–600. Springer, Heidelberg (1996)
4. Liao, H., Ishihara, H., Tran, H.H., Masamune, K., Sakuma, I., Dohi, T.: Fusion of Laser Guidance and 3-D Autostereoscopic Image Overlay for Precision-Guided Surgery. In: Dohi, T., Sakuma, I., Liao, H. (eds.) MIAR 2008. LNCS, vol. 5128, pp. 367–376. Springer, Heidelberg (2008)
5. Volonte, F., Pugin, F., Bucher, P., Sugimoto, M., Ratib, O., Morel, P.: Augmented Reality and Image Overlary Navigation with OsiriX in Laparoscopic and Robotic Surgery: Not Only a Matter of Fashion. J. Hepatobiliary Pancreat. Sci. 18, 506–509 (2011)
6. Marmurek, J., Wedlake, C., Pardasani, U., Eagleson, R., Peters, T.: Image-Guided Laser Projection for Port Placement in Minimally Invasive Surgery. Stud. Health Technol. Inform. 119, 367–372 (2006)
7. Gavaghan, K., Oliveira-Santos, T., Peterhans, M., Reyes, M., Kim, H., Anderegg, S., Weber, S.: Evaluation of a portable image overlay projector for the visualization of surgical navigation data: phantom studies. Int. J. Comp. Assis. Radio. Surg. 7, 547–556 (2012)
8. Enquobahrie, A., Cheng, P., Gary, K., Ibanez, L., Gobbi, D., Lindseth, F., Yaniv, Z., Aylward, S., Jomier, J., Cleary, K.: The image-guided surgery toolkit IGSTK: An open source C++ software toolkit. Journal of Digital Imaging 20(suppl. 1), 21–33 (2007)
9. Arun, K.S., Huang, T.S., Blostein, S.D.: Least-squares fitting of two 3-D point sets. IEEE Transactions on Pattern Analysis and Machine Intelligence 9(5), 698–700 (1987)
10. Pring, E.M., Adamczyk, M., Hosalkar, H.S., Bastrom, T.P., Wallace, C.D., Newton, P.O.: In situ screw fixation of slipped capital femoral epiphysis with a novel approach: a double-cohort controlled study. Journal of Children's Orthopaedics 4(3), 239–244 (2010)

Hierarchical HMM Based Learning of Navigation Primitives for Cooperative Robotic Endovascular Catheterization

Hedyeh Rafii-Tari[1], Jindong Liu[1], Christopher J. Payne[1],
Colin Bicknell[2], and Guang-Zhong Yang[1]

[1] The Hamlyn Centre for Robotic Surgery, Imperial College London, UK
[2] Academic Division of Surgery, Imperial College London, UK
{h.rafii-tari1,j.liu,g.z.yang}@imperial.ac.uk

Abstract. Despite increased use of remote-controlled steerable catheter navigation systems for endovascular intervention, most current designs are based on master configurations which tend to alter natural operator tool interactions. This introduces problems to both ergonomics and shared human-robot control. This paper proposes a novel cooperative robotic catheterization system based on learning-from-demonstration. By encoding the higher-level structure of a catheterization task as a sequence of primitive motions, we demonstrate how to achieve prospective learning for complex tasks whilst incorporating subject-specific variations. A hierarchical Hidden Markov Model is used to model each movement primitive as well as their sequential relationship. This model is applied to generation of motion sequences, recognition of operator input, and prediction of future movements for the robot. The framework is validated by comparing catheter tip motions against the manual approach, showing significant improvements in the quality of catheterization. The results motivate the design of collaborative robotic systems that are intuitive to use, while reducing the cognitive workload of the operator.

1 Introduction

Recent advances in steerable catheter technology and master/slave catheter navigation systems have aimed to improve standard catheterization practices by increasing the precision of motion, removing the operators from the radiation source, and providing added operator comfort [1]. However, most existing solutions have been designed without advanced ergonomic interfaces that utilize the natural skills of operators. Increased interest in robotic surgical systems and their growing presence offers new possibilities for real-time assistance through human-robot cooperation. Capturing the high-level structure of endovascular navigation by learning the primitive motions from few demonstrations of a catheterization task, and applying them to shared-control catheter navigation within different anatomical settings, can improve the quality of catheterization while reducing the cognitive workload of the operator.

P. Golland et al. (Eds.): MICCAI 2014, Part I, LNCS 8673, pp. 496–503, 2014.

Several commercial robotic platforms, such as the Magellan System (Hansen Medical, Mountain View, CA, USA), are used presently for endovascular intervention [2] while many research platforms have also been developed for remote control of standard catheters [1]. Most existing solutions, however, make use of multi-DoF haptic interfaces without considering conventional experience-related catheterization techniques. As a result, recent designs are moving towards more ergonomic master interfaces that replicate the natural motion patterns of operators [3]. An ideal human-robot interface aims to utilize the high-level decision making process of operators whilst providing the advantages of robotic control, including repeatability, precision and stability of motion. Learning of underlying navigation gestures, and the incorporation of these into the development of ergonomic shared-control robotic catheterization platforms, is important in ensuring that they are intuitive to use.

The increasing use of surgical robots offers new opportunities for autonomous and shared-control navigation, which has led to a growing interest in applying the learning-from-demonstration framework used in robotics [4] in different areas of minimally invasive surgery. These techniques have been applied towards complete automation of repetitive tasks [5], as well as low-level learning of motion trajectories for purposes of skill classification [6]. Higher level context learning has been applied to real-time recognition of operator intent to provide assistance in the form of virtual fixtures [7], and recognition of subtask completion for changing the control between operator and robot at certain steps of a procedure [8]. While in the field of endovascular intervention these techniques have been used for low-level learning and automation of optimum motion trajectories from multiple expert demonstrations [9], their application to model generalization and context-aware learning of complex tasks has not been explored.

This paper proposes a novel surgical human-robot cooperative system for endovascular intervention, based on learning-from-demonstration, by decomposing the procedure into a division of primitive motions and learning the model of each primitive as well as the higher-level structure of the task. In the proposed approach, Hidden Markov Models (HMMs) are used to model each movement primitive, while a higher abstraction level HMM is also learned to capture their sequential relationship. The learned models are applied towards generating sequences of motions, detecting operator input, and predicting future movements, using a hands-on robotic catheter driver with an ergonomic master interface that replicates standard bedside motions. Models learned from few demonstrations of a single catheterization task by an expert operator within a standard anatomy have been validated using the cooperative robotic system across multiple intermediate-level and novice operators, performing various complex tasks within different anatomical settings. The performance is evaluated by comparing catheter tip motion quality and navigation performance with the robot-assisted approach against manual catheterization. The learning framework addresses subject-specific anatomical variability by enabling intuitive human-robot collaborative navigation, and provides important insights into the design of shared-control robotic platforms that maintain the natural skills of operators.

2   Materials and Methods

2.1   Motion Primitive Learning and Hierarchical Modeling

The goal of this learning framework is to encode the high-level structure of a catheterization task, by decomposing it into a sequence of primitive motions and learning the model of each primitive and their sequential relationship, to enable human-robot cooperative catheter navigation. This will allow generalization of the learning capabilities, since many of the primitive manoeuvres performed by operators are common across different anatomies. The learned models are applied to generating motion sequences for the robotic driver, real-time recognition of operator input when correcting the motion of the robotic driver, and predicting future movements for the robot. Several mathematical frameworks for representing motion primitives have been employed in the past (e.g. neural networks, HMMs, dynamical models) [4]. This work uses HMMs to model the primitive movements, due to their ability to handle both spatial and temporal variability across multiple demonstrations, and since the same model can be used for generation of motion sequences as well as recognition of new motions.

The models were learned from few manual demonstrations of an expert operator (n=5, >100 endovascular procedures), cannulating the innominate artery of a silicone-based, anthropomorphic phantom of a healthy type I aortic arch (Elastrat Sarl, Switzerland, Fig. 1c). The two DoF axial (x) and rotational (θ) motion of the catheter applied by the operator was measured using a proximal position sensor, consisting of two contact-less magnetic rotary encoders and a roller-based mechanism [9]. Each dataset $\{x, \theta\}$ was manually segmented into three main primitive motions: a pushing motion, a pull and counterclockwise twist, and a clockwise twist. Each primitive gesture was modeled as a fully-connected HMM with N states. An HMM is represented by $\lambda = (\pi, A, B)$ consisting respectively of the initial state distribution, the state transition probability distribution, and the observation probability distribution [10]. Here a continuous observation model based on a Gaussian distribution was used: $b_i(o) = \mathcal{N}(o|\mu_i, \Sigma_i)$ where o is the observation vector and μ_i and Σ_i are the mean and covariance matrix in state i. The HMMs were trained using the Baum-Welch algorithm (based on Expectation Maximization (EM)), and the optimal number of states (N) for each HMM was selected using the Bayesian information criterion [11].

The HMMs were then used for on-line recognition of the operator's input gesture during the procedure, by calculating the log-likelihood between the input trajectory O and each of the primitive HMMs $\lambda_p \in \{\lambda_{p1}, \lambda_{p2}, \lambda_{p3}\}$ using the *forward-algorithm* of the HMMs [10], and classifying the gesture using the HMM with the maximum log-likelihood:

$$\underset{\lambda_p \in \{\lambda_{p1}, \lambda_{p2}, \lambda_{p3}\}}{\arg \max} \quad logP(O|\lambda_p). \tag{1}$$

In order to recreate a generalized version of the motion from the HMM corresponding to each primitive, the Viterbi algorithm was used to reconstruct the optimal sequence of state transitions [11]. The μ_i of the Gaussian distributions for each state was then used to extract a set of key-points at the mean time between two state transitions. By interpolating between these key-points (using piecewise cubic Hermite polynomials) and normalizing in time, a desired trajectory $\{x, \theta\}$ is extracted from the HMM of each primitive. These motions were then smoothed using a moving average filter (span=10) to enable smooth transitions for the robotic driver.

To represent the structure of movement patterns and how the motion primitives are sequenced, a second higher-level, fully-connected HMM (π^h, A^h, B^h) was learned, where each motion primitive corresponds to a single hidden state in the model [12]. For this model, the initial state distribution π^h represent the likelihood that a motion sequence will begin with a certain primitive, and the state transition probabilities A^h encapsulate the sequential relationship between the primitive motions. The output observation distribution for each state was defined as the likelihood that a motion sequence segment could have been generated by the model of that primitive:

$$b_i^h(O^s) = P(O^s|\lambda_i). \tag{2}$$

Here λ_i is the lower level HMM of the motion primitive at state i, O^s is an observation motion sequence segment, and the probability $P(O^s|\lambda_i)$ was computed using the *forward-algorithm* [10]. Using the set of motion primitives $[\lambda_{p1}, \lambda_{p2}, \lambda_{p3}]$ and the observed sequence of segmented motions from the demonstrations, the initial state distribution and the state transition probabilities were trained using the standard Baum-Welch algorithm [10]. The state transition probabilities A^h were then used to detect and monitor the input of the operator and predict the future movements of the robotic driver.

2.2   Experimental Setup

The learned model from the expert is used for human-robot cooperative catheterization of multiple arteries within different complex anatomical settings by inexperienced and intermediate-level operators, using a master-slave framework consisting of the proximal position sensing unit and a robotic catheter driver (Fig. 1). The catheter driver uses two servomotors that drive the catheter to follow a desired trajectories based on a PID controller [9]. The motions generated from the HMMs of each primitive are sent to the robotic driver sequentially based on the learned hierarchical model. A camera mounted on top of the phantom provides a 2D projected image for navigation. A graphical user interface (Labview, National Instruments Corp.) displays the current and upcoming motions of the robot to the operator at each stage, and allows the operator to indicate when they decide to correct the motion. During the correction phase the operator controls the master catheter at the proximal sensing unit and the robotic driver follows the motion of the operator. After the operator indicates that they are satisfied with the correction, the hierarchical model recognizes the primitive corresponding to the operator input and decides the future automated movement of the robotic driver. The framework was validated for cannulation of the left

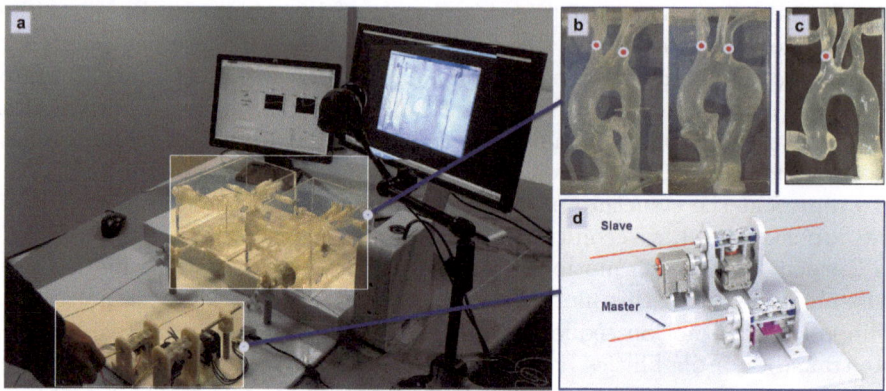

Fig. 1. Experimental setup of the proposed cooperative robot-assisted approach and the manual approach (a), phantoms of the aortic arch with aneurysm and stenosis for validation (b), phantom of the healthy arch used for learning the hierarchical model (c), intuitive master-slave framework (position sensing unit and robotic driver) (d).

subclavian (LSA) and the right common carotid (RCCA) arteries of two silicone-based, anthropomorphic phantoms of an aortic arch with an aneurysm, and a longer aortic arch with a re-created stenosis (Elastrat Sarl, Switzerland, Fig. 1b), and compared to completely manual catheterization. 5F shaped catheters and guidewires were used for this study, and guidewire manipulation was controlled manually by the operator. Information regarding catheter tip motion were obtained using six-DoF electromagnetic position sensors (Aurora, NDI) attached to the catheter tip. Fig. 1 shows the experimental setup used for validation.

The procedure was repeated multiple times across five novice operators (n = 10) and two intermediate-level operators (n = 8, ~ 10 simulator/endovascular procedures), on the LSA and RCCA of each phantom with each of the robot-assisted and manual approaches. Different performance metrics that were extracted for each cannulation through the position sensor attached to the catheter tip include: mean/maximum tip acceleration, smoothness of motion (corresponding to the change in slope of the tip displacement), and total catheter path length (corresponding to back and forth movements). Through these metrics the performance of the proposed robot-assisted approach was compared to the manual technique and differences were assessed using the non-parametric Wilcoxon rank-sum significance test ($P < 0.05$). Tip trajectory plots are also used to further demonstrate improvements in smoothness and stability of catheter motion. For this study all the processing and statistical analysis was performed in Matlab.

3   Results

Fig. 2 shows the lower level HMMs for each movement primitive, as learned from the expert operator's demonstrations. The generalized version of the motion extracted from each primitive is also displayed.

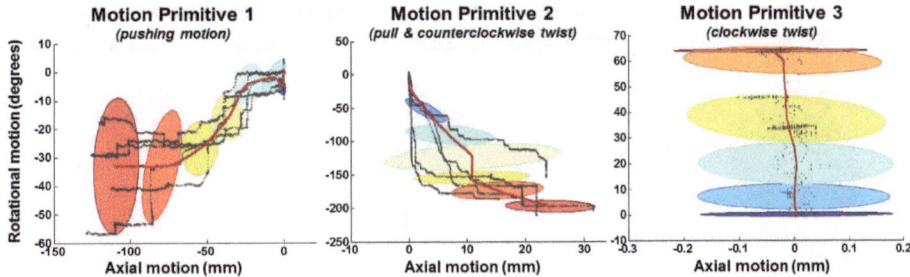

Fig. 2. Training data from the expert demonstrations (gray lines), learned HMMs, and the generalized form of the motion (red line) retrieved from the HMMs for each of the primitive motions. Different colors represent the states of each HMM, while the ellipses correspond to the covariances.

Table 1 shows the results of the non-parametric test, with median values for statistically significant differences ($P < 0.05$) between the manual approach and the cooperative robotic approach for each of the phantoms and arteries across the two experience levels. Significant performance differences can be seen for cannulation of each of the LSA and RCCA arteries within the two anatomies for the two experience levels. In each case, the robotic approach displays smoother and more stable catheter tip motion at lower accelerations. Smoother movements and a reduction in total path length correspond to a reduced number of back and forth movements at the catheter tip, which can translate into reduced vessel wall contact. This can have a significant impact on reducing complications that are caused as a results of interaction between the catheter and the arterial wall, including dissection, perforation, thrombosis and embolization, particularly in the presence of diseased vessels.

Table 1. Median values for statistically significant differences ($P < 0.05$) between the cooperative robotic approach vs. the manual approach, for cannulation of varying arteries within different anatomies across the two experience groups.

	Stenosis Model				Aneurysm Model			
	LSA		RCCA		LSA		RCCA	
Novice	Manual	Robot	Manual	Robot	Manual	Robot	Manual	Robot
mean accel. (mm/s^2)	2.1E3	**50.9**	1.9E3	**71.9**	1.6E3	**55.5**	2.4E3	**62.1**
max accel. (mm/s^2)	2.3E4	**1.4E4**	4.7E4	**1.0E4**	3.0E4	**5.3E3**	3.1E4	**6.0E3**
smoothness (mm)	2.5E3	**3.3E2**	3.6E3	**3.8E2**	4.6E3	**3.6E2**	4.1E3	**3.1E2**
path length (mm)	3.6E3	**5.5E2**	5.7E3	**7.1E2**	6.3E3	**5.8E2**	6.8E3	**6.0E2**
Intermediate	Manual	Robot	Manual	Robot	Manual	Robot	Manual	Robot
mean accel. (mm/s^2)	1.5E3	**64.6**	3.2e3	**84.5**	1.0e3	**49.5**	1.8E3	**67.8**
max accel. (mm/s^2)	2.3E4	**7.5E3**	3.4E4	**1.8E4**	1.9E4	**5.9E3**	2.9E4	**3.5E3**
smoothness (mm)	1.8E3	**2.7E2**	3.2E3	**3.3E2**	2.6E3	**2.6E2**	3.8E3	**2.7E2**
path length (mm)	2.9E3	**4.4E2**	4.4E3	**6.4E2**	6.0E3	**4.1E2**	6.2E3	**5.7E2**

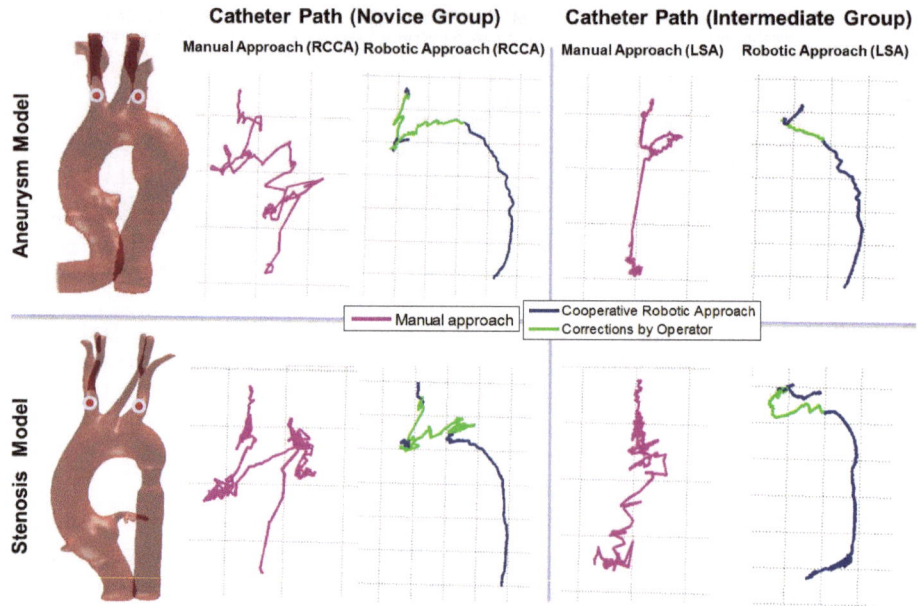

Fig. 3. Catheter path achieved by the robot-assisted approach vs. the manual approach within different models and arteries, across the two experience groups. The corrective motions of the operator are depicted with a different colour.

Fig. 3 displays examples of the catheter path during catheterization of different arteries and anatomies with the proposed robotic approach against the corresponding manual approach for each experience level. For the robot-assisted approach, the input and corrections of the operator are displayed in a different color. The results depict the improved quality of catheterization in terms of precision, smoothness, and stability of motion, compared to the manual approach, for both of the novice and intermediate experience levels.

4   Conclusion

In this paper a novel surgical human-robot cooperative system for endovascular catheterization, based on learning-from-demonstration, has been proposed. By learning the higher-level structure of task as a sequence of primitive motions, the framework allows for context-aware learning and generalization to different anatomical settings while addressing subject-specific variations. Models learned from few expert demonstrations of a single task have been validated across intermediate-level and inexperienced operators performing multiple catheterization tasks within different anatomical setting, using a hands-on robotic catheter driver and a proximal position sensing unit within an intuitive master-slave framework. The results depict significant improvements in the quality of catheterization in terms of stability and smoothness of motion and overall path length, compared to the manual approach, and further motivate the design of hands-on cooperative robotic platforms that utilize operator skill, while reducing the cognitive workload of the operator.

Acknowledgments. The authors would like to acknowledge Petros Giataganas and Drs. Su-Lin Lee and Tom Cundy for their contribution to this work.

References

1. Rafii-Tari, H., Payne, C.J., Yang, G.Z.: Current and emerging robot-assisted endovascular catheterization technologies: A review. Ann. Biomed. Eng. 42(4), 697–715 (2014)
2. Riga, C., Bicknell, C., Rolls, A., Cheshire, N., Hamady, M.: Robot-assisted fenestrated endovascular aneurysm repair (FEVAR) using the magellan system. J. Vasc. Interv. Radiol. 24(2), 191–196 (2013)
3. Payne, C., Rafii-Tari, H., Yang, G.Z.: A force feedback system for endovascular catheterisation. In: IEEE/RSJ International Conference on Intelligent Robots and Systems, pp. 1298–1304 (2012)
4. Argall, B.D., Chernova, S., Veloso, M., Browning, B.: A survey of robot learning from demonstration. Robot. Auton. Syst. 57(5), 469–483 (2009)
5. Berg, J.V.D., Miller, S., Duckworth, D., Hu, H., Wan, A., Fu, X.Y., Goldberg, K., Abbeel, P.: Superhuman performance of surgical tasks by robots using iterative learning from human-guided demonstrations. In: IEEE International Conference on Robotics and Automation, pp. 2074–2081 (2010)
6. Reiley, C.E., Plaku, E., Hager, G.D.: Motion generation of robotic surgical tasks: Learning from expert demonstrations. In: Annual International Conference of the IEEE Engineering in Medicine and Biology Society, pp. 967–970 (2010)
7. Kragic, D., Marayong, P., Li, M., Okamura, A.M., Hager, G.D.: Human-machine collaborative systems for microsurgical applications. Int. J. Robot. Res. 24(9), 731–741 (2005)
8. Padoy, N., Hager, G.: Human-machine collaborative surgery using learned models. In: IEEE International Conference on Robotics and Automation, pp. 5285–5292 (2011)
9. Rafii-Tari, H., Liu, J., Lee, S.L., Bicknell, C., Yang, G.Z.: Learning-based modeling of endovascular navigation for collaborative robotic catheterization. In: Mori, K., Sakuma, I., Sato, Y., Barillot, C., Navab, N. (eds.) MICCAI 2013, Part II. LNCS, vol. 8150, pp. 369–377. Springer, Heidelberg (2013)
10. Rabiner, L.: A tutorial on hidden markov models and selected applications in speech recognition. Proc. IEEE 77(2), 257–286 (1989)
11. Billard, A.G., Calinon, S., Guenter, F.: Discriminative and adaptive imitation in uni-manual and bi-manual tasks. Robot. Auton. Syst. 54(5), 370–384 (2006)
12. Kulic, D., Nakamura, Y.: Incremental learning of human behaviors using hierarchical hidden markov models. In: IEEE/RSJ International Conference on Intelligent Robots and Systems, pp. 4649–4655 (2010)

Towards Personalized Interventional SPECT-CT Imaging

José Gardiazabal[1,2], Marco Esposito[1], Philipp Matthies[1], Aslı Okur[1,2],
Jakob Vogel[1], Silvan Kraft[1,3], Benjamin Frisch[1],
Tobias Lasser[1], and Nassir Navab[1,4]

[1] Computer Aided Medical Procedures (CAMP)
[2] Department of Nuclear Medicine, Klinikum Rechts der Isar
[3] Department of Radiology, Klinikum Rechts der Isar
Technische Universität München, Germany
[4] Computer Aided Medical Procedures (CAMP),
Johns Hopkins University, USA

Abstract. The development of modern robotics and compact imaging
detectors allows the transfer of diagnostic imaging modalities to the operating room, supporting surgeons to perform faster and safer procedures.
An intervention that currently suffers from a lack of interventional imaging is radioembolization, a treatment for hepatic carcinoma. Currently,
this procedure requires moving the patient from an angiography suite for
preliminary catheterization and injection to a whole-body SPECT/CT
for leakage detection, necessitating a second catheterization back in the
angiography suite for the actual radioembolization. We propose an imaging setup that simplifies this procedure using a robotic approach to
directly acquire an interventional SPECT/CT in the angiography suite.
Using C-arm CT and a co-calibrated gamma camera mounted on a
robotic arm, a personalized trajectory of the gamma camera is generated
from the C-arm CT, enabling an interventional SPECT reconstruction
that is inherently co-registered to the C-arm CT. In this work we demonstrate the feasibility of this personalized interventional SPECT/CT imaging approach in a liver phantom study.

1 Introduction

Traditional medical imaging systems often employ a single contrast mechanism
like ultrasound reflection, X-ray transmission (CT), magnetic resonance (MRI),
single photon (SPECT) or positron emission (PET). These single-modality devices are able to provide medically useful pictures of almost any organ, but can
have unfavorable side effects such as limited resolution, sub-optimal contrast or
lack of anatomical references. In terms of interventional imaging, single-modality
devices such as robotic C-arm CT [1] or freehand SPECT [2] are used very successfully in clinical practice on a regular basis.

In the past 15 years, dual-modality systems that combine anatomic (like CT or
MRI) with functional imaging (like SPECT or PET) have become increasingly
common [3]. Such devices provide naturally co-registered datasets and enable

P. Golland et al. (Eds.): MICCAI 2014, Part I, LNCS 8673, pp. 504–511, 2014.

optimal fusion of information. The typical layout as whole-body gantry-based scanners, however, limits their use in organ-specific imaging and prevents most interventional applications, despite a number of possible scenarios where interventional dual-modality imaging would be highly desirable.

One particular example of such an interventional application is brachytherapy of unresectable liver tumors, like hepatocellular carcinoma (HCC). Brachytherapy in the form of radioembolization (Selective Internal RadioTherapy – SIRT) is an alternative to classical chemoembolization or chemotherapy [4]. In this case, microspheres loaded with ^{90}Y are injected into the hepatic arteries using a catheter for selective internal irradiation of the tumor cells. ^{90}Y mainly undergoes β^- decay, emitting electrons that are absorbed within at most 11 mm of tissue, making it possible to inject very high doses within a single treatment. It is, however, crucial to ensure that the radioactive compound remains confined to the injection site in order to irradiate only the surrounding cancer tissue. Any leakage to other parts of the liver or other organs, for example through a shunt to the lung, must be prevented.

The current practice is to inject ^{99m}Tc-MAA through a catheter first, which has demonstrated good prognostic value for the ^{90}Y distribution [5]. The patient is then transferred from the radiology department, where the catheterization and injection take place, to the nuclear medicine department for a whole-body SPECT scan, usually combined with CT, to monitor the ^{99m}Tc distribution. This process takes four to six hours on average and requires, if the result is positive, a second intervention in the radiology department with another catheterization for the actual radioembolization with ^{90}Y itself.

As shown by this example, the use of a diagnostic device incurs organizational complexity and prolongs the duration of the intervention. For this reason, we propose a novel approach to interventional SPECT/CT imaging consisting of a C-arm CT scanner and a robot-controlled gamma camera, where the latter's trajectory is optimized based on the patient's anatomy as extracted from the C-arm CT data. This approach enables clinicians to perform interventions like radioembolization on a single site and during a single procedure, substantially reducing patient stress and time commitment of the medical personnel. On top of this, the core imaging process also benefits from this fusion, as the required data can be collected very efficiently in a patient-specific manner, leading to equivalent medical information significantly faster and with similar accuracy as currently available in the state-of-the-art whole-body scenario.

This paper shows the feasibility of the combined interventional C-arm CT/robotic SPECT approach in an experimental liver phantom setting close to the clinical application.

2   Materials and Methods

2.1   Overview

As shown in Fig. 1, we extend an angiography suite by placing a robot-mounted multi-channel gamma camera next to the C-arm. Using appropriate calibration techniques as detailed in section 2.2, we can acquire all relevant data, X-ray transmission and gamma radiation, with respect to a single, common coordinate frame.

With this setup in place and calibrated, we first acquire a CT image of the volume of interest. Based on it, we extract the convex hull of the patient's (or phantom's) surface and compute an optimal trajectory for acquiring the SPECT images from minimal, but safe distances. Finally, we record the emission data by moving the gamma camera along the trajectory using the robotic arm and reconstruct the tracer distribution using likelihood-based tomographic reconstruction, as described in section 2.4.

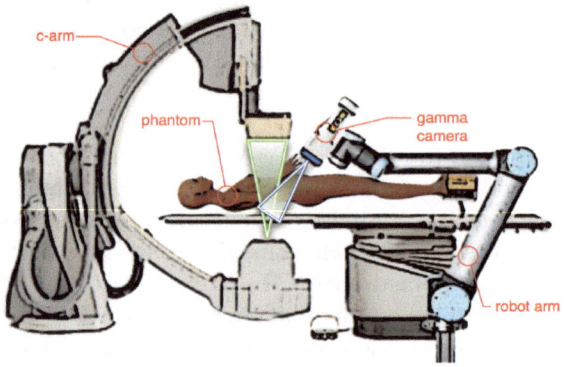

Fig. 1. Combined C-arm CT and robotic SPECT setup in the operating room

2.2   Coordinate Systems Calibration

In order to use the C-arm system without modifications, we assume its coordinate system as the reference. Consequently, we need to obtain the rigid transformation between the robot's base and the C-arm coordinate system.

For this purpose, we mount a custom-designed calibration target, shown in Fig. 2a, to the robot's wrist, as shown in Fig. 2b. The target contains highly visible spheres in a well-defined pattern, that can be segmented easily in the CT volume. Using point-based registration as suggested by Umeyama [6], we obtain the transformation between the CT image and the calibration target, which can be propagated to the robot's base thanks to the precisely known dimensions and joint angles via forward kinematics.

2.3   Trajectory Planning

The first step of the core acquisition protocol consists of recording the X-ray component of the joint signal by rotating the C-arm over 180° around the region of interest and reconstructing it into a 3D volume.

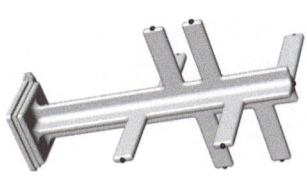

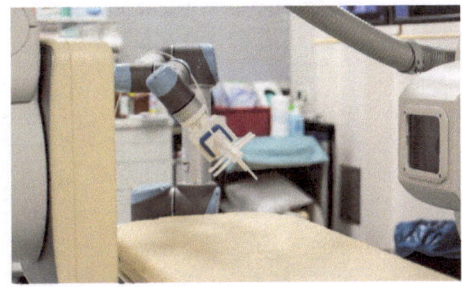

(a) Calibration tool   (b) Calibration setup

Fig. 2. a) CAD drawing of the calibration tool and b) setup used to map the C-arm coordinate system to the robot coordinate system. The spheres attached to the fins appear prominently in the CT volume and can be easily segmented.

In a second step, we compute a model of the patient's (or phantom's) surface from the CT image. As X-ray transmission through the surrounding air is significantly higher than through tissue, it is possible to distinguish both regions by applying a threshold. The convex hull is then a suitable mesh-model for the surface.

Finally, the trajectories are generated as three parallel scan-lines normal to the convex hull of the patient (up to a certain security distance, 1 cm in this case), as shown in Fig. 3. Note that, unlike a fixed gantry in diagnostic SPECT, the camera poses are much closer for a personalized trajectory with better detection statistics.

2.4 Image Reconstruction

Having collected the emission values by moving the camera along the acquisition trajectory, the final task is the reconstruction of the SPECT image. Considering the Poisson-distribution of the measured values m_j, we compute the maximum-likelihood estimate

$$\arg\max_{\mathbf{x}} \left(\sum_{j=1}^{m} m_j \log(\overline{m}_j(\mathbf{x})) - \overline{m}_j \right)$$

where $\overline{m}_j(\mathbf{x})$ denotes the expected measurement given a reconstruction $\mathbf{x}$. The solution to this optimization problem can be obtained in several ways, and we apply Maximum Likelihood Expectation Maximization (MLEM) as suggested by Shepp and Vardi [7]. An important aspect of this process is an accurate model of the camera's measurement probabilities, usually referred to as the forward model. We employ the procedure proposed in [8] that uses high-resolution lookup tables collected during long-term calibration measurements.

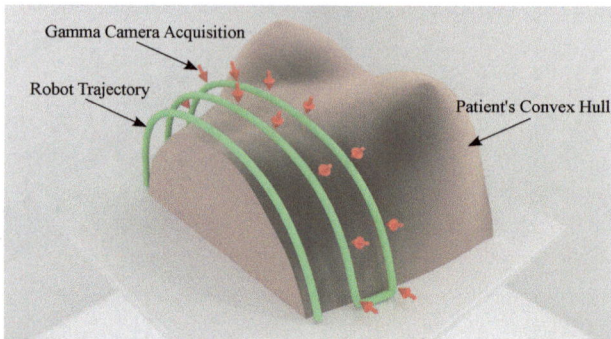

Fig. 3. Schematic representation of a personalized trajectory for the robot-guided gamma camera along the convex hull of the patient/phantom as extracted from CT. The green line represents the planned robot trajectory, that follows the convex hull plus the safety margin (1 cm), the red arrows indicate positions where the gamma camera acquires images.

The X-ray CT reconstruction is directly obtained from the software solution of the C-arm manufacturer, and is based on Feldkamp's variant of Filtered Back-Projection [9]. As the SPECT measurements have been collected relative to the C-arm's coordinate frame, the two volumetric images are inherently aligned.

3   Experiments

3.1   Setup

The imaging setup consists of a C-arm CT and a mini gamma camera mounted on a robotic arm, as illustrated in Fig. 1. The C-arm CT is a Philips Allura Xper FD20 set up in an angiography room. The mini gamma camera (Crystal Imager, Crystal Photonics, Germany) uses a $4 \times 4 \, cm^2$ CdZnTe crystal detector segmented into 16×16 pixels. The camera is mounted on a robotic arm (UR5, Universal Robots, Denmark) placed next to the C-arm, see Fig. 4b.

3.2   Experimental Procedure

Verification experiment. In a first experiment, we verify the quality of our calibration procedure. We attach a single ^{57}Co point source to a torso phantom and obtain a CT image. Based on the location of the point source segmented from the CT image, we instruct the robot with the gamma camera to acquire a single image centered on the point source. The expected result is a gamma camera image with the point source showing as a hotspot in the center.

Reconstruction experiment. In a second experiment, we place a human torso phantom with a liver model made out of candle gel (Ceraflex N 530 transparent,

Wachs- und Ceresinfabriken, Germany) on the exam table. Liver arteries are imitated by plastic tubes (4 mm diameter), filled with 4 MBq of ^{99m}Tc.

We obtain a CT image of the torso and compute the trajectory for the SPECT acquisition according to the procedure described in section 2.3. The emission data recorded by the robot-positioned gamma camera is reconstructed as an image inherently co-registered with the CT image. We expect to see the liver arteries in the reconstructed SPECT image embedded in the anatomical information from the CT.

4   Results

Verification experiment. Fig. 4a shows a planar scintigraphy of the ^{57}Co source, acquired with the gamma camera instructed to point its center at the source (see Fig. 4b), based on the source position as detected from the C-arm CT as well as the coordinate system calibration. The relocalization error, i.e. the offset from the hotspot's center of mass to the center of the image, is 1.6 camera pixels (corresponding to 3.9 mm).

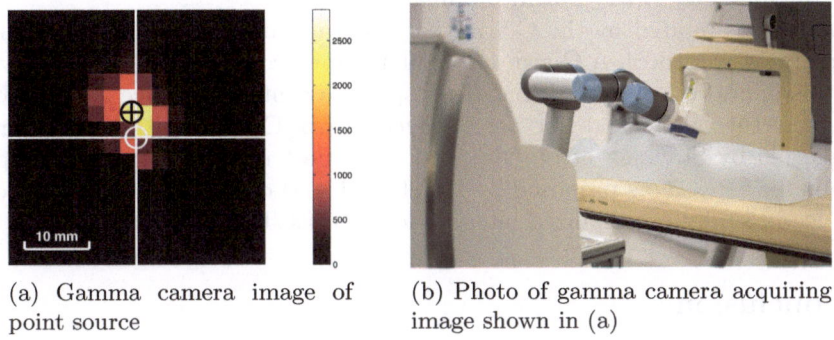

(a) Gamma camera image of point source

(b) Photo of gamma camera acquiring image shown in (a)

Fig. 4. Result of calibration verification experiment

Reconstruction experiment. Fig. 5a shows a 3D rendering of the robotic SPECT image of our phantom. The branching blood-vessels simulated by three activity-filled tubes are clearly distinguishable. The co-registered robotic SPECT/C-arm CT slice image in Fig. 5b shows that the offset between the tubes in the SPECT and the CT image is minimal.

5   Discussion

Calibration of the C-arm and gamma camera coordinate systems is a vital part of the imaging protocol. Our first experiment validates our approach, as the relocalization error is within the acceptable error limit for interventions. In addition to this, we performed a comparable experiment under guidance of an optical tracking system and only achieved considerably higher errors.

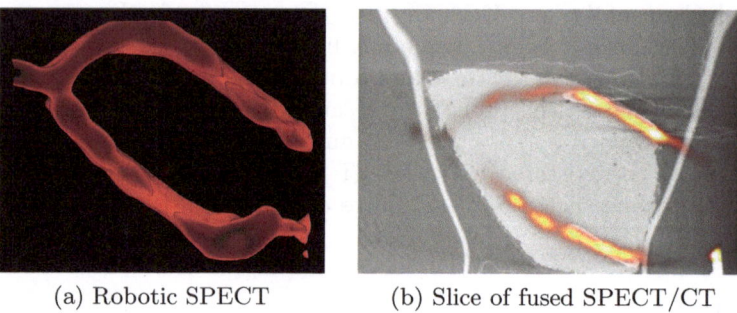

(a) Robotic SPECT   (b) Slice of fused SPECT/CT

Fig. 5. (a) 3D rendering of the SPECT image of the liver phantom with radioactive blood vessels and (b) slice of fused robotic SPECT/C-arm CT

The second experiment confirms the possibility of acquiring bi-modal interventional robotic SPECT and C-arm CT images in a clinical environment, with a realistic liver phantom. We were able to extract a patient-specific acquisition trajectory based on the convex hull of the torso and record a SPECT image that is naturally aligned to the C-arm CT image.

Our setup is limited by the C-arm that does not allow any customization of the acquisition protocol. A C-arm CT mounted on a robotic arm [1] would overcome this limitation, provided that the respective control interface is accessible. It would further allow to define personalized C-arm CT acquisition trajectories as suggested by Stayman et al. [10]. Also, the spectrum-based trajectory optimization for SPECT as proposed by Vogel et al. [11] could be considered. Both would lead to fully personalized interventional SPECT/CT acquisition.

6   Conclusion

This paper presents the first prototype for an interventional SPECT/CT scanner. We believe the quality is good enough to be used in an intra-operative scenario. In recent times, the community has shown considerable interest in such a device, and simulation studies have been published, for instance by Bowsher et al. [12] where a much heavier robot is used that cannot easily be removed or transferred. Our design is very light, thus meeting the accessibility and flexibility requirements of clinical practice.

The advantages of interventional SPECT/CT are obvious: the duration and complexity of interventions are substantially reduced, the progress can be monitored in an easy and flexible way (for instance, by acquiring a bremsstrahlung SPECT image [13]). The latter can also be used to quickly detect aberrations such as leaks, thus enabling effective quality control.

The suggested method is ready for further investigation in the operating room, opening the path for alternative applications, for example in the head and neck region.

Acknowledgements. This work was partially funded by the DFG cluster of excellence MAP, the TUM Institute for Advanced Study (funded by the German Excellence Initiative), and the Bayerische Forschungsstiftung (project Ro-BildOR). We want to thank Alexandru Duliu for his assistance with Blender.

References

1. Ganguly, A., Fieselmann, A., Marks, M., Rosenberg, J., Boese, J., Deuerling-Zheng, Y., Straka, M., Zaharchuck, G., Bammer, R., Fahrig, R.: Cerebral CT Perfusion Using an Interventional C-Arm Imaging System: Cerebral Blood Flow Measurements. Am. J. Neuroradiol. 32, 1525–1531 (2011)
2. Wendler, T., Herrmann, K., Schnelzer, A., Lasser, T., Traub, J., Kutter, O., Ehlerding, A., Scheidhauer, K., Schuster, T., Kiechle, M., Schwaiger, M., Navab, N., Ziegler, S.I., Buck, A.K.: First demonstration of 3-D lymphatic mapping in breast cancer using freehand SPECT. Eur. J. Nucl. Med. 37(8), 1452–1461 (2010)
3. Cherry, S.R., Sorenson, J.A., Phelps, M.E.: Physics in Nuclear Medicine. Elsevier Health Sciences (April 2012)
4. Sangro, B., Iñarrairaegui, M., Bilbao, J.I.: Radioembolization for hepatocellular carcinoma. Journal of Hepatology 56(2), 464–473 (2012)
5. Lam, M.G.E.H., Goris, M.L., Iagaru, A.H., Mittra, E.S., Louie, J.D., Sze, D.Y.: Prognostic Utility of 90Y Radioembolization Dosimetry Based on Fusion 99mTc-Macroaggregated Albumin-99mTc-Sulfur Colloid SPECT. Journal of Nuclear Medicine 54(12), 2055–2061 (2013)
6. Umeyama, S.: Least-squares estimation of transformation parameters between two point patterns. IEEE Transactions on Pattern Analysis and Machine Intelligence 13(4), 376–380 (1991)
7. Shepp, L.A., Vardi, Y.: Maximum Likelihood Reconstruction for Emission Tomography. Transactions on Medical Imaging MI-1(2), 113–122 (1982)
8. Matthies, P., Gardiazabal, J., Okur, A., Vogel, J., Lasser, T., Navab, N.: Mini Gamma Cameras for Intra-operative Nuclear Tomographic Reconstruction Medical Image Analysis (2014)
9. Feldkamp, L.A., Davis, L.C., Kress, J.W.: Practical cone-beam algorithm. Journal of the Optical Society of America A 1(6), 612–619 (1984)
10. Stayman, J., Siewerdsen, J.: Task-based trajectories in iteratively reconstructed interventional cone-beam CT, Lake Tahoe, CA, pp. 257–260 (2013)
11. Vogel, J., Lasser, T., Gardiazabal, J., Navab, N.: Trajectory optimization for intra-operative nuclear tomographic imaging. Medical Image Analysis 17(7), 723–731 (2013)
12. Bowsher, J., Yan, S., Roper, J., Giles, W., Yin, F.F.: Onboard functional and molecular imaging: a design investigation for robotic multipinhole SPECT. Medical Physics 41(1), 010701 (2014), PMID: 24387490 PMCID: PMC3888458
13. Ahmadzadehfar, H., Muckle, M., Sabet, A., Wilhelm, K., Kuhl, C., Biermann, K., Haslerud, T., Biersack, H.J., Ezziddin, S.: The significance of bremsstrahlung SPECT/CT after yttrium-90 radioembolization treatment in the prediction of extrahepatic side effects. European Journal of Nuclear Medicine and Molecular Imaging (October 2011), PMID: 21975832

Chest Modeling and Personalized Surgical Planning for Pectus Excavatum

Qian Zhao[1], Nabile Safdar[1], Chunzhe Duan[1],
Anthony Sandler[2], and Marius George Linguraru[1,3]

[1] Sheikh Zayed Institute for Pediatric Surgical Innovation,
Children's National Medical Center, Washington DC, USA
[2] Department of General and Thoracic Surgery,
Children's National Medical Center, Washington DC, USA
[3] School of Medicine and Health Sciences,
George Washington University, Washington DC, USA

Abstract. Pectus excavatum is among the most common major congenital anomalies of the chest wall whose correction can be performed via minimally invasive Nuss technique that places a pectus bar to elevate the sternum anteriorly. However, the size and bending of the pectus bar are manually modeled intraoperatively by trial-and-error. The procedure requires intense pain management in the months following surgery. In response, we are developing a novel distraction device for incremental and personalized PE correction with minimal risk and pain, akin to orthodontic treatment using dental braces. To design the device, we propose in this study a personalized surgical planning framework for PE correction from clinical noncontrast CT. First, we segment the ribs and sternum via kernel graph cuts. Then costal cartilages, which have very low contrast in noncontrast CT, are modeled as 3D anatomical curves using the cosine series representation and estimated using a statistical shape model. The size and shape of the correction device are estimated through model fitting. Finally, the corrected/post-surgical chest is simulated in relation to the estimated shape of correction device. The root mean square mesh distance between the estimated cartilages and ground truth on 30 noncontrast CT scans was 1.28±0.81 mm. Our method found that the average deformation of the sterna and cartilages with the simulation of PE correction was 49.71±10.11 mm.

Keywords: Pectus excavatum, personalized surgical planning, costal cartilage estimation, statistical shape models, correction device.

1   Introduction

Pectus excavatum (PE), involving posterior depression of the sternum and adjacent costal cartilages and ribs, is among the most common major congenital anomalies of the chest wall [1]. Severe deformities can cause cardiopulmonary impairment and reduction in lung volume. Anatomic evaluation of PE can be clinically performed using noncontrast CT with an index of severity (Haller Index) calculated based on measurements, electrocardiogram and cardiopulmonary exercise testing [1].

P. Golland et al. (Eds.): MICCAI 2014, Part I, LNCS 8673, pp. 512–519, 2014.

Surgical repair of PE can be performed via either an open operation or the minimally invasive Nuss technique. The Nuss procedure involves the placement of a substernal concave bar (pectus bar), which is passed behind the sternum through the chest and "flipped" into a convex position to elevate the sternum outward. However, the size and bending of the pectus bar are manually modeled intra-operatively by trial-and-error based on the patient's thoracic morphology (curvature). The process is slow, labor intensive and requires a high degree of expertise and experience. Another major disadvantage of the Nuss technique is the intensely painful post-surgical recovery.

To address the above challenges, we are developing a novel image-guided PE correction device that can be programmed to assume the desired chest shape and provide personalized treatment. The series of changes in the curvature and angulation that results in the final shape can be programmed to optimize the correction of the deformity. The device is intended to provide a personalized PE correction with minimal risk and pain, akin to orthodontic treatment using dental braces. The design of the device will be based on chest modeling (including the ribs, sternum and cartilages) from noncontrast CT data and simulation techniques.

Prior works on PE surgical planning are scarce. Vilaça et al. simulated the postsurgical cosmetic outcome in PE patients [2, 3]. The method focused on the skin simulation using a mass-spring model. However, it has been shown that the conventional pectus bar modeling based on the patient's skin profile is imprecise [4]. More recently, the same group evaluated a system simulating the pectus bar, but the design of the bar was not presented [5]. Wei et al. developed a biomechanical model of PE based on a finite element model using a single patient CT image [6], but the rib cage used to establish the model was manually segmented. Zhao et al. estimated the general cartilaginous region based on mesh contraction, but they did not estimate the results of surgical correction [7].

In this study, we propose an automatic method to personalize the surgical planning for PE correction by simulating the post-surgical results (which include for the first time the anatomy of the ribs, sternum and cartilages) and estimating the size and shape of the correction device. The severity analysis of PE is also assessed by comparing the preoperative and the estimated postoperative chest shape. We first automatically segment the ribs and sternum using kernel graph cuts, followed by skeletonization. Then the costal cartilages are estimated using a statistical shape model (SSM) based on cosine series representation of 3D anatomical curves, a key methodological contribution to allow the accurate analysis of cartilages which are otherwise difficult to visualize on noncontrast CT. To estimate the post-surgical or corrected chest, an ICA-based SSM of normal chests, built with healthy subjects, allows matching a patient's anatomy to its most similar normal subject. This allows precisely simulating the post-surgical results via registration and estimating the size and shape of the correction devices through model fitting. Finally, the severity of the deformations of the chest of PE patients is computed in relation to the estimated correction device. The technology is applicable to the design of both the Nuss/pectus bar and the novel incremental correction device.

2   Method

The method was evaluated on 30 thoracic CT scans of slice thickness 0.62 mm including 15 healthy subjects and 15 PE patients. The dataset consists of 25 male and 5 female patients with severe PE requiring corrective surgery (Haller index: 2.5-5.7) and average age of 14 years (range: 9-21). Each volumetric image consisted of axial images of size 512×512 pixels with in-plane resolution ranging from 0.59 to 0.82 mm. The manually segmented ribs, sterna, cartilages from CT scans were provided by a board certified radiologists as ground truth.

The ribs and sternum are first segmented using kernel graph cuts via kernel mapping (radial basis function used in this study) of the image data in the piecewise constant model of graph cuts [8]. However, this type of segmentation is not applicable to the cartilage, which is poorly, if at all, visible in noncontrast CT. After segmentation, the surface meshes are generated [9] and smoothed using Humphrey's Classes Laplacian smoothing [10].To model the rib cage, the skeletons of ribs and cartilages are extracted using a mesh contraction method [11] by using implicit Laplacian smoothing with global positional constraints.

2.1   Cartilage Estimation

The skeletons of ribs and cartilages are modeled as 3D curves and parameterized as coefficients of the cosine series expansion [12]. Unlike traditional splines, the cosine series representation does not have internal knots and explicitly models curves as a linear combination of the cosine basis. Modeling cartilages as 3D curves with cosine series representation does not require manually labeled landmarks or evenly-placed pseudo landmarks. Moreover, it allows different numbers of control points on 3D curves for different samples. We first map a 3D curve with n ordered control points $p_1, \ldots, p_n$ to the unit interval $[0, 1]$ based on the geodesic distance of the curve $p_j \to t_j = \frac{\sum_{i=1}^{j} \|p_i - p_{i-1}\|}{\sum_{i=1}^{n} \|p_i - p_{i-1}\|}$. Then the curve is parameterized using the cosine basis of the form $\psi_0(t) = 1, \psi_k(t) = \sqrt{2}\cos(k\pi t)$, where k is the degree of the cosine basis ($k = 19$ in the study). The curve reconstructed with k degree cosine basis is represented as $Y_{n \times 3} = \Psi_{n \times k} C_{k \times 3}$, where Ψ is the cosine basis and C the cosine coefficients. As the cosine series expansion is a compact representation of 3D curves, for a k degree cosine series expansion, there are only $3(k+1)$ parameters instead of $3n$ coordinates (usually $n \gg k$) for building the SSM. We build a SSM of C under the assumption of a Gaussian prior and therefore using principal component analysis (PCA): $C = \bar{C} + P \cdot b$, where $\bar{C}$ represents the mean coefficients, P the eigenvector matrix and b the shape parameters. Thus the SSM for 3D curves is $Y = \Psi\bar{C} + \Psi P b$. Fig. 1 (a) shows the first principal mode for the skeletons of ribs 1 through 7 and the corresponding cartilages.

For model fitting, we estimate each cartilage between the end point of the rib and the joint with the sternum (shown in Fig. 1 (b)) by minimizing the difference between the reconstructed rib skeleton and the real rib skeleton extracted from the ground truth in a least squares fashion:

$$b^* = \arg\min_{b} \left\| \Psi P b + \Psi \overline{C} - Y_{obs} \right\|, \text{ subject to} -2\sqrt{\lambda} < b < 2\sqrt{\lambda} \tag{1}$$

where Y_{obs} is the real rib skeleton (observation) and λ the eigenvalues corresponding to eigenvectors P.

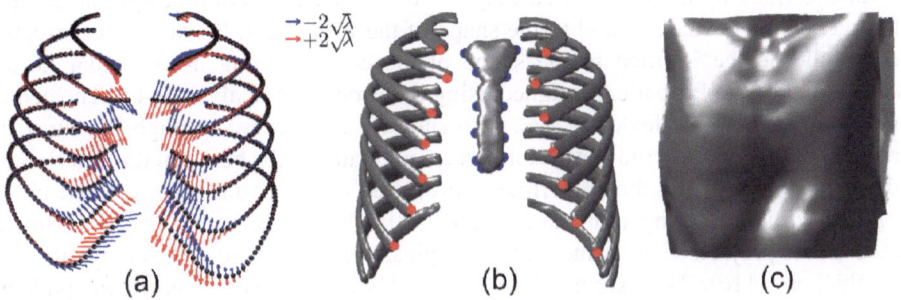

Fig. 1. The cartilages model, start and end points for estimating cartilages and the skin surface of a PE patient: (a) the first principal modes of variation for ribs and cartilages via PCA; the shape parameters are set to $\pm 2\sqrt{\lambda}$; (b) the end points of ribs (red dots) and the joints with the sternum (blue dots); and (c) the skin surface of a PE patient.

The final cartilages are generated as tubes centered on the cartilage centerlines. For each point on the centerline, an ellipse is generated. The distances between the centerlines and the surface mesh on ribs and sterna estimate the major and minor axes of the end points of cartilages. The major and minor axes of the intermediate points are assumed to vary linearly between the end points along the centerline of the cartilage.

2.2   Simulation of PE Correction and Estimation of Correction Device

ICA-Based Rib Cage Model Building
To create the multi-atlas of the normal chest (rib cage) shape, a SSM containing seven pairs of ribs (left and right) is built with data from 15 normal subjects. The model does not contain the cartilages or sterna, which can be severely deformed in PE patients, to allow matching the closest healthy chest shape to each PE case, as described below. For each rib, ten landmarks are uniformly sampled from the rib skeleton. The SSM is built using independent component analysis (ICA), instead of PCA, to model the local shape variations: $X = \bar{X} + A \cdot S$, where X are the training samples of the rib skeleton with mean shape $\bar{X}$, A the mixing matrix and S the independent components (ICs) regarded here as shape parameters. The ICs are ordered and selected using the method in [13] by using the entropy and the interquartile range to measure the sample variation. The cosine series method is not applicable here as we model the whole chest instead of individual ribs.

Correction Device Design and Rib Cage Correction
With the ICA-based SSM, the shape parameter of a PE patient's ribs s' is first calculated. Then the most similar normal chest/ribs of a PE patient's anatomy s^* from the healthy multi-atlas database is found using the Mahalanobis distance

$$s^* = \arg\min_{s^* \neq s'} \sqrt{(\mathbf{s} - \mathbf{s}')^T \Sigma^{-1} (\mathbf{s} - \mathbf{s}')}, \qquad (2)$$

where Σ is the covariance matrix of the normal rib cage samples.

The design (shape and size) of the correction device is estimated based on the costal surface fitted by the ribs and cartilages. For the pre-correction design (at the time of surgery), the device is fitted to the shape of the PE patient. For the post-correction design, the device is fitted to the shape of the corresponding most similar normal chest to that of the PE patient (aligned using the Procrustes analysis [14]). The centerline of the correction device is first estimated as a 3D curve through the most depressed points on the sternal posterior surface and lateral ribs between the anterior and midaxillary lines. Then the centerline is projected to the costal surface fitted by the ribs and cartilages using thin plate spline [15]. The correction device is estimated based on the projected centerline with the typical pectus bar size of 1.5cm width and 2 mm thickness [16]. The estimated correction device is personalized to PE patient's costal curvature instead of their skin profile, which is more precise and accurate especially for female patients. Finally, the PE patient's sternum, ribs and cartilages are deformed using a deformation field formed by the pre- and post-correction shape of the device based on B-spline registration [17] to simulate the corrected/post-surgical chest anatomy.

3   Experiments and Results

3.1   Cartilage Estimation

The Dice coefficient for the segmentation of ribs and sternum was 0.88±0.02 and (0.95±0.03 for sternum alone). One random normal case was selected as the template and its rib skeleton was registered to all other cases using non-rigid point registration to [18]. Before building the SSM of cartilages, all training samples were aligned using Procrustes analysis to remove the translation, rotation and scale [14]. One model was built for each skeleton. As mainly cartilages 4 through 7 are frequently affected in PE patients, we modeled ribs and cartilages 1 through 7 on both sides of the thorax (left and right) to a total of 14 models. The joints between cartilages and sternum were found by registering the testing sternum with the template. Note that for model training, the skeleton of both ribs and cartilages were extracted, while for model fitting, only the rib skeleton was used. Leave-one-out cross-validation was performed.

Three metrics were adopted to evaluate the method. One is the root mean square centerline distance error (RMSE-C) between the estimated cartilage centerlines and its ground truth, which was on average 2.50±0.80 mm. The RMSE-C for normal and PE cases were 2.04±0.44 mm and 2.74±0.85 mm, respectively. Another metric is the root mean square mesh distance error (RMSE-M) between the estimated cartilage mesh and the ground truth that was 1.28±0.81 mm. The RMSE-M for normal and PE cases were 1.20±0.34 mm and 1.14±0.38 mm, respectively. No significant difference of RMSE-M was recorded using the Wilcoxon test between normal subjects and PE

Table 1. The mean RMSE-C, RMSE-M and AMD errors for each pair of cartilages. Errors are larger on the inferior cartilages due to larger and complex shape variations. All values are in millimeters (mm).

Rib pair	1	2	3	4	5	6	7
RMSE-C	1.94±1.17	0.72±0.34	0.80±0.36	1.12±0.56	1.83±0.91	2.95±1.33	4.69±1.86
RMSE-M	1.47±1.39	0.64±0.68	0.49±0.43	0.43±0.30	0.48±0.36	0.79±0.52	2.4±1.05
AMDE	0.60±0.16	0.33±0.05	0.29±0.07	0.26±0.05	0.27±0.04	0.35±0.06	0.57±0.17

patients ($p=0.72$). The third metric is the average mesh distance error (AMDE) between the estimated cartilages and the ground truth, which was 0.38±0.16 mm. The RMSE-C, RMSE-M and AMDE of each pair of cartilages with the corresponding standard deviation are shown in Table 1. Fig. 2 shows the estimated cartilages of a PE case with the RMSE-M representing by the colormap. It can be seen that the errors of the cartilages 6 and 7 were generally larger that may be caused by their large shape variations and complex structures.

3.2   Rib Cage Correction and Correction Device Estimation

For correction device estimation, we performed experiments on the 15 retrospective CT data of PE patients. The average Mahalanobis distances between the shape parameters of the pre- and post-corrected ribcage and that of the closest normal were 5.58±1.08 and 4.50±0.78, respectively. Our reasoning is that the rib cage of the PE patient should be similar to that of the closest normal. The root mean square (RMS) distance between the pre- and post-correction ribs and the most similar normal anatomy were 11.15±2.68 and 10.02±2.49mm, respectively. Thus our method correctly identifies that there is no significant change in the shape of the ribs with the correction as observed clinically. Distinctively, the average deformation with correction of the sterna and cartilages was 49.71±10.11mm.

Since the conventional bar modeling and bending are based on the patient's skin surface morphology, we evaluated our method using the distance between our automatically estimated device (Fig. 3.d) and the surface of the chest convex hull (Fig. 3.e), which was 16.50±4.60 mm. This result reconfirms that the skin surface morphology is not a precise approximation of the shape of the rib cage; this is particularly relevant for overweight patients and females. Instead, our method evaluates the shape of the sternum, ribs and cartilages, the anatomical areas involved in PE correction. An example of corrected rib cage (post-surgery simulation) from a PE patient is shown in Fig. 3, with the color indicating severity of the PE deformation as the difference between the pre- and post-surgical rib cage.

For conventional Nuss surgery, the bar is fitted to the post-correction shape (Fig. 3.d), as the correction is done in a single but extremely painful step. For designing our new correction device, we require both the shape at the beginning of correction (Fig. 3.c) and at the end of correction (Fig. 3.d) to compute the incremental shape changes for PE correction. The intermediary steps are not addressed in this paper.

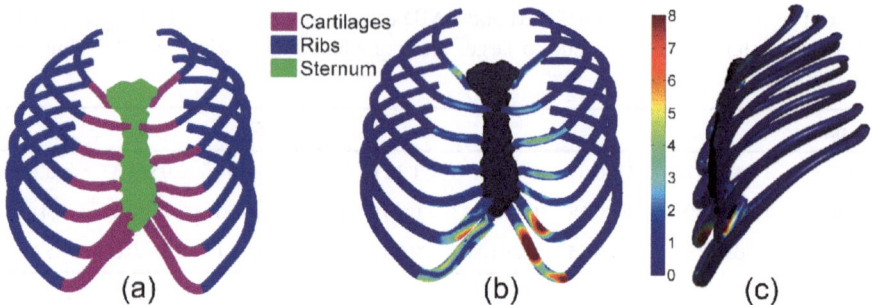

Fig. 2. The estimated cartilages of a PE patient: (a) the anatomy of the cartilages, ribs and sternum; (b) the estimated cartilages using a colormap indicating RMSE-M; and (c) the side view of (b). All values are in millimeters.

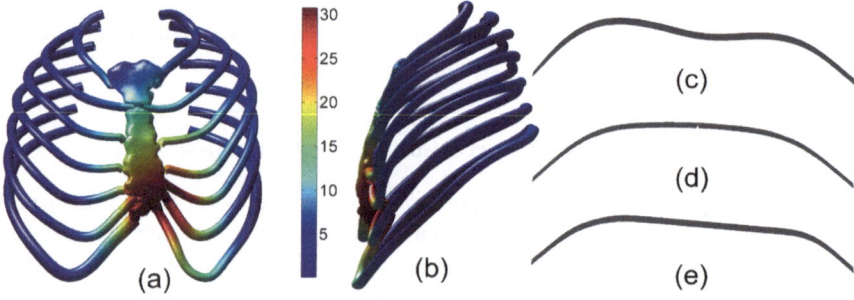

Fig. 3. The estimated corrected rib cage and the shape of correction device: (a) the corrected rib cage of the PE case shown in Fig.2 and the color indicates the severity of the PE deformation as the difference between the pre- and post-surgical (simulated) rib cage; (b) the side view of (a); (c) the shape of the device before correction (note the lifting of the chest compared to Fig. 2.c, as shown by colormap); (d) the shape of the device after correction using our method; and (e) the shape of the device estimated from the patient's skin profile. All values are in millimeters.

4   Conclusion

We proposed a personalized surgical planning method for PE correction using clinical noncontrast CT scans, which allows the modeling of the chest anatomy, including the ribs, sternum and cartilages, and simulating precise post-surgical results for the first time. As a methodological contribution, the skeletons of costal cartilages were modeled as 3D curves using the cosine series representation and estimated using a SSM built with the cosine coefficients to allow the accurate analysis of cartilages which are difficult to visualize on nonconstrast CT. Then the ICA-based SSM of the normal rib cage allowed matching a PE patient's anatomy to its most similar normal subjects and estimating the severity of the chest deformation. The average deformation of the sterna and cartilages with the simulation of PE correction was 49.71±10.11 mm. The technology is applicable to estimating the size and shape of both the Nuss/pectus bar, as in current clinical practice, and the design of the new correction device for optimal and incremental correction of PE in a less painful and controlled setting.

References

1. Jaroszewski, D., et al.: Current Management of Pectus Excavatum: A Review and Update of Therapy and Treatment Recommendations. The Journal of the American Board of Family Medicine 23, 230–239 (2010)
2. Moreira, A.H.J., et al.: Pectus excavatum postsurgical outcome based on preoperative soft body dynamics simulation. In: Proc. SPIE, pp. 83160K–83160K (2012)
3. Vilaça, J.L., et al.: Virtual simulation of the postsurgical cosmetic outcome in patients with Pectus Excavatum. In: Proc. SPIE, pp. 79642L–79642L (2011)
4. Lai, J.-Y., et al.: The measurement and designation of the pectus bar by computed tomography. Journal of Pediatric Surgery 44, 2287–2290 (2009)
5. Vilaça, J.L., et al.: Automatic Prebent Customized Prosthesis for Pectus Excavatum Minimally Invasive Surgery Correction. Surgical Innovation (2013)
6. Wei, Y., et al.: Pectus Excavatum Nuss Orthopedic finite element simulation. In: Biomedical Engineering and Informatics (BMEI), pp. 1236–1239 (2010)
7. Zhao, Q., et al.: Estimation of Cartilaginous Region in Noncontrast CT of the Chest. In: Proc. SPIE (in press, 2014)
8. Salah, M.B., et al.: Multiregion Image Segmentation by Parametric Kernel Graph Cuts. IEEE Transactions on Image Processing 20, 545–557 (2011)
9. Fang, Q., Boas, D.A.: Tetrahedral mesh generation from volumetric binary and grayscale images. In: ISBI 2009, pp. 1142–1145 (2009)
10. Vollmer, J., et al.: Improved Laplacian Smoothing of Noisy Surface Meshes. Computer Graphics Forum 18, 131–138 (1999)
11. Au, O.K.-C., et al.: Skeleton extraction by mesh contraction. ACM Trans. Graph. 27, 1–10 (2008)
12. Chung, M.K., et al.: Cosine series representation of 3D curves and its application to white matter fiber bundles in diffusion tensor imaging. Statistics and Its Interface 3, 69–80 (2010)
13. Zhao, Q., Okada, K., Rosenbaum, K., Zand, D.J., Sze, R., Summar, M., Linguraru, M.G.: Hierarchical Constrained Local Model Using ICA and Its Application to Down Syndrome Detection. In: Mori, K., Sakuma, I., Sato, Y., Barillot, C., Navab, N. (eds.) MICCAI 2013, Part II. LNCS, vol. 8150, pp. 222–229. Springer, Heidelberg (2013)
14. Gower, J.C.: Generalized procrustes analysis. Psychometrika 40, 33–51 (1975)
15. Bookstein, F.L.: Principal warps: thin-plate splines and thes decomposition of deformations. PAMI 11, 567–585 (1989)
16. Puri, B., et al.: Nuss procedure for pectus excavatum - An early experience. Medical Journal Armed Forces India 59, 316–319 (2003)
17. Besl, P.J., McKay, N.D.: A method for registration of 3-D shapes. PAMI 14, 239–256 (1992)
18. Myronenko, A., Xubo, S.: Point Set Registration: Coherent Point Drift. PAMI 32, 2262–2275 (2010)

A New 2.5D Representation for Lymph Node Detection Using Random Sets of Deep Convolutional Neural Network Observations

Holger R. Roth, Le Lu, Ari Seff, Kevin M. Cherry, Joanne Hoffman,
Shijun Wang, Jiamin Liu, Evrim Turkbey, and Ronald M. Summers

Imaging Biomarkers and Computer-Aided Diagnosis Laboratory,
Radiology and Imaging Sciences, National Institutes of Health Clinical Center,
Bethesda, MD 20892-1182, USA
holger.roth@nih.gov

Abstract. Automated Lymph Node (LN) detection is an important clinical diagnostic task but very challenging due to the low contrast of surrounding structures in Computed Tomography (CT) and to their varying sizes, poses, shapes and sparsely distributed locations. State-of-the-art studies show the performance range of 52.9% sensitivity at 3.1 false-positives per volume (FP/vol.), or 60.9% at 6.1 FP/vol. for mediastinal LN, by one-shot boosting on 3D HAAR features. In this paper, we first operate a preliminary candidate generation stage, towards ∼100% sensitivity at the cost of high FP levels (∼40 per patient), to harvest volumes of interest (VOI). Our 2.5D approach consequently decomposes any 3D VOI by resampling 2D reformatted orthogonal views N times, via scale, random translations, and rotations with respect to the VOI centroid coordinates. These random views are then used to train a deep Convolutional Neural Network (CNN) classifier. In testing, the CNN is employed to assign LN probabilities for all N random views that can be simply averaged (as a set) to compute the final classification probability per VOI. We validate the approach on two datasets: 90 CT volumes with 388 mediastinal LNs and 86 patients with 595 abdominal LNs. We achieve sensitivities of 70%/83% at 3 FP/vol. and 84%/90% at 6 FP/vol. in mediastinum and abdomen respectively, which drastically improves over the previous state-of-the-art work.

1 Introduction

Accurate detection and segmentation of enlarged Lymph Nodes (LNs) plays an important role for the staging of many diseases and their treatment, e.g. lung cancer, lymphoma and inflammation. These pathologies can cause affected LNs to become enlarged, i.e. swell in size. A LN's size is typically measured on Computed Tomography (CT) images following the RECIST guideline [1]. A LN is considered enlarged if its smallest diameter (along its short axis) measures more than 10 mm on an axial CT slice (see Fig. 1). Quantitative analysis plays a pivotal role for assessing the progression of certain diseases, accurate staging,

P. Golland et al. (Eds.): MICCAI 2014, Part I, LNCS 8673, pp. 520–527, 2014.

prognosis, choice of therapy, and follow-up examinations. Radiologists need to detect, quantitatively evaluate and classify LNs. This assessment is typically done manually and is error prone due to the fact that LNs can vary markedly in shape and size and can have attenuation coefficients similar to those of surrounding organs (see Fig. 1). Furthermore, manual processing is time-consuming and tedious and might delay the clinical workflow.

Previous work on computer-aided detection (CADe) systems for LNs mostly uses direct 3D information from volumetric CT images. State-of-the-art methods [2,3] perform boosting-based feature selection and integration over a pool of ∼50 thousand 3D Haar-like features to obtain a strong binary classifier for detecting LNs. Due to the limited availability of annotated training data and the intrinsic high dimensionality, modeling complex 3D image structures for LN detection is non-trivial. Particularly, lymph nodes have large within-class appearance, location or pose variations, and low contrast from surrounding anatomies over a patient population. This results in many false-positives (FP), to assure a moderately high detection sensitivity [4], or only limited sensitivity levels [2,3]. The good sensitivities achieved at low FP range in [2] are not directly comparable with the other studies since [2] reports on axillary, pelvic, and only some parts of the abdominal regions, while others evaluate only on mediastinum [5,3,4] or abdomen [6]. High numbers of FPs per image make efficient integration of CADe into clinical workflow challenging.

Our method employs a LN CADe systems [7,8] with high sensitivities as the first stage and focuses on effectively reducing FPs. In comparison, the direct one-shot 3D detection [2,3] saturates at ∼65% sensitivity at full FP range. Recently, the availability of large-scale annotated training sets and the accessibility of affordable parallel computing resources via GPUs has made it feasible to train deep Convolution Neural Networks (CNNs) and achieve great advances in challenging ImageNet recognition tasks [9,10]. Studies that apply deep learning and CNNs to medical imaging applications also show promise, e.g. [11], and classifying digital pathology [12]. Extensions of CNNs to 3D have been proposed, but computational cost and memory consumption are still too high to be efficiently implemented on today's computer graphics hardware units [11,13]. In this work, we investigate the feasibility of using CNNs as a highly effective of FP reduction. We propose to use 3D VOIs with a new 2.5D representation that may easily facilitate a generally-purposed 3D object detection by classification scheme.

2   Methods

2.1   LN Candidate Detection in Mediastinum and Abdomen

We use a preliminary CADe system for detecting LN candidates from mediastinal [7] and abdominal [8] CT volumes. In the mediastinum, lungs are segmented automatically and shape features are computed at voxel-level. The system uses a spatial prior of anatomical structures (such as esophagus, aortic arch, and/or heart) via multi-atlas label fusion before detecting LN candidates using a Support Vector Machine (SVM) for classification. In the abdomen, a random forest classifier is used to create voxel-level LN predictions. Both systems permit the combination of multiple statistical image descriptors and appropriate feature selection in order to improve LN detection beyond traditional enhancement filters. LN candidate generation is not a core topic of this paper. Currently, 94%-97% sensitivity level at the rates of 25-35 FP/vol. can been achieved [7,8]. Given sufficient training for the LN candidate generation step, close to 100% sensitivities could be reached in the future.

2.2   CNN Training on 2.5D Image Patches

In general computer vision, a CNN is typically designed to classify color images that contain three image channels: Red, Green and Blue (RGB). We map this set-up by assigning the axial, coronal and sagittal slices in a Volume-of-Interest (VOI) into to these three channels (see Fig. 1). Our approach is similar to [11] in that we use the three orthogonal slices (axial, coronal and sagittal) through the center of a CADe mark as the input patch. However, we aim to simplify the training of the CNN by jointly using three channel images. This differs from the approach of [11] that uses three individual and separately trained CNNs on each one of the orthogonal image slices, with a subsequent fusion of their predictions for image segmentation. The 3D CT data is resampled in order to extract VOIs at N_s different physical scales s (the edge length of each VOI), but with fixed numbers of voxels. In order to increase the training data variation and to avoid overfitting (analogous to the 2D data augmentation approach in [9]), each VOI is also translated along a random vector v in 3D space N_t times. Furthermore, each translated VOI is rotated around a randomly oriented vector v at its center N_r times by a random angle $\alpha = [0°, \ldots, 360°]$, resulting in $N = N_s \times N_t \times N_r$ random observation of each VOI (similar to [14]). This permits easy expansion of both the training and testing data for this type of neural net application. When classifying unseen data, the N random CNN predictions can be simply averaged at each VOI to compute a per-candidate probability:

$$p\left(x|\{P_1(x), ..., P_N(x)\}\right) = \frac{1}{N} \sum_{i=1}^{N} P_i(x), \tag{1}$$

where $P_i(x)$ is the CNN's classification probability for one individual image patch. The main purpose of this approach is to decompose the volumetric information from each VOI into a set of random 2D images (with three channels) that combine orthogonal slices at N reformatted orientations in 3D. Our relatively simple re-sampling of the 3D data circumvents using 3D CNN directly [13]. This not only greatly reduces the computational burden for training and testing, but more importantly, alleviates the curse-of-dimensionality problem. Direct training 3D deep CNN [13] for the volumetric object detection problem may not be feasible due to severe lack of sufficient training samples, especially in the medical imaging domain. CNNs generally need tremendous amounts of training examples to address overfitting, with respect to the large number of parameters. [9] uses translational shifting and mirroring of 2D image patches for

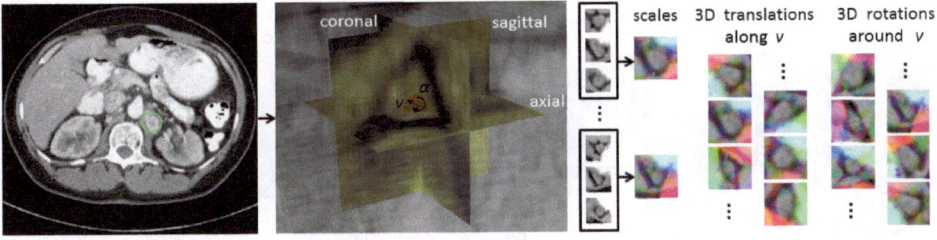

Fig. 1. Examples of lymph nodes (circled) in an axial CT slice of the abdomen. Image patches are generated from CADe candidates, using different scales, 3D translations (along a random vector v) and rotations (around a random vector v by a random angle α). Each image patch (visualized as RGB image) is composed of an axial (R), coronal (G), and sagittal slice (B) and centered at a LN candidate.

this purpose. Random resampling is an effective and efficient way to increase the amount of available training data. Our 2.5D representation is intuitive and applies the success of large scale 2D image classification, using CNN [9] effortlessly into 3D space. The above averaging process (i.e., Eq. 1) further improves the robustness and stability of 2D CNN labeling on random views (see Sec. 3).

The CNN architecture typically consists of several layers that apply convolutional filters to the input images (hence the name). The subsequent layers consist of max-pooling layers, fully-connected layers, and a final 2-way softmax layer for classification (see Fig. 2). In order to avoid overfitting, we use a recently published method called "DropConnect" that behaves as a regularizer when training the CNN [15]. DropConnect is a variation of the earlier proposed "DropOut" method. In order to allow efficient training of the CNN, we use a GPU-based open-source implementation by [9] with the DropConnect extension by [15]. Alongside the use of GPU acceleration, a speed-up in training has been achieved by using rectified linear units as the neuron model instead of the standard neuron model $f(x) = \tanh(x)$ or $f(x) = (1 + e^{-x})^{-1}$ [9]. At this time, the optimal architecture of CNNs for a particular image classification task is difficult to determine [10]. We evaluate several CNNs with slightly different layer architectures to choose the best CNN architecture for our classification task and find relatively stable behavior on our datasets. Hence, we fix the CNN architecture for the subsequent cross-validation performed in this study. A recent approach proposes to visualize the trained CNN model by deconvolution and in order aid understanding the behavior of CNNs [10]. These methods have the potential to allow better CNN design rather than using a heuristic approach as in this work.

3   Evaluation and Results

Radiologists labeled a total of 388 mediastinal LNs as positives' in CT images of 90 patients and a total of 595 abdominal LNs in 86 patients. In order to

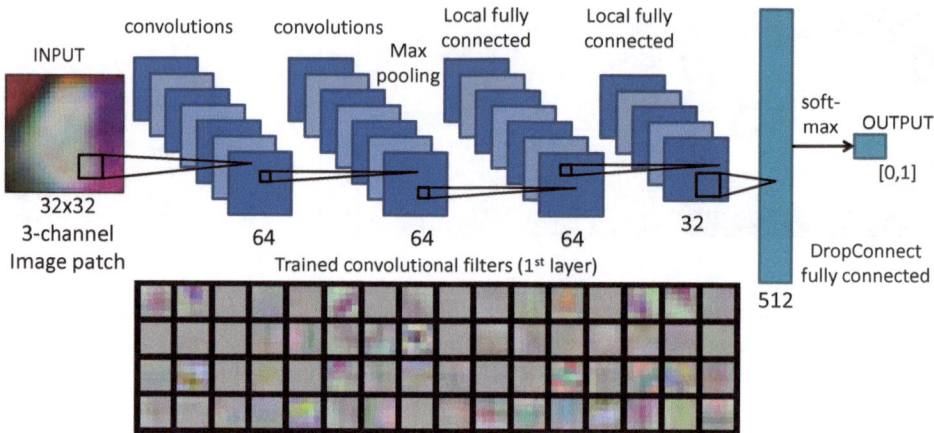

Fig. 2. Our convolution neural network consists of two convolutional layers, max-pooling layers, locally fully-connected layers, a DropConnect layer, and a final 2-way softmax layer for classification. The number of filters, connections for each layer, and the first layer of learned convolutional kernels are shown.

objectively evaluate the performance of our CNN based 2.5D detection module, 100% sensitivity at the LN candidate generation stage is assumed by injecting the labeled LNs into the set of CADe LN candidates (see Sec. 2.1). The CADe systems produce a total of 3208 false-positive detections (>15 mm away from true LN) in the mediastinum and 3484 in the abdomen. These false-positive detections are used as negative' LN candidate examples for training the CNNs. All patients are randomly split into three subsets (at the patient level) to allow a 3-folded cross-validation. We use different sample rates of positive and negative image patches to generate a balanced training set. This proves beneficial for training the CNN – no balancing is done during cross-validation. Each three-channel image patch is centered at a CADe coordinate with 32×32 pixels. All patches are sampled at 4 scales: $s = [30, 35, 40, 45]$ mm for the VOI edge length in physical image space, after iso-metric resampling of the CT image (see Fig. 1). We use a soft-tissue window level of [-100, 200 HU] as in [2]. Furthermore, all VOIs are $N = 100$ times randomly translated (up to 3 mm) and rotated at each scale ($N_s = 4$, $N_t = 5$ and $N_r = 5$). We train separate CNN models for mediastinum and for abdomen. Training each CNN model takes 9-12 hours on a NVIDIA GeForce GTX TITAN, while running the 2.5D image patch classification for testing runs in only circa 5 minutes. Image patch extraction from one CT volume takes around 2 minutes. We then apply the trained CNN to classify image patches from the testing datasets. Figure 3 shows a typical classification probability on a random subset of test VOIs. Averaging the N predictions at each LN candidate allows us to compute a per-candidate probability $p(x)$, as in Eq. 1. Varying a threshold parameter on this probability allows us to compute the free-response receiver operating characteristic (FROC) curves. FROC curves are compared in Fig. 4 for varying amounts of N. It can be seen that the classification performance

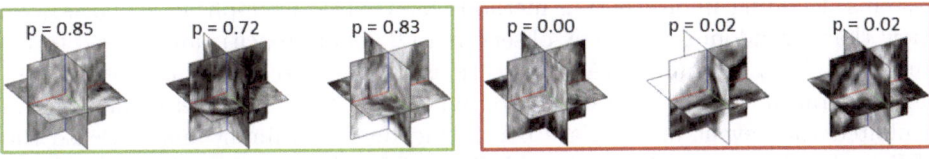

Fig. 3. Test probabilities of the CNN for being a lymph node on 'true' (left box) and 'false' (right box) lymph node candidate examples

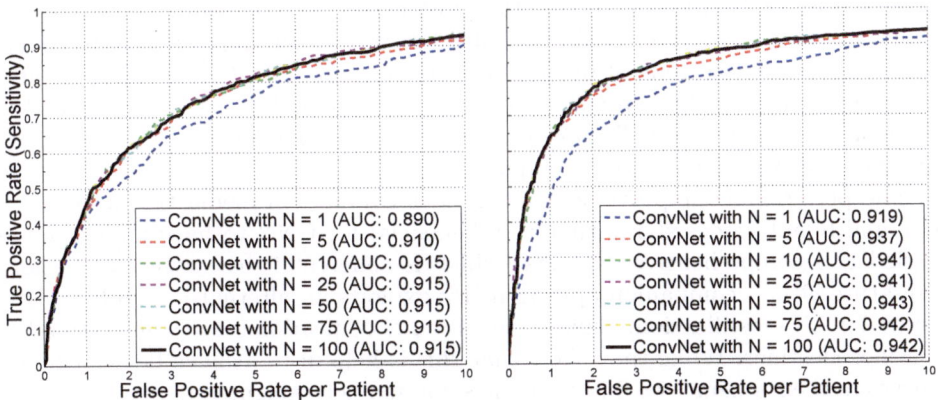

Fig. 4. Free-response receiver operating characteristic (FROC) curves for a 3-folded cross-validation using a varying number of N random CNN observers in 90 patients in the mediastinum (left) and 86 patients in the abdomen (right). AUC values are computed for corresponding ROC curves.

saturates quickly with increasing N. The classification sensitivity improves on the existing LN CADe systems [7,8] from 55% to 70% in the mediastinum and from 30% to 83% in the abdomen at a low rate of 3 FP per patient volume (FP/vol.) at $N = 100$. The area under the curve (AUC) improves from 0.76 to 0.942 in the abdomen, using the proposed false-positive reduction approach (AUC in the mediastinal was not available for comparison). At an operating point of 3 FP/vol., we achieve significant improvement: $p = 7.6 \times 10^{-3}$ and $p = 2.5 \times 10^{-14}$ in mediastinum and abdomen, respectively (Fisher's exact test). Further experiments show that performing a joint CNN model trained on both mediastinal and abdominal LN candidates together can improve the classification by ~10% to ~80% sensitivity improvement at 3 FP/vol. in the mediastinal set. The sensitivity level in the abdomen datasets remained stable.

4 Discussion and Conclusions

This work (among others) demonstrates that deep CNNs can be generalized to 3D/2D medical image analysis tasks, such as effective FP reduction in CADe systems. Building upon existing methods for CADe of lymph nodes (LNs), we show that a random set of CNN observers (a 2.5D approach) can be used to reduce FPs, from the initial CADe detections. Different scales, sampling through random translations and rotations around each of the CADe detections can be exploited to prevent or alleviate overfitting during training and increase the CNN's classification performance. AUC and FROC exhibit significant improvement on sensitivity levels at the range of clinically relevant FP/vol. rates. These results are a drastic improvement compared to the state-of-the-art methods. [3] reports 52.9% sensitivity at 3.1 FP/vol. in the mediastinum, while we achieve 70% at 3 FP/vol. In the abdomen, the most recent work [6] shows 70.5% sensitivity at 13.0 FP/vol. We obtain 83% at 3 FP/vol. (assuming ∼100% sensitivity at the LN candidate generation stage). Note that any direct comparison to another recent work is difficult since there are no common datasets available at the moment. Therefore, we will make our data[1] and supporting material[2] publicly available for convenient future comparison.

The performance improvement using joint training on mediastinum and abdominal lymph nodes shows that it is beneficial for CNN to have larger, more varied and comprehensive datasets (which is coherent to the computer vision literature [9]). A companion approach [16] exploits an alternative shallow hierarchy for LN classification, using a view-level classification score aggregation by another classifier. While they show that this is helpful to achieve better FROC curves in their scheme, we find that the same sparsely weighted fusion via learning does not improve over the simple average of Eq. 1. This probably indicates the high quality of our deep CNN predictions and shows this approach to be very effective and efficient. Future work will investigate more sophisticated methods of label fusion from the CNNs. The proposed 2.5D generalization of CNNs shows promise for a variety of applications in computer-aided detection of 3D medical images. For future work, the 2D views with the highest probability of being a LN could be used to present reformatted visualizations at that orientation (optimal to the CNN) to assist in radiologists' reading.

Acknowledgments. This work was supported by the Intramural Research Program of the NIH Clinical Center.

References

1. Therasse, P., Arbuck, S.G., Eisenhauer, E.A., Wanders, J., Kaplan, R.S., Rubinstein, L., Verweij, J., Van Glabbeke, M., van Oosterom, A.T., Christian, M.C., et al.: New guidelines to evaluate the response to treatment in solid tumors. JNCI 92(3), 205–216 (2000)
2. Barbu, A., Suehling, M., Xu, X., Liu, D., Zhou, S.K., Comaniciu, D.: Automatic detection and segmentation of lymph nodes from CT data. IEEE Transactions on Medical Imaging 31(2), 240–250 (2012)

---

[1] http://www.cc.nih.gov/about/SeniorStaff/ronald_summers.html
[2] https://sites.google.com/site/holgerrroth

3. Feulner, J., Kevin Zhou, S., Hammon, M., Hornegger, J., Comaniciu, D.: Lymph node detection and segmentation in chest ct data using discriminative learning and a spatial prior. MedIA 17(2), 254–270 (2013)
4. Feuerstein, M., Deguchi, D., Kitasaka, T., Iwano, S., Imaizumi, K., Hasegawa, Y., Suenaga, Y., Mori, K.: Automatic mediastinal lymph node detection in chest CT. SPIE Med. Imag., 72600V–72600V (2009)
5. Feuerstein, M., Glocker, B., Kitasaka, T., Nakamura, Y., Iwano, S., Mori, K.: Mediastinal atlas creation from 3-D chest computed tomography images: Application to automated detection and station mapping of lymph nodes. MedIA 16(1), 63–74 (2012)
6. Nakamura, Y., Nimura, Y., Kitasaka, T., Mizuno, S., Furukawa, K., Goto, H., Fujiwara, M., Misawa, K., Ito, M., Nawano, S., et al.: Automatic abdominal lymph node detection method based on local intensity structure analysis from 3D x-ray CT images. SPIE Med. Imag., 86701K (2013)
7. Liu, J., Zhao, J., Hoffman, J., Yao, J., Zhang, W., Turkbey, E.B., Wang, S., Kim, C., Summers, R.M.: Mediastinal lymph node detection on thoracic CT scans using spatial prior from multi-atlas label fusion. SPIE Med. Imag., 90350M–90350M (2014)
8. Cherry, K.M., Wang, S., Turkbey, E.B., Summers, R.M.: Abdominal lymphadenopathy detection using random forest. SPIE Med. Imag., 90351G–90351G (2014)
9. Krizhevsky, A., Sutskever, I., Hinton, G.: Imagenet classification with deep convolutional neural networks. In: NIPS, pp. 1106–1114 (2012)
10. Zeiler, M.D., Fergus, R.: Visualizing and understanding convolutional neural networks. arXiv:1311.2901 (2013)
11. Prasoon, A., Petersen, K., Igel, C., Lauze, F., Dam, E., Nielsen, M.: Deep feature learning for knee cartilage segmentation using a triplanar convolutional neural network. In: Mori, K., Sakuma, I., Sato, Y., Barillot, C., Navab, N. (eds.) MICCAI 2013, Part II. LNCS, vol. 8150, pp. 246–253. Springer, Heidelberg (2013)
12. Cireşan, D.C., Giusti, A., Gambardella, L.M., Schmidhuber, J.: Mitosis detection in breast cancer histology images with deep neural networks. In: Mori, K., Sakuma, I., Sato, Y., Barillot, C., Navab, N. (eds.) MICCAI 2013, Part II. LNCS, vol. 8150, pp. 411–418. Springer, Heidelberg (2013)
13. Turaga, S.C., Murray, J.F., Jain, V., Roth, F., Helmstaedter, M., Briggman, K., Denk, W., Seung, H.S.: Convolutional networks can learn to generate affinity graphs for image segmentation. Neural Computation 22(2), 511–538 (2010)
14. Göktürk, S.B., Tomasi, C., Acar, B., Beaulieu, C.F., Paik, D.S., Jeffrey, R.B., Yee, J., Napel, Y.: A statistical 3-D pattern processing method for computer-aided detection of polyps in CT colonography. IEEE Trans. on Med. Imag. 20, 1251–1260 (2001)
15. Wan, L., Zeiler, M., Zhang, S., Cun, Y.L., Fergus, R.: Regularization of neural networks using dropconnect. In: Proc. Int. Conf. Machine Learning (ICML 2013), pp. 1058–1066 (2013)
16. Seff, A., Lu, L., Cherry, K.M., Roth, H., Liu, J., Wang, S., Hoffman, J., Turkbey, E.B., Summers, R.M.: 2D view aggregation for lymph node detection using a shallow hierarchy of linear classifiers. In: Golland, P., Hata, N., Barillot, C., Hornegger, J., Howe, R. (eds.) MICCAI 2014. LNCS, vol. 8673, pp. 538–545. Springer, Heidelberg (2014)

Towards Automatic Plan Selection for Radiotherapy of Cervical Cancer by Fast Automatic Segmentation of Cone Beam CT Scans

Thomas Langerak[*], Sabrina Heijkoop, Sandra Quint, Jan-Willem Mens,
Ben Heijmen, and Mischa Hoogeman

Department of Radiation Oncology, Erasmus-MC Cancer Center,
Rotterdam, The Netherlands
{t.langerak,s.heijkoop,s.quint,j.w.m.mens,
b.heijmen,m.hoogeman}@erasmusmc.nl

Abstract. We propose a method to automatically select a treatment plan for radiotherapy of cervical cancer using a Plan-of-the-Day procedure, in which multiple treatment plans are constructed prior to treatment. The method comprises a multi-atlas based segmentation algorithm that uses the selected treatment plan to choose between two atlas sets. This segmentation only requires two registration procedures and can therefore be used in clinical practice without using excessive computation time. Our method is validated on a dataset of 224 treatment fractions for 10 patients. In 37 cases (16%), no recommendation was made by the algorithm due to poor image quality or registration results. In 93% of the remaining cases a correct recommendation for a treatment plan was given.

1   Introduction

One of the main treatment modalities for cervical cancer is External Beam Radiotherapy (EBRT) combined with brachytherapy and optionally chemotherapy. The aim of EBRT is to deliver an appropriate dose of radiation to the Clinical Target Volume (CTV), while minimizing the dose delivered to the Organs At Risk (OAR) that surround the CTV. For cervical cancer, the CTV typically consists of the upper part of the vagina, the cervix, the uterus and the nodal CTV. The most important OARs are the bladder in the anterior direction, the rectum in the posterior direction and the small bowels in the cranial direction (see Figure 1).

One of the main challenges when treating cervical cancer is that in the 23 treatment days the shape and position of the CTV exhibit a large day-to-day variation, depending on the amount of bladder filling (compare figure 1a to figure 1b). To ensure that the CTV is radiated, a large safety margin is used and as a result healthy tissue is unnecessarily irradiated. State-of-the-art treatment therefore uses a so-called Plan-of-the-Day procedure (Bondar et al., 2012) that selects at every treatment day the treatment plan that best fits the daily anatomy of the patient.

---

[*] Corresponding author.

P. Golland et al. (Eds.): MICCAI 2014, Part I, LNCS 8673, pp. 528–535, 2014.

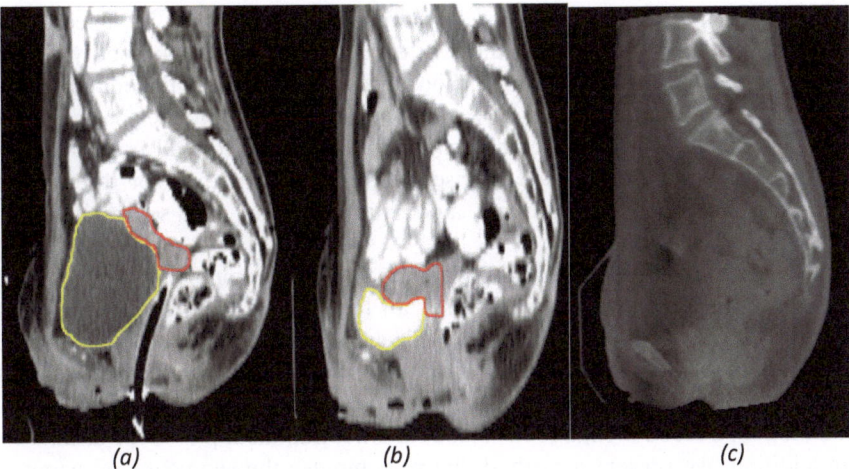

Fig. 1. Sagittal slices of CT scans of a patient (a) with a full bladder and (b) with an empty bladder. In both CT scans, both the bladder and the uterus are delineated. Figure c shows a CBCT scan of the same patient.

In our implementation of this procedure two treatment plans (TP_f and TP_e) are constructed prior to treatment based on two CT scans of the patient with varying bladder fillings. These scans were already part of normal clinical practice in order to be able to determine the extent of motion of the uterus as a result of the amount of bladder filling. Treatment plan TP_f can be used to treat the patient when the bladder is full to half-full; if the patient has an empty to half-full bladder, then TP_e can be used. It is not difficult to generate more treatment plan in the range from full to empty bladder, but the benefit of such a strategy has not been proven. In fact, existing research (Bondar et al., 2012) concludes that there is no significant benefit to more than two plans.

On the day of treatment, based on a Cone Beam CT (CBCT) scan that is acquired just before treatment, one of these two plans is then selected to be delivered to the patient. CBCT scans typically exhibit low soft tissue contrast, which makes it difficult to determine the exact location and shape of all relevant organs (see Figure 1c). Therefore, in our clinical procedure if no treatment plan can be reliably selected, a back-up plan (TP_b) is chosen that guarantees adequate coverage of the CTV but does not spare the OAR. As patients are typically treated in 23 treatment fractions, this procedure has to be performed 23 times. Although this is not part of the current clinical practice yet, after the delivery of the treatment the CBCT scan can be segmented to support a detailed analysis of the treatment up to that treatment day. In such an analysis the segmentation of each CBCT scan is coupled to the selected treatment plan in order to be able to determine what dose has been delivered to what organ. By accumulating this information over all treatment fractions it can be determined, at the end of treatment, what dose has been delivered to the target and to healthy tissues.

Selection of the correct treatment plan is currently done by a team of radiotherapy technicians (RTTs), who need to quickly interpret the daily CBCT scan using only visual assessment and identify the best treatment plan. Because they are under time pressure, RTTs tend to select the back-up treatment plan if they are uncertain about the treatment plan to use, for example as a result of poor image quality. Currently, there are only two treatment plans to choose from, which limits the complexity of the plan choice. In the future, however, we hope to further improve the sparing of healthy tissues by extending the number of treatment plans, such that all possible shapes of the target are better represented. Consequently, the complexity of the plan choice and time pressure will increase and automatic treatment plan selection becomes a necessity.

In this paper we present, to our knowledge, the first attempt to automate plan selection for cervical cancer. Our method uses all the images acquired on previous treatment days as an atlas in a multi-atlas-based segmentation procedure of the image that is acquired on the current day. A measure that is based on the agreement of the set of atlases expresses the confidence of the correctness of the segmentation. Based on this segmentation, a recommendation is made for what treatment plan to be used.

In addition, we present a method that re-computes the segmentation using only a subset of the atlases. Selection of the atlases is done based on the recommendation for a treatment plan. It can be expected that using a more dedicated atlas set leads to a more accurate segmentation that can be used for an interim or retrospective evaluation of the treatment. If the segmentation is of sufficient quality it can even form the basis for constructing a new treatment plan which can then be added to the treatment plan library, although this falls outside the scope of this paper.

In section 2 the existing literature on atlas selection is briefly reviewed as well as the literature on the Plan-of-the-Day procedure. Section 3 proposes the method, section 4 describes the data and experiments, section 5 presents the results and section 6 discusses our findings, suggests further research, and draws a conclusion.

2   Review of Existing Literature

Multi-atlas based segmentation was popularized in the first decade of this century by, amongst others, Heckemann et al., 2006, Aljabar et al., 2009, Rohlfing et al., 2005 and Klein et al., 2008. Following the initial investigations into the concept of multi-atlas-based segmentation in general, the focus of new research came to lie on the label fusion aspect of multi-atlas based segmentation. Most of these methods are based on the pioneering work by Warfield et al., 2004, on expectation maximization and include variants that use atlas selection (Langerak et al, 2010), local similarity measures (Asman, 2012; Commowick, 2012) and probabilistic models 13 et al., in press). Atlas selection has been proposed based on image similarity (Aljabar et al., 2009) and on segmentation similarity (Langerak et al., 2013)

Plan-of-the-day procedures have been described for radiotherapy treatment of cervical cancer (Bondar et al., 2012), bladder cancer (Murthy et al., 2011) and prostate cancer (Gill et al., 2013). In all of these cases, using a Plan-of-the-Day treatment is motivated by variable bladder- and rectum filling that influences the shape and position of the target.

3   Method

We assume that the first fraction CBCT scan, indicated as $CBCT_1$, was manually segmented by an expert and we use this scan to initialize both atlas sets A_f and A_e. It may seem more logical to use CT_f and CT_e to initialize the atlas sets, but these differ significantly from the CBCT scans, among others because a vaginal catheter is inserted to indicate the lower and upper part of the vaginal wall during the acquisition of the CT scans. This catheter is not present on the CBCT scans, which considerably hinders registration of the CT scans. Inserting a catheter during the acquisition of the CBCT scans to increase uniformity and make registration easier is not an option because of the decrease in patient comfort and a considerable increase in the time needed for treatment. Segmenting $CBCT_{i>1}$ was done using the following procedure:

1. $CBCT_1$ and $CBCT_i$ are registered in both directions using a rigid registration followed by a B-Spline driven non-rigid registration. Mutual information was used as the image similarity metric and we used a LBFGSB optimizer as provided by ITK.

2. The segmentations of all $CBCT_{j<i}$ are propagated to $CBCT_i$ indirectly, via $CBCT_1$. These propagated segmentations are denoted as S^0 to S^{i-1} and combined to a single result. To combine segmentations, the SIMPLE algorithm (Langerak et al., 2010) was used, but we do not expect any significant difference in outcome when using another label fusion method and therefore refer to the above mentiond paper for details of the label fusion method. The default parameters mentioned in the paper were used. The resulting segmentation is noted as S_i.

3. If the volume of the bladder $|B_i|$ in S_i is larger than $(|B_f|+|B_e|)/2$, then it is recommended to use TP_f for treatment. Otherwise TP_e is recommended. A confidence level is given by analyzing the variability of all individual atlas-based segmentations.

4. If the full bladder treatment plan was recommended then A_f is selected to be used in step 5, otherwise A_e is selected.

5. $CBCT_i$ is re-segmented using the selected atlas set. Note that this step hardly takes additional computation time because the necessary registrations were already computed in step 1. This is an automatic correction that differs from step 2 only in the fact that not all segmentations are used as an atlas, but only the subdivisions A_f and A_e.

6. $CBCT_i$ and its segmentation are manually corrected and approved by an RTT and added to the appropriate atlas set A_f or A_e.

The confidence level that is mentioned in step 3 is computed as the smallest agreement between any two propagated segmentations and is defined as $\min_{S1,S2\in[S_0,S_{i-1}]} DSC(S1,S2)$, where DSC is the Dice Similarity Coefficient. If the confidence level drops below a certain threshold, no recommendation for a treatment plan is given. In this case the segmentation is not added to either atlas set.

By using $CBCT_1$ as a reference image, this procedure only takes one forward and one backward registration per treatment fraction. The initial segmentation based on which a treatment plan is chosen is not necessarily very accurate because, due to the shape variation, some of the atlases will not register well to the target image. However, as it is not used as a final segmentation, but only to make a decision between the two atlas sets, it does not have to be very accurate. I.e. if bladder volumes vary between the full bladder volume $\left|B_f\right|$ and the empty bladder volume $\left|B_e\right|$ and n treatment plans are computed, then each treatment plan $T_{0\le m<n}$ covers the bladder volume range $[\left|B_e\right|+(\left|B_f\right|-\left|B_e\right|)\frac{m}{n},\left|B_e\right|+(\left|B_f\right|-\left|B_e\right|)\frac{m+1}{n,}]$, and therefore

segmentation volumes are allowed to be off by $\frac{(\left|B_f\right|-\left|B_e\right|)}{n}$, assuming that B_f fully overlaps B_e. In other words: the fewer sub-ranges and the larger the volume of the bladder in the full-bladder scan, the less accurate the segmentation needs to be to be able to choose the correct treatment plan.

4   Data and Experiments

In a retrospective study, we investigated a total of 234 treatment fractions for 10 patients: 9 patients were treated in 23 fractions and 1 patient was treated in 27 fractions. These patients were selected from our database because full- and empty-bladder treatment plans were available for these patients because the variations in bladder filling resulted in large motion of the uterus. In all CBCT scans three structures were manually segmented by an expert: the uterus, the bladder and the rectum. These segmentations served as a ground truth segmentation.

Not taking into account the first treatment fraction (in which the CBCT scan was manually delineated), in total 224 treatment plan decisions were made. For each patient i and fraction j, the chosen treatment plans were recorded as $TP_j^i \in \{TP_e, TP_f, TP_b\}$, where TP_e means that an empty-bladder treatment plan was used, TP_f stands for a full-bladder treatment plan and TP_b represents the back-up plan.

In 42 cases a back-up plan was chosen by the RTTs and no choice was made between an empty- or a full-bladder treatment plan. In these cases, a treatment plan decision was made retrospectively by an expert clinician.

First, the treatment plan that was recommended by our method was tested against the manual treatment plan decisions to validate the automatic treatment plan suggestion. In addition, it was tested whether the confidence measure correctly warned for inaccurate treatment plan recommendations. Finally, the accuracy of the re-segmentation using a dedicated atlas set was tested against the manual ground truth segmentation of the CBCT scans.

5   Results

Of the 224 treatment plan decisions, our method did not make a recommendation in 37 cases. A minimal confidence level of 0.3 was used that was experimentally determined. In 24 of these cases, the method would indeed have recommended the wrong treatment plan. For 173 of the remaining 187 cases, a correct recommendation was made, so our method achieved a 93% accuracy. A clinical investigation into whether the treatment plan suggestion supported the RTTs in their decision as a result of which the back-up plan was chosen less often is left for further research.

The refined segmentation that was computed with either the empty-bladder or the full-bladder atlas set was compared to the manual segmentations. The results are shown in Figure 2 in the form of a boxplot that indicates the median and the quartiles of the distribution of the accuracy. The DSC score for the bladder seems higher than for the Uterus and Rectum, but this is mainly due to the size of the bladder. Cases in which confidence levels were too low to recommend a treatment plan, whether correct or not, were not included in these results.

From this figure, it can be concluded that the segmentations that are computed are highly accurate, especially considering the fact that the underlying images are CBCT images, but not good enough for fully automatic segmentation. In our clinical practice, these segmentations are therefore used as an initial estimate that is manually corrected.

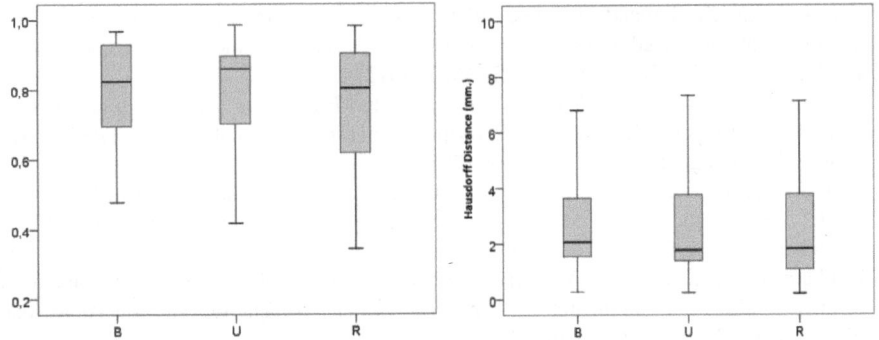

Fig. 2. Dice Similarity Coefficient (left) and Hausdorff distance in mm. (right) of the refined segmentations of the Bladder (B), Uterus (U), and Rectum (R).

6   Conclusions and Discussion

Given previous attempts to register images of cervical cancer patients, our results are encouraging but there are some limitations to our findings, mainly the fact that it is unknown what the inter- and intra-observer variability of manual segmentations is. Existing research suggests that the inter-observer variability is large when segmenting CBCT images, but this has only been investigated for prostate images. Our results show that the accuracy for atlas-based segmentation of the bladder is higher for the bladder than for the rectum and uterus. In the future we will therefore investigate a strategy to select atlases based on uterus shape and rectum filling in addition to bladder filling.

Furthermore, in section 3 we derived that the required accuracy of the rough initial segmentation increases with the number of available treatment plans. In our clinical practice only two treatment plans are used and this represents the easiest test case. It remains to be shown that our method also works in situations where more treatment plans are used, as a result of which the demands on the accuracy of the method become more strict.

In a visual inspection of the cases in which confidence was low, we noticed that in most cases where the low confidence was unjustified, it was caused by a single failed segmentation. In the future we plan to investigate whether it makes more sense to measure confidence as the average overlap between propagated atlas segmentations rather than the minimal overlap.

References

1. Aljabar, P., Heckemann, R.A., Hammers, A., Hajnal, J.V., Rueckert, D.: Multi-atlas based segmentation of brain images: atlas selection and its effect on accuracy. Neuroimage 46, 726–738 (2009)
2. Asman, A.J., Landman, B.A.: Formulating Spatially Varying Performance in the Statistical Fusion Framework. IEEE Trans. Med. Imaging 31(6), 1326–1336 (2012)
3. Bondar, M.L., Hoogeman, M.S., Mens, J.W., Quint, S., Ahmad, R., Dhawtal, G., Heijmen, B.J.: Individualized nonadaptive and online-adaptive IMRT treatment strategies for cervical cancer patients based on pre-treatment acquired variable bladder filling CT-scans. Int. J. Radiat. Oncol. Biol. Phys. 83(5), 1617–1623 (2012)
4. Commowick, O., Akhondi-Asl, A., Warfield, S.K.: Estimating a reference standard segmentation with spatially varying performance parameter: local MAP STAPLE. IEEE Trans. Med. Imaging 31(8), 1593–1606 (2012)
5. Gill, S., Pham, D., Dang, K., Bressel, M., Kron, T., Siva, S., Tran, P.K., Tai, K.H., Foroudi, F.: Plan of the day selection for online image-guided adaptive post-prostatectomy radiotherapy. Rad. Onco. 107(2), 165–170 (2013)
6. Heckemann, R.A., Hajnal, J.V., Aljabar, P., Rueckert, D., Hammers, A.: Automatic anatomical brain MRI segmentation combining label propagation and decision fusion. Neuroimage 33, 115–126 (2006)
7. Langerak, T.R., van der Heide, U.A., Kotte, A.N.T.J., van Vulpen, M., Viergever, M., Pluim, J.P.W.: Label fusion in atlas-based segmentation using a selective and iterative method for performance level estimation (SIMPLE). IEEE Transactions on Medical Imaging 29(12), 2000–2008 (2010)

8. Klein, S., van der Heide, U.A., Lips, I.M., van Vulpen, M., Staring, M., Pluim, J.P.W.: Automatic segmentation of the prostate in 3D MR images by atlas matching using localized mutual information. Medical Physics 35(4), 1407–1417 (2008)

9. Langerak, T.R., Berendsen, F.F., van der Heide, U.A., Kotte, A.N.T.J., Pluim, J.P.W.: Multi-atlas-based segmentation with preregistration atlas selection. Med. Phys. 40(9), 091701 (2013)

10. Murthy, V., Master, Z., Adurkar, P., Mallick, I., Mahantshetty, U., Bakshi, G., Tongaonkar, H., Shrivastava, S.: 'Plan of the day' adaptive radiotherapy for bladder cancer using helical tomotherapy. Radiother. Oncol. 99(1), 55–60 (2011)

11. Rohlfing, T., Brandt, R., Menzel, R., Russakoff, D.B., Maurer Jr., C.R.: Quo vadis, atlas-based segmentation? In: Suri, J.S., Wilson, D.L., Laxminarayan, S. (eds.) Handbook of Biomedical Image Analysis. Topics in Biomedical Engineering International Book Series, pp. 435–486 (2005)

12. Warfield, S.K., Zou, K.H., Wells, W.M.: Simultaneous truth and performance level estimation (STAPLE): an algorithm for the validation of image segmentation. IEEE Transactions on Medical Imaging 23(7), 903–992 (2004)

13. Wu, G., Wang, Q., Zhang, D., Nie, F., Huang, H., Shen, D.: A generative probability model of joint label fusion for multi-atlas based brain segmentation. Med. Image Anal. (in press)

Breast Cancer Risk Analysis Based on a Novel Segmentation Framework for Digital Mammograms

Xin Chen, Emmanouil Moschidis, Chris Taylor, and Susan Astley

Centre for Imaging Sciences, Institute of Population Health,
University of Manchester, Oxford Road, Manchester, M13 9PT, UK

Abstract. The radiographic appearance of breast tissue has been established as a strong risk factor for breast cancer. Here we present a complete machine learning framework for automatic estimation of mammographic density (MD) and robust feature extraction for breast cancer risk analysis. Our framework is able to simultaneously classify the breast region, fatty tissue, pectoral muscle, glandular tissue and nipple region. Integral to our method is the extraction of measures of breast density (as the fraction of the breast area occupied by glandular tissue) and mammographic pattern. A novel aspect of the segmentation framework is that a probability map associated with the label mask is provided, which indicates the level of confidence of each pixel being classified as the current label. The Pearson correlation coefficient between the estimated MD value and the ground truth is 0.8012 (p-value<0.0001). We demonstrate the capability of our methods to discriminate between women with and without cancer by analyzing the contralateral mammograms of 50 women with unilateral breast cancer, and 50 controls. Using MD we obtained an area under the ROC curve (AUC) of 0.61; however our texture-based measure of mammographic pattern significantly outperforms the MD discrimination with an AUC of 0.70.

Keywords: Digital mammogram, segmentation, breast cancer risk, mammographic density, texture analysis.

1 Introduction

A major focus of breast cancer imaging research in recent years has been the analysis of mammographic breast density. It has been shown that women with high percentage mammographic density (MD), measured as the proportion of the breast area occupied by dense fibroglandular tissue, have a two to six fold increased breast cancer risk compared to women with low MD [1,2]. Semi-automated computer based tools have been developed where the reader interactively sets thresholds for the breast region and for dense tissue, and the resulting MD is automatically calculated; the most widely used of these is Cumulus [3]. Whilst percentage density measured visually and by Cumulus have been related to cancer risk, these measures are subjective and area-based. Increasing interest in direct and objective measurement of volumes of fat and dense tissue has led to the development of automated volumetric methods such as Cumulus V [5] and Volpara^{TM} [6].

P. Golland et al. (Eds.): MICCAI 2014, Part I, LNCS 8673, pp. 536–543, 2014.

The categorical breast pattern assessment systems originally suggested by Wolfe [7] and Tabár [8] include more complex appearance patterns rather than simply estimating the relative proportion of dense tissue. In recent years, researchers have developed sophisticated texture extraction and analysis methods to characterize mammographic patterns, demonstrating the importance of using texture as a risk factor for breast cancer risk analysis [9].

In our previous work [10], we proposed a novel framework that is able to simultaneously segment the breast region, fatty tissue, pectoral muscle, glandular tissue and nipple region in digital mammograms. Building on this, one contribution of this paper is the development of an automatic MD estimation method, which we show to have discriminatory power for separating the mammograms of women with and without breast cancer. We then describe a texture extraction method for breast cancer risk analysis which outperforms the MD method.

In the following sections, we give a brief description of the segmentation framework followed by introducing the proposed methods for breast cancer risk analysis in section 3. A description of the evaluation methodology and results are given in section 4, and in section 5 we draw conclusions from our work to date, suggesting possible improvements and extensions to the techniques described in the paper.

2   Segmentation Framework

In machine learning method, image features and their associated labels are learnt from a training data set. When an unknown image feeds into the resulting model, the class of pixels in the new image can be estimated according to their corresponding feature descriptors. In [10], we described a system that combines the dual-tree complex wavelet transform (DT-CWT) and random forest (RF) classifier for the purpose of anatomic feature segmentation in mammograms. Here we briefly describe this method which forms the basis of the breast cancer analysis methods described in section 3.

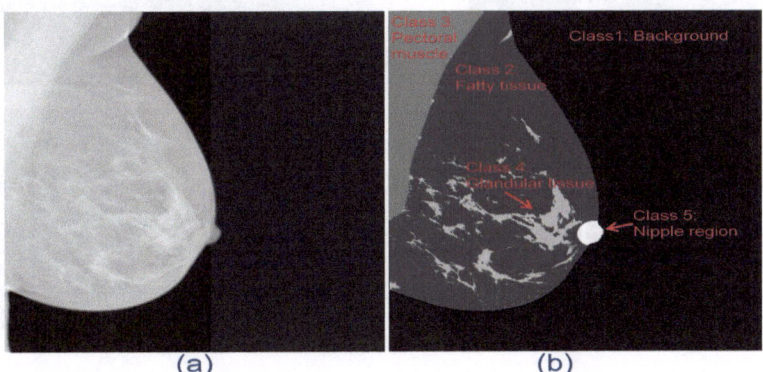

Fig. 1. (a) Logarithm of raw digital mammogram (b) Ground truth segmentation mask

In the training stage, medio-lateral oblique (MLO) view mammograms were segmented into five classes (1: background, 2: fatty tissue, 3: pectoral muscle, 4: glandular tissue, 5: nipple region). The ground truth segmentation was performed by a trained breast radiologist using a semi-automatic software interface; an example segmentation is shown in Fig. 1. For each training image, 500 pixels (as determined experimentally) were randomly selected from each of the five classes. To represent the features of each training pixel, the DT-CWT coefficients together with the normalised X-Y coordinates (origin at the top left corner) and the logarithm of the raw digital mammogram pixel value are used. The feature descriptor for each pixel is a 75-dimensional vector (magnitude and angle parts of DT-CWT × 6 orientations × 6 levels of image pyramid + 2 normalised x, y coordinates + 1 pixel value). Based on the feature vectors and their corresponding classes from all training images, we trained a RF model (200 trees) for classifying unseen mammograms.

When an unseen mammogram is analysed, the same method of calculating a feature vector for each pixel is used. By feeding the feature vector into the trained RF classifier, the probability that a pixel belongs to each of the five classes is obtained. For the input image shown in Fig. 2 (a), Fig. 2 (b)-(f) present the probability maps (brighter pixels represent higher probabilities) obtained for each of the five classes. By assigning the highest probability value of the five classes to each of the pixels, Fig. 2 (g) shows the combined probability map associated with the class labels in Fig. 2 (h). In Fig. 2(h), a small region below the nipple is inaccurately estimated as the nipple. However, the associated probability map (Fig. 2 (g)) shows that the pixels in the misclassified region have very low probabilities which reduce the confidence associated with classification to the assigned label. This smart functionality permits more effective application of the segmentation results in further analysis.

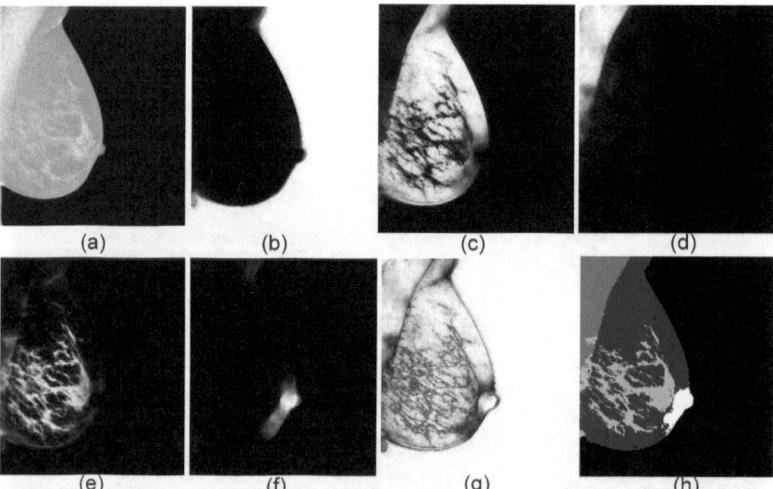

Fig. 2. (a) Input digital mammogram. Outputs from the proposed framework: (b) probability map of background (c) probability map of fatty tissue (d) probability map of pectoral muscle (e) probability map of glandular tissue (f) probability map of nipple region (g) combined probability map (h) label mask. Brighter pixels represent higher probabilities.

3   Breast Cancer Risk Analysis

3.1   Percentage Mammographic Density

A commonly used definition of mammographic density is the area of glandular tissue in a mammogram relative to the area of the breast (denoted as the breast region in this paper). One application of the segmentation framework described in section 2 is fully automatic estimation of MD. Based on the output segmentation mask (Fig. 2(h)), the total number of pixels in the glandular region is calculated and denoted as N_g. The breast region that excluding the pectoral muscle area can be calculated by summing the total number of pixels in the glandular region, fatty region and nipple region, represented by N_b. Hence, $\frac{N_g}{N_b} \times 100\%$ is the estimated MD. We have compared MD obtained automatically in this way with MD derived from the ground truth segmentation, and further investigated the capability to discriminate cancer and non-cancer subjects. The evaluation experiments and results are presented in section 4.

3.2   Mammographic Pattern Analysis

The DT-CWT has been shown to provide a suitable representation of linear structures in mammographic images [11]. We have also demonstrated that it is capable of discriminating different anatomical features in mammograms (section 2 and [10]). We therefore further investigate the use of the DT-CWT to characterize mammographic patterns for breast cancer risk analysis.

Similarly to the segmentation framework described in section 2, our method consists of a model training stage and a classification stage. In the training stage, the DT-CWT is applied to a number of selected pixel locations in the input training images. At each pixel location, the DT-CWT coefficients are calculated on 6 levels of the image pyramid and for 6 different orientations at each level. Therefore, a 72-element (2 magnitude and phase components of the DT-CWT$\times$ 6 orientations $\times$ 6 levels of image pyramid) feature descriptor is obtained for each selected pixel. Using the output of our segmentation method, the pixel selection process can be random sampling from the breast region, or selective sampling from the fatty and/or glandular regions depending on classification probability values. A comparison of different sampling strategies is given in section 4.3. By feeding the feature descriptors and their corresponding image types (cancer or non-cancer) to a RF classifier, a discrimination model can be trained. To determine whether an unseen image is likely to be from a woman with or without cancer, the same sampling strategy is used to extract a number of pixels. The same 72-element DT-CWT feature descriptor is calculated for each pixel and fed into the trained RF model. Based on the votes of trees from the RF model, the probability of each sample pixel belonging to a cancer (or non-cancer) mammogram can be calculated. The average probability of all the sample pixels is output as a breast cancer risk score.

4   Evaluation

4.1   Data and Pre-processing

We use a balanced case-control dataset of 50 cancer cases and 50 controls. All images are anonymised full-field digital screening mammograms obtained from GE Senographe Essential mammography systems with a pixel size of 94.1 μm. The cancer cases were selected randomly from the most recent available screen-detected malignant breast cancers identified, excluding interval cancers and mammograms showing bilateral breast cancer. The medio-lateral oblique (MLO) view of the contralateral breast was analysed as a surrogate for the prior mammogram. Controls were selected randomly from normal screening mammograms where a subsequent normal mammogram was available, using MLO views in the same ratio of left and right breasts as in the cancer cases. To minimise the effects of machine parameter variations and other image intensity variations, all the raw (unprocessed) digital mammograms were pre-processed by a normalisation algorithm that is embedded in the commercially available software Volpara^{TM} [6]. The density maps output by Volpara^{TM} are used as the input to our method. If not otherwise stated, all the experiments in section 4 were performed in a 5-fold cross validation manner. The dataset was randomly organised into five subgroups, each with 10 cancer cases and 10 controls. Four groups of images were used for training and testing was performed on the remaining group, repeating until all groups have been tested.

4.2   Evaluation of Automated Mammographic Density Estimation

We have compared MD from the automatic method described in section 3.1 with MD derived from the ground truth. The ground truth mask was obtained interactively as described in section 2, in a process similar to that used by Cumulus [3]. The Pearson correlation coefficient between the automated MD and their corresponding ground truth MD is 0.8012 (p-value <0.0001). A Bland-Altman plot and scatter plot of the two sets of values are shown in Fig. 3, which demonstrates the strong correlation between them. Additionally, by varying the threshold of the MD scores to assign images to cancer and non-cancer groups and comparing with known image classes, a receiver operating curve (ROC) can be generated which illustrates the capability of the method for determining whether a mammogram belongs to a cancer case or not. The area under the ROC curve (AUC) values for MD from the ground truth and from the automatic MD are 0.6160 and 0.5812 with the sensitivity and specificity at the equal-error-rate point of 60% and 57% respectively. These results are listed in Table 1 with the results obtained from the texture analysis method in section 4.3.

4.3   Evaluation of Mammographic Pattern Analysis

As described in section 3.2, based on the segmentation results, different sampling strategies can be used in the mammographic pattern analysis method. Here we compare different sampling strategies in terms of their discriminatory power for cancer

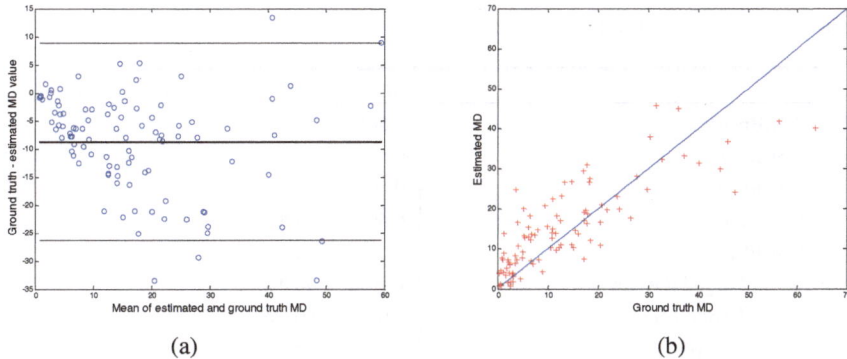

(a)   (b)

Fig. 3. Estimated MD vs. ground truth MD: (a) Bland-Altman plot (b) Scatter plot

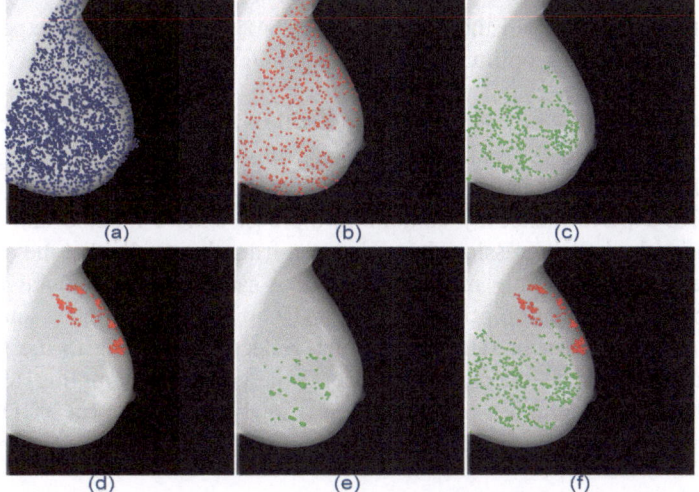

Fig. 4. Sampling strategies (total of 166639 pixels in the whole breast region in this example): (a) 3k random pixels in whole breast region (3KRBreast) (b) 500 random pixels in fatty region (0.5KRFat) (c) 500 random pixels in glandular region (0.5KRGla) (d) 500 pixels with highest probabilities in fatty region (0.5KPFat) (e) 500 pixels with highest probabilities in glandular region (0.5KPGla) (f) 500 pixels with highest probabilities in fatty region and 500 random pixels in glandular region (0.5KPFat_0.5KRGla).

risk analysis. As shown in Fig. 4, we have evaluated our methods using random sampling in the whole breast region, random sampling in the fatty region only, random sampling in the glandular region only, selective sampling in the fatty region (using pixels with a high probability of belonging to the fatty component of the breast), selective sampling in glandular region (using pixels with a high probability of belonging to the glandular component of the breast) and a combination of selective sampling in the fatty region and random sampling in the glandular region (combined the most successful sampling strategies from the two regions). The number of pixels for each

Table 1. ROC performance for breast cancer risk analysis by using different sampling strategies in texture analysis and MD scores

	AUC	Sensitivity/Specificity at EER
3KRBreast [a]	0.6050	54.0%
0.5KRFat [b]	0.6532	58.0%
0.5KRGla [c]	0.6032	56.0%
0.5KPFat [d]	**0.6912**	**66.0%**
0.5KPGla [e]	0.5508	56.0%
0.5KPFat_0.5KRGla [f]	**0.7052**	**66.0%**
Ground Truth MD	0.6160	60.0%
Automatic MD	0.5812	57.0%
0.5KPFat_0.5KRGla & Ground Truth MD	0.6800	64.0%

sampling strategy (shown in the caption of Fig. 4) was determined experimentally, with the aim of achieving optimum performance in terms of discriminatory power and computational time.

The ROC performance of each evaluation is listed in Table 1. The first column in Table 1 corresponds to the sampling methods illustrated in Figure 4, together with results for MD from the ground truth and the automatic MD. The last row in Table 1 shows the ROC performance by combining the best texture method and the ground truth MD using logistic regression. It can be seen from the results that the combination of selective sampling in fatty region and random sampling in glandular region produced the best discrimination power, with an AUC of 0.7052 and 66% sensitivity and specificity at the equal error rate (EER) point. Selective sampling in the fatty region alone produced almost as good performance as the combined sampling. We can also conclude that mammographic pattern (texture) analysis outperforms MD for breast cancer risk analysis, and linear combination of the two does not improve performance.

5   Conclusion and Discussions

In this paper, we presented a novel and effective framework for digital mammogram segmentation and breast cancer risk analysis. From this framework, the mammographic breast density can be estimated automatically, and has a strong correlation with the results from the ground truth (Pearson correlation coefficient of 0.8012). Automation is essential for use in breast screening, where throughput is high. Our method corresponds to the area based methods of estimating mammographic density which have, to date, shown the strongest relationship to cancer risk. Objective assessment of risk based on mammographic appearance has a texture component that has not been widely exploited in automated applications and commercial software, which tends to focus on the quantity of dense tissue within the breast rather than its pattern. We have developed an automated mammographic pattern analysis method which has achieved an AUC of 0.70 for discriminating between the contralateral mammograms of women with breast cancer and mammograms of women without breast cancer. This texture analysis method was found to have more discriminatory power than the well-established MD approach (AUC 0.61). The advantages seem to come from the sampling that concentrated on the fatty region rather than the selection of DT-CWT feature descriptor, since sampling over the entire breast or the glandular region performed no better than the MD. Presumably, such a sampling strategy might also work well with other texture measures. In the literature, AUC values reported for breast cancer risk analysis are in the range of 0.55 to 0.65, dependent on the data used for evaluation. We therefore claim that our methodology and evaluation as reported in this paper make a significant contribution to the problem of estimating breast cancer risk. Future work will concentrate on improving segmentation accuracy by investigating the contribution from each part of the feature descriptor, refining the sampling strategy. We will explore the underlying reason that fatty region contributes more than the glandular region for breast cancer analysis in an extended version of the paper, based on a larger dataset.

References

1. McCormack, V., dos, I., Silva, S.: Breast density and parenchymal patterns as markers of breast cancer risk: a meta-analysis. Cancer Epidemiol. Biomarkers Prev. 15(6), 1159–1169 (2006)
2. Boyd, N., Martin, L., Bronskill, M., Yaffe, M., Duric, N., Minkin, S.: Breast tissue composition and susceptibility to breast cancer. J. Natl. Cancer Inst. 102(16), 1224–1237 (2010)
3. Byng, J., Boyd, N., Fishell, E., Jong, R., Yaffe, M.: The quantitative analysis of mammographic densities. Phys. Med. Biol. 39(10), 1629 (1994)
4. Keller, B., Nathan, D., Wang, Y., Zheng, Y., Gee, J., Conant, E., Kontos, D.: Estimation of breast percent density in raw and processed full field digital mammography images via adaptive fuzzy c-means clustering and support vector machine segmentation. Phys. Med. Biol. 39(8), 4903–4917 (2012)
5. Alonzo-Proulx, O., Packard, N., Boone, J., Al-Mayah, A., Brock, K., Shen, S., Yaffe, M.: Validation of a method for measuring the volumetric breast density from digital mammograms. Phys. Med. Biol. 55(11), 3027–3044 (2010)
6. Jeffreys, M., Harvey, J., Highnam, R.: Comparing a New Volumetric Breast Density Method (Volpara^{TM}) to Cumulus. In: Martí, J., Oliver, A., Freixenet, J., Martí, R. (eds.) IWDM 2010. LNCS, vol. 6136, pp. 408–413. Springer, Heidelberg (2010)
7. Wolfe, J.: Breast patterns as an index of risk for developing breast cancer. Am. J. Roentgenol. 126(6), 1130–1137 (1976)
8. Gram, I., Funkhouser, E., Tabár, L.: "The Tabár classification of mammographic parenchymal patterns ". Eur. J. Radiol. 24(2), 131–136 (1997)
9. Nielsen, M., Karemore, G., Loog, M., Raundahl, J., Karssemeijer, N., Otten, J., Karsdal, M., Vachon, C., Christiansen, C.: A novel and automatic mammographic texture resemblance marker is an independent risk factor for breast cancer. Cancer Epidemiol. 35(4), 381–387 (2011)
10. Chen, X., Moschidis, E., Taylor, C., Astley, S.: A novel framework for fat, glandular tissue, pectoral muscle and nipple segmentation in full field digital mammograms. In: Fujita, H., Hara, T., Muramatsu, C. (eds.) IWDM 2014. LNCS, vol. 8539, pp. 201–208. Springer, Heidelberg (2014)
11. Berks, M., Chen, Z., Astley, S., Taylor, C.: Detecting and classifying linear structures in mammograms using random forests. In: Székely, G., Hahn, H.K. (eds.) IPMI 2011. LNCS, vol. 6801, pp. 510–524. Springer, Heidelberg (2011)

2D View Aggregation for Lymph Node Detection Using a Shallow Hierarchy of Linear Classifiers

Ari Seff, Le Lu, Kevin M. Cherry, Holger R. Roth, Jiamin Liu, Shijun Wang, Joanne Hoffman, Evrim B. Turkbey, and Ronald M. Summers

Imaging Biomarkers and Computer-Aided Diagnosis Laboratory,
Radiology and Imaging Sciences, National Institutes of Health Clinical Center,
Bethesda, MD 20892

Abstract. Enlarged lymph nodes (LNs) can provide important information for cancer diagnosis, staging, and measuring treatment reactions, making automated detection a highly sought goal. In this paper, we propose a new algorithm representation of decomposing the LN detection problem into a set of 2D object detection subtasks on sampled CT slices, largely alleviating the curse of dimensionality issue. Our 2D detection can be effectively formulated as linear classification on a single image feature type of Histogram of Oriented Gradients (HOG), covering a moderate field-of-view of 45 by 45 voxels. We exploit both max-pooling and sparse linear fusion schemes to aggregate these 2D detection scores for the final 3D LN detection. In this manner, detection is more tractable and does not need to perform perfectly at instance level (as weak hypotheses) since our aggregation process will robustly harness collective information for LN detection. Two datasets (90 patients with 389 mediastinal LNs and 86 patients with 595 abdominal LNs) are used for validation. Cross-validation demonstrates 78.0% sensitivity at 6 false positives/volume (FP/vol.) (86.1% at 10 FP/vol.) and 73.1% sensitivity at 6 FP/vol. (87.2% at 10 FP/vol.), for the mediastinal and abdominal datasets respectively. Our results compare favorably to previous state-of-the-art methods.

1   Introduction.

Lymph nodes (LNs) play a crucial role in disease progression and treatment. Enlarged lymph nodes in particular, considered by the widely followed RECIST criteria to be at least 10 mm in short axis diameter [1], are considered suspicious and can indicate metastatic cancer. Radiologists routinely assess lymph nodes in the vicinity of tumors to monitor patient response to various therapies. As a manual task, this can be highly time consuming and error prone. Thus, there have been intensive studies on automatic detection of lymph nodes on CT images in different sections of the body.

Previous work mostly leverages the direct 3D information from volumetric CT images. For instance, [2, 3] exploit the mixture of 3D Hessian blobness filter, directional difference filter, shape morphology and volume thresholds. The state-of-the-art methods [4, 5] perform boosting-based feature selection and integration over a pool of 50~60 thousands of 3D Haar wavelet features to finally obtain a strong binary

P. Golland et al. (Eds.): MICCAI 2014, Part I, LNCS 8673, pp. 544–552, 2014.

classifier on selected features. Due to the limited available training data and the intrinsic high dimensionality of modeling on complex 3D CT features, 3D LN detection is non-trivial. Particularly, lymph nodes have large within-class appearance/location/pose variations and low contrast from surrounding anatomy over a patient population. This results in many false positives to assure moderately high detection sensitivity [3, 6] or only limited sensitivity levels [5, 7]. The good sensitivities achieved at low FP range in [4] are not comparable with the other studies since [4] reports on axillary and pelvic + abdomen body areas, and others evaluate on either mediastinum [2, 5, 6] or abdomen [3, 7].

The essential idea of this work, LN detection by aggregating 2D views, assumes at least some portion of the 2D image patterns (on orthogonal slices) can be encoded and detected reliably for any true lymph node residing in a 3D volume of interest (VOI), while no or very weak 2D detections may be found for a false LN subvolume. The 2D view-based LN detection problem may contain labeling noise (as the label is given per VOI) but inhabits a lower dimensional feature space, with one order of magnitude more samples for training, compared with 3D detection. Our 2D detector is effectively implemented (following a 3D candidate generation preprocessing step) using Liblinear [8] on a single image feature type of Histogram of Oriented Gradients [9, 10]. We exploit max-pooling and sparse linear weighting schemes (Sec. 2.3) to softly aggregate these 2D detection scores for the final 3D LN detection. Importantly, we do not need to classify all 2D slices from a 3D lymph node VOI correctly or with an ultra high accuracy to obtain good results on LN detection. However any single detection error of 3D VOIs [4, 5] causes either a missing lymph node or a false positive count per case.

Our main contributions are three-fold. First, we present a new lymph node detection approach in 3D CT images by running a 2D detector on orthogonal slice views and aggregating their scores per VOI to compute the final LN classification confidence. Second, instead of deep cascade boosting classifiers [4, 5], our 2D detector works as a single shallow template matching step through the efficient inner-product between classifier and image in HOG feature space. Third, *to the best of our knowledge, we are the first to formulate the 3D lymph node classification problem as a sparse linear fusion of detections running only on 2D CT views.* Unlike [4, 5], our method does not need explicit segmentation for lymph node detection. Our method reports good performance on two datasets (90 patients with 389 mediastinal LNs and 86 patients with 595 abdominal LNs), and compares favorably to prior state-of-the-art work in mediastinal [2, 5, 6] and abdominal [3, 7] LN detection. The proposed method is suitable for detecting small, scattered anatomical objects in 3D scans, including lymph nodes.

2 Methods

2.1 Candidate Generation (CG) as Preprocessing

The first phase of the lymph node detection system involves the generation of a list of volumes of interest, containing all enlarged LNs as targeted objects (at the expense of low specificity), from any input 3D CT image. Within the body search region, four primitive types of voxel-level features are calculated at down-sampled grid space (every 3rd voxel in (x, y, z)): intensity, multiscale Hessian blobness scores, response values from multiscale DOG (Difference of Gaussian) filters, and the averages of these feature values from the neighborhoods of 3, 6, and 12 voxels as radii. In this way, multiscale low level image features are densely computed on the 3x3x3 grid voxels in CT volumes and used to further train a random forest [11] classifier, based on the manually segmented LN masks for classifying positive or negative class voxels (i.e., voxels inside an LN mask are treated as positive, and vice versa). Thus, a probability map is generated by the random forest (RF) for each CT scan which is thresholded and spatially grouped to obtain a set of detection candidates. The candidate location is recorded as the centroid of the grouped voxels. Each candidate is cropped as a cube VOI of $45 \times 45 \times 45$ voxels, centered at its found location and then assigned the label. If its location is inside a ground truth LN mask, the corresponding candidate is labeled as +1, otherwise -1. Through this step, close to 100% LN sensitivity can be achieved at 35~40 FPs per case by setting a moderately conservative threshold calibrated from the training RF Receiver operating characteristic (ROC) curve. Given sufficient training voxels and enough trees for the RF (e.g., 50~200), such a performance goal is feasible and may be possible through other ways of preprocessing, which is not the core topic in this paper. *Note that [5] boosts complex 3D HAAR wavelet features to form a one-shot LN detection system which has better sensitivity at low FP range, but their maximal sensitivity saturates at 65%. We use more primitive 3D Hessian/DOG features under a less greedy classifier to assure very high sensitivity only at high FP rates.*

2.2   3D Detection Decomposition as a Set of 2D Detections

View Sampling: From above, each candidate V has a computed centroid location (x, y, z) in 3D CT coordinates. From the center of V, for simplicity, we take 2D slices or views at 45×45 voxels along each of the three coordinate axes (i.e., axial, coronal and sagittal slices). After evenly sampling at 0, 1, 2, 3, ..., and k voxels away from the centroid we have 27 total image views $\{v_i\}_{i=1,2,...27}$ per candidate (without loss of generality, we set $k = 4$): stacking 9 sagittal, coronal, and axial slices from along x, y, and z-axes respectively. We also transfer the +1/-1 label from V to $\{v_i\}_{i=1,2,...27} \in V$ and attempt to build an effective detector on 2D views of $\{v_i\}_{i=1,2,...27}$ for all V, obtained from CG preprocessing. For generality, our detector will be learned by treating each v_i as an independent instance, regardless of its VOI and patient affiliations. Fig. 1 demonstrates an example of view sampling from a mediastinal lymph node candidate.

Feature Extraction: Detecting lymph node appearance against surrounding context in CT images is normally addressed by calculating 3D contrast filters such as 3D minimum directional difference filters [2, 3] or Haar features [4, 5]. In certain 2D views or slices, the intensity contrast pattern inside and outside of a lymph node can be effectively captured on the gradient domain as well, via multi-resolution Histogram of

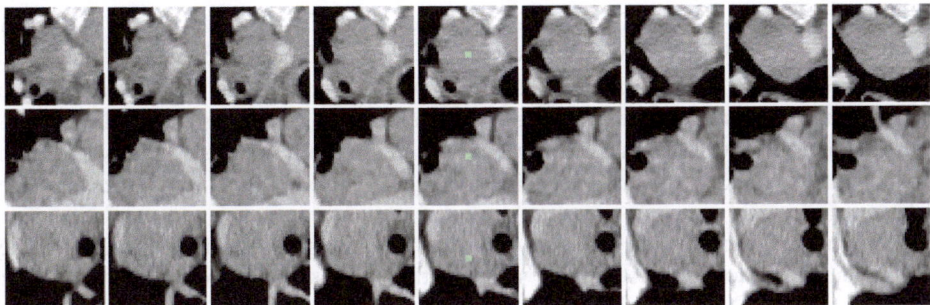

Fig. 1. Example mediastinal lymph node candidate with 9 consecutive axial (top row), coronal (middle row), and sagittal slices (bottom row). The candidate centroid is shown in green in the center column.

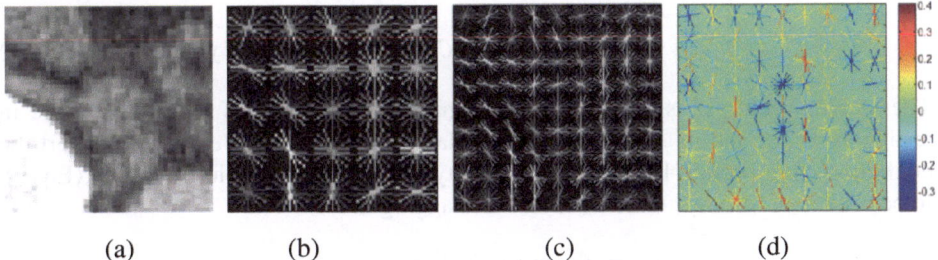

(a)   (b)   (c)   (d)

Fig. 2. Abdominal lymph node axial slice (a) and visual renderings of corresponding HOG features with 5×5 cells (b) and 9×9 cells (c) using VLFeat [10]. The learned feature weight vector ω in $\mathcal{C}_{9\times9}^{1}$ is also visualized in (d) for 9×9 cell HOG. The negative (blue) weights in the center of the abdominal LN model indicate expected low-magnitude intensity gradients.

Oriented Gradients (HOG) features [9, 12], as shown in Fig. 2. HOG features divide an image window to be encoded into square cells, delineating the quantized magnitude and orientation distributions of local intensity gradients for each cell. There are 13 HOG features after Principal Component Analysis-based compression, augmented with contrast sensitive and contrast insensitive features, leading to a 31-dimensional feature vector [9] per cell. Our multi-resolution HOG descriptor covers a moderately large 2D window of 45×45 voxels per view/slice, containing most lymph nodes of various sizes along with sufficient spatial context. The window can be configured with different cell sizes and numbers. For example, our implementation can extract 5×5 cells and 31 features per cell resulting in 775 features per image region, or 9×9 cells with 2511 features, mapping v_i into HOG feature space $x_i \in \mathcal{R}^d$. Illustrative examples of a CT slice and its HOG feature maps in different cell configurations are shown in Fig. 2.

Efficient Linear Classification: HOG features are normally coupled together with linear or non-linear (e.g., radial basis function (RBF) kernel) Support Vector Machine (SVM) classifiers for object detection [9, 12]. Taking our mediastinum dataset as an example, we have 4,168 VOIs from 90 patients after CG. By sampling 27 views per V, there are 112,536 2D view instances $\{x_i\}_{i=1,2,...,112536}$ for classification training and testing. However, 2D slice labels may be ambiguous and contain noise, requiring a robust classifier for effective handling as we simply label all slices from a TP-VOI as positive and vice versa. Some 2D views can be challenging to classify solely based on the local appearance, especially considering the CG process may not locate the true LN centroid.

For good efficiency and generality we enforce on linear classifiers, trained using Liblinear [8] which can effectively address the large-scale, robust linear classifier training issue. 2D view HOG feature vectors $\{x_i\}$ are treated as separate instances, looking to assign an individual confidence score to each. Given l training instances $x_i \in \mathcal{R}^d, i = 1,...,l$, and their corresponding $y_i \in \{-1,+1\}$ class labels, the L2-regularized and L2-loss linear SVM from Liblinear, $\mathcal{C}^1$, requires the minimization of the following cost:

$$\min_\omega \tfrac{1}{2}\omega^T\omega + C\sum_{i=1}^{l}(max(0, 1 - y_i\omega^Tx_i))^2 \qquad (1)$$

The weight vector ω is then used to assign confidence scores to each instance in testing as ω^Tx_i, and its sign indicates the classification label. We further convert the confidence to a pseudo-likelihood probability $\in [0,1]$ by Sigmoid transform (Eq. 2), to be used next for view classification score aggregation.

$$p_i = Sigmoid(\omega^Tx_i) = \frac{1}{1+\exp(-\omega^Tx_i)} \qquad (2)$$

Liblinear has shown to be very robust with respect to a range of C [8]. Our experimental results reported in this paper are based on $C = 1$. The feature weight vector ω learned for 9×9 cell HOG is visualized in Fig. 2-d. For comparison, a nonlinear RBF kernel SVM classifier, following a grid search for optimal parameters C and kernel width σ, is also trained [13]. It performs slightly better than our Liblinear model in training, but degenerates greatly in validation indicating poor generality.

2.3   Detection Aggregation by Max-Pooling or Sparse Linear Fusion

After Sec. 2.2, there are 27 scores $\{p_i\}$ per V. In the evaluation of various sparse coding models for object recognition, max-pooling shows the best result, analogous to the V1 area of the mammalian visual cortex [14]. Even though we only have a two-layer, shallow classification hierarchy, the maximum of the 27 confidence scores or probabilities can be reassigned to the candidate V as its probability of being a lymph node (+1).

$$\rho(V) = max_{i=1,2,...27}\{p_i\} \qquad (3)$$

Treating max-pooling as a special case, we propose to fit a sparse linear weighting function to the vector $P = [p_1, p_2,...p_{27}]^T$ and $\rho(P_k) = Sigmoid(\mathcal{W}^TP_k)$ where $\mathcal{W}$ is optimized according to Eq. 4 with a Gaussian prior $G(\mathcal{W}|0, \Sigma)$ and k=1,2,...,M is the index of VOIs. By mapping $y_k = -1$ to $y_k = 0$ for VOI labels,

$$W = \text{argmax}_W \left[[\textstyle\sum_{k=1}^{M} y_k \log(\rho(P_k)) + (1 - y_k)\log(1 - \rho(P_k))] - \frac{W^T \Sigma^{-1} W}{2} \right] \quad (4)$$

The hyper-parameters in Σ as a diagonal matrix control the variance of individual elements in W. When the jth diagonal coefficient $\sigma_j \to 0$ in Σ, the corresponding $W_j = 0$ due to the zero variance, and p_i becomes irrelevant for the final detection probability $\rho(P)$. This is known as the type-II maximum likelihood method in Bayesian statistics where Σ and W can be effectively solved by two-loop iterative optimization [15] to obtain the linear classifier C^2. In our shallow hierarchy, C^2 is trained using the outputs from view level C^1. Max-pooling is invariant to the view ordering in P from C^1. We also sort P ascendingly to align C^1 scores before C^2 training and testing.

In 6-fold CV (Sec. 3), the number of surviving non-zero coefficients in W varies $\in \{3, 4, ..., 8\}$ out of a total 27 dimensions which results in a sparse linear model. The reason for imposing the sparseness constraint on W is that elements of $P = [p_1, p_2,...,p_{27}]^T$ are highly inter-dependent since $\{v_i\}$ are sampled slice by slice.

3   Experiments

Data: We collect two datasets[1] for mediastinum and abdomen lymph node detection (summarized in Table 1). The population for study is selected from patients scanned within a four-month period in 2012, showing lymphadenopathy in either target region. A lymph node is defined as enlarged if its short axis diameter is $\geq 10mm$ [1]. CT slice thickness varies from 1 mm to 1.25 mm, and axial in-plane image resolution varies from 0.63 mm to 0.97 mm. The use of the data is IRB approved.

Table 1. Lymph node detection datasets

LN dataset	#Patients	#LNs	#TP Candidates	#FP Candidates
Mediastinal	90	389	960	3,208
Abdominal	86	595	1,005	3,484

Protocol: Six-fold cross validation (CV) is carried out by splitting the mediastinum and abdomen LN datasets separately into six disjoint sets at the patient level. Candidate generation (Sec. 2.1), trained previously, is not counted for this evaluation. Training classifiers C^1 and C^2 on 5 sets for a single CV iteration takes about 5 minutes. Processing time following candidate generation on a new testing patient case is generally $1 \sim 3$ seconds (with HOG feature computation).

Slice-Level C^1 Performance: At the slice level, 6,030 out of 25,920 positive class slice instances in the mediastinal dataset are classified correctly if taking $p_i = 0.5$ as a preliminary cutoff ($AUC = 0.719$). This results in a mean of 6.3 positively

---

[1] Datasets will be made publicly available at
http://clinicalcenter.nih.gov/drd/summers.html

classified slices per positive VOI, in contrast to 1.5 slices per negative VOI. We perform the Kolmogorov-Smirnov test on the $\mathcal{C}^1$ values between the positive and negative samples in validation. The obtained p-value is < 0.01, indicating a statistically significant difference. Thus, despite a relatively low recall (at slice-level), this layer of the classifer, $\mathcal{C}^1$, can weakly differentiate between positive and negative 2D views, paving the way for the next step, $\mathcal{C}^2$, to exploit slice score aggregation for VOI-level classification. In this layer, we evaluate varying spatial configurations of classifiers including $\mathcal{C}^1_{5\times5}$ and $\mathcal{C}^1_{9\times9}$ (illustrated in Fig. 2). Experimental results are reported using $\mathcal{C}^1_{5\times5}$.

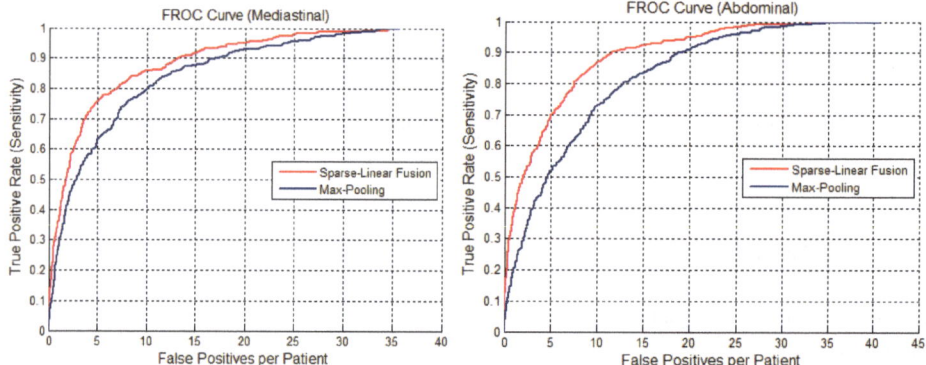

Fig. 3. Six-fold cross-validation FROC curves for the mediastinal (left) and abdominal (right) LN detection

Table 2. Comparison of our method with other previous work on lymph node detection

Method	Target Area	#Vol.	#LN	#TP	TPR(%)	FP/ vol.
Kitasaka[3]	Abdomen	5	221	126	57.0	58
Barbu [4]	Pelvic + Abdomen	54	569	455	80.0	3.2
Feuerstein[6]	Mediastinum	5	106	87	82.1	113
Feulner [5]	Mediastinum	54	289	153	52.9	3.1
Feulner [5]	Mediastinum	54	289	176	60.9	6.1
Nakamura [7]	Abdomen	28	95	28	70.5	13.0
Ours	Mediastinum	90	389	248	63.1	3.0
Ours	Mediastinum	90	389	305	78.0	6.0
Ours	Abdomen	86	595	419	70.1	5.1

VOI-Level $\mathcal{C}^2$ Performance & Comparison: As shown in Fig. 3, we report six-fold cross-validation (CV) FROC curves for both mediastinal and abdominal LN detection datasets. On validation, 63.1% sensitivity at 3 false positives/volume (FP/vol), 78.0% at 6 FP/vol, and 86.1% at 10 FP/vol are achieved for the mediastinal datasets. These correspond to 57.8% sensitivity at 3 FP/vol, 73.1% at 6 FP/vol and 87.2% at 10 FP/vol, for the abdominal datasets. Numerical comparison of our method to previous work [3, 4, 5, 6, 7] is given in detail in Table 2. Our results are demonstrated to have 10%~17% higher sensitivities (at 3, 6 FP/vol) than the recent state-of-the-art method in mediastinum [5], and ~21% higher (at 13 FP/vol)) than the most recent work [7] in abdomen. Note that the results in [4] are not directly comparable to the rest due to different target body regions. Sparse linear fusion by $\mathcal{C}^2$ dominates over the max-pooling scheme, which itself outperforms previous work, in the full range of the FROC curves.

4   Conclusion

We propose a novel approach to automated lymph node detection in CT images which exploits a hierarchy of classifiers trained on features extracted from 2D views of 3D candidate VOIs. In this manner, our detector circumvents expensive 3D feature computation during classification while still sufficiently capturing the spatial context necessary to recognize lymph node presence. Experimental results in both mediastinal and abdominal target regions demonstrate that our technique outperforms previous state-of-the-art methods for lymph node detection. A companion approach exploiting an alternative deep hierarchy for LN detection can be found in [16].

Acknowledgements. This work was supported in part by the Intramural Research Program of the NIH.

References

1. Eisenhauer, E.A., Therasse, P., Bogaerts, J., Schwartz, L.H., Sargent, D., Ford, R., Dancey, J., Arbuck, S., Gwyther, S., Mooney, M., Rubinstein, L., Shankar, L., Dodd, L., Kaplan, R., Lacombe, D., Verweij, J.: New response evaluation criteria in solid tumours: revised RECIST guideline (version 1.1). Eur. J. Cancer 45, 228–247 (2009)
2. Feuerstein, M., Glocker, B., Kitasaka, T., Nakamura, Y., Iwano, S., Mori, K.: Mediastinal atlas creation from 3-D chest computed tomography images: application to automated detection and station mapping of lymph nodes. Med. Image Anal. 16, 63–74 (2012)
3. Kitasaka, T., Tsujimura, Y., Nakamura, Y., Mori, K., Suenaga, Y., Ito, M., Nawano, S.: Automated extraction of lymph nodes from 3-D abdominal CT images using 3-D minimum directional difference filter. In: Ayache, N., Ourselin, S., Maeder, A. (eds.) MICCAI 2007, Part II. LNCS, vol. 4792, pp. 336–343. Springer, Heidelberg (2007)
4. Barbu, A., Suehling, M., Xun, X., Liu, D., Zhou, S.K., Comaniciu, D.: Automatic detection and segmentation of lymph nodes from CT Data. IEEE Transactions on Medical Imaging 31, 240–250 (2012)
5. Feulner, J., Zhou, S.K., Hammon, M., Hornegger, J., Comaniciu, D.: Lymph node detection and segmentation in chest CT data using discriminative learning and a spatial prior. Medical Image Analysis 17, 254–270 (2013)
6. Feuerstein, M., Deguchi, D., Kitasaka, T., Iwano, S., Imaizumi, K., Hasegawa, Y., Suenaga, Y., Mori, K.: Automatic mediastinal lymph node detection in chest CT. SPIE Medical Imaging, 72600–72611 (2009)

7. Nakamura, Y., Nimura, Y., Kitasaka, T., Mizuno, S., Furukawa, K., Goto, H., Fujiwara, M., Misawa, K., Ito, M., Nawano, S., Mori, K.: Automatic abdominal lymph node detection method based on local intensity structure analysis from 3D x-ray CT images. SPIE Medical Imaging, 86701–86707 (2013)
8. Fan, R., Chang, K., Hsieh, C., Wang, X., Lin, C.: LIBLINEAR: A library for Large Linear Classification. Journal of Machine Learning Research, 1871–1874 (2008)
9. Felzenszwalb, P.F., Girshick, R.B., McAllester, D., Ramanan, D.: Object detection with discriminatively trained part-based models. IEEE Transactions on Pattern Analysis and Machine Intelligence 32, 1627–1645 (2010)
10. Veldaldi, A., Fulkerson, B.: VLFeat: An open and portable library of computer vision algorithms (2008)
11. Breiman, L.: Random Forests. Machine Learning 45, 5–32 (2001)
12. Dalal, N., Triggs, B.: Histograms of oriented gradients for human detection. In: CVPR, vol. 1, pp. 886–893 (2005)
13. Chang, C., Lin, C.: LIBSVM: a library for support vector machines. ACM Transactions on Intelligent Systems and Technology 2, 27:21–27:27 (2011)
14. Boureau, Y.L., Le Roux, N., Bach, F., Ponce, J., LeCun, Y.: Ask the locals: Multi-way local pooling for image recognition. In: ICCV, pp. 2651–2658 (2011)
15. Raykar, V., Krishnapuram, B., Bi, J., Dundar, M., Rao, R.: Bayesian multiple instance learning: automatic feature selection and inductive transfer. In: ICML, pp. 808–815 (2008)
16. Roth, H.R., Lu, L., Seff, A., Cherry, K.M., Hoffman, J., Wang, S., Liu, J., Turkbey, E., Summers, R.M.: A new 2.5D representation for lymph node detection using random sets of deep convolutional neural network observations. In: Golland, P., Hata, N., Barillot, C., Hornegger, J., Howe, R. (eds.) MICCAI 2014. LNCS, vol. 8673, pp. 514–521. Springer, Heidelberg (2014)

Patient Specific Image Driven Evaluation of the Aggressiveness of Metastases to the Lung

Thierry Colin[1], François Cornelis[1,2], Julien Jouganous[1],
Marie Martin[1], and Olivier Saut[1]

[1] Institut de Mathématiques de Bordeaux, Université de Bordeaux
[2] Hôpital Pellegrin, CHU Bordeaux

Abstract. Metastases to the lung are a therapeutic challenge because some are fast-evolving while others evolve slowly. Any insight that can be provided for which nodule has to be treated first would help clinicians. In this work, we evaluate the aggressiveness but also the response to treatment of these nodules using a calibrated mathematical model. This model is a macroscopic model describing tumoral growth through a set of nonlinear partial differential equations. It has to be calibrated to a specific patient and a specific nodule using a temporal sequence of CT scans. To this end, a new optimization technique based on a reduced order method is developed. Finally, results on two clinical cases are presented that give satisfactory numerical prognosis of the evolution of a nodule during different phases: growth, treatment and post-treatment relapse.

Keywords: Tumor growth modeling, Medical imaging, Partial Differential Equations, Clinical data assimilation.

1 Introduction

The behavior of metastases to the lung is difficult to assess by clinicians. Some may grow rapidly while some stay stationary for years. This variation makes it difficult to decide when to treat especially when elderly and weak patients are concerned. In those cases, physicians try to restrict treatment to nodules that may become malignant. A numerical tool improving the prognosis of each nodule would be invaluable in this case.

Related Works. Currently, most applications of mathematical models in clinical oncology are somehow limited to models that neglect the spatial aspect of the cancer growth like [3]. These models cannot exploit all the information provided by medical imaging devices and must be used with statistical approaches. This prevents their applications for a specific patient as they only provide "average" answers. Furthermore, these mathematical models are not able to reproduce the observed evolution of a nodule just by using two or three measurements. As this is typically the number of images available for each patient, they are not relevant here. Newer works like [1,4,9] use image data with tumor growth models. They

P. Golland et al. (Eds.): MICCAI 2014, Part I, LNCS 8673, pp. 553–560, 2014.
© Springer International Publishing Switzerland 2014

are mostly targeting brain tumors, are simpler from a biological point of view and the way they are calibrated on patient data uses some very specific features of the model and can not be extended to our case. We built a spatial model in order to use, in a more relevant way, the information available from anatomical imaging. Here, we are concerned with metastases to the lung of a distant tumor. The metastases are not infiltrative and diffusion-type models are not well adapted. We introduce a system of nonlinear PDEs based on populations of cells, without diffusion, but including a micro model of angiogenesis, process by which the tumor drives the emergence of its own neo-vasculature.

Once an accurate model describing tumor growth is derived, its parameters have to be recovered for any patient-specific prognosis. This complex task is usually done by solving an inverse problem using medical images [1,2]. In this work, this calibration is solved using classical approaches combining stochastic and deterministic methods. This algorithm is neither model specific, contrary to the calibration method used in [4], nor computationally expensive like solving adjoint problems [2,9].

2   Mathematical Model

The model we use in this work is derived from the one described in [5]. We consider here only one kind of cancer cells. The tumor microenvironment, and in particular the quantity of nutrients available, is essential to explain its evolution. Consequently, instead of directly modeling the nutrient density, we use a very simplified angiogenesis model to take into account the process by which the tumor escapes the avascular stage.

Cell Behavior. The tumor cell density is denoted by P and evolves by

$$\frac{\partial P}{\partial t} + \nabla \cdot (\mathbf{v}P) = (\gamma_+ - \gamma_-)P, \tag{1}$$

where $\mathbf{v}$ is the velocity corresponding to the growth of volume created by the cellular division. Coefficients for proliferation and death by hypoxia, γ_+ and γ_-, are detailed in (2) and depend on the local vascularization denoted by M. Above a given threshold of nutrient supply M_{th}, cancer cells tend to proliferate whereas, below this threshold, they starve to death. The hyperbolic tangent in both γ_+ and γ_- expressions is used to smooth and regularize the threshold functions, and K is a fixed smoothing constant. These functions are given by:

$$\gamma_{+,-}(M) = \gamma_{0,1} \frac{1 \pm \tanh(K(M - M_{th}))}{2}, \tag{2}$$

where γ_0 is the proliferation rate of non hypoxic tumor cells and γ_1 is the death by hypoxia rate. We consider that the tissue is saturated, which gives us (see [8]) an equation on $\mathbf{v}$ (3)

$$\nabla \cdot \mathbf{v} = (\gamma_+ - \gamma_-)P. \tag{3}$$

To close the system of equations (see [8]), we consider that the velocity $\mathbf{v}$ is obtained through a Darcy law in Eq.(4): $\mathbf{v}$ is derived from a pressure or potential π in the tissue.

$$\mathbf{v} = -\nabla\pi. \tag{4}$$

Angiogenesis. At the end of the avascular stage, the tumor reaches such a size that its direct environment is not able to supply enough nutrients to allow it to keep on growing. At this point, cancer cells emit chemical signals which may result in the emergence of a neo-vasculature [6]. It is described by the equations (5) and (6). The scalar variable ξ describes the total amount of pro-angiogenic agents which are produced by quiescent cells (given by the expression $\int_\Omega (1 - \frac{\gamma_+}{\gamma_0})Pd\omega$, Ω being the computing domain), and eventually metabolized.

$$\frac{\partial\xi}{\partial t} = \alpha \int_\Omega (1 - \frac{\gamma_+}{\gamma_0})Pd\omega - \lambda\xi. \tag{5}$$

As we assume that the quantity of nutrient is proportional to the density of blood vessels in the tissue, we collect these two notions in one variable M that we shall call "vasculature". The vasculature M is damaged by tumor cells and produced where the quiescent cells are located proportionally to ξ by the term $\beta\xi(1 - \frac{\gamma_+}{\gamma_0})P$.

$$\frac{\partial M}{\partial t} = -\eta PM + \beta\xi(1 - \frac{\gamma_+}{\gamma_0})P. \tag{6}$$

Taking Therapeutical Effects into Account. The model architecture makes it easy to include different types of treatment. Chemotherapy effects can be simulated adding a death term $-\delta P$ on Eq.(1) which gives:

$$\frac{\partial P}{\partial t} + \nabla \cdot (vP) = (\gamma_+ - \gamma_-)P - \delta P. \tag{7}$$

To fulfill the saturation assumption Eq.(3) is modified as follows:

$$\nabla \cdot \mathbf{v} = (\gamma_+ - \gamma_- - \delta)P. \tag{8}$$

3   Calibration Method

As shown previously, the mathematical model has many parameters, namely α, β, γ_0, γ_1, η, λ and M_{th}, that must be determined through a complex inverse problem. Most of these parameters have no physical or biological meaning and cannot be recovered by experimental measurements. Furthermore, the medical images (CT scans) have to be processed to be used with this model.

Segmentation, Registration. Lung metastases are particularly interesting from a mathematical and technical point of view because of the quality of the imagery. Indeed, in CT scans of the lung, the tumor appears as white while healthy tissue (full of air) is mainly black. Delineating the tumor is therefore relatively easy and requires little intervention from clinicians. In practice, the segmentation is manually performed by the oncologist who choses a representative slice of the tumor. For each exam, this same slice of the tumor is segmented by the clinician. The slice is localized using physiological details such as blood vessels or bronchi. The patient is not in the same exact position for every exam. The targeted nodule is relocated to have a stationary center of gravity between scans. We made the reasonable assumption that the tumor is solid and its volume is not affected by patient's breath. The rotation of the abdomen between scans is also taken into account.

Formulation of the Inverse Problem. Given a sequence of medical images or snapshots of the tumor, we aim at finding a parameter set able to reproduce its observed behavior. Our approach is to use an objective function, which basically quantifies the difference between the observable data and the model simulation, and try to minimize it. There are different ways to measure this error and as a criterion we chose a combination of the comparison of the mass and the L^2 norm of the images. Mass is measured by integrating the cellular density P.

We need at least two images of the metastasis at different times to have a chance to personalize the model: the first one at $t_1 = 0$ is the initial condition for the tumor cell density and the other is used to parameterize the model. Whatever the minimization method, it is necessary to estimate many times the value of the objective function, and so to simulate the model for lots of parameter sets which could be quite expensive.

To make the calibration faster, we have developed a strategy based on a reduced order method called Proper Orthogonal Decomposition (POD).

Building a Reduced Order Model to Speed Up Computations. POD resolution method for dynamic systems consists in approaching partial differential equation systems with ordinary differential equations by decoupling efficiently the time and space variables (see [7]). The initial infinite dimension problem is thus replaced by a finite dimension problem.

Let us describe the POD use on the tumor cell density variable P. As we want to decouple space and time variables, we use the following representation for P (or any variable of interest): $P(X,t) = \sum_{i=1}^{d} a_i^P(t)\Phi_i^P(X) + \epsilon(X,t)$, where a_i^P are scalar functions depending on time and Φ_i^P are spatial functions called modes and represent the geometry of the variable P. The dimension of the reduced problem is denoted by d. The approximation error is denoted by $\epsilon(t,X)$. The goal of POD is to provide us with the best basis of spatial functions Φ_i^P to minimize the error.

These functions Φ_i^P are extracted from a database of admissible behaviors of P. To generate this database, we sample the parameter space using a cartesian grid, simulate the direct model for each parameter set thus obtained and keep several snapshots $(S_k^P)_k$ of the variable P. If the sample is correctly chosen, we have a representative set of geometrical configurations for the tumor cell density. Then we look for the functions Φ_i^P in the d-dimensional vectorial space generated by the snapshots from the database. They are, in other words, linear combinations of the snapshots. These functions are taken as an orthonormal basis minimizing the truncation error of the projection which allows us to use a few modes without losing too much precision. The POD approach is used on both the tumor cell density P and the pressure field π which are the two fields driven by PDEs in our system. Finally, the system of equations is projected along these modes and so approximated by an ODE system on the coefficients $(a_i^P(t))_i$ and a linear system on the coefficients $(a_i^\pi(t))_i$.

Complete Algorithm Used for the Inverse Problem. Replacing PDEs by ODEs makes the problem simpler and faster to solve so we use this reduced model for the inverse problem. Moreover, the modes, and the spatial derivatives associated, are computed once for all. Then we use a classical optimization strategy to minimize the distance between the model simulations and the observable. The first step is to find a reasonable parameter set via a particle swarm algorithm. A sensitivity analysis was performed on the model that shows the low influence of parameters α and β. Therefore, these two parameters are fixed and a gradient algorithm is used to refine the set of parameters.

4 Results and Discussions

4.1 Trying Our Method on a First Complete Test Case

Here is a typical case of a patient with lung nodules from a primary bladder tumor.

The method described previously is used on this first test case. Six CT scans are available (the first two of which are presented in Fig.1). The first three correspond to the tumor growth. Then the nodule reached a critical volume and the clinicians decided to treat it with a chemotherapy. The two following

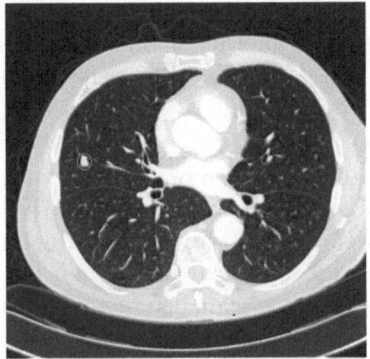 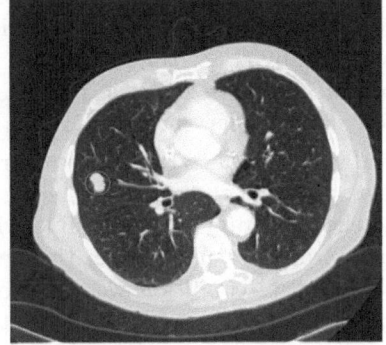

Fig. 1. Extract from a time sequence of CT scans showing the evolution of one nodule marked in red between 2008/06/07 (on the left) and 2008/09/22 (on the right)

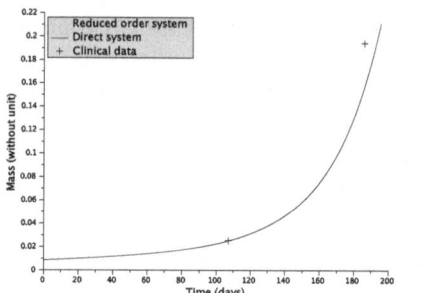 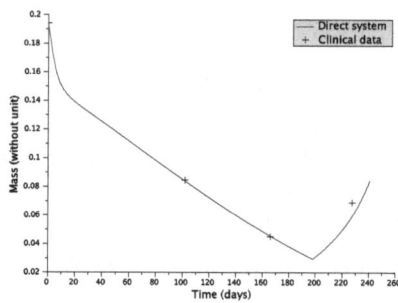

Fig. 2. Evolution of the tumoral masses as computed by our model after recovering its parameters during the growth (on the left) and after the beginning of the treatment (on the right). Tumoral masses measured on the CT scans by the clinicians are plotted with +, the reduced model simulation with dotted line and the direct model simulation with full line.

scans were used to control the response of the tumor to the treatment. Finally, a last control scan was planned after the end of the chemotherapy that showed a relapse as the tumor started growing again.

First, we use the first two scans (see Fig.1) to calibrate the model on the growth phase. Then the model is simulated up to the third scan date to see if the prediction is accurate. The tumor mass thus obtained by the model is compared to the medical data in Fig.2a.

As the model provides spatial information on the cells distribution, it is also interesting to evaluate the accuracy in shape of the results obtained with our method. For this, we used shape indicators such as the Volume Concordance (given by the expression $VC = 100 \times (1 - \frac{|P_{model} - P_{data}|}{|P_{data}|})$) and the DICE ($DICE = 100 \times (\frac{2*|P_{model} \cap P_{data}|}{|P_{model}| + |P_{data}|})$). We also compute a reference DICE between the first scan which is the initial condition of our system and the current scan. This represents the hypothesis of a non evolving tumor and gives a value of comparison. Moreover, the temporal prediction error is another significant indicator. If we denote by t_i the time of the ith exam and t'_i the time when the simulated tumor reaches the size of the real tumor at the ith exam; it is relevant to look at the delay between the simulation and the real case $t_i - t'_i$ and the normalized delay $100 \times \frac{t_i - t'_i}{t_i - t_0}$, $i = 1, 2$. These four indicators are given on Table 1.

Then, we tried to calibrate the treatment parameter δ to see if the response to the chemotherapy is predictable with our tool. Here only one parameter has to be determined which makes this second inverse problem easier than the first one. The initial condition we used for P is the last scan before treatment on 2008/12/10 and we used the first control scan during chemotherapy to calibrate the treatment parameter. The evolution of the tumor mass during the treatment provides a good insight into the therapeutical efficacy. It is given in Fig.2b and we can see that here again the model is predictive for this case and provides a

Table 1. Scalar indicators for the tumor growth of the first clinical case: DICE, Volume Concordance and delays

Date	2008/09/22	2008/12/10
DICE	90.96%	87.21%
reference DICE	54.94%	10.25%
Volume Concordance	82.54%	77.76%
Delay (days)	0	-6.7
Normalized Delay	0%	-3.6%

Table 2. Scalar indicators for the tumor under chemotherapy and rebound of the first clinical case: DICE, Volume Concordance and delays

Date	2009/03/21	2009/05/27	2009/07/27
DICE	92.26%	87.44%	84.79
reference DICE	57.63%	37.71%	52.78
Volume Concordance	84.4%	74.56%	69.9
Delay (days)	0.3	0.6	-6.4
Normalized Delay	0.1 %	0.2 %	-2.8%

Table 3. Scalar indicators for the tumor growth of the second test case: DICE, Volume Concordance and delays

Date	2010/03/11	2010/07/16
DICE	85.41%	88.69%
reference DICE	65.93%	38.09%
Volume Concordance	70.59%	76.45%
Delay (days)	0	5.6
Normalized Delay	0%	2.3%

good estimation of the response of the patient to this chemotherapy. Moreover, after the end of the treatment, the tumor started growing again and this relapse is also well predicted by the model. The same indicators that were used for the growth are given in Table 2. For the last exam, on 2009/07/27, the shape indicators are not relevant as the relapse is located at the periphery of the initial nodule and so the shape and location can not be predicted accurately.

4.2   A Second Test Case

The whole calibration method described previously is used on another case of tumoral growth. Here again, we use two scans at different time points to calibrate the model and a third image to quantify the accuracy of the prediction. The indicators are given in Table 3.

In this case, the growth is slower than in the previous one and the model is able to reproduce such a kind of dynamics. Indeed, the time error in prediction is about 6.4 days which, at the time scale we used and considering the tumor registration uncertainties, is a good result.

In each case, we always considered the same slice of the tumor. The same technique can be applied on the whole 3D volume reconstructed from the medical images which would enable us not to choose a particular slice. The complete method thus developed was successful to provide us with a relevant prognosis on the evolution of lung nodules for several clinical cases. A larger study on about 20 patients is ongoing to evaluate the quality of the prognosis on a larger scale.

References

1. Clatz, O., Sermesant, M., Bondiau, P.-Y., Delingette, H., Warfield, S.K., Malandain, G., Ayache, N.: Realistic simulation of the 3-d growth of brain tumors in mr images coupling diffusion with biomechanical deformation. IEEE Transactions on Medical Imaging 24(10), 1334–1346 (2005)
2. Hogea, C., Davatzikos, C., Biros, G.: An image-driven parameter estimation problem for a reaction–diffusion glioma growth model with mass effects. J. Math. Biol. 56(6), 793–825 (2008)
3. Simeoni, M., Magni, P., Cammia, C., Nicolao, G.D., Croci, V., Pesenti, E., Germani, M., Poggesi, I., Rocchetti, M.: Predictive pharmacokinetic-pharmacodynamic modeling of tumor growth kinetics in xenograft models after administration of anticancer agents. Cancer Res 64(3), 1094–1101 (2004)
4. Swanson, K.R., Alvord, E.C., Murray, J.D.: Virtual brain tumours (gliomas) enhance the reality of medical imaging and highlight inadequacies of current therapy. Br. J. Cancer 86(1), 14–18 (2002)
5. Colin, T., Iollo, A., Lombardi, D., Saut, O.: System identification in tumor growth modeling using semi-empirical eigenfunctions. Mathematical Models and Methods in Applied Sciences (2012)
6. Carmeliet, P., Jain, R.: Angiogenesis in cancer and other diseases. Nature (2000)
7. Kunisch, K., Volkwein, S.: Galerkin proper orthogonal decomposition methods for parabolic problems. Numer. Math, 117–148 (2001)
8. Ambrosi, D., Preziosi, L.: On the closure of mass balance models for tumor growth. Math. Mod. Meth. Appl. Sci 12(5), 737–754 (2002)
9. Liu, Y., Sadowski, S.M., Weisbrod, A.B., Kebebew, E., Summers, R.M., Yao, J.: Patient Specific Tumor Growth Prediction Using Multimodal Images. Medical Image Analysis (2014)

Multi-parametric 3D Quantitative Ultrasound Vibro-Elastography Imaging for Detecting Palpable Prostate Tumors

Omid Mohareri[1], Angelica Ruszkowski[1], Julio Lobo[1], Joseph Ischia[2],
Ali Baghani[3], Guy Nir[1], Hani Eskandari[1,3], Edward Jones[4], Ladan Fazli[4],
Larry Goldenberg[2], Mehdi Moradi[1], and Septimiu Salcudean[1]

[1] Department of Electrical and Computer Engineering, University of British
Columbia, Vancouver, BC, Canada
[2] Department of Urological Sciences, University of British Columbia,
Vancouver, BC, Canada
[3] Ultrasonix Medical Corporation, Richmond, BC, Canada
[4] Department of Pathology and Laboratory Medicine, University of British
Columbia, Vancouver, BC, Canada
{tims,omidm,moradi}@ece.ubc.ca

Abstract. In this article, we describe a system for detecting dominant prostate tumors, based on a combination of features extracted from a novel multi-parametric quantitative ultrasound elastography technique. The performance of the system was validated on a data-set acquired from $n = 10$ patients undergoing radical prostatectomy. Multi-frequency steady-state mechanical excitations were applied to each patient's prostate through the perineum and prostate tissue displacements were captured by a transrectal ultrasound system. 3D volumetric data including absolute value of tissue elasticity, strain and frequency-response were computed for each patient. Based on the combination of all extracted features, a random forest classification algorithm was used to separate cancerous regions from normal tissue, and to compute a measure of cancer probability. Registered whole mount histopathology images of the excised prostate gland were used as a ground truth of cancer distribution for classifier training. An area under receiver operating characteristic curve of 0.82 ± 0.01 was achieved in a leave-one-patient-out cross validation. Our results show the potential of multi-parametric quantitative elastography for prostate cancer detection for the first time in a clinical setting, and justify further studies to establish whether the approach can have clinical use.

1 Introduction

Prostate cancer is the most commonly diagnosed cancer among North American men. Even though trans-rectal ultrasound (TRUS) is used to guide prostate interventions because it can image the prostate, standard TRUS imaging is incapable of making a reliable differentiation between malignant and benign tissue

P. Golland et al. (Eds.): MICCAI 2014, Part I, LNCS 8673, pp. 561–568, 2014.
© Springer International Publishing Switzerland 2014

in the gland. Hence, its use is essentially limited to gland volume measurement and procedure guidance. An ideal imaging technique should accurately locate cancer foci in order to guide biopsies and focal therapy.

The use of tissue elasticity as a contrast mechanism to detect prostate tumors has been suggested in many previous studies, in the area of elastography imaging [1–4]. However, most clinical ultrasound elastography systems are based on a quasi-static tissue excitation, with major drawbacks such as dependency on operator skill and lack of reproducibility [5]. Hence, an absolute, quantitative elastography technique is highly desirable. Furthermore, the majority of tested real-time elastography systems are shown to have a high rate of false-positives [2, 6]. One major reason for this poor detection performance is hypothesized to be the fact that the current clinical elastography systems are only capable of producing an image that visualizes a single tissue physical parameter, such as stiffness or compliance, while cancerous tissues are complex and non-uniform and cannot be characterized using only one parameter.

Multi-parametric imaging is an emerging technology that combines information from different techniques, to improve detection rates beyond what can be achieved using any single imaging method. Brock *et al.* assessed a combination approach of ultrasound elastography and contrast enhanced ultrasound and showed that the multi-parametric approach decreased the false-positive value of real-time elastography alone from 34.9% to 10.3% [6]. Vibro-elastography - the multi-frequency tissue response over a wide excitation bandwidth [1, 7], as well as tissue nonlinear response as a function of applied displacements [3], are also shown to contain additional information that may increase the accuracy of cancer detection based on elastography.

In this article, *in vivo* 3D volumetric data acquired from multi-frequency quantitative vibro-elastography imaging is analyzed. This is the first report of such clinical data. We propose a novel set of features that combine the B-mode, strain, absolute elasticity, along with the frequency-dependent parameters that reveal tissue relaxation time and visco-elastic properties. A supervised classification framework is constructed and used to combine the multi-parametric features to separate cancerous and normal tissue and compute a cancer probability map.

2   Methods

Absolute Vibro-Elastography: A multi-frequency steady-state mechanical excitation is applied externally to generate tissue motion. A sequence of n_f frames of RF-data is acquired for each plane in an imaging volume by the ultrasound machine, and processed using a speckle tracking algorithm [8] to create a series of displacements per pixel as a function of time. With a linearity assumption, motion at each pixel has the same temporal frequency content as the input excitation, and therefore the tissue response can be described using complex exponentials (phasor: $p_i = A_i exp(j\phi_i)$) at each pixel for each frequency f_i. A single phasor displacement image is generated from n_f frames for each plane at each frequency and any traveling wave inside the tissue could be revealed from this image at each plane. Tissue strain could also be computed from this phasor image. The waves seen in phasor displacement images are only 2D projections of the actual traveling waves created by the steady state external excitations. Therefore, 2D phasor images are computed for a series of n_e planes creating a 3D volume. The Local Frequency Estimation (LFE) inversion algorithm [9] was used here for elasticity computation. This process is repeated for an entire volume producing N_E elastograms from N_p planes ($N_E = N_p - n_e + 1$).

System Implementation for Prostate Imaging: The main components of our prostate imaging system are depicted in Figure 1. A BK ultrasound machine (BK Medical, Herlev, Denmark) with a 8848 4-12 MHz biplane transducer was used for imaging the prostate and tissue displacement measurements. Raw In-phase Quadrature (IQ) data was captured at 42.66 Hz sampling rate and saved into an external PC through a DALSA Xcelera-CL PX4 Full frame grabber card (Teledyne DALSA, Waterloo, ON). A previously designed TRUS robot [10] was used to automatically control the rotation angle of the TRUS transducer and save location information of each image.

To ensure good wave penetration into the prostate in a noninvasive manner, we used transperineal excitation similar to the approach used in Magnetic Resonance elastography (MRE) [11]. An electromagnetic exciter in combination with an Agilent U2761A function generator (Agilent Technologies, Santa Clara, CA) was used to generate desired excitation frequencies. The excitation frequencies used for tissue motion generation in this study varied between 58 Hz to 180 Hz. Since we did not have external access to the image acquisition parameters of

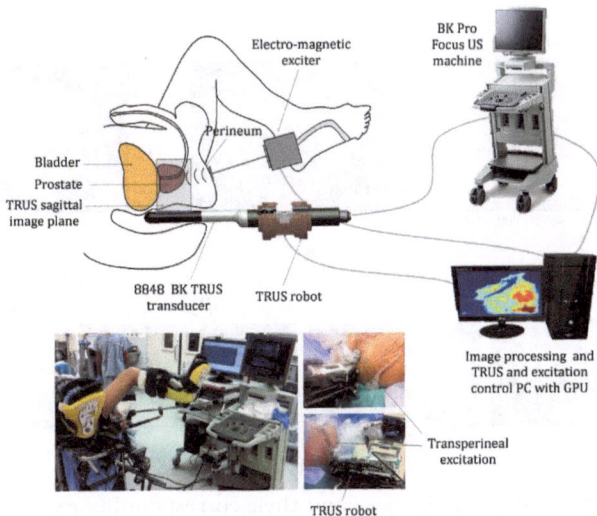

Fig. 1. Main components of the quantitative elastography imaging system with transperineal excitations and the data acquisition system in the clinical setting

the BK ultrasound machine, a band-pass sampling algorithm described in [12] was used here for phase and amplitude reconstruction with sampling frequencies that are lower than the excitation frequencies.

Patient Data Collection: Ten patients with clinically organ-confined prostate cancer (median patient age: 61 years, range: 52-70 and median baseline PSA: 6.4 ng/ml, range: 4.6-36.4) undergoing robotic radical prostatectomy at our institution agreed to participate in this study. For each patient, four to six volumes of multi-parametric data including time displacements, phasor displacement and elasticity data were acquired, for a variety of excitation frequencies. One of the acquired volumes for all patients was at an excitation frequency of 75 Hz and single frequency features were extracted from it. Data from other frequencies were used to compute frequency dependent parameters.

Whole-mount histopathology images of the excised prostate were used as ground truth for cancer detection validation. Each pathology slice was processed by a pathologist who marked the gland boundary, cancer regions and prostate anatomical zone boundaries. Approximately 75% of the cancer occurs in the peripheral zone (PZ). This zone was also segmented on the histopathology slides. Figure 2(a) shows an example pathology slide, and its corresponding acquired B-mode and absolute elastography image from one patient.

2.1 Data Analysis

Feature Extraction: To define regions of interests (ROI) for the classifier data, the acquired images were registered to the pathology images. A slice-to-surface, particle-filter-based registration technique [13] was used to register the

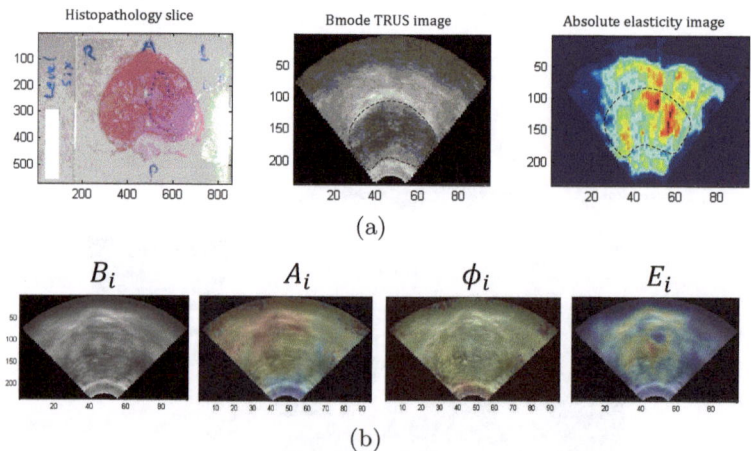

Fig. 2. (a) Example pathology images, and their corresponding reconstructed B-Mode and absolute elastography, (b) example slices of four types of volumetric images available for feature extraction: B-mode (B_i), displacement phasor magnitude (A_i) and phase (ϕ_i), and absolute elasticity (E_i). ($f_i = 75Hz$)

Table 1. Table of features

Data type	Featues per ROI							Index	Meaning
B_i	μ_B	σ_B	Max_B	Min_B	Med_B	$Kurt_B$	$Skew_B$	1-7	Brightness
E_i	μ_E	σ_E	Max_E	Min_E	Med_E	$Kurt_E$	$Skew_E$	8-14	Stiffness
A_i	μ_A	σ_A	Max_A	Min_A	Med_A	$Kurt_A$	$Skew_A$	15-21	Strain
ϕ_i	μ_ϕ	σ_ϕ	Max_ϕ	Min_ϕ	Med_ϕ	$Kurt_\phi$	$Skew_\phi$	22-28	
Frequency-response	m_ϕ							29	Relaxation-time
	m_E							30	Viscosity

stack of equispaced 2D pathology contours to the 3D surface extracted from the volumetric ultrasound images.

For each plane in each volume, four types of images are available for feature extraction: B-mode (B_i), displacement phasor magnitude (A_i) and phase (ϕ_i), and absolute elasticity (E_i). To identify ROIs, regions of interest were specified for both Class 1 (malignant cancer) and Class 0 (benign lesion) using the pathology markings which were registered to ultrasound data. A feature vector was created for each ROI corresponding to a whole tumor or a non-cancerous area. For each of the four data types (B_i, A_i, ϕ_i, E_i), seven statistical parameters of the pixel intensities within the ROI were calculated and used as features. These included the mean, standard deviation, maximum, minimum, median, kurtosis and skewness. Before extracting the features, histogram normalization was performed on the data across the data-set to map the intensities to the same dynamic rage for all cases. A feature vector with $n = 28$ components (described in Table 1) was created per ROI, all calculated from images with excitation at 75 Hz.

In order to leverage the multi-frequency data for each patient, two frequency dependent features were computed for each ROI and added to the feature vector. The displacement phasor phase (ϕ_i) and elasticity (E_i) frequency-response were analyzed for the range of frequencies available for each patient.

Assuming linearity, the tissue displacement transfer function could be formulated as: $G(j\omega) \cong \frac{X(j\omega)}{U(j\omega)} = \frac{1}{1+Tj\omega}$, where $X(j\omega)$ is the displacement measured at each pixel, $U(j\omega)$ is the input displacement from external excitation, and T is a time-constant. The phase of this transfer function is $\angle G(j\omega) = \arctan(T\omega)$, which is the same as the computed phasor phase ϕ_i at each frequency. Hence, the slope of a line fitted to the ϕ_i frequency-response will be T, an estimate of the tissue relaxation time. Such analysis was performed for each ROI in our data-set, and the slope of a line fitted to the ϕ_i frequency response was computed (m_ϕ) and added to the feature vector.

Tissue visco-elastic properties are reported to vary with the input excitation frequency [1] and the rate of such variations may yield more information about tissue characteristics. The frequency response of E_i was computed for each ROI and the slope of a line fitted to the curve (m_E), rate of change of elasticity with frequency, was included as another feature for each ROI. Using the combination of all described features, we incorporated the texture and intensity features from one common frequency and also used the multi-frequency content of the data.

Classification: Binary classification between malignant and benign lesions was performed using random forests [14] with bootstrapping of features and Gini Index. The following forest parameters were optimized using a grid-search method with a leave-one-patient-out cross-validation: (i) number of estimators/trees (N_e), (ii) maximum number of features considered when finding the best binary split (Max_{nf}), (iii) maximum depth of the tree (Max_{nt}).

To perform classifications consistent with the tissue types in the prostate gland, features were extracted twice: (i) only from the peripheral zone (PZ) of the prostate, (ii) from the whole gland (WG), since different regions in the prostate have inherently different elastic properties [15].

In order to demonstrate the performance of each group of features, four classification experiments with different feature vectors were performed: (i) multi-parametric and multi-frequency experiment ($n = 30$, feature index: 1-30 in Table 1), (ii) multi-parametric single-frequency experiment ($n = 28$, feature index: 1-28), (iii) multi-parametric and multi-frequency experiment without B-Mode features ($n = 23$, feature index: 8-30), (iv) single-frequency single-parametric experiment ($n = 7$, feature index: 8-14).

3   Results

The classification results in terms of sensitivity, specificity, accuracy and area under the ROC curve (AUC) for each experiments are presented in Table 2. In plotting the receiver operating characteristic (ROC) curve, a value of probability=0.5 was used as the cutoff between classes.

Comparison of Results in Each Prostate Region: For each of the experiments with different feature groups, the classification algorithms were tested once on ROIs extracted from the PZ, and once on ROIs from the WG. Results suggest that limiting the analysis to the PZ would consistently lead to better results in terms of AUC, specificity and accuracy (AUC changes from 0.79 ± 0.01 to 0.82 ± 0.01 in experiment (i)).

Comparison of Results for Different Feature Groups: Comparing the results of the multi-frequency multi-parametric experiment with single-frequency single-parameter elasticity imaging shows $\approx 10\%$ improvement in AUC and specificity in the PZ. Single-frequency single-parameter experiments represent the traditional single parameter elasticity imaging. Comparison between the results of experiment (i) and (ii) shows 4% improvement in an AUC and 7% improvement in the specificity in the PZ, when multi-frequency features are added to the feature vector. Without using features from B-Mode, the multi-frequency multi-parametric elasticity imaging could yield an AUC of 0.77 (compare the results of experiments (i), (iii)).

Table 2. Classification results. n: number of features, f-index: feature index, Zone: prostate region features extracted from, N_{ROI}: number of ROIs extracted, Param.: [N_e, Max_{nf}, Max_{nt}] for random forest, AUC: area under ROC curve. Results corresponding to PZ are colored in gray for easier comparison.

Random forest classification results								
Ex	n	f-index	Zone	N_{ROI}	Param.	Accuracy	Sensitivity	Specificity	AUC
i	30	1-30	PZ	164	[19, 19, 2]	0.72±0.01	0.61±0.02	0.82±0.04	0.82±0.01
			WG	231	[18, 14, 2]	0.67±0.01	0.63±0.03	0.74±0.02	0.79±0.01
ii	28	1-28	PZ	164	[17, 18, 2]	0.69±0.02	0.62±0.02	0.75±0.03	0.78±0.01
			WG	231	[17, 19, 2]	0.66±0.01	0.61±0.03	0.72±0.02	0.77±0.01
iii	23	8-30	PZ	164	[16, 17, 2]	0.65±0.02	0.61±0.02	0.72±0.03	0.77±0.01
			WG	231	[13, 4, 7]	0.64±0.02	0.60±0.04	0.68±0.02	0.75±0.02
iv	7	8-14	PZ	164	[19, 2, 2]	0.64±0.01	0.63±0.01	0.69±0.01	0.73±0.02
			WG	231	[18, 3, 2]	0.64±0.02	0.64±0.01	0.63±0.01	0.70±0.02

4   Discussions and Conclusions

Previous reports on the clinical application of elastography for prostate cancer detection all confirm its usefulness, but also agree on the fact that single parametric elasticity imaging alone is not sufficiently accurate to enable guidance for diagnosis and treatment. In the published clinical studies with whole mount histopathology validation, Brock et al., reported an overall sensitivity and specificity of 49% and 73.6% using shear-wave elastography [2]. Salomon et al. reported sensitivity and specificity of 75.4% and 76.6%, using quasi-static elastography [16]. We show that the combination of all features (experiment (i)) provides sensitivity of 61% and specificity of 82% and has a more efficient cancer detection performance than each method individually.

Nodular prostatic hyperplasia was observed inside the prostate transition zone for 80% of the cases. It causes changes in the tissue mechanical properties and could contribute to some of the false positive detections outside the PZ. Hence, the elasticity reconstruction is expected to perform better in the PZ region, leading to more accurate results.

Feature importance analysis from random forest classification shows that $Kurt_\phi$, $Kurt_A$, $Kurt_E$ have the highest importance rank in the classification results. Kurtosis is a measure of "peakedness" of the distribution of the parameters in each ROI. Such results reveal that a dominant tumor typically has a consistent intensity contrast with respect to the surrounding healthy tissue in elasticity and displacement phasor images.

A multi-parametric cancer detection framework based on quantitative vibro-elastography imaging was proposed in this paper. A unique set of features were computed based on the acquired data from 10 patients in a feasibility clinical study, and their detection performance was compared with traditional single parameter elastography. Promising detection results justify further clinical studies to prove the clinical usability of the system.

References

1. Salcudean, S.E., Sahebjavaher, R.S., et al.: Biomechanical modeling of the prostate for procedure guidance and simulation. In: Soft Tissue Biomechanical Modeling for Computer Assisted Surgery, vol. 11, pp. 169–198. Springer (2012)
2. Brock, M., Von Bodman, C., et al.: The impact of real-time elastography guiding a systematic prostate biopsy to improve cancer detection rate: A prospective study of 353 patients. J. Urol. 187(6), 2039–2043 (2012)
3. Zhang, M., Nigwekar, P., et al.: Quantitative characterization of viscoelastic properties of human prostate correlated with histology. Ultrasound Med. Biol. 34(7), 1033–1042 (2008)
4. Zhai, L., Madden, J., et al.: Acoustic radiation force impulse imaging of human prostates ex vivo. Ultrasound Med. Biol. 36(4), 576–588 (2010)
5. Ahmad, S., Cao, R., et al.: Transrectal quantitative shear wave elastography in the detection and characterisation of prostate cancer. Surg. Endosc. 27(9), 3280–3287 (2013)
6. Brock, M., Eggert, T., et al.: Multiparametric ultrasound of the prostate: adding contrast enhanced ultrasound to real-time elastography to detect histopathologically confirmed cancer. J. Urol. 189(1), 93–98 (2013)
7. Turgay, E., Salcudean, S., et al.: Identifying mechanical properties of tissue by ultrasound. Ultrasound Med. Biol. 32(2), 221–235 (2008)
8. Zahiri-Azar, R., Salcudean, S.E.: Motion estimation in ultrasound images using time domain cross correlation with prior estimates. IEEE Trans. Biomed. Eng. 53(10), 1990–(2000)
9. Muthupillai, R., Lomas, D.J.: Magnetic resonance elastography by direct visualization of propagating acoustic strain waves. Science 269(5232), 1854–1857 (1995)
10. Adebar, T., Salcudean, S., Mahdavi, S., Moradi, M., Nguan, C., Goldenberg, L.: A robotic system for intra-operative trans-rectal ultrasound and ultrasound elastography in radical prostatectomy. In: Taylor, R.H., Yang, G.-Z. (eds.) IPCAI 2011. LNCS, vol. 6689, pp. 79–89. Springer, Heidelberg (2011)
11. Sahebjavaher, R.S., Baghani, A., et al.: Transperineal prostate mr elastography: Initial in vivo results. Magn. Reson. Med. 69(2), 411–420 (2013)
12. Eskandari, H., Goksel, O., et al.: Bandpass sampling of high-frequency tissue motion. IEEE Trans. Ultrason. Ferroelectr. Freq. Control. 58(7), 1332–1343 (2011)
13. Nir, G., Salcudean, S.E.: Registration of whole-mount histology and tomography of the prostate using particle filtering. In: Proc. SPIE, vol. 8676, pp. 86760E–86760E–9 (2013)
14. Breiman, L.: Random forests. Mach. Learn. 45(1), 5–32 (2001)
15. McNeal, J.E., Redwine, A.E., et al.: Zonal distribution of prostatic adenocarcinoma. correlation with histologic pattern and direction of spread. Am. J. Surg. Pathol. 12(12), 897–906 (1988)
16. Salomon, G., Kollerman, J., et al.: Evaluation of prostate cancer detection with ultrasound real-time elastography: A comparison with step section pathological analysis after radical prostatectomy. Eur. Urol. 54(6), 1354–1362 (2008)

Multi-stage Thresholded Region Classification for Whole-Body PET-CT Lymphoma Studies

Lei Bi[1], Jinman Kim[1], Dagan Feng[1,2], and Michael Fulham[1,3,4]

[1] School of Information Technologies, University of Sydney, Australia
[2] Med-X Research Institute, Shanghai Jiao Tong University, China
[3] Department of Molecular Imaging, Royal Prince Alfred Hospital, Australia
[4] Sydney Medical School, University of Sydney, Australia

Abstract. Positron emission tomography computed tomography (PET-CT) is the preferred imaging modality for the evaluation of the lymphomas. Disease involvement in the lymphomas usually appear as foci of increased Fluorodeoxyglucose (FDG) uptake. Thresholding methods are applied to separate different regions of involvement. However, the main limitation of thresholding is that it also includes regions where there is normal FDG excretion and FDG uptake (NEUR) in structures such as the brain, bladder, heart and kidneys. We refer to these regions as NEURs (the normal excretion and uptake (of FDG) regions). NEURs can make image interpretation problematic. The ability to identify and label NEURs and separate them from abnormal regions is an important process that could improve the sensitivity of lesion detection and image interpretation. In this study, we propose a new method to automatically separate NEURs in thresholded PET images. We propose to group thresholded regions of the same structure with spatial and texture based clustering; we then classified NEURs on PET-CT contextual features. Our findings were that our approach had better accuracy when compared to conventional methods.

1 Introduction

Fluorodeoxyglucose positron emission tomography computed tomography (FDG PET-CT) is regarded as the imaging modality of choice for the evaluation staging, assessment of response / relapse of the lymphomas, where sites of disease usually display increased FDG uptake and the co-registered CT provides anatomical localization [6] [13]. A semiquanitative measure of FDG uptake is referred to as a standard uptake value (SUV), which is a radiotracer concentration normalized by patient mass [13]. The SUV is commonly used to describe regions of abnormal FDG uptake relative to other structures and SUV thresholding is the most common method to identify these in patients with lymphoma. Some investigators have proposed methods to calculate the threshold such as $50\%\text{SUV}_{max}$ or a SUV=2.5 [13]. A consequence of these methods is that when applied globally to the entire image, the FDG excretion by the kidneys and the normal high FDG such as cerebral uptake are delineated together with sites of

P. Golland et al. (Eds.): MICCAI 2014, Part I, LNCS 8673, pp. 569–576, 2014.
© Springer International Publishing Switzerland 2014

disease. Further, NEURs are often fragmented into a number of regions in a single structure, which make image interpretation more problematic. The ability to identify and label NEURs and separate them from sites of disease will improve lesion detection, interpretation and visualization.

In this study, we propose a multi-stage method to automatically label NEURs from thresholded PET images. PET-CT images were used to derive contextual image features with high discriminative attributes by taking advantage of the high PET sensitivity and anatomical localization data from CT. We used a spatial and texture based clustering algorithm to group the thresholded regions belonging to the same structure and then classified these grouped regions into one of the NEUR classes according to combined contextual features derived from PET-CT images.

1.1   Related Work

Our study relates to image classification techniques that attempt to separate and label different structures using image contextual features. We define related work into three main categories:

Abnormality detection research that attempted to detect only one type of abnormality, such as for liver tumors [11]. These methods rely on the selection of appropriate image features to separate abnormal and normal regions; they typically require segmentation to derive prior knowledge of the abnormalities, which adds complexity to the classification.

Multi-structure localization methods that detect and semantically label anatomical structures, such as the method proposed by Criminisi et al., [3]. These approaches generally only consider healthy normal structures, rather than abnormal structures.

Abnormality detection and multi-structure labeling methods label the structure and abnormalities usually in parallel. These methods rely on contextual features to separate normal from abnormal and rely exclusively on the localization of normal structures [14] [12].

Our study also uses contextual features to identify normal structures but we differ from previous work as follows: (1) we do not rely solely on contextual features because PET images have inconsistent localization information and have the inherent variability of FDG uptake among patients, NEURs are not consistent from patient to patient and, (2) we deal with whole-body PET-CT images rather than limited images of a particular region e.g. thorax or abdomen, which have greater clinical relevance than a limited assessment of the body.

2   Methods

2.1   Materials and Ground Truth Construction

Our dataset consists of 33 whole-body PET-CT studies from 10 lymphoma patients provided by the Department of Molecular Imaging, Royal Prince Alfred

(RPA) Hospital, Sydney; each patient had multiple scans (3 patients with 2 scans, 3 scans and 4 scans, each; 1 with 6 scans) during diagnosis and treatment of their lymphomas. All studies were acquired using a Siemens Biograph TruePoint PET-CT scanner (Siemens Medical Solutions, Hoffman Estates, IL, USA) with a PET resolution of 168×168 pixels at $4.07mm^2$ and CT resolution of 512×512 pixels at $0.98mm^2$ and slice thickness of $3mm$. The bed and linen were removed from CT by adaptive thresholding and image subtraction from a bed template [9].

Training data and ground truth data were constructed using the PET Response Criteria in Solid Tumors (PERCIST) thresholding method on each PET image (see Section 2.3). The resulting binary mask, consisting of NEUR was then manually labeled as belonging to the brain, bladder, heart, left kidney, right kidney or other structures. The other class contained regions of increased FDG uptake (identified from the clinical report) related uptake in brown fat and lymph node inflammation. A total of 503 thresholded regions were manually labeled and included 42 brain, 32 bladder, 35 heart, 73 left kidney, 75 right kidney and 246 other regions.

2.2 Multi-stage Classification Framework

Fig.1 shows the overview of the proposed classification framework; there are 4 main components: the PET image was thresholded based on PERCIST and its counterpart CT image was pre-processed to detect the bony skeleton (Section 2.3). The skeleton was then removed from the PET image and the remaining pixels were then grouped into individual regions via connected thresholding. A spatial and texture based clustering were then applied to group the fragmented regions into a structure (Section 2.4) prior to a contextual features based classification for NEURs labelling (Section 2.5).

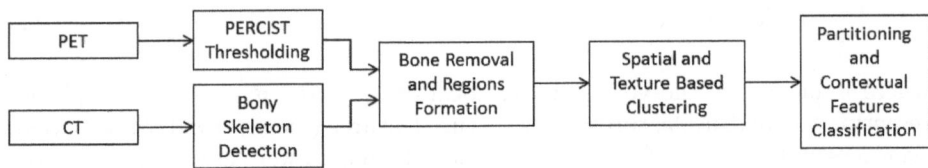

Fig. 1. Overview of our proposed multi-stage classification framework

2.3 Automatic PERCIST thresholding and Bony Skeleton Detection

PERCIST is a robust method for calculating the SUV threshold based on the combined use of a SUV normalized with lean body mass (SUV_{LBM}) together with a reference region of interest (ROI) [13]. We adopted the automated PERCIST calculation in Bi et al., [1] to generate a binary mask $T_{PERCIST}$. Here, the reference ROI was a sphere of diameter $3cm$ that was placed within the right lobe of the liver. We segmented the bony skeleton from CT and then removed these structures from the PERCIST thresholded PET image. A binary skeleton $T_{skeleton}$ mask was generated using a threshold of > 150 Hounsfield Units (HU) [7] on the CT image. $T_{skeleton}$ was subtracted from $T_{PERCIST}$. A morphological filter was applied on the resulting binary mask to remove noise.

2.4   Spatial and Texture Based Clustering

Thresholding methods typically result in a structure, e.g. the kidney, being fragmented into many regions. Such fragmentation increases the complexity of label classification (Section 2.5) since each region only partially represents a structure. Thus we grouped these fragmented regions, prior to classification, by identifying groups of similar structures according to their spatial location and texture image features.

Density-based spatial clustering (DBSC) was applied to find a number of clusters from estimated density distributions of regions in the dataset [4]. Formally, DBSC can be defined as a clustering algorithm based on the concept of density reachability (density-connected) where a region R is *directly density-reachable* from region R' if R' has at least κ number of neighbor regions (including R) residing within a given distance ϵ. R is further considered as *density-reachable* from R' if there is a sequence of regions $R_1, \cdots, R_n$ with $R_1 = R$ and $R_n = R'$, where R_{i+1} is *directly density-reachable* from R_i. Therefore, a density-based cluster is the maximum set of *density-reachable* (including directly and non-directly) regions. DBSC starts from a random region and iteratively visits all the regions. To avoid the false clustering of regions where only the spatial distance to each other was used, we incorporated a texture feature similarity between the regions denoted as:

$$D(R, R') = \omega_s \cdot min(\| p - p' \|) + \omega_t \cdot \sum_{i=1}^{n}(\| f_i(R) - f'_i \|_2) \qquad (1)$$

where p and p' are the voxels spatial locations $p \in R$, $p' \in R'$ and f, f' representing the texture features. Four texture features (mean, standard deviation, skewness and kurtosis), from the PET and CT images, were used to measure the similarities between the two regions; these features were selected for their proven performances in representing these images [11] [12]. To reduce the variability of FDG uptake across the PET scans when calculating texture similarity, we normalized the FDG uptake into SUV_{LBM}. ω_s and ω_t are the weights associated with the spatial distance and texture feature similarity terms. We set the minimum number of neighbor regions as $\kappa = 1$. This ensured that all regions may become a cluster and no fragmented regions were discarded. An equal weight was set to spatial distance and texture similarity. We calculated the distance $\epsilon = 10$ from the training data (plotting all the distances for individual region to its neighbors and then finding the distance that is able to group the maximum number of regions while having the minimum inhomogeneity within the cluster).

2.5   Whole-Body Partitioning and Contextual Features Classification

Prior to NEURs classification, whole-body PET-CT images were partitioned into three sections to reduce the search space: above lungs (AL), lungs (LA) and below lungs (BL). The lung structures were automatically segmented using an established adaptive thresholding method [7] to provide a coarse estimate of the sections.

Our classification was based on contextual features, which included combinations of region-level textures (RLT), scale-invariant features transform (SIFT) [10], and histogram of oriented gradients (HOG) [5]. RLT features were the same as in section 2.4 plus the addition of the average location in transverse, coronal and saggital planes (represented in percentages). RLT were used to describe the regions in a descriptive statistical manner representing a likelihood of a region at a spatial context. SIFT was used to describe the local features and can be considered to return important properties (key points) of the regions. The SIFT is robust for classification in different image scales or noise levels, which is a desired property for PET-CT. We sampled key points over the thresholded regions and a default 128 dimensional feature vector was used to represent each of these key points [10]. The HOG are similar to the SIFT, but they differ in that HOG compute on an overlapping squared cell, from which the edge orientations are measured. We used the same approach suggested by Felzenszwalb et al., [5] to set cell size equal to 8, with 9 directions in each cell. The HOG were sampled by using the cell over the thresholded regions and were represented via a 31 dimensional feature vector.

We used two separate bag-of-words (BoW) histograms to summarize the SIFT and HOG features, individually. Each of BoW histograms had 200 bins (100 bins for PET and CT). The two histograms, together with RLT features, were trained separately with a radial basis function (RBF) kernel to non-linearly map the data into a higher dimension space. This helps to make the training data more separable in a computationally efficient way, where a linear kernel usually has poor performance in a non-linear classification task while a polynomial kernel is computationally expensive [8]. The RBF kernel parameters were optimized with a default grid search analysis method in the LIBSVM described by Chang et al [2]. These features were then fitted into three separate multi-class support vector machine (SVM) (one-against-one) for classification, such that each SVM was optimized for different features. The probability score of region R to be classified as label m was calculated as the weighted combination of all the features defined as:

$$P(R) = \sum_{\varphi \in F} \gamma_\varphi \cdot \rho_\varphi(R), F = \{RLT, SIFT, HOG\} \tag{2}$$

where $m \in \{Brain, Bladder, Heart, L.kidney, R.kidney, Other\}$, φ is the contextual feature and $\rho_\varphi(R)$ is a probability matrix of different labels for given R and it is the output from SVM. γ_φ is the associate weight. We we used equal weights for this combination to avoid bias. The final labelling of region R was based on the matrix label with the highest probability.

3   Results and Discussion

We compared the labels assigned by our method with the labels of the ground truth. We used leave the same patient out cross-validation approach in our evaluation (leaving out all scans from the same patient to remove bias). In Fig. 2 we depict our classification results on 4 randomly selected patient studies. Our approach was able to separate NEUR classes; in Fig. 2(b) the kidneys are fragmented and in Fig. 2(a) there are multiple sites of disease in the left axilla and at the base of the left neck.

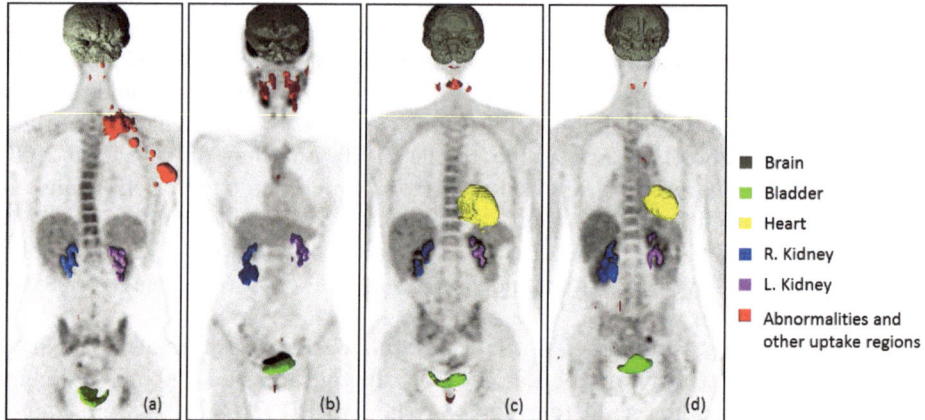

Fig. 2. Classification results from 4 randomly selected studies rendered on PET

We compared our method to two other approaches. The first was a conventional SVM method, similar to the work proposed by Wu et al., [14], where image features were extracted over regions from both PET and CT and fitted with an SVM. The second was based on a whole-body image partition (Section 2.5) and SVM (denoted as P+SVM), which resembles the approach in Song et al., [12]. The results are summarized in Table 1. Our method had higher classification accuracy, which we attribute to the grouping process; 5/5 studies had multiple heart fragments that were correctly grouped and there were 7/8 for the brain. P+SVM performed better compared to SVM, which was likely due to P+SVM restricting the search space during classification. The bladder was consistently classified by all methods, which was likely to be due to the bladder typically having the highest FDG value and in our data, without any fragmentation into multiple regions. The errors were mainly in the misclassification of the other regions. Two right kidney regions were wrongly classified as bladder, caused by

Table 1. Classification results of our method compared to a conventional SVM (SVM) and SVM applied to whole-body image partitions (P+SVM)

Methods (Overall)	Ground Truth	Prediction (%)					
		Other	Brain	Bladder	Heart	L.Kidney	R.Kidney
SVM	Other	**89.43**	-	0.41	1.22	4.47	4.47
(79.93%)	Brain	21.43	**73.81**	-	-	4.76	-
	Bladder	6.25	-	**93.75**	-	-	-
	Heart	40.00	-	-	**57.14**	2.86	-
	L.Kidney	36.99	-	1.37	-	**61.64**	-
	R.Kidney	30.67	-	1.33	-	-	**68.00**
P+SVM	Other	**91.87**	-	0.41	5.28	1.22	1.22
(89.01%)	Brain	23.81	**76.19**	-	-	-	-
	Bladder	6.25	-	**93.75**	-	-	-
	Heart	28.57	-	-	**71.43**	-	-
	L.Kidney	8.22	-	-	-	**91.78**	-
	R.Kidney	8.00	-	1.33	-	-	**90.67**
Our Method	Other	**93.90**	1.22	0.81	0.81	0.81	2.44
Grouping+P+SVM	Brain	9.52	**90.48**	-	-	-	-
(93.84%)	Bladder	6.25	-	**93.75**	-	-	-
	Heart	2.86	-	-	**97.14**	-	-
	L.Kidney	5.48	-	-	-	**94.52**	-
	R.Kidney	4.00	-	2.67	-	-	**93.33**

Table 2. Classification results using SIFT, HOG or RLT image features alone

Feature (Overall)	Prediction (%)					
	Other	Brain	Bladder	Heart	L.Kidney	R.Kidney
SIFT (84.10%)	80.08	97.62	93.75	97.14	76.71	86.67
HOG (85.69%)	93.09	90.48	93.75	85.71	61.64	78.67
RLT (88.67%)	93.90	78.57	78.13	71.43	90.41	88.00

sites of disease that involved the kidneys but this is a rare occurrence since the diseased regions would need to have similar contextual and spatial features from PET-CT.

We assessed the importance of the individual image features in the classification of NEURs by applying our method with only a specific feature of SIFT, HOG or RLT. In the results in Table 2, individual feature resulted in better classification of certain structures; indicating that heart can be better represented by SIFT and kidneys by RLT features for instance. When compared to the combined features in Table 1, the combination was able to make best use of the properties from all feature extraction algorithms.

4   Conclusion

In this study, we propose a new multi-stage classification method to classify and label regions of FDG excretion and normal uptake automatically from

PET-CT images. Our experiments with 33 clinical lymphoma PET-CT cases demonstrated that our approach had higher accuracy when compared to conventional methods. We suggest our approach will improve image interpretation and visualization.

References

1. Bi, L., Kim, J., Wen, L., Feng, D.D.: Automated and robust percist-based thresholding framework for whole body pet-ct studies. In: EMBC 2012, pp. 5335–5338. IEEE (2012)
2. Chang, C.-C., Lin, C.-J.: Libsvm: a library for support vector machines. ACM TIST 2(3), 27 (2011)
3. Criminisi, A., Shotton, J., Bucciarelli, S.: Decision forests with long-range spatial context for organ localization in ct volumes. In: MICCAI Workshop on Probabilistic Models for Medical Image Analysis (2009)
4. Ester, M., Kriegel, H.-P., Sander, J., Xu, X.: A density-based algorithm for discovering clusters in large spatial databases with noise. In: KDD, vol. 96, pp. 226–231 (1996)
5. Felzenszwalb, P.F., Girshick, R.B., McAllester, D., Ramanan, D.: Object detection with discriminatively trained part-based models. IEEE. T Pattern. Anal. 32(9), 1627–1645 (2010)
6. Freudenberg, L., Antoch, G., Schütt, P., Beyer, T., Jentzen, W., Müller, S.P., Görges, R., Nowrousian, M.R., Bockisch, A., Debatin, J.F.: Fdg-pet/ct in restaging of patients with lymphoma. Eur. J. Nucl. Med. Mol. I. 31(3), 325–329 (2004)
7. Hu, S., Hoffman, E.A., Reinhardt, J.M.: Automatic lung segmentation for accurate quantitation of volumetric x-ray ct images. IEEE. T. Med. Imaging. 20(6), 490–498 (2001)
8. Kakar, M., Olsen, D.R.: Automatic segmentation and recognition of lungs and lesion from ct scans of thorax. Comput. Med. Imag. Grap. 33(1), 72–82 (2009)
9. Kim, J., Hu, Y., Eberl, S., Feng, D., Fulham, M.: A fully automatic bed/linen segmentation for fused pet/ct mip rendering. In: Society of Nuclear Medicine Annual Meeting Abstracts, vol. 49, p. 387. Soc. Nuclear Med (2008)
10. Lowe, D.G.: Distinctive image features from scale-invariant keypoints. Int. J. Comput. Vision. 60(2), 91–110 (2004)
11. Pescia, D., Paragios, N., Chemouny, S.: Automatic detection of liver tumors. In: ISBI 2008, pp. 672–675. IEEE (2008)
12. Song, Y., Cai, W., Kim, J., Feng, D.D.: A multistage discriminative model for tumor and lymph node detection in thoracic images. IEEE. T. Med. Imaging. 31(5), 1061–1075 (2012)
13. Wahl, R.L., Jacene, H., Kasamon, Y., Lodge, M.A.: From recist to percist: evolving considerations for pet response criteria in solid tumors. J. Nucl. Med. 50(Suppl. 1), 122S–150S (2009)
14. Wu, B., Khong, P.-L., Chan, T.: Automatic detection and classification of nasopharyngeal carcinoma on pet/ct with support vector machine. IJCARS 7(4), 635–646 (2012)

fhSPECT-US Guided Needle Biopsy of Sentinel Lymph Nodes in the Axilla: Is it Feasible?

Aslı Okur[1,2,3], Christoph Hennersperger[1], Brent Runyan[1], José Gardiazabal[1,2], Matthias Keicher[4], Stefan Paepke[3], Thomas Wendler[4], and Nassir Navab[1,5]

[1] Computer Aided Medical Procedures, Technische Universität München, Germany
[2] Department of Nuclear Medicine, Technische Universität München, Germany
[3] Department of Gynecology, Technische Universität München, Germany
[4] SurgicEye GmbH, Munich, Germany
[5] Computer Aided Medical Procedures, Johns Hopkins University, USA

Abstract. Until now, core needle biopsy of the axillary sentinel lymph nodes in early stage breast cancer patients is not possible, due to the lack of a proper combination of functional and anatomical information. In this work we present the first fully 3D freehand SPECT - ultrasound fusion, combining the advantages of both modalities. By using spatial positioning either with optical or with electromagnetic tracking for the ultrasound probe, and a mini gamma camera as radiation detector for freehand SPECT reconstructions, we investigate the capability of the introduced multi-model imaging system, where we compare both 3D freehand SPECT and 3D ultrasound to ground truth for a realistic breast mimicking phantom and further analyze the effect of tissue deformation by ultrasound. Finally, we also show its application in a real clinical setting.

1 Introduction

Sentinel Lymph Node Biopsy (SLNB) is a standard surgical procedure in early breast cancer for determination of the cancer stage [1]. By injecting dedicated radiotracers (commonly a Tc-99m-colloid) close to the tumor, and using appropriate imaging techniques with dedicated gamma radiation detectors, such as scintigraphy or SPECT, it is possible to visualize the sentinel lymph node(s) (SLN(s)), which is/are the first node on the lymphatic drainage way and is/are most likely to have (micro-)metastasis in case the tumor has progressed.

During surgery, the breast surgeon can differentiate between the SLNs and non-radioactive lymph nodes (LNs) with small hand-held radiation detectors, called gamma probes. However, this is not an easy task, especially in patients where the SLN is too close to the actual injection site due to the collimation and sensitivity of the gamma probe as well as the shine-through and shadowing effect of the injection. It has been shown that freehand SPECT (fhSPECT) [2], an intra-operative 3D nuclear imaging technique based on tracked gamma probes, can improve the discrimination for breast cancer patients [3]. Furthermore, mini gamma cameras, providing realtime 2D images of the axilla, recently also have found their way into the operating room [4].

P. Golland et al. (Eds.): MICCAI 2014, Part I, LNCS 8673, pp. 577–584, 2014.

Until now, these solutions made the localization of the SLNs much more convenient for the surgeon, however, the excision of the SLN still takes place inside the operating room. The reason for this fact is that such nuclear images alone do only provide *functional*, but no anatomical information.

In contrast to this, US imaging is providing *anatomical* information and is also common practice for staging of lymph nodes. However, US can only detect metastatic LNs since these LNs are comparably bigger and appear conspicious in US images. In early stage breast cancer where the SLNB is indicated, metastasic and healthy LNs in axilla cannot be differentiated in US.

In order to be able to perform US-guided core needle biopsies of the radioactively labeled SLNs, one needs to combine the advantages of both modalities. The fusion of fhSPECT with US could thus help the physician to identify the SLNs on US images and eventually to perform core needle biopsies during US examination by using only local anesthesia.

In general, combining US with nuclear information has been proposed by [5], where optically tracked gamma probes were used, but did not include 3D SPECT-like reconstructions. Nowadays, there are solutions available, which allow quasi real-time fusion of 3D nuclear functional images with the US. Freesmeyer et al. [6] recently published their first clinical experience and results with such a system on thyroid patients. However, this work lacks on quantitave evaluation of the quality of the 3D reconstructions and uses a non-diagnostic version of fhSPECT (lower image resolution and sensitivity).

In this work, we investigate for the first time the fusion of the fhSPECT and US data for the application in breast cancer. To do so, we propose a system using optically tracked 3D fhSPECT based on gamma cameras instead of probes to increase image quality, and 3D freehand US data either with optical (OP) or electromagnetic (EM) tracking. We compare both to ground truth SPECT/CT obtained for a realistic breast mimicking phantom and analyze the effect of tissue deformation by US. Finally we also show results of such a system on real patients.

2   Materials and Methods

Hardware Setup. For our study we used a Sonix RP US system (Ultrasonix, MA, USA) with an linear US probe (L14-5 GPS) (Fig. 1(a)), which incorporates a sensor for the EM tracking system (3D Guidance driveBAY 2, Ascension Technology Corporation, VT, USA). To compare the accuracy of the EM to the optical tracking for US, we mount a reference target on the probe (Fig. 1(b)).

The fhSPECT images are generated using a declipseSPECT Imaging Probe system (SurgicEye GmbH, Munich, Germany), which uses a 2D mini gamma camera (Crystal Photonics, Berlin, Germany) for radiation detection (Fig. 1(c)) and an infrared optical tracking system (Polaris Vicra, Northern Digital Inc., Ontario, Canada) for spatial positioning. The 3D fhSPECT images are reconstructed using the declipseSPECT software. The US images and the meta data with the US settings are saved synchronized with the tracking information from both of the localization systems.

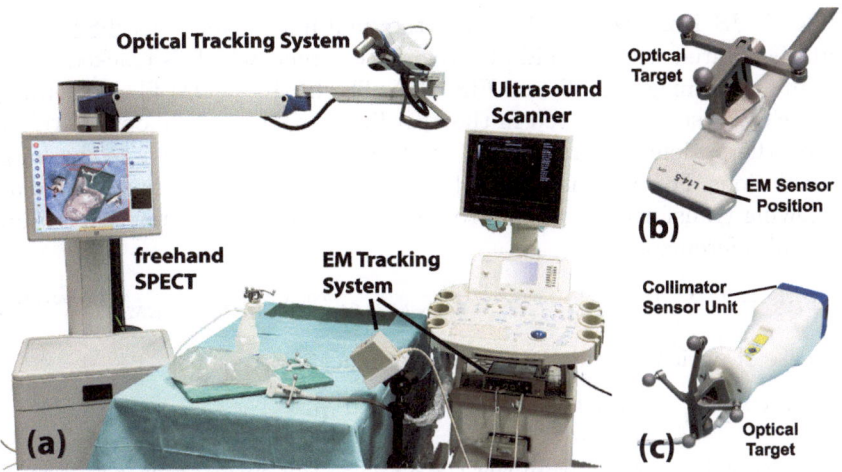

Fig. 1. (a) Hardware setup. (b) Ultrasound probe. (c) Mini gamma camera.

fhSPECT Reconstruction. The fhSPECT system uses position information from the optical tracking system in addition to nuclear information from the attached radiation detector, in our case the mini gamma camera. This information is then combined with calibration data specific for the detector to produce an input data set. The input data set is then processed using a standard Maximum Likelihood Expectation Maximization (MLEM) solver. Post processing options can include Gaussian filtering, if desired.

US Calibration. To calibrate the US probe for both tracking systems, a calibration phantom similar to the one in [7], is constructed. It consists of a pyramidal aluminum frame, where its three faces are covered with a thin nylon layer. In contrast to [7], the three faces all join at the same vertex with face angles of 90°, resulting in a trirectangular tetrahedron, whose three edges form a local coordinate system. For calibration, an US sequence of the pyramid is acquired such that the intersection of the US image plane and the pyramid forms a triangle. Based on the pyramid coordinate system, direct point correspondences from 2D image points in the US plane to the corresponding positions in 3D space can be established, and used to obtain the transformation from the US plane to the coordinates of the tracking system, cf. [8].

US Compounding. As vizualization is of crucial importance for the fusion of fhSPECT to 3D ultrasound data, we employ an volume compounding step, i.e. an interpolation of the acquired, irregularly sampled US data on a rectangular grid, yielding a 3D volume. Following [9], we apply compounding as a backward-warping normalized convolution directly on the ultrasound scanlines. As this system provides fast compounding and resulting volumes of high quality, it is suitable for direct fusion with fhSPECT images.

fhSPECT-US Fusion. The fusion of the final images for both fhSPECT and US data is assured with the aid of a reference target, which is tracked both optically and electomagnetically, cf. Fig. 2(a). The final DICOM files generated by the fhSPECT system are saved in the coordinate system of the optical reference target on the patient. Therefore, we use this coordinate system as the base for our calculations. For a point in US plane, in the case of dual tracking, we apply the following transformation chain to get its positions in the reference frame of the optical reference target

$$^{refOP}\mathbf{T}_{US} = {}^{refOP}\mathbf{T}_{refEM} \cdot {}^{refEM}\mathbf{T}_{worldEM} \cdot {}^{worldEM}\mathbf{T}_{probeEM} \cdot {}^{probeEM}\mathbf{T}_{US}$$

In the case of optical tracking only, the sequence shortens to

$$^{refOP}\mathbf{T}_{US} = {}^{refOP}\mathbf{T}_{worldOP} \cdot {}^{worldOP}\mathbf{T}_{probeOP} \cdot {}^{probeOP}\mathbf{T}_{US},$$

where the transformations from the US plane to the optical target $^{probeOP}\mathbf{T}_{US}$, as well as to the EM sensor on the US probe $^{probeEM}\mathbf{T}_{US}$ are calculated as mentioned before. Furthermore, the transformation between the optical tracking target, serving as a reference for the patient, and the electromagnetic sensor rigidly attached to it, is known from precision manufactured target construction files. Alternatively, a calibration of the reference target w.r.t. EM and optical system can be achieved by hand-eye calibration [8].

3   Experiments and Results

Phantom Design. In order to demonstrate the technical feasibility of the system, possible phantom designs were discussed with experienced breast surgeons and nuclear medicine physicians to model the clinical scenario in the best possible way. With the goal of a realistic biopsy phantom for the axilla region, we cut from a plastic female torso mannequin the region of one breast and the axilla and use this as a mold for a phantom. As tissue mimicking material, Ceraflex N530 gel (C Tromm GmbH, Germany) is used, as it is well suited for US, SPECT and CT imaging, and additionally deforms in a realistic way when pressure is applied to the surface (Fig. 2(a)). Thus the phantom does not only allow for an evaluation of the US-SPECT fusion by itself, but also for an analysis of the changes in accuracies due to tissue deformation.

To evaluate the fusion scenario with the goal of finding SLNs to biopsy, 4 spheres with similar sizes as the SLNs (240-300 ml) are placed in the phantom. One of spheres is filled with 1.1 MBq of Tc-99m before insertion into the phantom to represent a SLN, while the others are filled with water representing non-radioactive LNs in the same region.

Data Acquisition. We scanned our phantom with both the fhSPECT and the 3D US system in 5 different configurations with varying positions and orientations of one or both tracking systems w.r.t the breast phantom (cf. Fig. 1). In each configuration, we scanned the phantom at least once with fhSPECT for

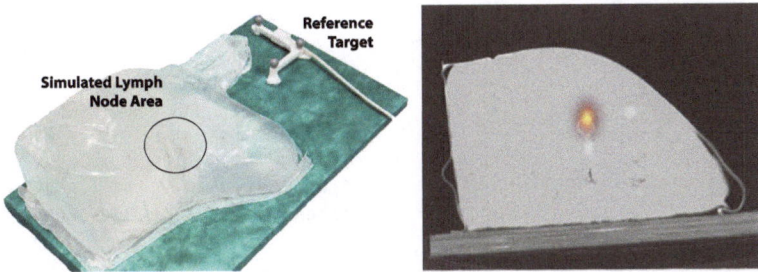

Fig. 2. (a) Tissue mimicking breast phantom, where the spheres represent LNs. (b) SPECT/CT fusion of the radioactive sphere in the phantom.

about 2 minutes. Furthermore, at least 2 sweeps were acquired with the 3D US system for each configuration, trying to cover all spheres. To evaluate the quality of the 3D US system on its own, both EM and OP tracking systems were used simultaneously for the acquistions, enabling a direct comparison of the resulting accuracies for both systems. Furthermore, the impact of deformation changes was evaluated separately using 4 US acquisitions with varying pressure applied to the breast phantom surface.

All phantom acquisitions for both fhSPECT and US were performed by the same person to avoid user-dependent variation. Finally, a SPECT/CT (Siemens Symbia T6) of the phantom was acquired to enable direct comparison of the acquired data ground truth image data (Fig. 2 (b)).

Offline Evaluation. We evaluated the fhSPECT and US images separately to the CT, by comparing the centroids of the spheres placed in the phantom w.r.t. the optical reference target. For this, we first calculated the transformation from CT coordinates to the reference target coordinates by the means of point based registration. This is achieved by using the coordinates of the centers of the retroreflective spheres on the reference target in the CT image and their corresponding known coordinates based on its CAD design. The RMS registration error for our transformation was calculated as 0.8 mm.

For each of the fhSPECT reconstructions we then segmented the hotspot with an automatic region growing algorithm using the global maximum as the seed and 50% as threshold. Later, we computed the centroid of the segmented hotspot and calculated its coordinates w.r.t. the patient reference frame using the meta information of the DICOM tags of the reconstruction.

The online reconstructions with 3 mm voxel size resulted in 2.17 mm average localization error (ALE) (stdev: 1.04 mm) for fhSPECT reconstructions. We additionally reconstructed the same acquisitions with 1 mm voxelsize for the same volume. These had an average error of 1.73 mm (stdev: 0.67 mm) instead. As a reference for fhSPECT quality, we calculated the fusion error between SPECT and CT centroids as 3.5 mm, cf. Fig 2(b).

For all US scans, we manually segmented the spheres in the acquired 3D US scans for both optical and EM tracking. Average localization errors of the sphere

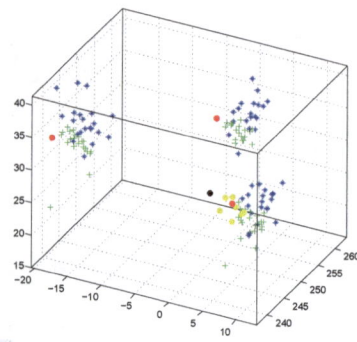

	EM		Optical	
	Mean	Std	Mean	Std
Sphere1	4.95	1.21	5.88	1.74
Sphere2	5.20	1.51	5.24	1.23
Sphere3	5.75	1.67	5.23	1.52
Sphere4	3.88	0.73	3.97	1.66

Fig. 3. (a) Segmented sphere centroids compared for ground truth CT (red), fhSPECT (yellow), US EM (blue) and US optical (green). (b) Localization errors in mm calculated for US and ground truth (CT).

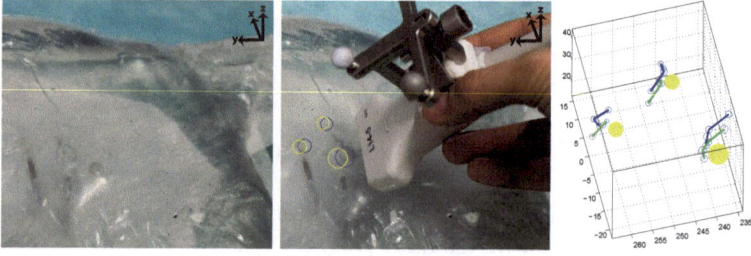

Fig. 4. Effect of deformation on phantom. Phantom position as used for fhSPECT (a) and Ultrasound (b) show noticeable deformation (marked circles). (c) Extracted centroids for trajectories with increasing pressure for US EM (blue) and US OP (green) in relation to the CT (yellow).

centroids from 3D-US to ground truth yielded 5.36 mm (stdev: 1.56 mm) for optical and 5.22 mm (stdev: 1.49 mm) for EM tracking respecetively. Results for the average errors to the 4 individual spheres are given in Fig. 3. From the 3D visualization, a systematic error of both tracking systems in direction of the US probe orientation can be observed. We also evaluated the deviations from ground truth regarding varying pressure applied during acquisition. Exactly this *pressure* was found to be the main cause for localization errors, as with increased pressure, the errors increase similarily for both tracking systems due to higher deformation (mean ALE 5.16 mm for normal pressure, 10.46 mm for high pressure), cf. Fig. 4.

Patient Studies. We also scanned 7 patients preoperatively right after radiotracer injection and scintigraphy imaging. Since our system with optical tracking of the US probe is not yet clinically approved, we used a GE Logiq E9 US system (GE Milwaukee, USA) with built-in EM tracking instead, which is the same as our previous setup. This US system can also visualize on-site the imported 3D fhSPECT DICOM images fused on the 2D image plane of the tracked US probe.

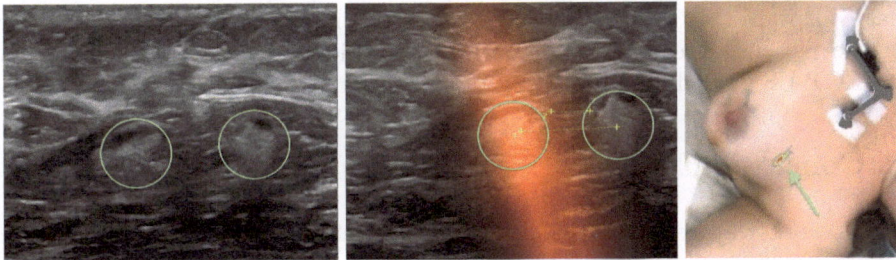

Fig. 5. (a) US image of two LNs in the axilla of the patient. (b) Fused image of fhSPECT and US. Left LN is identified as the sentinel. The distance of the two LNs is from centers 11.7 mm (1), from borders 4.7 mm (2). (c) fhSPECT reconstruction overlaid on the patient.

In order to experience the clinical challenges posed by an interventional usage of such a fused fhSPECT-US system, we scanned one patient additionally once more before surgery inside the OR. (Fig. 5). The accuracy was enough for the surgeon to determine the SLN on US images and he was confident that he would be even able to perform the fhSPECT-US-guided core needle biopsy, if approved.

4   Discussion

Although fhSPECT has much smaller detector sizes than the conventional SPECT, it achieved better localization scores. We believe that this is due to smaller distances between the actual radiation source and the detector and therefore provides better detection statistics with the mini gamma camera. Another reason could be its smaller voxel size (1 mm for fhSPECT, 4.8 mm for SPECT).

The localization error for US is considered to be mainly due to the deformation of the phantom during scanning. This is crucial for the fusion of the two images in real scenarios, as small movements of the patient might easily interfere with the reliability of the fusion. In an intervention using local anesthesia this can easily happen between two scans and needs to be taken into account. However, new scanning protocols can be suggested for compensation of the deformation effect, such as a preceding scan without any pressure applied as reference, prior to the actual US scan.

For US, both tracking systems achieved comparable scores, where both have their own advantages and disadvantages. EM provides easier handling of the US probe than the optical tracking and therefore, final solutions using EM tracking might ease the acceptance by the end users. However, since the fhSPECT system already uses optical tracking and integrated augmented reality visualization, optical tracking of the US probe might be beneficial in final fhSPECT-US solutions in terms of visualization and integration into one system.

Despite the deformation of soft tissue, results were satisfactory in regard to the clinical application towards fhSPECT-US guided core needle biopsies of SLNs. In our patient studies, we could identify one LN to be the sentinel on the fused images. However, to clinically approve this, an interventional study, investigating the patient outcome by comparison of radio-guided surgical SLNBs and fhSPECT-US guided core needle SLNBs is essential.

5   Conclusion

In this work we presented the first fully 3D fhSPECT-US fusion using mini gamma cameras and optional EM or optical tracking. Our evaluation showed that both optical and EM tracking systems are suitable for such multi-modal data fusion within clinical settings. This might allow actual needle biopsies of SLNs in the future and reduce the number of comparably invasive SLNB procedures.

Acknowledgements. We would like to thank the Bayerische Forschungsstiftung (Project RoBildOR) and SurgicEye GmbH.

References

1. Vidal-Sicart, S., Olmos, R.V.: Sentinel node mapping for breast cancer: Current situation. Journal of Oncology 2012, e361341 (2012)
2. Wendler, T., Herrmann, K., Schnelzer, A., Lasser, T., Traub, J., Kutter, O., Ehlerding, A., Scheidhauer, K., Schuster, T., Kiechle, M., Schwaiger, M., Navab, N., Ziegler, S.I., Buck, A.K.: First demonstration of 3-D lymphatic mapping in breast cancer using freehand SPECT. EJNMMI 37(8), 1452–1461 (2010)
3. Bluemel, C., Schnelzer, A., Okur, A., Ehlerding, A., Paepke, S., Scheidhauer, K., Kiechle, M.: Freehand SPECT for image-guided sentinel lymph node biopsy in breast cancer. EJNMMI 40(11), 1656–1661 (2013)
4. Bricou, A., Duval, M.-A., Charon, Y., Barranger, E.: Mobile gamma cameras in breast cancer care - a review. EJSO 39(5), 409–416 (2013)
5. Wendler, T., Feuerstein, M., Traub, J., Lasser, T., Vogel, J., Daghighian, F., Ziegler, S.I., Navab, N.: Real-time fusion of ultrasound and gamma probe for navigated localization of liver metastases. In: Ayache, N., Ourselin, S., Maeder, A. (eds.) MICCAI 2007, Part II. LNCS, vol. 4792, pp. 252–260. Springer, Heidelberg (2007)
6. Freesmeyer, M., Opfermann, T., Winkens, T.: Hybrid integration of real-time US and freehand SPECT: proof of concept in patients with thyroid diseases. Radiology, 132–415 (January 2014)
7. Liu, J., Gao, X., Zhang, Z., Gao, S., Zhou, J.: A new calibration method in 3d ultrasonic imaging system. In: Proc. of the 20th Ann. Int. Conf. of the IEEE Engineering in Medicine and Biology Society, vol. 2, pp. 839–841. IEEE (1998)
8. Tsai, R.Y., Lenz, R.K.: A new technique for fully autonomous and efficient 3D robotics hand/eye calibration. IEEE Transactions on Robotics and Automation 5(3), 345–358 (1989)
9. Hennersperger, C., Karamalis, A., Navab, N.: Vascular 3D+T freehand ultrasound using correlation of doppler and pulse-oximetry data. In: Stoyanov, D., Collins, D.L., Sakuma, I., Abolmaesumi, P., Jannin, P. (eds.) IPCAI 2014. LNCS, vol. 8498, pp. 68–77. Springer, Heidelberg (2014)

Gland Ring Morphometry for Prostate Cancer Prognosis in Multispectral Immunofluorescence Images

Richard Scott, Faisal M. Khan, Jack Zeineh,
Michael Donovan, and Gerardo Fernandez

Icahn School of Medicine at Mount Sinai
1425 Madison Avenue, New York, NY 10029
{richard.scott,faisal.khan,jack.zeineh,
michael.donovan,gerardo.fernandez}@mssm.edu

Abstract. Morphometric features characterizing the fusion and fragmentation of the glandular architecture of advanced prostate cancer have not previously been based upon the automated segmentation of discrete gland rings, due in part to the difficulty of extracting these structures from the H&E stained tissues. We present a novel approach for segmenting gland rings in multi-spectral immunofluorescence (IF) images and demonstrate the utility of the resultant features in predicting cancer recurrence in a cohort of 1956 images of prostate biopsies and prostatectomies from 679 patients. The proposed approach is evaluated for prediction of actual clinical outcomes of interest to physicians in comparison with previously published gland-unit features, yielding a concordance index (CI) of 0.67. This compares favorably to the CI of 0.66 obtained using a semi-automated segmentation of the corresponding H&E images from the same patients. This work presents the first algorithms for segmentation of gland rings lacking a central lumen, and for separation of touching epithelial units, and introduces new gland adjacency features for predicting prostate cancer clinical progression across both biopsy and prostatectomy images.

Keywords: Gleason, prostate, segmentation, watershed, Voronoi, gland.

1   Introduction

Prostate cancer is primarily assessed by the Gleason grading system which classifies the tissue architecture into five patterns of increasing severity. In the lower risk grades of 1 through 3, the architecture consists primarily of isolated or touching gland rings surrounded by fibromuscular stromal tissue. Each gland is composed of a ring of epithelial cells surrounding a duct, the lumen. The connected glandular cytoplasm, or "epithelial unit", contains just one gland ring. As the cancer progresses to grade 4, epithelial units fuse together creating chains of gland rings, or "cribriform" sheets of rings. A second axis of variation in grade 4 and 5 disease is the increasing fragmentation of rings resulting in sheets of isolated cells and non-ring epithelial fragments (the terms "glandular" and "epithelial" are interchangeable).

P. Golland et al. (Eds.): MICCAI 2014, Part I, LNCS 8673, pp. 585–592, 2014.
© Springer International Publishing Switzerland 2014

This progression introduces two new challenges for automated segmentation that have not previously been addressed directly. First is the problem of separating epithelial units that are touching but not fused to each other. Second is identifying discrete glandular rings without dependence on a central lumen. Successful segmentation of these components would better capture architectural patterns and lead to significantly improved morphometric features for predicting prostate cancer prognosis.

The Gleason grade is assessed by pathologists in light microscopy images of tissue stained using conventional H&E. While common in clinical practice, such images often present significant challenges in automated analysis of glandular objects due to uneven contrast between glands and stroma, and the frequent tearing of the tissue.

In multispectral IF [3] microscopy, multiple proteins in the tissue specimen are simultaneously labeled with different fluorescent dyes. Each dye has a distinct emission spectrum and binds to its target protein within a tissue compartment (ie nuclei or cytoplasm). The tissue is imaged with a multispectral camera, then spectrally unmixed, with one image per dye. Two common dyes that reveal the tissue structure are DAPI (a nuclear stain) and CK18 (stains epithelial cytoplasm). Nuclear objects are segmented and then separated using a co-localization scheme into epithelial nuclei positive for both DAPI and CK18 and stromal nuclei positive for DAPI but not CK18.

Because of its highly specific identification of molecular components and accurate delineation of tissue compartments, as compared to the stains in (H&E) light microscopy, multiplex IF microscopy offers the advantage of more reliable and accurate image segmentation and consequent feature extraction.

This work presents one of the first endeavors in segmenting and extracting predictive features of glandular objects such as rings in multispectral IF microscopy and furthermore correlates the resulting features with clinical progression outcomes relevant to physicians.

1.1   Related Work

There has been significant prior work on deriving architectural features from unsegmented graphs such as Minimum Spanning Trees (MST), Voronoi diagrams and Delaunay triangulation in analyzing individual nuclei in both H&E and IF images [1], [5], [10]. While glandular morphometry has been analyzed in whole prostate H&E images [6, 7], analysis of microscopic H&E images has been a recent development [2], [8], [9], [11]. Most of the literature has focused on cancer vs. benign classification with limited sets of images, often less than 100, and evaluates the morphometric features with respect to tumor architecture [8, 9], rather than clinical outcomes of progression. Of note, [2] presented analysis of H&E images from 1027 patients yielding a set of "gland unit" features derived from semi-automated seeding of lumens. However, this paper presents the first effort in automated glandular analysis in microscopic IF images.

2   Gland Ring Segmentation Approach

The proposed gland ring segmentation approach executes on two IF biomarker images, CK18 for epithelial cytoplasm (Fig. 1a and 2a) and DAPI for epithelial and stromal nuclei (Fig. 1c and 2c). These images are segmented, leveraging an approach previously developed by researchers in a cohort of over 900 prostate biopsy images [3], to produce labeled masks of connected epithelial areas and nuclei (Fig. 1d and 2d). Next, adjacent/touching CK18 units are separated (Fig. 1b and 2b), followed by segmentation of epithelial units into distinct gland rings (Fig. 1e and 2e), concluding with a final classification of the gland ring type which leads to predictive features. Fig. 1 to 3 in the following sections are 0.25 micron/pixel regions clipped from the 1280x1024 IF images to illustrate the algorithmic detail.

2.1   Separation of Touching CK18 Gland Units and Lumen Detection

Touching or almost touching CK18 (epithelial cytoplasm) areas contain visible cytoplasm membranes around the outer boundary of the area, which form a dark, low-contrast linear ridge in the image values (Fig. 1a). We propose a method of enhancing these ridges by leveraging a fast-marching algorithm [4] to propagate the initial CK18 border (white edges in Fig. 1b). Fast marching takes as input a propagation speed image, which we create by adding together the CK18 edge strength (morphological edge filter) and the ridge edge strength (bottom hat filter), then inverting and multiplying by the original image values. The propagation is initialized with low values along the original borders and high values elsewhere, which causes the fast marching output image to contain low values along edges reachable by rapid propagation. In many cases this image can be thresholded at a low value to extract the ridge edges, but this approach is not robust. Instead, we use watershed segmentation of the inverted propagation image (high values along ridges) to extract the ridges (yellow edges in Fig. 1b).

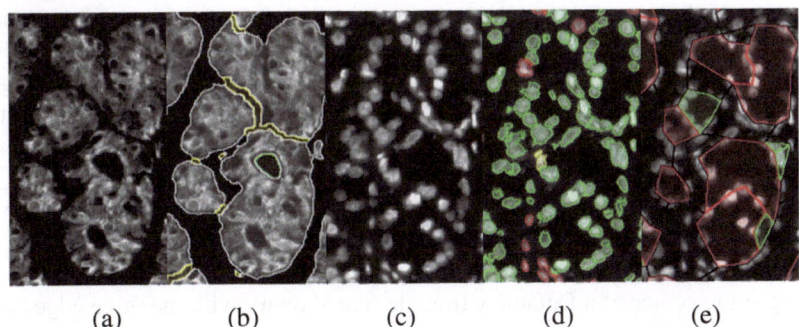

(a)   (b)   (c)   (d)   (e)

Fig. 1. Fully automated segmentation of Gleason grade 4. Inputs (a), (c) and outputs (b), (d), (e). CK18 stain (a), epithelial unit separation (yellow lines) (b), DAPI stain (c), epithelial nuclei segmented in green, stromal nuclei in red (d), and polygonal gland rings (red) and fragments (green) (e). The upper epithelial unit in (b) has no lumens, but has 2 rings in (e), while the lower right epithelial unit in (b) has 2 lumens (one outlined in green), and 2 rings in (e).

In the CK18 image both lumen and stromal regions are dark and it is important to distinguish them to generate meaningful architectural features. Not all stromal regions contain DAPI nuclei, especially in small stromal islands between tightly pack glands, and conversely some lumens contain epithelial nuclei sloughed-off or cut through an indented gland. Additionally, when separation edges touch a region, the region can be classified as stromal, as seen, for example in small dark area where the three separation edges meet in Fig. 1b.

A heuristic lumen decision rule combines information about the number of nuclei, touching separation edges, and the size of the area to classify dark CK18 regions as lumen or stroma. A minimum lumen size is set to be larger than the nuclei holes in the CK18 staining. Fig. 2 shows a number of lumens in a fused, cribriform gland.

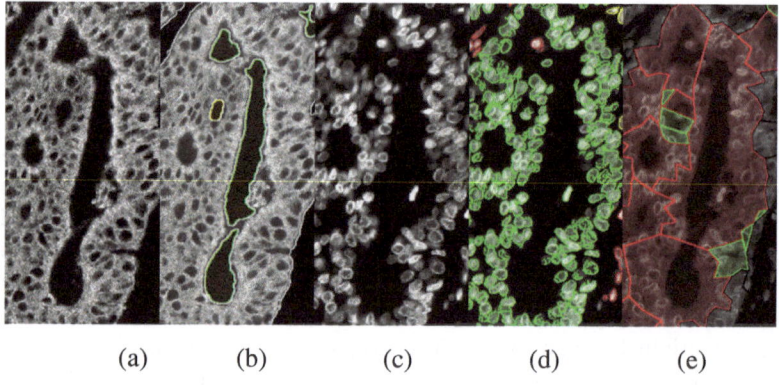

(a)   (b)   (c)   (d)   (e)

Fig. 2. Segmentation of fused glands in cribriform pattern Gleason 4 with multiple rings in the same epithelial unit (e). Input CK18 (a), epithelial unit separation (b), input DAPI (c), nuclei segmentation in (d), and final gland rings in (e).

2.2   Segmentation of Epithelial Nuclei into Discrete Gland Rings

Given the coordinates of the nuclei in each epithelial unit, the next stage in our proposed approach is to cluster the nuclei into rings using a graph-based algorithm. A ring is detected when the nuclei around the border are tightly spaced, with larger inter-nuclei gaps in the interior. One way to segment these regions would be to initialize a distance transform from the nuclei, followed by watershed segmentation to separate rings. Instead, we use a custom watershed merging algorithm on the Delaunay triangulation/Voronoi graph because a graph-based algorithm is better able to keep track of the intermediate regions' shape information and thus enables better merging rules. Figure 3 shows an example of a Voronoi graph, where each vertex can be thought of as sitting at the center of a Delaunay triangle (not shown), with the three edges at each vertex representing the connectivity of touching Delaunay triangles.

The watershed algorithm scans through the Delaunay triangles in order of the size of the longest triangle edge, and at each step decides whether to merge with each of the three neighbors, keeping track of the size and shape of merged polygonal regions. The algorithm starts with the longest triangles, at the center of potential rings, and grows to convex or near-convex regions, stopping when the length of the touching edge is significantly shorter than the longest edges in both regions. This rule causes separate rings to be detected when part of a gland is pinched, as in the leftmost ring in Figure 3. The decision rule also avoids merging rings in different epithelial units, and does merge rings which cross over lumen areas.

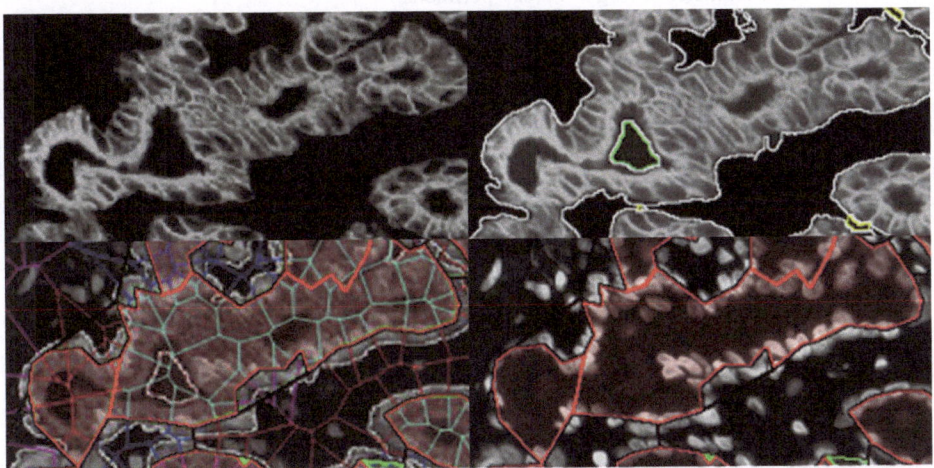

Fig. 3. Segmentation of gland rings in Gleason grade 3; in the bottom left the Voronoi diagram is overlayed with the resulting rings. The single epithelial unit has four small lumens (top left), but only two gland rings (bottom right). This sausage-link pattern of lumens without surrounding nuclei can be caused by snaking of the lumen channel within the gland, above and below the plane of the cut tissue and so does not represent fused glands.

2.3   Ring Classification and Prognostic Feature Development

Table 1 and Figure 4 present lower level structural metrics used in a series of heuristic decision rules (eg a ring has at least 4 epithelial nuclei) to classify polygonal rings as either gland ring, gland fragments, stromal, under-segmented, or touching the image border.

Table 2 presents our novel approach to building families of prognostic image features from ring metrics and other variables. In consultation with an expert pathologist, gland ring features were defined by analyzing proportions of epithelial nuclei in several categories. Our new ring adjacency features are based on the observation that the fusion and fragmentation of gland rings tends to reduce the proportion of gland nuclei adjacent to stroma and lumens.

The features are parameterized in four ways to explore the feature space: by statistic (ratio or mean), by region type (7 combinations of ring/fragment/stroma), by weighting factor (8+ alternatives including area of epithelial nuclei in the ring, etc.) and by variable (20+ alternatives, including Stouch and Ltouch, see Table 1, with a range of thresholds), creating features which systematically sample the glandular architectural feature space.

Table 1. Ring Metrics. These six metrics (based on D, d and b in Figure 4) characterize the shape of the gland ring and the degree to which the ring is adjacent to stroma and lumen areas. These metrics are used to define a novel family of ring adjacency features (Table 2).

Metric	Description
D	Outer diameter of ring = 4 area / perimeter
d	Inner clearing free of nuclei = 2nd largest chord in nuclei triangulation
b	Border gap = 2nd largest gap between nuclei around ring border
L	Lumen or clearing diameter = excess of inner diameter over border gap = d – b
Ltouch	Lumen touch = proportion of ring inner border touching inner clearing = L/D
Stouch	Stromal touch = proportion of ring outer border touching stroma
Density	Density of the border nuclei gaps compared to the interior gaps = d/b (good rings have dense nuclei around the border compared to the interior)

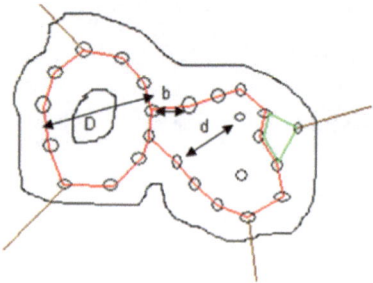

Fig. 4. Illustration of gland ring metrics described in Table 1

Table 2. Family of image features defined for gland ring adjacency

Ratio = weighted average of the adjacency variable within regions of type r, normalized over all regions. Region type r is a subset of: {1,2,3: ring, fragment, stroma}. Weight is based on factors including nuclear area.	$$\frac{\sum_{j=1}^{num\_regions} regionflag_{rj}\ weight_j\ variable_j}{\sum_{j=1}^{num\_regions} weight_j}$$ $regionflag_{rj}$ is an indicator function: =1 if region j has region type r, or = 0 otherwise
Mean = mean of the weighted adjacency metric over a set of regions	$$\frac{\sum_{j=1}^{num\_regions} regionflag_{rj}\ weight_j\ variable_j}{\sum_{j=1}^{num\_regions} regionflag_{rj}}$$

3   Experimental Design and Results

We developed our features in a cohort of 1030 IF images of prostatectomy samples from 373 patients. Due to acute clinical need of biopsy based prognostic tools for treating newly diagnosed patients, we then validated our approach in a separate set of 926 biopsy IF images from 306 patients. All results below are on the biopsy set.

Segmentation accuracy was evaluated against a manually annotated ground truth on a randomly selected subset of 266 images (due to limited pathologist availability for ground truth annotation). Epithelial unit separation is a relatively difficult task due to the low contrast of the edges and existence of other confusing edges such as nuclear membranes or low stain uptake on the gland periphery. Nevertheless, the separation sensitivity was 89%, specificity 93% with a Dice score of 84%. Lumen classification had a sensitivity of 96%, specificity 98% and Dice score of 92%. Gland ring segmentation accuracy was also good, with a sensitivity of 88%, specificity of 96% and Dice score of 89%.

We then evaluated the prognostic and predictive correlation of the features with clinical outcome (the time to significant disease progression including metastasis and/or death-of-disease) by the concordance index (CI) [2], [5] in the full set of 906 biopsy images. We compared this performance to established features in the literature by executing those techniques on the same set of patients; in particular MST features [5] and one of the best H&E glandular predictive features from [2]. The results with two of our representative features are presented in Table 3.

Table 3. Clinical progression prediction of two new representative ring adjacency features as compared to previously published IF [5] and H&E [2] morphometric gland features

Feature	Description	CI
Ratio_AreaEN_Ring_StG40_DeG15	Proportion of epithelial nuclear area in "good" rings with Stouch greater than 40 and density greater than 1.5	0.67
MeanLtouchRingSoftStG50	Mean of the SoftStG50 variable (stromal touching percentage > 50%) weighted by the lumen touching proportion. This feature responds strongly to rings with relatively large lumens	0.67
MST proportion of nuclei with 2 edges	Proportion of epithelial nuclei with 2 edges in a MST [5]	0.65
Relative Area of Epithelial Nuclei Outside Gland Unit	H&E Feature from [2]: Proportion of the epithelial nuclei in symmetrical gland-unit areas around lumens	0.66

The morphometric features from our proposed approach correlated well with the clinical Gleason grade, a common endpoint in the literature (Pearson's correlation coefficients of approximately -0.47 with a p-value < 0.0001). However, Gleason is an indirect assessment of disease severity, and our proposed features not only predict clinical outcomes with good performance, they are competitive with (even outperforming) previously published approaches.

4   Conclusions

We have identified two new targets for segmentation algorithms in multispectral IF images, namely epithelial unit and gland ring segmentations, and demonstrated the utility of morphometric features resulting from our proposed algorithms to predict prostate cancer progression in over 1900 images.   This effort presents one of the first approaches for the morphological analysis of glandular objects in IF microscopy and is competitive with, even outperforming, similar efforts in H&E light microscopy. The approaches are robust to real-world variations in patient processing and wet-lab biases as they were trained on a set of 326 prostatectomy patients and validated in a separate cohort of 306 biopsy patients.

References

1. Doyle, S., Hwang, M., Shah, K., Madabhushi, A., Feldman, M., Tomaszeweski, J.: Automated grading of prostate cancer using architectural and textural image features. In: Proc. IEEE Int. Symp. Biomed. Imaging, pp. 1284–1287 (2007)
2. Fogarasi, S., Khan, F., Pang, H., Mesa-Tejada, R., Donovan, M., Fernandez, G.: Glandular Object Based Tumor Morphometry in H&E Biopsy Samples for Prostate Cancer Prognosis. In: Proc. SPIE (2011)
3. Ajemba, P., Scott, R., Ramachandran, J., Liu, Q., Khan, F., Zeineh, J., Fernandez, G.: Iterative approach to joint segmentation of cellular structures. In: Proc. SPIE (2011)
4. Sethian, J.: Level Set Methods and Fast Marching Methods. Cambridge University Press (1996)
5. Tabesh, A., Vengrenyuk, Y., Teverovskiy, M., Khan, F., Sapir, M., Powell, D., Mesa-Tejada, R., Donovan, M., Fernandez, G.: Robust Tumor Morphometry in Multispectral Fluorescence Microscopy. In: Proc. SPIE (2009)
6. Naik, S., Madabhushi, A., Tomaszeweski, J., Feldman, M.: A Quantitative Exploration of Efficacy of Gland Morphology in Prostate Cancer Grading. In: IEEE 33rd North East Bioengineering Conference, pp. 58–59 (2007)
7. Naik, S., Doyle, S., Madabhushi, A., Tomaszewski, J., Feldman, M.: Gland Segmentation and Gleason Grading of Prostate Histology by Integrating Low-, High-level and Domain Specific Information. In: Workshop on Microscopic Image Analysis with Applications in Biology (2007)
8. Sparks, R., Madabhushi, A.: Statistical shape model for manifold regularization: Gleason grading of prostate histology. Computer Vision and Image Understanding 117(9), 1138–1146 (2013)
9. Nguyen, K., Sabata, B., Jain, A.K.: Prostate cancer grading: Gland segmentation and structural features. Pattern Recognition Letters 33(7), 951–961 (2012)
10. Lopez, C.M., Agaian, S., Sanchez, I., Almuntashri, A., Zinalabdin, O., Rikabi, A.A., Thompson, I.: Exploration of efficacy of gland morphology and architectural features in prostate cancer gleason grading. In: IEEE Int. Conf. on SMC, pp. 2849–2854 (2012)
11. Rashid, S., Fazli, L., Boag, A., Siemens, R., Abolmaesumi, P., Salcudean, S.E.: Separation of Benign and Malignant Glands in Prostatic Adenocarcinoma. In: Mori, K., Sakuma, I., Sato, Y., Barillot, C., Navab, N. (eds.) MICCAI 2013, Part III. LNCS, vol. 8151, pp. 461–468. Springer, Heidelberg (2013)

Automated Detection of New or Evolving Melanocytic Lesions Using a 3D Body Model

Federica Bogo[1,2], Javier Romero[1], Enoch Peserico[2], and Michael J. Black[1]

[1] Max Planck Institute for Intelligent Systems, Tübingen, Germany
[2] Università degli Studi di Padova, Padova, Italy

Abstract. Detection of new or rapidly evolving melanocytic lesions is crucial for early diagnosis and treatment of melanoma. We propose a fully automated pre-screening system for detecting new lesions or changes in existing ones, on the order of $2 - 3$mm, over almost the entire body surface. Our solution is based on a multi-camera 3D stereo system. The system captures 3D textured scans of a subject at different times and then brings these scans into correspondence by aligning them with a learned, parametric, non-rigid 3D body model. This means that captured skin textures are in accurate alignment across scans, facilitating the detection of new or changing lesions. The integration of lesion segmentation with a deformable 3D body model is a key contribution that makes our approach robust to changes in illumination and subject pose.

1 Introduction

Malignant melanoma is an aggressive form of skin cancer, the incidence of which is rapidly increasing worldwide. Early detection promptly followed by excision is the key to a favorable prognosis [2]. Unfortunately, in its early phases, a melanoma is often indistinguishable from a benign melanocytic lesion (a common mole). A sensitive sign of a malignant melanocytic lesion is its *evolution*; the appearance of a new lesion or changes in an existing one suggest an increased probability of a melanoma [2]. Digital imaging systems allow a dermatologist to compare pictures of a patient's body taken at different times [4]. However, manual comparison remains challenging (due to changes in the pose or illumination between scanning sessions) and time-consuming when applied to the whole body (many patients have hundreds of lesions). To improve early detection and comprehensive skin surface analysis, we develop an automated image acquisition and analysis system that provides a first level of surveillance; putative changes can then be evaluated by a dermatologist. The system can also find use in the acquisition and analysis of data for epidemiological studies.

Specifically, relying on the framework introduced in [1], we propose a fully automated pre-screening system to detect new or changing melanocytic lesions using a learned, deformable, parametric 3D body shape model. The approach is summarized in Fig. 1. First, we capture a 3D triangulated mesh, or "scan", using 22 pairs of high-resolution stereo cameras that capture body shape and 22 color cameras that capture skin texture. Acquisition is rapid (a few milliseconds

P. Golland et al. (Eds.): MICCAI 2014, Part I, LNCS 8673, pp. 593–600, 2014.

per scan) and the system does not require patients to accurately hold a specific pose. Given scans of a patient taken on different days there will be changes in pose, shape, lighting, hair and skin texture. Our novelty lies in using a 3D body model to accurately register (align) such scans across time, correct for lighting, and to build a "map" of the skin surface that can be used for analysis. This involves several key technologies. First, we use a learned statistical model of body shape variation, constructed from thousands of detailed 3D scans of different people. This model accounts for variations in body shape and pose between scans. Second, we define a method that uses the 3D shape information together with image texture information to accurately align scans with the model. This brings every scan of the patient into correspondence. Once scans are aligned, we compare them across time to identify changes. To that end, we define a basic segmentation algorithm that detects putative lesions in the scan images; such lesions are then compared across scans using the registration.

In a pilot study using synthetic lesions, the method detects new lesions or changes in existing ones on the order of 2–3mm. The system is robust to changes in body pose, illumination, presence or absence of sparse body hair etc. Our segmentation scheme takes advantage of multiple camera views to robustly detect lesions by using consistency across views; artifacts tend not to be consistent. This goes beyond previous work to use many cameras to see most of the body at once and to integrate all this information into a coherent 3D model of body shape and appearance that enables lesion detection over time.

Related work. Most previous work on lesion change detection addresses the problem in high-magnification images of small regions surrounding a lesion obtained with a dermatoscope (see [4] for a survey). Tracking multiple lesions, however, is a challenging problem that has received surprisingly little attention [4].

The task can be subdivided into two parts: segmentation/detection and registration/matching. Segmentation/detection approaches usually identify a set of lesion candidates using simple image processing methods [7, 9–11] and then filter the results using unsupervised [7, 9] or supervised [10] classification. Matching lesions in images taken at different times is challenging and approaches take many forms. The diameter of a lesion is generally small compared to its displacement between different images, making matching hard. One approach solves for a rigid 2D transformation between images given user-provided matches [8]. In [5], back torso images are mapped to a common 2D template. Pose variation and non-rigid changes in body shape cause non-linear, anisotropic deformations of the skin, further complicating matching. Other approaches focus on the topological relations between lesions and use graph-matching methods to find the relationship between images [3, 5, 6]. While able to produce robust matchings, these approaches have difficulty with large numbers of lesions.

Voigt and Classen [11] perform both segmentation and registration. Images of the patient's front and back torso are acquired with a single camera and a positioning framework for adjusting the patient's pose. Lesion borders are detected by thresholding the output of a Sobel operation; due to the large number of skin features easily mistaken for lesions, such as hair, this can lead to poor

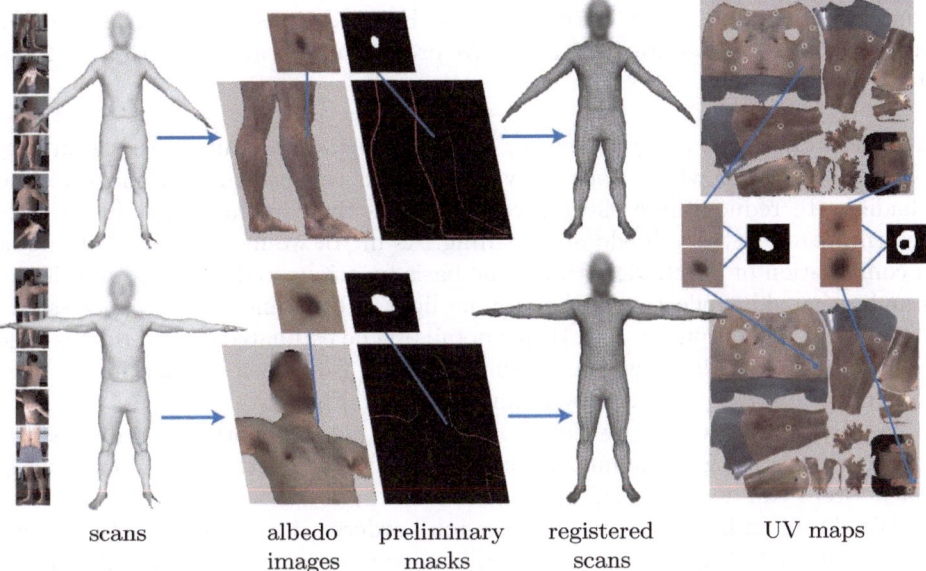

| scans | albedo images | preliminary masks | registered scans | UV maps |

Fig. 1. Overview of our approach. After scan capture, we preprocess camera images in order to eliminate shadows and obtain a preliminary lesion segmentation. We bring scans into alignment with a 3D body model, that normalizes for pose and shape variations. Once scans are registered, we compare them and identify changes in the parameterized space defined by the model.

performance. The precise positioning of the patient attempts to remove the registration problem but, in practice, humans are deformable and there will always be non-rigid changes in pose and shape.

Virtually all previous segmentation and registration techniques are evaluated only on a small part of the body, commonly the back or front torso. These methods do not provide a solution to the full-body analysis/screening problem. In contrast, we consider the entire body surface (or most of it) at once, simplifying the acquisition process for both the patient and doctor.

2   Method

Our method proceeds in four steps (see Fig. 1): 1) acquisition of a textured 3D scan of the subject; 2) albedo extraction and preliminary lesion segmentation; 3) scan registration to a 3D body model (with coherent topology across scans and subjects); 4) segmentation refinement and skin surface tracking in the parameterized space defined by the model.

1. Scan acquisition. Our acquisition system is a full-body 3D stereo capture system (3dMD, Atlanta, GA) with 22 modular, medical standard scanning units. Each unit contains a pair of grayscale stereo cameras and one or two speckle projectors, plus a single RGB camera for texture extraction. A set of 20 flash units illuminate the body during capture. Each scan results in a triangulated, high-resolution, non-watertight mesh. We process images at a resolution of 1224×1024 pixels.

2. Albedo extraction and preliminary lesion segmentation. Automated lesion segmentation on the whole body may suffer from the presence of shadows and shading. To reduce these effects, we preprocess the camera images in order to discriminate between albedo and shading. As in [1], we model scene lighting as a combination of 9 Spherical Harmonic basis functions under the assumption of Lambertian skin reflectance. We assume light is constant across scan sessions, and simply precompute it (see [1] for details). The estimated light model is used for computing shadows, which are then removed from each original image I_j to produce the corresponding albedo image A_j (see Fig. 1).

In each image, we isolate skin from background and clothing by means of a simple thresholding of the hue. We choose a conservative threshold, since subsequent steps can deal with skin false positives.

We obtain an initial estimation of lesion borders using Laplacian-of-Gaussian (LoG) filtering [9, 10]. Since lesion radii can vary depending on the subject and camera viewpoint, the LoG filter is applied at five different scales. Linear Discriminant Analysis (LDA) is used to classify each pixel in A_j into a lesion binary mask M_j based on the output of the multi-scale LoG filter. LDA classification produces, for each albedo image A_j, a binary mask M_j, marking each pixel as lesional or non-lesional.

Facial features and occlusion boundaries, due to their high second-derivative response, may be erroneously identified as lesional (red pixels in preliminary masks, Fig. 1). However, these artifacts tend to be elongated, while lesions are spatially compact. We postprocess M_j in order to keep only compact connected components. For each connected component in M_j, we consider its minimum bounding box; if the ratio between its major and minor side is too high, or fewer than half of the pixels inside it are lesional, the component is discarded.

3. Scan registration. We register scans of the same subject captured in different sessions by aligning each scan S with a common, triangulated template mesh T^*. In this process, T^* is aligned (i.e. deformed) to S, giving a registered scan T. Our registration technique exploits both 3D shape and appearance information, and relies on a learned, statistical 3D human body model. It is similar, in many respects, to that described in [1]; we briefly review it here for completeness.

Our model factorizes body deformations into a set of pose-dependent transformations (parameterized by pose θ) and a set of identity-dependent transformations, D. The appearance of each subject is modeled through a high-resolution UV map, U. We learn the pose-dependent transformations from a corpus of registered scans of different people [1]. D and U are learned by registering an initial set of scans of the subject [1]; these scans need to be captured only once, during the first session (see Sec. 3 for details about the initialization).

The quality of the correspondence between T and S is measured in terms of an error with three components: E_S, E_U and E_C. E_S expresses how close the mesh surfaces are in 3D space, while E_U enforces similarity between their color appearance; E_C encourages deformations that are consistent with the learned body model. Mathematically, we minimize the following energy function:

$$E(T, \boldsymbol{\theta}; S, U, D) = \lambda_S E_S(T; S) + \lambda_U E_U(T; U, \{A_j\}, \{M_j\}) + \lambda_C E_C(T, \boldsymbol{\theta}; S, D) \tag{1}$$

where λ_S, λ_U and λ_C represent weights assigned to the different terms.

With respect to the formulation provided in [1], we slightly modify the appearance term E_U to give more importance to appearance consistency around lesions. More precisely, given U, T and the calibration parameters of camera j, we render a synthetic image $\bar{A}_j$ (Fig. 2(b)). E_U encourages consistency between each albedo image A_j and the corresponding synthetic image $\bar{A}_j$:

$$E_U(T; U, \{A_j\}, \{M_j\}) = \sum_{\text{cams } j} \sum_{\text{pixels } \boldsymbol{y}} w_{M_j}(\boldsymbol{y})(\Gamma_{\sigma_1, \sigma_2}(A_j)[\boldsymbol{y}] - \Gamma_{\sigma_1, \sigma_2}(\bar{A}_j)[\boldsymbol{y}])^2 \tag{2}$$

where $w_{M_j}(\boldsymbol{y})$ is a weighting function assigning higher weight to pixel $\boldsymbol{y}$ if $\boldsymbol{y}$ is marked as lesional in M_j, and $\Gamma_{\sigma_1, \sigma_2}$ defines a Ratio of Gaussians (RoG) of parameters σ_1 and σ_2.

4. Lesion segmentation refinement and change detection. The presence of sparse hair, small skin artifacts or generic image noise may affect the performance of the pre-segmentation described above, producing a high number of false positives. Using more restrictive classification thresholds or artifact removal algorithms (as in [10]) may produce false negatives, i.e. discard actual lesions. Crucially, these artifacts tend to be mistaken as lesions only from specific viewpoints. We exploit our multi-camera capture framework to filter out lesions that are not consistently detected by a number of relevant (i.e. with a good viewpoint) cameras. More formally, for any template surface point $\boldsymbol{x}$, denote by $uv(\boldsymbol{x})$ its mapping from 3D to UV space, and by $\pi_j(\boldsymbol{x})$ its projection onto the image plane defined by camera j. $M_j[\pi_j(\boldsymbol{x})]$ equals 1 if $\boldsymbol{x}$ is classified as lesional according to camera j, 0 otherwise. For each camera j, denote by $\omega_{\boldsymbol{x},j}$ the cosine of the angle between the surface normal at $\boldsymbol{x}$ and the ray from $\boldsymbol{x}$ to the camera's center. We denote the set of cameras for which $\boldsymbol{x}$ is visible by $J(\boldsymbol{x})$. Pixel $uv(\boldsymbol{x})$ is classified as lesional if and only if

$$\frac{\sum_{\text{cams } j \in J(\boldsymbol{x})} M_j[\pi_j(\boldsymbol{x})] \max(\omega_{\boldsymbol{x},j}, 0)}{\sum_{\text{cams } j \in J(\boldsymbol{x})} \max(\omega_{\boldsymbol{x},j}, 0)} > \delta \tag{3}$$

where δ is a system parameter. This corresponds to computing a weighted average of the classifications provided by different cameras – where the contribution of each camera is weighted according to the quality of its viewpoint. Figure 2 shows how the final segmentation varies depending on δ: artifacts like sparse hair tend not to be consistently detected across different cameras, and are therefore filtered out; lesions exhibit more consistency (see e.g. the bottom of the back and the right shoulder). We quantitatively evaluate the sensitivity of the system to the value of δ in Sec. 3.

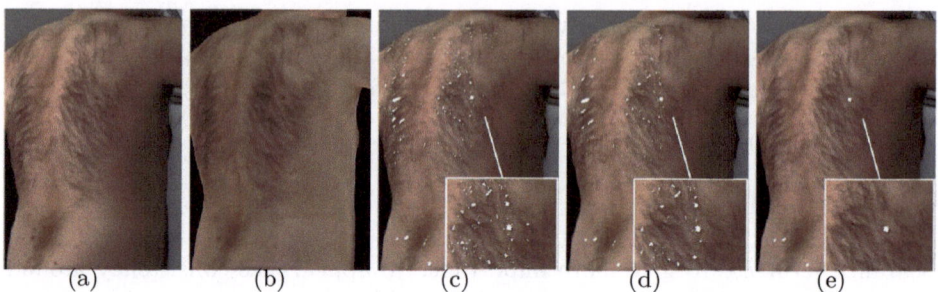

Fig. 2. A real (a) and a synthetic albedo (b) image of a subject's back. Figures (c)-(e) show the final segmentation obtained by setting δ in Eq. 3 to 0, 0.2 and 0.5, respectively.

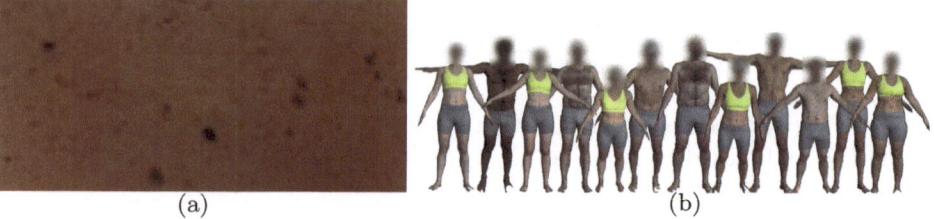

Fig. 3. (a) Skin patch exhibiting a synthetic lesion (large lesion towards upper left). (b) Scans of subjects, showing varied skin phenotype and pose.

Detected lesions are integrated into a full-body UV map (see Fig. 1). This greatly simplifies the tracking of changes in lesions compared to using multiple single images. Each UV map pixel is associated with the same template surface point, independently of subject pose and shape. UV maps from different times are therefore directly comparable. A detection that does not overlap with one in a previous map reveals a new lesion; a detection that does overlap, but comprises a higher number of pixels, is likely to reveal a lesion that has grown.

3   Experimental Evaluation

We evaluated our system on a set of 6 male and 6 female subjects of ages 23 to 44 years, height 160 to 186 cm, and weight 55 to 82 kg. There was considerable variation in terms of skin tone, number of melanocytic lesions, and presence of sparse body hair (Fig. 3(b)). We trained the LDA classifier (Sec. 2) on a set of 50 images of 10 different subjects, captured from different viewpoints; there is no overlap between the subjects used for evaluation and those used for training.

For this pilot study, we artificially created and altered lesions by drawing with a marker on the subjects' skin. Note that these synthetic lesions look realistic at the resolution of our images, as seen in Fig. 3(a).

Each subject was scanned in 2 poses, respectively with arms held horizontally, and pointing downwards at an angle (Fig. 3(b)). For each subject, we captured two initial scans in order to learn D and U (Sec. 2). After the initial scans, for

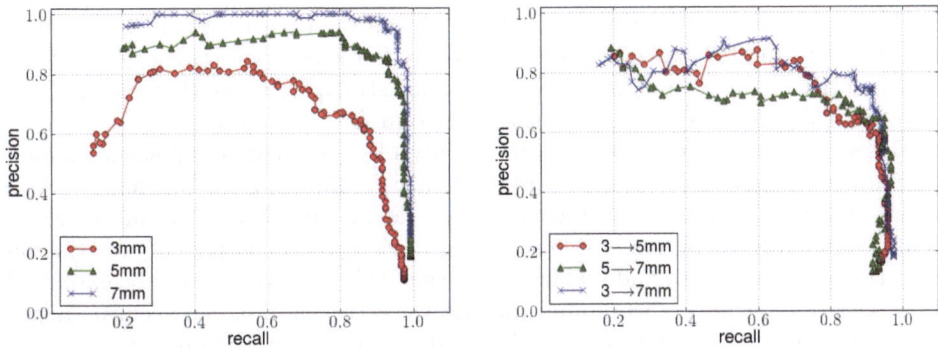

Fig. 4. Precision/recall curves for detecting new lesions (left) and increased lesion sizes (right), for 100 values of the parameter δ evenly spaced between 0 and 1. Precision and recall values are computed by aggregating the values obtained for all the subjects.

each subject we created 10 synthetic lesions with a diameter of 3mm, and rescanned them in the 2 poses. We then expanded each synthetic lesion first to a diameter of 5mm, and then to a diameter of 7mm, re-scanning the subjects in the 2 poses each time. This yielded 4 timepoints with increasing lesion diameter (0, 3, 5 and 7mm): 3 pairs of timepoints ($0 \rightarrow 3$mm, $0 \rightarrow 5$mm, $0 \rightarrow 7$mm) correspond to the appearance of new lesions of different diameters, while the other 3 pairs ($3 \rightarrow 5$mm, $3 \rightarrow 7$mm, $5 \rightarrow 7$mm) correspond to changes in existing lesions. For each pose, and pair of timepoints, our system identifies a set of "suspect" lesions – lesions deemed either new or modified. For different values of δ (Sec. 2), our system yields different values of precision (the fraction of suspect lesions that were actually new or modified lesions) and recall (the fraction of new or modified lesions that were reported as suspect lesions).

Figure 4 reports the results for the "arms downward" pose, since it was the most comfortable for all subjects. The results for the other pose are almost identical. On average, a high recall ($> 90\%$) was achieved for all pairs of timepoints, with a precision $> 50\%$ in the case of small (3mm) new lesions, $> 80\%$ in the case of larger new lesions (5mm and 7mm), and $60 - 80\%$ in the case of changes in existing lesions. Note that, while high precision is desirable, high recall is more important since the consequences of missing a potential melanoma are much direr than those of a false alarm.

The acquisition of each scan requires a few milliseconds. Further processing (scan generation, alignment, UV map analysis) can be performed off-line; in our experiments, it required a few minutes per scan on a common desktop machine.

4   Conclusions

We have proposed a novel solution for "full-body" screening of melanocytic lesions. A multi-camera stereo system captures the 3D shape and skin texture of a subject. Given two such scans of the same subject, taken at different times, we bring them into registration by aligning each scan with a learned, parametric 3D body model. Once scans are registered, we compare them across time and identify changes in skin lesions. In a pilot study, we show that our method automatically detects changes on the order of a few millimeters.

Based on our results, a longitudinal study of dermatological patients should be pursued. Future work should explore higher-resolution RGB imagery and the effect of varying number/resolution of cameras on detection. Another research line would explore less expensive scanning devices (e.g. the Kinect) for the acquisition of the 3D data and texture. Here the 3D body model could be exploited to integrate information from multiple poses (cf. [12]) and, given accurate alignment, image super-resolution could be used to obtain high-quality texture.

Acknowledgments. F. Bogo and E. Peserico were supported in part by MIUR proj. AMANDA, prot. 2012C4E3KT_001.

References

1. Bogo, F., Romero, J., Loper, M., Black, M.: FAUST: Dataset and evaluation for 3D mesh registration. In: IEEE Conference on Computer Vision and Pattern Recognition, CVPR (2014)
2. Dunki-Jacobs, E., Callender, G., McMasters, K.: Current management of melanoma. Current Problems in Surgery 50, 351–382 (2013)
3. Huang, H., Bergstresser, P.: A new hybrid technique for dermatological image registration. In: IEEE International Conference on BioInformatics and BioEngineering (BIBE), pp. 1163–1167 (2007)
4. Korotkov, K., Garcia, R.: Computerized analysis of pigmented skin lesions: A review. Artificial Intelligence in Medicine 56(2), 69–90 (2012)
5. Mirzaalian, H., Hamarneh, G., Lee, T.: A graph-based approach to skin mole matching incorporating template-normalized coordinates. In: IEEE Conference on Computer Vision and Pattern Recognition (CVPR), pp. 2152–2159 (2009)
6. Mirzaalian, H., Lee, T., Hamarneh, G.: Uncertainty-based feature learning for skin lesion matching using a high order MRF optimization framework. In: Ayache, N., Delingette, H., Golland, P., Mori, K. (eds.) MICCAI 2012, Part II. LNCS, vol. 7511, pp. 98–105. Springer, Heidelberg (2012)
7. Perednia, D., White, R., Schowengerdt, R.: Automated feature detection in digital images of skin. Computer Methods and Programs in Biomedicine 34, 41–60 (1991)
8. Perednia, D., White, R., Schowengerdt, R.: Automatic registration of multiple skin lesions by use of point pattern matching. Computerized Medical Imaging and Graphics 16, 205–216 (1991)
9. Pierrard, J., Vetter, T.: Skin detail analysis for face recognition. In: IEEE Conference on Computer Vision and Pattern Recognition (CVPR), pp. 1–8 (2007)
10. Taeg, S., Freeman, W., Tsao, H.: A reliable skin mole localization scheme. In: IEEE International Conference on Computer Vision (ICCV), pp. 1–8 (2007)
11. Voigt, H., Classen, R.: Topodermatographic image analysis for melanoma screening and the quantitative assessment of tumor dimension parameters of the skin. Cancer 75, 981–988 (1995)
12. Weiss, A., Hirshberg, D., Black, M.: Home 3D body scans from noisy image and range data. In: IEEE International Conference on Computer Vision (ICCV), pp. 1951–1958 (2011)

Bone Tumor Segmentation on Bone Scans Using Context Information and Random Forests

Gregory Chu[1], Pechin Lo[1], Bharath Ramakrishna[1], Hyun Kim[1]
, Darren Morris[2], Jonathan Goldin[1], and Matthew Brown[1]

[1] Center for Computer Vision and Imaging Biomarkers, UCLA Radiology, USA
[2] MedQIA Imaging CRO, USA

Abstract. Bone tumor segmentation on bone scans has recently been adopted as a basis for objective tumor assessment in several phase II and III clinical drug trials. Interpretation can be difficult due to the highly sensitive but non-specific nature of bone tumor appearance on bone scans. In this paper we present a machine learning approach to segmenting tumors on bone scans, using intensity and context features aimed at addressing areas prone to false positives. We computed the context features using landmark points, identified by a modified active shape model. We trained a random forest classifier on 100 and evaluated on 73 prostate cancer subjects from a multi-center clinical trial. A reference segmentation was provided by a board certified radiologist. We evaluated our learning based method using the Jaccard index and compared against the state of the art, rule based method. Results showed an improvement from 0.50 ±0.31 to 0.57 ±0.27. We found that the context features played a significant role in the random forest classifier, helping to correctly classify regions prone to false positives.

1   Introduction

Metastasis to bone occurs in nearly all patients with advanced forms of the most common human cancers – breast, lung, and prostate [1]. The extent of bone metastasis strongly associates with shorter survival times as well as a degradation in quality of life [2,3]. Whole-body bone scan is a highly sensitive nuclear medicine technique for visualizing bone tumors and is the accepted standard imaging modality for assessment. Recent studies have shown nontrivial differences in physician interpretation of bone scans [4]. This motivates the need for an automated bone tumor segmentation method aimed at reducing the significant time and variability of hand-annotated bone scan analysis. The aim is to provide a method for objective and reproducible bone scan tumor measurements, and a foundation for their potential correlation with other clinical measures.

Interpretation can be difficult due to the highly sensitive but non-specific nature of bone tumor appearance on bone scans [5]. There are several factors to this. Firstly, the image intensity is proportional to the osteoblastic activity in bones. This is a marker for bone tumor growth – however, it is also a marker for degenerative joint disease (DJD), bone fractures, and bone infections. DJD

P. Golland et al. (Eds.): MICCAI 2014, Part I, LNCS 8673, pp. 601–608, 2014.
© Springer International Publishing Switzerland 2014

is very common and can manifest as high intensity in the jaws, neck, shoulders, spine, pelvis, elbows, knees, and ankles. Secondly, the appearance and intensity of a given tumor is bone and location dependent [6,7]. For example, on a given patient scan, a tumor in the humerus may appear fainter than the intensity of that patient's tumor-free spine. Thirdly, a non-trivial proportion of the radioactive tracer often remains in the kidneys, bladder, sinus cavities, thyroid, and catheters. These three factors, combined with the lack of depth discrimination inherent to the two-dimensional nature of the imaging modality, make accurate tumor segmentation challenging. Visual bone scan diagnosis recommendations advise the physician to use contextual information when evaluating an area of high intensity. For example, for a given area of high intensity, if it exists near a joint or the thyroid, it is less likely to be a tumor. Additionally, if the joint has a symmetric counterpart (e.g. shoulders), and if the counterpart has a similar appearance, both areas are likely to be DJD [5,7].

Brown et al. published a region based thresholding method for segmenting tumors on bone scans, and used it to compute a tumor area measure that has since been adopted as a primary outcome measure in several phase II and III clinical drug trials [8,9]. Chu et al. extended this method by adding several rules to remove false positives and demonstrated state of the art performance [10].

In contrast to the rule based method in the literature, we propose a unified model that uses both intensity and context features in a random forest classifier to segment bone tumors on bone scans. The intensity features, computed at multiple Gaussian scales, describe local neighborhood information. The context features describe a pixel's location relative to the rest of the body, and relative differences in local intensity features between two points. The location information is relative to a set of landmark points on the bone scan. We identify the landmark points by a modified active shape model (ASM) algorithm with histogram of oriented gradient (HOG) features [11,12].

2   Methods

We built a Random Forest classifier to segment metastatic bone tumors using intensity and context features. The steps in the pipeline include pre-processing, landmark detection, feature computation using the landmarks, and classification.

Due to the variation in image sizes and resolutions, we pre-processed the scans by standardizing the resolution by segmenting the whole-body using histogram analysis as described in [10], and resampling the image within a bounding box of the segmentation to a standard space (800 by 200 pixels). We used this resampled image for all subsequent steps.

2.1   Landmark Detection Using an Active Shape Model

We defined 31 landmark points for anterior (AP) and posterior (PA) bone scans that marked salient areas, e.g. the top of the head, the shoulders, the hip joints, the knees, etc. The landmarks are shown in Fig. 1a.

To train the point distribution model (PDM), we first applied a Procrustes analysis to align the shapes, followed by a principal component analysis (PCA) to the set of M aligned shapes. Each shape x was described by 31 points. The mean shape $\bar{x}$, covariance matrix S, the matrix of reduced eigenvectors P, and the vector of parameters b, were calculated as described in [11]. To reduce the noise in the model, we retained only 90% of the eigenvectors. The PDM was represented by

$$b = P^T(x - \bar{x}) \tag{1}$$

To train the template matching ASM, we modified the work in [11], using HOG descriptors [12] to capture the different set of gradient directions for each landmark. The HOG descriptor was calculated at 8 orientations on a 17 by 17 pixel patch around a landmark. The patch was split into 2 by 2 cells of size 8 by 8 pixels. We computed the descriptor as described in [12] using the VLFeat library [13]. We trained the ASM with HOG descriptor at 3 image resolutions: full, half, and quarter. Due to the sparse nature of the HOG descriptor, we reduced the dimensionality using PCA, retaining 90% of the eigenvectors.

When applying the ASM to a new image, the task at each iteration was to find the best suggested movement for each landmark point based on HOG descriptor matching. To do so, we searched horizontally, vertically, and diagonally in a 9 by 9 pixel patch centered on the point. The best new point was defined as the test point that minimized the Mahalanobis distance between this test point's HOG descriptor and the landmark point's trained HOG descriptor. Subsequently, we constrained the set of the suggested new landmark points, contained in b, to within the limits of $\pm 1.5\sqrt{\lambda_i}$, where λ_i is the eigenvalue for the ith principal component. We searched at 3-resolutions, with 15 iterations at each resolution, in the following order: quarter, half, full resolution,

2.2   Intensity and Context Features

Due to the relative nature of the image intensity units across scans, we normalized the intensity prior to feature computation. We defined a mask containing the legs and upper arms of the patient, and computed the 75th centile of the intensity histogram in that mask, defined as the normalization intensity value n, similar to [10]. We created the mask by defining rectangular regions using the landmark points as vertices. The intersection of this mask and the whole-body segmentation is shown in Fig. 1b. We then linearly rescaled the entire image by $f(I_i) = (r/n) \times I_i$, where $i = 1, 2..., N$, N is the number of pixels, r is the reference intensity value, I_i is the original intensity at pixel i, and $f(I_i)$ is the normalized intensity. In our experiments we set r to 15.

For each pixel p, we computed a set of 12 common local intensity features including the output of Gaussian filters up to the second order derivatives $(L, L_x, L_y, L_{xx}, L_{yy}, L_{xy})$, the gradient magnitude, the Laplacian, eigenvalues of the Hessian matrix ($k1, k2$, where $k1 > k2$), $k1/k2$, and the L2-norm of $k1$ and $k2$. Radiologists observed that tumors appeared focal and benign uptake appeared diffuse and textured. To capture this, we computed the mean and range of 4 of the most common gray level co-occurrence matrix (GLCM) properties, i.e. contrast, correlation, energy, and homogeneity, as described in [14]. We computed the GLCM on patches of size 11x11, with intensity values quantized into 8 bins between the minimum and maximum intensity of the patch, at 4 orientations, symmetrically, and with offset distances of a single pixel. To ensure representation of objects with varying size, we computed the previous features on 3 Gaussian smoothed images ($\sigma = 1, 2, 4$ pixels). The use of Gaussian derivatives at multiple scales to describe local image structure was motivated by scale-space theory [15].

The context features consisted of 1) an offset vector between a given pixel, p, and each of the landmark points, q_i, 2) a difference in intensity at p and each of the q_i, and 3) the difference in the set of 12 intensity features between p, and the reflected point about the midline p'. We computed the context features of type (2) and (3) at 3 Gaussian scales ($\sigma = 1, 2, 4$ pixels). We computed p' by 1) reflecting the pixel p across the midline, which we obtained by fitting a line to 8 landmark points associated with the superior-inferior axis, and 2) searching a 17 by 17 pixel patch for the closest match to p. We defined the closest match to be the minimum absolute difference in intensity on a smoothed image ($\sigma = 4$ pixels).

In total, we computed 60 intensity and 191 context features.

2.3   Sampling

Our task was to classify pixels into two classes: tumor (positive) and non-tumor (negative). We obtained the positive samples by randomly sampling pixels from the reference segmentation, while enforcing a minimum distance constraint of 5 pixels between samples in order to reduce the amount of correlation between samples.

An issue with our data was that the number of negative samples, which was everything in the image besides tumor, was very large compared to the number of positive samples. To prevent the classifier from biasing toward the negative cases, we needed to enforce equal numbers of negative and positive samples. Since the number of negative samples was small, we ideally preferred negative samples prone to being false positives, namely, samples corresponding to non-tumor pixels with high intensity.

We constructed a probability map of pixels prone to being false positives, shown in Fig. 1d. To construct the map, we created a mask containing areas excluding tumor but of high intensity, for each image in the training set. The probability map was the normalized sum of the masks across all images in the training set. We set the target number of negative samples per image, K, to be equal to the average number of positive samples per image in the training set. Then, we selected K negative samples per image where each sample was selected using the probability map as the sampling distribution. This resulted in a higher frequency of samples in regions prone to false positives.

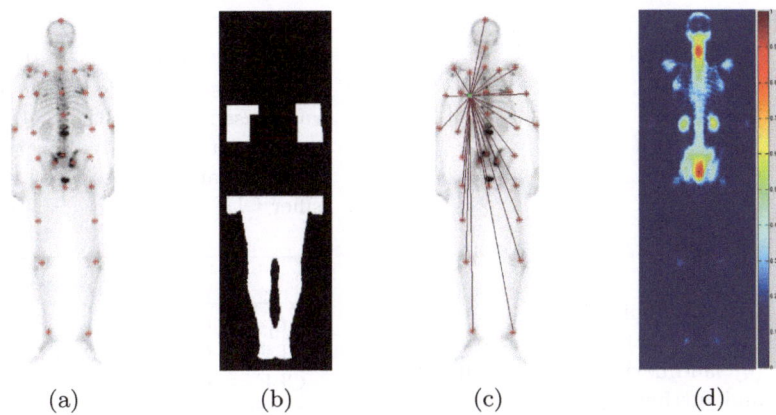

| (a) | (b) | (c) | (d) |

Fig. 1. (a) 31 landmark points on a PA scan. (b) Mask of upper arms and legs. (c) 31 offset vectors from point p (green) to all landmark points. (d) Probability map of regions prone to false positives.

2.4   Random Forest Classification and Segmentation

We used the random forest classifier from the sci-kit learn library to discriminate between classes of tumor and non-tumor [16]. To train the classifier, we first standardized the features by subtracting the mean and dividing by the standard deviation. The classifer used 100 trees, 20 random features at each split, and the Gini impurity measure as a splitting criteria, motivated by [17].

To obtain a segmentation, we thresholded the classifier's probability output. To train the threshold value, we split the training set into two subsets, set A and B. We trained a classifier on set A using the sampling method in Sect. 2.3, and then tested the classifier on all pixels in the images in set B. We then found the threshold that yielded the optimal Jaccard index (JI).

3   Experiments and Results

Our dataset consisted of 213 pairs of anterior (AP) and posterior (PA) bone scans from different subjects, collected from 56 different sites in a large multi-center metastatic prostate cancer drug trial. All scans were acquired 2-4 hours post injection of Tc-MDP. The pixel spacings in our data prior to resampling ranged from 2 to 3 mm. All 213 subjects had a reference tumor segmentation. An initial segmentation was provided by the method in [10], and subsequently, manually edited and reviewed by a board certified radiologist. We randomly split the dataset into a training set of 140 subjects and a testing set of 73 subjects. For 60 of the 140 training subjects, we manually annotated 31 landmark points.

To verify our landmark detection method, we ran a 3-fold cross validation experiment. The mean distance between the points after applying the ASM and the annotated landmarks was 6.3 pixels across all landmarks points and all 60

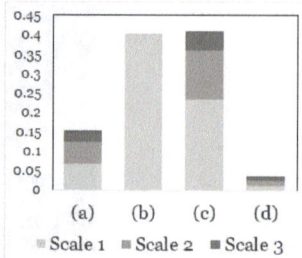

Fig. 2. Gini feature importance by type: (a) intensity, (b) offset, (c) landmark, and (d) symmetry, and further subdivided by Gaussian scale

Table 1. Mean±SD of JI and A_z across all subjects for the rule based state of the art [10], a classifier w/o context features $CLF_{w/o}$, and the proposed classifier CLF

	JI	A_z
[10]	0.50±0.31	-
$CLF_{w/o}$	0.49±0.26	0.91±0.05
CLF	0.57±0.27	0.96±0.03

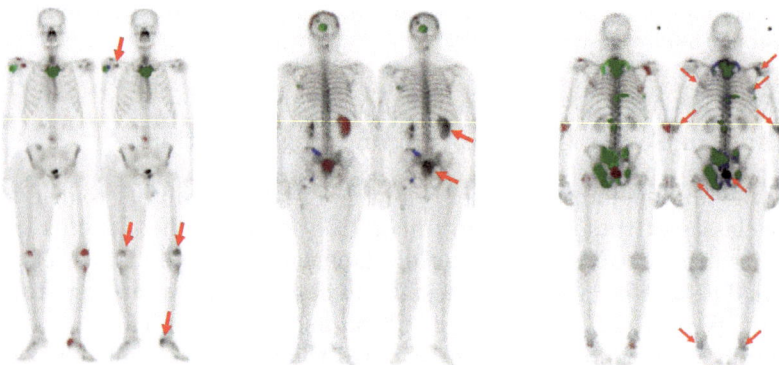

Fig. 3. Segmentations of 3 subjects, showing the rule based method [10] on the left, and the proposed, machine learned method on the right. True positives are shown in green, false positives in red, and false negatives in blue. Areas incorrectly classified by [10] and correctly classified by the proposed method as non-tumor are highlighted with red arrows. Note the ability for the proposed classifier to perform well in areas with tumor and high intensity non-tumor in close proximity, e.g. in the right shoulder of case 1, and the bladder in case 3.

scans. As a point of reference, we annotated the 31 landmarks a second time on 15 patients, and the mean distance between the first and second annotation was 3.1 pixels.

We trained two classifiers for AP and PA images. To train the threshold used to segment the probability output of the classifier, we used 100 subjects for set A and 40 subjects for set B. For the AP and PA classifier, the threshold was 0.87 and 0.81, respectively.

To test the classifiers, we classified all pixels in the image on 73 AP/PA image pairs, and evaluated the segmentation by computing the JI per subject.

We excluded from evaluation a 1-pixel rim on the inside and outside of the reference segmentation. This was to reduce the effect of partial voluming and a bias towards the segmentation output from [10], which we used to initialize the reference segmentation. We also performed a supplemental classification evaluation on a subset of pixels (limited by the number of positives) from each subject, sampled using the method described in Sect. 2.3. This method ensured an equal number of positive and negative samples. By varying the threshold on the probability, we computed the area under the ROC curve, A_z. To account for the randomness in the sampling, we repeated the evaluation 10 times.

We compared the mean performance across the AP and PA scans, and across the 73 test subjects, using the method in [10], a trained classifier without context features ($CLF_{w/o}$), and our proposed classifier with context features (CLF). Results are summarized in Table 1. We built the $CLF_{w/o}$ classifier in order to evaluate the influence of context features on the classification.

4 Discussion and Conclusion

In Fig. 2, we see that the random forest classifier found the context features (offset and landmark type features) to be highly important, equaling 81% of the total Gini feature importance. Furthermore, in Table 1, when we compare the JI and A_z for $CLF_{w/o}$ and the proposed CLF, we observe an increase in JI from 0.49 to 0.57, and a significant increase in A_z from 0.91 to 0.96. This indicates that the context features played an important role in bone tumor classification. We also see that the state of the art performed similarly to $CLF_{w/o}$, with a JI of 0.50 and 0.49, respectively, suggesting that the context features may have been a significant factor in the overall improvement over the rule based method.

Fig. 3 shows the segmentations of 3 subjects, displaying the state of the art on the left and the proposed method on the right. We see that regions prone to false positives like the shoulders, scapula, elbows, kidneys, bladder, knees and heels are properly classified as non-tumor. Note, in particular, the ability for the proposed classifier to perform well in areas with tumor and high intensity non-tumor in close proximity. This improvement may be due to the restrictiveness of a rule based approach compared to a learning based approach.

Bone tumor segmentation on bone scans is a new area of research with significant clinical impact. In this work, we developed a random forest classifier to segment tumors on bone scans using intensity and context features aimed at addressing areas prone to false positives. We found that context features played a critical role in the classification process. This learning based method demonstrates incremental improvement over the state of the art, rule based bone tumor segmentation method. In future work, we plan to investigate the use of more intelligent methods to segment the classifier probability output.

References

1. Mundy, G.: Metastasis to Bone: Causes, Consequences and Therapeutic Opportunities. Nat. Rev. Cancer. 2, 584–593 (2002)
2. Coleman, R.: Clinical Features of Metastatic Bone Disease and Risk of Skeletal Morbidity. Clin. Cancer Res. 12, 6243s (2006)
3. Sonpavde, G., Pond, G., Berry, W., Wit, R., Eisenberger, M., Tannock, I., Armstrong, A.: The Association Between Radiographic Response and Overall Survival in Men with Metastatic Castration-Resistant Prostate Cancer Receiving Chemotherapy. Cancer 117, 3963–3971 (2011)
4. Sadik, M., Suurkula, M., Hoglund, P., Jarund, A., Edenbrandt, L.: Quality of Planar Whole-body Bone Scan Interpretations – A Nationwide Survey. Eur. J. Nucl. Med. Mol. Im. 35(8), 1464–1472 (2008)
5. Bombardieri, E., Aktolun, C., Baum, R., Maffioli, L., Moncayo, R., Mortelmans, L., Reske, S.: Bone Scintigraphy: Procedure Guidelines for Tumour Imaging. Eur. J. Nucl. Med. Mol. Im. 30, 99–106 (2003)
6. Larson, S., Nelp, W.: The Radiocolloid Bone Marrow Scan in Malignant Disease. J. Surgical Onc. 3(6), 685–697 (1971)
7. Holder, L., Collier, D., Fogelman, I.: An Atlas of Planar and SPECT Bone Scans. CRC Press (2000)
8. Brown, M., Chu, G., Kim, H., Allen-Auerbach, M., Poon, C., Bridges, J., Vidovic, A., Ramakrishna, B., Ho, J., Morris, M., Larson, S., Scher, H., Goldin, J.: Computer-Aided Quantitative Bone Scan Assessment of Prostate Cancer Treatment Response. Nucl. Med. Commun. 33(4), 384–394 (2012)
9. Scher, H., Smith, M., Sweeney, C., Corn, P., Logothetis, C., Vogelzang, N., Smith, D., Hussain, M., George, D., Bono, J., Higano, C., Small, E., Goldin, J., Brown, M., Aftab, D., Noursalehi, M., Weitzman, A., Basch, E.: An Exploratory Analysis of Bone Scan Lesion Area, Circulating Tumor Cell change, Pain Reduction, and Overall Survival in Patients with Castration-Resistant Prostate Cancer Treated with Cabozantinib. J. Clin. Onc. 31(15), 5026 (2013)
10. Chu, G., Lo, P., Kim, H., Auerbach, M., Goldin, J., Henkel, K., Banola, A., Morris, D., Coy, H., Brown, M.: Preliminary Results of Automated Removal of Degenerative Joint Disease in Bone Scan Lesion Segmentation. In: Proc. SPIE 8670 Medical Imaging, 867007 (2013)
11. Cootes, T., Taylor, C., Cooper, D., Graham, J.: Active Shape Models - Their Training and Application. Comp. Vis. and Im. Und. 61(1), 38–59 (1995)
12. Dalal, N., Triggs, B.: Histogram of Oriented Gradients for Human Detection. In: CVPR, pp. 886–893 (2005)
13. Vedaldi, A., Fulkerson, B.: VLFeat: An Open and Portable Library of Computer Vision Algorithms, http://www.vlfeat.org/
14. Haralick, R., Shanmugam, K., Dinstein, I.: Textural Features for Image Classification. IEEE Trans. Sys. Man and Cyb. 6, 610–621 (1973)
15. Lindeberg, T.: Scale-Space Theory in Computer Vision. Kluwer Academic Publishers (1994)
16. Pedregosa, F., Varoquaux, G., Gramfort, A., Michel, V., Thirion, B., Grisel, O., Blondel, M., Prettenhofer, P., Weiss, R., Dubourg, V., Vanderplas, J., Passos, A., Cournapeau, D., Bruncher, M., Perrot, M., Duchesnay, E.: Scikit-learn: Machine learning in Python. J. of Mach. Learn. Res. 12, 2825–2830 (2011)
17. Breiman, L., Friedman, J., Stone, C., Olshen, R.: Classification and Regression Trees. Chapman and Hall/CRC (1984)

Automated Colorectal Tumour Segmentation in DCE-MRI Using Supervoxel Neighbourhood Contrast Characteristics

Benjamin Irving[1], Amalia Cifor[1], Bartłomiej W. Papież[1], Jamie Franklin[2],
Ewan M. Anderson[2], Sir Michael Brady[3], and Julia A. Schnabel[1]

[1] Institute of Biomedical Engineering,
Department of Engineering Science, University of Oxford, UK
`benjamin.irving@eng.ox.ac.uk`
[2] Department of Radiology, Oxford University Hospitals NHS Trust, Oxford, UK
[3] Department of Oncology, University of Oxford, UK

Abstract. Dynamic contrast-enhanced magnetic resonance imaging
(DCE-MRI) is a powerful protocol for assessing tumour progression from
changes in tissue contrast enhancement. Manual colorectal tumour delineation is a challenging and time consuming task due to the complex
enhancement patterns in the 4D sequence. There is a need for a consistent approach to colorectal tumour segmentation in DCE-MRI and
we propose a novel method based on detection of the tumour from signal enhancement characteristics of homogeneous tumour subregions and
their neighbourhoods. Our method successfully detected 20 of 23 cases
with a mean Dice score of 0.68 ± 0.15 compared to expert annotations,
which is not significantly different from expert inter-rater variability of
0.73 ± 0.13 and 0.77 ± 0.10. In comparison, a standard DCE-MRI tumour segmentation technique, fuzzy c-means, obtained a Dice score of
0.28 ± 0.17.

1 Introduction

Dynamic contrast-enhanced magnetic resonance imaging (DCE-MRI) is becoming a key modality for monitoring of tumour progression and response to therapy. DCE-MRI scans show contrast uptake in tissue, and, in principle, provide
information about the perfusion and vascularity. A bolus of contrast agent is
injected into a peripheral vein and travels through the circulatory system and
into the extravascular-extracellular space (EES) – leading to characteristic tissue signal enhancement curves. These can be parameterised by pharmacokinetic
(PK) models [9] and provide a measurement of tumour changes to monitor patient outcomes [2]. It is increasingly recognised that tumour heterogeneity is
present in colorectal tumours due to the structure of the vasculature, hypoxia
and necrosis, and that it is key to assessing the likely efficacy of therapy.

Accurate tumour segmentations are required for DCE-MRI in order to correctly characterise these changes. This is a challenging and time consuming task

P. Golland et al. (Eds.): MICCAI 2014, Part I, LNCS 8673, pp. 609–616, 2014.
© Springer International Publishing Switzerland 2014

to perform manually, partly because of the complex signal enhancement patterns, limited soft tissue contrast and low resolution of the 4D DCE-MRI scan. Alternatively, high resolution T2-weighted images can be acquired, manually annotated and non-rigidly registered to the DCE-MRI, but this is also time consuming. Instead, DCE-MRI contrast uptake curves potentially offer tumour specific features for automated segmentation.

In DCE-MRI, PK models [9] are popular methods of quantifying contrast enhancement but results are sensitive to the choice of compartment model, which in turn depends on the tissue. In practice, no single model may be adequate for the whole region, and Hamy et al. [6] use principal component analysis (PCA). To-date DCE-MRI colorectal tumour segmentation remains relatively unexplored. Fuzzy c-means has become established as a method to segment tumours in DCE-MRI images [3], which has the advantage that it is unsupervised. It iteratively assigns a fuzzy label to each voxel based on the distance of the enhancement curve from each cluster centre. However, the complex anatomy of the lower abdomen renders unsupervised clustering less effective. Fulkerson et al. [5] use a quick-shift superpixel representation of a 2D image for object recognition using a support vector machine classifier with features extracted from each superpixel and its neighbours. Mahapatra et al. [8] also develop a supervoxel approach for localisation of regions contraining Crohn's disease in conventional 3D MRI. Both [5], [8] use 2D and 3D supervoxel representations. However, unlike previous analysis, we develop a method for 4D contrast varying imaging using novel PCA and SLIC coupling using heterogeneous local neighbourhood characteristics.

We propose a novel method to automatically segment colorectal tumours from DCE-MRI scans as a key first step toward representing and quantifying heterogeneity. The method generates a supervoxel representation of the dynamic image and detects supervoxel regions that contain tumour based on features of the supervoxel and neighbourhood characteristics. Our contributions include: a novel method to automatically segment colorectal tumours from DCE-MRI (the authors are not aware of any existing method), robust learning from poorly defined masks, extension of simple iterative clustering (SLIC) [1] to 4D DCE-MRI, and supervoxel neighbourhood based learning for encoding tumour characteristics. Sec. 2 outlines the dataset, in Sec. 3 our segmentation method is introduced, and the method is evaluated on 23 colorectal cancer cases in Sec. 4.

2   Materials

T1-weighted DCE-MRI scans were acquired from 23 patients with rectal adenocarcinomas using a 1.5 T GE scanner with a gradient echo, fat-suppressed sequence (LAVA) (TR=4.5 ms, TE=2.2 ms and flip angle 12°). The scans were acquired prior to downstaging chemo-radiotherapy. Multihance^{TM}was injected just after the scan start, and images were acquired every 12 s for between 20 and 25 successive periods at a resolution of $0.78 \times 0.78 \times 2.0$ mm. High resolution small FOV axial-oblique T2-weighted images were acquired prior to the DCE-MRI scan with a resolution of $0.39 \times 0.39 \times 3.30$mm (TR=14ms, TE=12ms, flip

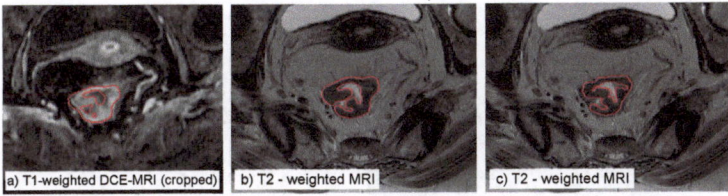

Fig. 1. Colorectal MRI images with annotations a) DCE-MRI axial slice (with tumour annotation) b,c) Corresponding T2 MRI showing inter-rater variability

angle 40°). Scans were acquired axial to the tumour at the point of invasion in order to minimise partial volume effects.

Colorectal tumours were delineated on the high resolution T2-weighted scans by a radiologist and registered to the DCE-MRI scans. The T2 and DCE-MRI scans were acquired consecutively and the majority of the alignment is performed using the DICOM coordinates. The T2 scans were then resampled and registered to the baseline DCE-MRI (prior to contrast) to correct for minor abdominal motion in the time between scans [7]. Using this transformation, masks could be aligned to the DCE-MRI volume, and were checked by a radiologist. However, manual segmentation of colorectal tumours is a challenging task because of: partial volume effects in the axial plane, complex anatomy in the lower rectum making it difficult to delineate normal anatomical structures, wall thickening due to venous congestion, and mucinous tumours. Fig. 1 shows a single axial slice of the T1-weighted DCE-MRI (at a fixed time) and the T2-weighted MRI. Two annotations are shown to illustrate expert variability, and this sets a fundamental limit on the evaluation of any method against the radiologist "ground truth".

3   Method

Our colorectal tumour segmentation method uses a PCA representation of the contrast uptake curves as input to an n-feature Simple Linear Iterative Clustering (SLIC) algorithm of the heterogeneous tumour and surrounding tissue in DCE-MRI. This section describes the preprocessing, supervoxel extraction, derivation of features from the supervoxels, and the segmentation of unseen cases.

Preprocessing: A subregion is defined by detecting the MRI foreground based on Otsu thresholding to find the patient boundary. The patient boundary was used to automatically crop the DCE-MRI to an ROI surrounding tumour (approximately 25% of the original volume) based on the general location of the rectum. **Processed tumour volume-of-interest.** The registered DCE-MRI tumour annotation provides the ground truth to learn to characterise the tumour in the image. Small failures in the ground truth result in poor learning and, therefore, supervoxels entirely contained within the annotation were used with linear discriminant analysis (LDA) to assign a posterior probability to each

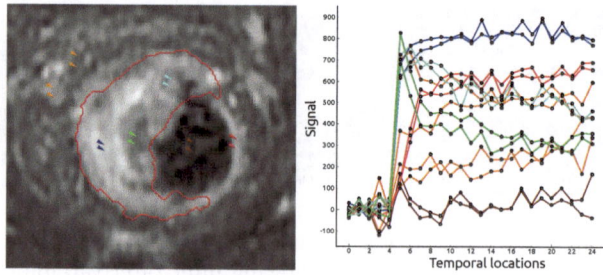

Fig. 2. Signal enhancement curves for the tumour and surrounding tissue where shape relates to tissue perfusion and vascularity. *Green, blue* and *cyan* are selected from regions of the tumour, *red* shows the rectal wall and mucosa, *orange* shows surrounding tissue, and *brown* the lumen. This figure illustrates the heterogeneity in the tumour, as well as similarities between subregions of the tumour.

voxel of being part of the tumour. Supervoxels containing at least 20% of the annotation with a high tumour probability were classified as tumour. This provided a more robust ground truth for training (Fig. 3). **Injection time and image normalisation.** Injection time may vary between scans and was detected from the steepest gradient in contrast enhancement in the image (contrast in the arteries). Signal enhancement curves were also normalised by the 80th percentile of the maximum contrast.

Supervoxel Representation: Fig. 2 shows signal enhancement curves for regions in the tumour (red mask) and surrounding tissue – illustrating the heterogeneity in the tumour, as well as similarities within subregions. Examples such as this motivate use of a supervoxel representation to cluster consistent subregions and extract the connectivity between subregions of the tumour, lumen and wall.

PCA applies a linear transform to project corresponding points into uncorrelated space and for dimensionality reduction. The eigenvectors from the covariance matrix of the features are used to apply this projection: $\mathbf{b} = \Phi^T (\mathbf{x} - \bar{\mathbf{x}})$ where $\mathbf{x}$ is the signal enhancement curve, $\mathbf{b}$ is the representation in uncorrelated space and Φ^T is the transposed eigenvectors of the covariance. A single enhancement curve is represented as the mean shape and a linear combination of each principal component by $\mathbf{x} \approx \bar{\mathbf{x}} + \Phi\mathbf{b}$. Standard deviation of each mode is given by the eigenvalue $\sigma_i = \sqrt{\lambda_i}$. The enhancement curves are represented by the first 5 principal modes (99% of the variation). Fig. 3a shows variation of the curves with two standard deviations from the curve mean ($\mu \pm 2\sigma_i$).

SLIC [1] typically generates superpixels from an image using an adaptation of k-means clustering and penalising distance from the cluster centre. SLIC has been shown to be a fast method with good performance [1]. SLIC initialises k cluster centres by sampling the grid regularly with distance $S = \sqrt{(N/k)}$, where N denotes the number of voxels. A distance function is defined that usually combines a color/intensity distance and spatial distance measure, and voxels are assigned to the closest cluster by searching a 2S x 2S x 2S neighbourhood (3D

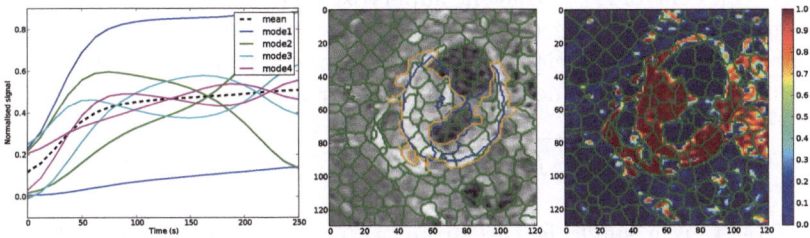

Fig. 3. SLIC supervoxel generation a) Two standard deviations of the first 4 modes of variation from the mean enhancement curve b) Supervoxels shown on a single slice and at a single time point of the 4D DCE-MRI volume (registered tumour mask in blue and preprocessed in orange) c) Posterior probabilities used for mask preprocessing.

volume). We have extended SLIC to an n-feature image to enable extraction of supervoxels from a DCE-MRI image based on the features of the enhancement. The feature distance (d_f) and spatial distance(d_s) are defined as:

$$d_f^2 = \frac{1}{n} \sum_k^n (b_{jk} - b_{ik})^2, \quad d_s^2 = \sum_k^3 (x_{jk} - x_{ik})^2 \qquad (1)$$

where b_{jk} is the kth principal component of the jth voxel, and (x_{j1}, x_{j2}, x_{j3}) is the 3D coordinate of the jth voxel in mm. As discussed, we use n=5 components. The range of each principal component is normalised between $[0, 1]$ for the volume. The distances can be combined as a relative distance measure by:

$$D = \sqrt{d_f + (d_s/r)} \qquad (2)$$

where $r = \frac{S}{\text{compactness}}$ is a weight. *Compactness* was chosen to be 0.05 and the average cluster size was chosen be 400 voxels by qualitatively assessing the ability of the supervoxel algorithm to correctly separate thin structures such as mucosal walls for the first 4 cases. Fig. 3 shows the modes of variation used to characterise the curves and a 2D axial slice of the 3D supervoxel representation.

Features from Supervoxel Neighbourhoods: Principal components are found for the voxel contrast enhancement curves, and n-feature SLIC was used to generate supervoxel clusters (v_i). The mean and standard deviation of the PCA modes (b_i) in each supervoxel (v_i) were used as features ($\mathbf{f}_i$) to characterise the enhancement. Features were all normalised between $[0, 1]$. Superpixel connectivity is used by Fulkerson et al. [5] to capture neighbourhood variation. We use rotationally invariant supervoxel feature magnitude of the gradient to capture changes related to the tumour, because the tumour can be characterised as a contiguous region, with structure in the tumour heterogeneity, that may abut lumen that contains non-enhancing air or stool, and a thin rectal wall/mucosa (Fig. 2). The supervoxel adjacency graph $G(V, E)$ was found where each supervoxel $v_i \in V$ and edges (E) connect adjacent supervoxels (v_i, v_j). The vector

(d_{ij}) between centroids of adjacent supervoxels (v_i, v_j) and the unit vector $\hat{d}_{ij}$ was then calculated. Using G, rotationally invariant descriptors related to the gradient magnitude the neighbouring supervoxel features were used to encode neighbourhood variation and approximated for each feature by:

$$f_{\nabla i} = \sqrt{(f_{x+1} - f_{x-1})^2 + (f_{y+1} - f_{y-1})^2 + (f_{z+1} - f_{z-1})^2} \qquad (3)$$

where $f_i \in \mathbf{f}_i$ is a single feature from six neighbouring supervoxels with $\hat{d}_{ij}$ most representative of the six-connected neighbour orientations. Therefore, each supervoxel is represented by 10 features from the mean and standard deviation of the modes of each supervoxel, and 10 features from the neighbourhood.

Classification and Evaluation: To date we have evaluated two classifiers: LDA and random forests, which are increasingly used in medical imaging applications [8]. Patients 1-4 were used for parameter tuning and leave-one-out cross validation (LOOCV) was used to evaluate the algorithm by testing on each patient and training on the remainder. The classifier was trained on all training set supervoxels and used to classify supervoxels in a test case. Finally, connected region size and the central moment of inertia are used to exclude additional smaller regions (shown in Fig. 4). These results were compared to the standard fuzzy c-means algorithm for DCE-MRI tumour segmentation [3].

4   Results

The registered expert annotations from the T2 images provide the ground truth in order to train and evaluate our algorithm on DCE-MRI. The tumour centre is accurate but edges may vary making annotation preprocessing an important step (Sec. 3). Variability in the T2 manual annotations and registration error were assessed to quantify the uncertainty. Ten cases were relabelled by two radiologists and inter-rater voxelwise Dice scores of 0.73 ± 0.13 and 0.77 ± 0.10 were found when comparing to the original annotations. Registration error was quantified by an expert correcting the registered mask on the DCE-MRI using the T2 as reference for four cases (case 1-4). The Dice score between the registered mask and corrected mask was 0.94 ± 0.01. Fig. 4 shows the original annotations, tumour probabilities assigned to each supervoxel during classification, and the final segmentation for two cases. Segmentations are consistent but with variability on the border which agrees with inter-observer variability. Our method successfully detected 20 cases but failed to detect 3 cases (16, 18, 20), which showed slower tumour contrast uptake. The detected cases were segmented with a voxelwise mean Dice score of 0.68 ± 0.15 (compared to the processed ground truth), and 0.56 ± 0.13 for the original ground truth. The mean Dice scores for the automated algorithm were not significantly different from either of the experts (p=0.33 and p=0.06 using a Wilcoxon rank sum test). Fuzzy c-means [3] was considerably poorer with 0.28 ± 0.17 and 0.19 ± 0.14 for the processed and original masks,

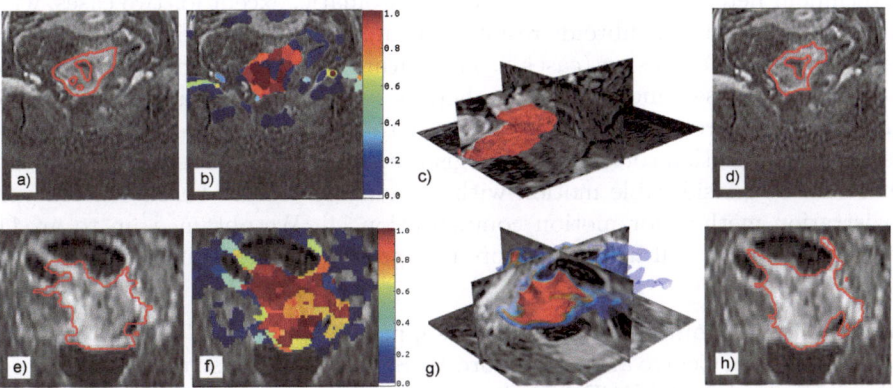

Fig. 4. A single slice through tumour example segmentations, a-d) case 6 axial slice, e-h) case 2 sagittal slice: Expert segmentations (a, e), Tumour probabilities assigned to the supervoxels during classification (transparent has $prob < 0.02$) (b, f), and (d, h) segmentations from our method. 3D representations are also shown of d) and f).

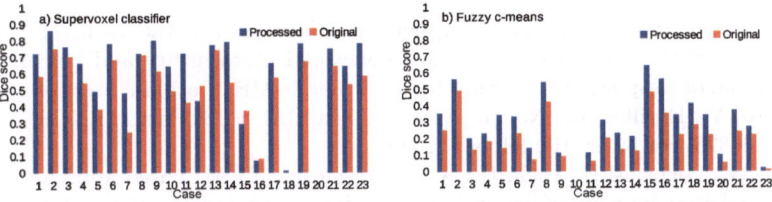

Fig. 5. Dice score for the supervoxel classification method and fuzzy c-means method compared to the processed ground truth and the original ground truth

respectively. Fig. 5 shows the Dice score for each case using our supervoxel classifier and fuzzy c-means, compared to the preprocessed mask and original mask. RF achieved poorer results than the LDA results implemented here, which was probably due to the limited size of the training set leading to more sophisticated classifiers overfitting to the training set. This method was developed in Python and C++, and took an average of 3.7 ± 2.4 minutes to segment an unseen case (4 times faster than an expert of approximately 15 minutes).

5   Discussion

We introduced, a novel method to segment colorectal tumours directly from 4D DCE-MRI scans using the signal enhancement patterns of the tumour and surrounding regions. This has not been previously addressed, achieves results equivalent to the inter-observer variability in segmentation for most cases, and is considerably better than the standard fuzzy c-means technique. It also demonstrates the potential of contrast enhancement curves to quantify tissue differences and tumour heterogeneity. Our method is automatic, except for two cases, where the presence of uterine fibroids resulted in similar appearance in DCE-MRI, and required manual exclusion (cases 8, 11). Future research will apply this method to a larger dataset, including post-therapy cases, and include a more explicit model-based representation of the tumour to distinguish fibroids. As an initial assessment of motion correction, we registered the DCE-MRI temporal sequences that showed considerable motion with an adapted feature-based diffeomorphic registration method for motion compensation [4]. We obtained up to an 11% improvement and will further explore this potential increment in future work.

Acknowledgements. This research is supported by the CRUK/EPSRC Oxford Cancer Imaging Centre and the Oxford EPSRC IAA. We also thank Prof. Fergus Gleeson as lead of the DCE-MRI imaging trial.

References

1. Achanta, R., Shaji, A., Smith, K., Lucchi, A.: SLIC superpixels compared to state-of-the-art superpixel methods. IEEE Trans. Pattern Anal. Mach. Intell. 34, 2274–2281 (2012)
2. Bhushan, M., Schnabel, J.A., Chappell, M., Gleeson, F., Anderson, M., Franklin, J., Brady, S.M., Jenkinson, M.: The Impact of Heterogeneity and Uncertainty on Prediction of Response to Therapy Using Dynamic MRI Data. In: Mori, K., Sakuma, I., Sato, Y., Barillot, C., Navab, N. (eds.) MICCAI 2013, Part I. LNCS, vol. 8149, pp. 316–323. Springer, Heidelberg (2013)
3. Chen, W., Giger, M.L., Bick, U.: A fuzzy c-means (FCM)-based approach for computerized segmentation of breast lesions in dynamic contrast-enhanced MR images.. Acad. Radiol. 13, 63–72 (2006), doi:10.1016/j.acra.2005.08.035
4. Cifor, A., Risser, L., Chung, D., Anderson, E.M., Schnabel, J.A.: Hybrid feature-based diffeomorphic registration for tumor tracking in 2-d liver ultrasound images. IEEE Trans. Med. Imag. 32, 1647–1656 (2013)
5. Fulkerson, B., Vedaldi, A., Soatto, S.: Class segmentation and object localization with superpixel neighborhoods. IEEE Int. Conf. Comput. Vis., 670–677 (2009)
6. Hamy, V., Dikaios, N., Punwani, S., Melbourne, A., Latifoltojar, A., Makanyanga, J., Chouhan, M., Helbren, E., Menys, A., Taylor, S., Atkinson, D.: Respiratory motion correction in dynamic MRI using robust data decomposition registration - Application to DCE-MRI. Med. Image Anal. 18, 301–313 (2014)
7. Heinrich, M.P., Jenkinson, M., Bhushan, M., Matin, T., Gleeson, F.V., Brady, M., Schnabel, J.A.: MIND: modality independent neighbourhood descriptor for multi-modal deformable registration. Med. Image Anal. 16, 1423–1435 (2012)
8. Mahapatra, D., Schuffler, P.J., Tielbeek, J.A.W., Makanyanga, J.C., Stoker, J., Taylor, S.A., Vos, F.M., Buhmann, J.M.: Automatic Detection and Segmentation of Crohn's Disease Tissues From Abdominal MRI. IEEE Trans. Med. Imag. 32, 2332–2347 (2013)
9. Tofts, P.S., Brix, G., Buckley, D.L., Evelhoch, J.L., Henderson, E., Knopp, M.V., Larsson, H.B., Lee, T., Mayr, N.A., Parker, G., et al.: Estimating kinetic parameters from dynamic contrast-enhanced T 1-weighted MRI of a diffusable tracer: standardized quantities and symbols. J. Magn. Reson. Imaging 10, 223–232 (1999)

Real-Time Visualisation and Analysis of Internal Examinations – Seeing the Unseen

Alejandro Granados[1], Niels Hald[1], Aimee Di Marco[2], Shahla Ahmed[2],
Naomi Low-Beer[2], Jenny Higham[2], Roger Kneebone[1], and Fernando Bello[1]

[1] Simulation and Modelling in Medicine and Surgery, Department of Surgery and Cancer
St. Mary's Hospital, Imperial College London, UK
[2] Imperial College Healthcare NHS Trust
St. Mary's Hospital, Imperial College London, UK
a.granados@imperial.ac.uk

Abstract. Internal examinations such as Digital Rectal Examination (DRE) and bimanual Vaginal Examination (BVE) are routinely performed for early diagnosis of cancer and other diseases. Although they are recognised as core skills to be taught on a medical curriculum, they are difficult to learn and teach due to their unsighted nature. We present a framework that combines a visualisation and analysis tool with position and pressure sensors to enable the study of internal examinations and provision of real-time feedback. This approach is novel as it allows for real-time continuous trajectory and pressure data to be obtained for the complete examination, which may be used for teaching and assessment. Experiments were conducted performing DRE and BVE on benchtop models, and BVE on Gynaecological Teaching Assistants (GTA). The results obtained suggest that the proposed methodology may provide an insight into what constitutes an adequate DRE or BVE, provide real-time feedback tools for learning and assessment, and inform haptics-based simulator design.

Keywords: Internal Examinations, Digital Rectal Examination, Bimanual Vaginal Examination, Prostate Cancer, Rectal Cancer, Vaginal Abnormalities, Cervix Abnormalities.

1   Introduction

Physical examination through Digital Rectal Examination (DRE) or bimanual Vaginal Examination (BVE) plays a key role in the early diagnosis and detection of anorectal [1,2], prostate [3], vaginal and cervix [4] abnormalities. Despite this importance, teaching and assessment of DRE and BVE is often inadequate as visual cues are minimal – both learner and trainer are unable to see what each other is doing. The intimate nature of these examinations results in patients being unwilling to be examined by junior trainees.

In addition, there is a lack of understanding of what are the pressure and palpation techniques that lead to an adequate examination. Previous attempts have focused on computing performance metrics from pressure sensors embedded on an instrumented

P. Golland et al. (Eds.): MICCAI 2014, Part I, LNCS 8673, pp. 617–625, 2014.

prostate [5,6], or on a pelvic benchtop model [7]. The main objective of such studies has been the validation of the proposed simulator by comparing the performance of experts and novices. However, by using a discrete number of sensors on fixed anatomical locations, the proposed systems not only fail to capture other important regions such as the rectum and vaginal walls, but are also unable to offer a continuous pressure map across the anatomy to be examined, which may help better understand how to properly conduct a DRE or BVE.

In this paper we describe a framework that is able to continuously capture real-time pressure and position information during a DRE or BVE, playback an examination, as well as provide tools for the analysis of pressure and palpation techniques. Using a previously published Cognitive Task Analysis (CTA) that decomposes the examination into a series of steps or tasks [8,9], we have annotated these steps with a range of properties computed from the sensor data. Our hypothesis is that our system will enable better understanding and assessment of DRE and BVE by quantifying and analysing trajectories and forces. First, the sensor setup, 3D visualisation, task decomposition, task properties and experimental studies are described. Results of the three studies for DRE and BVE are then presented, followed by a discussion and conclusions.

2   Methods

2.1   Position Tracking and Pressure Sensing

A position sensor coil (Aurora Micro 6DOF 0.8mmx9mm) was placed on the nail of the expert's examining finger(s) and tracked with an electromagnetic tracker (NDI Aurora, tracking volume 50x50x50mm) located next to the DRE / BVE benchtop model or Gynaecological Teaching Assistant (GTA). A capacitive pressure sensor pad (Pressure Profile System FingerTPS) located on the fingerprint was used to capture pressure during the examination (Fig. 1). Both Application Programming Interfaces (APIs) from NDI and PPS were integrated into a single-thread-based application using Qt and libQGLViewer, capturing each examination at a 40Hz sampling rate. This configuration allows for continuous data recording (position, orientation and pressure) while palpating any internal structure during the examination.

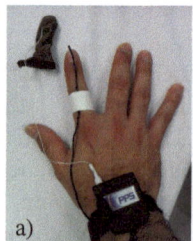 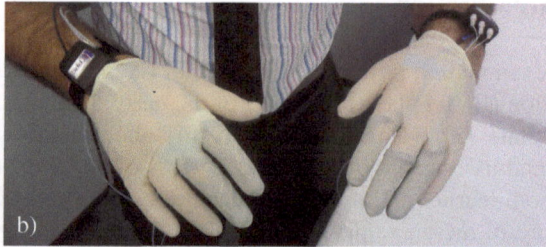

Fig. 1. a) DRE: a Micro 6DOF position sensor coil on the nail of the index finger with a capacitive pressure sensor next to it. b) BVE on GTAs: a consultant wearing position sensors (index and middle fingers of both hands) with five pressure sensor sheaths (one additional next to middle finger of external hand).

2.2   3D Visualisation

The DRE and BVE benchtop models were CT scanned to produce reference anatomical models to be used during the visualisation. 3D surface models were constructed using marching cubes in VTK. Before performing the examination, four anatomical landmarks were touched by the expert using one of the tracked index fingers. These landmarks were used to register the 3D surface models with the corresponding benchtop model using the standard Iterative Closest Point (ICP) algorithm in VTK (Fig. 2).

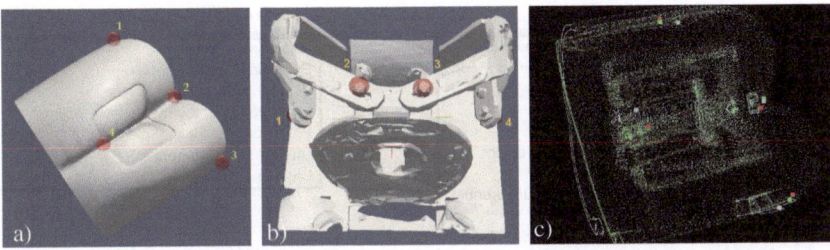

Fig. 2. 3D Surface models and landmarks of a) DRE and b) BVE benchtop models in VTK; c) Results of ICP landmark-based registration of DRE model are shown in green (mesh before registration in grey and landmarks from sensors in red).

Our framework allows real-time visualisation during recording, as well as retrospective playback of a DRE or BVE. 3D DRE models of a specific prostate type (N – normal, UB – unilateral benign, BB – bilateral benign, UC – unilateral carcinoma, BC – bilateral carcinoma) or 3D BVE models may be loaded and registered. A 3D mesh representation of the examining finger is shown for visual purposes only and it is translated and rotated according to the position sensor, as well as colour-coded to indicate the amount of pressure recorded by the relevant pressure sensor at that particular anatomical location. A real-time pressure plot indicates the applied pressure at each time point (Fig. 3).

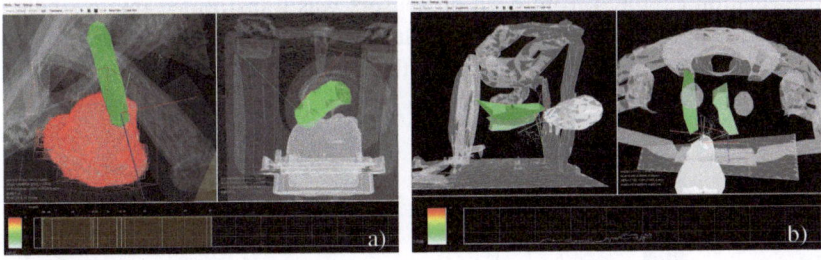

Fig. 3. a) DRE with a unilateral carcinoma prostate (left - prostate with collision detection tree). b) BVE model with a position sensor embedded in the movable uterus, index and middle fingers.

2.3   Task Decomposition and Annotation

During playback, the pressure plot is used to label/annotate all relevant steps pertaining to the internal stage of DRE and BVE (Table 1) by selecting the initial and finishing time intervals of each task. These labels were then used to compute a series of properties (see section 2.4): duration, anatomical coverage, finger(s) orientation, and palpation primitives. The annotated tasks form the cornerstone of our data analysis.

Table 1. *Left*: physical and sensorial tasks for the internal examination stage during DRE [8]. *Right*: palpation and discrete finger movement examination tasks for BVE [9].

Task	DRE task	Task	BVE task (discrete sections)
23	Position pad of right index finger on anus	4	Insertion of fingers
24	Apply gentle pressure with finger pad on anus for a few seconds	5	Examination of the cervix
		6	Test for cervical excitation
26	Insert finger with pad posteriorly	7	Examination of the uterus
27	Assessment of sphincter tone	8	Palpation of adnexae
28	Insert finger beyond sphincter into rectum	9	Uterosacral ligaments
29	Coccyx is reached	10	Closing
32	Rectal wall palpation: start circumferential palpation at level of coccyx		
33	Rectal wall palpation: systematic, full 360 degree sweep		
34	Prostate palpation		
45	Remove finger		

2.4   Task Properties

For simplicity and due to space constraints, we only describe the properties obtained for the DRE tasks as an example of the type of properties that may be generated with our framework. Using Dickinson's subdivision of the prostate [10], together with position tracking data of a 7mm-radius sphere representation of the fingertip (centre located 7mm under the nail) and a collision detection algorithm based on an Axis Aligned Bounding Box (AABB) tree representation of the prostate, it is possible to label each triangle of the 3D mesh during playback as it is palpated, according to the region to which it belongs. Each region was assigned a state (normal, enlarged or carcinoma) according to the type of prostate being examined and its location. Quaternion information captured from position sensors was transformed into a single scalar representing finger orientation [-90,90] during palpation by computing the cross product of the tangent of the sensor data to the normal of the triangle (see Fig. 4).

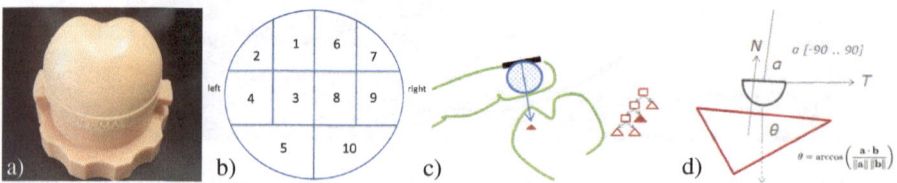

Fig. 4. a) DRE benchtop model (normal prostate). b) Region labelling. c) Collision detection between finger and prostate. d) Finger orientation obtained during collision detection based on the normal of colliding triangles and tangent vectors computed from sensor quaternion data.

The rectum was subdivided in a similar way based on finger orientation and insertion depth, with location data represented in polar coordinates (Fig. 5).

Palpation primitives refer to the fundamental elements of finger movement. They include: a) abduction/adduction, b) flexion/extension, c) supination/pronation and d) compliance. These primitives describe tasks during internal examination [8,9] and are inferred from position data. By computing the frequency of occurrence of palpation primitives (rectum and prostate), we expect to correlate frequencies with examination styles across models and experts (Table 2).

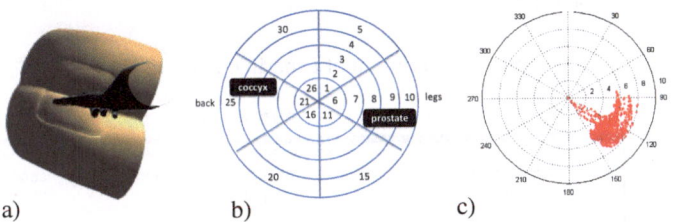

a)   b)   c)

Fig. 5. Subdivision of the rectum: a) DRE benchtop model with a finger pointing downwards (180°) just before insertion (0cm). b) 30 regions defined in polar coordinates based on finger orientation (sectors subdivision every 60°) and insertion depth (concentric rings every 2cm). c) An example of an examination performed by a urologist.

Table 2. Computing frequency of palpation primitives for the prostate (abduction/adduction, flexion/extension, compliance) and for the rectum (supination/pronation and compliance)

	Definition	**Frequency**
Abduction/Adduction	Lateral movement between adjacent regions (Fig. 4b)	On occurrence while palpating adjacent regions
Flexion/Extension	Upward and downward movement between adjacent regions belonging to the base (1,2,6,7), mid (3,4,8,9) and apex (5,10) sections of the prostate	On occurrence while palpating adjacent regions
Supination/Pronation	Movement relative to the orientation of the finger/hand	When the hand is rotated ± 45° (Fig. 5b)
Compliance	Movement related to the exertion of forces in a single region	When the standardised pressure is ≥1 standard deviation of applied pressure

2.5   Experimental Studies

Three different experimental studies (Table 3) were designed to develop and validate the use of our visualisation and analysis tool: a) DRE on a benchtop model, b) BVE on a benchtop model and c) BVE on GTAs (Fig. 6). Ethics approval was obtained from the NHS National Patient Safety Agency Research Ethics Committee.

The aim of the first study (DRE on benchtop model) was to establish an adequate sensor calibration protocol, validate the registration process, and assess the quality of the recorded data. It also allowed us to integrate the annotation of CTA-based tasks, validate the collision model of the prostate and devise an analysis pipeline. The purpose of the second study (BVE on benchtop model) was to extend our framework to

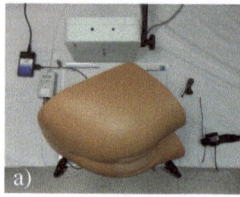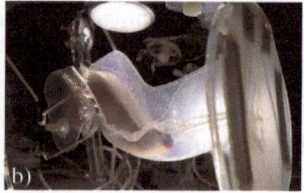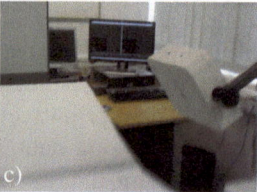

Fig. 6. Experimental setup. a) DRE benchtop model. b) Internal view of bespoke BVE benchtop model. c) BVE on GTAs.

Table 3. Description of experimental studies

	DRE benchtop	BVE benchtop	BVE on GTAs
Subjects	N, UB, BB, UC, BC[1]	Movable uterus and ovaries	4 GTAs
Participants	1 colorectal consultant	10 gynaecology consultants	2 gynaecology consultants
Examinations	2 per subject	2 per subject	1 per subject
Total	10	20	8
Position sensors	internal (1)	internal (2)	internal (2)
		uterus (1)	external (2)
Pressure sensors	internal (1)	internal (2)	internal (2)
			external (3)

[1] Prostate types: normal (N), unilateral benign (UB), bilateral benign (BB), unilateral carcinoma (UC), bilateral carcinoma (BC)

multiple position and pressure sensors, including a position sensor to track the movement of the uterus. The intention of the third study (BVE on GTAs) was to pilot the use of our framework on real subjects.

3   Results

In order to compare pressure across experiments, the pressure data was normalised using a sample version of the Z-score to compute an estimate for the number of standard deviations a given pressure is from the mean. IBM SPSS Statistics was used to obtain descriptive statistics and run univariate ANOVA tests.

3.1   DRE on a Benchtop Model

Regarding pressure, we found no significant differences between the average standardised pressures applied to normal, enlarged or carcinoma regions across prostates. A significant difference ($p<.01$) was found between the average standardised pressure applied to normal ($\mu=-0.03$) and carcinoma ($\mu=0.48$) regions of the UC prostate type.

When comparing across tasks (Table 1), task 34 (prostate palpation) exhibited the highest average standardised pressure as well as the largest variability ($\mu=0.52$, $\sigma=0.81$). Large variability was also observed during task 33 (rectum palpation – $\mu=-0.78$, $\sigma=0.57$), task 26 (finger insertion – $\mu=-0.55$, $\sigma=0.59$) and task 45 (finger removal – $\mu=-0.64$, $\sigma=0.62$). In terms of average duration, task 34 took twice as long as task 33, with an average 60% of the prostate being palpated against only 35% of the rectum.

With respect to movement primitives during prostate palpation (Table 2), on average, abduction/adduction and compliance were done the most in the BC prostate (10 and 3 times, respectively), whilst flexion/extension was done the most in BB and UC prostates (8 times). Related to the rectum, we studied movement primitives for the whole examination based on polar coordinates (Fig. 5b). On average, supination was performed the most during UB examinations (19.5 times), whilst compliance was performed the most during UB and UC examinations (5.5 and 4.5 times respectively).

3.2   BVE on a Benchtop Model

The use of multiple sensors allowed us to study the behaviour of the fingers, as well as the movement of the uterus during the examination. On average, the distance between the position tracking sensors of the internal examining fingers was the closest during task 7 (palpating the uterus – 32.37mm), with a slight increase during task 5 (palpating the cervix – 37mm) and task 8 (palpating the adnexae – 38.98mm). The smallest average distance between the sensor in the uterus and the sensor in the index finger was during task 7 (μ=33.38mm) followed by task 5 (μ=35.11mm).

Regarding the movement of the uterus, the sensor in the uterus moved on average the most during task 5 within a distance of 23.73mm (pull/push), 26.51mm (upward/downward) and 19.14mm (sideways), whilst it moved in a reduced space during task 7 within an average distance of 18.6mm, 22.3mm and 16.33mm, respectively. Considering the initial position of the sensor in the uterus, the uterus was pushed a maximum distance of 27.16mm and lifted a maximum distance of 10.43mm during task 5, compared to 26.72mm and 12.44mm during task 7.

3.3   BVE on GTAs

We studied the behaviour of the fingers of both hands and the pressure applied during examination of real subjects. The average distance between the sensors on the external fingers (index and middle) during task 5 was 24.8mm, whilst the average distance between the sensors on the internal fingers was 49.6mm, and between the sensors on the index fingers of both hands was 159.1mm. During task 7, we observed that the palpation of the uterus was occasionally performed with one finger. When two fingers were used, the minimum distance was 22.96mm. The external average distance was 22.6mm, whilst the average distance between the hands was 116.3mm. During task 8, the average distances were 22.27mm, 36.59mm and 94.76mm.

Regarding pressure, the average standardised pressure measured by the sensors on the ring, middle and index fingers of the external hand during task 5 was -0.73, -0.64, -0.59, whilst the standardised pressure recorded on the index and middle fingers of the examining hand was, on average, -0.18 and -0.14. During task 7, the average standardised pressures were 0.53, 0.24, 0.31 for the external hand, and 0.16 and -0.18 for the examining hand. During task 8, the average standardised pressures were 0.72, 0.82, 0.63 for the external hand, and 0.66 and 0.87 for the examining hand. A significant difference (p<.01) was found between the averages of these five pressure sensors during task 5 (μ=-0.46), task 7 (μ=0.21) and task 8 (μ=0.74).

4   Discussion and Conclusions

We have developed a framework for visualisation and analysis of internal examinations through real-time continuous position and pressure sensor data. Findings from three studies confirm our hypothesis of enabling better understanding and assessment of DRE and BVE by unveiling the unseen through playback and analysis of task-based information that includes quantitative measures such as pressure, duration, finger position and orientation, and movement primitives.

DRE on a benchtop model – the fact that a significant difference was only found between the average pressure applied to normal and carcinoma regions of the UC prostate type suggests that the pressure applied to normal and enlarged regions is within a similar range. The potential of using movement primitives to better understand and analyse palpation patterns has been illustrated by the different frequency of such primitives depending on prostate type.

BVE on a benchtop model – the use of multiple sensors allows the observation and study of the behaviour of internal fingers during the examination, as well as movement of the uterus. Coordinated bimanual interaction when lifting the uterus resulted in a small distance between fingers and between fingers and the uterus. Also, during palpation of adnexae, the internal fingers appear to slightly separate in order to lift the adnexae and be able to palpate them externally. Results also suggest that the uterus is not only lifted, but also pushed during bimanual interaction.

BVE on GTAs – a similar behaviour of internal and external fingers was observed on real subjects, together with a reduction in the distance between hands for tasks 5, 7 and 8 (larger to smaller). Average standardised pressure was significantly different across these tasks, with the highest pressure applied during adnexae palpation. This variation in pressure applied and finger behaviour suggests that different palpation patterns are used when examining the uterus, cervix and adnexae.

Compared to other studies, our approach allows us to understand pressure applied to specific organs continuously, as well as the movement of examining fingers throughout the examination. There is significant potential for our framework to be used as a teaching and learning tool for unsighted examinations, offering trainees detailed feedback, allowing them to see what the trainers are doing, and allowing the trainers to objectively assess performance during a DRE or BVE.

Future work includes recruiting more participants from specialities that typically conduct DRE in order to investigate differences in performance and emphasis. A study on human subjects (Rectal Teaching Assistance) will follow. Further studies using a linear progression model will allow us to correlate quantitative task properties with adequate and competent performance for both DRE and BVE.

References

1. Bharucha, A.E., Rao, S.S.: An Update on Anorectal Disorders for Gastroenterologists. Gastroenterology 146, 37–45 (2014)
2. Wong, R.K., et al.: The digital rectal examination: a multicenter survey of physician's and students' perceptions and practice patterns. Am J Gastroenterol 107, 1157–1163 (2012)
3. American Cancer Society. Prostate Cancer: Early Detection (2013)
4. Henderson, J.T., Harper, C.C., Gutin, S., et al.: Routine bimanual pelvic examinations: practices and beliefs of US obstetrician-gynecologists. Am. J. Obstet. Gynecol. 208, 109.e1-7 (2013)
5. Balkissoon, R., et al.: Lost in translation: unfolding medical students' misconceptions of how to perform a clinical digital rectal examination. Am. J. of Surg. 197(4), 525–532 (2009)
6. Wang, N., et al.: Using a prostate exam simulator to decipher palpation techniques. Simulation in healthcare. Journal of the Society for Simulation in Healthcare 5(3), 60–152 (2010)
7. Pugh, C.: Use of a Mechanical Simulator to Assess Pelvic Examination Skills. JAMA: The Journal of the American Medical Association 286(9), 1021-a-1023 (2001)
8. Low-Beer, N., et al.: Hidden practice revealed: using task analysis and novel simulator design to evaluate the teaching of digital rectal examination. AJS 201(1), 46–53 (2011)
9. Gale, C.: Can a CTA be developed that is likely to be useful for teaching vaginal examination? MEd in Surg. Edu. Thesis. Imperial College London, Faculty of Medicine (2012)
10. Dickinson, L., et al.: MRI for the detection, localisation, and characterisation of prostate cancer. European urology 59(4), 477–494 (2011)

Tracing Retinal Blood Vessels by Matrix-Forest Theorem of Directed Graphs

Li Cheng[1,3], Jaydeep De[1,2], Xiaowei Zhang[1], Feng Lin[2], and Huiqi Li[4]

[1] Bioinformatics Institute, A*STAR, Singapore
[2] School of Computer Engineering, Nanyang Technological University, Singapore
[3] School of Computing, National University of Singapore, Singapore
[4] Beijing Institute of Technology, China

Abstract. This paper aims to trace retinal blood vessel trees in fundus images. This task is far from being trivial as the *crossover* of vessels are commonly encountered in image-based vessel networks. Meanwhile it is often crucial to separate the vessel tree structures in applications such as diabetic retinopathy analysis. In this work, a novel directed graph based approach is proposed to cast the task as label propagation over directed graphs, such that the graph is to be partitioned into disjoint sub-graphs, or equivalently, each of the vessel trees is traced and separated from the rest of the vessel network. Then the tracing problem is addressed by making novel usage of the matrix-forest theorem in algebraic graph theory. Empirical experiments on synthetic as well as publicly available fundus image datasets demonstrate the applicability of our approach.

1 Introduction

Topological and geometrical properties of retinal blood vessels in fundus images can provide valuable clinical information in diagnosing diseases. In particular, vascular anomaly in retina is one of the clinical manifestations of retinal diseases such as diabetic retinopathy, glaucoma, and hypertensive retinopathy. Take diabetic retinopathy as an example, it is a leading cause of blindness in the working-age population of most developed countries. Diabetic retinopathy is the result of progressive damage to the network of tiny blood vessels that supply blood to the retina. Proliferative diabetic retinopathy is specifically characterized by the formation of newly formed vessels in the retina [1]. This thus requires the description of blood vessel tree structure in clinical diagnosis, and as a result, calls for the tracing and separation of each vessel tree in the fundus images.

Existing efforts in retinal vessel analysis can be roughly categorized into segmentation-based and tracking-based. The segmentation-based methods (e.g.[2]) often use pixel classification to produce a binary segmentation (i.e a pixel is classified into vessel or non-vessel). The tracking-based methods (e.g. [3]) usually start with a seed, and track the intended vessel based on local intensity or texture information. Segmentation-based methods tend to produce many disconnected and isolated segments, less favourable for retaining the important

P. Golland et al. (Eds.): MICCAI 2014, Part I, LNCS 8673, pp. 626–633, 2014.
© Springer International Publishing Switzerland 2014

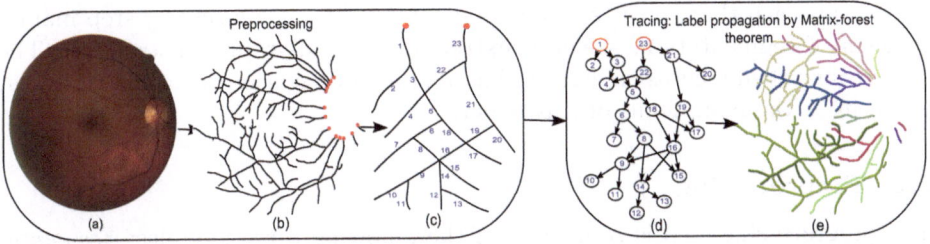

Fig. 1. Overview of our tracing pipeline where our focus is the tracing step

topological properties of vessel networks. Meanwhile vessel tracking methods often better preserve the connectivity structure of vessel segments. Nonetheless they encounter great difficulties with the occurrence of *crossover* at the junction points. Current methods often fail to trace properly, as it is nontrivial to predict whether the vessel segments at a junction point belong to one tree or multiple trees, and for the later case, to which tree each segment belongs. In this paper, we dedicate our attention to addressing this bottleneck *crossover* issue.

We consider a different tracing approach that can take into account both local and global contextual information of the vessel network, as summarized below: After initial pixel-based segmentation and skeleton extraction, a novel *directed graph* (or digraph) representation is formed, where each segment in the skeleton map becomes a node, and a direct contact between two adjacent segments corresponds to an edge of the two corresponding nodes. The segments in the skeleton map touching the optic disk area are considered as the root nodes. The number of trees to-be-found in the the vessel network thus equals the number of root nodes. The tracing problem is now formulated as label propagation on directed graphs or digraphs: The goal is to propagate tree labels from known root nodes to the rest of the graph, such that the digraph will be split into disjoint sub-graphs, which corresponds to trees of the vessel network. This allows us to consider and make novel usage of the recent development of matrix-forest theorem [4] studied in algebraic digraph theory.

In term of major contributions, our approach offers a principled way of addressing the tracing with crossover problem. By connecting to the well-established algebraic directed graph theory [4], local and global contextual information can be both considered explicitly. We expect the digraph theoretical representation can open the door to some insightful understanding of the characteristics of crossover sections in vessel networks. Finally, our algorithm is also simple and easy to implement.

2   Our Approach

The problem of vessel tracing is to trace blood vessels by separating them into disjoint vessel trees, each starting from a unique root segment within the optic disk, as illustrated in red dots at Figure 1(b). Figure 1 describes the pipeline of our approach that consists of *two* main steps: The *preprocessing* step mainly consists of segmentation, skeleton extraction, and digraph construction; The *tracing* step then focuses on digraph-based label propagation using Matrix-forest theorem — the main focus of this paper.

2.1 Preprocessing

The preprocessing step is comprised of the following three modules: *Segmentation*: As illustrated in Figure 1 (a)→(b), an input retinal image is segmented into a binary image, with vessel pixels being foreground and the rest as background. Note this step is skipped for synthetic retinal images as they are already binary images. *Skeleton map*: Build a skeleton map from the binary image, and remove the optic disk area as marked within red ellipse in Figure 1(b). The cusps attached to the removed optic disk are the tips of root segments, which are also presented as red dots in Figure 1(c), a zoom-in subset of (b). *Skeleton to digraph*: A segment is defined in the skeleton as the group of connected pixels that ends in either a junction or a tip. This segment corresponds to a node in the resulting digraph, as shown in Figure 1(c)→(d). Two nodes are then linked with a directed edge, when the two coinciding segments from the skeleton map contact and satisfy the ordering criteria, a modification of the well-known stream ordering method from the hydrology community (http://en.wikipedia.org/wiki/Strahler_number). More details can be found at our previous work [5].

2.2 Tracing by Matrix-Forest Theorem on Digraphs

The tracing problem becomes that of separating the vessel trees with only tree roots known, which can be equivalently formulated as a digraph-based label propagation problem with one labeled node per class (vessel tree). That is, all the source nodes are labeled in this problem, each with a unique label (tree), and the task is to make predictions on the remaining unlabeled nodes by propagating the class labels following the underlying digraph structure.

Problem Set-up. Let $G = (\mathcal{V}, \mathcal{E}, W)$ denote a digraph, where $\mathcal{V} = \{v_1, v_2, \ldots v_n\}$ is the set of nodes, $\mathcal{E}$ the set of directed edges each connecting two adjacent nodes, and $W = [w_{ij}] \in \mathbb{R}^{n \times n}$ the asymmetric non-negative matrix with $w_{ij} \geq 0$ being the weight of the directed edge from v_i to v_j. The out-degree of each node v_i is computed as $d_i^+ = \sum_{j=1}^n w_{ij}$. Denote the out-degree matrix $D = \mathrm{Diag}(d_1^+, \cdots, d_n^+)$, that is, $D = \mathrm{Diag}(W\mathbf{1})$, with $\mathbf{1}$ an all-one column vector. Define the digraph Laplacian $L = D - W$. A row-stochastic transition probability matrix $P = [p_{ij}]$ can be constructed as $p_{ij} = \frac{w_{ij}}{d_i^+}$, or equivalently as $P = D^{-1}W$. Note undirected graphs can be regarded as special digraphs characterized algebraically by their symmetric weight matrix W, i.e. the symmetric pair w_{ij} & w_{ji} correspond to bi-directional edges with equal weights. We focus here on a transductive inference scenario where labels from the set of few labeled nodes $\mathcal{V}_l$ are to be propagated to the rest unlabeled nodes $\mathcal{V}_u$, with $\mathcal{V} = \mathcal{V}_l \cup \mathcal{V}_u$. The labels are multiclass, each corresponds to a separate vessel tree. To simplified the notation we assume $\mathcal{V}_l$ contains the first l nodes, $\mathcal{V}_l = \{v_1, \ldots, v_l\}$. To accommodate label information, define a label matrix Y of size $n \times K$ (assuming there are K class labels available), with each entry Y_{ik} containing 1 if node i belongs to $\mathcal{V}_l$ and is labeled with class k, and 0 otherwise. Also define the length n ground-truth label vector $\mathbf{y}$ that includes two disjoint parts $\mathbf{y}_l$ and $\mathbf{y}_u$: $\mathbf{y}_l$ is the input label vector of length l over the set of labeled nodes, with each entry y_i for the input class assignment of node $v_i \in \mathcal{V}_l$; $\mathbf{y}_u$ is the hold-out ground-truth label for the unlabeled nodes, i.e. a vector of length $n - l$. Similarly, define the initial label vector $\hat{\mathbf{y}}$ containing also two parts, $\hat{\mathbf{y}}_l := \mathbf{y}_l$ and $\hat{\mathbf{y}}_u = \mathbf{0}$, where $\mathbf{0}$ is an all-zero vector of length $n - l$. Define the prediction vector $\mathbf{y}^*$ with also two parts $\mathbf{y}_l^* := \mathbf{y}_l$, as well as $\mathbf{y}_u^*$ of length $n - l$, containing the prediction results, where each y_i^* denotes the predicted class assignment for a node $v_i \in \mathcal{V}_u$.

The proposed label propagation algorithm (shown in Algorithm 1 and referred to as MFTD) is derived based on matrix-forest theorem [4] of algebraic digraph theory [6], as follows. Let w_{max} denote the entry in W containing the strongest signal, i.e. $w_{\max} = \max_{i,j} |w_{ij}|$. The forest matrix is defined as

$$S_1 := (I + \alpha L)^{-1}, \tag{1}$$

a normalized forest matrix where each (i, j)-th entry denotes the number of trees rooted at node i that also include the j-th node, as in Theorem 4 of [4]. It can be viewed as a generalization of the celebrated matrix-tree theorem (e.g. [7]) for undirected graphs to digraphs. Further, let $\tilde{L} := \lim_{\alpha \to \infty} (I + \alpha L)^{-1}$, which is a matrix of normalized spanning forests. Both S_1 and $\tilde{L}$ has a number of interesting properties [8]: Each entry of both matrices is non-negative, and both matrices are row-stochastic; $\tilde{L}$ resides in the null space of digraph Laplacian L, as $L\tilde{L} = \tilde{L}L = 0$; $\text{rank}(L) = n - \text{rank}(\tilde{L})$; $L + \beta\tilde{L}$ is non-singular for any $\beta > 0$, and is the "complementary perturbation of L" [9]. Indeed, this brings forward the second forest matrix,

$$S_2 := (L + \beta\tilde{L})^{-1}, \tag{2}$$

which is also termed the matrix of dense forest in [4]. As presented in what follows, varying the preprocessing schemes of normalizing W, we have two variants: MFTD$_a$ starts with a preprocessing effort to normalize W, $W \leftarrow \frac{W}{w_{\max}}$; MFTD$_b$ considers a different normalization of W as $W \leftarrow D^{-1}W$ instead, i.e. $P = W$.

Proposition 1. *Under normalization scheme of $W \leftarrow D^{-1}W$, the forest matrix becomes $S_1 = (1 - \tau)(I - \tau P)^{-1}$, with $\tau = \frac{\alpha}{1+\alpha}$.*

When applied on the second forest matrix S_2 using (2), this clearly leads to two additional variants that are denoted as MFTD$_c$ & MFTD$_d$, respectively.

One can interpret the (i, j)-th entry S_{ij} of the forest matrix S (being either $S := S_1$ or $S := S_2$) as quantifying the accessibility of a particle from a node v_i to visit node v_j along the digraph structure. This provides a notion of affinity from state i to j. The intuition is, if a state j is close to the initial state i in terms of graph structure, it will be visited by the particle more often than if it is far away from initial state, i.e., we visit our close relatives more often than our

Algorithm 1. Label Propagation by Matrix-Forest Theorem of Digraphs (MFTD)

Input: A digraph $G = (\mathcal{V}, \mathcal{E}, W)$, label information Y, $\mathbf{y}_l$, and $\alpha \in (0, 1)$.
Output: $\mathbf{y}_u^*$
Compute the out-degree matrix D.
Compute the affinity matrix by $A = SY$ and (1) (or (2)).
Predict $\mathbf{y}_u^*$: Compute the i-th entry by (3), for any unlabeled node $v_i \in \mathcal{V}_u$.

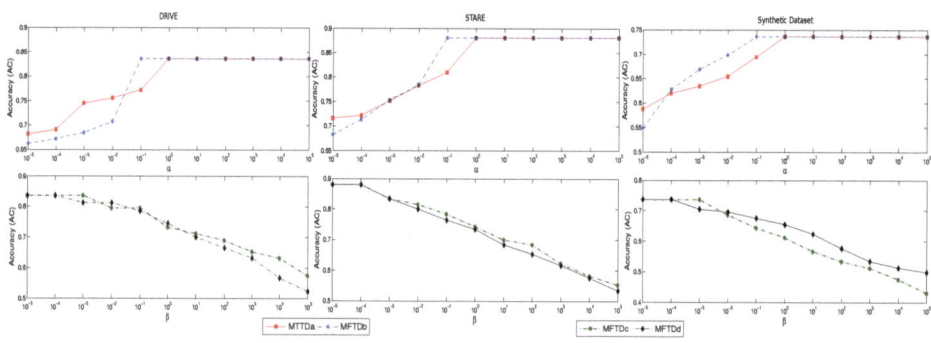

Fig. 2. Performance (AC) as a function of varying α or β of MFTD$_{a-d}$

distant ones. Now define the affinity matrix as $A = SY$, a matrix of size $n \times K$, with each entry a_{ik} being associated with an affinity score of state i belonging to class k. To infer $\mathbf{y}_u^*$ of the unlabeled states $\mathcal{V}_u$, our algorithm predicts each entry's class assignment by identifying a label with the largest affinity score,

$$\mathbf{y}_i^* = \arg\max_k a_{ik}, \qquad \forall v_i \in \mathcal{V}_u. \tag{3}$$

PAC-Bayesian Label-propagation Bound. We report an investigation of the generalization bound of our approach on unseen data, which is an adaptation of [10]. We start by reformulating our algorithm (i.e. both (1) and (2)) as an equivalent representation $\mathbf{h} = S\hat{\mathbf{y}}$, where $\hat{\mathbf{y}}$ is the initial label vector with partial labels $\hat{y}_i \in \{\pm 1\}$ for $v_i \in \mathcal{V}_l$, and $\hat{y}_i = 0$ otherwise. The obtained $\mathbf{h}$ is the "soft" label vector with h_i being the "soft" label for node v_i, which will be assigned with class label sign(h_i) when making predictions. The hypothesis space is defined as $\mathcal{H} := \left\{ \mathbf{h} \mid \mathbf{h} = S\hat{\mathbf{y}}, \|\hat{\mathbf{y}}\|_2 \leq \sqrt{l} \right\}$. For any label vector $\mathbf{h}$, define the *test error* as $\mathcal{L}_{l,n}(\mathbf{h}) := \frac{1}{n-l} \sum_{i=l+1}^{n} \ell(h_i, y_i)$ w.r.t. its 0/1 loss function ℓ satisfying $\ell(h_i, y_i) = 1$ if $h_i \neq y_i$ and 0 otherwise, and let the *empirical error* of $\mathbf{h}$ be $\hat{\mathcal{L}}_{l,n}(\mathbf{h}) := \frac{1}{l} \sum_{i=1}^{l} \ell(h_i, y_i)$.

Theorem 1. *For any $\delta \in (0, 1)$, with probability at lest $1 - \delta$ over random draws of $\mathcal{V}_l$ from $\mathcal{V}$, the following bound holds for any $\mathbf{h} \in \mathcal{H}$*

$$\mathcal{L}_{l,n}(\mathbf{h}) \leq \hat{\mathcal{L}}_{l,n}(\mathbf{h}) + \sqrt{\left(\frac{2\hat{\mathcal{L}}_{l,n}(\mathbf{h})n}{n-l}\right) \frac{ln\frac{1}{\delta} + 7ln(n+1)}{l-1}} + \frac{2\left(ln\frac{1}{\delta} + 7ln(n+1)\right)}{l-1}.$$

Table 1. Comparison with leading label propagation methods. See text for details.

Synthetic Dataset

	CDRN	WVRN	CTK$_d$	CTK$_u$	SGL	MFTD
AC	0.63	0.65	0.63	0.71	0.71	0.74
DS	0.62	0.62	0.61	0.68	0.64	0.71

DRIVE [11]

	CDRN	WVRN	CTK$_d$	CTK$_u$	SGL	MFTD
AC	0.69	0.67	0.73	0.79	0.76	0.83
DS	0.68	0.64	0.72	0.74	0.75	0.77

STARE [12]

	CDRN	WVRN	CTK$_d$	CTK$_u$	SGL	MFTD
AC	0.71	0.73	0.75	0.83	0.79	0.88
DS	0.68	0.69	0.74	0.78	0.76	0.82

3   Experiments

Our approach is evaluated in our in-house synthetic dataset[1], as well as two
testbeds, DRIVE [11] and STARE [12]. The synthetic dataset contains $17,000$
synthesized retinal images with varying densities of blood vessels. Meanwhile,
DRIVE dataset contains 40 retinal fundus images, and STARE has 20 fundus
images. Exemplar images of the three datasets are illustrated in Figure 3.

Our approach is compared with the following label propagation methods:
Class Distribution Relational Neighbor classifier (CDRN) [13], Weighted Vote
Relational Neighbor classifier (WVRN) [13], Digraph variant of the Commute
Time Kernel classifier (CTK$_d$), and the original Commute Time Kernel classifier for undirected graphs (CTK$_u$) [14], and Symmetrized Graph Laplacian
(SGL) [15]. To summarize, CTK$_u$ is an undirected graph-based method, CTK$_d$,
SGL, and the proposed MFTD are digraph-based methods, while the rest methods are not graph-theoretical. To ensure fair evaluations, the internal parameters
of the comparison methods are either set to as is from the authors' original source
code, or as suggested in the papers. In terms of evaluation metric, the micro-
averaged accuracy (AC)is utilized, which is the sum of all true positive counts
divided by the total number of instances. Besides, the DIADEM score (DS) [16]
is also employed, being a dedicated measure that has been widely used by the
biological tracing community.

Effect of Varying α (or β) of Our Approach. Our first experiment is to evaluate the effect of varying the value of our algorithmic parameter, namely α in
MFTD$_{a-b}$, or β in MFTD$_{c-d}$. This is performed on all three datasets. As presented in Figure 2, the performance (AC) is displayed as a function of varying
parameter value (α in row 1 & β in row 2) of our proposed algorithms MFTD$_{a-d}$,
with x-axis being in log-scale. Surprisingly, all four variants of our MFTD framework produces exactly the same results when $\alpha \geq 1$ and $\beta \leq 10^{-4}$, which is also

---

[1] Downloadable at `http://web.bii.a-star.edu.sg/~jaydeepd/tracing.htm`

verified under the AC criterion as in the figure. This is very interesting as despite their differences in algebraic forms and graph-theoretical interpretations, effectively these variants are *equivalent* characterized by their ability of tracing retinal blood vessels. To avoid redundancies, we will collectively refer to the performance of all these four variants as MFTD, and fix $\alpha = 1$ and $\beta = 10^{-4}$ during the rest experiments.

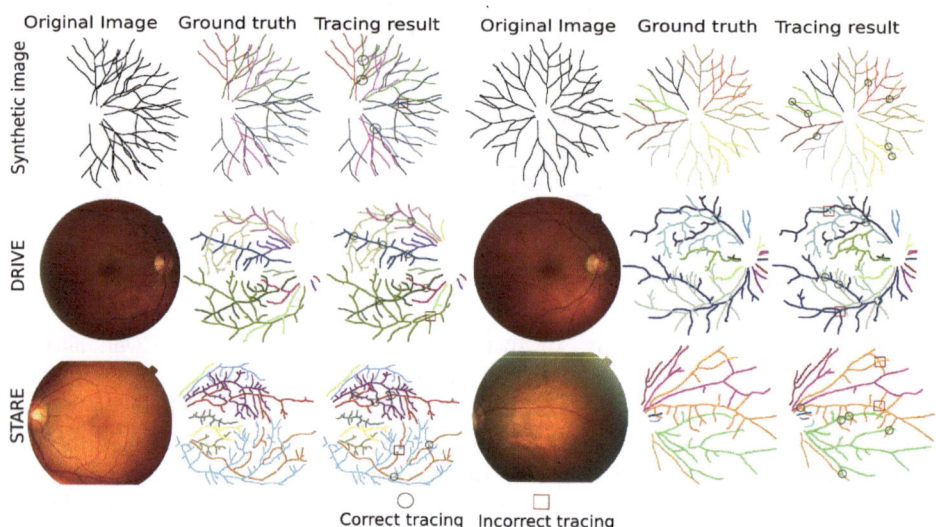

Fig. 3. Each row presents two exemplar retinal tracing results on Synthetic dataset, DRIVE, and STARE, respectively. Segments with the same color form a distinct vessel tree. Thus the number of colors equal to the number of classes (vessel trees). Selected correct (wrong) tracing segments are shown in green circles (red squares).

Comparison with the State-of-the-art Label Propagation Methods. The performance of our approach is evaluated on three scenarios and is compared with nine label propagation methodsas reported in Table 1.Overall our approach consistently outperforms the other methods by a large margin. The second best performer is usually CTK_u, which are followed by SGL and CTK_d. To facilitate visual inspection, Figure 3 presents exemplar images and comparison results. It suggests that empirically our approach delivers visually plausible tracing results when comparing to the ground-truths side-by-side, and the errors occur at those challenging spots that are often also difficult for human observers.

Comparison with State-of-the-art Tracing Systems. We also compare with GOGP of [3] on DRIVE. DIADEM scores (DS) of the proposed MFTD on image no. 19 of DRIVE is 0.81, which is significantly higher than that of 0.71 obtained on the same image by [3]. We note in the passing that MFTD slightly outperforms the 0.765 of our earlier work [5], meanwhile we expect further gain would be achieved with the adoption of a better skeleton to digraph conversion.

4 Conclusion and Outlook

A novel approach is proposed for tracing vessels in fundus images. The tracing problem is solved by utilizing matrix-forest theorem of digraphs. Empirical evaluation demonstrates the superior performance of our approach. For future direction we plan to work with broader applications such as neurite tracing.

Acknowledgements. This research was partially supported by A*STAR JCO grants, as well as NSFC (No. 81271650) and NCET-10-0041.

References

1. Viswanath, K., McGavin, D.: Diabetic retinopathy: Clinical findings and management. Community Eye Health 16(46), 21–24 (2003)
2. Becker, C., Rigamonti, R., Lepetit, V., Fua, P.: Supervised feature learning for curvilinear structure segmentation. In: Mori, K., Sakuma, I., Sato, Y., Barillot, C., Navab, N. (eds.) MICCAI 2013, Part I. LNCS, vol. 8149, pp. 526–533. Springer, Heidelberg (2013)
3. Turetken, E., Gonzalez, G., Blum, C., Fua, P.: Automated reconstruction of dendritic and axonal trees by global optimization with geometric priors. Neuroinformatics 9, 279–302 (2011)
4. Agaev, R.P., Chebotarev, P.Y.: Spanning forests of a digraph and their applications. Automation and Remote Control 62(3), 443–466 (2001)
5. De, J., Li, H., Cheng, L.: Tracing retinal vessel trees by transductive inference. BMC Bioinformatics 15(20), 1–20 (2014)
6. Harary, F., Norman, R., Cartwright, D.: Structural models: an introduction to the theory of directed graphs. Wiley (1965)
7. Brualdi, R., Ryser, H.: Combinatorial Matrix Theory. Cambridge Uni. Press (1991)
8. Chebotarev, P.Y., Agaev, R.P.: Forest matrices around the laplacian matrix. Linear Algebra and its Applications 356(1-3), 247–253 (2002)
9. Meyer, C., Stadelmaier, M.: Singular m-matrices and inverse positivity. Linear Algebra and its Applications 22, 139–156 (1978)
10. Derbeko, P., El-Yaniv, R., Meir, R.: Explicit learning curves for transduction and application to clustering and compression algorithms. J. Artif. Intell. Res. 22, 117–142 (2004)
11. Staal, J., Abramoff, M., Niemeijer, M., Viergever, M., van Ginneken, B.: Ridge based vessel segmentation in color images of the retina. IEEE Trans. Med. Imag. 23(4), 501–509 (2004)
12. Hoover, A., Kouznetsova, V., Goldbaum, M.: Locating blood vessels in retinal images by piecewise threshold probing of a matched filter response. IEEE Trans Med Imag 19(3), 203–210 (2000)
13. Macskassy, S., Provost, F.: Classification in networked data: A toolkit and a univariate case study. JMLR 8, 935–983 (2007)
14. Fouss, F., Francoisse, K., Yen, L., Pirotte, A., Saerens, M.: An experimental investigation of kernels on graphs for collaborative recommendation and semisupervised classification. Neural Network 31, 53–72 (2012)
15. Zhou, D., Huang, J., Schölkopf, B.: Learning from labeled and unlabeled data on a directed graph. In: ICML (2005)
16. Gillette, T.A., Brown, K.M., Ascoli, G.A.: The diadem metric: comparing multiple reconstructions of the same neuron. Neuroinformatics 9(2-3), 233–245 (2011)

Learning Fully-Connected CRFs for Blood Vessel Segmentation in Retinal Images

José Ignacio Orlando[1,2,3] and Matthew Blaschko[1,4]

[1] Équipe Galen, INRIA Saclay, Île-de-France, France
[2] Consejo Nacional de Investigaciones Científicas y Técnicas, CONICET, Argentina
[3] Pladema Institute, UNCPBA, Argentina
[4] Center for Learning and Visual Computing, École Centrale Paris, France

Abstract. In this work, we present a novel method for blood vessel segmentation in fundus images based on a discriminatively trained, fully connected conditional random field model. Retinal image analysis is greatly aided by blood vessel segmentation as the vessel structure may be considered both a key source of signal, e.g. in the diagnosis of diabetic retinopathy, or a nuisance, e.g. in the analysis of pigment epithelium or choroid related abnormalities. Blood vessel segmentation in fundus images has been considered extensively in the literature, but remains a challenge largely due to the desired structures being thin and elongated, a setting that performs particularly poorly using standard segmentation priors such as a Potts model or total variation. In this work, we overcome this difficulty using a discriminatively trained conditional random field model with more expressive potentials. In particular, we employ recent results enabling extremely fast inference in a fully connected model. We find that this rich but computationally efficient model family, combined with principled discriminative training based on a structured output support vector machine yields a fully automated system that achieves results statistically indistinguishable from an expert human annotator. Implementation details are available at http://pages.saclay.inria.fr/matthew.blaschko/projects/retina/.

Keywords: Blood vessel segmentation, Fundus imaging, Conditional Random Fields, Structured Output SVM.

1 Introduction

Retinal images–also known as fundus images or retinographies–are projective color images of the inner surface of the human eye (Figure 1). They allow physicians to observe the retina and its internal parts, including the vascular tree, the optic disc, the fovea, etc. [1]. Retinal blood vessels provide useful information for several applications, including medical diagnosis and screening of ophthalmological and cardiovascular diseases. The vessels tortuosity, for instance, can be used to characterize hypertensive retinopathy, and the measurement of vessels diameter is utilized to diagnose hypertension [2]. Changes in the vasculature distribution are also interpreted as a possible symptom of diabetic retinopathy [1]. Moreover, vessels are used to assist laser surgeries [3] and as landmarks for image registration [4]. All these applications require the segmentation of the retinal vasculature. In current best practice, trained specialists delineate

P. Golland et al. (Eds.): MICCAI 2014, Part I, LNCS 8673, pp. 634–641, 2014.
© Springer International Publishing Switzerland 2014

the vessels manually, although this is a particularly tedious and time-consuming task. Difficulties in the imaging process–such as the inadequate contrast between vessels and background, and uneven background illumination–increase the variability among segmentations performed by different human observers. These facts motivate the development of automatic strategies for blood vessel segmentation without human intervention.

In the last two decades, several approaches have been introduced to solve this problem, but none of them have yet proved to be accurate enough to be assumed as a standard by the medical community [1]. These segmentation algorithms can be classified into two general categories, supervised and unsupervised. Supervised methods require a set of labeled training samples to learn a model. These samples are composed of pixels with known annotations and their features. Most of the effort in supervised segmentation involves finding new features for training, or better classifiers to perform the pixel classification task. For instance, Ricci and Perfetti [5] combine a linear support vector machine (SVM) with a line detector feature. Becker *et al.* [6] learn the features in a supervised way, based on a gradient boosting framework. Unsupervised methods usually involve systems based on clustering, region-oriented approaches [7, 8] or thresholding after vessel enhancement with filters [2, 9], line detectors [5, 10] or morphological operators [11]. More complex image processing operations have been combined with vessel centerline detection at different scales to obtain the final segmentation [11, 12]. The main advantage of unsupervised methods is that they do not need to be trained using manual annotations. However, they have reported worse results than supervised approaches [10].

Conditional Random Fields (CRFs) have been widely utilized to solve segmentation problems in several applications [13]. To the best of our knowledge, however, they have not been yet applied to retinal blood vessel segmentation in fundus images. This is likely due to that standard pairwise potentials such as in a Potts model assign a low prior to the elongated structures that comprise a vessel segmentation. We overcome this by using a much richer class of potentials.

The main contribution of our paper consists of an automatic method for blood vessels segmentation in retinal images based on fully-connected CRFs. We follow the efficient inference approach proposed in [14], and we learn its configuration in a supervised way, using a Structured Output SVM (SOSVM) [15]. We validate the approach on the main benchmark data set for vessel segmentation in fundus images, the DRIVE data set [16]. In contrast with several published works, no test data was utilized to adjust the parameters of the method. Instead, we randomly split the original training data into two subsets, one for training and the other for validation. Once we found the best configuration using the validation set, we applied it over the images in the test set. In this statistically principled setting, we report a fully-automated system that achieves a performance statistically indistinguishable from an expert human annotator.

The remainder of this paper is organized as follows: the formulation of the fully-connected CRF is described in Section 2; in Section 3 we explain how we learn the CRF model using a SOSVM. In Section 4 we include our results and a comparison against other state-of-the-art works. Finally, Section 5 concludes the paper.

2   Fully-Connected CRF Segmentation

We pose the segmentation task as an energy minimization problem in a fully-connected conditional random field (CRF). In the original definition of CRFs, images are mapped to graphs, where each pixel represents a node, and every node is connected with an edge to its immediate neighbors [13]. In the fully-connected version, each node is assumed to be a neighbor of every other. Following this approach the method is able to take into account not only neighboring information but also long-range interactions between pixels. This property improves the segmentation accuracy, but makes the inference process computationally expensive. Recently, however, Krähenbühl and Koltun [14] have introduced an efficient inference approach under the restriction that the pairwise potentials are a linear combination of Gaussian kernels over a Euclidean feature space. This approach, which is based on taking a mean field approximation of the original CRF, is able to provide accurate segmentations in less than a second.

We denote $\mathbf{y} = \{y_i\}$ as a labeling over all pixels of the image in the label space $\mathcal{L} = \{-1, 1\}$, where 1 is associated to blood vessels and -1 to any other class. Its corresponding energy function is given by the sum of its unary energy ψ_u and its pairwise energy ψ_p:

$$E(\mathbf{y}) = \sum_i \psi_u\left(y_i, \mathbf{x}_i\right) + \sum_{i<j} \psi_p\left(y_i, y_j, \mathbf{f}_i, \mathbf{f}_j\right) \tag{1}$$

where $\mathbf{x}_i$ and $\mathbf{f}_i$ are the unary and pairwise features, respectively. Unary potentials define a log-likelihood over the label assignment $\mathbf{y}$, and they are traditionally computed by a classifier [14]. Pairwise potentials define a similar distribution but considering only the interactions between pixels features and their labels. Parameters for both potentials are learned using a Structured Output SVM, as we explain in detail in Section 3.

Unary Potentials: We obtain the unary potentials according to the following expression:

$$\psi_u\left(y_i, \mathbf{x}_i\right) = -\langle \mathbf{w}_{u_{y_i}}, \mathbf{x}_i \rangle - \beta_{y_i} \tag{2}$$

where $\mathbf{w}_{u_{y_i}}$ is a weight vector and β_{y_i} is a bias term, respectively, both associated to the label y_i.

Pairwise Potentials: Following the restriction imposed by the inference approach we use, our pairwise potentials are obtained as follows:

$$\psi_p\left(y_i, y_j, \mathbf{f}_i, \mathbf{f}_j\right) = \mu(y_i, y_j) \sum_{m=1}^{M} w_p{}^{(m)} k^{(m)}\left(f_i^{(m)}, f_j^{(m)}\right) \tag{3}$$

where each $k^{(m)}$ is a Gaussian kernel over an arbitrary feature $f^{(m)}$, $w_p{}^{(m)}$ is a linear combination weight, and $\mu(y_i, y_j)$ represents a label compatibility function. In general, our pairwise kernels have the following form:

$$k^{(m)}\left(f_i^{(m)}, f_j^{(m)}\right) = \exp\left(-\frac{|\mathbf{p}_i - \mathbf{p}_j|^2}{2\theta_p^2} - \frac{\left|f_i^{(m)} - f_j^{(m)}\right|^2}{2\theta_{(m)}^2}\right) \tag{4}$$

where $\mathbf{p_i}$ and $\mathbf{p_j}$ are the coordinate vectors of pixels i and j. We include positions in order to increase the effect of close pixels over distant ones. Parameters θ_p and $\theta_{(m)}$ control the degree of relevance of the two parts of the kernels into the expression. The scale value $\theta_{(m)}$ is estimated as the median of the distances over pairs $(f_i^{(m)}, f_j^{(m)})$ [17]. In the same way, θ_p is obtained using $f^{(m)} = \mathbf{p}$. The compatibility function μ is given by the Potts model, $\mu(y_i, y_j) = [y_i \neq y_j]$. It penalizes nearby similar pixels that are assigned to different labels.

3   Learning CRF's Parameters Using Structured Output SVM

Our goal is to learn a vector $\mathbf{w} = (\mathbf{w}_u, \mathbf{w}_\beta, \mathbf{w}_p)$, where $\mathbf{w}_u$, $\mathbf{w}_\beta$ and $\mathbf{w}_p$ are the weights for the unary features, for the bias term and for the pairwise kernels, respectively. We obtain it in a supervised way, using the 1-slack formulation of the Structured Output SVM with margin-rescaling presented in [15].

Let the training set $S = \{(s^{(1)}, y^{(1)}), ..., (s^{(n)}, y^{(n)})\}$, where n is the number of training images. Each $y^{(i)}$ corresponds to the ground truth of the i-th image in the training set. Each set $s^{(i)} = \{x^{(i)}, B, f^{(i)}\}$ contains the set $x^{(i)}$ of unary feature vectors, a bias constant B, and the set $f^{(i)}$ of pairwise features for every pixel in the image.

The weights $\mathbf{w}$ are obtained by solving:

$$\min_{\mathbf{w}, \xi \geq 0} \frac{1}{2} \|\mathbf{w}\|^2 + C\xi \tag{5}$$

$$\text{s.t.} \forall \left(\bar{y}^{(1)}, ..., \bar{y}^{(n)} \right) : \sum_{i=1}^{n} \langle \mathbf{w}, \varphi(s^{(i)}, y^{(i)}) - \varphi(s^{(i)}, \bar{y}^{(i)}) \rangle \geq \sum_{i=1}^{n} \Delta(y^{(i)}, \bar{y}^{(i)}) - \xi$$

where C is a regularization constant; ξ is a slack variable shared across all the constraints $\bar{y}^{(i)}$; $\varphi(s, y)$ is a feature map function that relates a given set s with a given labeling y; and $\Delta(y, \bar{y})$ is a loss function that evaluates the difference between a ground truth y and a constraint $\bar{y}$. In this work, we define Δ as the typical Hamming loss:

$$\Delta(y, \bar{y}) = \sum_{i} [y_i \neq \bar{y}_i] \tag{6}$$

Our feature map is defined as follows:

$$\varphi(s, y) = \left(\sum_{k} \varphi_u(\mathbf{x}_k, y_k), \sum_{k} \varphi_\beta(B, y_k), \sum_{k} \sum_{j<k} \varphi_p(y_k, y_j, \mathbf{f_k}, \mathbf{f_j}) \right) \tag{7}$$

where the components represent the sum of the unary feature map, the bias feature map and the pairwise feature map, respectively, for all the pixels in the image. We make precise the definitions of φ_u, φ_β, and φ_p in the sequel.

We define a binary vector $\varphi_y(y_i) \in \{0, 1\}^{|\mathcal{L}|}$ such that:

$$\varphi_y(y_i) \begin{cases} (1, 0) \text{ if } y_i = -1 \\ (0, 1) \text{ if } y_i = 1 \end{cases} \tag{8}$$

The individual feature maps are obtained as follows:

$$\varphi_u(\mathbf{x}_k, y_k) = \mathbf{x}_k \otimes \varphi_y(y_k) \qquad (9)$$

$$\varphi_\beta(B, y_i) = B\varphi_y(y_i) \qquad (10)$$

$$\forall m : [\varphi_p(y_k, y_j, \mathbf{f}_k, \mathbf{f}_j)]_m = \mu(y_i, y_j)k^{(m)}(f_i^{(m)}, f_j^{(m)}) \qquad (11)$$

where $\otimes$ is the Kronecker product. Eq. (5) is solved using a cutting-plane approach [15].

4   Validation and Results

We validate our method using the publicly available data set DRIVE [16]. DRIVE is widely utilized in the state-of-the-art to quantify blood vessel segmentation performance. The data set is divided into two sets: one for training and one for test, each of them containing 20 images. The test set provides two manual segmentations generated by two different experts for each image. The selection of the first observer is accepted as ground truth and used for performance evaluation in literature. The training set includes a set of manual segmentations made by the first observer.

We performed the evaluation of our method in terms of sensitivity (Se) and specificity (Sp):

$$Se = \frac{TP}{TP + FN}, \quad Sp = \frac{TN}{TN + FP}, \qquad (12)$$

where TP, TN, FP and FN represent the number of true positives, true negatives, false positives and false negatives, respectively. Sensitivity and specificity are indicators of the capability of the algorithm to identify blood vessels and to exclude all other classes, respectively.

The value of C and the combination of features utilized to compute the unary and pairwise energies of the CRF were selected without using test data. We have divided the original training set into two new subsets, *training** and *validation*, containing 75% and 25% of the images, respectively. We utilized *training** to train the model, and *validation* to optimize the combination of parameters. We then used the selected parameters to re-train on the *training** set, and we evaluated the final model on the test set. During model selection, we used a criterion that minimized the distance with respect to the Se and Sp of the second human observer.

Several state-of-the-art features were considered, including wavelets [18], line [5,10] and ridge detectors [8], matched filter responses [19], vessel enhancers [20–24], gradient module, Huffman's entropy and image intensities. A forward selection process was followed to select the best combination. All features are obtained over preprocessed images. We first select the green band of the original color image. Then we extend the borders of the FOV [18], and finally we subtract an estimated background for bias correction using a median filter with square windows of length 25. For each combination of features, values of $C = 10^i$, with $i = \{0, 1, ..., 5\}$, were explored. The best configuration we found for the unary features utilize 2-D Gabor wavelets [18], line detectors [5]

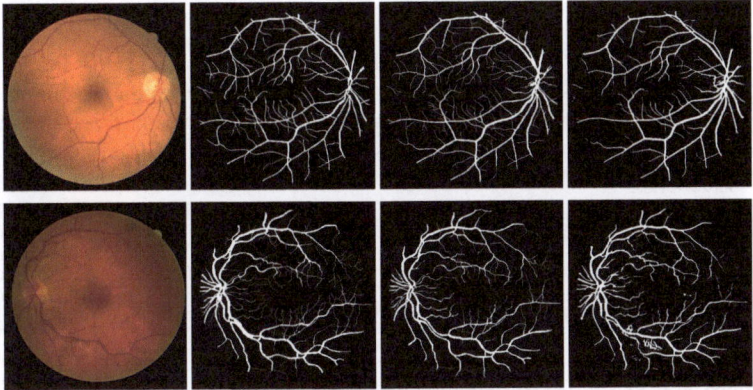

Fig. 1. Examples of results obtained on healthy (top) and pathological (bottom) images from DRIVE. From left to right: original images, ground truth labelings, 2nd human observer labelings, our segmentations.

and the vessel enhancement process proposed in [22]. The vessel enhanced image obtained after applying the process proposed in [23] is utilized as a pairwise feature.

Two segmentation examples, obtained over a healthy and a pathological image, are included in Figure 1. We also include the ground truth labeling and the labeling performed by the second observer for qualitative comparison.

We have performed an extensive comparison of our method with state-of-the-art automated methods that report their results in terms of Se and Sp, and that are not trained on the test set. Figure 2 shows a scatter plot of the competing methods as well as the performance of the human observer, in terms of Se and Sp. We also include results obtained following the same principled discriminative training but using a local-neighborhood based CRF. The numerical values are listed in Table 1.

5   Conclusions

In this work, we have presented a discriminatively trained segmentation model based on a fully connected CRF for the purpose of blood vessel segmentation in fundus images. Conditional random fields have not been previously applied in this setting, likely due to standard pairwise potentials (such as in a Potts model) leading to poor performance in the presence of thin, branching structures. In contrast, our approach is able to achieve high accuracy by considering a much more expressive, fully connected graph structure. The benefits of this approach are demonstrated empirically.

Extensive comparison with state-of-the-art methods has shown that our approach performed best and is a fully-automated segmentation algorithm that achieves results on par with a human annotator as measured by sensitivity and specificity. Our method is statistically tied with the expert annotator for both measures. This is in part due to previous studies focusing on raw pixel accuracy, which ignores the fact that the number of pixels occupied by blood vessels is a relatively small fraction of the image. As a result, competing methods suffer as measured by sensitivity. In contrast, our method closely

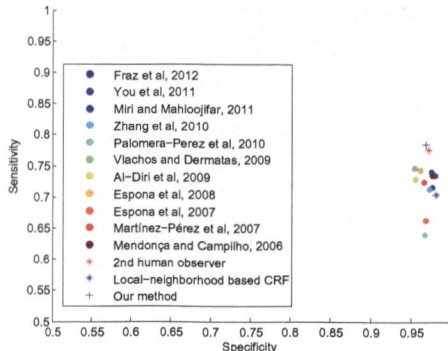

Fig. 2. Scatter-plot of Se vs. Sp, comparing existing methods, local-neighborhood based CRF, the proposed method, and the human annotator, based on DRIVE data set. Our method is statistically tied with the performance of the expert annotator and achieves a much higher sensitivity than all other segmentation systems.

Table 1. Comparison of Se and Sp of our method with respect to the existing blood vessel segmentation algorithms and the human observer, based on DRIVE data set.

Method	Sensitivity	Specificity
Fraz et al., 2012 [11]	0.7152	0.9769
You et al., 2011 [25]	0.741	0.9751
Miri and Mahloojifar, 2011 [2]	0.7352	0.9795
Zhang et al., 2010 [9]	0.712	0.9724
Palomera-Pérez et al., 2010 [26]	0.64	0.967
Vlachos and Dermatas, 2009 [12]	0.747	0.955
Al-Diri et al., 2009 [27]	0.7282	0.9551
Espona et al., 2008 [28]	0.7436	0.9615
Espona et al., 2007 [29]	0.6634	0.9682
Martínez-Pérez et al., 2007 [8]	0.7246	0.9655
Mendonca and Campilho, 2006 [7]	0.7344	0.9764
Local-neighborhood based CRF	**0.7042±0.049**	**0.9815±0.005**
Our method	**0.785±0.045**	**0.967±0.007**
2nd human observer	**0.776±0.059**	**0.973±0.008**

matches the performance of an expert human both in sensitivity and specificity, and achieves a substantially higher sensitivity than all other competing methods. Sensitivity is particularly important as it reflects an accurate estimation of the vessel pixels, the primary goal in vessel segmentation for fundus image analysis. Additional implementation details are available at `http://pages.saclay.inria.fr/matthew.blaschko/projects/retina/`.

Acknowledgements. This work is partially funded by ERC Grant 259112, and FP7-MC-CIG 334380.

References

1. Fraz, M.M., Remagnino, P., Hoppe, A., Uyyanonvara, B., Rudnicka, A.R., Owen, C.G., Barman, S.A.: Blood vessel segmentation methodologies in retinal images–a survey. Computer Methods and Programs in Biomedicine 108(1), 407–433 (2012)
2. Miri, M.S., Mahloojifar, A.: Retinal image analysis using curvelet transform and multistructure elements morphology by reconstruction. IEEE T-BME 58(5), 1183–1192 (2011)
3. Kanski, J.J., Bowling, B.: Synopsis of Clinical Ophthalmology. Saunders Limited (2012)
4. Li, Y., Gregori, G., Knighton, R.W., Lujan, B.J., Rosenfeld, P.J.: Registration of OCT fundus images with color fundus photographs based on blood vessel ridges. Optics Express 19(1), 7 (2011)
5. Ricci, E., Perfetti, R.: Retinal blood vessel segmentation using line operators and support vector classification. IEEE T-MI 26(10), 1357–1365 (2007)
6. Becker, C., Rigamonti, R., Lepetit, V., Fua, P.: Supervised feature learning for curvilinear structure segmentation. In: Mori, K., Sakuma, I., Sato, Y., Barillot, C., Navab, N. (eds.) MICCAI 2013, Part I. LNCS, vol. 8149, pp. 526–533. Springer, Heidelberg (2013)
7. Mendonca, A.M., Campilho, A.: Segmentation of retinal blood vessels by combining the detection of centerlines and morphological reconstruction. IEEE T-MI 25(9) (2006)

8. Martinez-Perez, M.E., Hughes, A.D., Thom, S.A., Bharath, A.A., Parker, K.H.: Segmentation of blood vessels from red-free and fluorescein retinal images. Medical Image Analysis 11(1), 47–61 (2007)
9. Zhang, B., Zhang, L., Zhang, L., Karray, F.: Retinal vessel extraction by matched filter with first-order derivative of Gaussian. Computers in Biology and Medicine 40(4), 438–445 (2010)
10. Nguyen, U.T., Bhuiyan, A., Park, L.A., Ramamohanarao, K.: An effective retinal blood vessel segmentation method using multi-scale line detection. Pattern Recognition (2012)
11. Fraz, M.M., Remagnino, P., Hoppe, A., Uyyanonvara, B., Rudnicka, A.R., Owen, C.G., Barman, S.A.: Ensemble classification system applied for retinal vessel segmentation on child images containing various vessel profiles. Image Analysis and Recognition (2012)
12. Vlachos, M., Dermatas, E.: Multi-scale retinal vessel segmentation using line tracking. Computerized Medical Imaging and Graphics 34(3), 213–227 (2010)
13. Li, S.Z.: Markov Random Field Modeling in Image Analysis, 3rd edn. Springer (2009)
14. Krähenbühl, P., Koltun, V.: Efficient inference in fully connected CRFs with Gaussian edge potentials. In: NIPS (2012)
15. Joachims, T., Finley, T., Yu, C.N.J.: Cutting-plane training of structural SVMs. Machine Learning 77(1), 27–59 (2009)
16. Staal, J., Abràmoff, M.D., Niemeijer, M., Viergever, M.A., van Ginneken, B.: Ridge based vessel segmentation in color images of the retina. IEEE T-MI 23(4), 501–509 (2004)
17. Schölkopf, B.: Support Vector Learning. PhD thesis, Oldenbourg Verlag, Munich (1997)
18. Soares, J.V., Leandro, J.J., Cesar, R.M., Jelinek, H.F., Cree, M.J.: Retinal vessel segmentation using the 2-d Gabor wavelet and supervised classification. IEEE T-MI 25(9) (2006)
19. Al-Rawi, M., Qutaishat, M., Arrar, M.: An improved matched filter for blood vessel detection of digital retinal images. Computers in Biology and Medicine 37(2), 262–267 (2007)
20. Frangi, A.F., Niessen, W.J., Vincken, K.L., Viergever, M.A.: Multiscale vessel enhancement filtering. In: Wells, W.M., Colchester, A.C.F., Delp, S.L. (eds.) MICCAI 1998. LNCS, vol. 1496, pp. 130–137. Springer, Heidelberg (1998)
21. Marín, D., Aquino, A., Gegúndez-Arias, M.E., Bravo, J.M.: A new supervised method for blood vessel segmentation in retinal images by using gray-level and moment invariants-based features. IEEE T-MI 30(1), 146–158 (2011)
22. Sinthanayothin, C., Boyce, J.F., Cook, H.L., Williamson, T.H.: Automated localisation of the optic disc, fovea, and retinal blood vessels from digital colour fundus images. British Journal of Ophthalmology 83(8), 902–910 (1999)
23. Saleh, M.D., Eswaran, C.: An efficient algorithm for retinal blood vessel segmentation using h-maxima transform and multilevel thresholding. Computer Methods in Biomechanics and Biomedical Engineering 15(5), 517–525 (2012)
24. Zana, F., Klein, J.-C.: Segmentation of vessel-like patterns using mathematical morphology and curvature evaluation. IEEE TIP 10(7), 1010–1019 (2001)
25. You, X., Peng, Q., Yuan, Y., Cheung, Y.-M., Lei, J.: Segmentation of retinal blood vessels using the radial projection and semi-supervised approach. Pattern Recognition 44(10) (2011)
26. Palomera-Pérez, M.A., Martinez-Perez, M.E., Benítez-Pérez, H., Ortega-Arjona, J.L.: Parallel multiscale feature extraction and region growing: application in retinal blood vessel detection. IEEE T-ITB 14(2), 500–506 (2010)
27. Al-Diri, B., Hunter, A., Steel, D.: An active contour model for segmenting and measuring retinal vessels. IEEE T-MI 28(9), 1488–1497 (2009)
28. Espona, L., Carreira, M.J., Penedo, M.G., Ortega, M.: Retinal vessel tree segmentation using a deformable contour model. In: ICPR (2008)
29. Espona, L., Carreira, M.J., Ortega, M., Penedo, M.G.: A snake for retinal vessel segmentation. In: Martí, J., Benedí, J.M., Mendonça, A.M., Serrat, J. (eds.) IbPRIA 2007. LNCS, vol. 4478, pp. 178–185. Springer, Heidelberg (2007)

Feature Space Optimization for Virtual Chromoendoscopy Augmented by Topography

Germán González[1], Vicente Parot[1], William Lo[2],
Benjamin J. Vakoc[2], and Nicholas J. Durr[1,*]

[1] Madrid-MIT M+Vision Consortium,
Massachusetts Institute of Technology, Cambridge MA 02139, USA
{ggonzale,vparot,ndurr}@mit.edu
[2] Wellman Center for Photomedicine, Harvard Medical School and
Massachusetts General Hospital, Boston MA 02114, USA
william_lo@hms.harvard.edu, vakoc.benjamin@mgh.harvard.edu

Abstract. Optical colonoscopy is the preferred modality for the screening and prevention of colorectal cancer. Chromoendoscopy can increase lesion detection rate by highlighting tissue topography with a colored dye, but is too time-consuming to be adopted in routine colonoscopy screening. We developed a fast and dye-free technique that generates virtual chromoendoscopy images that incorporate topography features acquired from photometric stereo endoscopy. We demonstrate that virtual chromoendoscopy augmented by topography achieves similar image quality to conventional chromoendoscopy in ex-vivo swine colon.

Keywords: optical colonoscopy, chromoendoscopy, photometric stereo endoscopy, topography.

1 Introduction

Colonoscopy screening reduces the risk of mortality from colorectal cancer by finding and removing precancerous lesions in the large intestine. However, the protective value of colonoscopy screening is limited because endoscopists frequently miss lesions [1, 2]. Chromoendoscopy is a technique that enhances tissue contrast in endoscopy by spraying and rinsing a dye over a tissue surface. Indigo carmine is often used as a chromoendoscopy dye for colonoscopy. As a nonabsorbed dye, indigo carmine increases lesion contrast by highlighting topographical irregularities in the colon mucosa [3]. Unfortunately, even though chromoendoscopy with indigo carmine is known to significantly improve adenoma detection rates [4, 5], it is not used in routine colonoscopy screening because the process of iteratively spraying and rinsing the dye dramatically increases the procedure timbale [1]. Thus there is a need for alternative techniques that increase the contrast from topographical features of the mucosa without increasing procedure time [6].

---

* This work has been financially supported by the Comunidad de Madrid through the Madrid-MIT M+Visión Consortium.

P. Golland et al. (Eds.): MICCAI 2014, Part I, LNCS 8673, pp. 642–649, 2014.
© Springer International Publishing Switzerland 2014

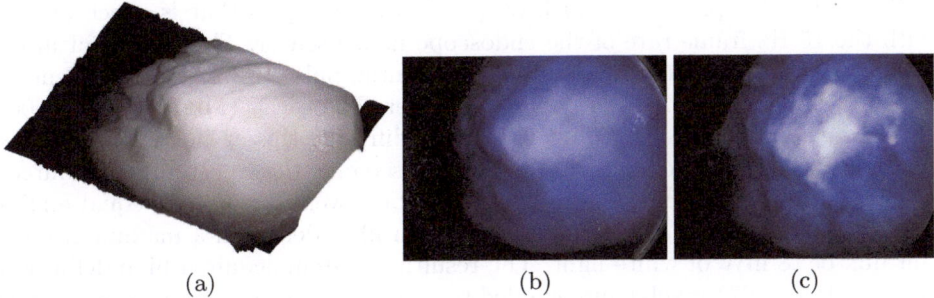

(a)   (b)   (c)

Fig. 1. (a) Image and topography obtained by PSE. (b) Virtual chromoendoscopy calculated by incorporating features from the image and topography of the same field of view as in (a). (c) Dye-based chromoendoscopy image performed in the same field of view as (a).

There have been several efforts to develop dye-free techniques for rapid virtual chromoendoscopy that would be practical for use in routine colonoscopy screening. For instance, Olympus, Pentax, and Fujinon have introduced Narrow Band Imaging (NBI), i-Scan, and Fujinon intelligent chromoendoscopy (FICE), respectively, as spectral approaches to emphasize superficial tissue structure and vascular patterns. All of these techniques create a non-photorealistic image using a combination of selected wavelength channels [7]. However, unlike dye-based chromoendoscopy, these virtual chromoendoscopy techniques have failed to show a convincing improvement in colonoscopy adenoma detection rates [8–10]. A major limitation of existing virtual chromoendoscopy approaches is that the origin of the contrast in these techniques (the optical properties of the tissue) is fundamentally different than that of dye-based chromoendoscopy (the tissue topography).

In this paper, we present a virtual chromoendoscopy technique that, unlike previous approaches, enhances contrast based on topographical features. We use photometric stereo endoscopy (PSE) [11], to acquire both the conventional uniform illumination images and high-frequency topographical images of the field-of-view. Though the low-frequency spatial information is not captured with PSE, the high-frequency topography is more clinically relevant. In fact, dye-based chromoendoscopy also preferentially highlights the sharp topographical changes in the mucosa surface. Our approach, called Virtual Chromoendoscopy Augmented with Topography (VCAT), produces images that are comparable to those obtained with dye-based chromoendoscopy (Figure 1).

2   Experimental Setup

Videos of tissue illuminated from a sequence of four alternating white-light sources were acquired using a Pentax gastroscope (EG-2990i) that was modified for clinical PSE in a similar manner to a previous report [12]. We used a Pentax

EPK-i5010 video processor which outputs a digital signal that is synchronized with the 15 Hz frame rate of the endoscope image sensor. The synchronization pulses were converted to a cycle of four sequential pulse trains that were sent to an LED driver via an Arduino microcontroller. The LEDs (Mightex FCS-0000-000) were coupled to 1mm light guides with diffusing tips at the distal end. We turned off the conventional light sources and used only these custom LED sources to illuminate the sample. The four optical fibers were oriented at equal angles about the center of the gastroscope tip. Each fiber delivered a maximum radiant flux of 18 mW of white light. The resulting system acquired high-definition images (1230 x 971 pixels) and enabled topographical reconstructions every four frames (3.75 Hz) in a system that has the same outer diameter (14 mm) as conventionally-used colonoscopes.

The high frequency topography of the field of view was calculated using a photometric stereo endoscopy method which reduces errors arising from an unknown working distance by assuming constant source vector directions and high-pass filtering the calculated topography map (11). The underlying assumption is that the error incurred in the fixed estimation of light source positions changes slowly from pixel to pixel, and can thus be corrected by filtering the shape gradients with a spatial frequency high-pass filter. The four source vectors for all pixels in the image were assumed to be equal to that of a pixel in the center of the field-of-view, for which source vectors were calculated assuming a 40 mm working distance. The resulting x and y gradients calculated by photometric stereo were high-pass filtered by subtracting a low-pass image resulting from blurring gradients with a 100 pixel Gaussian kernel with $\sigma = 100$ pixels. A height map is estimated from the high-pass filtered gradients using a multigrid solver for the Poisson equation that minimizes integration errors (11).

To demonstrate and validate the potential of topography-based virtual chromoendoscopy, we imaged three ex-vivo swine colons. Each of them was cleaned, cut, and spread open on a flat surface. The PSE endoscope was fixed above the tissue and images were acquired before and after spraying and rinsing an approximately 0.5% solution of indigo carmine chromoendoscopy dye. Although there are no accessible swine models for colorectal cancer, swine colon do exhibit a range of surface topographies that are qualitatively similar to normal and abnormal regions in the human colon.

3   Virtual Chromoendoscopy Augmented with Topography

We use PSE to simultaneously acquire conventional white light images and topography information. Specifically, we calculate the uniformly illuminated image I_u, the surface normal maps $\mathbf{N}$, and the tissue height maps h from the PSE images. VCAT combines information from the conventional, uniformly-illuminated image and topographical measurement to emulate the dye accumulation in topographical features in dye-based chromoendoscopy (Algorithm 1).

Data: Photometric Stereo Images **I**. Weight vector w
Result: Virtual Chromoendoscopy Image I_{VCAT}
while *New Image I_n* **do**

　　－ remove specular reflections from $I_n \rightarrow I_n^c$
　　－ perform PSE to compute the normal and height maps
　　　$\mathbf{I}^c = \{I_n^c, I_{n-1}^c, I_{n-2}^c, I_{n-3}^c\} \rightarrow \{h, \mathbf{N}\}$
　　－ estimate a uniformly illuminated image from $\mathbf{I}^c \rightarrow I_u$
　　－ equalize the image to match the color and intensity properties of a canonical
　　　chromoendoscopy image $I_u \rightarrow I_e$
　　－ generate features from $\{I_e, h, \mathbf{N}\} \rightarrow \mathbf{f}$
　　－ combine the features to generate the VCAT image $I_{VCAT} = f(\mathbf{f})$

end

Algorithm 1. Virtual chromoendoscopy augmented with topography

3.1   Removal of Specular Reflections

We use a photometric stereo algorithm that assumes that the object has a Lambertian surface remittance. Consequently, specular reflections from the wet tissue surface create artifacts in the topographical reconstruction. These errors create artificial dips and bumps that may be highlighted by virtual chromoendoscopy. Since the fiber optics of our photometric stereo system closely represent point sources and the surface of the colon varies smoothly, specular reflections appear in our images as circular-like shapes of high brightness. To detect them we use a scale-space approach based on the Laplacian of a Gaussian filter. For each image I_n we compute its convolution with a Laplacian of Gaussian filters at different scales σ and normalize them with σ^2. We then project the scale-space approach into a single 2-dimensional image $I_L = \max_\sigma (I_n * LoG_\sigma)\sigma^2$. Pixels that have a greater value than the mean plus three standard deviations in I_L are considered specular reflections and removed from the image. The values of the corrected image I_n^c at those locations are estimated by solving Laplace's equations from its boundary pixels.

3.2   Features for computing VCAT

For each set of images **I**, we compute features that are combined to generate a virtual chromoendoscopy luminance image. We compute five features that are based on both the image information as well as the topography:

Equalized uniformly illuminated image I_e: We compute I_e as the L channel of the mean value of the four sequential images acquired by the PSE system, after correcting for specular reflections and converting it into Lab color space. $\bar{I} = (I_n^c + I_{n-1}^c + I_{n-2}^c + I_{n-3}^c)/4$. We adjust the brightness and contrast of the uniformly illuminated image so that it matches those of a canonical chromoendoscopy image.

Height map: We decompose the height map obtained from PSE into two features: **pits** and **crevices**, depending on whether the height map is positive or negative.

θ: Angle of the surface normal with respect to the z direction.

Image offset: A vector of ones added to compensate for image offsets.

3.3 Feature Combination

The goal of virtual chromoendoscopy is to replicate as faithfully as possible an objective chromoendoscopy image I_{ch}. Towards that end, we estimate the luminance of the VCAT image as a linear combination of image and topological features $\mathbf{f}$. We use a minimization process to obtain the weight vector $\hat{w}$ that optimally combines the features, using as a cost function the squared error between the estimated luminance image and the luminance of the real chromoendoscopy image I_{ch}^{L},

$$\hat{w} = \underset{w}{\operatorname{argmin}} ||I_{ch}^{L} - \mathbf{f} \cdot w||. \tag{1}$$

This linear problem can be solved by applying Moose-Penrose pseudoinversion of the feature matrix and multiplying it by the objective image:

$$\hat{w} = pinv(\mathbf{f}) \cdot I_{ch}^{L}. \tag{2}$$

The same process can be applied when estimating the weighting vector $\hat{w}$ with several images by changing the objective image I_{ch} and the features $\mathbf{f}$ in Eq. 1 for a concatenation of the images and features.

3.4 Virtual Chromoendoscopy Image Estimation

Given an input image I_n, its features $\mathbf{f}$, and the weight vector computed previously $\hat{w}$, the luminance of the virtual chromoendoscopy image I_{VCAT}^{L} is estimated as a linear combination of the features, using as weights $\hat{w}$:

$$I_{VCAT}^{L} = \mathbf{f} \cdot \hat{w}. \tag{3}$$

The color components of the virtual chromoendoscopy image are obtained by equalizing the chrominance of the original image I_n to match the chrominance of the canonical chromoendoscopy image.

4   Evaluation

We equalized the brightness and contrast of each I_{ch} acquired in three different swine colons to reduce illumination artifacts. We evaluated the VCAT by comparing I_{VCAT}^{i} with I_{ch}^{i}.

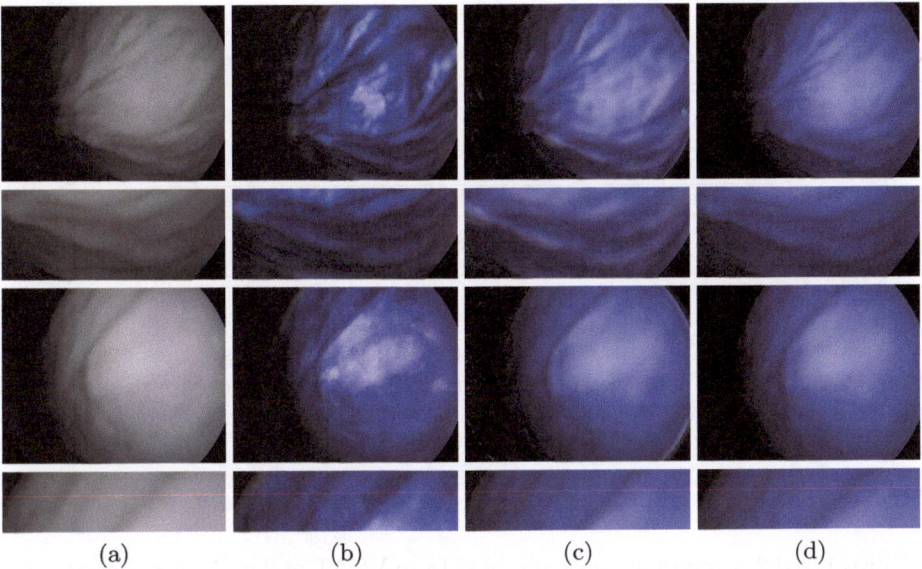

(a)   (b)   (c)   (d)

Fig. 2. First and third samples of our training images. Second and fourth rows show zoomed in regions of the samples. (a) Original images after removing specular reflections. (b) Image of same field of view as left column after applying dye-based chromoendoscopy. (c) VCAT. (d) Virtual chromoendoscopy by equalizing the color statistics of the conventional image in the left column to that of the chromoendoscopy image in the middle-left column. Qualitatively, the VCAT technique appears to enhance regions with ridges in the same way that real chromoendoscopy does, as highlighted in the second and fourth rows.

4.1 Evaluation Methodology

We performed leave-one-out cross-validation to estimate the performance of the system on unseen images. For each image sample i, we compute the weighting vector $\hat{w}_i$ with the remaining pair of PSE images and real chromoendoscopy and reconstruct the estimated I^i_{VCAT}.

In order to evaluate if the topographical features described in Section 3.2 help on the generation of realistic VCAT images, we generate virtual chromoendoscopy images without using the topographical features: I^i_{vc}. We do so by adjusting the brightness, contrast and color channels of the uniformly illuminated images to that of the canonical chromoendoscopy image. We compare those two sets of virtual chromoendoscopy images, $\{I^i_{VCAT}\}$ and $\{I^i_{vc}\}$, to the objective image, $\{I^i_{ch}\}$, using two similarity measurements: root mean squared error (RMSE) and the structural similarity index (SSIM) [13]. The SSIM index is a framework for image comparison as a function of their luminance, contrast, and structural similarity. Since we are minimizing the norm of the difference between $\{I^i_{VCAT}\}$ and $\{I^i_{ch}\}$, the RMSE will correspondingly decrease within the training set. However, since we are performing leave-one-out cross-validation the RMSE from the test image is a valid metric for evaluation.

Table 1. Quantification of the similarity between real chromoendoscopy, the proposed virtual chromoendoscopy, and virtual chromoendoscopy by color equalization for the two evaluation metrics: RMSE and SSIM

Measure	RMSE				SSIM			
Sample	S1	S2	S3	p-value	S1	S2	S3	p-value
I_{VCAT}	3.06	6.32	4.12	0.08	0.882	0.747	0.848	0.026
I_{vc}	3.21	6.68	4.28		0.815	0.704	0.771	

We further demonstrate our system in three different videos of the porcine colon. However, we can not quantify the effects of virtual chromoendoscopy in such videos since we do not have registered real chromoendoscopy frames to them.

5   Results

Figures 1 and 2 compare images obtained from VCAT and real chromoendoscopy. As expected, images from VCAT incorporate topographical contrast by highlighting the ridges and darkening the pits in the colon mucosa. Figure 2 also shows virtual chromoendoscopy obtained by color equalization. Color equalization is done by scaling and shifting the a and b components of the image in *Lab* color space to match those of a canonical chromoendoscopy image. Qualitatively, VCAT produces images that are more similar to real chromoendoscopy than virtual chromoendoscopy by color equalization, as highlighted in the second and fourth rows of Fig. 2.

The quantification of the image improvement is shown in Table 1. Incorporating topographical features results in both lower RMSE and higher SSIM. We performed a student t-test on the results to show their statistical significance. Although we have only three points in our dataset, the improvement p-value for the SSIM metric is statistically significant.

6   Discussion

While PSE can reconstruct the 3D topography of the colon surface, the interpretation of this additional information may require a steep learning curve for the gastroenterologist. Chromoendoscopy, on the other hand, highlights features from the colon topography in a way that is intuitive and familiar to gastroenterologists. In this paper we have proposed a method to generate images that are similar to chromoendoscopy but incorporate the 3D topography of the field of view that is easily and quickly acquired from PSE. We have showcased and quantified the technology in a dataset of three registered images of three ex-vivo swine colon, demonstrating that virtual chromoendoscopy images that include topographical information more closely resemble real chromoendoscopy images than those that do not include topographical information. This technique could enable gastroenterologists improve their lesion detection rates in routine colonoscopy by incorporating the clinically-valuable topographical contrast obtained by PSE in a familiar representation. The evaluation of the performance of VCAT in ex-vivo and in-vivo human colon tissue is underway.

References

1. Rex, D.K.: Maximizing detection of adenomas and cancers during colonoscopy. The American Journal of Gastroenterology 101(12), 2866–2877 (2006)
2. Pohl, H., Robertson, D.J.: Colorectal cancers detected after colonoscopy frequently result from missed lesions. Clinical Gastroenterology and Hepatology: the Official Clinical Practice Journal of the American Gastroenterological Association 8(10), 858–864 (2010), PMID: 20655393
3. Song, L.M.W.K., Adler, D.G., Chand, B., Conway, J.D., Croffie, J.M.B., DiSario, J.A., Mishkin, D.S., Shah, R.J., Somogyi, L., Tierney, W.M., Petersen, B.T.: Chromoendoscopy. Gastrointestinal Endoscopy 66(4), 639–649 (2007)
4. Brooker, J.C., Saunders, B.P., Shah, S.G., Thapar, C.J., Thomas, H.J.W., Atkin, W.S., Cardwell, C.R., Williams, C.B.: Total colonic dye-spray increases the detection of diminutive adenomas during routine colonoscopy: A randomized controlled trial. Gastrointestinal Endoscopy 56(3), 333–338 (2002)
5. Hurlstone, D.P., Cross, S.S., Slater, R., Sanders, D.S., Brown, S.: Detecting diminutive colorectal lesions at colonoscopy: a randomised controlled trial of pan-colonic versus targeted chromoscopy. Gut 53(3), 376–380 (2004), PMID: 14960519
6. Durr, N.J., Gonzlez, G., Parot, V.: 3D imaging techniques for improved colonoscopy. Expert Review of Medical Devices 11(2), 105–107 (2014), PMID: 24387658
7. Pohl, J., May, A., Rabenstein, T., Pech, O., Ell, C.: Computed virtual chromoendoscopy: a new tool for enhancing tissue surface structures. Endoscopy 39(1), 80–83 (2007), PMID: 17252465
8. Adler, A., Pohl, H., Papanikolaou, I.S., Abou-Rebyeh, H., Schachschal, G., Veltzke-Schlieker, W., Khalifa, A.C., Setka, E., Koch, M., Wiedenmann, B., Rösch, T.: A prospective randomised study on narrow-band imaging versus conventional colonoscopy for adenoma detection: does narrow-band imaging induce a learning effect? Gut 57(1), 59–64 (2008), PMID: 17681999
9. Nass, J.P., Connolly, S.E.: Current status of chromoendoscopy and narrow band imaging in colonoscopy. Clinics in Colon and Rectal Surgery 23(1), 21–30 (2010), PMID: 21286287 PMCID: PMC2850163
10. Rex, D.K., Helbig, C.C.: High yields of small and flat adenomas with high-definition colonoscopes using either white light or narrow band imaging. Gastroenterology 133(1), 42–47 (2007), PMID: 17631129
11. Parot, V., Lim, D., Gonzlez, G., Traverso, G., Nishioka, N.S., Vakoc, B.J., Durr, N.J.: Photometric stereo endoscopy. Journal of Biomedical Optics 18(7), 076017-1–076017-7 (2013), PMID: 23864015
12. Durr, N.J., Gonzalez, G., Lim, D., Traverso, G., Nishioka, N.S., Vakoc, B.J., Parot, V.: System for clinical photometric stereo endoscopy. In: Advanced Biomedical and Clinical Diagnostic and Surgical Guidance Systems XII, San Francisco, CA, vol. 8935(51). SPIE (February 2014)
13. Wang, Z., Bovik, A.C., Sheikh, H.R., Simoncelli, E.P.: Image quality assessment: from error visibility to structural similarity. IEEE Transactions on Image Processing 13(4), 600–612 (2004)

Multi-frame Super-resolution with Quality Self-assessment for Retinal Fundus Videos

Thomas Köhler[1,2], Alexander Brost[1], Katja Mogalle[1],
Qianyi Zhang[1], Christiane Köhler[3], Georg Michelson[2,3],
Joachim Hornegger[1,2], and Ralf P. Tornow[3]

[1] Pattern Recognition Lab, Friedrich-Alexander-Universität Erlangen-Nürnberg,
Erlangen, Germany
[2] Erlangen Graduate School in Advanced Optical Technologies (SAOT),
Erlangen, Germany
thomas.koehler@fau.de
[3] Department of Ophthalmology, Friedrich-Alexander-Universität
Erlangen-Nürnberg, Erlangen, Germany

Abstract. This paper proposes a novel super-resolution framework to reconstruct high-resolution fundus images from multiple low-resolution video frames in retinal fundus imaging. Natural eye movements during an examination are used as a cue for super-resolution in a robust maximum a-posteriori scheme. In order to compensate heterogeneous illumination on the fundus, we integrate retrospective illumination correction for photometric registration to the underlying imaging model. Our method utilizes quality self-assessment to provide objective quality scores for reconstructed images as well as to select regularization parameters automatically. In our evaluation on real data acquired from six human subjects with a low-cost video camera, the proposed method achieved considerable enhancements of low-resolution frames and improved noise and sharpness characteristics by 74 %. In terms of image analysis, we demonstrate the importance of our method for the improvement of automatic blood vessel segmentation as an example application, where the sensitivity was increased by 13 % using super-resolution reconstruction.

1 Introduction

Fundus imaging is one of the most routinely used modalities in clinical practice to diagnose retinal diseases. High-end fundus cameras provide color photographs of high spatial resolution captured from the background of the human eye. Despite their broad application for diagnostic purposes, e. g. for diabetic retinopathy or glaucoma, fundus cameras are limited to the acquisition of single or stereo images. In this context, novel video camera systems provide a complementary technology that enables the acquisition of fast temporal changes for new applications such as time course measurement of fundus reflections to examine the cardiac cycle [1]. However, inherent limitations for diagnostic applications are the lower spatial resolution as well as the inferior conditions in terms of signal-to-noise ratio (SNR) and image contrast due to technological or economical constraints.

Methods used for image enhancement in fundus video imaging include denoising techniques, e. g. temporal averaging schemes [2]. Additionally, blind

P. Golland et al. (Eds.): MICCAI 2014, Part I, LNCS 8673, pp. 650–657, 2014.
© Springer International Publishing Switzerland 2014

deconvolution has been proposed for image restoration [3]. However, this technique is applied to pairs of photographs acquired in a longitudinal examination rather than video data and does not increase the spatial resolution in terms of pixel sampling. To overcome this issue, multi-frame super-resolution algorithms [4] reconstruct a high-resolution (HR) image with improved SNR from multiple low-resolution (LR) frames by exploiting sub-pixel motion in an image sequence. Established methods formulate super-resolution from a Bayesian perspective as maximum a-posteriori (MAP) estimation [4] or employ marginalization to reconstruct HR images [5]. As super-resolution is an ill-posed problem and sensitive to the accuracy of the motion estimate, robust algorithms have been introduced, e. g. in the work of Farsiu et al. [6]. Super-resolution methods have also been utilized for various medical imaging modalities [7]. In terms of retinal imaging, Murillo et al. [8] have presented a first super-resolution approach for scanning laser ophthalmoscopes. However, to the best of our knowledge, this method has not been investigated for fundus video imaging. In particular, it does not consider specific aspects of fundus images such as heterogeneous illumination.

This paper proposes a novel super-resolution framework to reconstruct HR images from LR video sequences in retinal imaging. In our approach, natural eye movements during an examination are used as a cue for super-resolution. The major contribution of our work is threefold. First, we incorporate retrospective illumination correction for photometric registration to the underlying imaging model to compensate spatially and temporally heterogeneous illumination on the fundus. Second, we utilize no-reference quality assessment for fundus images to provide objective image quality scores and to select reconstruction parameters automatically. Finally, our experimental evaluation demonstrates the importance of our method towards diagnostic applicability of fundus video cameras.

2 Proposed Method

2.1 Multi-frame Super-resolution Reconstruction

We exploit LR frames denoted as $\boldsymbol{y}^{(1)}, \ldots, \boldsymbol{y}^{(K)}$ where the luminance channel of the k-th frame ($k = 1 \ldots K$) is reorganized into a vector $\boldsymbol{y}^{(k)} \in \mathbb{R}^M$. Due to eye motion during image acquisition, each frame $\boldsymbol{y}^{(k)}$ is warped with respect to the unknown HR image $\boldsymbol{x} \in \mathbb{R}^N$ according to a geometric transformation. Each warped $\boldsymbol{y}^{(k)}$ is a blurred and downsampled version of $\boldsymbol{x}$ due to the camera point spread function (PSF) and the finite pixel size. Furthermore, spatially and temporally heterogeneous illumination is a common issue in retinal imaging and results in photometric differences between $\boldsymbol{x}$ and $\boldsymbol{y}^{(k)}$. Finally, each frame is affected by additive noise $\boldsymbol{\epsilon}^{(k)}$. We utilize a generative model [6] extended with a photometric transformation to define the relation between $\boldsymbol{x}$ and each $\boldsymbol{y}^{(k)}$:

$$\boldsymbol{y}^{(k)} = \boldsymbol{\gamma}_m^{(k)} \odot \boldsymbol{D}\boldsymbol{B}^{(k)}\boldsymbol{M}^{(k)}\boldsymbol{x} + \gamma_a^{(k)}\boldsymbol{1} + \boldsymbol{\epsilon}^{(k)}, \tag{1}$$

where $\boldsymbol{D}$, $\boldsymbol{B}^{(k)}$ and $\boldsymbol{M}^{(k)}$ models sub-sampling, blur and the geometric transformation of $\boldsymbol{x}$ for the k-th frame, respectively. $\boldsymbol{\gamma}_m^{(k)}$ represents the bias field which affects the k-th frame in a multiplicative illumination model, where $\odot$ denotes the element-wise vector product. The additive term $\gamma_a^{(k)}\mathbf{1}$ for the all-one vector $\mathbf{1}$ models varying brightness over time. Assuming a fixed and space invariant PSF $K(\mathbf{u})$ resulting in a fixed blur kernel $\mathbf{B} = \mathbf{B}^{(k)}$, the different transformations $\mathbf{D}$, $\mathbf{B}$ and $\mathbf{M}^{(k)}$ are combined to a sparse system matrix $\mathbf{W}^{(k)}$ [5]:

$$\mathbf{W}^{(k)} = \mathbf{D}\mathbf{B}\mathbf{M}^{(k)} \text{ with } W_{ij} = K\left(||\mathbf{u}_i - \mathbf{M}^{(k)}(\mathbf{v}_j)||_2\right), \tag{2}$$

where $\mathbf{u}_i$ are the coordinates of the i-th pixel in $\mathbf{x}$ and $\mathbf{M}^{(k)}(\mathbf{v}_j)$ are the coordinates of the j-th pixel $\mathbf{v}_j$ in $\mathbf{y}^{(k)}$ warped to $\mathbf{x}$ using the transformation $\mathbf{M}^{(k)}$.

Geometric and Photometric Registration. Image registration is decomposed into two stages for photometric and geometric transformations. The photometric transformation is modeled by the bias field $\gamma_m^{(k)}$ which is assumed to be spatially smooth and temporal changes in brightness modeled by $\gamma_a^{(k)}$. To estimate $\gamma_m^{(k)}$, we employ a retrospective correction based on a B-spline approximation [9] of $\mathbf{y}^{(k)}$. Once the bias field $\gamma_m^{(k)}$ is determined, the associated illumination corrected frame $\tilde{\mathbf{y}}^{(k)}$ is obtained by inverting the illumination model:

$$\tilde{\mathbf{y}}^{(k)} = \gamma_m^{(k)-1} \odot \mathbf{y}^{(k)}, \tag{3}$$

where $\gamma_m^{(k)-1}$ denotes the pixel-wise inverted bias field. Then, the illumination corrected frames $\tilde{\mathbf{y}}^{(1)},\ldots,\tilde{\mathbf{y}}^{(K)}$ are photometrically registered up to an offset $\gamma_a^{(k)}$ which is determined by the temporal changes of the median brightness:

$$\gamma_a^{(k)} = \text{Median}(\tilde{\mathbf{y}}^{(k)}) - \text{Median}(\tilde{\mathbf{y}}^{(r)}). \tag{4}$$

For geometric registration, we focus on steady acquisitions, where eye motion is given by small random movements excluding saccades occurring in wider intervals. Therefore, eye motion is modeled by a 2-D homography in $\mathbf{M}^{(k)}$ as perspective distortions caused by the retina curvature are negligible. The homography is estimated by means of affine registration [10] in a robust coarse-to-fine scheme from the photometrically registered frame $\tilde{\mathbf{y}}^{(k)}$, where $\tilde{\mathbf{y}}^{(1)}$ is used as reference.

Image Reconstruction. After geometric and photometric registration, the system matrices $\mathbf{W}^{(k)}$ are assembled from the transformation parameters according to Eq. (2). Multi-frame super-resolution is formulated as unconstrained minimization problem using the L_p norm as data fidelity measure:

$$\hat{\mathbf{x}} = \arg\min_{\mathbf{x}} \left\{ \sum_{k=1}^{K} \left|\left| \mathbf{y}^{(k)} - \gamma_m^{(k)} \odot \mathbf{W}^{(k)}\mathbf{x} - \gamma_a^{(k)} \right|\right|_p^p + \lambda \cdot R(\mathbf{x}) \right\}, \tag{5}$$

where $R(\mathbf{x})$ weighted by λ regularizes the HR estimate $\mathbf{x}$ to enforce smoothness. In order to make super-resolution robust to the registration uncertainty, we chose $p = 1$ and adopted L_1 norm minimization [6], which corresponds to a MAP estimate for $\mathbf{x}$ if $\epsilon^{(k)}$ is Laplacian noise. For $R(\mathbf{x})$, the edge preserving bilateral total variation (BTV) with window size L and weight α is employed:

$$R(\mathbf{x}) = \sum_{m=-L}^{L} \sum_{n=-L}^{L} \alpha^{|m|+|n|} ||\mathbf{x} - \mathbf{S}_v^m \mathbf{S}_h^n \mathbf{x}||_1, \tag{6}$$

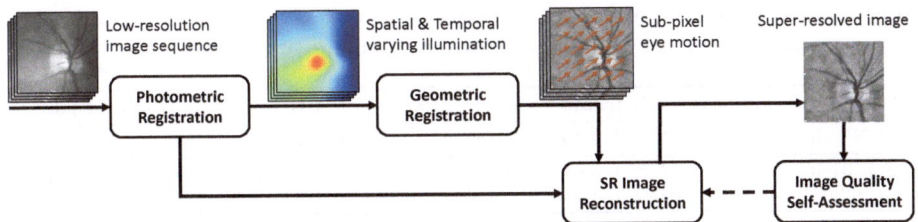

Fig. 1. Flowchart of the proposed multi-frame super-resolution framework

which compares $\boldsymbol{x}$ to its shifted versions in vertical and horizontal direction defined in matrix notation by $\boldsymbol{S}_v^m$ and $\boldsymbol{S}_h^n$, respectively. The objective function in Eq. (5) is minimized employing iterative Scaled Conjugate Gradient (SCG) optimization to enhance the convergence compared to steepest descent minimization [6]. The temporal median of the geometrically and photometrically registered LR sequence bicubic upsampled to the HR grid is used as initial guess for SCG.

2.2   Image Quality Self-assessment and Parameter Selection

Super-resolution relies on the initialization of the regularization weight λ and is affected by residual noise in case of too small λ, whereas a large λ leads to over-smoothing. Parameter selection typically involves cross validation procedures based on simple measures such as the mean squared error [5]. However, these measures do not correlate with visual perception for diagnostic purposes. In this paper, the content-based no-reference quality metric Q_v [11] for fundus images is utilized. Q_v quantifies noise and sharpness for an image $\boldsymbol{x}$ according to:

$$Q_v(\boldsymbol{x}) = \sum_{\boldsymbol{p}_i \in \mathcal{P}(\boldsymbol{x})} \sigma_i \cdot q(\boldsymbol{p}_i), \qquad (7)$$

where $q(\boldsymbol{p}_i)$ measures the local quality for an anisotropic patch $\boldsymbol{p}_i$, which is combined to $Q_v(\boldsymbol{x})$ based on spatially adaptive weights σ_i. The set of patches $\mathcal{P}(\boldsymbol{x})$ is indicated by a dominant intensity gradient orientation determined by statistical significance testing and σ_i denotes the local variance of a vessel probability map in $\boldsymbol{p}_i$ estimated via blood vessel segmentation. To obtain unbiased scores, all patches $\boldsymbol{p}_i$ and weights σ_i are computed for the temporal median of the registered sequence $\tilde{\boldsymbol{y}}^{(1)}, \ldots, \tilde{\boldsymbol{y}}^{(K)}$. As $Q_v(\boldsymbol{x})$ depends on the number of patches, quality assessment is normalized by the reference frame $\boldsymbol{y}^{(r)}$ according to $\tilde{Q}_v(\boldsymbol{x}) = (Q_v(\boldsymbol{x}) - Q_v(\boldsymbol{y}^{(r)}))/Q_v(\boldsymbol{y}^{(r)})$ to quantify the relative improvement. We combine super-resolution with a data-driven selection of the regularizer weight according to:

$$\hat{\lambda} = \arg\max_{\lambda} Q_v(\boldsymbol{x}_\lambda), \qquad (8)$$

where $\boldsymbol{x}_\lambda$ denotes the super-resolved image reconstructed according to Eq. (5) with weight λ. In order to find an optimal weight, we perform a grid search with equidistant step size $\Delta \log \lambda$ in the interval $[\log \lambda_l, \log \lambda_u]$ of the log-transformed

Table 1. Peak-signal-to-noise ratio (PSNR) along with sensitivity and specificity of vessel segmentation for LR frames, temporal median and super-resolution

	LR frame	Median image	SR image	Ground truth
PSNR (in dB)	31.09 ± 3.10	31.41 ± 3.28	**31.92 ± 3.39**	-
Sensitivity (%)	57.59 ± 6.01	67.83 ± 4.96	**70.37 ± 5.00**	72.85 ± 6.70
Specificity (%)	94.31 ± 1.40	94.80 ± 1.19	**93.99 ± 1.26**	94.57 ± 1.34

range of λ chosen as initialization. For a fixed λ, a few SCG iterations are performed to check whether it improves the super-resolved image. For the selected $\hat{\lambda}$, a super-resolved image is estimated according to Eq. (5) by running SCG until convergence. The overall flowchart of our framework is outlined in Fig. 1.

3   Experiments and Results

We adjusted all parameters experimentally based on real fundus video data used in our experiments[1]. For BTV regularization, we chose $\alpha = 0.7$ and $L = 1$ with $\log \lambda_l = -2.0$, $\log \lambda_u = 0$ and step size $\Delta \log \lambda = 0.2$ to select an optimal weight. For quality self-assessment, anisotropic patches of size 8×8 were analyzed.

Synthetic Data. We generated synthetic image sequences with $K = 16$ frames for 40 images taken from the DRIVE database [12], by applying our model defined in Eq. (1) in forward direction. The frames were related to the reference frame by a uniformly distributed random translation (-2 to $+2$ pixels) to simulate eye motion, affected by Gaussian noise ($\sigma_n = 0.01$), blurred by an isotropic Gaussian PSF ($\sigma = 1.0$) and sub-sampled by a factor of 2. For super-resolution, we considered the green color channel as in fundus imaging the red and blue ones are typically over- and under-saturated, respectively. Super-resolved images were assessed using the peak-signal-to-noise ratio (PSNR). Additionally, we investigated blood vessel segmentation [13] as application of our method to compare an automatic segmentation to a manually created gold standard. Quantitative measures are summarized in Table 1 and the associated qualitative results are presented in Fig. 2. Our framework improved the mean PSNR by 0.8 dB compared to LR images. In terms of vessel segmentation, the sensitivity was enhanced by 13 % as fine vessels were reconstructed by our method. Both increases achieved by super-resolution compared to LR frames and the temporal median were statistically significant ($p < 0.05$) based on a Wilcoxon signed-rank test. The specificity was comparable to segmentation on the ground truth.

Real Data. We acquired monochromatic fundus video data with a low-cost camera prototype developed by Ralf P. Tornow, FAU Erlangen-Nürnberg, Germany. The system is based on a CCD camera (640×480 px) equipped with LED illumination and covers a field of view (FOV) of $20°$. As frame rate we chose 12.5 Hz. The left eye from six healthy subjects was examined. Additionally, we examined the subjects with a Kowa nonmyd camera (1600×1216 px, $25°$ FOV)

---

[1] Supplementary material is available online http://www5.cs.fau.de/research/software/

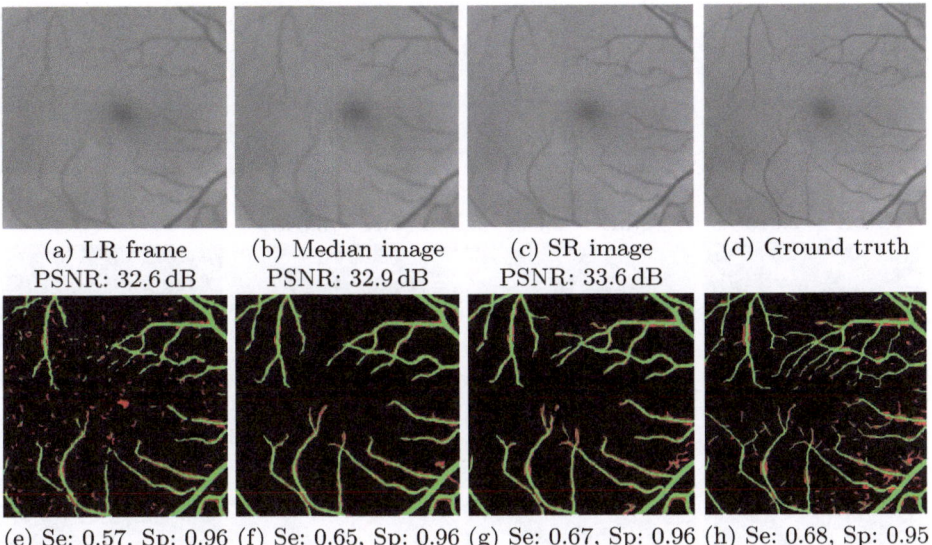

(a) LR frame   (b) Median image   (c) SR image   (d) Ground truth
PSNR: 32.6 dB   PSNR: 32.9 dB   PSNR: 33.6 dB

(e) Se: 0.57, Sp: 0.96 (f) Se: 0.65, Sp: 0.96 (g) Se: 0.67, Sp: 0.96 (h) Se: 0.68, Sp: 0.95

Fig. 2. Synthetic images with peak-signal-to-noise ratio (PSNR) for LR data (a), temporal median (b) and super-resolved data (c) in comparison to the ground truth (d). We evaluated sensitivity (Se) and specificity (Sp) for vessel segmentation where true-positive and false-positive pixels shown in (e) - (h) are color-coded in green and red.

used in clinical practice to acquire HR images for comparison. We considered two regions of interest (ROI) as shown in Fig. 3: (i) One ROI (256×256 px) showing the optic nerve head was processed to evaluate the ability to super-resolve anatomical structures such as optic disk and cup. (ii) A second ROI (120×120 px) containing small blood vessels was analyzed to assess the reconstruction of fine structures. We used $K = 8$ frames with a magnification factor of 2 and an isotropic Gaussian PSF ($\sigma = 1.0$).

We compared super-resolved images to the green channel of HR data acquired with the Kowa camera. Both image types were registered based on manually selected feature points and a projective transformation. For the sake of comparison between the Kowa image and video data, we also corrected the bias filed of the Kowa image. Visually, we obtained substantial enhancements of structures such as blood vessels by means of super-resolution while noise was suppressed as depicted in Fig. 3. Opposed to raw video data, photometric registration utilized in our framework compensated heterogeneous illumination. The similarity to the registered Kowa image was assessed using the normalized mutual information (NMI). Super-resolution yielded the highest similarity with NMI = 0.048. Additionally, we applied our framework in a sliding window scheme based on K successive frames for each window. The relative quality measures $\tilde{Q}_v$ for ten consecutive windows per subject and both ROIs are summarized as boxplots in Fig. 4. On average, the proposed framework yielded $\tilde{Q}_v = 1.6$ and further improved the quality score by 0.74 compared to temporal median filtering.

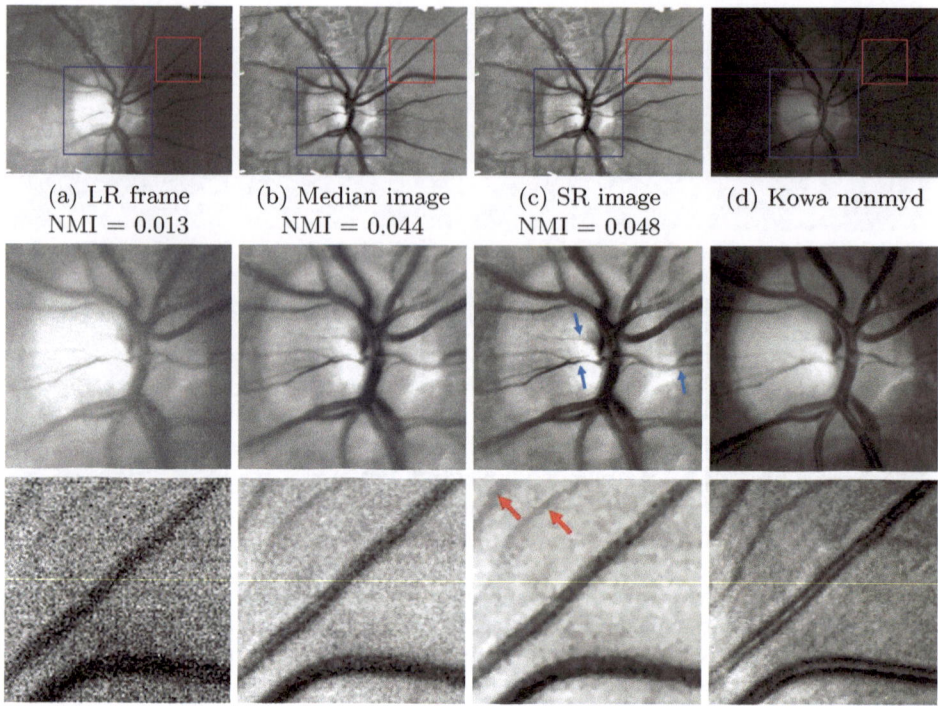

Fig. 3. Results obtained from the low-cost camera: Low-resolution frame (a), temporal median used as initial guess (b), final super-resolved image (c) and green channel of Kowa nonmyd image for the same subject (d). We assessed the similarity to the registered Kowa image using the normalized mutual information (NMI).

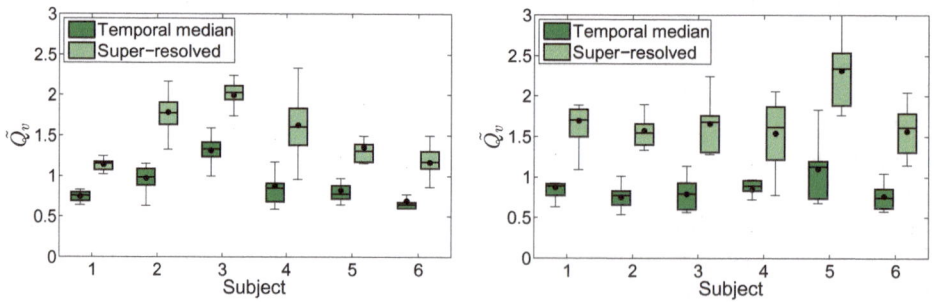

Fig. 4. Boxplot of $\tilde{Q}_v$ for temporal median filtering and super-resolution in image regions showing the optic nerve (left) and blood vessels (right) as depicted in Fig. 3

4   Conclusion and Future Work

This paper proposes a novel super-resolution framework for fundus video imaging. Multi-frame super-resolution exploits natural eye movements during an examination by means of affine registration to reconstruct a motion-compensated HR image from LR video data. The underlying model considers photometric registration to account for heterogeneous illumination. We also employ quality self-assessment for automatic parameter selection and to provide an objective quality score for reconstructed images. Our method is able to achieve an image quality for super-resolved images generated with a low-cost fundus camera that is comparable to a high-resolution commercially available camera. The investigation of super-resolution for an analysis of disease-specific anomalies to improve the reliability of medical diagnoses is ongoing research. We will also study the impact of the proposed method in large-scale studies, e. g. in glaucoma screening.

Acknowledgments. The authors gratefully acknowledge funding of the Erlangen Graduate School in Advanced Optical Technologies (SAOT) by the German National Science Foundation (DFG) in the framework of the excellence initiative.

References

1. Tornow, R., Kopp, O., Schultheiss, B.: Time course of fundus reflection changes according to the cardiac cycle. Invest. Ophthalmol. Vis. Sci. 44, 1296 (2003)
2. Köhler, T., Hornegger, J., Mayer, M., Michelson, G.: Quality-guided denoising for low-cost fundus imaging. In: Proceedings BVM 2012, pp. 292–297 (2012)
3. Marrugo, A.G., Sorel, M., Sroubek, F., Millán, M.S.: Retinal image restoration by means of blind deconvolution. J. Biomed. Opt. 16(11), 116016 (2011)
4. Milanfar, P.: Super-resolution imaging. CRC Press (2010)
5. Pickup, L.C., Capel, D.P., Roberts, S.J., Zisserman, A.: Overcoming Registration Uncertainty in Image Super-resolution: Maximize or Marginalize? EURASIP J. Adv. Signal Process., 1–15 (2007)
6. Farsiu, S., Robinson, M.D., Elad, M., Milanfar, P.: Fast and robust multiframe super resolution. IEEE Trans. Image. Process. 13(10), 1327–1344 (2004)
7. Greenspan, H.: Super-resolution in Medical Imaging. Comput. J. 52(1), 43–63 (2008)
8. Murillo, S., Echegaray, S., Zamora, G., Soliz, P., Bauman, W.: Quantitative and qualitative image quality analysis of super resolution images from a low cost scanning laser ophthalmoscope. In: Proc. SPIE Medical Imaging, pp. 79624T (2011)
9. Kolar, R., Odstrcilik, J., Jan, J., Harabis, V.: Illumination Correction and Contrast Equalization in Colour Fundus Images. In: Proc. EUSIPCO 2011, pp. 298–302 (2011)
10. Evangelidis, G.D., Psarakis, E.Z.: Parametric image alignment using enhanced correlation coefficient maximization. IEEE Trans. Pattern. Anal. Mach. Intell. 30(10), 1858–1865 (2008)
11. Köhler, T., Budai, A., Kraus, M.F., Odstrcilik, J., Michelson, G., Hornegger, J.: Automatic no-reference quality assessment for retinal fundus images using vessel segmentation. In: Proceedings CBMS 2013, pp. 95–100 (2013)
12. Staal, J., Abràmoff, M.D., Niemeijer, M., Viergever, M.A., van Ginneken, B.: Ridge-based vessel segmentation in color images of the retina. IEEE Trans. Med. Imaging 23(4), 501–509 (2004)
13. Budai, A., Bock, R., Maier, A., Hornegger, J., Michelson, G.: Robust vessel segmentation in fundus images. Int. J. Biomed. Imaging, 154860 (2013)

An Automated System for Detecting and Measuring Nailfold Capillaries

Michael Berks, Phil Tresadern, Graham Dinsdale, Andrea Murray, Tonia Moore, Ariane Herrick, and Chris Taylor

University of Manchester, Manchester, United Kingdom
michael.berks@manchester.ac.uk

Abstract. Nailfold capillaroscopy is an established qualitative technique in the assessment of patients displaying Raynaud's phenomenon. We describe a fully automated system for extracting quantitative biomarkers from capillaroscopy images, using a layered machine learning approach. On an unseen set of 455 images, the system detects and locates individual capillaries as well as human experts, and makes measurements of vessel morphology that reveal statistically significant differences between patients with (relatively benign) primary Raynaud's phenomenon, and those with potentially life-threatening systemic sclerosis.

1 Introduction

Systemic sclerosis (SSc) is a connective tissue disorder which can lead to morbidity and mortality, often in young people – with a reported prevalence among adults of 250 per million [1]. Clinically, it results in fibrosis and microvascular abnormality, leading to ischaemic injury (e.g. ulceration, scarring, and gangrene), particularly in the fingers and toes. The commonest presenting feature is Raynaud's phenomenon (episodic colour change and pain in the fingers, usually in response to cold), but this is also a symptom of the more common, and relatively benign, primary Raynauds phenomenon (PR).

There is thus a clinical need to distinguish between PR and SSc-related Raynauds phenomenon. There is also a pressing need for quantitative biomarkers for monitoring SSc response to treatment, both clinically and in clinical trials, where existing endpoints (eg digital ulceration) are unreliable, leading to a limited evidence base [2, 3]. Nailfold capillaroscopy, a non-invasive technique for imaging capillaries at the base of the fingernails (see Figure 1), is already used clinically to assess the degree of microvascular abnormality, and has the potential to provide quantitative biomarkers for SSc. Standardised protocols for qualitative grading of nailfold images exist [4], but do not provide quantitative data. (Semi-)Manual measurements of capillary spacing, vessel width at the tops of loops (apices) and vessel tortuosity have been shown to have potential as quantitative biomarkers for SSc [5], but are too time-consuming and open to subjective factors for routine use. There is thus a clear rationale for developing automated methods for analysing nailfold images.

In this paper we describe and evaluate a fully automated system for detecting and measuring capillaries in nailfold images, adopting a machine learning approach, and building on experience with existing semi-automated systems [5, 6]. Specifically, our

P. Golland et al. (Eds.): MICCAI 2014, Part I, LNCS 8673, pp. 658–665, 2014.

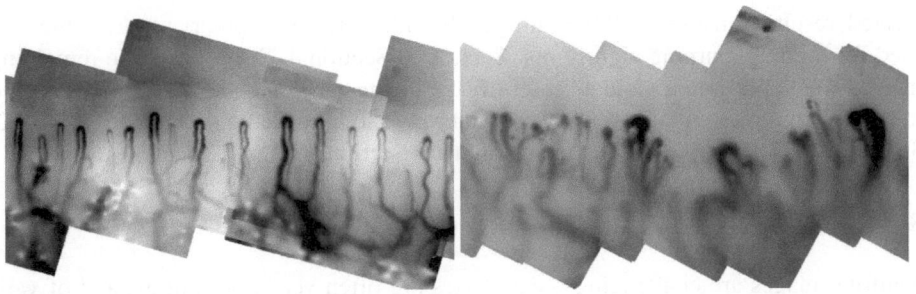

Fig. 1. Sections from two nailfold mosaics: one from a healthy control subject (left) and one from a patient with SSc (right) showing enlargement, distortion and irregular spacing of capillaries

contributions are: (a) a method for detecting vessels and estimating their width and orientation; (b) a method for generating candidate capillary apices; (c) a method for refining candidate capillary apices and measuring apical width and tortuosity; (d) a large-scale evaluation of performance, compared to human experts and; (e) initial results for classifying patients based on image level summary statistics of the automated capillary measurements.

In summary we show that our automated system is indistinguishable from human experts in detecting and locating capillary apices, and that there are statistically significant differences, at the population level, between automated capillary measurements for SSc patients and normal or PR subjects.

2   Nailfold Capillaroscopy Data

Our images were acquired by a capillaroscopy system in a tertiary referral centre for patients with SSc. Patients gave informed consent. High magnification, 768×576, 8-bit monochome pixel video frames were captured at a resolution of $1.25 \mu m$ per pixel. Images captured along the nailbed were registered and compounded into a single mosaic (similarly to [7]) showing the whole nailfold (Figure 1).

In normal subjects, capillary loops are all similar, arranged regularly and approximately vertical. Current clinical practice confines attention to the distal row of capillaries, whose apices lie on a smooth, approximately horizontal line near the top of the image. This pattern is disrupted in SSc by structural damage to the microvasculature (Figure 1).

We have used a set of 990 mosaics, manually annotated as part of a separate clinical study, involving three subject groups: healthy controls (HC), subjects with PR, and patients with SSc. Each image was annotated independently by two expert observers, one of whom (Observer 1) was the same for every image, with the other drawn from a pool of experts. In each image, the observers attempted to mark the locations and apical widths of all distal capillaries. This is a challenging and subjective task for which perfect agreement is rare (see Section 6).

In a subset of 80 images, Observer 1 provided a precise demarcation of the inner and outer edges of the distal capillaries. Regions of interest around these capillaries were created, resulting in a set of 450 training RoIs with matching capillary masks, which we used for training learning algorithms (Section 3, Section 4, Section 5). The remaining images were split into a validation set of 456 images (104 HC, 83 PR, 269 SSc) used to locate capillaries and determine the distal row, and a test set of 455 images (104 HC, 83 PR, 268 SSc) used to evaluate performance (Section 6).

3   Vessel Detection and Characterisation

Nailfold images are challenging – capillaries are often very low contrast and of variable width ($10 - 300\mu m$) and appearance, whilst significant artefacts can be present. Although previous work on automated capillaroscopy is limited, we can draw on the extensive literature on curvilinear structure detection in medical images (eg [8–10]. In particular, we adopt the well-established machine learning approach to predict, at each pixel, the probability that it belongs to a vessel (vesselness) [9], and the local orientation and width [10]. In the following sections we explain the features we used to describe local image structure, and the learning methods we used to obtain vesselness, orientation and width models.

3.1   Image Features

To characterise local structure at each training pixel, we use a feature vector of responses to symmetric (even) and asymmetric (odd) filters across scale and orientation. Specifically, we use a steerable filter bank [11] of directional second order derivatives of a Gaussian kernel [8] and their (approximate) Hilbert transforms so that responses at any orientation can be computed efficiently. From an initial scale $\sigma = 1$ pixel we compute even and odd responses at six angles $\theta_i = {}^{i\pi}/6$ over five scales, in each case keeping σ fixed whilst downsampling the image by a factor of 2 in each direction (i.e. the coarsest scale is equivalent to $\sigma = 16$ at the original image resolution). For the coarser scales, we use bilinear interpolation to approximate the responses at the finest scale. At each pixel the responses at that pixel, along with its 8-connected neighbours, are concatenated into a feature vector without further manipulation. These features are designed to accommodate the wide range in size, shape and orientation of imaged capillaries.

3.2   Learning Vesselness, Orientation and Width Models

We treat vessel detection as a supervised classification problem, and orientation and width prediction as regression problems, all based on the features outlined in the previous section. We have used Random Forests [12], due to their ease of training, flexibility, relative robustness to over-fitting and strong performance in comparable learning tasks, but we do not believe the choice of learning method is critical.

For training, we used the 80 fully annotated images described in Section 2 each of which provides a binary vessel mask for training a vesselness classifier. To provide ground-truth for orientation and width regression, we skeletonised the binary masks, measured orientation and width at each centreline point, and propagated the measurements back to every point on the binary vessel mask using a simple nearest pixel interpolation. For orientation regression, we represented orientation as a unit vector in the complex plane, $t = \cos 2\theta + i \sin 2\theta$, doubling the angle θ to make orientation invariant to direction [13], and avoiding wraparound problems that arise if angle is used directly.

We trained three random forests (RFs), each containing 100 trees: one classifier on background versus labelled vessel pixels, and one regressor each for orientation and width. Although orientation and width are only defined for the vessel points, to ensure we generate unbiased, random predictions in the background of unseen images, we include background points with uniformly sampled random widths and orientations in training the regressors.

To make predictions in an unseen image we apply the separable basis filters, compute the interpolated, steered responses and extract feature vectors, before feeding the vectors through the trees in each forest and computing the mean, pooled over all leaf nodes, as the prediction output. For orientation, the unit vectors are converted back to radians. The result for each input image is a map of vesselness (V_v), orientation (V_θ) and width (V_w) (Figure 2(a-b)). Note that predictions of width and orientation made in this manner are significantly more accurate than analytic estimates, and, by reusing the same features as extracted for V_v, requires minimal additional computation.

4   Locating Candidate Capillary Apices

The maps V_v, V_θ and V_w provide an approximate segmentation of vessels and their low-level properties. However to extract meaningful measurements we need to detect and localise the apices of individual capillaries. Treating this as an object detection problem, we again adopt a learning approach in which each vessel pixel votes for the location of a nearby apex. Specifically, we use RF regression, trained using patches sampled near annotated capillary apices in the training data, to encode observed relationships between appearance and location [14].

To train the RF, we thin V_v by applying non-maximal suppression along the line normal to the estimated vessel orientation. We then extract 64×64 training patches, centred at local maxima in V_v and scaled and rotated according to the estimated width and orientation. If a patch contains a marked apex and is also centred at a vessel pixel in the original training masks, we label the patch as positive and record the offset to the apex; otherwise, we label the patch as negative. For each patch, a histogram of gradients (HoG) feature vector is formed by concatenating weighted histograms of gradient direction, computed for overlapping blocks in the patch [15]. A 100 tree RF classifier is then trained to distinguish between positive and negative patches, whilst a regression forest is trained to predict the offset associated with each positive patch.

For an unseen image, we extract a scale- and rotation-normalised patch about each local maximum in V_v (Figure 2(b)) and pass these through the classification forest. The output labels at each leaf node are pooled and averaged, forming $\alpha(p)$, the probability that the patch contains an apex. The regression forest then predicts the offset to the nearest apex, and therefore the apex location in the image. A Gaussian kernel – centred at the apex, scaled by $\sigma = V_w(a)$ and weighted by $\alpha(p)$ – is added to a vote map of apex locations A. Here the classifier plays a crucial role in weighting the regressor votes, so that only patches in which an apex is visible significantly contribute to A. The local maxima of A are the candidate locations for capillary apices (Figure 2(c)).

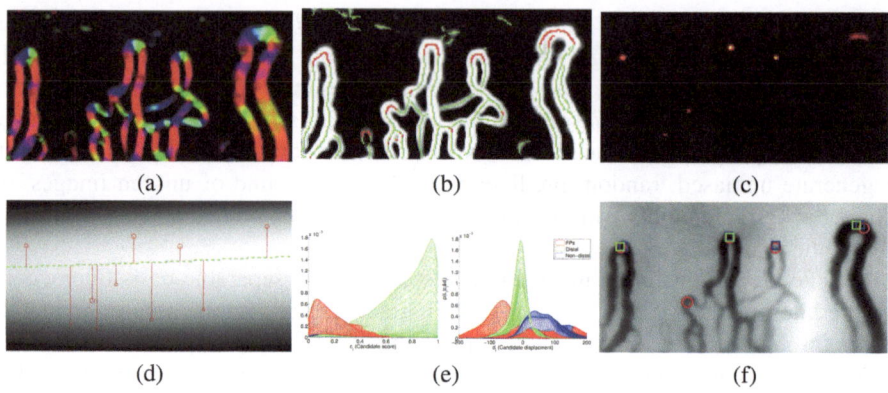

Fig. 2. Detecting nailfold capillaries (a) Estimated vessel orientation V_θ, displayed using an hue/intensity color-map for angle/prediction confidence; (b) Vesselness V_v with oriented local maxima marked by green dots. Red dots have $\alpha(q) > 0.5$ and vote for apex locations; (c) Vote map A of apex locations; (d) Estimated distal row (green line), from weighted kernel density of maxima in A. Candidate capillary locations are shown as red circles (scaled by candidate appearance score) with y displacements to estimated distal line; (e) Mesh plots of the joint class conditional distribution over candidate displacement and appearance score, viewed from score axis (left) and displacement axis (right): false positves (red), distal capillaries (green), non-distal capillaries (blue); (f) Capillaries selected by our method (red circle) and experts observers (blue and green squares), solid markers show distal capillaries.

5   Refining Candidate Apices and Making Measurements

Given a set of candidate apex locations as training data, we can now train a new classifier that better discriminates between true apices and false positives, and between distal and non-distal apices. We do so in two ways: first, we reclassify each candidate, now using patches located only at candidate apex locations; second, we exploit the fact that capillaries should lie in a single, approximately horizontal line across the image.

To train the new classifier, we used candidate apices computed for the set of 441 validation images. Each candidate (x_i, y_i) was labelled as positive only if it fell within a circle centred at a marked apex with diameter equal to the marked apical width. Of the 13,492 positive and 24,369 negative samples, the positive samples were further split into 9,735 distal and 3,757 non-distal capillaries. A 100 tree RF classifier was trained as before, using HoG features from scale- and rotation-normalised patches extracted about each sampled candidate from the original image (rather than V_v). The outputs of the trees were pooled to give a single appearance score, $c_i \in [0, 1]$, for each candidate, allowing us to define each candidate as the tuple of its location and score, (x_i, y_i, c_i). In addition to the final appearance score, the location of a candidate relative to the other candidates in any image can indicate its likelihood of being a distal row apex. Specifically, we assume the ideal distal row to be a smooth line running across the mosaic and passing through every true distal capillary apex. If we can estimate this line in an unseen image, we can use the vertical displacement of each candidate to the line to classify it as distal or nondistal.

To achieve this, we compute a density map of candidate locations by summing a Gaussian kernel centred at each discrete candidate location. Each kernel is weighted by the candidate's appearance score, c_i, so that strong candidates contribute more to the density. The density for each location in the mosaic can thus be computed as

$$D(u, v) = Z \sum_{i=1}^{N} c_i \exp\left[-\frac{(u - x_i)^2}{2\sigma_x{}^2}\right] \exp\left[-\frac{(v - y_i)^2}{2\sigma_y{}^2}\right] \tag{1}$$

where there are N candidates in the image, Z is a normalisation constant so that D sums to unity, and σ_x, σ_y are functions of the variances of x_i, y_i. Each apex's displacement from the distal row is then given by

$$d_i = y_i - \arg\max_v D(x_i, v) \tag{2}$$

Using the observers' annotations, each candidate $C_i = (x_i, y_i, c_i, d_i)$ in the validation images is assigned a label $L_i \in [1, 2, 3]$ for false positives, distal capillaries and non-distal capillaries respectively. Figure 2(e) shows a kernel estimate of the class-conditional probability density $P(c_i, d_i|L_i)$. The class priors for each label type $P(L_i)$ can be estimated empirically from the data, allowing Bayes' rule to be used to compute the class probability, $P(L_i|c_i, d_i)$, of each candidate, given its appearance score and displacement.

Each candidate is rejected, or labelled as either a distal or non-distal capillary. For each kept candidate C_i we record its width $V_w(x_i, y_i)$, and use V_θ and V_v to compute the entropy of an orientation histogram of pixels connected to C_i as a measure of tortuosity. Finally, we compute capillary density as the mean distance between the distal apexes.

6   Results

We applied our detection method (O_3) to the set of 455 test images, and compared the selected capillaries to the annotations of the two human observers (O_1 and O_2). In total, 15,391 capillaries were selected by at least one of the three observers. The results illustrate the difficulty of the task. For example, of the 7047 distal capillaries (DCs) marked by O_1, only 56% were also marked by O_2, whilst 74% were marked by the automated system (O_3). Defining true positives via consensus between the experts, of the 3913 DCs marked by both O_1 and O_2, 84% were marked by O_3, which is a probably a workable performance level. Given the level of disagreement between the experts, false positives are even harder to assess. Of the 7913 DCs marked by O_3, 27% were marked by neither O_1 nor O_2. On the other hand, of the 7047 DCs marked by O_1, 17% were marked by neither O_2 nor O_3, and 44% were not marked by O_2.

Overall, the results suggest similar performance between O_1, O_2 and O_3. To test this formally, we considered the capillaries (both distal and non-distal) selected by each observer as truth and assessed how well each of the two observers detected these capillaries. Table 1 shows the precision, recall and F-measure for each pair of observers. To test the labelling of capillaries as distal or non-distal, we considered all capillaries jointly selected by each pair of observers, and computed accuracy and Cohen's kappa

Table 1. Pairwise agreement between observers. For each row O_i v O_j denotes the performance of observer i using j as ground truth. O_1, O_2 denotes consensus of the two human observers. Precision, recall and F-measures are given for vessel detection, classification accuracy and Cohen's Kappa statistic for labelling capillaries as distal or not.

Observers	Capillary detection			Distal v Non-distal	
	Precision	Recall	F-measure	Accuracy	Cohen's κ
O_2 v O_1	70.7 ± 1.3	46.2 ± 1.8	55.8 ± 1.4	89.5 ± 0.8	0.613 ± 0.025
O_3 v O_1	66.8 ± 1.1	59.6 ± 0.9	63.0 ± 0.8	90.8 ± 0.9	0.574 ± 0.028
O_3 v O_2	51.7 ± 1.9	70.5 ± 1.0	59.6 ± 1.3	87.2 ± 1.2	0.557 ± 0.028
O_3 v O_1, O_2	64.1 ± 1.8	80.9 ± 0.7	71.5 ± 1.1	93.6 ± 1.0	0.690 ± 0.034

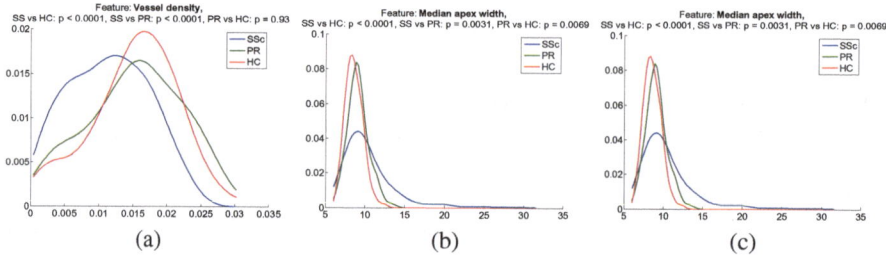

Fig. 3. Distributions of capillary measurements by subject group: (a) Capillary density; (b) Median apical width; (c) Median capillary tortuosity

statistic to quantify agreement. Accuracy and kappa statistics were not computed for capillary detection because there is no defined true negative class for the task (this is effectively the space of all images not containing a capillary). In addition to the pairwise tests, we computed equivalent values for the software versus the consensus of the two humans.

Standard errors for each value were computed from 1,000 bootstrap samples of the test images. For the F-measures and Cohen's kappa statistics we computed the difference between the agreement of O_1 and O_2 and the average of their individual agreement with O_3. 95% confidence intervals of $(-7.01, -3.90)$ and $(-0.019, 0.12)$ respectively, suggest there was no significant reduction between the software's performance and either human on the two tasks (if anything the software showed greater agreement to the humans individually than the humans did to each other on the detection task).

Finally, we present initial results for disease status characterisation, based on the measurements extracted for the detected capillaries. Distributions of capillary measurements (capillary density, median width and median tortuosity) for the three groups HC (104 images), RP (83 images), and SSc (268 images) are shown in Figure 3. To test for differences between the distributions we used the non-parametric Wilcoxon rank sum test. Tests for all measurements between all groups showed significant differences at the 0.01 confidence level (at least), except for the comparison between RP and HC for vessel density – an expected result given that we would not expect the RP group to show any signs of capillary loss.

7   Conclusions

We have presented a fully automated system for measuring vessel morphology from nailfold capillaroscopy images. Evaluation on a large data set suggests that our system performs as well as experts in detecting vessels, and initial results for automated measurement suggest that we can detect significant differences between disease groups. Further work will involve refining apex detection, adding more sophisticated measurements, and combining measurements to make useful predictions for individuals.

Acknowledgements. This work was funded by the Wellcome Trust. We are grateful to all the observers that annotated images used in the study.

References

1. Mayes, M., Lacey, J., Beebe-Dimmer, J., Gillespie, B., Cooper, B., Laing, T., Schottenfeld, D.: Prevalence, incidence, survival, and disease characteristics of systemic sclerosis in a large us population. Arthritis Rheum 48, 2246–2255 (2003)
2. Herrick, A.L.: Contemporary management of raynaud's phenomenon and digital ischaemic complications. Current Opinion in Rheumatology 23, 555–561 (2011)
3. Herrick, A.L., Roberts, C., Tracey, A., Silman, A., Anderson, M., Goodfield, M., McHugh, N., Muir, L., Denton, C.P.: Lack of agreement between rheumatologists in defining digital ulceration in systemic sclerosis. Arthritis & Rheumatism 60(3), 878–882 (2009)
4. Cutolo, M., Pizzorni, C., Secchi, M.E., Sulli, A.: Capillaroscopy. Best Practice and Research Clinical Rheumatology 22(6), 1093–1108 (2008)
5. Murray, A.K., Moore, T.L., Manning, J.B., Taylor, C., Griffiths, C.E.M., Herrick, A.L.: Non-invasive imaging techniques in the assessment of scleroderma spectrum disorders. Arthritis Rheum 61(8), 1103–1111 (2009)
6. Paradowski, M., Markowska-Kaczmar, U., Kwasnicka, H., Borysewicz, K.: Capillary abnormalities detection using vessel thickness and curvature analysis. KES 2, 151–158 (2009)
7. Anderson, M.E., Allen, P.D., Moore, T., Hillier, V., Taylor, C.J., Herrick, A.L.: Computerized nailfold video capillaroscopy – A new tool for assessment of raynauds phenomenon. J. Rheumatology, 841–848 (2005)
8. Staal, J., Abràmoff, M.D., Niemeijer, M., Viergever, M.A., van Ginneken, B.: Ridge-based vessel segmentation in color images of the retina. IEEE Trans. Med. Imag. 23(4), 501–509 (2004)
9. Soares, J.V.B., Leandro, J.J.G., Jr., R.M.C., Jelinek, H.F., Cree, M.J.: Retinal vessel segmentation using the 2-D Gabor wavelet and supervised classification. IEEE Trans. Med. Imag. 25(9), 1214–1222 (2006)
10. Berks, M., Chen, Z., Astley, S., Taylor, C.: Detecting and classifying linear structures in mammograms using random forests. In: Székely, G., Hahn, H.K. (eds.) IPMI 2011. LNCS, vol. 6801, pp. 510–524. Springer, Heidelberg (2011)
11. Freeman, W.T., Adelson, E.H.: The design and use of steerable filters. IEEE Trans. Pattern Anal. Mach. Intell. 13(9), 891–906 (1991)
12. Breiman, L.: Random forests. Mach. Learn. 45, 5–32 (2001)
13. Mardia, K.V., Jupp, P.E.: Directional Statistics. Wiley (2000)
14. Criminisi, A., Shotton, J., Robertson, D., Konukoglu, E.: Regression forests for efficient anatomy detection and localization in CT studies. In: Menze, B., Langs, G., Tu, Z., Criminisi, A. (eds.) MICCAI 2010. LNCS, vol. 6533, pp. 106–117. Springer, Heidelberg (2011)
15. Dalal, N., Triggs, B.: Histograms of oriented gradients for human detection. In: Proc. IEEE Conf. on Comp. Vis. and Patt. Recog. (2005)

Geodesic Patch-Based Segmentation

Zehan Wang[1], Kanwal K. Bhatia[1], Ben Glocker[1], Antonio Marvao[2],
Tim Dawes[2], Kazunari Misawa[3], Kensaku Mori[4,5], and Daniel Rueckert[1]

[1] Biomedical Image Analysis Group, Department of Computing,
Imperial College London, London, UK
[2] Institute of Clinical Sciences, Imperial College London, London, UK
[3] Aichi Cancer Center, Nagoya, Japan
[4] Department of Media Science, Nagoya University, Nagoya, Japan
[5] Information and Communications Headquarters, Nagoya University, Nagoya, Japan

Abstract. Label propagation has been shown to be effective in many
automatic segmentation applications. However, its reliance on accurate
image alignment means that segmentation results can be affected by any
registration errors which occur. Patch-based methods relax this dependence by avoiding explicit one-to-one correspondence assumptions between images but are still limited by the search window size. Too small,
and it does not account for enough registration error; too big, and it
becomes more likely to select incorrect patches of similar appearance for
label fusion. This paper presents a novel patch-based label propagation
approach which uses relative geodesic distances to define patient-specific
coordinate systems as spatial context to overcome this problem. The approach is evaluated on multi-organ segmentation of 20 cardiac MR images
and 100 abdominal CT images, demonstrating competitive results.

1 Introduction

Accurate segmentation in medical imaging plays a crucial role in many applications from patient-specific diagnosis to population studies. The ability to perform
this task without human intervention is particularly desirable for large datasets.
Multi-atlas label propagation approaches [7],[10],[1], in which labels from multiple atlases are propagated to target images after registration, have been shown to
be highly effective. However, dependence on image registration for these methods can be problematic as inaccurate alignment adversely affects segmentation
quality. Additionally, finding suitable (fixed) registration parameters that yield
accurate non-linear correspondences on different images can be a challenge on its
own, particularly for anatomies that are highly variable. Patch-based methods
for label propagation [3],[11] can help alleviate this dependence since they do
not rely on explicit one-to-one correspondences between images, and are often
able to use affine rather than non-rigid registration, yet still produce comparable
results.

Patch-based segmentation assumes that patches with similar intensities and
from similar local neighbourhoods are likely to be the part of the same anatomical structure. Traditionally, this locality is enforced by a sliding search window

P. Golland et al. (Eds.): MICCAI 2014, Part I, LNCS 8673, pp. 666–673, 2014.

of a fixed size (typically $< 11^3$ voxels). Label fusion then determines spatially-varying weights for each label according to the similarity of the corresponding patches within each voxel neighbourhood. This neighbourhood, when defined as a fixed size search window, imposes a hard restriction on tolerance to any registration errors that occur. Increasing the size increases the tolerance to registration errors but also increases the computational requirements and may yield patches with similar appearance but from different anatomical structures. Using hierarchical frameworks [5], [15] partly addresses these restrictions, however these approaches still use a fixed search window size. More recently, several methods have reformulated the standard patch-based approach to consider the local neighbourhood for each voxel globally based on k nearest neighbours (kNN) [13] or a trained neighbourhood approximation [8] rather than using a fixed search window size. This alleviates the computational burden, whilst the selection of patches are regularised by different approaches to apply spatial context and consistency. Another approach uses random forests trained on individual atlases with spatially varying representation of patches instead of fixed patch sizes [16].

The use of spatial context regularises the patch selection process by comparing spatial similarities between patches as well as their appearance similarity. This enables locally similar patches of different structures to be distinguished when larger search windows are used and also increases the tolerance with regards to variability between images in intensities for the same structures. One approach to incorporating spatial context is to use spatial coordinates and euclidean distances between labelled structures [13], [6]. However, this does not take into account the context of the image such as the boundaries between structures and is sensitive to anatomical variability when comparing between subjects. In this paper, we propose instead to use geodesic distances within the image to provide spatial context which is able to contribute information on the locality of structure boundaries. The use of geodesic distances has been shown to be effective in interactive segmentation [4] and we adopt this within an automated patch-based segmentation method, formulating a multi-resolution approach based on adaptive, anatomically-specific coordinates in order to leverage its use. We implement this within a kNN framework using fast-building kNN data structures, so that these adaptive spatial features can be applied at run time. We evaluate our proposed methods on multi-structure and multi-organ segmentation of 20 cardiac MR images and 100 abdominal CT images, respectively.

2 Methods

Our framework is intended to extend the ability of patch-based segmentation methods to tolerate potential registration errors. Increasing this tolerance requires patch comparisons to be made within a search space that can encompass the margin of error but also maintain the sense of "locality" which restricts the comparison to relevant patches. To do this, we define the local neighbourhood for each patch by its kNN in terms of both spatial context and intensity similarity, so as to distinguish between similar patches from different structures. This allows the search space of patches to be global whilst maintaining the sense of locality, thus removing the requirement for a fixed search window size to be set.

2.1   Adaptive Coordinate System as Spatial Context

When dealing with potentially large misalignments between images, spatial context based on explicit image coordinates can be unreliable. Spatial context should therefore be defined in a way that is robust to misregistrations. To this end, we introduce the concept of *relative distances*. If we can establish any reference points or an initial rough segmentation, we can then use a distance transform on the labelled structures to create a non-Cartesian, *patient-specific coordinate system* that is invariant to how anatomical structures are positioned within the image (Fig. 1a, 1b). For a voxel x, we define the spatial context $S(x)$ as a vector $[d(x, r_1), d(x, r_2), ..., d(x, r_n)]$ where $d(.)$ is the distance and $r_1, ..., r_n$ are labelled structures or landmarks.

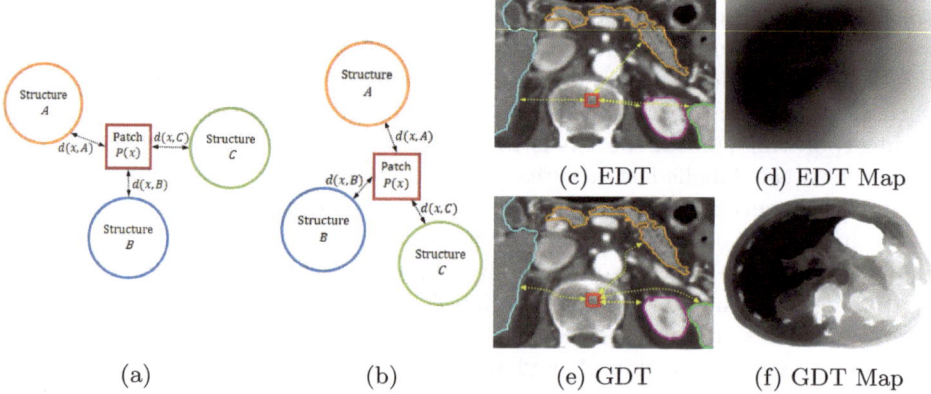

Fig. 1. (a) and (b) shows how spatial context for x can be provided by the distances to structures regardless of how they are positioned within the image. (c) and (e) provide an example where this type of spatial context can be used and how the distances will be different. (d) and (f) show the respective distance maps using EDT and GDT from the liver, where distances are shown as being proportional to the intensity.

In principle, at least three reference points are required to localise a point in 3D space, but useful information can still be obtained with less. For example, relative distances from two structures can localise a curve, whilst distances from a single structure can provide enough spatial context for a surface. This may be enough to distinguish between patches of similar intensities from different structures.

One possible approach for relative distances is to use the Euclidean Distance Transform (EDT), however the EDT does not take information present within the image into account, such as visible boundaries between structures, and may be insufficient when high anatomical variation exists (see Fig. 1). To improve localisation, we propose to additionally include information from visible boundaries, given by image gradients, between structures.

2.2 Geodesic Distance Transform (GDT)

To overcome the shortfalls of the EDT in providing adaptive spatial context, we propose the use of a geodesic distance transform (GDT), which takes into account image gradients and describes distances between structures using the shortest path along the image intensities rather than just through physical (empty) space [4]. In general, the geodesic distance between two points x, y within an image I is defined as follows:

$$d(x,y) = \inf_{\mathbf{\Gamma} \in \mathbf{P}_{x,y}} \int_0^{l(\mathbf{\Gamma})} \sqrt{1 + \gamma^2 (\nabla I(s) \cdot \mathbf{\Gamma}'(s))^2} ds \qquad (1)$$

where $\mathbf{\Gamma}$ is a path in the set of all paths, $\mathbf{P}_{x,y}$ between x and y and is parametrised by its arclength $s \in [0, l(\mathbf{\Gamma})]$. The EDT can be considered a special case of the GDT, since these are equivalent when γ is set to 0. To calculate the GDT, we use the approach from [12] which was also used in [4] and demonstrated to have good performance with linear computational requirements.

2.3 Spatially Weighted Label Fusion

With the inclusion of spatial context, the label fusion for voxel x is determined as follows - let $P(x)$ be a vector of intensities for the patch at voxel x and let $\{y_{L,i} : i \in 1, ..., k\}$ represent potential matches from the atlas library for each label L. A weighting w_L for each label L is determined by comparing the k nearest patches from the atlas library with regards to both intensities $P(x)$ and spatial context $S(x)$ - and as such no search window is used:

$$w_L(x) = \sum_{i=1}^{k} w(x, y_{L,i}) \qquad (2)$$

where

$$w(x,y) = e^{\dfrac{-\{||P(x) - P(y)||_2^2 + \alpha ||S(x) - S(y)||_2^2\}}{h^2(x)}} \qquad (3)$$

and similarly to [3], $h^2(x)$ is determined by the minimum distance:

$$h^2(x) = \min\{||P(x) - P(y_i)||_2^2 + \alpha ||S(x) - S(y_i)||_2^2\} \qquad (4)$$

A spatial weighting α balances the relative importance between the spatial and intensity components. The final label $\hat{L}$ at voxel x is decided by majority vote, i.e. $\hat{L}(x) = \arg\max_L w_L(x)$.

2.4 Framework Implementation

As an overall segmentation framework, we propose applying a multi-resolution approach with the core methods described above in an iterative process where only the boundaries, defined by the difference between the dilation and erosion of each segmentation, are refined as the segmentation is propagated through higher resolutions [13]. Multiple resolutions of each image can be created offline by constructing a Gaussian image pyramid. This reduces the computational cost compared to processing directly at the native resolution.

The GDT is always calculated in the native resolution (and downsampled if required) so that the same spatial weighting α can be used at all resolutions. There are several options for an initial segmentation to enable the use of the GDT for spatial context. For instance, the intersections of the atlases can be used if this does not yield an empty set. However this may not always occur, in which case, a coarse segmentation can be established in the lowest resolution using coordinates as spatial context [14] or another segmentation technique. These can be eroded, and relative distances can be calculated from eroded versions of each structure to reduce the initial error. Successive refinements of the boundary regions reduces the dependence on the initial segmentation.

For patch selection, it is highly desirable to have an efficient kNN data structure, since performing global kNN search can be a computational bottleneck. In our implementation, ball trees were used since they (and metric trees in general) have been shown to have better performance in higher dimensional spaces (> 20) compared to space-partitioning structures like the kd-tree [9].

3 Experiments and Results

3.1 Cardiac MR Dataset

We applied our proposed approach and compared it to using voxel coordinates and the EDT as spatial context, in addition to the standard patch-based approach from [3] (Coupé) in segmenting the left ventricle, myocardium and right ventricle in end diastole frames of 20 subjects under a single breath-hold. The MR images were captured from a 1.5T Philips Achieva system and have a native resolution of $256 \times 256 \times 64$ voxels with voxel sizes of $1.25 \times 1.25 \times 2 \text{mm}^3$.

In total, 3 resolution levels were used by our approach, with the lowest resolution at $5 \times 5 \times 5 \text{mm}^3$ voxel sizes and the intermediate level at $2.5 \times 2.5 \times 2.5 \text{mm}^3$ voxel sizes. Images were aligned using affine registration with 6 manually placed landmarks, and the intersections of the atlases were used as initial segmentations. We evaluated each method using leave-one-out cross validation and used the all available atlases (19) to segment each test image. A patch size of $5 \times 5 \times 5$ voxels was used for all resolutions and k was fixed at 40 for the kNN methods. For the different approaches to spatial context, α was selected in the lowest resolution and then applied for all subsequent resolutions whilst γ was set at 100 for GDT. The values for k and γ were not tuned.

Table 1 and Fig. 3 summarises the final segmentation accuracy and examples of segmented images using our proposed method are presented in Fig. 2.

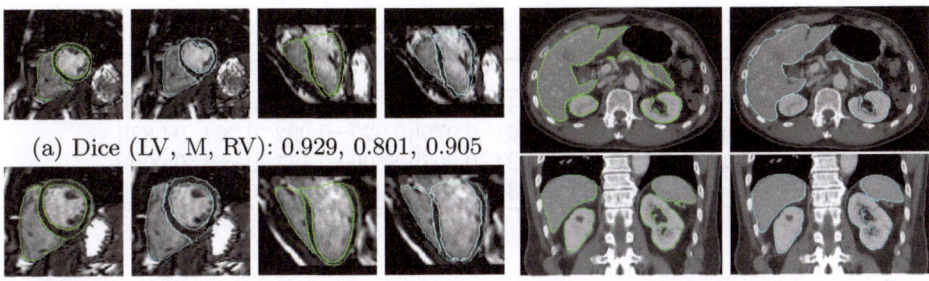

(a) Dice (LV, M, RV): 0.929, 0.801, 0.905

(b) Dice (LV, M, RV): 0.953, 0.838, 0.934   (c) Dice (L, S, P, K): 0.947, 0.955, 0.826, 0.924

Fig. 2. Examples from using our approach (in cyan) for the Left Ventricle (LV), Myocardium (M) and Right Ventricle (RV) in (a) and (b), and Liver (L), Spleen (S), Pancreas (P), Kidneys (K). Reference segmentations are outlined in green.

Table 1. Overall Dice Coefficients shown as mean (median) ±standard deviation

Method/Description	Left Ventricle	Myocardium	Right Ventricle
Coordinates $\alpha = 7$	0.931 (0.934) ±0.016	0.763 (0.763) ±0.049	0.871 (0.879) ±0.037
EDT $\alpha = 13$	0.938 (0.938) ±0.017	0.806 (0.814) ±0.049	0.882 (0.893) ±0.047
GDT $\alpha = 5$	0.934 (0.941) ±0.019	0.797 (0.803) ±0.039	0.901 (0.904) ±0.021
[3] window size = 7^3	0.931 (0.936) ±0.020	0.773 (0.787) ±0.053	0.889 (0.902) ±0.035

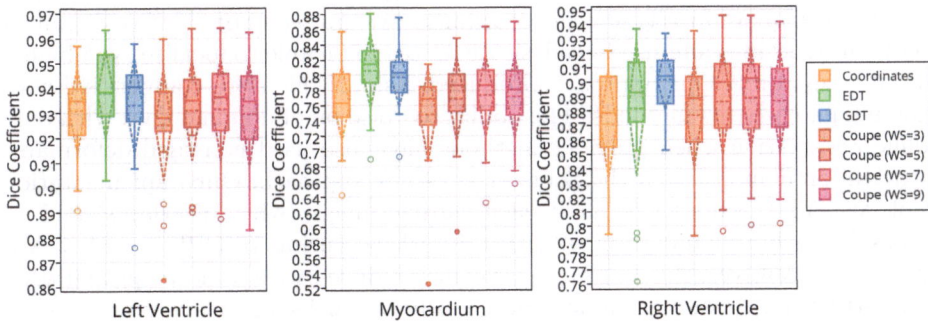

Fig. 3. Comparison of segmentation accuracy with regards to different spatial context and different search window sizes (WS=x). Solid line represents the median, the dashed lines represents the mean and standard deviation.

3.2 Abdominal CT Dataset

We also evaluated our method on 100 abdominal CT scans which have an in plane resolution of 512×512 voxels with voxel sizes ranging from 0.55 to 0.82mm and contain between 263 to 538 slices with spacing ranging from 0.4 to 0.8mm depending on the field of view and the slice thickness. For each scan, manual segmentations of the liver, spleen, pancreas and the kidneys were generated by a single trained rater.

Table 2. Overall Dice Coefficients shown as mean±standard dev. [worst, best]

Organ	Ours	[15]
Liver	0.945±0.025 [0.842, 0.977]	0.940±0.028 [0.814, 0.974]
Spleen	0.925±0.084 [0.461, 0.979]	0.920±0.092 [0.264, 0.982]
Pancreas	0.655±0.186 [0.024, 0.902]	0.696±0.167 [0.069, 0.909]
Kidneys	0.924±0.077 [0.334, 0.982]	0.925±0.072 [0.515, 0.982]

For our approach, four resolutions levels were used, ranging from 4mm^4 to 1mm^3 voxel sizes. For each test image, affine registration (without landmarks) was used to align the atlases, with the 50 nearest chosen using sum of squared differences as the distance measure. Initial coarse segmentations were established by using coordinates as spatial context [14] with $\alpha = 3$, whilst subsequent refinements using GDT as spatial context used $\alpha = 7$. Our results are presented in Table 2 alongside those from [15] where affine registration followed by additional organ level non-rigid deformable registrations were used. Similarly to [15], we apply graph cuts [2] as post processing to obtain the final segmentation.

4   Discussion and Conclusion

This paper has presented a new patch-based segmentation approach which uses spatial context to provide robustness to misregistrations. To do this, we defined an adaptive, anatomically-specific coordinate system based on relative distances between structures and used geodesic distances to be able to localise even highly variable anatomy. Our approach produced results which are competitive with existing patch-based methods. The ability to do so on abdominal data with only affine registration when previous methods have also used non-rigid deformable registration demonstrates the robustness of our approach. Our implementation took around 4 hours to segment each cardiac image (with 19 atlases) and 14 hours for each abdominal image (with 50 atlases) using 16 CPU cores clocked at 2.8Ghz. However, this can be significantly reduced with a more optimal kNN data structure. Also, our framework is easily parallelisable, since voxels are labelled independently, and is very scalable with parallel hardware. Furthermore, kNN patch search for each atlas is performed independently, enabling usage of distributed networks. Overall this approach shows much potential, particularly in more challenging datasets where achieving accurate registration is difficult.

References

1. Aljabar, P., Heckemann, R.A., Hammers, A., Hajnal, J.V., Rueckert, D.: Multi-atlas based segmentation of brain images: Atlas selection and its effect on accuracy. NeuroImage 46(3), 726–738 (2009)
2. Boykov, Y., Veksler, O., Zabih, R.: Fast Approximate Energy Minimization via Graph Cuts. IEEE PAMI 23(11), 1222–1239 (2001)

3. Coupé, P., Manjón, J.V., Fonov, V., Pruessner, J., Robles, M., Collins, D.L.: Patch-based segmentation using expert priors: Application to hippocampus and ventricle segmentation. NeuroImage 54(2), 940–954 (2011)
4. Criminisi, A., Sharp, T., Blake, A.: GeoS: Geodesic Image Segmentation. In: Forsyth, D., Torr, P., Zisserman, A. (eds.) ECCV 2008, Part I. LNCS, vol. 5302, pp. 99–112. Springer, Heidelberg (2008)
5. Eskildsen, S.F., Coupé, P., Fonov, V., Manjón, J.V., Leung, K.K., Guizard, N., Wassef, S.N., Østergaard, L.R., Collins, D.L.: BEaST: brain extraction based on nonlocal segmentation technique. NeuroImage 59(3), 2362–2373 (2012)
6. Glocker, B., Pauly, O., Konukoglu, E., Criminisi, A.: Joint Classification-Regression Forests for Spatially Structured Multi-object Segmentation. In: Fitzgibbon, A., Lazebnik, S., Perona, P., Sato, Y., Schmid, C. (eds.) ECCV 2012, Part IV. LNCS, vol. 7575, pp. 870–881. Springer, Heidelberg (2012)
7. Heckemann, R.A., Hajnal, J.V., Aljabar, P., Rueckert, D., Hammers, A.: Automatic anatomical brain MRI segmentation combining label propagation and decision fusion. NeuroImage 33(1), 115–126 (2006)
8. Konukoglu, E., Glocker, B., Zikic, D., Criminisi, A.: Neighbourhood approximation using randomized forests. Medical Image Analysis 17(7), 790–804 (2013)
9. Kumar, N., Zhang, L., Nayar, S.K.: What Is a Good Nearest Neighbors Algorithm for Finding Similar Patches in Images? In: Forsyth, D., Torr, P., Zisserman, A. (eds.) ECCV 2008, Part II. LNCS, vol. 5303, pp. 364–378. Springer, Heidelberg (2008)
10. Rohlfing, T., Brandt, R., Menzel, R., Maurer, C.R.: Evaluation of Atlas Selection Strategies for Atlas-Based Image Segmentation with Application to Confocal Microscopy Images of Bee Brains. NeuroImage 21(4), 1428–1442 (2004)
11. Rousseau, F., Habas, P., Studholme, C.: A Supervised Patch-Based Approach for Human Brain Labeling. IEEE TMI 30(10), 1852–1862 (2011)
12. Toivanen, P.J.: New geodosic distance transforms for gray-scale images. Pattern Recognition Letters 17(5), 437–450 (1996)
13. Wang, Z., Donoghue, C., Rueckert, D.: Patch-based segmentation without registration: Application to knee MRI. In: Wu, G., Zhang, D., Shen, D., Yan, P., Suzuki, K., Wang, F. (eds.) MLMI 2013. LNCS, vol. 8184, pp. 98–105. Springer, Heidelberg (2013)
14. Wang, Z., Wolz, R., Tong, T., Rueckert, D.: Spatially Aware Patch-Based Segmentation (SAPS): An Alternative Patch-Based Segmentation Framework. In: Menze, B.H., Langs, G., Lu, L., Montillo, A., Tu, Z., Criminisi, A. (eds.) MCV 2012. LNCS, vol. 7766, pp. 93–103. Springer, Heidelberg (2013)
15. Wolz, R., Chu, C., Misawa, K., Fujiwara, M., Mori, K., Rueckert, D.: Automated abdominal multi-organ segmentation with subject-specific atlas generation. IEEE TMI 32(9), 1723–1730 (2013)
16. Zikic, D., Glocker, B., Criminisi, A.: Atlas Encoding by Randomized Forests for Efficient Label Propagation. In: Mori, K., Sakuma, I., Sato, Y., Barillot, C., Navab, N. (eds.) MICCAI 2013, Part III. LNCS, vol. 8151, pp. 66–73. Springer, Heidelberg (2013)

Tagged Template Deformation

Raphael Prevost[1,2,*], Rémi Cuingnet[1], Benoit Mory[1],
Laurent D. Cohen[2], and Roberto Ardon[1]

[1] Philips Research Medisys, Suresnes, France
[2] CEREMADE UMR 7534, Universite Paris Dauphine, Paris, France

Abstract. Model-based approaches are very popular for medical image segmentation as they carry useful prior information on the target structure. Among them, the implicit template deformation framework recently bridged the gap between the efficiency and flexibility of level-set region competition and the robustness of atlas deformation approaches. This paper generalizes this method by introducing the notion of tagged templates. A tagged template is an implicit model in which different subregions are defined. In each of these subregions, specific image features can be used with various confidence levels. The tags can be either set manually or automatically learnt via a process also hereby described. This generalization therefore greatly widens the scope of potential clinical application of implicit template deformation while maintaining its appealing algorithmic efficiency. We show the great potential of our approach in myocardium segmentation of ultrasound images.

1 Introduction

Segmentation of medical images is an important part of clinical workflow, typically used to assess anatomical information such as the volume or the shape of an organ. Leveraging the strong anatomical priors available for medical images, model-based approaches are particularly effective and popular. In a number of clinical applications, methods based on atlas deformation achieve state-of-the-art performance results [16]. Yet, they suffer from a high computational burden and can only be employed for images with a standardized acquisition protocol (such as CT or MR images). Very recently though, the *implicit template deformation* framework [12,15] bridged the gap between level-set region competition [4] and atlas deformation approaches. Its unique properties (computational efficiency, topology preservation, compatibility with user interactions) were employed to achieve fast and reliable segmentation of different kinds of medical images [6,8,13]. However, even if an advanced shape prior can be embedded within this framework [14], it still assumes that appearance can be globally defined, which is a strong constraint. In this paper, we present a method to use an enriched model that couples prior information on the object's appearance with its shape.

Elaborated appearance models have been already proposed in other frameworks. One of the earliest was the well-known *active appearance model* [3] that

---

* Raphael Prevost is now affiliated to ImFusion GmbH (Munich, Germany).

P. Golland et al. (Eds.): MICCAI 2014, Part I, LNCS 8673, pp. 674–681, 2014.

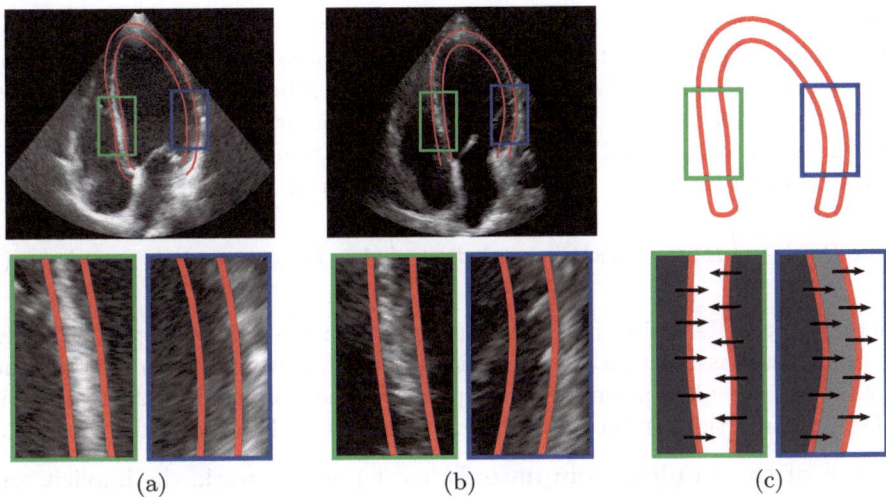

(a)   (b)   (c)

Fig. 1. The appearance of an object (here the myocardium) may vary (a) between different regions (*e.g* green and blue). However, this variation is consistent across subjects (b) so it can be embedded as a prior information within the model (c). For each edge of the model, we know what direction the image gradient (black arrows) should have.

however suffers from the usual problems of explicit methods. Level-set approaches were also extended to take into account variations in the appearance prior. In [11], the appearance model is a function of the distance to the shape boundary and in [5] a labeling function balancing the contribution of the data-fidelity term with respect to the regularization term is introduced. While this allows a better representation than a global appearance prior, it is still too constrained for many medical applications. Our work can be thought of as a generalization and extension of both ideas. Finally, an extension of the *MetaMorph* framework was proposed in [9]. This work aimed at learning jointly the shape and the appearance of the organ to be segmented. However, this results in a mutual information registration problem that needs to be solved at test time, which would be too time-consuming in 3D for our target applications.

The main contributions of this article are essentially methodological and consist in (i) an interpretation of template deformation as a flux minimization problem, (ii) an enrichment of the shape template with an appearance model that is able to exploit specific image features with various confidence levels, (iii) a method to automatically learn such enhanced models.

2   Segmentation by Implicit Template Deformation

Implicit template deformation [12,14] is a variational framework for image segmentation that consists in finding an implicit function $\phi : \Omega \to \mathbb{R}$ whose zero level-set will be the segmentation boundary. The key particularity is that the set of admissible implicit functions is defined with respect to an initial *implicit template* $\phi_0 : \Omega_0 \to \mathbb{R}$ as the set of functions obtained by deforming ϕ_0 with a geometric transformation ψ. Provided some constraints on ψ, the template ϕ_0 can be considered as a shape model: if ψ is a diffeomorphism, then ϕ and ϕ_0 will have the same topology. The transformation ψ is sought as the minimum of a region competition energy and a regularization term:

$$\min_{\psi} \; \mathcal{R}(\psi) + \int_{\Omega} H(\phi_0 \circ \psi(\mathbf{x})) \; r_{int}(\mathbf{x}) \; d\mathbf{x} + \int_{\Omega} (1 - H(\phi_0 \circ \psi(\mathbf{x}))) \; r_{ext}(\mathbf{x}) \; d\mathbf{x} \quad (1)$$

where H is the Heaviside step function, and $r_{int} : \Omega \to \mathbb{R}^+$ and $r_{ext} : \Omega \to \mathbb{R}^+$ are pointwise classification error functions in the foreground (resp. background) region. $\mathcal{R}$ is a regularization term that penalizes the magnitude and irregularities of local deformations induced by ψ, typically set to a Free-Form deformation.

Choice of the implicit template. In most previous work, the implicit template ϕ_0 was either set to the signed distance function of a simple geometric shape [13] or to a given pre-segmented shape [15]. However, another (and better) strategy is to learn ϕ_0 as the mean of a training set [14].

Regularization prior. The regularization term can be defined as $\mathcal{R}(\psi) = \frac{1}{2}\|\psi - \mathbf{Id}\|_\sigma^2$, where $\|x\|_\sigma^2 = \langle x, K_\sigma^{-1} * x \rangle$ and K_σ a Gaussian kernel. When a learning database is available, this term can be generalized to $\mathcal{R}(\psi) = \frac{1}{2}\|\psi - P_\mathbb{L}\psi\|_U^2$ where $P_\mathbb{L}$ is the operator that projects a deformation onto the space $\mathbb{L}$ of the first variation modes of a PCA analysis [14].

Appearance prior. The image-based functions r_{int} and r_{ext} are usually defined as logarithms of probabilities, following maximum likelihood principles. Such probabilities can be learnt via classifiers, such as random forests [6]. However they are estimated using only local image features and are therefore *independent from the shape model*. In Figure 1, we show a clinical application in which this approach is too restrictive. Indeed, the appearance of the target organ may vary (depending on the location with respect to the model).

3   Tagged Template Deformation

A flux minimization problem. The image-based term in (1) is a volume integral and can be written as $E(\psi) = \int_{\Omega} H(\phi_0 \circ \psi(\mathbf{x})) \; (r_{int} - r_{ext})(\mathbf{x}) \; d\mathbf{x}$ plus a constant term that is neglected in the minimization. However, under simple regularity assumptions, this energy can be reformulated as a surface integral:

$$E(\psi) = \int_{(\phi_0 \circ \psi)^{-1}(0)} \langle \mathbf{f}(\mathbf{x}), \mathbf{n}(\mathbf{x}) \rangle \; d\mathbf{x} \quad (2)$$

with $\mathbf{n}$ the normal of the current segmentation and $\mathbf{f} = \mathcal{G} * (r_{int} - r_{ext})$ the convolution of the image term with the Green function $\mathcal{G}$ of Poisson equation [1]. E is therefore the flux of the vector field $\mathbf{f}$ across the segmentation boundary.

In a number of clinical applications such as ultrasound, we may only assume what contrast the target object should have (*e.g* it is brighter than its neighborhood). A convenient choice for $\mathbf{f}$ is then the gradient of the image $\boldsymbol{\nabla} I$ (or its opposite, depending on the contrast of the target object). As pointed out in [10], the corresponding image-based functions are the image Laplacian $r_{int}(\mathbf{x}) = \pm \Delta I(\mathbf{x})$ and $r_{ext}(\mathbf{x}) = 0$. Our proposed model encompasses this case and even goes beyond by considering any surface or region-based feature.

Flux minimization with tagged model. Let us assume that we have a set of K such vector fields $(\mathbf{f}_k)_{k=1...K}$. Instead of encoding the appearance of the whole target object, each $\mathbf{f}_k$ can be specialized to describe a particular region of the structure to be segmented. This region is defined via a *tag* function T_k : $\Omega_0 \rightarrow [-1, 1]$. The absolute value of T_k is a fuzzy indicator of the region, while its sign indicates whether the flux of $\mathbf{f}_k$ should be minimized or maximized. Note that T_k, as it is defined in the template referential Ω_0 rather than the image referential Ω, will have to be warped by ψ as well. The tagged implicit template deformation energy therefore reads:

$$E(\psi) = \sum_{k=1}^{K} \int_{(\phi_0 \circ \psi)^{-1}(0)} T_k \circ \psi(\mathbf{x}) \ \langle \mathbf{f}_k(\mathbf{x}) , \mathbf{n}(\mathbf{x}) \rangle \ d\mathbf{x} = \sum_{k=1}^{K} E_k(\psi) \qquad (3)$$

Numerical optimization. After applying the divergence theorem, the derivative of E with respect to a parameter $\mathbf{p}_i$ of the transformation ψ reads:

$$\boldsymbol{\nabla}_{\mathbf{p}_i} E_k(\psi) = \int_{\Omega} \delta(\phi_0 \circ \psi) \left\langle \boldsymbol{\nabla} \phi_0 \circ \psi \ , \ \frac{\partial \psi}{\partial p_i} \right\rangle \ (T_k \circ \psi \ . \ div(\mathbf{f}_k) \ + \ \langle \boldsymbol{\nabla}(T_k \circ \psi), \mathbf{f}_k \rangle)$$

$$+ \int_{\Omega} H(\phi_0 \circ \psi) \left(\left\langle \boldsymbol{\nabla}(T_k \circ \psi) \ , \frac{\partial \psi}{\partial \mathbf{p}_i} \right\rangle div(\mathbf{f}_k) + \left\langle \boldsymbol{\nabla}^2(T_k \circ \psi) \ . \frac{\partial \psi}{\partial \mathbf{p}_i}, \mathbf{f}_k \right\rangle \right)$$

Here the factor $\delta(\phi_0 \circ \psi)$ gives a small support to the first integrand, therefore computations are done only on the zero level-set of $\phi_0 \circ \psi$ instead of the whole volume (we refer the reader to [12] for details on implementation). The second integrand is however defined over the whole volume represented by $H(\phi_0 \circ \psi)$ and thus potentially represent a computational burden. Yet we point out that its dependence on the derivatives of T allows to reduce this overhead: If T has a sparse gradient (*e.g* is a piecewise-continuous function), these terms can also be computed from a small number of contributions.

Relationship with atlas deformation methods. Tagged template deformation is closely related to atlas deformation method since the segmentation is obtained by registering a template. The great benefits of such methods are their robustness as well as topology preservation [16]. Our proposed framework yields the same advantages but the difference is that our tagged template is defined in a piecewise manner. This yields a much more efficient algorithm since image-based forces within the gradient computation are only computed on surfaces instead of the whole volume: our C++ implementation currently allows a segmentation of a 3D image in only a few seconds on a standard laptop. It is also more flexible due to the possibility of choosing the image features $(\mathbf{f}_k)_k$ which makes it applicable to non-standardized modalities such as ultrasound.

4   Learning a Tagged Model from a Database

In this section we infer the tags from an annotated database and a set of possible features $(\mathbf{f}_k)$. We assume that we have a set of images $(I_n)_{n=1...N}$ and their associated set of features $(\mathbf{f}_{n,k})_{k=1...K}$. As a pre-processing step, all images are registered to the model referential Ω_0; the features will be transported by the same transformations $(\psi_n)_{n=1...N}$. Such registrations do not need to be precise everywhere but in the neighborhood of the zero level-set of ϕ_0.

A feature $\mathbf{f}_k$ is significant at point $\mathbf{x}$ (*i.e.* has a high tag absolute value) if it is locally in agreement with the ground truth (*i.e.* it is aligned with the normal of the ground truth) across the whole training set. The function S_k defined below quantifies this significance:

$$S_k(\mathbf{x}) = \frac{1}{N} \sum_{n=1}^{N} \left\langle \frac{\boldsymbol{\nabla}\phi_0(\mathbf{x})}{|\boldsymbol{\nabla}\phi_0(\mathbf{x})|}, \ \mathbf{f}_{n,k} \circ \psi_n(\mathbf{x}) \right\rangle \tag{4}$$

We are mainly interested in the values of S on the zero level-set of ϕ_0. At such points, $\frac{\boldsymbol{\nabla}\phi_0(\mathbf{x})}{|\boldsymbol{\nabla}\phi_0(\mathbf{x})|}$ represents the inward unit normal of the hypersurface represented by ϕ_0. To better understand (4), let us consider the case $\mathbf{f}_{n,k} = \boldsymbol{\nabla}I_n$. If the point $\mathbf{x}$ belongs to an edge of the image I_n that follows the boundary of the model, then the image gradient $\boldsymbol{\nabla}I_n(\mathbf{x})$ will be collinear to the normal and their scalar product will be high (in absolute value). Therefore $S_k(\mathbf{x})$ will have a large magnitude where there is a consistent edge across the images of the database (positive for bright-to-dark edges and vice versa). Conversely, at points where the interior of the model is sometimes brighter and sometimes darker than its exterior (*i.e.* image edges that are not reliable), S_k will be close to zero. It will also vanish when the model boundary crosses a perpendicular edge. While S_k may seem as a good tag function candidates, their gradient has no reason to be sparse. As mentioned in Section 3, the efficiency of our method is directly dependent on this sparsity. We therefore rather define the tags as

$$T_k^* = \arg\min_{T} \int_{\Omega_0} \left(\frac{1}{2}\|T(\mathbf{x}) - S_k(\mathbf{x})\|^2 + \nu\|\boldsymbol{\nabla}T_k(\mathbf{x})\| \right) d\mathbf{x} \tag{5}$$

which is the usually called a *total-variation regularization* of S. Indeed the L_1-norm of the gradient has the interesting property of favoring piecewise-constant functions. Problem (5) is solved with the method described in [2]. Results of such a process will be given hereafter for myocardium in ultrasound images.

5   Application to Myocardium Segmentation in US Images

Ultrasound imaging is widely used to diagnose and understand cardiac heart diseases. However myocardium segmentation, because of its complex appearance, is very challenging and only interactive methods have been proposed so far [7].

Our dataset is composed of 42 images coming from 14 subjects (both healthy volunteers and patients). The considered images are 2D long-axis, taken from a 4-chamber view of the heart, with a spatial resolution of 0.5 mm × 0.5 mm.

Learned tags for myocardium in US images. The result T^* of the tag learning process is presented in Figure 2. Here the mean model is defined as a closed curve including both the internal and external contours, and was estimated via the shape learning process described in [14]. For the sake of simplicity and clarity, we only used one feature which is the smoothed image gradient $\mathbf{f} = \nabla I_\sigma$. The most significant and consistent edges (in the region of the septum for instance) are detected. The pixels at the apex are also clustered into a sub-region, but with lower confidence. Furthermore, we notice a tag inversion between the inner and outer boundary at the apex and the bottom-right of the model. Others areas (*e.g* at each part of the apex) are completely neglected: the segmentation will solely be interpolated by the shape prior without taking the image into account.

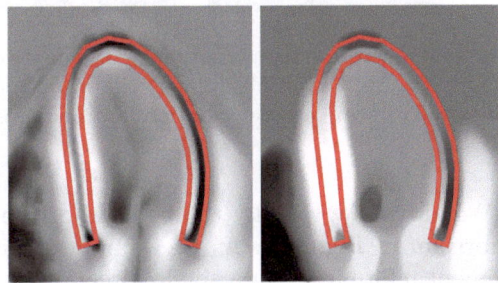

Fig. 2. Tags learning for myocardium segmentation in US in the referential of the mean model shown in red. Black represents -1, grey 0 and white 1. (Left) Mean scalar product map S. (Right) Tags T^* obtained after total-variation regularization of S. Different zones are detected, as expected from the images in Figure 1.

Evaluation of the myocardium segmentation. A clinician clicked on 3 points in each image within the myocardium: one at the apex and one at each valve. The three points are used to initialize the position and size of the mean model (see left image in Figure 3). Besides, it is naturally possible with implicit template deformation to indicate some points that should lie inside or outside the segmentation (see [12]). We therefore also use these points as inner constraints.

The validation has been performed with a leave-one-patient-out strategy. We evaluate our approach by computing for each image (*i*) the mean absolute distance, (*ii*) the maximum distance and (*iii*) the Dice coefficient, between the segmentation and the ground truth. The results are summarized in Table 1. For comparison purposes, we also indicate the scores obtained with the initial contour (placed with 3 points) and with the baseline method (constant positive tags). All reported metrics are significantly better with the new tagged template deformation method (p-value ≤ 0.0001 with a Wilcoxon signed rank test).

The distance-based metrics (3.15 for the mean absolute distance and 9.76 for the maximum distance) are slightly higher than [7], namely 1.18 and 4.41. However, their method needed 6 points *on the contour*, while we only need 3 points *inside* the myocardium. Besides, their validation database was solely composed of healthy subjects. Images from patients with pathologies are more difficult to segment since the learning is less reliable.

Table 1. Results for the myocardium segmentation averaged over the 42 images, reported in mm. Figures in brackets indicate standard-deviations.

	Mean distance	Max distance	Dice coeff.
Initialization	4.87 mm (1.53)	15.17 mm (3.65)	0.59 (0.17)
Standard temp. def.	5.10 mm (0.49)	16.65 mm (3.48)	0.59 (0.08)
Tagged temp. def.	**3.15 mm** (0.88)	**9.76 mm** (2.29)	**0.77** (0.06)

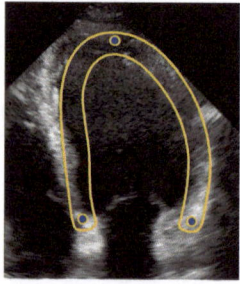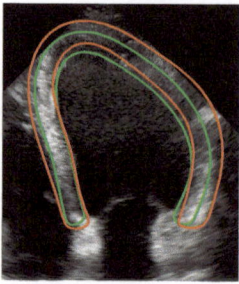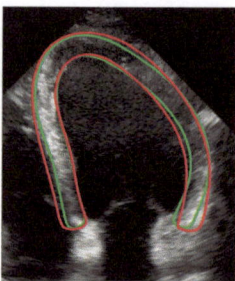

Fig. 3. Myocardium segmentation in US images compared to the ground truth in green. From left to right: Initialization of the mean model with 3 points, segmentation with the standard template deformation approach (orange) and the new model (red).

We also show visually the benefits of the tagged template over the baseline algorithm in Figure 3. As the standard template can only take into account gradient information in a single direction, it may segment correctly the septum but then cannot capture the correct boundary at the apex. Furthermore, it takes too much into account the image information at some points of the model (typically on both sides of the apex). The results might then be even worse than the initialization, as shows Table 1. Conversely, the segmentation obtained with the tagged model has a better behavior and is much closer to the ground truth.

6   Conclusion

By introducing tagged models, we have greatly enriched the prior information that is exploited in the promising framework of implicit template deformation. This extension widens the scope of potential clinical applications of this segmentation method; we indeed showed that major improvements were achieved over the standard approach in the context of myocardium segmentation in US images. Note however that this new framework is completely generic and valid both in 2D and 3D thanks to the implicit representation of shapes. It therefore paves the way for multi-organ segmentation: several organs can be represented by an implicit function, each of them being tagged in order to be attached to a dedicated image-based energy. It therefore represents a further step towards atlas-based methods, with a much more efficient and flexible approach though.

References

1. Arfken, G.B., Weber, H.J., Ruby, L.: Mathematical methods for physicists, vol. 6. Academic Press, NY (1985)
2. Chambolle, A., Pock, T.: A first-order primal-dual algorithm for convex problems with applications to imaging. JMIV 40(1), 120–145 (2011)
3. Cootes, T.F., Edwards, G.J., Taylor, C.J.: Active appearance models. IEEE Transactions on Pattern Analysis and Machine Intelligence 23(6), 681–685 (2001)
4. Cremers, D., Rousson, M., Deriche, R.: A review of statistical approaches to level set segmentation: integrating color, texture, motion and shape. International Journal of Computer Vision 72(2), 195–215 (2007)
5. Cremers, D., Sochen, N., Schnr, C.: Towards recognition-based variational segmentation using shape priors and dynamic labeling. In: Griffin, L.D., Lillholm, M. (eds.) Scale-Space 2003. LNCS, vol. 2695, pp. 388–400. Springer, Heidelberg (2003)
6. Cuingnet, R., Prevost, R., Lesage, D., Cohen, L.D., Mory, B., Ardon, R.: Automatic detection and segmentation of kidneys in 3D CT images using random forests. In: Ayache, N., Delingette, H., Golland, P., Mori, K. (eds.) MICCAI 2012, Part III. LNCS, vol. 7512, pp. 66–74. Springer, Heidelberg (2012)
7. Dietenbeck, T., Alessandrini, M., Barbosa, D., D'hooge, J., Friboulet, D., Bernard, O.: Detection of the whole myocardium in 2D-echocardiography for multiple orientations using a geometrically constrained level-set. MIA 16(2), 386–401 (2012)
8. Gauriau, R., Cuingnet, R., Prevost, R., Mory, B., Ardon, R., Lesage, D., Bloch, I.: A generic, robust and fully-automatic workflow for 3D CT liver segmentation. In: Yoshida, H., Warfield, S., Vannier, M.W. (eds.) Abdominal Imaging 2013. LNCS, vol. 8198, pp. 241–250. Springer, Heidelberg (2013)
9. Huang, X., Li, Z., Metaxas, D.: Learning coupled prior shape and appearance models for segmentation. In: Barillot, C., Haynor, D.R., Hellier, P. (eds.) MICCAI 2004. LNCS, vol. 3216, pp. 60–69. Springer, Heidelberg (2004)
10. Kimmel, R., Bruckstein, A.M.: Regularized Laplacian zero crossings as optimal edge integrators. International Journal of Computer Vision 53(3), 225–243 (2003)
11. Leventon, M.E., Faugeras, O., Grimson, W.E.L., Wells III, W.M.: Level set based segmentation with intensity and curvature priors. In: Workshop on Mathematical Methods in Biomedical Image Analysis, pp. 4–11. IEEE (2000)
12. Mory, B., Somphone, O., Prevost, R., Ardon, R.: Real-time 3D image segmentation by user-constrained template deformation. In: Ayache, N., Delingette, H., Golland, P., Mori, K. (eds.) MICCAI 2012, Part I. LNCS, vol. 7510, pp. 561–568. Springer, Heidelberg (2012)
13. Prevost, R., Mory, B., Correas, J.M., Cohen, L.D., Ardon, R.: Kidney detection and real-time segmentation in 3D contrast-enhanced ultrasound images. In: Proceedings of IEEE ISBI 2012, pp. 1559–1562 (2012)
14. Prevost, R., Cuingnet, R., Mory, B., Cohen, L.D., Ardon, R.: Incorporating shape variability in image segmentation via implicit template deformation. In: Mori, K., Sakuma, I., Sato, Y., Barillot, C., Navab, N. (eds.) MICCAI 2013, Part III. LNCS, vol. 8151, pp. 82–89. Springer, Heidelberg (2013)
15. Saddi, K., Chefd'hotel, C., Rousson, M., Cheriet, F.: Region-based segmentation via non-rigid template matching. In: Proceedings of ICCV, pp. 1–7 (2007)
16. Wolz, R., Chu, C., Misawa, K., Mori, K., Rueckert, D.: Multi-organ abdominal CT segmentation using hierarchically weighted subject-specific atlases. In: Ayache, N., Delingette, H., Golland, P., Mori, K. (eds.) MICCAI 2012, Part I. LNCS, vol. 7510, pp. 10–17. Springer, Heidelberg (2012)

Segmentation of the Right Ventricle Using Diffusion Maps and Markov Random Fields

Oliver Moolan-Feroze[1], Majid Mirmehdi[1],
Mark Hamilton[2], and Chiara Bucciarelli-Ducci[2]

[1] Visual Information Laboratory, University of Bristol, BS8 1UB
[2] Bristol Heart Institute, Bristol, BS2 8HW
oliver.moolan-feroze@bristol.ac.uk, majid@cs.bris.ac.uk

Abstract. Accurate automated segmentation of the right ventricle is difficult due in part to the large shape variation found between patients. We explore the ability of manifold learning based shape models to represent the complexity of shape variation found within an RV dataset as compared to a typical PCA based model. This is empirically evaluated with the manifold model displaying a greater ability to represent complex shapes. Furthermore, we present a combined manifold shape model and Markov Random Field Segmentation framework. The novelty of this method is the iterative generation of targeted shape priors from the manifold using image information and a current estimate of the segmentation; a process that can be seen as a traversal across the manifold. We apply our method to the independently evaluated MICCAI 2012 RV Segmentation Challenge data set. Our method performs similarly or better than the state-of-the-art methods.

1 Introduction

The role of magnetic resonance imaging (MRI) of the left ventricle (LV) in the diagnosis of cardiovascular disease is well established. This has resulted in a large body of research into automated LV segmentation [1], a necessary precursor to the extraction of cardiac parameters. Although research in right ventricular (RV) segmentation is comparatively sparse, recent work [2] has highlighted the importance of RV function to cardiac health. This has resulted in a push within the community to establish accurate and effective methods for RV segmentation and a reflection of this is the 2012 MICCAI challenge on RV segmentation [3].

Accurate RV segmentation is difficult. Even in healthy patients, challenges include inter-patient morphological differences, lack of contrast at cavity borders, obliquity of the tricuspid valve annulus, ventricular trabeculation, and shape variation between apical and basal slices. Responding to these difficulties, researchers have tended towards the inclusion of prior knowledge of the RV to inform segmentation. Often this has taken the form of cardiac atlases or statistical shape models.

Segmentation with cardiac atlases requires the non-rigid registration of a single or multiple expert labellings to the target image; an increased number of

P. Golland et al. (Eds.): MICCAI 2014, Part I, LNCS 8673, pp. 682–689, 2014.

which provide robustness to shape variation. An optimal segmentation is then decided through a system of consensus voting or statistical measures [4]. Zaluga et al. [5] implement a multi-atlas method with a course-to-fine strategy. The prevention of mis-registration is also tackled in [6], where intermediate label results are incorporated into atlas-target registrations to improve alignment. Although proven effective, these methods are slow as a result of the multiple non-rigid registrations required to align the atlases.

The statistical model approach encodes expected shape variation typically using some form of principal component analysis (PCA). Both Mitchell et al. [7], and Ordas et al. [8] construct Point Distribution Models (PDM) of both ventricles before applying them in an active appearance/shape model framework [9]. Forgoing the requirement for corresponding landmarks – a lengthy and error prone process needed for PDMs – Grosgeorge et al. [10] construct their model using PCA of signed distance functions. By generating highly deformed shapes, a static prior map is created that encompasses the extent of the variation found within the training data. Although not applied to RV segmentation, distance functions are used in [11]. Through Expectation-Maximisation, shape priors that are increasingly better fitted to the target image are generated.

Although PCA models have proven effective in many applications, recent research has investigated the ability of shape-based Diffusion Maps [12] – a type of manifold learning method – to represent the intrinsic non-linearity found in many medical datasets [13]. Detailing a method for embedding new shapes into a manifold, and providing a solution to the Diffusion Map pre-image problem, this work has paved a way for the practical use of these models for segmentation. This is evidenced in [14] where a Diffusion Map shape prior is combined with a level-set segmentation with good results.

In this work, we explore the role of a Diffusion Map shape model in application to RV segmentation. We propose that such a model will be better able to represent the complex variations displayed by the RV. The main contribution is in the novel combination of a Diffusion Map shape model with a Markov Random Field (MRF) 2D segmentation framework. Through an iterative method, image data and segmentation results from the MRF are used to generate shapes from the model that increasingly resembles the target image – a process that can be seen as a traversal over a shape manifold. The generated shapes in turn influence the MRF in the form of prior probability maps. In Sect. 2, we detail our method including both MRF formulation and Diffusion Map shape generation. In Sect. 3, we first evaluate the ability of the Diffusion Map model to represent the complex shapes within an RV dataset in comparison to a typical PCA model. This is followed by an assessment of our overall segmentation method when applied to the independently evaluated MICCAI RV Segmentation Challenge dataset.

2   Proposed Method

The proposed segmentation method consists of two steps, iteratively applied until convergence. The first is *Segmentation* (Sect. 2.1) in which we generate an estimation of the segmentation using an MRF framework combined with a prior probability map generated from a manifold shape model. For the initial iteration, the prior is generated from a mean shape and is aligned to the target using manually placed landmarks. The second step is *Prior Update* (Sect. 2.2) where we combine the current estimate of the segmentation with image information to update the prior through a process of manifold traversal. The method terminates when the difference in segmentation estimation between two iterations falls below a threshold.

Integral to the overall process is the manifold shape model. We define a shape as a signed distance function s. The Diffusion Map is constructed over the set of training shapes $\Gamma = \{s_i\}$ where $i \in 1, \dots, p$ following the method outlined in [13]. To measure shape similarity, we use the distance proposed in [15],

$$d^2\left(s_i, s_j\right) = \sum_{x \in \Omega_s} \left(H(s_i(x)) - H(s_j(x))\right)^2 , \qquad (1)$$

where $H(.)$ is the Heaviside function. This benefits from being fast, as well as being positive, symmetric, and obeying the triangle inequality. The result of this process is our shape model - an embedding $\Phi(s) = y$, $y \in \mathrm{R}^m$ where m is the dimensionality of the reduced space.

2.1 Segmentation Using MRFs and Manifold Shape Priors

We model the segmentation as an MRF. The field is a graph $\mathcal{G} = \langle \mathcal{V}, \mathcal{E} \rangle$ where $\mathcal{V}$ is the set of n image pixels $I = (x_1, \dots, x_n)$ and $\mathcal{E}$ the edges that connect them with their neighbours. A set of labels $\alpha \in \{O, B\}$ represent the object and background classes. The labelling $\boldsymbol{\alpha} = (\alpha_1, \dots, \alpha_n)$ applied over the graph constitutes a segmentation. Each label assignment incurs a cost specified by the energy function

$$E_\omega(I, \boldsymbol{\alpha}) = E_\omega^{\mathrm{d}}(I, \boldsymbol{\alpha}) + E_\omega^{\mathrm{b}}(I, \boldsymbol{\alpha}) + E_\omega^{\mathrm{p}}(I, \boldsymbol{\alpha}, M_\omega) . \qquad (2)$$

The optimal labelling is when E_ω is at its minimum. The first term E_ω^{d} is a data term which measures the sum of the individual labelling costs at each node in $\mathcal{V}$. This is computed using the local image information and a foreground and background Gaussian Mixture Model (GMM), with 1 and 2 modes respectively

$$E_\omega^{\mathrm{d}}(I, \boldsymbol{\alpha}) = \sum_{i \in \mathcal{V}} - \log p(x_i | \alpha_i, \boldsymbol{\mu}, \boldsymbol{\sigma}) , \qquad (3)$$

where $P(x_p | \alpha_i, \boldsymbol{\mu}, \boldsymbol{\sigma})$ is the probability of the pixel belonging to either the foreground or background given the GMM parameters $\boldsymbol{\mu}$ and $\boldsymbol{\sigma}$.

The second term of the energy function, E_ω^{b}, encourages a smooth labelling over the graph by penalising pairs of nodes (i, j) that have differing label assignments, such that

$$E_\omega^{\mathrm{b}}(I, \boldsymbol{\alpha}) = \sum_{\alpha_i \neq \alpha_j, i, j \in \mathcal{E}} \exp\left(-\frac{(x_i - x_j)^2}{2\sigma_{\mathrm{b}}^2}\right) \cdot \frac{1}{dist(i, j)} . \qquad (4)$$

σ_b is varied to compensate for an expected amount of signal noise in the image and $dist(i,j)$ represents the Euclidean distance between the two nodes.

The final term E_ω^p incorporates prior shape information into the MRF. A shape generated from the Diffusion Map $\hat{s}$ is transformed into a probabilistic atlas image M_ω

$$M_\omega(i) = \begin{cases} 1 & \text{if} \quad \hat{s}(i) \le 0 \\ \exp\left(-\hat{s}(i)/\gamma\right) & \text{if} \quad \hat{s}(i) > 0 \end{cases} \tag{5}$$

where the value γ controls the 'spread' of the influence of the prior outside the boundaries of the zero-level set of $\hat{s}$. The prior term is then defined as

$$E_\omega^p(I, \boldsymbol{\alpha}, M_\omega) = \sum_{i \in \mathcal{V}} - \begin{cases} \log M_\omega(T(i)) & \text{if} \quad \alpha_i = \text{O} \\ \log(1 - M_\omega(T(i))) & \text{if} \quad \alpha_i = \text{B} \end{cases} \tag{6}$$

where T is a rigid transform that aligns the model with the target image. The MRF is optimised using the graph cut method of Boykov et al. [16].

2.2   Prior Update through Manifold Traversal

Using the learned manifold and the image data from the segmentation target we present a method of generating patient specific shape priors. This technique of iterative prior generation can be seen as a traversal over the manifold where each iteration produces a shape that increasingly resembles the target. An example of the manifold traversal can be seen in Fig. 1. To drive the traversal, we take the signed distance function of our current estimate of the segmentation s^* and transform it into the space of the model using T^{-1}. This is used to query into the manifold. As Diffusion Maps do not provide a simple way of embedding new data into a learned manifold, we use the Nyström extension [13]. This provides an operator $\hat{\Phi}(T^{-1}(s^*)) = y^*$ where y^* represents the coordinates in the space of the manifold. We take y^* as an estimate of the coordinates that would be produced by embedding the true segmentation and find the nearest neighbours $\mathcal{N}$. The shapes that constitute these neighbours are the templates from which a new shape $\hat{s}$ can be generated. This is done by taking their linear combinations $\hat{s} = \sum_{i \in \mathcal{N}} \theta_i s_i$, where $\theta_i \ge 0$ and $\sum_{i \in \mathcal{N}} \theta_i = 1$. By varying the values in θ we influence the generated shape $\hat{s}$.

To ensure that the generated shape $\hat{s}$ resembles the segmentation target we aim to satisfy two conditions: (a) that it resembles our current 'best guess' at the segmentation s^* and, (b) that it fits to the target image, compensating for inaccuracies in s^*. We encode these two conditions in the energy function

$$E_\eta(\hat{s}, s^*, I, T, \lambda_\eta) = E_\eta^d(\hat{s}, T^{-1}(s^*)) + \lambda_\eta E_\eta^h(I) \ . \tag{7}$$

The first term is d^2 from (1) and will penalise $\hat{s}$ from deviating from s^*. Similar to [11], the second term is a measure of the entropy inside and outside of the image region enclosed by $T(\hat{s})$, such that

$$E_\eta^h(I) = \sum_{x_i \in I} - ((p_O(x_i) \log p_O(x_i)) + (p_B(x_i) \log p_B(x_i))) \ , \tag{8}$$

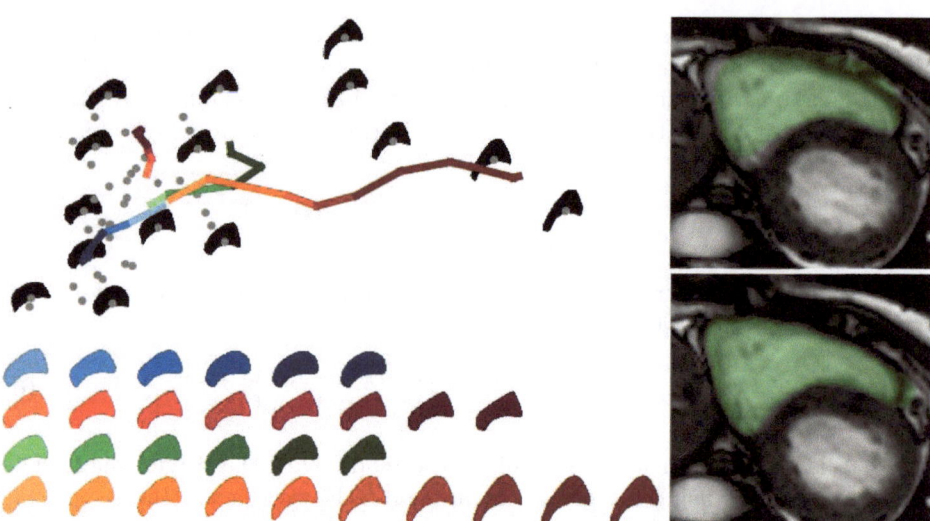

Fig. 1. Visualisation of Manifold Traversal. (Left) Image displaying a learned manifold with traversals overlaid. Black shapes are taken from the training data. Coloured paths map the traversal across the manifold during segmentation. Images below the manifold show the changing shape of the generated prior at each iteration of the segmentation with colours corresponding to their paths. (Right) Example of initial prior (top) and prior at the end of manifold traversal (bottom)

where p_O and p_B are the probability of image value x_i being found in the foreground or background respectively. These are computed by generating histograms of the image intensity values in the corresponding regions of $T(\hat{s})$. The value λ_η is a weighting term which varies the influence of the entropy calculation. To find the optimal prior, we define the functional $S_{\mathcal{N},\theta} = \sum_{s_i \in \mathcal{N}} \theta_i s_i$ and compute the optimal transform $\hat{T}$ and shape parameters $\hat{\theta}$ using Powell's method [17],

$$\underset{\theta,T}{\operatorname{argmin}}\ E_p(S_{\mathcal{N},\theta}, s^*, I, T, \lambda_\eta)\ . \tag{9}$$

3   Evaluation

To evaluate the performance of the proposed method we applied it to the MIC-CAI 2012 RV Segmentation Challenge dataset [3]. This data was acquired from 32 patients with diagnosed cardiac pathologies, where for each examination, two volumes representing end-diastole (ED) and end-systole (ES) were manually labelled by a cardiac radiologist. The data was split into two sets of 16 examinations, one for training and one for testing. Due to the shape variation between both apical and basal slices and between ED and ES, we split the training data into 11 sets - 6 models at ED and 5 at ES. For all our experiments, the dimensionality of the manifold model was 3.

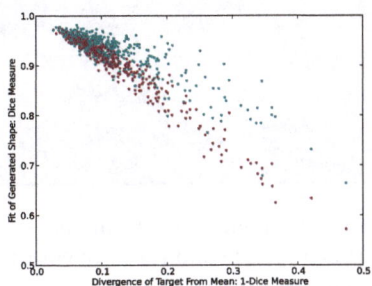

Fig. 2. Plot of manifold (blue) and PCA with 30 modes (red) performance against the divergence of the target from the mean

Table 1. Table showing the DM mean (μ) and standard deviation (σ) from the first experiment

		DM ($\mu \pm \sigma$)
Propsed	ED	0.94 ± 0.03
Method	ES	0.92 ± 0.05
	Total	**0.93 ± 0.04**
PCA	ED	0.93 ± 0.04
10 modes	ES	0.88 ± 0.08
	Total	**0.91 ± 0.06**
PCA	ED	0.93 ± 0.04
30 modes	ES	0.89 ± 0.08
	Total	**0.91 ± 0.06**

Model Shape Generation Comparison – The first experiment compared the ability of our model against a typical PCA model to represent the complex shapes exhibited by the RV. For both methods, we generated a series of shape models using leave-one-out cross validation across all 11 groupings of training data. The manifold model was built as in Sect. 2, and the PCA models were built by applying PCA to the set of aligned training shapes. The top 10 and 30 modes we retained, which accounted for 97.7% and 99.9% of the variation found within the data. To test our model, we generated a new shape $\hat{s}$ from the test shape s_t by optimising (9) with $\lambda_\eta = 0$ and fixing T as the identity matrix. For the PCA method, we extracted the shape parameters by transforming s_t into the PCA space, regularised them to be within $\pm 3\sigma$ of the learned variation and reconstructed the shape $\hat{s}$ in the typical manner.

Table 1 displays the Dice Metric (DM) over the target s_t and generated shape $\hat{s}$. It shows that all models are able to represent new shapes well, with the manifold model performing slightly better. Also of interest are the results in Fig. 2, where the performance of both our model and the 30 mode PCA model is plotted against the dissimilarity of s_t from the mean shape. This shows that our method is better able to adapt to the extremities of the data variation.

Evaluation on MICCAI 2012 RV Segmentation Dataset – We applied the proposed method to segmentation using the MICCAI RV challenge dataset. We learned the manifold models as described previously. In addition, GMMs were generated for each model to capture the intensity variations between the basal and apical slices. Together, these were applied to the 16 test-set examinations. The results generated by our method were independently evaluated by the organisers of the challenge. As in [10], minimal manual input provided an initial alignment for the model. This consisted of two landmarks at the junction of the RV and LV. Since we optimise the transform T during segmentation, the method is somewhat robust to initial landmark placement.

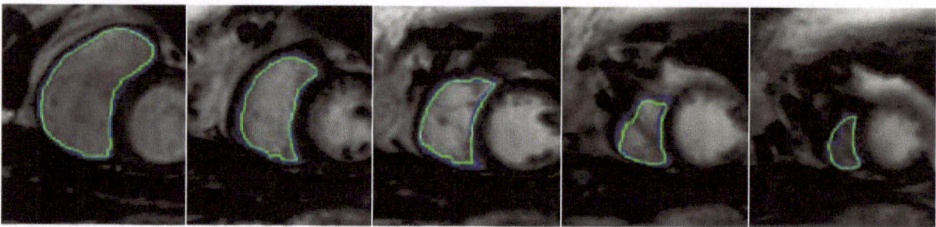

Fig. 3. Example output of our segmentation method. All images are from the same examination at ED. The manual segmentation is outlined in blue and the segmentation produced by the proposed method is outlined in green.

Table 2. Results from RV segmentation and comparison with the state-of-the-art

	Phase	Dice Metric	Haussdorf Distance
Proposed Method	ED	**0.86 ± 0.10**	8.40 ± 4.21
	ES	**0.75 ± 0.18**	**10.02 ± 5.78**
Grosgeorge et al. [10]	ED	0.83 ± 0.15	9.48 ± 5.41
	ES	0.70 ± 0.22	10.56 ± 5.54
Bai's et al. [6]	ED	0.86 ± 0.11	**7.70 ± 3.75**
	ES	0.69 ± 0.25	11.16 ± 5.53

For each slice segmented, both the DM and Haussdorf Distance (HD) were computed. The results can be seen in Table 2 where they are compared against Grosgeorge et al. [10] and Bai et al. [6]. Example output can be seen in Fig. 3. The results show that our method performed similarly or slightly better than the state-of-the-art in most metrics, with greatest improvement during ES. This, coupled with the results in Table 1 lends support to our argument that a manifold model is well suited for dealing with the complex RV shapes. The code was written in C++ with little optimisation. Segmentation of a single volume takes between 7-10 minutes depending on the speed of convergence. The tests were run on an Intel Core i7 CPU @ 2.80GHz with 16Gb of memory.

4   Conclusions and Future Work

We proposed a novel method of combining shape priors generated from a learned manifold into a Markov Random Field segmentation framework. By alternating between segmentation and improving the prior, we have shown that the manifold is able to generate priors that fit to the shape of target even when the morphology is complex. We have tested the performance of our method with an independently evaluated dataset with results that are comparable with the state-of-the-art methods.

For future work we intend to implement the method in 3D to be able to use the improved accuracy of the basal segmentations to influence the more difficult apical slices. In addition, we aim to improve our manifold traversal method by better utilising the underlying geometry of the data. This will allow us to extrapolate, increasing the amount of shape variation that the model can fit to.

References

1. Petitjean, C., Dacher, J.N.: A review of segmentation methods in short axis cardiac MR images. Medical Image Analysis 15(2), 169–184 (2011)
2. Caudron, J., Fares, J., Lefebvre, V., Vivier, P.H., Petitjean, C., Dacher, J.N.: Cardiac MRI assessment of right ventricular function in acquired heart disease: factors of variability. Academic Radiology 19(8), 991–1002 (2012)
3. Petitjean, C., Ruan, S., Grosgeorge, D.: Right Ventricle Segmentation in Cardiac MRI: a MICCAI 2012 Challenge (2012)
4. Warfield, S., Zou, K., Wells, W.: Simultaneous truth and performance level estimation (STAPLE): an algorithm for the validation of image segmentation. IEEE Trans. Medical Imaging 23(7), 903–921 (2004)
5. Zuluaga, M.A., Cardoso, M.J., Modat, M., Ourselin, S.: Multi-atlas propagation whole heart segmentation from MRI and CTA using a local normalised correlation coefficient criterion. In: Ourselin, S., Rueckert, D., Smith, N. (eds.) FIMH 2013. LNCS, vol. 7945, pp. 174–181. Springer, Heidelberg (2013)
6. Bai, W., Shi, W., O'Regan, D.P., Tong, T., Wang, H., Jamil-Copley, S., Peters, N.S., Rueckert, D.: A probabilistic patch-based label fusion model for multi-atlas segmentation with registration refinement: application to cardiac MR images. IEEE Trans. Medical Imaging 32(7), 1302–1315 (2013)
7. Mitchell, S.: Multistage hybrid active appearance model matching: segmentation of left and right ventricles in cardiac MR images. IEEE Trans. Medical Imaging 20, 415–423 (2001)
8. Ordas, S., Boisrobert, L., Huguet, M., Frangi, A.: Active shape models with invariant optimal features (IOF-ASM) application to cardiac MRI segmentation. Computers in Cardiology, 633–636 (2003)
9. Cootes, T., Taylor, C.: Active shape models-their training and application. CVIU 61, 38–59 (1995)
10. Grosgeorge, D., Petitjean, C., Dacher, J.N., Ruan, S.: Graph cut segmentation with a statistical shape model in cardiac MRI. CVIU 117(9), 1027–1035 (2013)
11. Zhu-Jacquot, J., Zabih, R.: Graph Cuts Segmentation with Statistical Shape Priors for Medical Images. In: Signal-Image Technologies and Internet-Based System, pp. 631–635 (2007)
12. Coifman, R.R., Lafon, S.: Diffusion maps. Applied and Computational Harmonic Analysis 21(1), 5–30 (2006)
13. Etyngier, P., Segonne, F., Keriven, R.: Shape Priors using Manifold Learning Techniques. In: IEEE ICCV, pp. 1–8 (2007)
14. Thorstensen, N., Étyngier, P., Ségonne, F., Keriven, R.: Diffusion maps as a framework for shape modeling. CVIU 115(4), 520–530 (2011)
15. Chan, T., Zhu, W.: Level Set Based Shape Prior Segmentation. IEEE CVPR 2, 1164–1170 (2005)
16. Boykov, Y., Veksler, O., Zabih, R.: Fast approximate energy minimization via graph cuts. IEEE PAMI 23(11), 1222–1239 (2001)
17. Powell, M.: Direct search algorithms for optimization calculations. Acta Numerica (1998)

Differential and Relaxed Image Foresting Transform for Graph-Cut Segmentation of Multiple 3D Objects

Nikolas Moya[1], Alexandre X. Falcão[1],
Krzysztof C. Ciesielski[2,3], and Jayaram K. Udupa[3]

[1] Institute of Computing, University of Campinas, Campinas, SP, Brazil
[2] Department of Mathematics, West Virginia University, Morgantown, WV, USA
[3] Department of Radiology, University of Pennsylvania, Philadelphia, PA, USA

Abstract. Graph-cut algorithms have been extensively investigated for interactive binary segmentation, when the simultaneous delineation of multiple objects can save considerable user's time. We present an algorithm (named DRIFT) for 3D multiple object segmentation based on seed voxels and Differential Image Foresting Transforms (DIFTs) with relaxation. DRIFT stands behind efficient implementations of some state-of-the-art methods. The user can add/remove markers (seed voxels) along a sequence of executions of the DRIFT algorithm to improve segmentation. Its first execution takes linear time with the image's size, while the subsequent executions for corrections take sublinear time in practice. At each execution, DRIFT first runs the DIFT algorithm, then it applies diffusion filtering to smooth boundaries between objects (and background) and, finally, it corrects possible objects' disconnection occurrences with respect to their seeds. We evaluate DRIFT in 3D CT-images of the thorax for segmenting the arterial system, esophagus, left pleural cavity, right pleural cavity, trachea and bronchi, and the venous system.

Keywords: Image segmentation, differential image foresting transform, boundary smoothing, graph-cut algorithms.

1 Introduction

This work studies the segmentation algorithm which, given an image (3D, medical) and $M \geq 1$ desired objects, returns a label map L from the image domain D into $\{0, \ldots, M\}$, where the label 0 designates the background and voxels in the ith object are assigned to label $1 \leq i \leq M$. Although some algorithms do not need more input (e.g., those based on the Mumford-Shah model [1]), they are neither efficient nor accurate. Therefore, we will focus on the algorithms that require the object location as input, in a format of the seed sets $\lambda^{-1}(0), \ldots, \lambda^{-1}(M)$ (see e.g. [2–5]), where λ is a function from $S \subset D$ into $i \in \{0, \ldots, M\}$.

Even with seeds indicating object location, the state-of-the-art segmentation methods rarely provide satisfactory results in a single execution, asking for the user's assistance to add seeds and improve segmentation. These steps can be

P. Golland et al. (Eds.): MICCAI 2014, Part I, LNCS 8673, pp. 690–697, 2014.

repeated several times until user's satisfaction is reached. Most algorithms, however, are limited to binary segmentation, when the simultaneous segmentation of multiple objects can save the user's time considerably.

Figure 1 illustrates the interactive 3D segmentation of multiple objects using Differential Image Foresting Transforms (DIFTs) [6]. Markers (seed sets, represented by distinct colors) propagate their labels to the most strongly connected voxels in the image. The image is interpreted as a graph, with arcs given by an *adjacency relation* between voxels, and each voxel is conquered by a seed which offers an optimum path to it. The result is an *optimum-path forest* with labeled trees, where each object is the union of the trees painted with the same color (the label map). The forest is used to correct segmentation, since it connects markers to their influence zones in the image. This algorithm takes time proportional to the number of voxels in the first execution, but subsequent segmentation corrections (marker addition and/or removal) usually take time proportional to the size of the modified regions (i.e., sublinear time). The label map is also a graph cut that minimizes the maximum arc-weight along the cut, given seeds as constraints (i.e., the DIFT is a GC_{max} algorithm [7]). The DIFT is part of the Image Foresting Transform (IFT) methodology [8], which accepts as input either an image or an optimum-path forest resulting from a previous execution.

A crucial requirement in the above procedure is an interactive response time to the user's actions (i.e., a few seconds or, preferably, instantaneous response). The DIFT meets the speed requirement for large medical images and stands behind efficient implementations of GC_{max} methods, such as Iterative Relative Fuzzy Connectedness [7] and Watershed Transforms [6]. A negative aspect of

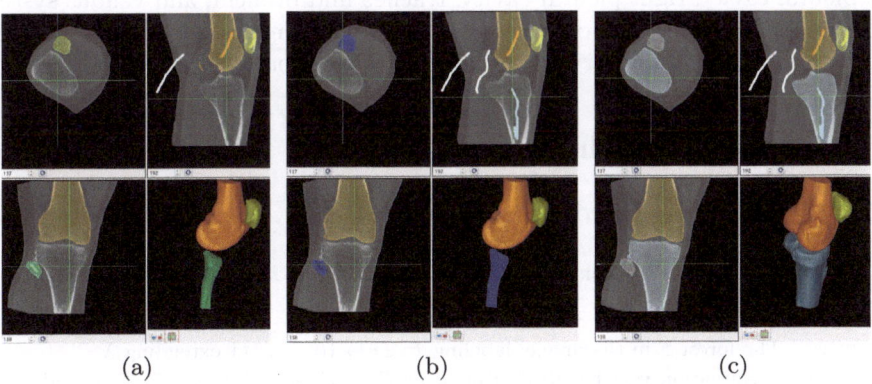

(a)   (b)   (c)

Fig. 1. (a) By examining orthogonal slices, the user draws green, yellow and orange markers (seed voxels) in three bones and white marker in the background. The bottom-right part displays the 3D rendition of the resulting label map. (b) The user can change mind, pick any voxel in the influence zone of the green marker to remove the bone (dark blue indicates marked for removal). At the same time, the user can insert new markers (cyan for a new bone and white for background) to adjust segmentation. (c) The algorithm removes the green bone and creates a new result with the other three selected bones.

such methods, however, is the lack of regularity of the segmented object boundaries (the "leaking problem"). Boundary smoothness can be enforced by postprocessing. In [9], for instance, the IFT results were adjusted by the max-flow algorithm and in [10], a version of diffusion was used for boundary smoothing, resulting into the "relaxed IFT algorithm" (RIFT).

In this paper, we revisit the RIFT algorithm [10] to correct its inconsistency in segmentation and to propose its differential version with a considerably faster boundary smoothing process, which applies diffusion while the boundary between distinct labels is expanded inward the objects (and background) through a few iterations (e.g., 10). The initial boundary is also found during the DIFT computation, when wavefronts from distinct labels meet each other. Given that any post-processing for boundary smoothing might disconnect a part of an object from its most strongly connected seed, such inconsistency is corrected as follows: We find (in a fully automatic way) a modified set of seeds and use the DIFT algorithm with these seeds to create a new forest, which induces the segmentation closed to the one produced by the smoothing step, while removing any objects' disconnection occurrences. This second forest-induced segmentation is the one that the user examines and either accepts, or continues to improve.

One can use the boundary smoothing and connectivity correction (second DIFT module) steps after each application of the first DIFT module or only once, at the end of the process. In preliminary tests, we found the latter less accurate in most cases, since it does not give the chance to correct the process. Therefore, we evaluate the first solution, named *Differential and Relaxed IFT* (DRIFT), in comparison with the DIFT [6] and the Dynamic Graph-Cut (DGC) algorithms [11] for segmenting 3D CT-images of the thorax into: arterial system, esophagus, left pleural cavity, right pleural cavity, trachea and bronchi, and venous system. The segmentation of these objects is especially challenging due to their different shapes and lack of boundary information in several parts.

2   The Details of the Algorithm

The DRIFT Algorithm can be presented as follows.

Algorithm 1 – DRIFT ALGORITHM

INPUT: The image $I: D \to \mathbb{R}^m$ and seeds' labeling $\lambda: S \to \{0, \ldots, M\}$.
OUTPUT: The forest $\mathbb{F}$ in the image; labeling $L: D \to \{0, \ldots, M\}$ extending λ.
AUXILIARY: Termination variable *flag* initiated as *FALSE*, boundary set $B \subset D$, and dilated boundary set $B_d \subset D$.

1. *Run DIFT with I and λ to get the forest $\mathbb{F}$, label map L, and boundary set B.*
2. **While** *flag* = *FALSE* **do**
3.   *Smooth L from B, returning new labeling L' and dilated set $B_d \supset B$.*
4.   *Run DIFT from B_d to get new $\mathbb{F}$ and associated labeling L consistent with L'.*
5.   **If** *User is satisfied with L* **then**
6.   └ *Set flag* ← *TRUE.*
7.   **Else**

8.   ⌊   ⌊   *Get correcting labeling λ' from the user.*
9.   ⌊   ⌊   *Run DIFT for λ' to get new forest $\mathbb{F}$, labeling L, and set B.*

In the rest of these section we will explain in more details what stands behind the lines 1, 3, 4, 8, and 9.

Details on DIFT. We assume that $D \subset \mathbb{Z}^3$ and its voxels are the nodes of a graph G, whose arcs $\{s,t\} \subset \mathcal{A} \subset D \times D$ satisfy $0 < \|t - s\| \leq \sqrt{3}$ (adjacency relation). We also say that $\mathcal{A}(s)$ is the set $\{t \in D : 0 < \|t - s\| \leq \sqrt{3}\}$. The graph G is weighted on the arcs by $w(s,t) = K\omega(t)$, where $K > 0$ is an integer and ω is defined to assign lower values on object boundaries than elsewhere:
$$\omega(s) = 1 - \frac{1}{|\mathcal{A}(s)|} \sum_{t \in \mathcal{A}(s)} \frac{\|I(t) - I(s)\|}{I_{\max}}, \quad I_{\max} = \max_{s \in D} \|I(s)\|.$$
The *DIFT* algorithm can be run for: any subgraph G' of G induced by the vertices $D' \subset D$; any set $S' \subset D'$ of seeds such that for each $t \in D'$ there is a path in G' from t to S'; any labeling $\lambda \colon S' \to \{0, \ldots, M\}$; and any initial seed-strength map $\mu \colon S' \to [0, K]$. Then, *DIFT* returns a forest $\mathbb{F}$ in G' rooted at S', that is, a family of paths in G' such that: any initial segment of a $p \in \mathbb{F}$ is also in $\mathbb{F}$; every $p \in \mathbb{F}$ contains precisely one seed from S'; and for each $t \in D'$ there is a $p_t \in \mathbb{F}$ from $s_t \in S'$ to t. The paths in $\mathbb{F}$ are indicated by the predecessor map $P \colon D' \setminus S' \to D'$, where $P(t)$ is a predecessor of t in p_t. Since the map P uniquely determines $\mathbb{F}$, we will identify $\mathbb{F}$ with P, wherever convenient. The forest $\mathbb{F}$ returned by *DIFT* is optimal in the following sense. For a path $\pi = \langle t_0, \ldots, t_n \rangle$ from S' we define its strength as $f(\pi) = \min_{i<n}\{\mu(t_0), w(t_i, t_{i+1})\}$. Then for any path $\pi = \langle t_0, \ldots, t_m, t \rangle$ in G' with $\langle t_0, \ldots, t_m \rangle \in \mathbb{F}$ and $t \notin S'$, either $f(p_t) > f(\pi)$ or both $f(p_t) = f(\pi)$ and $\lambda(s_t) \leq \lambda(t_0)$.

Line 1. We run *DIFT* with $D' = D$, $S' = S$, λ provided by the user, and $\mu(s) = K$ for all $s \in S'$ and for $s \in D' \setminus S'$, $\mu(s) = -\infty$. The output labeling L is defined as $L(t) = \lambda(s_t)$ and the boundary set B is $\{s \in D : \exists t \in \mathcal{A}(s), L(t) \neq L(s)\}$.

Line 3. The smoothing is a diffusion filtering on the label map L, starting from B, that takes a fix number T of iterations (e.g., $T = 10$). At each iteration, B generates a dilated set $B_d = B \cup \{t \in D \setminus B, t \in \mathcal{A}(s), s \in B\}$, which turns to be the set B for the next iteration. The final set B_d is also returned and it contains the voxels that might have changed labels during diffusion.

For every $s \in D$, put $W(s) = \frac{1}{1+\alpha(1-\omega(s))}$, where $\alpha \in [0, 1]$ is a fixed smoothing factor, and define a normalization factor as $N(s) = \sum_{t \in \mathcal{A}(s)} W(t)$. (For sake of efficiency, the maps W and N should be computed only once and used as input).

Put $L_0 = L$ and for every $t \in B_d$ and $l \in \{0, 1, \ldots, M\}$ define $\mu_0(l, t) = 1$ if $l = L_0(t)$ and $\mu_0(l, t) = 0$, otherwise. Then, recursively, for $i \in \{1, \ldots, T\}$ and $s \in B$, we find $\mu_i(l, s) = \frac{1}{N(s)} \sum_{t \in \mathcal{A}(s),\, L_{i-1}(t)=l} \mu_{i-1}(l, t) W(t)$. Note that $\sum_{l=1}^{M} \mu_i(l, s) = 1$ for every $i \in \{0, \ldots, T\}$ and $s \in B$. Define the labeling L_i by putting $L_i(s) = l$ when for every $l' \in \{0, 1, \ldots, M\}$ either $\mu_i(l, s) > \mu_i(l', s)$ or both $\mu_i(l, s) = \mu_i(l', s)$ and $l \leq l'$. At the end, $L' = L_T$.

Line 4. Let $U_0 = \{t \in B_d \colon L'(t) \neq L(t)\}$ be the set of voxels that changed labeling and U be the subtrees of the voxels in U_0. That is, U is the set of all $t \in D$ for which the path $p_t \in \mathbb{F}$ contains a voxel from U_0. The voxels in U were influenced (w.r.t. $\mathbb{F}$) by the change of labeling and they need to be "reconquered." Define the frontier set S' as $s \in D \setminus U$ for which there exists a $t \in \mathcal{A}(s) \cap U$ with $L(s) = L'(t)$. This is the new set of seeds, that will compete for the voxels in U.

For this we put $D' = U \cup S'$ and define, for every $s \in S'$, $\lambda(s) = L(s)$ and $\mu(s) = f(p_s)$, where $p_s \in \mathbb{F}$, and for every $s \in U$, $\mu(s) = -\infty$. Run DIFT with this setup.

Of course, the forest $\mathbb{F}'$ that is returned is defined only on D'. However, if $P' \colon U \to D'$ is a predecessor map for $\mathbb{F}'$, then the new predecessor map defined as P' on U, as an old predecessor map on $D \setminus U$, determines full predecessor map on D and the new forest $\mathbb{F}$ (for, possibly decreased, set $S \setminus U$ of seeds). It is worth to notice that, this new forest need not to be optimal in the sense discussed above.

Line 8. The correcting labeling λ' is a map from $W \subset D$ into $\{-1, 0, \ldots, M\}$. The meaning of a label $\lambda'(s) \in \{0, \ldots, M\}$ is straightforward: it means that the user assigns s as a seed for the ith object (background). (Note that assignment makes sometimes sense even when we previously had $\lambda(s) = i$, as this changes the connectivity strength between s and the seed set.) The assignment $\lambda(s) = -1$, on the other hand, is for removing the marker, whose influence zone (its forest) contains s. Given that the user can make mistakes, marker deletion is a desirable feature.

Line 9. Let $W_0 = \{s \in W \colon \lambda'(s) = -1\}$ and $W_1 = W \setminus W_0$. From W_0, the predecessor map identifies a set U_0 with the roots of all trees selected for removal and, as for line 4, let U be the subtrees of the voxels in U_0.

Define the frontier set F as those $s \in D \setminus U$ for which there exists a $t \in \mathcal{A}(s) \cap U$. Put $S' = W_1 \cup F$ and $D' = D$. Define λ and μ on S' as follows. For $s \in W_1$ we put $\lambda(s) = \lambda'(s)$ and $\mu(s) = K$. For $s \in F$ we put $\lambda(s) = L(s)$ and $\mu(s) = f(p(s))$. For $s \in U \setminus W_1$ we put $\mu(s) = -\infty$. Then, we run $DIFT$ with this setup to get a forest $\mathbb{F}'$ on D'. We recreate from it the new forest $\mathbb{F}$ and label map L, as in Line 4, and the boundary set B, as in Line 1.

3   Experiments

The experiments evaluate the accuracy and efficiency of the DRIFT (as an IRFC implementation [7]), DIFT [6], and DGC [11] algorithms running on the same input graph (nodes are voxels) from 40 3D CT-images of the thorax to segment: the arterial system (AS), esophagus (E), left pleural cavity (LPS), right pleural cavity (RPS), trachea and bronchi (TB), and venous system (VS). Since DGC is constrained to segment object by object, we present the total mean number of executions and the sum of the mean times spent per execution on each object. The ground-truth (GT) images were created by several experts, as described in [12]. The images were acquired with voxel size $0.5 \times 0.5 \times 5mm^3$, so they were interpolated to $158 \times 158 \times 116$ voxels with $2.5 \times 2.5 \times 2.5mm^3$ each.

Seeking to reduce costs and biases associated with evaluation by real users, we used geodesic robot users to generate the seed sets [13]. Given the GT image, the geodesic robot adds a given number of seeds along the executions in the error components, until they are too small for new marker selection. The markers were spheres whose radius varied proportionally with the size of the error components within $[1, 10]$ voxels. A maximum of 56 makers per execution was used (8 markers per object plus 8 for the background), the number of smoothing iterations $T = 10$, and the smoothing factor $\alpha = 0.5$.

The error values in Table 1 are in mm and they correspond to the mean error over the 40 images according to the average symmetric absolute surface distance between GT and segmentation[1].

Table 1. Mean error and standard deviation in mm per object after convergence, using 8 seeds per object (background) and 10 smoothing iterations

Algorithm	AS	E	LPS	RPS	TB	VS	Mean
DRIFT	2.6±2.19	1.3±0.58	1.0±1.91	0.8±1.36	0.8±0.33	1.6±0.86	1.4±0.95
DIFT	3.4±1.43	2.2±2.14	0.7±0.24	0.7±0.24	0.7±0.24	2.1±1.25	1.6±0.52
DGC	4.8±0.95	3.4±0.63	1.2±0.13	1.1±0.15	1.3±0.74	4.2±0.72	2.0±0.57

For a statistical significance level of 95%, DRIFT is more accurate than DGC in all cases and than DIFT for AS, E, and VS (sparse objects). On average, it required less executions for convergence (i.e., it should not affect the user's control over segmentation) and its response time was about 4.6s per execution (Table 2).

Table 2. Mean number of executions and mean time per execution (s) and their standard deviations

Algorithm	# of executions			Time per execution (s)		
	DRIFT	DIFT	DGC	DRIFT	DIFT	DGC
Thorax	13.8±4.95	15.5±5.0	48.1 ± 13.16	4.6 ±0.96	2.5±0.61	8.5 ± 2.4

Figure 2 also illustrates for the most accurate methods, DIFT and DRIFT, that irrespective to their accuracy differences, the results with boundary smoothing seem to match better with the users' expectations. All these aspects involving real users need to be investigated.

---

[1] http://mbi.dkfz-heidelberg.de/grand-challenge2007/sites/eval.htm

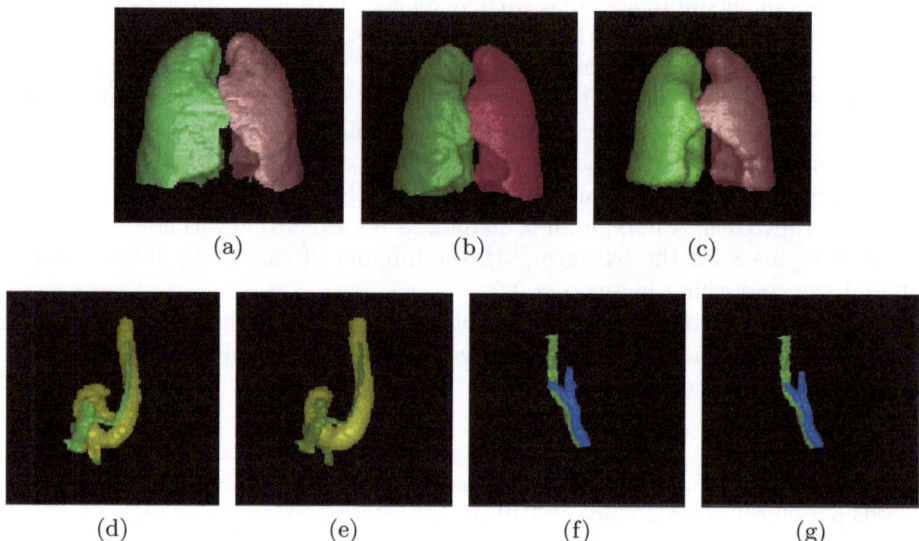

Fig. 2. RPS and LPS: (a) GT, (b) DIFT, and (c) DRIFT. AS and VS: (d) DIFT and (e) DRIFT. E and TB: (f) DIFT and (g) DRIFT.

4 Conclusion

We presented the DRIFT algorithm for interactive segmentation of multiple 3D objects using optimum-path forests and boundary smoothing. DRIFT can provide better accuracies than the DIFT and DGC algorithms, with interactive response time to the user's actions, being much faster and correct with respect to the RIFT algorithm. DRIFT can be used to devise new segmentation methods, by choice of other connectivity functions [8], as well as to implement state-of-the-art methods [7] more efficiently. The algorithm was tested on 40 3D CT-images of the thorax, presenting accuracy gains and visual results that seem to better match with the users' expectations. From Table 2, DRIFT required only about 63s of computational time, on average, to complete segmentation of 6 objects, considerably outperforming the DGC algorithm in accuracy and speed.

Future research is required to extend DRIFT to supervoxel graphs for further speed-up gains and assess it on other datasets, possibly involving distinct imaging modalities, with different arc-weight functions, and in practical situations involving multiple experts.

Acknowledgments. The authors thank FAPESP (2013/17991-0), CAPES, CNPq (303673/2010-9,479070/2013-0).

References

[1] Mumford, D., Shah, J.: Optimal approximations by piecewise smooth functions and associated variational problems. Communications on Pure and Applied Mathematics 42(5), 577–685 (1989)

[2] Boykov, Y., Jolly, M.P.: Interactive graph cuts for optimal boundary & region segmentation of objects in N-D images. In: International Conference on Computer Vision, vol. 1(1), pp. 105–112 (2001)

[3] Sinop, A., Grady, L.: A seeded image segmentation framework unifying graph cuts and random walker which yields a new algorithm. In: Proceedings of ICCV (2007)

[4] Ciesielski, K., Udupa, J., Saha, P., Zhuge, Y.: Iterative relative fuzzy connectedness for multiple objects, allowing multiple seeds. Computer Vision and Image Understanding 107(3), 160–182 (2007)

[5] Couprie, C., Grady, L., Najman, L., Talbot, H.: Power watersheds: A unifying graph-based optimization framework. IEEE Transactions Pattern Analysis and Machine Inteligence 33(7), 1384–1399 (2011)

[6] Falcão, A., Bergo, F.: Interactive volume segmentation with differential image foresting transforms. IEEE Transactions on Medical Imaging 23(9), 1100–1108 (2004)

[7] Ciesielski, K., Udupa, J., Falcão, A., Miranda, P.: Fuzzy connectedness image segmentation in graph cut formulation: A linear-time algorithm and a comparative analysis. Journal of Mathematical Imaging and Vision 44(3), 375–398 (2012)

[8] Falcão, A., Stolfi, J., Lotufo, R.A.: The image foresting transform: theory, algorithms, and applications. IEEE Transactions on Pattern Analysis and Machine Intelligence 26(1), 19–29 (2004)

[9] Ciesielski, K., Udupa, J., Miranda, P., Falcão, A.: Joint graph cut and relative fuzzy connectedness image segmentation algorithm. Medical Image Analysis 17(8), 1046–1057 (2013)

[10] Malmberg, F., Nyström, I., Mehnert, A., Engstrom, C., Bengtsson, E.: Relaxed image foresting transforms for interactive volume image segmentation. In: Proceedings of SPIE-The International Society for Optical Engineering, vol. 23(1), pp. 40–51 (2010)

[11] Kohli, P., Torr, P.H.S.: Dynamic graph cuts for efficient inference in markov random fields. IEEE Transactions on Pattern Analysis and Machine Intelligence 29(12), 2079–2088 (2007)

[12] Udupa, J., Odhner, D., Tong, Y., Matsumoto, M.M.S., Ciesielski, K.C., Vaideeswaran, P., Ciesielski, V., Saboury, B., Zhao, L., Mohammadianrasanani, S., Torigian, D.: Fuzzy model-based body-wide anatomy recognition in medical images. In: Proceedings SPIE on Medical Imaging, vol. 8671, pp. 86712B–86712B-7 (2013)

[13] Kohli, P., Nickisch, H., Rother, C., Rhemann, C.: User-centric learning and evaluation of interactive segmentation systems. Int. J. Computer Vision 100(3), 261–274 (2012)

Segmentation Based Denoising of PET Images: An Iterative Approach via Regional Means and Affinity Propagation*

Ziyue Xu, Ulas Bagci**, Jurgen Seidel, David Thomasson,
Jeff Solomon, and Daniel J. Mollura

Department of Radiology and Imaging Sciences,
National Institutes of Health (NIH), Bethesda, MD 20892, USA
ulas.bagci@nih.gov

Abstract. Delineation and noise removal play a significant role in clinical quantification of PET images. Conventionally, these two tasks are considered independent, however, denoising can improve the performance of boundary delineation by enhancing SNR while preserving the structural continuity of local regions. On the other hand, we postulate that segmentation can help denoising process by constraining the smoothing criteria locally. Herein, we present a novel iterative approach for simultaneous PET image denoising and segmentation. The proposed algorithm uses generalized Anscombe transformation priori to non-local means based noise removal scheme and affinity propagation based delineation. For non-local means denoising, we propose a new regional means approach where we automatically and efficiently extract the appropriate subset of the image voxels by incorporating the class information from affinity propagation based segmentation. PET images after denoising are further utilized for refinement of the segmentation in an iterative manner. Qualitative and quantitative results demonstrate that the proposed framework successfully removes the noise from PET images while preserving the structures, and improves the segmentation accuracy.

Keywords: PET Denoising, PET Segmentation, Regional Means, Affinity Propagation, Generalized Anscombe Transformation.

1 Introduction

Positron emission tomography (PET) reveals metabolic activities by detecting gamma photon pairs caused by positron annihilation from radiotracers localized to specific regions. It provides diagnostic and therapeutic interpretation for evaluation of many diseases. As compared with anatomical imaging techniques of computed tomography (CT) and magnetic resonance imaging, PET images are known by their high sensitivity and low spatial resolution. Moreover, PET images suffer from noise caused by random and scattered coincidences, and has low signal-to-noise ratios (SNRs).

---

* This research is supported by CIDI, the intramural research program of the National Institute of Allergy and Infectious Diseases (NIAID) and the National Institute of Biomedical Imaging and Bioengineering (NIBIB).
** Corresponding author.

P. Golland et al. (Eds.): MICCAI 2014, Part I, LNCS 8673, pp. 698–705, 2014.

Quantitative measurements of PET images such as mean and maximum standardized uptake value (SUV_{max} and SUV_{mean}) and metabolic tumor volume (MTV) are strongly affected by the denoising and segmentation. For instance, noise distribution in PET images (non-Gaussian) [1] degrades the sensitivity of SUV-based quantitative metrics and affects the correct boundary of lesions. Meanwhile, object information through delineation can help promoting the denoising performance. However, joint interaction between denoising and delineation is often ignored by conventional approaches [2,3]. For denoising, the major challenge is to reduce noise while preserving the small structures under low resolution condition. Incorporating knowledge of small structures can address this challenge. Therefore, segmentation can improve the performance of denoising by introducing additional constraints for smoothing process. For segmentation, on the other hand, the challenge is to robustly extract the regions under low SNR. Hence, denoising can promote the accuracy of segmentation by increasing SNR as long as there is no resolution loss. In order to address this coupled problem, an efficient segmentation algorithm is required to estimate boundaries of metabolically active uptake regions; and an accurate denoising method is desirable to enhance SNR.

Current approaches in PET denoising focus on Gaussian smoothing, adaptive diffusion filtering [2], filtering in transformation domain with anatomical information [3], and soft thresholding method [1]. Since Gaussian smoothing and adaptive diffusion filtering rely on neighboring voxels, they are only able to catch local similarities. As PET images are low resolution, such methods are not optimal and cause local blurring and information loss. Incorporation of anatomical information can help defining the candidate structures, however, it may create artifacts due to the fact that anatomical-functional correspondence does not always hold for all locations. Soft thresholding methods have been shown to be effective in noise removal; however, accurately modeling noise distribution is a challenging problem. Recently, non-local means method [4] gained increasing attention for its effectiveness in noise reduction and structure preservation of low SNR images by considering global similarity measurement instead of intensity gradient alone.

Detailed noise characteristics of PET images are still unknown. A Poisson model is proposed recently [1] where noise is transformed to Gaussian using variance stabilizing transform (VST). In this study, we assume both multiplicative and additive noise component in a mixed Poisson-Gaussian model because pure Poisson modeling may be suboptimal either. Next, the generalized Anscombe transformation (GAT) with its optimal inversion [5] were utilized for variance stabilization.

To address all challenges described above, in this paper, we propose an iterative approach for simultaneous PET image denoising and segmentation by (1) stabilizing noise under mixed Poisson-Gaussian model with GAT, (2) estimating local uptake regions using affinity propagation (AP) clustering, (3) removing Gaussianized noise using regional means within the non-local means framework by incorporating class information from segmentation, and (4) applying the optimal inverse GAT (IGAT) to obtain denoised PET images. Steps (2) and (3) are utilized in an iterative manner to enhance the performance of each other and final segmentation result is the clustering result of (2) at convergence. The proposed method can be performed on either 2-D or 3-D, and the presented results are using 3-D algorithm. A flowchart for the presented scheme is shown in Fig. 1. In the next section, the proposed framework is presented in detail.

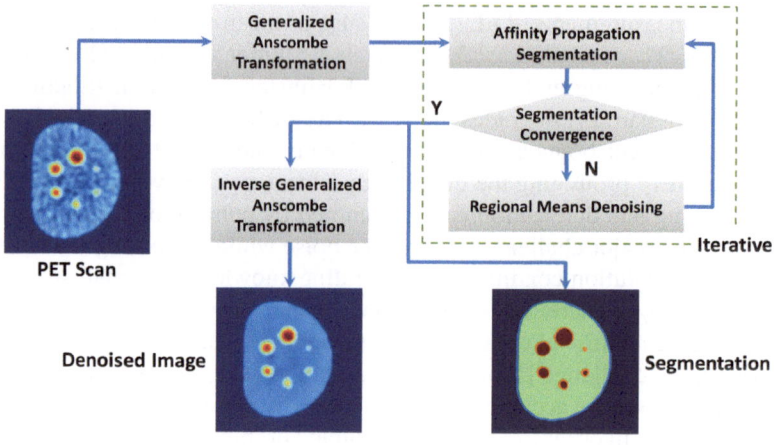

Fig. 1. Flowchart of the iterative segmentation based denoising algorithm

2   Methods

In the proposed framework, we incorporate the region information from segmentation process for promoting the performance of denoising and the resulting image with higher SNR can enhance the performance of segmentation in an iterative manner.

Generalized Anscombe Transformation and Optimal Inverse: GAT is the general version of the classical Anscombe transformation designed for stabilizing the noise variance assuming a mixed Poisson-Gaussian model. According to the theorem, intensities are modeled as a scaled Poisson variable corrupted by additive Gaussian noise. Let p denote the Poisson variable with variance λ, α denote the scale parameter, and n denote the Gaussian noise with mean μ and standard deviation σ, we have the voxel intensity as

$$x = \alpha p + n \tag{1}$$

where $p \sim \mathcal{P}(\lambda)$ and $n \sim \mathcal{N}(\mu, \sigma^2)$. Noise stabilization can further be achieved by GAT as

$$GAT(x) = \begin{cases} \frac{2}{\alpha}\sqrt{\alpha x + \frac{3}{8}\alpha^2 + \sigma^2 - \alpha\mu}, & x > -\frac{3}{8}\alpha - \frac{\sigma^2}{\alpha} + \mu \\ 0, & \text{otherwise,} \end{cases} \tag{2}$$

so that the resulting $y = GAT(x)$ has approximately unity variance. Once the PET images are transformed with GAT, Gaussianized noise can be removed with the proposed method, leading to a better delineation performance. Final step is the inverse GAT to transform the denoised PET images back to original image domain. Herein, we use the the exact unbiased inverse of the GAT [5] to recover the intensity information.

Affinity Propagation Based PET Image Segmentation: We propose an iterative way to tackle delineation of uptake regions in PET images by combining the power of a robust segmentation and structure preserving denoising algorithms. For a robust and accurate segmentation algorithm, we use affinity propagation (AP) algorithm [6] recently shown to be very effective for PET images [7]. Other PET segmentation techniques can instead be used for this purpose as long as highly accurate delineation results are guaranteed. Due to page limitation, we refer our readers the original AP paper in [7] that we follow in our study for the details of the novel similarity functions and delineation steps. Briefly, AP clustering is utilized to find optimal thresholding levels that separate the PET image into several regions.

Regional Means Denoising: AP clustering yields a robust estimation of uptake regions, although the group separation can be inaccurate locally due to intensity variation under low SNR. This information serves as a "pre-screening" for non-local means denoising, and hence we introduce the notion "regional means" for this technique. The key idea is to enhance SNR while preserve the true uptake regions, so that the enhanced image can help AP to generate a better segmentation result that in turn benefit the denoising in the next iteration. The basic formulation for non-local means [4] filtering is that for a point in image, its estimated value after filtering is the weighted average of all the points in the image instead of only its neighbors. The method can be performed on both 2-D and higher dimensional images. In the following, without loss of generality, we present a 3-D formulation for the proposed method with which the results were generated. The basic non-local means algorithm utilizes the redundant information of structural patterns within the image by considering the similarity between local patches with size $N \times N \times N$, which provides a more reliable reduction of noise than the conventional local intensity schemes, as it enables more robust comparison than conventional neighborhood filters. However, for computational purposes, the search of similar patches is usually restricted in a larger "search window" of $M \times M \times M (M > N)$. Therefore, from implementation perspective, the information utilization is restricted. Since approximate region estimation can be efficiently performed by AP, it is possible to remove this computation restriction of search window. Instead of searching the entire image or restricted within local neighborhood, we propose the regional means scheme as follows.

For point u in GAT transformed image $J = GAT(I)$, its intensity is $J(u)$ and class label given by AP segmentation is $L(u)$ with corresponding group size $G(L(u))$. Class labels are ordered consecutive natural number such that $L(u) > L(v)$, if $J(u) > J(v)$. In order to determine its similar patches over the image, we search the following regions Ω:

1. Local search window of size $M \times M \times M$,
2. Random sample $\min\{M^3, G(L(u))\}$ points in the regions with class label $L(u)$ (candidate region),
3. Random sample $\min\{M^3, G(L(u) - 1)\}$ points in the regions with class label $L(u) - 1$ (neighbor region I) if $L(u) > 1$,
4. Random sample $\min\{M^3, G(L(u) + 1)\}$ points in the regions with class label $L(u) + 1$ (neighbor region II) if $L(u) < \max_u L(u)$.

Last step is to apply regional means to point u as

$$RM(J(u)) = \sum_{v \in \Omega} w(u, v) J(v), \qquad (3)$$

where the weights $w(u, v)$ depend on the similarity between the two patches $\mathcal{A}_u$ and $\mathcal{A}_v$ centered at point u and v as

$$w(u, v) = \frac{1}{\mathcal{Z}(u)} e^{-||\mathcal{A}_u - \mathcal{A}_v||^2 / h^2} \tag{4}$$

where $||\mathcal{A}_u - \mathcal{A}_v||$ represents the Euclidean distance between the two intensity vectors from the two patches. $\mathcal{Z}(u)$ is the normalizing constant such that

$$\mathcal{Z}(u) = \sum_v e^{-||\mathcal{A}_u - \mathcal{A}_v||^2 / h^2} \tag{5}$$

so that the weighting parameter satisfies the weighting conditions of $0 \leq w(u, v) \leq 1$ and $\sum_v w(u, v) = 1$, parameter h determines the degree of filtering. In this way, the resulting Ω is not restricted to local areas anymore, but with the expense of increased computational complexity by the order of four. With the information from segmentation, our technique is able to cover sufficient points that can contribute to the denoising at point u.

3   Experiments and Results

In order to evaluate both denoising and segmentation performance, we used 20 PET-CT images on two different NEMA phantoms with different reconstruction parameters. The first phantom contains six spheres with diameters of 10, 13, 17, 22, 28, and 37 mm, background concentration is 0.44 uCi/ml, and hot sphere concentration is 1.75 uCi/ml. The spatial resolution is $128 \times 128 \times 47$ with spacing $2.73 \times 2.73 \times 3.27$ mm, and the image is in units of Bq/ml. The second phantom has five spheres with diameters of 4, 5, 6, 8, and 10 mm. The true activities are 32.2 mCi/ml in the spheres and 6.2mCi/ml in the background. The spatial resolution is $256 \times 256 \times 95$ with spacing $0.95 \times 0.95 \times 1.90$ mm, and the image is in units of mCi/ml. In addition to phantom images, 20 MRI-PET images relating to different diseases were collected with IRB approval from 20 patients. The spatial resolution is 172×172 in plane with slice number from 189-211, and spacing $4.17 \times 4.17 \times 2.00$ mm. The denoising performance of the proposed iterative regional means method is compared with commonly used methods including Gaussian filtering, anisotropic diffusion, non-local means, and block matching [8] methods. All methods for comparison were performed over the image after GAT stabilization. The segmentation performance is compared with CT ground truth for phantom images, and manual reference for patient images.

Evaluation of Denoising: Using phantom images, the boundaries between each uptake region and background can be accurately defined from CT scans. For patient scans, 20 regions with lesions were manually determined from all subjects by experts. Statistics of noise reduction performance, including SNR and max/mean uptake value, were then computed for all uptake regions from several ROIs within each of them (the convention for PET image measurements). The ROIs were identical among original and filtered images for comparison.

Qualitative results at sample slices from both phantom and human images are shown in Fig. 2 with the original image (A), the corresponding CT/MRI (B), the filtering result

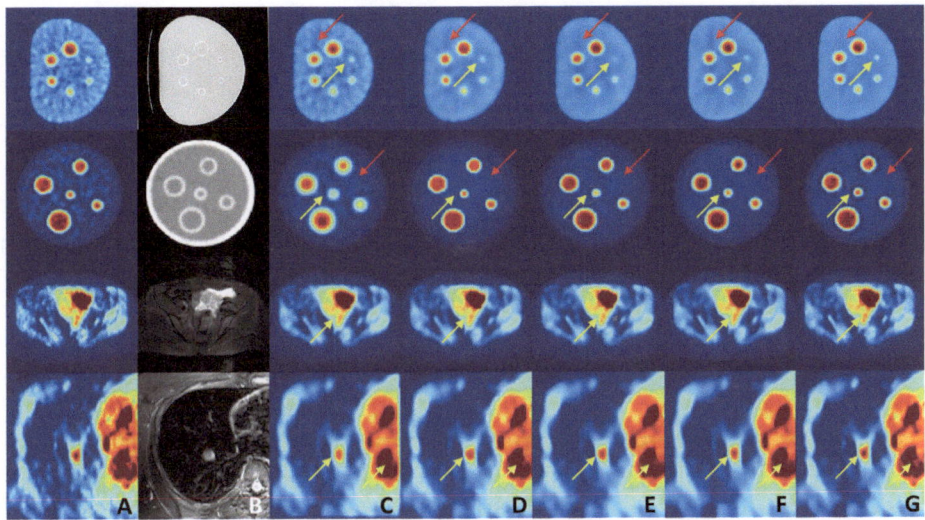

Fig. 2. Qualitative results for denoising: the original image (A), the corresponding CT/MR image (B), the filtering result of Gaussian filtering (C), anisotropic diffusion (D), non-local means (E), block matching (F), and the proposed method (G). Yellow arrows point out the small uptake regions and red arrows shows the residual noise regions.

of Gaussian filtering (C), anisotropic diffusion (D), non-local means (E), block matching (F), and the proposed method (G). The red arrows show noise reduction areas where other methods show limited success; while the yellow arrows point out the preserved fine details with the proposed method where other methods over-smooth and blur the small structures.

Quantitative analysis confirms the qualitative observation that the proposed method effectively removed the noise from PET image and preserved the fine details of small regions. As shown in Fig. 3 A/D, ROIs were divided into high uptake regions (blue) and low uptake regions (red). Low uptake background regions are not influenced by partial volume effect; thus, provide reliable estimation of overall Signal-to-Noise Ratio (SNR). Further, relative contrast (RC) were calculated for high uptake regions and compared with low uptake regions, measuring object-to-background contrast relative to the noise in each region.

$$SNR = \mu_{\mathcal{L}}/\sigma_{\mathcal{L}},$$
$$RC = |\mu_{\mathcal{H}} - \mu_{\mathcal{L}}|/\sqrt{\sigma_{\mathcal{H}}\sigma_{\mathcal{L}}}, \tag{6}$$

where $\mu_{\mathcal{H}}$, $\mu_{\mathcal{L}}$, $\sigma_{\mathcal{H}}$, and $\sigma_{\mathcal{L}}$ denote the mean and standard deviation of high / low uptake regions. For denoising methods to be effective, two most commonly used markers for PET images, SUV_{max} and SUV_{mean}, should not be changed significantly before and after denoising. Fig. 3 C/E illustrates an intensity profile along a sample line within the PET image Fig. 3 B/D, as compared with the block matching method (blue), which is the state-of-the-art for denoising, the proposed algorithm (red) successfully preserved the intensity level for different objects and minimized the noise from the original

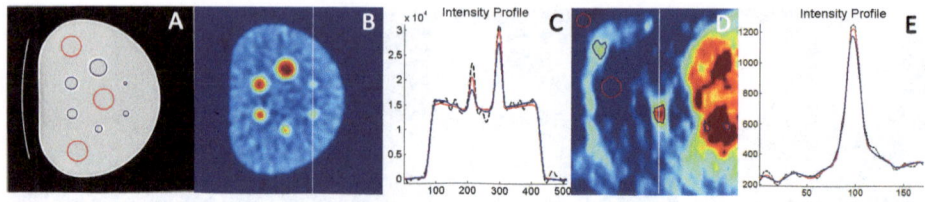

Fig. 3. (A, D) ROI distribution in high uptake regions (blue) and low uptake regions (red), (B, D) original image showing sample line location, and (C, E) intensity profile on the sample line for original image (black), block matching method (blue), and proposed method (red).

Table 1. Statistics of denoising performance for different methods. P: phantom; H: human.

	SNR		RC		Max RR		Mean RR		OR	BR
	P	H	P	H	P	H	P	H	P	P
Original	11.73	7.08	11.32	34.14	0%	0%	0%	0%	59.28%	85.02%
Gaussian	15.62	7.01	12.88	27.76	11.08%	9.27%	9.55%	5.51%	53.99%	85.21%
Diffusion	21.05	7.25	16.38	33.98	13.20%	7.20%	7.37%	3.37%	55.99%	85.72%
Non-Local Means	21.88	7.69	13.70	37.67	13.27%	7.04%	11.03%	3.61%	54.41%	85.89%
Block Matching	20.36	9.92	14.02	39.97	7.32%	6.96%	6.87%	3.59%	56.27%	85.41%
Proposed	35.55	11.82	19.15	52.40	2.97%	3.55%	2.61%	1.29%	58.24%	86.26%

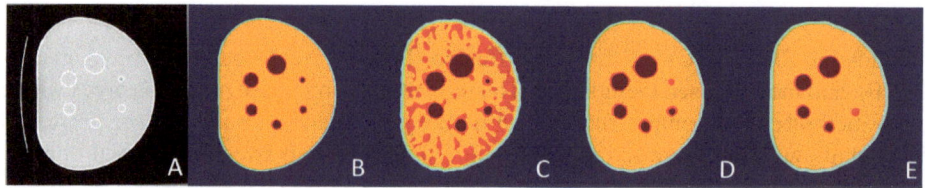

Fig. 4. Segmentation results: (A) corresponding CT image, (B) ground truth from CT image, (C) initial segmentation result, (D) final segmentation result given by proposed method, (E) final segmentation result from image denoised by block matching method.

image (black). Table 1 presents the quantitative results of SNR, RC, max and mean value reduction rate (RR) of the ROIs as well as the ratio of uptake values as compared with phantom ground truth for object and background regions - object ratio (OR), and background ratio (BR). Our experimental results show that the proposed method outperforms other methods in all measurements for the task of PET image denoising. Note that for human subjects (H), OR and BR are not available because the true local uptake value is not known unlike in phantom case (P).

Evaluation of Segmentation: Fig. 4 illustrates the segmentation result given by AP over the phantom image and denoised results. The regions (B) defined by CT image (A) are used as ground truth for assessing segmentation performance. As shown, initial segmentation result (C) can include redundant thresholding levels due to the noise, while the final result recovers the information by enhancing the image (D). Other denoising techniques are also able to reduce the noise, however, local structures are not preserved (E). Dice similarity coefficient (DSC), and Hausdorff distance (HD) are calculated for further evaluation, and the result are 92.75% for DSC and 3.14 mm for HD (pixel size 2.73 x 2.73 mm).

4   Discussion and Conclusion

In this study, we presented an effective tool for PET image denoising and segmentation. The proposed algorithm adopts affinity propagation for estimating different uptake regions, this information is further incorporated within a regional means denoising technique to enhance the SNR, which in turn helps promoting the accuracy of segmentation algorithm in an iterative manner. We also utilized generalized Anscombe transformation and its optimal inverse before and after the denoising-segmentation procedure, in order to Gaussianize the noise in PET images under mixed Poisson-Gaussian model. Experimental results demonstrated that the proposed framework effectively removes the noise from PET images while the structures are preserved, especially for small uptake regions.

References

1. Bagci, U., Mollura, D.J.: Denoising PET images using singular value thresholding and stein's unbiased risk estimate. In: Mori, K., Sakuma, I., Sato, Y., Barillot, C., Navab, N. (eds.) MICCAI 2013, Part III. LNCS, vol. 8151, pp. 115–122. Springer, Heidelberg (2013)
2. Tauber, C., Stute, S., Chau, M., Spiteri, P., Chalon, S., Guilloteau, D., Buvat, I.: Spatio-temporal diffusion of dynamic PET images. Physics in Medicine and Biology 56(20), 65–83 (2011)
3. Turkheimer, F.E., Boussion, N., Anderson, A.N., Pavese, N., Piccini, P., Visvikis, D.: PET image denoising using a synergistic multiresolution analysis of structural (MRI/CT) and functional datasets. Journal of Nuclear Medicine 49(4), 657–666 (2008)
4. Buades, A., Coll, B., Morel, J.M.: A non-local algorithm for image denoising. In: IEEE Computer Society Conference on Computer Vision and Pattern Recognition, vol. 2, pp. 60–65 (2005)
5. Makitalo, M., Foi, A.: Optimal inversion of the generalized Anscombe transformation for Poisson-Gaussian noise. IEEE Transactions on Image Processing 22(1), 91–103 (2013)
6. Frey, B.J., Dueck, D.: Clustering by passing messages between data points. Science 315, 972–976 (2007)
7. Foster, B., Bagci, U., Xu, Z., Dey, B., Luna, B., Bishai, W., Jain, S., Mollura, D.: Segmentation of PET images for computer-aided functional quantification of tuberculosis in small animal models. IEEE Transactions on Biomedical Engineering 61(3), 711–724 (2014)
8. Dabov, K., Foi, A., Katkovnik, V., Egiazarian, K.: Image denoising by sparse 3-D transform-domain collaborative filtering. IEEE Transactions on Image Processing 16(8), 2080–2095 (2007)

Detection and Registration of Ribs in MRI Using Geometric and Appearance Models

Golnoosh Samei*, Gábor Székely, and Christine Tanner

Computer Vision Laboratory, ETH Zurich, 8092 Zurich, Switzerland

Abstract. Magnetic resonance guided high intensity focused ultrasound (MRgHIFU) is a new type of minimally invasive therapy for treating malignant liver tissues. Since the ribs on the beam path can compromise an effective therapy, detecting them and tracking their motion on MR images is of great importance. However, due to poor magnetic signal emission of bones, ribs cannot be entirely observed in MR. In the proposed method, we take advantage of the accuracy of CT in imaging the ribs to build a geometric ribcage model and combine it with an appearance model of the neighbouring structures of ribs in MR to reconstruct realistic centerlines in MRIs. We have improved our previous method by using a more sophisticated appearance model, a more flexible ribcage model, and a more effective optimization strategy. We decreased the mean error to 2.5 mm, making the method suitable for clinical application. Finally, we propose a rib registration method which conserves the shape and length of ribs, and imposes realistic constraints on their motions, achieving 2.7 mm mean accuracy.

1 Introduction

MRgHIFU is a relatively new and promising therapy, which locally ablates the tissues by focusing ultrasound beams on the target region. This form of therapy has already been successfully applied to static organs such as brain tumours and uterine fibroids. Yet, its applicability to organs in the abdomen, such as the liver is limited due to the motion caused by respiration.

There has been extensive work on modeling the respiratory motion of abdominal and thoracic organs e.g. [12,8]. Yet, for an effective therapy, knowledge of the accurate position of the organs on the beam path, as well as the position of the target, is required. In particular, the ribcage poses an important challenge, as it encloses parts of the liver and the absorption and reflections of ultrasound at bones can cause overheating at the ribs and their surrounding [7,14].

Currently, no imaging device is fast enough to allow real-time acquisition and quantification of the 3D motion of the ribcage and the target organ. Hence, partial observations need to be complemented by prior knowledge about the expected 3D motion. MR is the available image modality in MRgHIFU and also has the advantage that long acquisitions can be performed without any known

---

* We acknowledge the grant n° 270186 from the EU's Seventh Framework Programme.

P. Golland et al. (Eds.): MICCAI 2014, Part I, LNCS 8673, pp. 706–713, 2014.

adverse effects on the volunteers. Therefore, to quantify the respiratory motion of the ribcage and its correlation with that of the liver in 4D MRIs, it is necessary to detect and register the ribs in this modality.

While hardly investigated in MRI, detecting ribs in CT has been extensively explored, e.g. [6,11]. Staal et al. [11], find local CT image structures, by means of ridge detection, and classify these into ribs and non-ribs. Eventually, full ribs are formed by grouping these rib structures. The general steps of this method have been applied to MR images [9]. However, the results from 5 volunteers on high resolution MRIs show quite noisy extractions and confusion between ribs.

Recently, we proposed a method [10] where the idea of combined use of a geometric ribcage model from CT and an MR appearance model was presented. Being built on a relatively small dataset, the models could not capture the variation in the population adequately, which led to high mean errors relative to the intercostal distances. In this work, we improve our previous method by using more sophisticated appearance features, reducing the redundancy between the different attribute models, increasing the flexibility of the ribcage model in adapting to a new subject, and enhancing the strategy for finding optimal ribcage parameters. These improvements reduced the errors from 8.1 mm to 2.5 mm, making the rib detection method suitable for clinical application.

In addition to rib detection, we require an MR rib registration method to study the ribs motion. Initial attempts with an elastic image registration method lead to unrealistic rib deformations. Avoiding these was another motivation for creating the geometric ribcage model. In this work we propose the incorporation of the ribcage model into a rib registration method, such that shape and length of the ribs are conserved and anatomically plausible results are achieved.

2 Materials

We used two abdominal image datasets. The **CT-Dataset** consists of high resolution CT images of end-inspiration (EI) breath-holds (BH). The images were acquired from 20 healthy volunteers, with a resolution of $1.37 \times 1.37 \times 1\,\text{mm}^3$, in the anterior-posterior (AP), left-right (LR), and inferior-superior (IS) direction, respectively. The images were acquired and used in accordance with the local institutional review board regulations and were made available to us by the authors of [3]. The **MR-Dataset** consists of free-breathing 4D MRIs [13] obtained from 10 healthy volunteers ($1.33 \times 1.33 \times 5\,\text{mm}^3$ in AP, IS, LR direction). Additionally, we have 5 BH 3D MR images in EI, and end-expiration (EE) with half (2.5 mm) slice-thickness. We applied our rib detection method to the EE images, as they show less artifacts in the reconstructed 4D MRIs.

3 Method

We built a ribcage model for ribs enclosing the liver, namely the right ribs number 7 to 10. Each rib was defined by its shape, length and orientation. The attributes of each rib are highly correlated with each other and with those of other ribs. By building a statistical population model of these attributes, we extracted the main modes of variation of the ribcage geometry. Moreover, this model allowed us to generate anatomically plausible ribs using a few parameters. For detection all of these attributes had to be determined while for registration only the rotation angles were optimized to ensure shape and length preservation.

3.1   Ribcage Model

We built our ribcage model from CT data similar to [10]. First, the ribs were segmented in the CT images using a simple region growing algorithm in the 3D Slicer software [4]. To include full ribs, they were separated from the vertebral column at their joints and not as previously at the tubercle.

The centerline and natural coordinate system (NCS) of each rib were found, and a rotation from the NCS of each rib to the world coordinate system (WCS) was computed [10]. The corresponding 3 Euler angles constitute the rotation parameters. Finally, we established inter-subject correspondence between all ribs by locating the anatomical landmark, *angle point*, as the most posterior point in WCS, and using it to divide the ribs into two segments. Each segment was uniformly subdivided into a fixed number of points (100 points in total).

Shape Model. All ribs were normalized to have equal length and the 3D position vectors of all the 100 points of a rib were concatenated to form a 300D vector. The resulting vectors for ribs number 7 to 10 of all subjects formed a population of 80 ribs in total. By performing principle component analysis (PCA) on these vectors, we captured the high correlation between the elements of these vectors, with the first 2 PCs covering 96% of the variation. Hence, we chose our shape parameters to be the projection of the 300D vector of each rib onto these 2 PCs.

Ribcage Parameters. Each rib has 6 parameters, namely 2 shape parameters, 3 Euler angles and 1 length value. To model the correlation between these parameters for all the ribs, we performed another PCA on 20 instances of the resulting 24D vectors, with 6 PCs capturing 96% of the population variation. This allowed us to generate the centerlines of the ribs 7-10 approximately by 6 parameters $\mathbf{h} = [h_1..h_6]$. However, due to the relatively small training dataset, the population model might not capture the whole variability. Therefore, we reintroduce some local flexibility to the model to further adjust the generated ribcage to the given MR image, see Sec. 3.2 Optimization Strategy.

3.2   Rib Detection

The parameter vector $\mathbf{h}$ defined in Sec. 3.1, is used to represent a ribcage, and for detection we need to determine values for $\mathbf{h}$ such that the reconstructed ribs $r_{\mathbf{h}}$, are located on the rib centerlines in the given MR image. Therefore, we need a method which determines the likelihood of a given image location being on the centerline of a rib (referred to as *ribness* hereafter), a cost function for a set of generated ribs based on these likelihoods, and a strategy to find the optimal set of ribs according to the cost function.

Appearance Model. For a set of generated rib centerlines, we want to determine their ribness probability given an MRI. Hence, we create an appearance model which computes the ribness probability of a point based on the intensities of its neighbourhood. To that end, we used RF classifiers [1] trained on MRI sagittal patches similar to [10]. However, in [10], feature vectors were based merely on image intensities, which make the model sensitive to intensity range changes. Moreover, slight changes in the structures (such as the size of the rib cross sections), would result in very dissimilar features, necessitating a large training set to learn all the variations. To overcome these shortcoming, we used more robust features namely $\mathcal{F}_{\mathbf{p}} = (F_{\mathbf{p}}^1...F_{\mathbf{p}}^6)$, with 6 channels for a point $\mathbf{p} = [x_{\mathbf{p}}, y_{\mathbf{p}}, z_{\mathbf{p}}]$, as in [2]. These channels were comprised of raw intensity values, normalized intensity values, Canny and Soble edge detector responses, outputs of morphological operators (erosion and dilation) on the intensity, and the response of a Gabor filter bank with eight different rotations and four different phase shifts. Each $\mathcal{F}_{\mathbf{p}}$ was constructed from neighbourhood $N_{\mathbf{p}}^w(i,j) = I(x_{\mathbf{p}} + i, y_{\mathbf{p}} + j, z_{\mathbf{p}})$, around point $\mathbf{p}$ with $i, j \in \{-w, .., w\}$ and $I(x, y, z)$ the interpolated MR intensity at position $[x, y, z]$. Furthermore, we assumed that the ribness probability of $\mathbf{p}$ conditioned on patch $N_{\mathbf{p}}^{15}$, is independent of the rest of the image I, and therefore obtained $P(\mathbf{p}|I) \approx P(\mathbf{p}|N_{\mathbf{p}}^w)$. Additionally we used RF thresholds on comparison features [2], rather than on the original features as done previously in [10]. We trained our RF on positive features, $\mathcal{F}_{\mathbf{p}_R}$, extracted from points on the manually determined rib centerlines ($\mathbf{p}_R$) and negative features, $\mathcal{F}_{\mathbf{p}_N}$, from randomly selected points ($\mathbf{p}_N$) with a distance of $\geq 10\,$mm from all $\mathbf{p}_R$. To obtain more discriminative classifiers, we trained 4 RFs for regions along the ribs with different appearances on sagittal slices. The first one (C1) was built for the points that had an AP distance of 5 mm from the angle point. The second one (C2), was trained on the points within an LR distance of 5 mm (slice thickness) from the most lateral rib point. The third and fourth classifiers (C3, C4) were trained on the points between the angle point and the most lateral rib points, and the remaining points, respectively.

Cost Function. Similar to [10], we adapt a Bayesian framework where the cost function, $C(\mathbf{h})$, is based on the conditional negative log-likelihood of the parameters $\mathbf{h}$, given the MR image I. However, the cost function utilized in [10], sharply increases with distance to rib centers, making it very hard to optimize. An ideal cost measure for efficient solving of our optimization problem should be proportional to the distance to rib centers with a smooth gradient. Therefore we employed a cost function that incorporates the ribness evidence from the neighbouring voxels by spatially smoothing the RF log-likelihood with a Gaussian kernel:

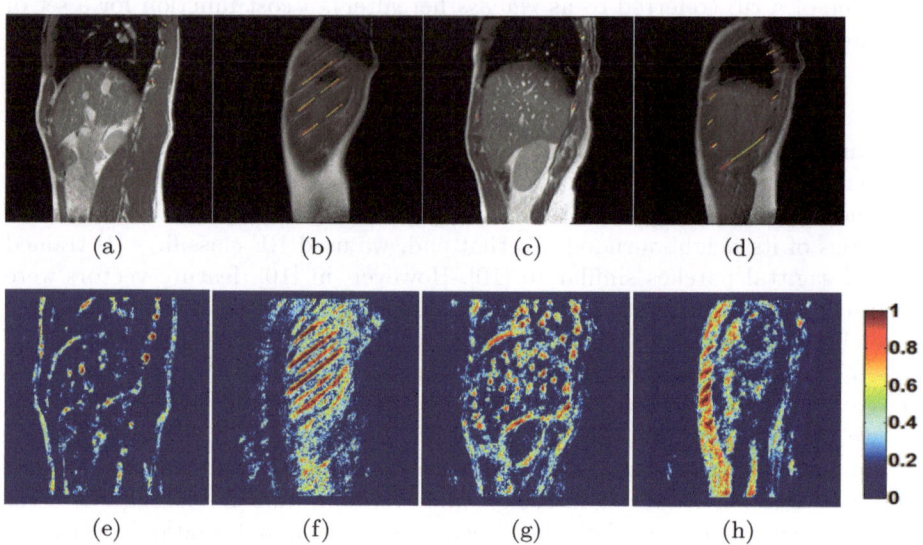

Fig. 1. (a-d) The detected (yellow) and the ground truth centerlines (red) on 4 sagittal slices. (e-h) The probability heat maps for the slices shown in (a-d) obtained from classifiers (e) C1, (f) C2, (g) C3 and (h) C4.

$$C(\mathbf{h}|I,\sigma) = -\sum_{\mathbf{p} \in r_{\mathbf{h}}} \sum_{\mathbf{q} \in S_{\mathbf{p}}^{3\sigma}} log(P(\mathbf{q}|N_{\mathbf{q}}^{w})) \cdot G^{\sigma}(\mathbf{q} - \mathbf{p}), \qquad (1)$$

where G^{σ} is a Gaussian kernel with variance σ^2, $S_{\mathbf{p}}^{3\sigma}$ is a spherical neighbourhood around $\mathbf{p}$ with radius 3σ, and $r_{\mathbf{h}}$ is the rib associated with parameters $\mathbf{h}$.

Optimization Strategy. We positioned a generated centerline in the image using the location of a so-called starting point, which is manually selected in the vicinity of the rib's joint to the vertebral disk. It defines the position of one of the first rib points (exactly which one is determined during optimization). Furthermore, we reject any solution which exceeds the bounding box of the ribcage defined as in [10]. Optimization is based on grid search and a multi-resolution approach. First, we draw hypotheses h by uniformly sampling the interior of a 6-D hyper-ellipsoid which covers 95% of the multidimensional Gaussian distribution associated with the PCA model. From these, further hypotheses are created by uniformly changing the proposed orientation for all ribs within $\pm 20^{\circ}$ in steps of 5°, by assigning the starting point to one of the first points up to the angle point. Then we calculate $C(r_{\mathbf{h}}|I, 5)$ for all hypotheses in the bounding box and keep the $k = 5$ best results. In the next steps, we divide σ and the rotation range by 3 and modify the rib orientations and the starting point. We repeat this process until either the change in cost function is below a threshold $\tau = 12$, or a maximum number of 3 iterations has been reached.

3.3 Rib Registration

A global rigid registration of the image volume cannot capture the individually different rotations of the ribs around their joints to the vertebral column. Also, an unconstrained non-rigid registration would introduce too many degrees of freedom. Therefore, we use our ribcage model to track the ribs by exploiting the fact that the shape and length of the ribs do not change. Hence, our detection framework and the optimization scheme of Sec. 3.2 can be simplified to find only the optimal rotation angles of the ribs and fixing all other parameters.

As a faster alternative to computing the RF cost measure, we used registration after the first detection step as follows. For a given rotation of the moving rib, we determined for each point on the fixed (i.e detected) rib the corresponding point on the moving rib. Then we calculate the negative normalized cross correlation (-NCC) between their associated two 2D patches. Finally, we chose the rotation with the lowest mean -NCC value over all rib points.

4 Experiments and Results

We generated our ground truth (GT) rib centerlines from manually selected points as in [10]. Since we used the same MR dataset for building the appearance models as for evaluating our method, we performed leave-one-out experiments. An example result is shown in Fig. 1, where the closeness of GT and detected centerlines can be observed. Moreover, the RF classifier falsely assigned high probabilities to the intercostal space (Fig. 1b,1f) and the liver vessels (Fig. 1c,1g), which indicates the importance of the constraints from the geometric model.

We report three error measures to describe the location accuracy (DistanceError), the accuracy in detecting the whole rib (LengthError), and the clinically relevant error (OutOfPlaneError). DistanceError was defined as the closest Euclidean distance between a point on the detected centerline and the GT. LengthError denotes the difference in length of the detected centerline and the GT. DistanceError and LengthError are 3D errors, while only the 2D error projected onto the ribcage surface matters clinically when deciding which elements of the HIFU transducer should be active for treatments through the ribcage [5]. Hence, we define OutOfPlaneError as the projection of the DistanceError on the z axis (LR direction) of the GT rib's NCS, see Table 1 for detection results summary.

The rib registration algorithm was evaluated on BH images at EE and EI. The LengthError is the same for registration and detection, as the ribs' length do not change in registration. The mean DistanceError is marginally lower for RF (see Table 2), however, NCC requires substantially lower computation time. Note that DistanceError of NCC also includes the detection error, as the registration is initialized with the detected and not the GT centerline.

Table 1. Statistics (mean ± std (95%)) of rib detection errors in mm

Subject	OutOfPlaneError	DistanceError	LengthError
1	0.64 ± 0.51 (1.64)	1.66 ± 0.91 (3.36)	14.70 ± 7.98 (24.66)
2	1.04 ± 0.93 (2.60)	2.27 ± 1.38 (5.05)	13.70 ± 12.03 (29.86)
3	1.03 ± 1.20 (3.08)	2.08 ± 1.23 (3.86)	9.52 ± 8.45 (19.52)
4	0.97 ± 1.19 (3.53)	2.80 ± 1.60 (5.85)	25.38 ± 7.29 (30.91)
5	1.37 ± 1.37 (4.14)	2.31 ± 1.53 (5.36)	23.22 ± 7.74 (31.20)
6	1.50 ± 1.34 (4.55)	3.15 ± 1.66 (6.33)	11.00 ± 9.65 (19.78)
7	1.67 ± 2.13 (6.62)	2.74 ± 2.08 (7.38)	16.49 ± 12.49 (27.93)
8	1.02 ± 1.24 (3.86)	2.22 ± 1.40 (5.18)	7.45 ± 5.29 (13.49)
9	1.34 ± 1.61 (5.14)	2.40 ± 1.65 (5.74)	7.54 ± 9.44 (18.40)
10	1.87 ± 3.16 (8.85)	3.58 ± 3.09 (9.87)	37.88 ± 4.56 (41.76)
11	0.93 ± 0.97 (3.06)	2.65 ± 1.98 (7.30)	21.12 ± 4.77 (26.49)
12	1.37 ± 1.37 (4.15)	2.63 ± 1.81 (5.71)	7.07 ± 5.14 (12.46)
13	0.99 ± 1.00 (3.20)	2.10 ± 1.41 (4.80)	9.95 ± 4.89 (16.44)
14	1.29 ± 1.08 (3.56)	2.64 ± 1.55 (5.66)	7.95 ± 8.58 (20.57)
15	1.03 ± 0.92 (3.04)	2.27 ± 1.01 (4.20)	9.78 ± 7.78 (20.35)
all	1.20 ± 1.48 (4.09)	2.49 ± 1.73 (5.67)	14.87 ± 11.09 (35.09)

Table 2. Statistics (mean ± std (95%)) of rib registration error and motion in mm

Sbj	NCC		RF	Respiratory
	OutOfPlaneError	DistanceError	DistanceError	motion
11	1.04 ± 0.96 (3.41)	4.60 ± 2.20 (7.89)	3.33 ± 2.58 (9.65)	4.06 ± 2.91 (9.85)
12	0.73 ± 0.65 (2.10)	2.14 ± 1.11 (4.23)	2.21 ± 1.08 (4.37)	5.82 ± 4.16 (13.02)
13	0.81 ± 0.77 (2.43)	2.47 ± 1.16 (4.30)	2.84 ± 3.43 (9.61)	9.46 ± 5.31 (17.75)
14	1.65 ± 1.53 (5.17)	2.98 ± 1.32 (5.06)	2.85 ± 1.45 (5.47)	6.06 ± 3.68 (12.54)
15	1.78 ± 1.71 (4.51)	3.54 ± 2.35 (8.62)	2.56 ± 2.01 (6.01)	9.73 ± 5.79 (18.78)
all	1.20 ± 1.28 (3.90)	3.07 ± 1.87 (6.81)	2.72 ± 2.26 (5.90)	6.27 ± 4.94 (16.39)

5   Discussion and Conclusion

In this study we showed that, despite their poor visibility, ribs can be detected in MRI by combining geometric and appearance ribcage models learned from CT and MR respectively. We substantially improved our previous results [10], reducing mean errors from 7.2 mm to 2.4 mm for the shared subset of the two studies (subject 1-10).

We also proposed a constrained non-rigid rib registration method based on our ribcage model, and implemented two registration schemes with clinically suitable errors using the RF and -NCC cost measures.

Future work will be on improving the implementation of our algorithm for faster detection and registration. One approach can be to build a regression RF to predict the distance of points to rib centerlines, which would give $C(\mathbf{h}|I, \sigma)$ directly without the need for convolution.

While the mean errors along the ribs were low (2.5 mm), the anterior part of the detected ribs were on average 14 mm shorter than the ground truth. This was possibly caused by the fact that due to the difficulty in distinguishing cartilage from the bones in MR, some of the manual rib landmarks may have been placed on the cartilage, whereas the CT geometric model did not include them. In future, cartilage will be included in both models for creating an accurate method for the entire ribcage. Obtaining a dataset of MR and CT of the same subjects, will provide a better ground truth for evaluating our method.

References

1. Breiman, L.: Random forests. Mach. Learn. 45(1), 5 (2001)
2. Dantone, M., Gall, J., Fanelli, G., Van Gool, L.: Real-time facial feature detection using conditional regression forests. In: CVPR, pp. 2578–2585. IEEE (2012)
3. Donner, R., Menze, B., Bischof, H., Langs, G.: Global localization of 3D anatomical structures by pre-filtered Hough forests and discrete optimization. Med. Image. Anal. 17(8), 1304–1314 (2013)
4. Fedorov, A., Beichel, R., Kalpathy-Cramer, J., Finet, J., et al.: 3D slicer as an image computing platform for the quantitative imaging network. Magn. Reson. Imaging 30(9), 1323–1341 (2012)
5. Gao, J., Volovick, A., Pekelny, Y., Huang, Z., Cochran, S., Melzer, A.: Focusing through the rib cage for MR-guided transcostal FUS. In: AIP Conf. Proc., vol. 1481(1), pp. 94–99 (2012)
6. Lee, J., Reeves, A.P.: Segmentation of individual ribs from low-dose chest CT. In: SPIE Med. Imaging, p. 76243J (2010)
7. Li, F., Gong, X., Hu, K., Li, C., Wang, Z.: Effect of ribs in HIFU beam path on formation of coagulative necrosis in goat liver. In: AIP Conf. Proc., vol. 829(1), pp. 477–480 (2006)
8. McClelland, J.R., Hawkes, D., Schaeffter, T., King, A.: Respiratory motion models: A review. Med. Image. Anal. 17(1), 19–42 (2013)
9. Noorda, Y.H., Bartels, L.W., Viergever, M.A., Pluim, J.P.W.: Rib detection in 3D MRI using dynamic programming based on vesselness and ridgeness. In: Yoshida, H., Warfield, S., Vannier, M.W. (eds.) Abdominal Imaging 2013. LNCS, vol. 8198, pp. 212–220. Springer, Heidelberg (2013)
10. Samei, G., Tanner, C., Székely, G.: Rib detection in MR images using shape priors and appearance models. In: ISBI, pp. 798–801. IEEE (2014)
11. Staal, J., van Ginneken, B., Viergever, M.A.: Automatic rib segmentation and labeling in computed tomography scans using a general framework for detection, recognition and segmentation of objects in volumetric data. Med. Image. Anal. 11(1), 35 (2007)
12. Tanner, C., Boye, D., Samei, G., Szekely, G.: Review on 4D models for organ motion compensation. Crit. Rev. Biomed. Eng. 40(2), 135 (2012)
13. Von Siebenthal, M., Székely, G., Gamper, U., Boesiger, P., Lomax, A., Cattin, P.: 4D MR imaging of respiratory organ motion and its variability. Phys. Med. Biol. 52, 1547 (2007)
14. Wu, F., Wang, Z., Chen, W., Zhu, H., Bai, J., Zou, J., Li, K., Jin, C., Xie, F., Su, H.: Extracorporeal high intensity focused ultrasound ablation in the treatment of patients with large hepatocellular carcinoma. Ann. Surg. Oncol. 11(12), 1061–1069 (2004)

Patient-Specific Semi-supervised Learning for Postoperative Brain Tumor Segmentation

Raphael Meier[1], Stefan Bauer[1,2], Johannes Slotboom[2],
Roland Wiest[2], and Mauricio Reyes[1]

[1] Institute for Surgical Technologies and Biomechanics,
University of Bern, Switzerland
[2] Inselspital, Bern University Hospital, Switzerland
raphael.meier@istb.unibe.ch

Abstract. In contrast to preoperative brain tumor segmentation, the problem of postoperative brain tumor segmentation has been rarely approached so far. We present a fully-automatic segmentation method using multimodal magnetic resonance image data and patient-specific semi-supervised learning. The idea behind our semi-supervised approach is to effectively fuse information from both pre- and postoperative image data of the same patient to improve segmentation of the postoperative image. We pose image segmentation as a classification problem and solve it by adopting a semi-supervised decision forest. The method is evaluated on a cohort of 10 high-grade glioma patients, with segmentation performance and computation time comparable or superior to a state-of-the-art brain tumor segmentation method. Moreover, our results confirm that the inclusion of preoperative MR images lead to a better performance regarding postoperative brain tumor segmentation.

1 Introduction

Brain tumors are a rather rare but fatal disease. The most common type of primary brain tumors are gliomas, where the Glioblastoma (GBM) is its most aggressive form with a median patient survival that ranges from 12.2 to 15.9 months [1].

The current approach for treatment of glioma patients involves primary tumor surgery (resection) followed by combined radio- and chemotherapy. The imaging modality of choice is Magnetic Resonance Imaging (MRI). Recent clinical studies, such as e.g. [2], use manual, image-based volumetric analysis rather than diameter-based measures for assessing the outcome of tumor surgery. Lately, it has been shown that manual segmentation of postoperative GBM images is being subject to large interobserver variability [3]. Fully-automatic segmentation methods have the potential to resolve this issue.

High-grade gliomas such as GBMs can be subdivided into four different tumor subcompartments: enhancing tumor, non-enhancing tumor, necrosis and edema [5]. We are interested in segmenting residual enhancing tumor since knowledge about its location and volume is of great clinical relevance. In radiation therapy the enhancing tumor is used for defining the gross tumor volume to be

P. Golland et al. (Eds.): MICCAI 2014, Part I, LNCS 8673, pp. 714–721, 2014.

targeted. Furthermore, the volume of residual enhancing tumor serves as an inclusion criteria for chemotherapy [4] and correlates with patient survival [2]. The segmentation of postoperative brain tumor images is more challenging than segmenting preoperative images for various reasons such as:

- Hemorrhages (caused by surgery) may appear hyperintense on T_1-weighted MR images which can lead to confounding with enhancing tumor.
- Depending on the amount of blood degradation products contained in the resection cavity, the appearance of the cavity can be confounded with the appearance of necrosis or edema.
- The appearance of the postoperative image is influenced by factors that can not be straightforwardly included in a computational model (such as e.g. the experience and skill of the neurosurgeon). From a statistical learning-based point of view these additional (when compared to preoperative images), external influences can be seen as additional dimensions of our feature space. Informally, one can then say that for having the same predictive performance on postoperative images as for preoperative images, a larger number of training samples is needed (curse of dimensionality).

In this work, we rely on multimodal MR images for discriminating hemorrhages from enhancing tumor. We do not attempt to model external influences on the image appearance. However, we try to minimize the overall complexity by employing a machine learning-based model that is *patient-specific*. In other words, we try to solve the present image segmentation by direct inference (i.e. solving it for one patient at a time) rather than induction (i.e. inferring a 'general' rule).

The problem of segmenting postoperative brain tumor images (compared to preoperative images, e.g. see [6]) has received little attention so far. In 2002, Moonis et al. [7] proposed a method based on fuzzy-connectedness for segmenting postoperative MR images. Their approach is semi-automatic and requires the manual definition of seed points. Kanaly et al. [8] proposed a semi-automatic method based on thresholding of the difference image between T_1-weighted pre- and postcontrast images. Recently, Kwon et al. [9] developed a preoperative and post-recurrence brain tumor registration, which included the segmentation of (postoperative) post-recurrence images using a Bayesian joint registration and segmentation framework. In contrast, we segment the initial postoperative scan where recurrences are usually absent and circumvent the need for time-consuming registration procedures via the use of semi-supervised learning. Semi-supervised learning has been used previously in the context of brain tumor segmentation. Lee et al. [10] proposed a semi-supervised discriminative random field. They also employed a patient-specific model for segmenting enhancing tumor. However, they applied their model only on two-dimensional, preoperative images. Caban et al. [11] proposed a framework of sequential transductive and inductive learning based on conditional mixture Naive Bayes and Support Vector Machines. Their framework was designed for annotating edema in multi-modal, temporal MRI studies of patients with high-grade gliomas.

Our contribution is a fully-automatic method for segmenting the enhancing tumor in postoperative multimodal MR images. We introduce a patient-specific semi-supervised learning approach that is resilient to the presence of hemor-rhages by combining information from pre- and postoperative images without the need of registering them.

2 Methods

We approach the problem of segmenting postoperative multimodal MR images of brain tumor patients from a machine learning-based point of view. Hence, we consider it as a classification problem in which we seek a hypothesis h that maps a voxel in an image to its corresponding tissue class label. Voxels are represented by a feature vector $\mathbf{x} \in \mathbb{R}^n$. The target tissue class label $y \in \{0, 1\}$ is a bi-nary variable, representing enhancing tumor ($y = 1$) and remaining brain tissue ($y = 0$) respectively. Furthermore, for every patient we are given a preoperative multimodal image $\Omega_{pre} = \{\omega_{T1}, \omega_{T1c}, \omega_{T2}, \omega_{FLAIR}\}$ and a postoperative image Ω_{post} also consisting of T_1-weighted, T_1-weighted post-contrast, T_2-weighted and $FLAIR$-weighted MR images. Those four modalities are considered standard in clinical acquisition protocols. We further rely on a training set $\mathcal{S}$, which will be used to infer h (=training). A previously unseen voxel i can then be classified via $h(\mathbf{x}^{(i)}) : \mathbf{x}^{(i)} \rightarrow y^{(i)}$ (=testing).

2.1 Features

Before extracting voxel-wise feature vectors, a multimodal image is preprocessed. This step encompasses noise-reduction, intensity normalization and bias field correction (corresponds to the pipeline proposed in [12]). The features to be extracted can be subdivided into appearance- and context-sensitive features. Appearance-sensitive features are the voxel-wise monomodal intensity values, voxel-wise intensity difference between pre- and post-contrast T_1-weighted im-ages, first-order statistics (extracted over a 26-voxel neighborhood) and gradi-ent magnitude textures (local mean and variance) of the respective modalities. Context-sensitive features are symmetric intensity differences computed between the contralateral hemispheres. The axis of symmetry has been defined as the mid-sagittal plane in an atlas. For increasing the robustness of the symmetric features, we smooth the images with a Gaussian kernel ($\sigma = 3.0$) before extracting them. In the end, we obtain a 45-dimensional feature vector $\mathbf{x}$.

2.2 Patient-Specific Semi-supervised Learning

For solving our classification problem, we make two assumptions: First, we as-sume that for every preoperative image Ω_{pre} a corresponding label map can be generated. Ideally, such a map consists of labels for the healthy tissues (CSF, GM, WM) and four tumoral subcompartments (enhancing tumor, non-enhancing tumor, necrosis and edema). Second, we assume that the enhancing tumor and its residual appear *sufficiently* similar in the pre- and postoperative images (im-plying proximity in the feature space).

Regarding the first assumption, considerable improvement on segmenting pre-operative brain tumor images has been achieved the last two years (see the MICCAI BRATS challenges 2012 & 2013 [5]). Hence, such a label map can be automatically created by a segmentation algorithm. We think that the second assumption holds for pre- and postoperative images of the same patient. Those two assumptions form together with the requirement that the postoperative image Ω_{post} to be segmented is available during training the basis of our approach.

In supervised learning, we are given a fully-labeled training set $\mathcal{S} = \{(\mathbf{x}^{(i)}, y^{(i)}):$ $i = 1, ..., |\mathcal{S}|\}$ ($|\cdot|$ representing the cardinality of a set), whereas in a semi-supervised setting only a subset ($\mathcal{S}_\ell \subseteq \mathcal{S}$) of the training data is labeled. This setting can now be translated to our situation, where we have for every patient j a fully-labeled preoperative image $\Omega_{pre,j}$ and an unlabeled postoperative image $\Omega_{post,j}$. The main idea is now to train a model both on the labeled preoperative image data as well as on the unlabeled postoperative data of the *same* patient. This way, information from the pre- and postoperative image can be combined through a common feature space, omitting an error-prone and time-consuming registration step. The final aim is that the model estimates for every voxel in the postoperative image the corresponding tissue class label. Since test data (postoperative image) is already available during training the labels can be propagated from the labeled to unlabeled data, which is also known as *transduction*. Consequently, our transductive model tries to solve the classification problem directly for the available data rather than inferring a general rule h.

2.3   Semi-supervised Decision Forest

Decision Forests are an increasingly popular discriminative model mainly used for solving classification and regression problems. A thorough introduction into decision forests in the context of computer vision and medical image analysis can be found in the book of Criminisi et al. [13]. In [13] a semi-supervised variant of the decision forest model has been proposed, yet only applied to two-dimensional toy datasets. We adopt this model for solving our problem of postoperative brain tumor segmentation.

During training of a supervised decision forest, for each decision tree, data is passed down from the root to the leafs. In doing so, data is split such that for every internal (=split) node k of the respective decision tree an objective function is maximized. We consider the information gain IG_k defined as

$$IG_k(\mathcal{S}_k, \theta_k) = H(\mathcal{S}_k) - \sum_{i \in \{L,R\}} \frac{|\mathcal{S}_k^i|}{|\mathcal{S}_k|} H(\mathcal{S}_k^i) \tag{1}$$

where $H(\mathcal{S}_k)$ denotes the entropy, $\mathcal{S}_k^i$ the training data after the split and $\{L, R\}$ index the left and right child node respectively.

In every split node k, we choose the parameters θ_k of a weak learner $h_k(\mathbf{x}, \theta_k)$ such that the information gain is maximized, i.e. $\theta_k^\star = \arg\max_{\theta_k \in \Theta} IG_k(\mathcal{S}_k, \theta_k)$, where Θ denotes the parameter space. In other words, an optimal split is a decision boundary which separates the training data such that the resulting empirical class distributions of the children show minimal entropy. Optimization is performed by exhaustive search over a randomly selected subspace of Θ. In this work, we consider h_k to be an axis-aligned hyperplane. For handling unlabeled training data the information gain defined in equation (1) is extended by an unsupervised term $IG_{k,u}$ resulting in

$$IG_k(\mathcal{S}_k, \theta_k) = IG_{k,u}(\mathcal{S}_k, \theta_k) + \alpha \cdot IG_{k,s}(\mathcal{S}_{k,\ell}, \theta_k) \qquad (2)$$

where $IG_{k,s}$ corresponds to equation (1), $\mathcal{S}_{k,\ell}$ denotes the labeled subset of the training data in node k and $IG_{k,u}$ is defined as

$$IG_{k,u}(\mathcal{S}_k, \theta_k) = \log(\det \Sigma(\mathcal{S}_k)) - \sum_{i \in \{L,R\}} \frac{|\mathcal{S}_k^i|}{|\mathcal{S}_k|} \log(\det \Sigma(\mathcal{S}_k^i)). \qquad (3)$$

The sets $\mathcal{S}_k$, $\mathcal{S}_k^i$ refer to the complete (labeled and unlabeled) training data before and after the split and Σ is a $n \times n$ covariance matrix, respectively. The coefficient α controls the influence of the labeled data. Above formulation corresponds to the one proposed in [13].

A decision forest establishes a partitioning of the feature space. Since we are considering axis-aligned weak learners, we obtain rectangularly shaped partitions. A regular decision forest uses data in such a partition to estimate the respective leaf statistics. In the particular case of semi-supervised decision forests we are dealing with unlabeled data as well as labeled data. This has the consequence that some of the data points or even all data points affiliated with a leaf are unlabeled. However, for estimating leaf statistics all the training data points need a label. Thus, we have to propagate class labels from the labeled subset in a meaningful way. As suggested in [13], this can be realized by finding the closest labeled point in terms of a geodesic distance G. In the present case, G corresponds to the shortest geodesic path along data points, starting and ending at an unlabeled and labeled data point respectively. The local distance function between data points is chosen to be the symmetric Mahalanobis distance [13] (results from the assumption that the leaf density follows a multivariate Gaussian distribution, cf. equation (3)). Since performing label propagation for each data point separately is computationally not feasible, the forest model approximates it by conducting it for the leaf centroids only. Therefore, we compute the geodesic distance between the means associated with the gaussian partitions. Leafs are represented as nodes in a graph. The shortest (discrete) geodesic distance can then be determined by solving the all-pairs shortest path problem for this particular graph, which can be achieved by the Floyd-Warshall algorithm. The closest leaf statistics are then propagated to the respective unlabeled leaf.

After propagation of leaf statistics, the posterior probability $p(y|\mathbf{x}_u)$ for an unlabeled feature vector corresponds to an average over the whole forest: $p(y|\mathbf{x}_u) = 1/T \sum_{t=1}^{T} p_t(y|\mathbf{x}_u)$, where $p_t(y|\mathbf{x}_u)$ is computed based on the empirical class-histogram stored in the leaf of tree t containing vector $\mathbf{x}_u$. The assignment of an unlabeled voxel i to its most probable tissue class $\tilde{y}^{(i)}$ is then performed according to the MAP-rule: $\tilde{y}^{(i)} = \arg\max_y p(y^{(i)}|\mathbf{x}_u^{(i)})$.

3   Results

For evaluating our method, we relied on image data of 10 high-grade glioma patients (images resampled to 1 $[mm]$ isotropic resolution, mean preoperative contrast-enhancing tumor volume in $[ml]$: 13.7 ± 11.2). This encompasses pre- and postoperative multimodal images of four modalities ($T_1, T_{1c}, T_2, FLAIR$). For five patients a complete resection of contrast-enhancing tumor has been performed, whereas for the other five patients a residual tumor volume is present. Before the evaluation, all the images were skullstripped and rigidly registered. The (pre- and postoperative) ground truth was defined by manual expert segmentation.

For comparison, we chose one of the top-ranked segmentation methods (which is based on [12]) of the BRATS Challenge [5]. The method, primarily designed for segmenting preoperative low- and high-grade gliomas, employs a supervised decision forest classifier followed by a spatial regularization using a Conditional Random Field. We think that due to the methodological similarity between our approach and the one chosen for comparison, the influence of semi-supervised learning may be more apparant. Class imbalance is taken into account via undersampling of the majority class ($y = 0$). Our method, which we refer to as *SSDF* (Semi-Supervised Decision Forest), is trained and evaluated on the labeled preoperative and unlabeled postoperative image of one patient at a time. The supervised method, which we simply refer to as *DF*, is once trained on labeled preoperative images only (*DFPRE*), once trained and evaluated (leave-one-out cross-validation) on labeled postoperative images (*DFPOST*) and finally trained and evaluated using both labeled pre- and postoperative images (leave-one-out cross-validation) (*DFPREPOST*).

Our method has been implemented using C++ and the Sherwood library [13]. We fixed the number of trees T to 40 and α to 1.0. The computation time is mainly defined by the number of leafs, i.e. by the depth D of the forest, and the size of the image volume. The number of leafs l correspond to the number of nodes in the all-shortest path problem to be solved for label propagation. Since the Floyd-Warshall algorithm has a time complexity of $O(l^3)$, computation time increases drastically with D. We found that a depth of $D = 8$ resulted in a good trade-off between performance and computation time.

For quantitative evaluation of the segmentation results, we chose to measure sensitivity, specificity, positive predictive value (PPV) and absolute volume error in $[ml]$. We chose not to estimate the Dice coefficient due to the small size of the residual tumor segments, which results in drastic changes of overlap measures. Results are depicted in table 1. Sensitivity and PPV can be computed for the patients with residual tumor volume only. Specificity and absolute volume error for all 10 patients. We further defined a true positive value of zero for a particular method and image to be a 'miss' and counted the total number of missed instances (#MISSED) per method. The average computation time of *SSDF* (training + testing) is about 3.5 minutes, which is less than the average testing time for *DF* of about 5 minutes.

Table 1. Results of quantitative evaluation. Performance measures are described by the tuple (median, range) due to the small sample size.

Method	Sensitivity	Specificity	PPV	Abs. volume error [ml]	#MISSED
SSDF	$(0.16, 0.27)$	$(0.99, 0.08)$	$(0.24, 0.93)$	$(0.24, 4.72)$	1
DFPRE	$(0.26, 0.61)$	$(0.96, 0.26)$	$(0.15, 0.93)$	$(2.38, 11.24)$	0
DFPOST	$(0, 0.12)$	$(0.99, 0.01)$	$(0, 0.92)$	$(0.15, 6.49)$	3
DFPREPOST	$(0.19, 0.26)$	$(0.99, 0.06)$	$(0.25, 0.92)$	$(0.48, 5.87)$	1

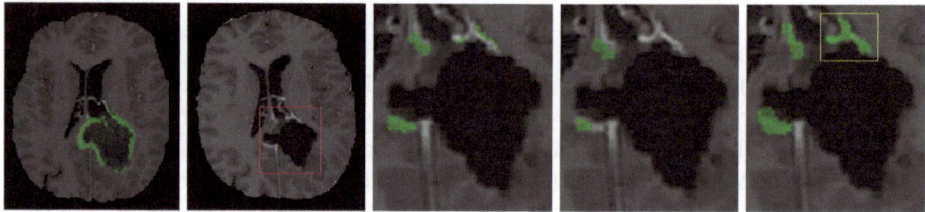

Fig. 1. Exemplary case, T_{1c}-weighted images (green = enhancing tumor), from left to right: Preoperative image, Postoperative image (relevant area is magnified), result for *SSDF*, result for *DFPREPOST*, ground truth. In this specific case, part of the choroid plexus (yellow box) has been infiltrated by the tumor which was correctly detected by our approach.

4   Discussion and Conclusion

When analyzing the segmentation results qualitatively as well as quantitatively, we make several observations. First, *DFPRE* tends to oversegment the residual enhancing tumor. This is reflected in the high sensitivity, low specificity (compared to other approaches), highest absolute volume error and zero misses. The oversegmentation is caused by the inability of the model to properly discriminate between hemorrhage and enhancing tumor. In contrast, *DFPOST* tends to undersegment the residual enhancing tumor and completely misses three cases. The performance of our approach *SSDF* seems superior to *DFPRE* which indicates that in other preoperative images lies no relevant information for segmenting a particular postoperative image. The results of the combined model *DFPREPOST* are comparable to *SSDF* which suggests that information from pre- and postoperative images is truly complementary for segmenting postoperative images. In favor of *SSDF* is the smaller error in volume. An exemplary case supporting our idea of patient-specificity is shown in figure 1. However, due to the small sample size these observations are of preliminary nature. The advantage of *SSDF* over *DFPREPOST* is that it can discriminate residual enhancing tumor from hemorrhages without requiring postoperative ground truth data. The generation of ground truth data for postoperative images is subject to large inter-observer variability [3] and even more time-consuming than for preoperative images.

We presented a fully-automatic method for segmenting residual enhancing tumor in postoperative MR images, which is important to assess surgical outcome and make further treatment decisions. Our approach allows information from pre- and postoperative images to be integrated without the necessity to register them. We think that our initial results provide a basis for further research of this important yet rarely approached segmentation problem.

Acknowledgments. This project has received funding from the European Union's Seventh Programme for research, technological development and demonstration under grant agreement No [600841], from the Swiss Cancer League and the Swiss National Science Foundation.

References

1. Zinn, P.O., Colen, R.R.: Imaging genomic mapping in glioblastoma. Neurosurgery 60, 126–130 (2013)
2. Sanai, N., Polley, M.Y., McDermott, M.W., et al.: An extent of resection threshold for newly diagnosed glioblastomas. J. Neurosurg. 115(1), 3–8 (2011)
3. Kubben, P.L., Postma, A.A., Kessels, A.G.H., van Overbeeke, J.J., van Santbrink, H.: Intraobserver and interobserver agreement in volumetric assessment of glioblastoma multiforme resection. Neurosurgery 67(5), 1329–1334 (2010)
4. Newton, H.: Handbook of Brain Tumor Chemotherapy. Academic Press (2006)
5. B. Menze, et al.: The Multimodal Brain Tumor Image Segmentation Benchmark (BRATS) (submitted, 2014)
6. Bauer, S., Wiest, R., Nolte, L.P., Reyes, M.: A survey of MRI-based medical image analysis for brain tumor studies. Phys. Med. Biol. 58(13), 97–129 (2013)
7. Moonis, G., Liu, J., et al.: Estimation of tumor volume with fuzzy-connectedness segmentation of MR images. AJNR 23(3), 356–363 (2002)
8. Kanaly, C.W., Ding, D., Mehta, A.I., Waller, A.F., Crocker, I., Desjardins, A., Reardon, D.A., Friedman, A.H., et al.: A novel method for volumetric MRI response assessment of enhancing brain tumors. PLoS One 6(1) (2011)
9. Kwon, D., Niethammer, M., Akbari, H., Bilello, M., Davatzikos, C., Pohl, K.: PORTR: Pre-Operative and Post-Recurrence Brain Tumor Registration. IEEE TMI 33(3), 651–667 (2014)
10. Lee, C.H., Wang, S., et al.: Learning to Model Spatial Dependency: Semi-Supervised Discriminative Random Fields. In: Schölkopf, B., Platt, J., Hofmann, T. (eds.) NIPS 2006, vol. 19, pp. 793–800. MIT Press, Cambridge (2006)
11. Caban, J.J., Lee, N., Ebadollahi, S., Laine, A.F., Kender, J.R.: Concept Detection in Longitudinal Brain MR Images Using Multi-Modal Cues. In: IEEE ISBI, pp. 418–421. IEEE Press, New York (2009)
12. Bauer, S., Fejes, T., Slotboom, J., Wiest, R., Nolte, L.P., Reyes, M.: Segmentation of Brain Tumor Images Based on Integrated Hierarchical Classification and Regularization. In: Proceedings of MICCAI-BRATS 2012, pp. 10–13 (2012)
13. Criminisi, A., Shotton, J.: Decision Forests for Computer Vision and Medical Image Analysis. Springer, London (2013)

Robust Cortical Thickness Measurement
with LOGISMOS-B

Ipek Oguz and Milan Sonka

The University of Iowa, Department of Electrical and Computer Engineering, Iowa City, USA

Abstract. Cortical thickness (CT) is an important morphometric measure that has implications for psychiatric and neurologic processes. We propose a novel approach for automatically computing CT in an accurate and robust manner using LOGISMOS-B: Layered Optimal Graph Image Segmentation of Multiple Objects and Surfaces for the Brain. LOGISMOS-B is a cortical surface segmentation method based on LOGISMOS graph segmentation and generalized gradient vector flows. We evaluate our method on two different datasets ($n = 83$ total). The results show that LOGISMOS-B is more accurate than the popular FreeSurfer (FS) method and provides more reliable thickness measurements across a variety of challenging images. LOGISMOS-B accurately recovers known CT patterns, both across cortical lobes and locally, such as between the banks of the central sulcus, in healthy subjects and MS patients. Manual landmarks indicate a signed surface distance of 0.081 ± 0.447mm for WM and 0.018 ± 0.498mm for LOGISMOS-B, compared to 0.263 ± 0.452mm for WM and -0.167 ± 0.556mm for GM for FS, highlighting the surface placement accuracy of LOGISMOS-B. Finally, a regresion study shows that LOGISMOS-B provides strong correlation with age and plausible annual thinning rates across the cortex, with locally discerning thinning patterns, in agreement with the literature.

Keywords: LOGISMOS, cortical thickness, optimal multi-surface segmentation, cortical reconstruction, generalized gradient vector flow.

1 Introduction

Cortical thickness (CT) is an important morphometric measure used to describe the local thickness of the layers of the cerebral cortex. It has been implicated in many diseases and disorders, such as autism, schizophrenia and Huntington's disease. The longitudinal trajectory of CT in healthy development and aging is also of interest.

Despite its considerable significance in neuroscience, measurement of CT from in vivo MRI data is challenging. Manual CT measurements are time-consuming and often inaccurate and irreproducible, given the intrinsically 3-D nature of the CT measure and the highly folded anatomy of the human cerebral cortex. Volumetric and surface-based approaches have been developed for automated thickness analysis [1]. Volumetric approaches such as ANTS [16], Laplacian methods [6,13] and GAMBIT [17] often suffer from partial voluming effects. Surface-based approaches such as FreeSurfer (FS) [3], CLASP [8] and CRUISE [4] have to address the difficult and computationally expensive problem of resolving topological inconsistencies. Given the lack of a gold standard, validation of CT algorithms has to rely on either imperfect independent standards such as

P. Golland et al. (Eds.): MICCAI 2014, Part I, LNCS 8673, pp. 722–730, 2014.
© Springer International Publishing Switzerland 2014

slice-based manual measurements, postmortem measurements and synthetic datasets, or indirect measures such as stability and power analysis.

One of the most common CT analysis tools is FreeSurfer. The cortical reconstruction in FS is based on a surface deformation method using a spring-like term for regularization and an intensity-based term for attracting the boundary to the desired intensity profiles [3]. Gradient descent is used for optimizing this deformation energy along with adaptive step sizes to avoid self-intersections. Once the white and gray matter (WM/GM) surfaces are reconstructed, the CT measurement is based on symmetric closest point matching. In particular, for each GM vertex v, the CT is given by:

$$Thickness(v) = \frac{d(v, f(v)) + d(f(v), g(f(v)))}{2},\tag{1}$$

where $f(v)$ is the closest WM vertex to GM vertex v, $g(v)$ is the closest GM vertex to WM vertex v, and $d(a, b)$ is Euclidean distance between two points.

We propose a novel CT analysis approach based on the LOGISMOS graph segmentation framework [19] and its more recent LOGISMOS-B[1] variant for accurate cortical reconstruction [11], followed by Laplacian-based thickness measurement. LOGISMOS-B is an accurate and computationally efficient cortical segmentation approach that relies on generalized gradient vector flows for handling the complex geometry of the cortical surface. Paired with the theoretically appealing Laplacian-based thickness measurement method, our pipeline offers a robust CT analysis approach.

2 Methods

Our CT measurement pipeline consists of 3 main steps: 1) accurate cortical reconstruction using LOGISMOS-B, 2) thickness computation using the Laplace equation, and 3) atlas-based cortex parcellation for regional analysis.

2.1 Cortical Reconstruction with LOGISMOS-B

LOGISMOS-B is a recently reported [11] cortical reconstruction algorithm. The input consists of a single T1w image. This image is used for atlas-based tissue classification and bias-field correction using the BRAINSABC suite [7]. The tissue classification results are used for skullstripping. The brain is then split into hemispheres by detecting the plane of maximal symmetry. The WM tissue segmentation is topologically corrected by removing handles and holes, including subcortical structures, ventricles and artifacts.

This initial WM segmentation is used to build a properly-ordered multicolumn graph. The mesh representation of the WM segmentation forms the base graph in the LOGISMOS framework [19]. From each vertex of this base graph, a column is built to represent the local search space. The choice of the method for column construction is crucial for determining the behavior of the segmentation. Starting at each vertex of the base graph, LOGISMOS-B follows the streamlines of the generalized gradient vector flow (GGVF) [18] computed on the gradient f of the bias-corrected T1w image.

The GGVF field $\tilde{\mathbf{v}}$ is given by the equilibrium solution of $\mathbf{v}_t = g(|\nabla f|)\nabla^2 \mathbf{v} - h(|\nabla f|)(\mathbf{v} - \nabla f)$. The smoothing term produces a smoothly varying vector field while

---

[1] B for Brain.

the data term penalizes against large deviations from the input. The weighting functions g and h are chosen to allow reduced smoothing near strong gradients, as in [18].

The WM and GM surfaces are treated as mutually interacting surfaces of the same object. In the LOGISMOS framework, this is represented by two copies of the same graph that are connected together. There are three types of arcs in this composite graph: the intra-column arcs provide the appropriate graph structure for the minimum-cost closed set algorithm, the inter-column arcs enforce surface smoothness constraints and inter-surface arcs enforce inter-surface separation constraints.

As an important extension of the original LOGISMOS-B approach [11], we newly incorporate regionally-dependent parameters in the form of anatomy-derived minimum surface separation constraints. For the regions that are known a priori to have thin cortices, we allow for a reduced minimum surface separation. In particular, for the visual cortex and the postcentral sulcus, among the thinnest in the cortex [2], the minimum inter-surface separation constraint was set to 2mm, while it was set to 2.5mm for the rest of the brain. The definitions of regions for this purpose is obtained using an atlas-based approach. The atlas mapping created during the BRAINSABC tissue classification is used to carry the atlas labels to the subject space. Each graph column is assigned a label by considering the label at the pre-segmentation mesh vertex. If this point falls outside the cortex, then the label of a second node that corresponds to the minimum separation constraint between the two surfaces is considered. Any graph columns still without assigned labels are labeled via majority voting from neighboring columns.

Once the graph construction is complete, $s - t$ cut graph optimization is used for finding the minimum-cost closed set of this graph, which within the LOGISMOS framework is equivalent to optimal multi-surface segmentation. The cost functions reflect the gradient magnitude of the bias-corrected and smoothed T1w image for the WM surface, and a weighted sum of the first and second order gradients for the GM surface. Finally, the brainstem and cerebellum are removed using a mask mapped from the atlas.

2.2   Laplacian-Based Cortical Thickness Computation

When cortical surfaces are known, thickness computation methods based on the Laplace equation [6] proved both popular and relevant. In this volumetric approach, the Laplace equation is set up using the input WM and GM surfaces as boundary conditions ($u(x) = 1$ and $u(x) = -1$, respectively), such that $\nabla^2 u(x) = 0$. The smooth gradient of u, $v = \frac{\nabla u}{||\nabla u||}$ is used to compute streamlines, which are guaranteed to not intersect each other and provide a one-to-one correspondence between the two surfaces. The length of each streamline is reported as the thickness measurement.

In particular, we use an implementation of the approach described in [13], which uses a boundary element method (BEM) approach for improved accuracy. We scan-convert the final LOGISMOS-B surfaces, with the brainstem and cerebellum intact, to high-resolution (0.5mm) images to use as input for this purpose. The CT measurements are pulled back to the final surfaces (after the removal of the brainstem and cerebellum) by looking up thickness values at the GM mesh vertex locations; in case these vertices fall outside the valid domain (due to discretization), the corresponding WM mesh vertex is used instead. Keeping the brainstem and cerebellum in place for the thickness computation prevents any topological defects or sharp features at the removal site and provides a more stable thickness measurement for the cortical areas in this region.

2.3   Regional Parcellation

In order to facilitate regional CT measurements, we create a parcellation of the cortex into regions of interest (ROI's), again using the atlas ROI's mapped to the subject space. While a coarse parcellation is previously computed during the graph construction, this is done in the absence of the final surface reconstructions and is therefore prone to errors. After the LOGISMOS-B segmentation is finalized, cortical parcellation labels are improved by considering the final WM and GM vertices for label assignment.

3   Experimental Methods

Datasets. The first dataset from Johns Hopkins University (JHU)[2] [15] has an isotropic resolution of $(1mm)^3$ for the healthy controls ($n = 5$) and $(0.83mm)^3$ for the MS patients ($n = 5$). Manual landmarks are identified by 2 independent raters in 7 clusters on both WM and GM surfaces. Each cluster (calcarine, central sulcus, cingulate, parieto-occipital, sup. frontal, sup. temporal, Sylvian fissure) has 30 landmarks per hemisphere. A total of 7 clusters × 2 hemispheres × 2 surfaces × 30 landmarks × 2 raters = 1680 landmarks are available per subject, or 16,800 landmarks total. The second dataset consists of 73 healthy subjects from the publicly available IXI[3] database, collected at the IoP in London. These images have a resolution of $0.937 \times 0.937 \times 1.2mm^3$.

Manual thickness. We compute closest-point matching between the WM and GM landmarks. Points that have multiple matches are discarded to avoid inaccurate thickness measurements. Euclidean distance between remaining pairs serves as manual CT. Note that this is far from being a gold standard. The landmarks were chosen for a cortical reconstruction validation study; as such, they are not meant to provide accurately paired points for CT measurement. This may cause over- or under-estimation of CT.

LOGISMOS-B surface reconstruction and Laplacian CT measurement. The same cortical reconstruction parameters as presented in [11] are used. The atlas in the BRAINS package was used for tissue classification and regional parcellation, including 70 cortical ROI's. 20,000 graph columns per hemisphere were used, each containing 120 nodes, with a node spacing of 0.1mm. The step size is 0.015625 for solving the Laplace equation and 0.125 for the transport equation, which allow for a stable solution [13]. The transport equation is run for 100 iterations (50 backward and 50 forward).

FS surface reconstruction and thickness measurement. FS currently represents the most commonly used approach for CT analysis; version 5.1 was used.

Symmetric closest point (SCP) thickness on LOGISMOS-B surfaces. To separate the effect of cortical reconstruction accuracy from thickness measurements, we also report the thickness measures computed using Eqn. 1 on the LOGISMOS-B surface reconstructions. We refer to this method as LOGISMOS-B + SCP.

Evaluation Strategy. The LOGISMOS-B surface reconstruction and positioning algorithm was previously validated [11]; therefore, in this manuscript, we focus on the evaluation and validation of the thickness measurements given the surfaces.

---

[2] http://www.iacl.ece.jhu.edu/Cortical_data/
[3] http://biomedic.doc.ic.ac.uk/brain-development

Table 1. Left, Mean ± std. deviation of whole-brain CT. Right, Mean and std. dev. of distance between manual landmarks and reconstructed surfaces (JHU). * indicates statistical significance.

	JHU		IXI			LOGISMOS-B	FreeSurfer
	Left	Right	Left	Right			
FreeSurfer	3.154 ± 0.798	3.038 ± 0.760	2.824 ± 0.987	2.853 ± 0.996	Signed WM	*0.081 ± 0.447	0.263 ± 0.452
LOGISMOS-B	2.626 ± 1.151	2.700 ± 1.168	2.946 ± 1.259	2.998 ± 1.255	Signed GM	*0.018 ± 0.498	-0.167 ± 0.556
LOGISMOS-B + SCP	2.232 ± 0.654	2.276 ± 0.662	2.315 ± 0.799	2.363 ± 0.810	Unsigned WM	*0.579 ± 0.264	0.611 ± 0.302
					Unsigned GM	0.681 ± 0.298	0.703 ± 0.331

First, we use the JHU dataset to compare the automated CT measurements to the Manual thickness per landmark cluster. We also use the landmark locations, which represent the gold standard for surface placement, to assess the error and bias for each method; signed distance to the landmarks measures surface placement bias, whereas unsigned distance measures bulk error in placement.

Next, we compare the automated CT measurements on both datasets to known patterns from the literature. Specifically, the post-central gyrus is markedly thinner than the pre-central gyrus [10]. The frontal and temporal lobes are thicker than the occipital lobe. MS patients have thinner cortices overall, and in particular in the frontal and temporal lobes, compared to healthy subjects [14]. The brain is relatively symmetric, but asymmetric regions are known to exist such as the superior temporal gyrus [9].

Next, we present the regression of CT against subject age in the large IXI dataset. Similar to [16], we normalize the CT measurements by brain size, estimated by the volume of the skullstrip mask. We compare the findings to known patterns from literature: it is well established that the frontal, insular, temporal and parietal GM shrinks throughout healthy aging, whereas the occipital cortex is largely spared and remains relatively stable across the lifespan (e.g., [12] and the many references therein). Hutton et al. [5] report a CT decrease of up to 0.02mm/yr. in select regions of the cortex, especially in frontal and temporal areas, with the whole-brain average thinning of 0.009mm/yr.

4 Results

Tab. 1 summarizes the whole brain CT measurements. Two-tailed paired t-tests reveal that all pairs of methods are significantly different from each other (for JHU, $p \ll 0.001$ for all pairs; for IXI, $p = 0.05$ between LOGISMOS-B + SCP and Laplacian, $p \ll 0.001$ for all other pairs). Tab. 1 also summarizes the landmark errors for the JHU dataset. LOGISMOS-B surface placement is significantly more accurate than FS.

Tab. 2 shows the average CT measurements per cluster and the amount of asymmetry in CT measurements for each method for the JHU dataset. Overall, most clusters show high symmetry; however, the superior temporal sulcus (ST) is found to exhibit a strong asymmetry with the LOGISMOS-B approach, consistent with literature [9].

Table 2. Left, average CT per cluster (JHU). Right, asymmetry in CT measurements computed as the difference between left and right hemisphere CT. All units are mm.

CT	Manual	FreeSurfer	LOGISMOS-B	LOGISMOS-B + SCP	Asymmetry	Manual	FreeSurfer	LOGISMOS-B	LOGISMOS-B + SCP
CALC	2.432	2.281	2.068	1.535	CALC	0.020	-0.061	-0.196	0.003
CING	3.356	3.441	3.049	2.267	CING	0.053	-0.063	-0.053	0.054
CS	2.796	2.964	2.270	2.157	CS	0.169	0.162	-0.003	-0.004
PO	2.665	2.877	2.300	2.072	PO	-0.220	0.236	0.024	0.009
SF	2.782	3.143	2.906	2.557	SF	-0.346	0.070	-0.231	-0.154
ST	3.193	3.352	3.116	2.671	ST	-0.041	0.099	-0.206	-0.111
SYL	3.083	3.359	2.965	2.415	SYL	0.240	0.062	-0.067	-0.020

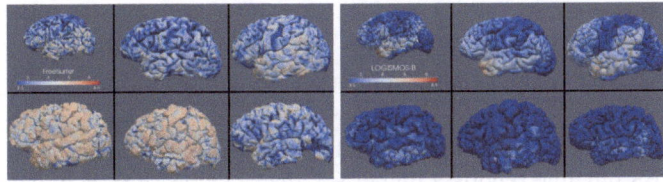

Fig. 1. FS and LOGISMOS-B CT(JHU). Top row, healthy, bottom, MS patients.

LOGISMOS-B reports lower CT measurements in the postcentral gyrus (2.1mm for JHU, 2.2mm for IXI) than in the precentral gyrus (2.4mm for both JHU and IXI), consistent with literature. Tab. 3 compares the healthy and MS groups. The FS measurements disagree with the known fact that MS patients exhibit cortical thinning ([14] and references therein). LOGISMOS-B, in contrast, follows this expected pattern. In fact, in addition to the diffuse overall thinning in the whole brain, LOGISMOS-B reports a marked focal thinning in the frontal and temporal lobes, in close agreement with [14].

Fig. 1 shows representative FS and LOGISMOS-B CT results in the JHU dataset for qualitative evaluation. We observe that the FS surface reconstruction is less than ideal especially for the MS patients; note the missing chunk of tissue for the rightmost subject near the inferior temporal gyrus, as well as the fused appearance of the gyri throughout the brain for all MS subjects, especially in comparison to the LOGISMOS-B surfaces.

Tab. 4 presents the summary statistics per lobe for the IXI dataset. In Tab. 3 and 4, consistent with the literature, the LOGISMOS-B CT measurements are higher in the frontal and the temporal lobes than in the occipital lobe. In Tab. 4, FS reports a low cingulate thickness, by as much as 2mm. Note that the 1.6mm CT reported by FS is not very credible, considering the cingulate CT of over 3mm reported in many in vivo studies (e.g., [16]) and $2.7 - 3.0$mm in postmortem specimen [2], which is expected to be lower than in vivo MRI measurements due to shrinkage during fixation of the brain. LOGISMOS-B reports a cingulate thickness of 3.4mm, consistent with the literature.

Tab. 4 presents the regression analysis of CT against subject age. Overall, LOGISMOS-B reports a more rapid thinning per year (as indicated by the slope) and a stronger correlation with age than FS. In particular, LOGISMOS-B reports average thinning of 0.022mm/yr. in the frontal lobe, but a low correlation and only 0.002mm/yr. thinning in the occipital lobe, closely matching the literature. FS-reports only 0.008mm/yr. thinning in the frontal lobe and 0.005mm/yr. thinning and a rather strong correlation in the occipital lobe. The similarity of these two rates and its mismatch with published literature indicate that FreeSurfer is either overestimating occipital thinning or underestimating frontal thinning, or, likely, both.

Table 3. Lobar CT (JHU). Mean ± std. deviation are reported in mm.

	Healthy			MS		
	FreeSurfer	LOGISMOS-B	LOGISMOS-B + SCP	FreeSurfer	LOGISMOS-B	LOGISMOS-B + SCP
Cingulate	3.273 ± 0.742	3.250 ± 1.057	2.460 ± 0.916	3.467 ± 0.747	2.755 ± 2.909	2.081 ± 0.860
Frontal	3.037 ± 0.624	3.271 ± 0.905	2.694 ± 0.611	3.439 ± 0.821	2.502 ± 0.787	2.259 ± 0.505
Insular	3.298 ± 0.971	3.121 ± 0.990	2.368 ± 0.893	3.451 ± 1.015	2.515 ± 2.324	1.956 ± 0.775
Occipital	2.575 ± 0.686	2.326 ± 1.735	1.918 ± 0.541	2.672 ± 0.789	2.089 ± 0.535	1.757 ± 0.506
Parietal	2.674 ± 0.683	2.603 ± 0.755	2.278 ± 0.480	3.152 ± 0.842	2.216 ± 0.458	2.076 ± 0.401
Temporal	3.314 ± 0.735	3.133 ± 1.290	2.496 ± 0.798	3.381 ± 0.815	2.502 ± 1.081	2.103 ± 0.651
Whole brain	2.939 ± 0.737	2.929 ± 1.180	2.414 ± 0.692	3.246 ± 0.864	2.381 ± 1.068	2.085 ± 0.574

5 Discussion

We observe that SCP underestimates thickness. The LOGISMOS-B + SCP measurements are consistently lower than the Laplacian measurements on the same surfaces and lower than the manual measurements (Tab. 1-2), by as much as 15% on average. Despite this bias, the FS pipeline reports a higher CT than LOGISMOS-B in the JHU dataset (Tab. 1-2), suggesting that the FS surface reconstruction must be over-compensating. This is also supported by Tab. 1, which shows bias in FS surface placement. Clearly, over-estimating in one module and under-estimating in another is not an ideal way for reliable measurement. LOGISMOS-B has excellent surface reconstruction accuracy [11], which should inevitably lead to higher accuracy for *any* meaningful thickness measurement approach. The Laplacian method is one such approach.

The inaccurate FS reconstruction for MS subjects, especially the artificially enlarged GM segmentation (Fig. 1), leads to higher reported CT in the MS patients compared to healthy subjects (Tab. 3). The robust LOGISMOS-B accurately captures the thinning in MS patients, both diffusely and focally.

The FS cingulate measurements in Tab. 4 are inconsistent with literature, unlike LOGISMOS-B findings. The LOGISMOS-B + SCP results represent the midway point between the two methods. This indicates that the SCP measurement bias is only partially responsible for the observed cingulate CT discrepancy. This suggests that the LOGISMOS-B surface placement is superior to FS in the IXI dataset, just like for JHU.

LOGISMOS-B findings regarding age effects on CT (Tab. 4) are closely consistent with the literature, unlike FS results. LOGISMOS-B also shows a greater range of these age effects on thickness, which should translate into higher statistical power in studies compared to FS, which report relatively homogeneous thinning rates.

The improved accuracy in LOGISMOS-B is largely due to its graph-based segmentation which guarantees a globally optimal solution and is therefore extremely robust to local image artifacts. LOGISMOS-B used the same parameters on both datasets, indicating its robustness against different acquisition parameters and a large variety of subjects, including healthy volunteers and MS patients and a large age range. Furthermore, while the current experiments used only T1w images for a fair comparison with FS, it is straightforward to extend LOGISMOS-B to use additional images such as T2w scans by simply adapting the cost function, which may further improve the accuracy.

It is also important that the CT is measured along non-intersecting paths. The Laplacian-based methods inherently guarantee this. The closest-point matching in the FS approach often leads to intersecting paths in the tightly folded cortex.

Table 4. Left, Mean ± std. deviation of CT. Right, CT vs. age regression (IXI).

Lobar CT	FreeSurfer	LOGISMOS-B	LOGISMOS-B + SCP
LCingulate	1.526 ± 1.668	3.429 ± 1.116	2.675 ± 0.913
LFrontal	3.037 ± 0.693	3.296 ± 1.269	2.622 ± 0.804
LInsular	3.326 ± 0.997	3.196 ± 1.937	2.323 ± 0.920
LOccipital	2.549 ± 0.790	2.274 ± 1.342	1.803 ± 0.574
LParietal	2.763 ± 0.686	2.605 ± 0.877	2.074 ± 0.589
LTemporal	3.283 ± 0.821	3.166 ± 1.155	2.423 ± 0.838
RCingulate	1.703 ± 1.676	3.359 ± 1.182	2.519 ± 0.955
RFrontal	3.073 ± 0.702	3.337 ± 1.404	2.649 ± 0.830
RInsular	3.157 ± 1.243	3.126 ± 1.689	2.211 ± 0.916
ROccipital	2.626 ± 0.818	2.311 ± 0.968	1.869 ± 0.565
RParietal	2.775 ± 0.691	2.653 ± 0.853	2.146 ± 0.586
RTemporal	3.339 ± 0.813	3.325 ± 1.184	2.556 ± 0.860

Regression	LOGISMOS-B		FreeSurfer	
	Correlation	Slope	Correlation	Slope
LCingulate	-0.219	-0.006	-0.418	-0.003
LFrontal	-0.710	-0.022	-0.570	-0.007
LInsular	-0.575	-0.017	-0.421	-0.006
LOccipital	-0.164	-0.002	-0.436	-0.005
LParietal	-0.639	-0.012	-0.568	-0.006
LTemporal	-0.586	-0.013	-0.541	-0.007
RCingulate	-0.364	-0.011	-0.350	-0.003
RFrontal	-0.716	-0.023	-0.581	-0.008
RInsular	-0.702	-0.019	-0.500	-0.009
ROccipital	-0.230	-0.002	-0.422	-0.005
RParietal	-0.671	-0.013	-0.553	-0.007
RTemporal	-0.504	-0.011	-0.435	-0.006

6   Conclusion

The reported cortical thickness measurement algorithm, using LOGISMOS-B cortical reconstruction and Laplacian-based thickness measurement, is based on a highly accurate cortical reconstruction by extending the LOGISMOS graph segmentation framework using generalized gradient vector flows. Compared to the current state-of-the-art, LOGISMOS-B offers improved accuracy and robustness in cortical thickness studies.

Acknowledgments. This research was funded, in part, by NIH-NIBIB grant R01-EB004640. The authors would like to thank Jerry Prince and Peter Calabresi for providing the JHU dataset [15], and Marc Niethammer and Joohwi Lee for the Laplacian-based thickness implementation.

References

1. Clarkson, M., Cardoso, J., Ridgway, G., Leung, K., Rohrer, J., Fox, N., Ourselin, S.: A comparison of voxel and surface based CT estimation methods. NeuroImage 57, 856–865 (2011)
2. von Economo, C.: The Cytoarchitectonics of the Human Cerebral Cortex. Oxford Univ. Press, London (1929)
3. Fischl, B., Dale, A.: Measuring the thickness of the human cortex from MRI. PNAS (2000)
4. Han, X., Pham, D., Tosun, D., Rettmann, M., Xu, C., Prince, J.: CRUISE. NeuroImage (2004)
5. Hutton, C., Draganski, B., Ashburner, J., Weiskopf, N.: A comparison between VBCT and VBM in normal aging. Neuroimage 48, 371–380 (2009)
6. Jones, S., Buchbinder, B., Aharon, I.: 3D mapping of CT using Laplace's equation. HBM 11(1), 12–32 (2000)
7. Kim, E.Y., Johnson, H.J.: Robust multi-site MR data processing: Iterative optimization of bias correction, tissue classification, and registration. Front Neuroinform 7(29), 1–18 (2013)
8. Kim, J.S., Singh, V., Lee, J.K., Lerch, J., Ad-Dab'bagh, Y., MacDonald, D., Lee, J.M., Kim, S.I., Evans, A.C.: Automated 3D extraction and eval. of the inner and outer cortical surfaces using a Laplacian map and partial volume effect classification. NeuroImage 27, 210–221 (2005)
9. Luders, E., Narr, K., Thompson, P., Rex, D., Jancke, L., Toga, A.: Hemispheric asymmetries in CT. Cereb Cortex 16, 1232–1238 (2006)
10. Meyer, J., Roychowdhury, S., Russell, E., Callahan, C., Gitelman, D., Mesulam, M.: Location of the CS via CT of the precentral and postcentral gyri on MR. Am. J. Neuroradiol. 17 (1996)
11. Oguz, I., Sonka, M.: LOGISMOS-B: Layered optimal graph image segmentation of multiple objects and surfaces for the brain. IEEE Trans. Med. Imaging 33, 1–16 (2014)
12. Park, D.C., Reuter-Lorenz, P.: The adaptive brain: Aging and neurocognitive scaffolding. Annu. Rev. Psychol. 60(1), 173–196 (2009)
13. Pichon, E., Nain, D., Niethammer, M.: A Laplace equation approach for shape comparison. SPIE Medical Imaging (2006)
14. Sailer, M., Fischl, B., Salat, D., Tempelmann, C., Schönfeld, M., Busa, E., Bodammer, N., Heinze, H., Dale, A.: Focal thinning of the cerebral cortex in MS. Brain 126, 1734–1744 (2003)
15. Shiee, N., Bazin, P., Cuzzocreo, J., Ye, C., Kishore, B., Carass, A., Calabresi, P., Reich, D., Prince, J., Pham, D.: Robust reconstruction of the human brain cortex in the presence of the WM lesions: Method and validation. HBM (2013)

16. Tustison, N.J., Avants, B.B., Cook, P.A., Song, G., Das, S., Strien, N.V., Stone, J.R., Gee, J.C.: The ANTS CT processing pipeline. SPIE Medical Imaging (2013)
17. Vachet, C., Hazlett, H.C., Niethammer, M., Oguz, I., Cates, J., Whitaker, R., Piven, J., Styner, M.: Group-wise automatic mesh-based analysis of CT. SPIE Medical Imaging (2011)
18. Xu, C., Prince, J.: GGVF external forces for active contours. Sig. Proc. 71, 131–139 (1998)
19. Yin, Y., Zhang, X., Williams, R., Wu, X., Anderson, D.D., Sonka, M.: LOGISMOS: cartilage segmentation in the knee joint. IEEE TMI 29, 2023–2037 (2010)

Label Inference with Registration and Patch Priors

Siqi Bao and Albert C.S. Chung

Lo Kwee-Seong Medical Image Analysis Laboratory,
Department of Computer Science and Engineering,
The Hong Kong University of Science and Technology, Hong Kong

Abstract. In this paper, we present a novel label inference method that integrates registration and patch priors, and serves as a remedy for labelling errors around structural boundaries. With the initial label map provided by nonrigid registration methods, its corresponding signed distance function can be estimated and used to evaluate the segmentation confidence. The pixels with less confident labels are selected as candidate nodes to be refined and those with relatively confident results are settled as seeds. The affinity between seeds and candidate nodes, which consists of regular image lattice connections, registration prior based on signed distance and patch prior from the warped atlas, is encoded to guide the label inference procedure. For method evaluation, experiments have been carried out on two publicly available data sets and it only takes several seconds for our method to improve the segmentation quality significantly.

1 Introduction

Due to poor contrast condition and intensity inhomogeneity in brain magnetic resonance (MR) images, it is challenging to provide a reliable segmentation result. Manual labelling is tedious and time-consuming, which also suffers from inter- and intra-labeler variability [13]. Various automatic labelling methods have been proposed and atlas-based segmentation approaches become widely used owing to the relatively high accuracy. With manually labelled atlas, the label map for the target image can be propagated from the atlas based on nonrigid registration [9]. To obtain a reasonable deformation field, smoothness or regularization term is conventionally enforced during registration [6,14]. However, because of the anatomical variability among subjects, the enforcement of regularization can lead to labelling errors near the object surfaces.

Patch-based method is first introduced for image denoising [4] and later employed in medical image segmentation. In [11], with the similarity values calculated from a kernel function as weights, the small patches inside a region weighted vote for the labels of the target image. In this process, no nonrigid registration is required and all information provided by the small patches will be utilized. To reduce the adverse impact from dissimilar patches, an extension is proposed in [3], by first ranking these small patches based on structure similarity and then combining the selected ones together for the final labelling.

P. Golland et al. (Eds.): MICCAI 2014, Part I, LNCS 8673, pp. 731–738, 2014.

As pointed out in [15], patch-based methods can fail to provide accurate labels close to boundaries and one label inference approach based on Gaussian processes has been proposed by estimating contour-driven distribution over label maps. However, as a result of poor contrast and weak boundaries, the contour is difficult to extract in brain MR images. In this paper, we present a novel label inference method integrated with registration and patch priors, to help correct the label errors around structural boundaries. Experiments on two public data sets indicate that the proposed label refinement method (label inference) can improve the segmentation quality significantly and efficiently.

2   Methodology

In this paper, label inference is formulated on an undirected weighted graph, with nodes selected automatically from the target image based on confidence evaluation. Besides the typical image lattice connections, registration prior based on signed distance and patch prior from the warped atlas image are encoded to assist the refinement procedure. Under the framework of Random Walker, label inference can be viewed and solved as the discrete Dirichlet problem.

2.1   Confidence Evaluation

In Fig. 1, the segmentation result for the left hippocampus provided by one benchmark registration method ANTs is shown in blue. As compared with the ground truth displayed in red, it can be observed that label errors mainly lie around the boundary of the subcortical structure. In other words, the segmentation results for pixels or voxels close to the structural border have low confidence level as compared with those far away from the perimeter. In this paper, a new label inference method is proposed to improve the atlas-based extraction of one subcortical structure in brain MR images. Signed Distance Function (SDF) [12] is employed as shape representation and utilized to help evaluate the segmentation confidence of the warped label map. The SDF for one binary image can be constructed by calculating the Euclidean distance between one pixel and its nearest pixel on the object boundary. Each pixel in the image has its corresponding signed distance and negative or positive value indicates inside (foreground) or outside (background) the object respectively.

For one pixel located around the boundary, the absolute value of its signed distance approaches 0 and its confidence of the current label is relatively low. In our approach, we assume that the segmentation confidence of one pixel is proportional to the absolute value of its signed distance. Given one positive value ρ, the pixels with signed distance $-\rho < d < \rho$ are regarded as candidate nodes, whose labels have low confidence level and need to be refined. The labels for the pixels with signed distance $d \geq \rho$ or $d \leq -\rho$ are regarded as confident results and these pixels can be viewed as foreground or background seeds.

We use x_i to represent the probability that one node belongs to the foreground ($x_F = 1$ for the foreground seed and $x_B = 0$ for the background seed). By

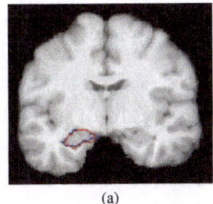
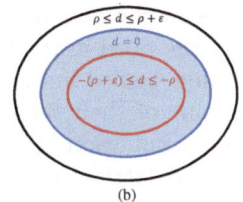

(a)   (b)

Fig. 1. (a) Comparison of segmentation results from ANTs (Blue) and manually labelled ground truth (Red). (b) Blue curve: boundary of the object with signed distance $d = 0$; Red curve: the layer inside the object with signed distance $-(\rho + \varepsilon) \le d \le -\rho$; Black curve: the layer outside the object with signed distance $\rho \le d \le \rho + \varepsilon$.

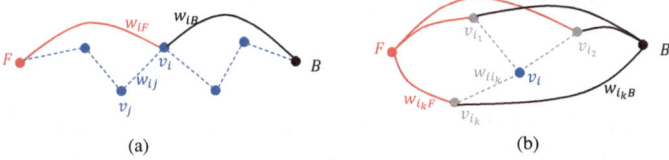

(a)   (b)

Fig. 2. (Colour Image) (a) Illustration of encoding lattice connections (blue dashed lines) and registration prior (red and black lines). (b) Illustration of encoding patch prior from the atlas (gray dashed lines) and rater reliability (red and black lines). Virtual nodes v_{i_k} $(k = 1, \cdots, K)$ are associated with candidate node v_i.

encoding the relationship between candidate nodes and seeds into one graph $G = (V, E)$, we try to seek the optimal solution for x_i and improve the current segmentation quality. V refers to the set of nodes, which consists of nodes selected from the target image (foreground seeds V_F, background seeds V_B and candidate nodes V_C) and virtual nodes V_V generated from the warped atlas. The foreground seeds V_F are obtained by selecting pixels with signed distance $-(\rho+\varepsilon) \le d \le -\rho$, and the background seeds V_B are chosen from the pixels with signed distance $\rho \le d \le \rho+\varepsilon$, as shown in Fig. 1(b). To balance the influence from foreground and background seeds on candidate nodes, we randomly select background seeds to make the numbers of two kinds of seeds equal. As for the virtual nodes V_V, they act as mediators between candidate nodes and seeds, which will be illustrated in detail later. $E \subseteq V \times V$ refers to the set of edges connecting two nodes i and j, with w_{ij} as edge weight.

2.2   Registration Prior

With the foreground and background seeds settled, we can propagate the influence of seeds to candidate nodes through image lattice. For the candidate node $v_i \in V_C$, we consider the affinity between v_i and its neighbors, with the edge weight w_{ij} assigned with the common Gaussian function,

$$\forall \, v_j \in \mathcal{N}(v_i), \quad w_{ij} = \exp(-\beta_1(I_T(v_i) - I_T(v_j))^2), \qquad (1)$$

where $\mathcal{N}(v_i)$ refers to the 6-nearest neighbors of v_i in 3-D images, $I_T(\cdot)$ is the intensity value for the pixel in the target image and β_1 is one tuning parameter. In Fig. 2(a), the blue dashed lines refer to the edges connecting candidate nodes (blue dots) and some of their 6-connected lattice neighbors, with edge weights which are defined in Equation (1).

Besides the regular lattice connections, registration prior is also exploited to guide the label inference procedure according to the signed distances of candidate nodes. For one node with a smaller signed distance, more impacts are supposed to be received from the foreground seed and vice versa. To involve the registration prior in the graph, direct edges between the candidate node and seeds are appended, as the red and black lines shown in Fig. 2(a). The red dot is one foreground seed ($F \in V_F$) and the black dot is one background seed ($B \in V_B$). We define w_{iF} and w_{iB} using the sigmoid function,

$$w_{iF} = \frac{1}{1 + e^{d_i}}, \quad w_{iB} = \frac{1}{1 + e^{-d_i}}, \tag{2}$$

in which d_i is the signed distance for candidate node v_i. With the definitions above, $0 < w_{iF} < 1$, $0 < w_{iB} < 1$, $w_{iF} + w_{iB} = 1$ can be inferred. To some extent, w_{iF} can represent the probability implied by registration prior that v_i belongs to the foreground, similarly for w_{iB}. For the candidate nodes located at the boundary ($d_i = 0$), the impacts of registration prior from the foreground and background seeds are equal and then other prior knowledge can dominate the label inference of these nodes, in such way the boundary errors can be suppressed. In our approach, the SDF can help choose candidate nodes to be refined and assist the utilization of the registration prior accordingly.

2.3 Patch Prior

Based on the deformation field determined in the registration procedure, the label map of the atlas can be deformed to provide the segmentation result for the target image. At the same time, the intensity profile of the atlas can also be warped based on the deformation field. Due to regularization or smoothness term utilized during registration, the warped intensity profile of the atlas differs with that of the target image. As such, it is reasonable to see that the warped label map is inaccurate for the target image at some pixels, especially around the structural boundaries. In this paper, we propose to use patch prior from the warped atlas to assist the label inference procedure of the target image and to relax the constraint brought by regularization during registration.

For one candidate node v_i in the target image, the intensity information around it, in terms of patch, $\mathcal{P}_1(v_i)$ is taken into consideration. Similar patches for $\mathcal{P}_1(v_i)$ are searched inside a larger patch $\mathcal{P}_2(v_i)$ in the warped atlas image. In 3-D MR image segmentation, the sizes of $\mathcal{P}_1$ and $\mathcal{P}_2$ are $(2r_1+1)^3$ and $(2r_2+1)^3$ respectively, where $r_2 > r_1 > 0$. The similarity between two patches is defined as follows,

$$\forall\, \mathcal{P}_1(v_{i_k}) \subset \mathcal{P}_2(v_i), \quad S(v_i, v_{i_k}) = \sum_{x \in \mathcal{P}_1(v_i),\ y \in \mathcal{P}_1(v_{i_k})} (I_T(x) - I_A(y))^2, \tag{3}$$

where I_T and I_A are the intensity profiles of the target image and warped atlas respectively, v_{i_k} is one pixel in the warped atlas such that patch $\mathcal{P}_1(v_{i_k})$ is inside the larger patch $\mathcal{P}_2(v_i)$. After performing sorting on the similarity values, we can pick up K patches $\mathcal{P}_1(v_{i_k})$ $(k = 1, \cdots, K,\ K \geq 2)$ which are similar with $\mathcal{P}_1(v_i)$, to decrease the adverse impact from dissimilar patches. The central pixels v_{i_k} of these similar patches are added as virtual nodes to the graph, connected with corresponding candidate node v_i, as shown in Fig. 2(b). The edge weight w_{ii_k} between candidate node v_i and one of its virtual nodes v_{i_k} is defined based on the patch similarity,

$$\forall\ v_{i_k} \in V_V(v_i), \quad w_{ii_k} = \frac{1}{Z(v_i)} S(v_i, v_{i_k})^{-\beta_2}, \tag{4}$$

where $V_V(v_i)$ is the set of virtual nodes associated with v_i. As experimentally demonstrated in [1], the above weight gives better performance as compared with other related similarity metrics. β_2 is one tuning parameter and $Z(v_i)$ is a normalization constant to guarantee $\sum_{k=1}^{K} w_{ii_k} = 1$.

To deal with the manual labelling inconsistency [13] for the prior provided by the warped atlas, we introduce one term α to encode this kind of uncertainty. The edge weights between the virtual point and the seeds are given as follows,

$$w_{i_k F} = \alpha L(v_{i_k}), \quad w_{i_k B} = 1 - \alpha L(v_{i_k}), \tag{5}$$

where α is one tuning parameter related to the rater reliability, $L(\cdot)$ is the label of a node, with 1 or 0 standing for foreground or background respectively.

2.4   Label Inference

The basic energy function for target image segmentation [10] is given as follows,

$$
\begin{aligned}
E(x) &= E_{unary}(x) + E_{binary}(x), \\
&= \sum_{v_i} (w_{iF}^q |x_i - 1|^p + w_{iB}^q |x_i - 0|^p) + \sum_{e_{ij}} w_{ij}^q |x_i - x_j|^p,
\end{aligned} \tag{6}
$$

where the first unary term measures the data cost of each node independently and the second term is the pair-wise potential through edges. By assigning various values to p and q, the general energy function can be deformed to different models, like Graph Cut, Random Walker, Power Watershed, etc. Considering shrunk surface emerged in Graph Cut and rough boundary acquired by Power Watershed, we herein choose to model label inference under the framework of Random Walker, with p and q set to 2. By combining the two graphs shown in Fig. 2, the objective function of the label inference problem can be written as,

$$
\begin{aligned}
\min_{x} \quad & \sum_{v_i} [w_{iF}^2 (x_i - 1)^2 + w_{iB}^2 x_i^2] + \sum_{e_{ij}} w_{ij}^2 (x_i - x_j)^2 + \\
& \sum_{v_{i_k}} [w_{i_k F}^2 (x_{i_k} - 1)^2 + w_{i_k B}^2 x_{i_k}^2] + \sum_{e_{ii_k}} w_{ii_k}^2 (x_i - x_{i_k})^2,
\end{aligned} \tag{7}
$$

$s.t.\quad x_F = 1,\ x_B = 0.$

The first term involves the registration prior based on signed distance and the second term is the nodal affinity through 6-connected image lattice. As for the third and forth terms, the patch prior from the warped atlas is introduced as virtual points, setting up intermediate connections between candidate nodes and seeds. According to Equation (7), label inference is a discrete Dirichlet problem and can be solved as the Laplace equation with Dirichlet conditions using Graph Analysis Toolbox [7]. With the unique solution obtained for x_i, the labels of candidate nodes can be updated, $L(v_i) = 1$ if $x_i \geq \frac{1}{2}$ and $L(v_i) = 0$ otherwise.

It is worth noting that the proposed label refinement method is not limited to single-atlas based segmentation and it can be extended to multi-atlas based segmentation with minor changes in the following two steps. Since multiple atlases can produce different label maps, majority voting is first carried out to obtain the initial segmentation result for the target image. As for the selection of virtual nodes, we will take the patch similarity values from all atlases into consideration and select K similar patches after ranking.

3 Experiments

The performance of our label inference (LI) method has been evaluated on two publicly available data sets – IBSR (www.cma.mgh.harvard.edu/ibsr) and LPBA40 (www.loni.ucla.edu/Atlases/LPBA40). IBSR consists of 18 T1-weighted MR brain images with 84 labeled structures and LPBA40 includes 40 subjects with 56 structures delineated. Given various modes existed in a large population [2], we first divided each data set into subgroups based on Affinity Propagation (AP) clustering [5] using Mutual Information and selected the central image of each cluster as the atlas. For the rest of the images in each subgroup, histogram matching with Insight Toolkit (www.itk.org) and affine transformation using FLIRT [8] were carried out as pre-processing.

In the experiments, our LI method was applied to the initial label maps provided by two benchmark methods – ANTs and IRTK, which rank high in the evaluation of 14 nonrigid registration methods [9]. During implementation, the intensity distance $(I_T(v_i) - I_T(v_j))^2$ in w_{ij} has been normalized to $[0, 1]$ and the parameter settings used in the evaluation are listed as follows, $\beta_1 = 5$, $\beta_2 = 0.5$, $\rho = 2$, $\varepsilon = 1$, $\alpha = 0.9$ and $K = 2$.

Dice Coefficient (DC) was employed to assess the labelling accuracy on subcortical structures and each structure was divided into left/right, with DC values calculated respectively. Quantitative segmentation results measured with DC on two data sets are listed in Table 1 and Table 2, with the highest value written in bold. It can be observed that with the assistance of LI, the segmentation accuracy of ANTs and IRTK can be improved considerably (1.8% and 2.9% on IBSR, 3.0% and 2.9% on LPBA40).

To provide a comprehensive evaluation, we tested the performance of our extended label inference (ELI) method in multi-atlas based segmentation. The parameter settings were remained unchanged expect for K, which was set to the number of atlases. To fuse the label maps generated by multiple atlases,

Table 1. Label Inference on IBSR data set

Methods	Thalamus	Caudate	Putamen	Pallidum	Hippocampus	Amygdala	Average
ANTs	0.870-0.868	0.822-0.794	0.851-0.856	0.780-0.790	0.741-0.756	0.677-0.660	0.789±0.028
ANTs+LI	0.884-0.883	0.851-0.824	0.864-0.878	0.789-0.805	0.769-0.779	0.684-0.672	0.807±0.026
IRTK	0.855-0.840	0.792-0.759	0.786-0.763	0.684-0.666	0.687-0.678	0.609-0.573	0.724±0.106
IRTK+LI	0.873-0.863	0.825-0.780	0.811-0.793	0.717-0.696	0.722-0.715	0.638-0.599	0.753±0.097

Table 2. Label Inference on LPBA40 data set

Methods	Putamen	Caudate	Hippocampus	Average
ANTs	0.794-0.803	0.756-0.751	0.779-0.782	0.777±0.040
ANTs+LI	0.824-0.832	0.790-0.785	0.805-0.807	0.807±0.040
IRTK	0.777-0.778	0.766-0.763	0.773-0.761	0.770±0.042
IRTK+LI	0.811-0.810	0.794-0.790	0.799-0.788	0.799±0.044

Table 3. Extended Label Inference on IBSR data set

Methods	Thalamus	Caudate	Putamen	Pallidum	Hippocampus	Amygdala	Average
ANTs+MV	0.894-0.896	0.839-0.826	0.884-0.888	0.825-0.826	0.794-0.807	0.742-0.719	0.828±0.023
ANTs+WV	0.894-0.899	0.850-0.837	0.887-0.889	0.819-0.821	0.793-0.805	0.737-0.709	0.828±0.016
ANTs+ELI	0.906-0.910	0.870-0.859	0.893-0.901	0.831-0.839	0.814-0.825	0.757-0.738	0.845±0.017
IRTK+MV	0.873-0.868	0.820-0.802	0.847-0.831	0.767-0.752	0.753-0.750	0.702-0.662	0.786±0.053
IRTK+WV	0.874-0.870	0.820-0.805	0.854-0.839	0.768-0.756	0.756-0.758	0.699-0.663	0.788±0.044
IRTK+ELI	0.892-0.887	0.857-0.840	0.873-0.863	0.794-0.781	0.789-0.787	0.730-0.694	0.816±0.039

Table 4. Extended Label Inference on LPBA40 data set

Methods	Putamen	Caudate	Hippocampus	Average
ANTs+MV	0.862-0.858	0.828-0.821	0.841-0.835	0.841±0.028
ANTs+WV	0.861-0.857	0.834-0.828	0.840-0.836	0.843±0.029
ANTs+ELI	0.867-0.863	0.845-0.841	0.847-0.842	0.851±0.025
IRTK+MV	0.845-0.838	0.832-0.825	0.827-0.814	0.830±0.035
IRTK+WV	0.844-0.837	0.833-0.828	0.830-0.817	0.832±0.035
IRTK+ELI	0.859-0.852	0.845-0.841	0.840-0.828	0.844±0.030

we utilized classic majority voting (MV), with the results of intensity weighted voting (WV) provided for reference. As shown in Table 3 and Table 4, our ELI method can obtain better DC values consistently. All experiments were run on a 3.30 GHz, Dual-Core CPU with 20 GB RAM. Given the average computation time consumed by pair-wise deformation, 32 minutes for ANTs and 22 minutes for IRTK, it only takes around 9 seconds to finish the label inference procedure, which demonstrates that the proposed method can improve the segmentation quality efficiently.

4   Conclusion

In atlas-based image segmentation, the quality of labels around structural boundaries is usually poor. To deal with this problem, in this paper, we propose a novel
method to refine these labels. By employing signed distance function to evaluate
the initial label map, we can pick up the nodes whose labels need to be refined
and select nodes with confident results as seeds. Registration prior based on
signed distance and patch prior generated from the warped atlas are encoded in
the label inference procedure, together with the nodal affinity through lattice in
the target image. Experimental results on two public data sets indicate that the
proposed method can improve the labelling quality effectively and efficiently.

References

1. Artaechevarria, X., Munoz-Barrutia, A., Ortiz-de Solorzano, C.: Combination
   strategies in multi-atlas image segmentation: Application to brain mr data. IEEE
   TMI 28(8), 1266–1277 (2009)
2. Blezek, D.J., Miller, J.V.: Atlas stratification. MedIA 11(5), 443–457 (2007)
3. Coupé, P., Manjón, J.V., Fonov, V., Pruessner, J., Robles, M., Collins, D.L.: Patch-
   based segmentation using expert priors: Application to hippocampus and ventricle
   segmentation. NeuroImage 54(2), 940–954 (2011)
4. Coupé, P., Yger, P., Prima, S., et al.: An optimized blockwise nonlocal means denoising filter for 3-d magnetic resonance images. IEEE TMI 27(4), 425–441 (2008)
5. Frey, B.J., Dueck, D.: Clustering by passing messages between data points. Science 315(5814), 972–976 (2007)
6. Glocker, B., Komodakis, N., Tziritas, G., Navab, N., et al.: Dense image registration
   through mrfs and efficient linear programming. MedIA 12(6), 731–741 (2008)
7. Grady, L., Schwartz, E.: The graph analysis toolbox: Image processing on arbitrary
   graphs. CAS/CNS Technical Report Series (021) (2003)
8. Jenkinson, M., Bannister, P., Brady, M., Smith, S.: Improved optimization for
   the robust and accurate linear registration and motion correction of brain images.
   NeuroImage 17(2), 825–841 (2002)
9. Klein, A., Andersson, J., et al.: Evaluation of 14 nonlinear deformation algorithms
   applied to human brain mri registration. NeuroImage 46(3), 786–802 (2009)
10. Lézoray, O., Grady, L.: Image Processing and Analysis with Graphs: Theory and
    Practice. CRC Press (2012)
11. Rousseau, F., Habas, P.A., Studholme, C.: A supervised patch-based approach for
    human brain labeling. IEEE TMI 30(10), 1852–1862 (2011)
12. Sethian, J.A.: Level set methods and fast marching methods. CUP (1999)
13. Shattuck, D.W., Mirza, M., Adisetiyo, V., et al.: Construction of a 3d probabilistic
    atlas of human cortical structures. NeuroImage 39(3), 1064–1080 (2008)
14. Sotiras, A., Komodakis, N., Glocker, B., Deux, J.-F., Paragios, N.: Graphical mod-
    els and deformable diffeomorphic population registration using global and local
    metrics. In: Yang, G.-Z., Hawkes, D., Rueckert, D., Noble, A., Taylor, C. (eds.)
    MICCAI 2009, Part I. LNCS, vol. 5761, pp. 672–679. Springer, Heidelberg (2009)
15. Wachinger, C., Sharp, G.C., Golland, P.: Contour-driven regression for label infer-
    ence in atlas-based segmentation. In: Mori, K., Sakuma, I., Sato, Y., Barillot, C.,
    Navab, N. (eds.) MICCAI 2013, Part III. LNCS, vol. 8151, pp. 211–218. Springer,
    Heidelberg (2013)

Automated 3D Segmentation of Multiple Surfaces with a Shared Hole: Segmentation of the Neural Canal Opening in SD-OCT Volumes

Bhavna J. Antony[1], Mohammed S. Miri[1], Michael D. Abràmoff[2,3,1],
Young H. Kwon[2], and Mona K. Garvin[3,1]

[1] Electrical & Computer Engineering, The University of Iowa, Iowa City, IA USA
[2] Ophthalmology & Visual Sciences, The University of Iowa, Iowa City, IA USA
[3] Iowa City VA Healthcare System, Iowa City, IA USA
mona-garvin@uiowa.edu

Abstract. The need to segment multiple interacting surfaces is a common problem in medical imaging and it is often assumed that such surfaces are continuous within the confines of the region of interest. However, in some application areas, the surfaces of interest may contain a shared hole in which the surfaces no longer exist and the exact location of the hole boundary is not known *a priori*. The boundary of the neural canal opening seen in spectral-domain optical coherence tomography volumes is an example of a "hole" embedded with multiple surrounding surfaces. Segmentation approaches that rely on finding the surfaces alone are prone to failures as deeper structures within the hole can "attract" the surfaces and pull them away from their correct location at the hole boundary. With this application area in mind, we present a graph-theoretic approach for segmenting multiple surfaces with a shared hole. The overall cost function that is optimized consists of both the costs of the surfaces outside the hole and the cost of boundary of the hole itself. The constraints utilized were appropriately adapted in order to ensure the smoothness of the hole boundary in addition to ensuring the smoothness of the non-overlapping surfaces. By using this approach, a significant improvement was observed over a more traditional two-pass approach in which the surfaces are segmented first (assuming the presence of no hole) followed by segmenting the neural canal opening.

1 Introduction

Many medical imaging applications exist for which it is desirable to segment multiple interacting three-dimensional surfaces. Example approaches for enabling the optimal segmentation of multiple surfaces include a graph-theoretic approach [1], which transforms the multiple surface segmentation problem into that of obtaining a minimum-closure in a constructed graph, and the graph-cut approach [2] which transforms a multi-object labeling problem (with geometric constraints) directly into that of obtaining a minimum-cost *s-t* cut in a constructed graph. However, in some applications, a set of interacting surfaces have

P. Golland et al. (Eds.): MICCAI 2014, Part I, LNCS 8673, pp. 739–746, 2014.
© Springer International Publishing Switzerland 2014

a shared "hole" in which the surfaces do not exist. An example of such an application is that of segmenting the neural canal opening (NCO, the boundary of a "hole") and the surrounding surfaces within spectral-domain optical coherence tomography (SD-OCT) volumes (Figs. 1(a)-(c)). The NCO is an important structure relevant to glaucoma [3,4] as it can provide a stable reference by which to monitor structural changes of the optic nerve head [3].

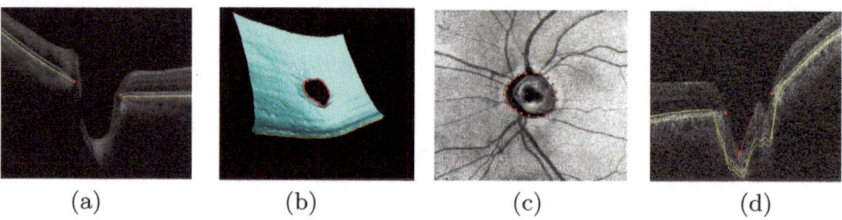

    (a)   (b)   (c)   (d)

Fig. 1. The surfaces and the NCO depicted on (a) a central xz-slice from a human OCT image and (b) a 3D rendering of the segmented surfaces. (c) The xy-location of the NCO depicted on a projection image. (d) An example where the segmented surfaces are "pulled" away from the NCO by deeper structures (indicated by the arrow).

Previously, a Markov model based approach [5] was proposed for the segmentation of the optic disc and cup margins in time-domain OCT images. More recently, a two-step graph-theoretic approach [4] was proposed for the same in SD-OCT images. The method began by segmenting the surrounding surfaces while ignoring the fact that the surfaces do no exist inside the NCO, and subsequently segmenting the projected location of the NCO (i.e., projected boundary of the hole) in a projection image. The fact that the initial multiple-surface segmentation ignored the existence of the hole makes the segmentation more prone to errors in this region due to a deeper structure (indicated by the red arrow in Fig. 1(d)) inside of the NCO "pulling" the surfaces away from their actual locations near the boundary of the hole. Furthermore, they were only able to quantitatively evaluate their algorithm in the x-y plane using projected manual tracings of the optic disc, and thus, it is difficult to assess the accuracy of the neural canal opening points in the z-direction (i.e., depth direction).

    In this work, we present an approach for simultaneously segmenting multiple surfaces with a hole and apply the approach for the segmentation of the NCO in 3D and the surrounding surfaces from the SD-OCT volumes of glaucoma patients. This contrasts with prior 3D work which has focused on using a single two-step approach. In particular, the general framework of our approach reflects an extension of the graph-theoretic approach [1] proposed for simultaneous segmentation of multiple surfaces (without a hole). The overall cost function was extended to incorporate the hole boundary and new boundary constraints were included to ensure the feasibility of the set of surfaces. The proposed method was also compared to the previously proposed [4] two-step approach, where it showed a significant improvement ($p < 0.001$) in the accuracy of the segmentation of the NCO boundary location. We also demonstrated the ability to measure important parameters such as the minimum rim width (MRW) using these segmentations, where the measurements obtained did not significantly differ from those obtained using the manual delineations.

2   Method

Formulation of the Surfaces with a Shared Hole Problem. Assume we have a volume of dimensions $X \times Y \times Z$ and wish to find n layered surfaces with a shared hole as illustrated in Fig. 1. The presence of the hole, divides the volume into three regions (see Fig. 2) namely the outside $\mathcal{O}$, the boundary $\mathcal{B}$ and the inside of the hole $\mathcal{H}$. Intuitively, we will consider a surface set with a shared hole feasible if 1) individual surface smoothness constraints are satisfied outside the hole, 2) the surfaces obey minimum and maximum surface distance constraints outside the hole, 3) the surfaces come together at the hole boundary, and 4) the hole boundary satisfies its own set of smoothness constraints.

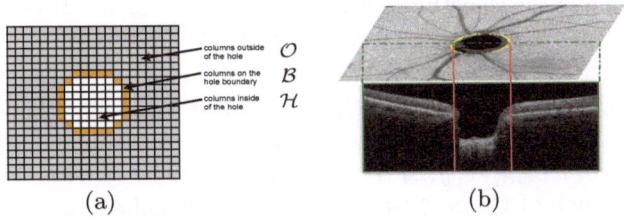

(a)   (b)

Fig. 2. (a) The 2D overview of the division of columns into the three sets: the hole boundary, the hole itself and the region outside the hole. (b) An example of the 2D segmentation of the NCO boundary that is used to define set $\mathcal{B}$.

Each of the n surfaces $\{f_1(x,y), \ldots, f_n(x,y)\}$ are defined over the columns in $\mathcal{O} \cup \mathcal{B}$, where the smoothness constraint for each surface i is defined by:

$$|f_i(x+1,y) - f_i(x,y)| \leq \Delta_{x_i} \quad \text{and} \quad |f_i(x,y+1) - f_i(x,y)| \leq \Delta_{y_i}, \quad (1)$$

where Δ_{x_i} (Δ_{y_i}) is the x-smoothness (y-smoothness) parameter for surface i (see Figs. 3(a) and (b)). For each of the columns in $\mathcal{O}$, each i–$(i+1)$ pair of surfaces (where surface $i+1$ is directly "above" surface i) is also constrained by the surface distance constraints, where $\delta_{i,i+1}^l \leq f_{i+1}(x,y) - f_i(x,y) \leq \delta_{i,i+1}^u$, where $\delta_{i,i+1}^l$ and $\delta_{i,i+1}^u$ are the minimum and maximum allowed distance between the surfaces, respectively. Note that these two feasibility constraints are defined similarly as in the standard multiple surface segmentation problem (without a hole) [1].

We also require that the x-y projection of the hole boundary be representable using a function defined in polar coordinates $f_b(\theta)$ (i.e., having one intersection per sampled angular ray) and that this projected boundary be sufficiently smooth: $|f_b(\theta) - f_b(\theta + \Delta_\theta)| \leq \Delta_r$ where Δ_θ is the angular distance between sampled rays and Δ_r is the smoothness parameter specifying the maximum change in radial position between angular rays. Furthermore, for columns in $\mathcal{B}$, we require that the minimum and maximum distance between all surfaces be equal to 0 (i.e., the surfaces come together at any column on the shared hole boundary), as depicted in Figs. 3(c) and (d).

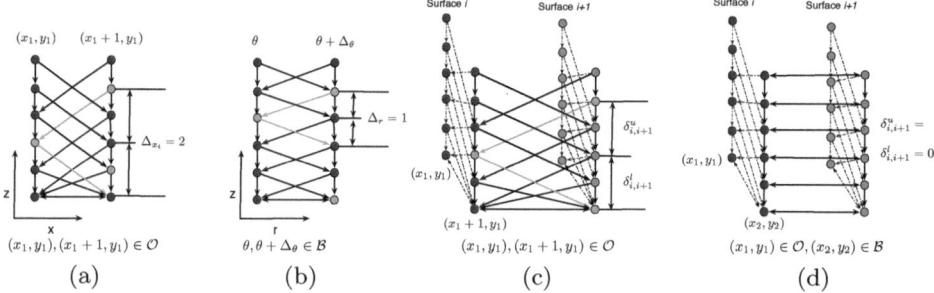

Fig. 3. Illustration of the smoothness constraints within regions (a) $\mathcal{O}$ and (b) $\mathcal{B}$, and the surface-interaction constraints within regions (c) $\mathcal{O}$ and (d) $\mathcal{B}$

Cost of a feasible surface set with a shared hole. For the segmentation of the surfaces and the shared hole, every voxel in the volume will be assigned $n+1$ costs: one cost, $c_{\mathrm{surf}_i}(x, y, z)$ $(i = 1, \ldots, n)$, associated with the unlikeliness of belonging to each of the n surfaces and one cost, $c_b(x, y, z)$, associated with belonging to the boundary of the shared hole. Then, the cost of a feasible surface set with a shared hole (given $\mathcal{O}$, $\mathcal{B}$) is defined as follows:

$$C_T = \sum_{i=1}^{n} \sum_{(x,y) \in \mathcal{O}} c_{\mathrm{surf}_i}(x, y, f_i(x, y)) + \lambda \sum_{(x,y) \in \mathcal{B}} c_b(x, y, f_1(x, y)), \qquad (2)$$

where the first term is associated with the "on-surface" costs in region $\mathcal{O}$ and the second term is associated with the cost of the shared hole boundary points.

Segmentation of Multiple Surfaces with a Shared Hole. The iterative approach proposed for the segmentation of surfaces and the NCO is illustrated in Fig. 4. As an initialization step, the original formulation of the graph-theoretic approach [1,6] (where the existence of the hole is ignored) is used to segment the junction of the inner and outer segments (IS/OS line) (marked in blue in Fig. 1(a)) of the photoreceptors and the Bruch's membrane (BM) (marked in yellow in Fig. 1(a)) in the volumetric image. Next, the following two steps (labeled Iteration A and Iteration B) are repeated until achieving convergence of the segmented boundary column-set $\mathcal{B}$. In the first step (Iteration A), we create a projection image and update our estimate of the projected boundary columns $\mathcal{B}$ of the NCO by finding a minimum-closure in a graph. In the second step (Iteration B), given this estimate of $\mathcal{B}$, we find the corresponding optimal (see

Eq. 2) set of feasible surfaces that meet at the hole boundary in the volumetric image by solving another single minimum-closure problem in a constructed graph. Further details of each step are provided below.

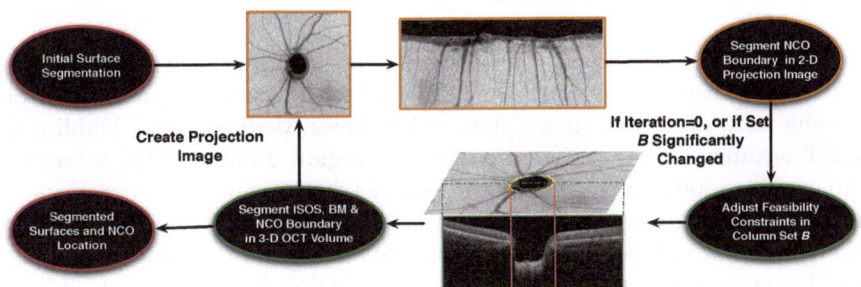

Fig. 4. Schematic showing the segmentation process

Iteration A: Segmentation of projected hole boundary columns. The projection image was created by averaging 20 pixels above and below the BM surface. This projection image was then polar transformed and the NCO was segmented using a graph-theoretic approach that incorporated shape priors [7].

Iteration B: Simultaneous segmentation of the surfaces and the NCO shared hole. Before computing the cost functions for the regions $\mathcal{B}$, $\mathcal{O}$ and $\mathcal{H}$, the volumetric image was also polar-transformed with an angular spacing of $1°$. In the volumetric images, the NCO can be difficult to identify at the upper and lower regions of the NCO where the end points get closer together and the large blood vessels that characterize these regions of the retina also cast large vessels shadows. However, in the polar-transformed scans, the NCO's continuity is maintained, making it easier to visualize and delineate.

The cost function for the regions $\mathcal{O}$ and $\mathcal{H}$ consisted of on-surface cost terms derived from Gaussian-derivative filters, while the cost function for $\mathcal{B}$ incorporated textural features learned from a training set. As the NCO boundary can be modeled as a "corner", the textural features used to learn the properties of the NCO boundary points included corner detectors such as Harris and SUSAN [8] as well as first order steerable Gaussian derivatives at scales $\sigma = \{1, 2, 3, 4, 5\}$ and orientations $\theta = \{0°, \pm30°, \pm60°, \pm90°\}$, computed in 2D and 3D.

The training set (described further in Section 3) utilized here consisted of 25 radial volumes that each contained 180 slices, where the NCO was identified in all of the slices. The background samples were limited to a random selection of five samples near the NCO per slice. A random forest, an ensemble classifier [9], was then trained to identify the NCO boundary points in the volumetric image. The individual feature significances were used to select a smaller set of features, where the final set of 20 features only contained those that contributed at least 2% to the overall feature significance.

Finally, two surfaces, the IS/OS line and Bruch's membrane, and their shared hole were segmented simultaneously in the polar coordinate space using the above defined feasibility constraints and cost functions. The value of λ was set to 8 to emphasize the hole boundary cost.

3   Experimental Methods

The data used in this experiment consisted of 44 optic nerve head SD-OCT scans obtained from 44 patients that presented with varying stages of glaucoma. The scans were obtained on a Cirrus (Carl Zeiss Meditec, Inc., Dublin, CA) SD-OCT scanner and were acquired from a region 2mm x 2mm x 6mm and contained 200 x 200 x 1024 voxels. The volumetric scans were converted into the polar coordinate space where the slices were 1° apart. Manual delineations were obtained from an independent expert (trained to detect the NCO boundary in SD-OCT images) on 10 randomly selected radial slices from each of the 44 scans. These tracings were then verified by a second independent expert, with a third and final verification being performed by a glaucoma specialist to give us our consensus manual tracings. The 25 independent datasets used to train the NCO classifier were also obtained from human patients on a Cirrus SD-OCT scanner, using the same imaging protocol described above.

The segmentation accuracy obtained using the proposed method (Approach III) was statistically compared (using a paired t-test) to results obtained when using a two-step approach, where the projected location of the NCO was computed using 1) a pixel classification approach (Approach I) [6] and, 2) a graph-theoretic approach (Approach II) [4]. These two boundary column-set estimates were then projected down onto the initial segmentation of the Bruch's membrane to give us the 3D location of the NCO.

The metrics used to gauge the accuracy of the segmentation consisted of the unsigned difference between 1) the 2D segmentation in the projection image and the manual delineations, 2) the z locations of the automated segmentation and the manual delineations, and 3) the 3D Euclidean distance between the automated segmentation and the manual delineations.

Additionally, the minimum rim width (MRW) [10], a metric associated with the progression of glaucoma and defined as the minimum distance from the NCO to the internal limiting membrane (ILM), was also computed using the proposed method and statistically compared to values obtained using the manual tracings.

4   Results

Table 1 shows the complete summary of the accuracy assessment conducted using the three metrics described above. The 3D Euclidean distance (in microns) between the manual delineations and the segmented NCO for Approaches I, II and III were found to be 139.67 ± 61.68 μm, 136.77 ± 38.24 μm and 55.29 ± 33.97 μm, respectively. The errors noted in Approaches I and II for all 3 metrics were found to be significantly larger ($p < 0.001$) than those obtained using the proposed method.

Table 1. Summary of accuracy assessment of the NCO segmentation. The errors are expressed in microns (and voxels).

	2D	z	3D
Pixel Classification (Approach I)	128.36 ± 61.23 (4.28 ± 2.04)	46.85 ± 30.21 (23.99 ± 15.47)	139.67 ± 61.68
Two-step Graph Method (Approach II)	62.28 ± 26.74 (2.08 ± 0.89)	117.21 ± 43.14 (60.01 ± 22.09)	136.77 ± 38.24
Proposed Iterative Method (Approach III)	46.05 ± 28.40 (1.54 ± 0.95)	29.58 ± 20.24 (15.15 ± 10.36)	55.29 ± 33.97

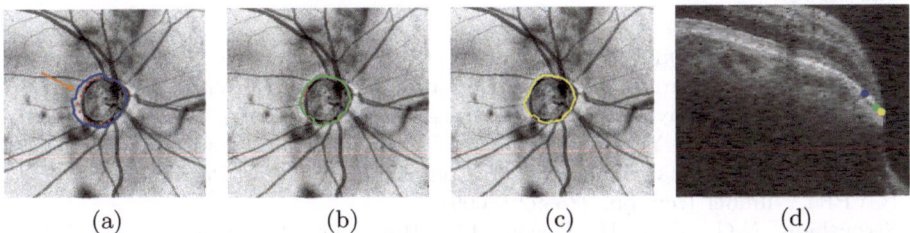

(a)   (b)   (c)   (d)

Fig. 5. An example of the segmentation result obtained after the (a) first (blue), (b) second (green) and (c) third (yellow) iteration. The manual tracings are marked in red. (d) The 3D location of the segmented NCO and the manual tracings for the location indicated on (a).

Fig. 5 show the iterative results obtained on a dataset. As shown, the error in the location of the NCO substantially reduces from iteration to iteration, until the final result coincides with the manually delineated point. The mean MRW computed using the manually delineated points was found to be 179 ± 81.46 μm. The MRW computed using Approaches I, II and III were 247.23 ± 74.95 μm, 241.50 ± 103.94 μm and 184.09 ± 84.06 μm, respectively. The MRW measurements obtained using Approaches I and II were found to significantly ($p < 0.0001$) differ from those obtained using the manual tracings, while the MRW measurements obtained using Approach III was not significantly different ($p > 0.05$) from those obtained using the manual tracings.

5   Conclusion and Discussion

We have presented an iterative graph-based method for the automated simultaneous segmentation of surfaces with a shared hole. A graph-theoretic approach [1] was reformulated to meet the new requirements of surfaces that meet at a shared hole boundary, thereby allowing for the boundary of the hole to be detected in 3D. The proposed method was applied to the segmentation of the NCO in SD-OCT images obtained from patients that presented with varying stages of glaucoma, where it showed good accuracy in the 2D plane as well as in 3D, as well as a significant improvement over existing approaches.

Furthermore, this method allows for the computation of the minimum rim width in 3D. This provides an objective measure that could be used to augment the subjective planimetry assessments that are currently used to assess the progression of the disease.

Acknowledgements. This work was supported, in part, by the Department of Veterans Affairs (CDA-2 IK2RX000728) and the National Institutes of Health (R01 EY018853 and R01 EY023279).

References

1. Garvin, M.K., Abràmoff, M.D., Wu, X., Russell, S.R., Burns, T.L., Sonka, M.: Automated 3-D intraretinal layer segmentation of macular spectral-domain optical coherence tomography images. IEEE Trans. Med. Imag. 28(9), 1436–1447 (2009)
2. Delong, A., Boykov, Y.: Globally optimal Segmentation of multi-region objects. In: IEEE International Conference on Computer Vision and Pattern Recognition (CVPR), Number Iccv, pp. 285–92 (2009)
3. Strouthidis, N.G., Yang, H., Downs, J.C., Burgoyne, C.F.: Comparison of clinical and three-dimensional histomorphometric optic disc margin anatomy.. Invest. Ophthalmol. Vis. Sci. 50(5), 2165–2174 (2009)
4. Hu, Z., Abràmoff, M.D., Kwon, Y.H., Lee, K., Garvin, M.K.: Automated Segmentation of Neural Canal Opening and Optic Cup in 3D Spectral Optical Coherence Tomography Volumes of the Optic Nerve Head. Invest. Ophthalmol. Vis. Sci. 51(11), 5708–5717 (2010)
5. Boyer, K.L., Herzog, A., Roberts, C.: Automatic recovery of the optic nervehead geometry in optical coherence tomography. IEEE Trans. Med. Imag. 25(5), 553–570 (2006)
6. Lee, K., Niemeijer, M., Garvin, M.K., Kwon, Y.H., Sonka, M., Abràmoff, M.D.: Segmentation of the optic disc in 3D-OCT scans of the optic nerve head. IEEE Trans. Image Process. 29(1), 159–168 (2009)
7. Song, Q., Bai, J., Garvin, M.K., Sonka, M., Buatti, J.M., Wu, X.: Optimal multiple surface segmentation with shape and context priors. IEEE Trans. Med. Imag. 32(2), 376–386 (2013)
8. Smith, S.M., Brady, J.M.: SUSAN - A New Approach to Low Level Image Processing. International Journal of Computer Vision 23, 45–78 (1995)
9. Breiman, L.: Random forests. Machine Learning 45(1), 5–32 (2001)
10. Reis, A.S.C., Sharpe, G.P., Yang, H., Nicolela, M.T., Burgoyne, C.F., Chauhan, B.C.: Optic disc margin anatomy in patients with glaucoma and normal controls with spectral domain optical coherence tomography. Ophthalmology 119(4), 738–747 (2012)

Coupled Sparse Dictionary for Depth-Based Cup Segmentation from Single Color Fundus Image*

Arunava Chakravarty and Jayanthi Sivaswamy

Center for Visual Information Technology,
International Institute of Information Technology Hyderabad, India

Abstract. We present a novel framework for *depth* based optic cup boundary extraction from a *single* 2D color fundus photograph per eye. Multiple depth estimates from shading, color and texture gradients in the image are correlated with Optical Coherence Tomography (OCT) based depth using a coupled sparse dictionary, trained on image-depth pairs. Finally, a Markov Random Field is formulated on the depth map to model the relative depth and discontinuity at the cup boundary. Leave-one-out validation of depth estimation on the *INSPIRE* dataset gave average correlation coefficient of 0.80. Our cup segmentation outperforms several state-of-the-art methods on the *DRISHTI-GS* dataset with an average F-score of 0.81 and boundary-error of 21.21 pixels on test set against manual expert markings. Evaluation on an additional set of 28 images against OCT scanner provided groundtruth showed an average rms error of 0.11 on Cup-Disk diameter and 0.19 on Cup-disk area ratios.

1 Introduction

Glaucoma, a sight-threatening disease, is characterized by the deformations in the optic disk (OD) in retina. The OD is a bright elliptic region with a central depression (called the optic cup) devoid of retinal nerve fibers surrounded by a neuro-retinal rim, where the nerve fibers bend into the cup region (Fig 1(a)). Glaucoma destroys optic nerve fibers causing neuro-retinal rim thinning and cup enlargement which is widely measured quantitatively via the vertical Cup-Disk diameter ratio (CDR). Deriving CDR from fundus images requires accurate OD and the cup boundaries and hence their segmentation has received much attention. Majority of the existing methods perform OD segmentation in 2 stages: OD localization using intensity and shape based template matching such as Hough transform [1][2], followed by boundary extraction using ellipse fitting [3] or specially adapted deformable models [1],[2].Though most methods report good performance in OD segmentation, cup segmentation remains a challenging problem. The optic cup boundary (OCB) is largely characterized by change in depth of the retinal surface in the OD region and hence methods for cup segmentation rely on (i) explicit measurement of depth or (ii) appearance features

---

* This work is partly funded by the Department of Science and Technology, Govt. of India, under Grant DST/INT/NL/Biomed/P(3)/2011(G).

P. Golland et al. (Eds.): MICCAI 2014, Part I, LNCS 8673, pp. 747–754, 2014.
© Springer International Publishing Switzerland 2014

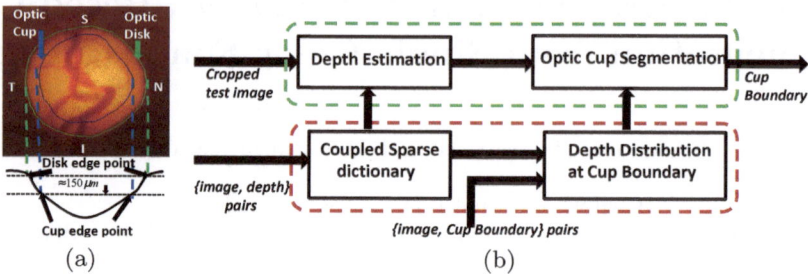

(a)   (b)

Fig. 1. (a) Sample OD sub-image with a sketch of corresponding depth. (b) System for cup segmentation. Top green box - online system; bottom red box - offline system.

which provide depth cues. In (i), depth information is obtained either from 3D imaging modalities such as OCT [4] or derived using stereo image pairs [5] [1]. Though better suited for accurate OCB extraction, the availability, portability and cost of these imaging devices inhibits their use in a glaucoma screening. In (ii) high level depth cues are extracted from single color fundus images based on pallor intensity and vessel bends [2] in addition to superpixels [3] and graph cut [6] based approaches. In absence of depth information, these features are susceptible to shape, color variabilities and indistinct OCB. Further, sparse distribution of vessels in the nasal, temporal sides and occurrence of vessel bends at non-OCB locations makes its detection challenging.

To deal with above mentioned challenges, we propose a *depth* based OCB extraction framework from *single* color fundus image per eye in which multiple depth estimates from shading, color and texture gradients are extracted from the image and correlated with OCT based depth values using a coupled sparse dictionary pre-trained on a set of image-depth pairs. Finally, OCB is extracted using a novel contour point detection based MRF formulation defined on the depth map to model the relative depth and discontinuity at OCB while reducing computation by lowering the number of sites to be labeled. We leverage the fact that in a clinical setting, OCT and fundus imaging are possible while for screening, only fundus imaging may be possible in the field. While supervised methods for estimating depth from single images have been recently used in computer vision [7] [8], such strategy remains unexplored in the medical domain.

2   Methodology

A square region around the OD center is automatically extracted using a Hough transform based OD localization [2]. The region is aligned based on symmetry in vessel density (in the nasal-temporal and superior-inferior regions) and resized to a standard size of 393×393 pixels. The proposed method shown in Fig. 1(b) comprises of 2 stages: depth map estimation from single image per eye (sec. 2.1) and OCB extraction from the estimated depth map (sec. 2.2).

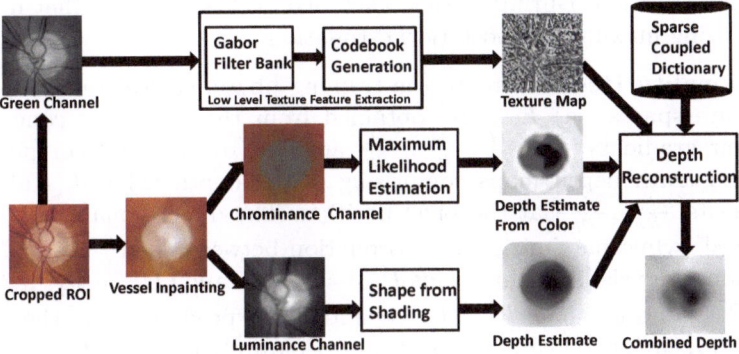

Fig. 2. Block diagram of the proposed supervised depth estimation

2.1 Depth Estimation

As noted in [1], different clinical studies have defined OCB as 50 microns below the retinal surface, $\frac{1}{2}$ or $\frac{1}{3}$ drop in depth from the OD edge to the deepest point. This indicates that *relative depth estimates rather than absolute depth values define the OCB*. Hence, we obtain depth maps defined up to an arbitrary scale factor rather than absolute depth values.

The proposed depth estimation (Fig. 2) comprises of extraction of chrominance (C), luminance (L) and texture word map (T) features, followed by individual depth map estimates d_c and d_l from C and L respectively. d_l and d_c suffer from inaccuracies due to the lack of 1-1 correspondence between C and d, simplified assumptions in shape from shading (SFS)and treating each pixel independent of its neighborhood. To obtain a more accurate and robust depth map, 8×8 image patches are extracted and represented in a feature space P_{cca} and correlated to OCT based depth estimates Q_{cca} using coupled sparse dictionaries U and V to obtain the final depth map. Details are provided below.

Feature Extraction: (a) T : 30 energy responses of a Gabor filter bank (6 orientations, 5 scales) [9] along with their 1st and 2nd order derivatives along two directions ($30 \times (2 + 2) = 120$) are combined to obtain a 150-D feature vector for each pixel which is clustered (during training) into 60 words. Each pixel is represented by the nearest word index [10] to obtain T. For remaining features, diffusion based inpainting is first applied to suppress vessels.(b) C : At each pixel, the color values r,g,b are normalized as $j/(r+g+b)$; j is r,g,b respectively to obtain 3-D feature C. (c) L: The luminance information is obtained by suppressing high color gradients in intensity channel using [11].

Individual Depth Estimates: d_l is obtained from L by complementing the output from a simple but fast SFS algorithm [12]. d_c is obtained from C using a supervised approach;for each depth value $d \in [0, 255]$, $P(C \mid d)$ is learnt from a training set of image-depth pairs, using a 3-D Gaussian Mixture Model with number of Gaussians selected in the range 1-6 that maximizes the Akaike information criterion. During testing, each pixel is assigned a d that maximizes $P(d \mid C)$ using maximum a posteriori estimation.

Dimensionality Reduction: In the training phase, each pixel is represented in 2 feature spaces: (a) $F \in R^7$ obtained from the image by concatenating d_l, d_c, their gradients $\frac{\partial d_l}{\partial x}, \frac{\partial d_l}{\partial y}, \frac{\partial d_c}{\partial x}, \frac{\partial d_c}{\partial y}$ and T, (b) $G \in R^3$ computed from the ground truth depth maps comprising of the depth value d_{oct} along with it's gradients $\frac{\partial d_{oct}}{\partial x}, \frac{\partial d_{oct}}{\partial y}$ at the pixel position. The dimensionality of F and G are reduced (while maximizing the correlation between them) using Canonical Correlation Analysis [13]. This yields $P_{cca} = \phi_{img}^T.F$ and $Q_{cca} = \phi_{depth}^T.G$, where $\phi_{img} \in R^{7 \times 3}$ and $\phi_{depth} \in R^{3 \times 3}$ (x^T denotes transpose of x) are the canonical factors. Now, each pixel can be represented separately in $P_{cca}, Q_{cca} \in R^3$ spaces extracted from image and depth map respectively. Only P_{cca} is computed using pre-trained ϕ_{img} during testing.

Coupled Sparse Dictionary Training: From each image-depth pair in training dataset, 8×8 overlapping patches(1 pixel apart) are extracted and represented in 2 feature spaces: $P, Q \in R^{192}$ obtained by concatenating the 3-D features of each of the 64 pixels of the patch in P_{cca} and Q_{cca} space respectively. The objective is to learn two, overcomplete (each consisting of 1100 basis vectors), coupled sparse dictionaries U and V in the P and Q feature space, such that the same sparse code α is shared in the two representations: $P = U.\alpha$ and $Q = V.\alpha$ for all the training patches. This is done by concatenating the corresponding vectors [14][8] for each training patch, $Z = \{z_i = (p_i^T, q_i^T)^T\}$, $p_i \in P$ and $q_i \in Q$. An online dictionary learning algorithm[1] [15] was used for learning the sparse dictionary $W \in R^{384 \times 1100}$ from the feature set Z using batch size of 600, sparsity coefficient $\lambda = 0.6$ and max-iteration$= 800$. The learnt basis vectors W was split into U and V by taking the first and last 192 rows of W.

Coupled Sparse Dictionary Testing. Once U and V are learnt, given a new test image, its representation P_{test} can be extracted from the image and sparse code α^* can be estimated by solving the LASSO problem. The desired Q_{est} is then obtained by projecting α onto the depth basis V [16].

$$\alpha^* = argmin_\alpha ||U.\alpha - P_{test}||_2^2 \quad s.t. \quad ||\alpha||_1 \leq \lambda \qquad (1)$$

$$Q_{est} = V.\alpha^* \qquad (2)$$

After reconstructing the 3-channel D' from Q_{est}, we backproject it to obtain $D_{est} = (\phi_{depth})^{-1}.D'$, D_{est} consisting of the depth value d and its gradients $\frac{\partial d}{\partial x}$ and $\frac{\partial d}{\partial y}$ at each pixel. The refined depth value is taken as the average of d and the depth estimated from $\frac{\partial d}{\partial x}$ and $\frac{\partial d}{\partial y}$ using inverse gradient methods [11].

2.2   Optic Cup Boundary Extraction

The depth map computed by stage 1 is used to extract its boundary as described next. Consider a circular ROI centered at $r_0 = (x_0, y_0)$ with radius R. We denote

---

[1] Implemented using SPAMS available at `http://spams-devel.gforge.inria.fr/`

the depth profile along a ray in direction θ_j from r_0 by $d_j(r)$, where $r \in [0, R]$. Let the closed curve B be the desired boundary, centred at r_0, required to be detected from the depth map. B is uniformly sampled to obtain an ordered set of boundary points $b_j; j = 0, ..J$. Note that this sampling is aligned to the orientation θ_j about r_0. We take a probabilistic approach to finding B by determining the likelihood that a point in $d_j(r)$, belongs to B. Let $B = \{b_j | 0 \leq j \leq (J)\}$, be a random field where each b_j is associated with $d_j(r)$, such that $P(b_j = r)$ represents the probability that $b_j = r$ is a boundary point on $d_j(r)$. The set of labels associated with b_j is $L = 0, 1...R$. Assuming a pairwise Markovian property that each b_i is only affected by its immediate adjacent neighbors, we define the Neighbour set $N = \{(b_j, b_{j+1}) | 0 \leq j \leq (J-1)\} \bigcup \{(b_J, b_0)\}$. We define a Markov Random Field based energy function $E(X)$ which is minimized to get the optimal labelling.

$$E(B) = \sum_{b_j \in B} D_{b_j}(b_j) + \lambda \sum_{(b_j, b_l) \in N} V_{b_j b_l}(b_j, b_l) \qquad (3)$$

The data term $D_{b_j}(b_j)$ defines how well the labelling of b_j fits the probability distribution learnt from the boundary points on profile $d_j(r)$ from a set of training images. Both d and r values are normalized to $[0, 1]$ along each direction separately. We define $D_{b_j}(b_j)$ as

$$D_{b_j}(b_j = k) = 1 - P(k|b_j) \qquad (4)$$

$P(k|b_j)$ represents the probability of assigning label k to the random variable b_j associated with profile $d_i(r)$. A Gaussian model is used to parameterize the distribution, since the $d_j(r)$ on cup boundaries tend to cluster around a single mode. The pairwise term $V_{b_j b_l}(b_j, b_l)$ captures the shape constraints in terms of the relative position of the boundary points in adjacent profiles.

$$V_{b_j b_l}(b_j = m_j, b_l = m_l) = 1 - P_j(|m_j - m_l|) \qquad (5)$$

$|m_j - m_l|$ is the absolute difference in distance of the boundary points from r_0 in the adjacent profiles d_j and d_{j+1}. During training, the probability distribution (assumed to Gaussian) $P_j(|m_j - m_l|)$ between every adjacent boundary points is learnt from the ground truth data. Eqn.3 is solved using a multi-label graph cut approach with tree-reweighted message passing algorithm.

3   Experimental Results

Depth Estimation: The proposed depth estimation method was validated on 30 monocular color fundus images from INSPIRE dataset, obtained at a resolution of 4096×4096, cropped to a region of interest centered at OD. Corresponding depth maps obtained using SD-OCT scans in $200 \times 200 \times 1024$ mode [5] are available as ground truth. Due to limited availability of data, a leave-one-out cross validation analysis is done using correlation coefficient ρ to quantitatively measure the similarity in the overall trends of the estimated depth maps d and

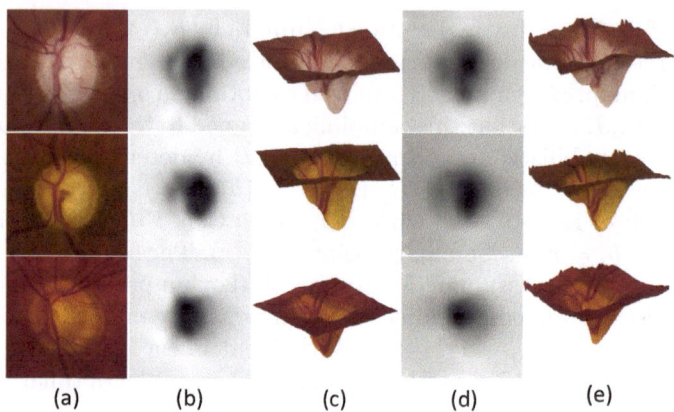

(a)   (b)   (c)   (d)   (e)

Fig. 3. OD regions from 3 sample images (column a) with corresponding depth estimates visualised as greysacle image where depth increases from white to black and topographical surface. Columns (b,c): ground truth; (d,e): computed results.

the ground truth D; $\rho(d, D) = \dfrac{\sum_m \sum_n (d_{m,n} - \bar{d})(D_{m,n} - \bar{D})}{\sqrt{(\sum_m \sum_n (d_{m,n} - \bar{d}))^2 (\sum_m \sum_n (D_{m,n} - \bar{D}))^2}}$ with $\bar{d}$ and $\bar{D}$ representing the mean values of d and D. m,n represents pixel locations in d and D. The mean ρ was found to be 0.80 ± 0.12.

Optic Cup Segmentation: The method for optic cup segmentation was validated on DRISHTI-GS dataset [17] which consists of 50 training and 51 test images obtained using 30 degree FOV at a resolution of 2896×1944. The ground truth OD and cup segmentation masks were obtained by a majority voting of manual markings by 4 ophthalmologists. Quantitative evaluation is based on the F-score to measure the extent of region overlap and the absolute pointwise localization error (measured in the radial direction) in the computed boundary as against the ground truth as reported in [2]. Both metrics were derived using a 10 fold cross validation approach, where for each of the 5 images, the parameters of the Gaussian distributions where learnt from the remaining 45 images. Performance evaluation on the test set is derived after training the system on an independent training set. The quantitative results have been provided in Table 1. Cup segmentation results are also reported for methods based on vessel bends [2], superpixels [3] and that provided along with the benchmark dataset in [17] for comparison. The tabulated figures show that the proposed method outperforms all the methods including [17] which relies on multiple input images. Results of cup segmentation on sample images are shown in figure 4.

Finally, we compare the results of the proposed method against OCT scanner provided values for CDR and cup to disc area ratios (CAR). Color fundus images for 28 eyes (18 Normal, 10 Glaucoma) were obtained at a resolution of 2896×1944 and 30 degree FOV along with OCT imaging whose reports provided ground truth CDR, CAR values. While the proposed method was used for cup segmentation, method in [2] was used for disc segmentation. The root mean square (rms) error for CDR was found to be 0.11 ± 0.08 for and 0.10 ± 0.05

Table 1. F-score and average boundary error in pixels

| | Optic Cup | | | |
| | F-score | | Boundary error(px) | |
	Train	Test	Train	Test
R-bend[2]	0.74 ± 0.20	0.77 ± 0.20	33.91 ± 25.14	30.51 ± 24.80
Superpixel[3]	0.67 ± 0.12	0.63 ± 0.13	37.04 ± 16.96	41.00 ± 16.50
Multiview [17]	0.77 ± 0.17	0.79 ± 0.18	24.24 ± 16.90	25.28 ± 18.00
Proposed method	0.80 ± 0.18	0.81 ± 0.16	22.10 ± 19.47	21.21 ± 15.09

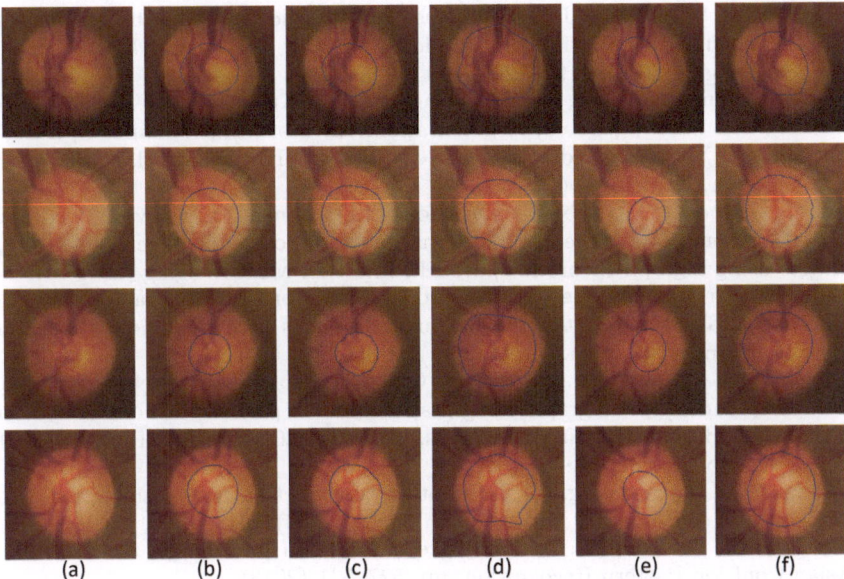

(a)　　(b)　　(c)　　(d)　　(e)　　(f)

Fig. 4. Qualitative results; a: Input image ; b: ground truth cup marking; Cup boundaries computed using c: proposed method d: R-bend e: Superpixel and f: Multiview

while rms error in CAR was 0.17 ± 0.12 and 0.21 ± 0.11 for Normal and Glaucoma cases, respectively. While CDR error is uniformly low for both classes, it is marginally higher for the glaucoma class for CAR.

4 Discussion and Conclusion

Inspired by the clinical significance of depth information of the retinal surface in the OD region and its use for cup segmentation in 3D imaging modalities (like OCT, HRT) and stereo image pairs, we have proposed a novel, supervised method for depth-based cup segmentation. The method relies on a dictionary trained on fundus image-depth map pairs. Although exact estimation of depth from single view images is a highly underconstrained problem, the performance of the proposed method (avg. correlation coefficient of 0.8 against ground truth) indicates that there is sufficient potential in the method. Since this was achieved with a moderate sized training set (30 pairs) it is possible to improve the results with a larger training set. Future work will explore ways to combine pallor and vessel kink information to further improve the reported results.

References

1. Xu, J., Chutatape, O., Sung, E., Zheng, C., Kuan, P.C.T.: Optic disk feature extraction via modified deformable model technique for glaucoma analysis. Pattern Recognition 40(7), 2063–2076 (2007)
2. Joshi, G.D., Sivaswamy, J., Krishnadas, S.R.: Optic disk and cup segmentation from monocular color retinal images for glaucoma assessment. IEEE Trans. on Medical Imaging 30(6), 1192–1205 (2011)
3. Cheng, J., Liu, J., Tao, D., Yin, F., Wong, D.W.K., Xu, Y., Wong, T.Y.: Superpixel classification based optic cup segmentation. In: Mori, K., Sakuma, I., Sato, Y., Barillot, C., Navab, N. (eds.) MICCAI 2013, Part III. LNCS, vol. 8151, pp. 421–428. Springer, Heidelberg (2013)
4. Hu, Z., Niemeijer, M., Lee, K., Abràmoff, M.D., Sonka, M., Garvin, M.K.: Automated segmentation of the optic disc margin in 3-d optical coherence tomography images using a graph-theoretic approach. In: SPIE Med. Imaging (2009)
5. Tang, L., Garvin, M.K., Lee, K., Alward, W.L., Kwon, Y.H., Abràmoff, M.D.: Robust multiscale stereo matching from fundus images with radiometric differences. IEEE Pattern Anal. Mach. Intel. 33(11), 2245–2258 (2011)
6. Zheng, Y., Stambolian, D., O'Brien, J., Gee, J.C.: Optic disc and cup segmentation from color fundus photograph using graph cut with priors. In: Mori, K., Sakuma, I., Sato, Y., Barillot, C., Navab, N. (eds.) MICCAI 2013, Part II. LNCS, vol. 8150, pp. 75–82. Springer, Heidelberg (2013)
7. Saxena, A., Chung, S., Ng, A.: 3-d depth reconstruction from a single still image. Intl. Journal of Computer Vision 76(1), 53–69 (2008)
8. Agrawal, H., Namboodiri, A.: Shape reconstruction from single relief image. In: Asian Conf. on Pattern Recognition, pp. 527–531 (2013)
9. Kruizinga, P., Petkov, N.: Nonlinear operator for oriented texture. IEEE Trans. on Image Processing 8(10), 1395–1407 (1999)
10. Malik, J., Belongie, S., Shi, J., Leung, T.: Textons, contours and regions: Cue integration in image segmentation. In: ICCV. vol. 2, pp. 918–25 (1999)
11. Funt, B., Drew, M., Brockington, M.: Recovering shading from color images. In: Sandini, G. (ed.) ECCV 1992. LNCS, vol. 588, pp. 124–132. Springer, Heidelberg (1992)
12. Tsai, P., Shah, M.: Shape from shading using linear approximation. Image and Vision Computing 12, 487–498 (1994)
13. Weenink, D.: Canonical correlation analysis. In: Inst. of Phonetic Science, Univ. of Amsterdam, vol. 25, pp. 81–99 (2003)
14. Tang, Y., Yuan, Y., Yan, P., Li, X.: Single-image super-resolution via sparse coding regression. In: Intl. Conf. on Image and Graphics. pp. 267–272 (2011)
15. Mairal, J., Bach, F., Ponce, J., Sapiro, G.: Online dictionary learning for sparse coding. In: Intl. Conf. on Machine Learning, pp. 689–696 (2009)
16. Vondrick, C., Khosla, A., Malisiewicz, T., Torralba, A.: Hoggles: Visualizing object detection features. In: Intenl. Conf. on Computer Vision, pp. 1–8 (2013)
17. Sivaswamy, J., Krishnadas, K., Joshi, G.D., Jain, M., Ujjwal, Abbas, T.S.: Drishti-GS: retinal image dataset for optic nerve head(ONH) segmentation. In: Int. Symp. on Biomed. Eng. (2014)

Topo-Geometric Filtration Scheme for Geometric Active Contours and Level Sets: Application to Cerebrovascular Segmentation

Helena Molina-Abril and Alejandro F. Frangi

Centre for Computational Imaging and Simulation Technologies in Biomedicine, Mechanical Engineering Department, University of Sheffield, UK

Abstract. One of the main problems of the existing methods for the segmentation of cerebral vasculature is the appearance in the segmentation result of wrong topological artefacts such as the kissing vessels. In this paper, a new approach for the detection and correction of such errors is presented. The proposed technique combines robust topological information given by Persistent Homology with complementary geometrical information of the vascular tree. The method was evaluated on 20 images depicting cerebral arteries. Detection and correction success rates were 81.80% and 68.77%, respectively.

1 Introduction

Accurate segmentation of the cerebral vasculature is important as part of several advanced radiological and interventional procedures; e.g. in making more objective detection of vascular pathologies (carotid stenosis, cerebral aneurysm, malformations), quantification (of stenosis grading, aneurysm measurements), personalised hemodynamic modelling, and interventional planning of endovascular procedures. Automated analysis of the cerebral vessels, however, remains challenging as it has to be robust to limited image resolution, artefacts in image acquisition, image noise, complex vascular morphologies even in healthy conditions as well as morphological alterations due to pathological conditions.

Several methods have been proposed in the literature for the segmentation of cerebral vasculature [9]. One of the main problems of the existing methods is that they are not robust to recover and preserve the topology of the underlying vascular tree. This is particularly problematic when trying to recover the full or large portions of the cerebral vasculature. Missing (e.g. due to poor image resolution or artefacts) or kissing vessels (i.e. when two distinct but parallel running vessels cannot be distinguished) can easily mislead vascular segmentation algorithms so that the final result contains missing or fused vascular segments.

In particular, due to their large presence in cerebral vasculature segmentation results, several segmentation methods address the kissing vessel problem by using shape priors that aim to prevent their formation [11,8,13]. However, these methods either require a trade-off between geometrical accuracy and topological correctness, or cannot guarantee topological correctness nor the absence

P. Golland et al. (Eds.): MICCAI 2014, Part I, LNCS 8673, pp. 755–762, 2014.

of kissing vessels. Due to the fact that the vast majority of kissing vessels introduce topological alterations in the resulting vascular network, more general methods incorporating topological restrictions in the segmentation process could be considered a solution to the problem. Chen and Freedman [6] proposed an approach that enforces specific topological constrains within the level-set segmentation framework (called C&F method in the sequel). This method is a general approach that allows topological control within a level set evolution by using Persistent Homology [7], which is a concept borrowed from algebraic topology. Given a known initial topology of the object to be segmented, the method is able to correct every topological error within a given segmentation. To the best of our knowledge the C&F method has never been tested to quantitatively demonstrate its effectiveness on any clinical application. From our experience, the main drawback of this method is that the manipulations required for correcting the topology of the object may alter its geometry in an undesired manner leading to incorrect segmentations.

Our work builds upon the C&F method, which is extended to enable automatic detection and semi-automatic correction of kissing vessels in cerebrovascular image segmentations. We believe that this is the first method specifically dealing with the detection and correction of such artefacts. This is particularly relevant in view of population imaging efforts where one is interested in extracting quantitative image information from large image databases, and where manual detection and correction have a huge impact in terms of reproducibility and processing time.

2   Persistent Homology for Segmentation Errors Correction

Given a segmentation result, the C&F method makes use of the concepts of homology groups and persistent homology to detect and eliminate incorrect topological features that are present in the initial segmentation. This approach is based in geometric active contours (GAC) [5] that is an image-based object modelling approach based on the theory of curve/surface evolution and level set frameworks. In GAC, contours are represented implicitly using the zero-level set of a higher-dimension function called the level set function. Given a known initial topology of the object to be segmented, the C&F method automatically drives the evolving contour within the GAC framework towards the correct object's topology. Let us introduce some of the concepts, coming from homology theory, that are used in this method.

Homology groups are efficiently computable topological invariants that have already proved their usefulness in different applications and their potential in multidimensional digital image analysis [7]. The homology groups $H(O)$ of an n–dimensional digital object O provide information on the number of connected components and holes of various dimensions. For instance, in a $3D$ image, 0–holes can be seen as connected components, 1–holes as handles, and 2–holes as voids in the image. These topological features of the image are algebraically represented by the so-called homology classes. Intuitively, if we focus on a canonical basis of the vector space formed by the group of homology classes, we could think of having one homology class for each topological feature in the image. For example, if we think on the vessels in Fig. 1 (a) as solid tubes, there is one connected component and two handles, that is one 0–dimensional homology class and two 1–dimensional homology classes (algebraically independent). The C&F method makes use of these concepts to remove the topological errors of a given segmentation. That is, knowing the correct topology of the object to be segmented, the method assures the elimination of the undesired homology classes. This elimination is performed by an automatic evolution of the object's contour that is based on its homological information. The contour of the object is implicitly represented as the zero level set $\phi : \Omega \to \mathbb{R}$ where Ω is the domain of interest and ϕ is the signed distance function. The method uses *Persistent Homology* for the homology computation of the domain Ω. Persistent homology is a technique for computing topological features of a given topological space, which at the same time provides meaningful measurements of its topological properties. Given a domain Ω and a function $\phi : \Omega \to \mathbb{R}$ for each $t \in \mathbb{R}$, the persistent homology algorithm grows the sublevel set $\phi^{-1}(-\infty, t]$ from the empty set to the entire domain. Throughout this process, the algorithm detects the points (called *critical points*) in which homology changes (the number of p–dimensional algebraically independent homology classes increases or decreases).

Once the critical points are computed, and supposing that the contour we are segmenting is homeomorphic to a d–sphere, the C&F method makes use of the concept of *robustness* [3]. Roughly speaking, given a homology class $\alpha \in H(O)$ of an object O, its robustness $\rho_\phi(\alpha)$ is a measure of how much ϕ needs to be modified to get rid of the topological feature represented by α. Formally, the robustness $\rho_\phi(\alpha)$ is the minimal r such that there exists an r–perturbation of ϕ on which α disappears in the perturbed object $h^{-1}(\infty, 0]$. An r–perturbation, h of ϕ, is the real-valued function h such that $\|h - \phi\|_\infty = max_{x \in \Omega}|h(x) - \phi(x)| \leq r$. The total robustness is defined as: $Rob_k(O) = \sum_{\alpha \in H(O)}^{n} \rho_\phi(\alpha)^k - (max_{\alpha \in H(O)}\rho_\phi(\alpha))^k$, where n is the number of homology classes in O. The evolution of a flow that drives the contour C and its signed distance function ϕ towards the minimum total robustness allows the elimination of its homology classes. The final evolution equation (considering for instance degree $k = 3$ robustness) is the following:

$$\tfrac{\partial E}{\partial \phi} = 3\left(\sum_{\alpha \in H(O), c_\alpha \neq c_{min}} \delta(x - c_\alpha)\right) sign(\phi(x))\phi^2(x) \tag{1}$$

where δ is a Dirac delta function, c_α is the critical point associated to a homology class $\alpha \in H(O)$, and c_{min} is the critical point associated with the most robust homology class (the only homology class we want to keep that is representing the connected component of the object). In practice, δ is implemented as a Gaussian with variance σ^2. The effect of this evolution is the modification of the contour within a small neighbourhood (defined by the Gaussian) of each critical point. This modification leads to the elimination of the topological feature associated to the corresponding critical point.

3   Methodology

By analysing segmentation results of the cerebral vasculature, one can realize that most of the topological errors are due to kissing vessels that emerge from poor or limited image resolution. The automatic detection of these errors is not trivial, and to the best of our knowledge no effective solution is currently available for their correction. Other topological errors such as disconnected components or voids are easier to detect and correct using connected component algorithms.

Taking into consideration that the method described in Section 2 is designed for the correction of topological errors, we could contemplate its application to the automatic detection and correction of the kissing vessels in cerebral vasculature segmentations. One example of the application of the C&F method can be seen in Fig. 1 (b)-(d) where two kissing vessels are correctly removed after applying C&F (critical points are represented as black dots). However, even if the C&F method assures a correct topology of the result, the algorithm provides a solution that is in many occasions far from the desired one. There are two main reasons for that: First, the location of critical points does not correspond in general with the location of the kissing vessel. Second, the evolution of the contour within a predefined neighbourhood (determined by the variance of the Gauss function that approximates the Dirac function in (1)) does not respect the correct geometry of the vascular tree (see Fig. 1 (c)-(e)). In Section 3.1 we propose a new method in which, by including geometrical information of the vascular tree within the C&F method, the localization of kissing vessels is drastically improved. In Section 3.2, a correction framework that avoids the incorrect results of the type of those shown in Fig. 1 (e) is proposed. The algorithm described in [4] has been used for the initial segmentations.

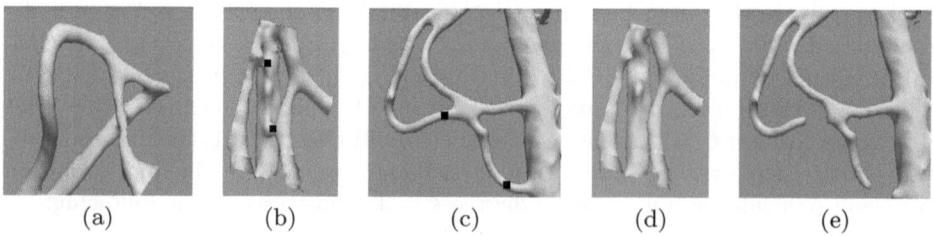

| (a) | (b) | (c) | (d) | (e) |

Fig. 1. (a) Part of the cerebral vasculature. (b) - (c) Initial segmentations. (d) Correct result and (e) incorrect result after applying the C&F method.

3.1   Detection Method

Simplicial Complexes and Filtrations. A topological space for which we want to compute Persistent Homology can be represented using different structures. *Simplicial complexes* are convenient representations of topological spaces, specially for computer implementations, consisting of a collection of simplices that are glued together in a structured manner. A *q–simplex* in $\mathbb{R}^k$ is defined to be a set of the form: $\{\sum_{j=0}^{q} a_j v_j : 0 \leq a_j \leq 1 \text{ for } j = 0, \ldots, q \text{ and } \sum_{j=0}^{q} a_j = 1\}$

where v_j are affinely independent points. For example, a 0–simplex is a vertex, a 1–simplex and edge, a 2–simplex a triangle, and a 3–simplex a tetrahedron. Let K be a simplicial complex. A *filtration* is a nested sequence of subcomplexes: $\emptyset = K_0 \subset \cdots \subset K_n = K$. We may think of a filtration as a description of how to construct K by adding blocks at a time. We can now focus in the topological evolution of a filtration of complexes by the corresponding sequence of homology groups. Since $K_{i-1} \subset K_i$, the inclusion map defined by $f(x) = x$ induces a homomorphism between the homology groups $f_* : H_p(K_{i-1}) \rightarrow H_p(K_i)$. The nested sequence of complexes corresponds to sequences of homology groups connected by homomorphisms, $0 = H_p(K_0) \rightarrow H_p(K_1) \rightarrow \cdots \rightarrow H_p(K_n) = H_p(K)$, one for each dimension p. Given a filtration, the persistent homology algorithm considers this last sequence and detects when a new homology class is born and when an existing class dies as we proceed forward through the filtration [7]. Therefore, the definition of the filter function $\phi : K \rightarrow \mathbb{R}$, is crucial within this method. If there are two simplexes whose inclusion creates a new homology class, the one that is first introduced in the filtration will be selected as critical point. In the C&F method, the filter function is defined by the signed distance function. The main idea of the work presented here consists of obtaining additional geometrical information that could guide the definition of a more appropriate filtration scheme. Using this information, we create a geometry-driven filtration that gives priority to points that belong to kissing vessels to be selected as critical points.

Geometrical Properties of Kissing Vessels. The first step for incorporating geometrical information is to compute the skeleton of the segmented vasculature. We use the algorithm presented in [2] for this purpose. The skeleton of a vascular tree can be seen as a graph where the centerlines are edges and their intersections are the vertices of the graph. The geometrical properties of the kissing vessels are based on the following observations (see Fig. 2 (a)-(d)): (1) They correspond with short centerlines in the vasculature skeleton, (2) its corresponding centerline are often perpendicular to its neighbouring centerlines and (3) they often cause drastic changes in the vessel radius with respect to its neighbouring centerlines. Taking into account these observations, we define a *kissingness measure* for each centerline c of the skeleton: $KS(c) = (\pi(c) + \alpha(c))/l(c)$, where: (1) $\pi(c) = \frac{1}{n}\sum_{i=1}^{n}(r_c - r_i)^2$ depends on the radius of c and its neighbouring centerlines. r_c is the normalized radius of c and r_i the normalized radius of its n neighbouring centerlines, for $i \in \{1 \ldots n\}$, (2) $\alpha(c) = \frac{1}{n}\sum_{i=1}^{n}\sin(\theta(i,c))$ depends on the angle of c with its neighbouring centerlines, where $i \in \{1 \ldots n\}$ are the neighbouring centerlines of c and $\theta(i,c)$ is the minimum angle between the centerlines i and c, and (3) $l(c)$ is the normalized length of c. The set of edges with maximal kissingness value is defined as the *suspicious kissing* set.

Geometry-Driven Filtration. As mentioned before, our aim is to give priority in the filtration process to the points that are close to the edges that belong to kissing vessels. Using the set of suspicious kissing edges, the idea consists in decreasing the values of the signed distance function around them, and then use this modified signed distance function as the filter function for the persistent homology algorithm. Having smaller filter values around the suspicious kissing edges, makes the points around them more probable to be selected as critical points (because they will be considered earlier in the persistent homology algorithm). For each suspicious kissing edge, we define a spring force [12] that acts to pull the contour toward the kissing edge middle point. Then the level set function of the initial segmentation is evolved under the influence of these forces (Fig. 2 (c)-(e)). This evolution is performed using the topological control evolution presented in [10], which guarantees the preservation of the initial contour's topology. Once this modification is done, the persistent homology of the domain delineated by the resulting contour can be computed following the filtration defined by the modified signed distance function. The set of critical points obtained after this computation are the points detected as kissing vessels.

Algorithm 1: Kissing points detection method

Require: Signed distance function ϕ, suspicious edges set S, spring forces $F_s(x) = 0$
> for each edge $e_j \in S$ **do**
>> $x_c \leftarrow MiddlePoint(e_k)$
>> for each point $x_d \in e_k$ **do**
>>> $F_s(x_d) = F_s(x_d) + d(x_c, x_d)$ $\qquad\qquad$ ▷ Spring forces F_s, Euclidean distance d
>> while No topological change occurs **do** $\qquad\qquad\qquad\qquad$ ▷ Contour evolution
>>> Evolve ϕ following $\frac{\partial \phi}{\partial t}(x, t) = F_s(x)$
> **return** $CriticalPoints \leftarrow PH(\phi)$ $\qquad\qquad\qquad$ ▷ Persistent Homology PH

3.2 Correction Framework

Once the kissing vessels are detected, we could correct the topological errors in the mesh by minimizing the energy term in Equation (1). However, the correction result depends on the width of the approximation of the Dirac delta function, that is the neighbourhood of the critical point on which the evolution will have effect. Due to the wide variety of kissing vessel's shapes and locations, their automatic correction leads to geometrically incorrect results (Fig. 2 (f)-(h)). We propose here a semi-automatic correction framework in which the user can iteratively modify the segmentation results via a simple, easy-to-use graphical interface. Once the critical points have been automatically detected, instead of using a predefined neighbourhood (as in C&F), we use adjustable ellipsoids to define the neighbourhood for Equation (1). For each critical point, we create an ellipsoid centred at it. The framework allows the user to modify its axes, position and inclination. After the user has finished adjusting it to the concrete kissing vessel, the method automatically eliminates the kissing vessel applying Equation (1) within the neighbourhood defined by the ellipsoid (Fig. 2 (i)-(j)).

4   Results

The proposed method was compared with the C&F method using twenty patients scanned with 3D rotational X-ray angiography. Diagnostic images were acquired as part of the @neurIST project [1]. The persistent homology algorithm that is core to the C&F method requires $O(m^3)$ operations in the worst

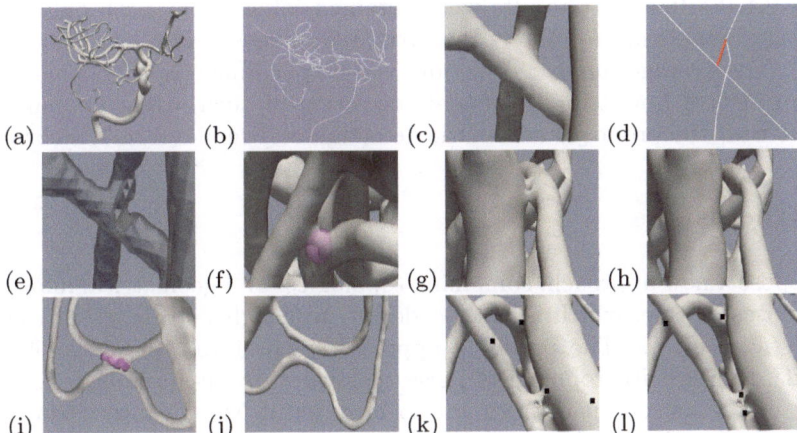

Fig. 2. (a) Initial segmentation and (b) its skeleton. (c) Kissing vessel (d) its skeleton (the red centerline is suspicious) and (e) the signed distance function after the spring forces evolution. (f) The influence of the Gaussian for $\sigma^2 = 0.4$. (g) Segmentation result and (h) correction result for $\sigma^2 = 0.1$. (i) Ellipsoidal neighbourhood. (j) Correction result. (k) Points detected with the C&F method and (l) with the proposed method.

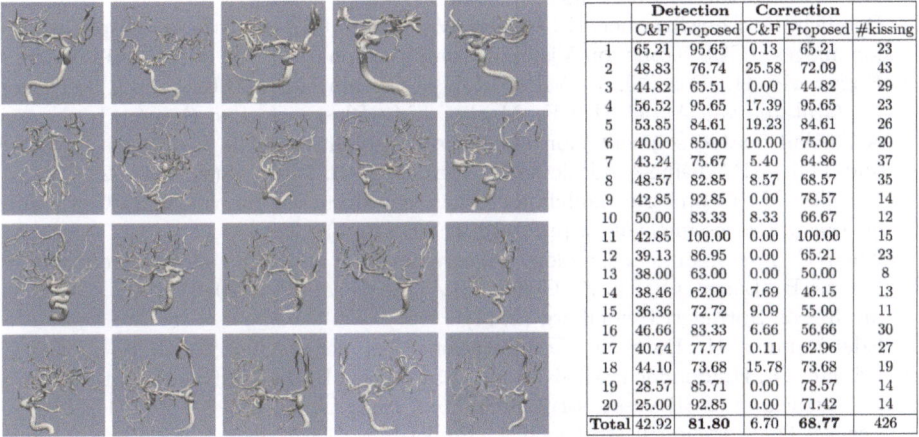

	Detection		Correction		
	C&F	Proposed	C&F	Proposed	#kissing
1	65.21	95.65	0.13	65.21	23
2	48.83	76.74	25.58	72.09	43
3	44.82	65.51	0.00	44.82	29
4	56.52	95.65	17.39	95.65	23
5	53.85	84.61	19.23	84.61	26
6	40.00	85.00	10.00	75.00	20
7	43.24	75.67	5.40	64.86	37
8	48.57	82.85	8.57	68.57	35
9	42.85	92.85	0.00	78.57	14
10	50.00	83.33	8.33	66.67	12
11	42.85	100.00	0.00	100.00	15
12	39.13	86.95	0.00	65.21	23
13	38.00	63.00	0.00	50.00	8
14	38.46	62.00	7.69	46.15	13
15	36.36	72.72	9.09	55.00	11
16	46.66	83.33	6.66	56.66	30
17	40.74	77.77	0.11	62.96	27
18	44.10	73.68	15.78	73.68	19
19	28.57	85.71	0.00	78.57	14
20	25.00	92.85	0.00	71.42	14
Total	42.92	**81.80**	6.70	68.77	426

Fig. 3. Segmentation results. Detection, correction rates and number of initial kissings.

case, where m is the number of simplices. The inclusion of the geometrical filtration takes $O(m)$ and hence introduces negligible extra computational cost. The initial segmentations and the percentage of correctly located kissing vessels for both methods are shown in Fig. 3. The rate increases from 42.92% with the C&F method to 81.80% with our approach. An example is shown in Fig. 2 (k)-(l), where our method allowed a correct location of every kissing vessel and using the C&F method only two out of four were correctly located. With respect to the correction method, we run the C&F algorithm for three different values of $\sigma = 0.1, 0.5, 0.9$. Best results were obtained for $\sigma = 0.5$ with only 6.7% of the kissing vessels appropriately removed. We increased the correction rate to 68.77%. The average number of kissing vessels per image is 21.8. This number gives an idea of how tedious manual correction of such artefacts could be in contrast with the proposed automatic detection and semi-automatic correction.

5   Conclusions

We propose a new approach, combining topological and geometrical information of the vascular tree, which is able to detect in a high percentage of cases the kissing vessel errors. The proposed approach outperforms the state-of-the-art methods dealing with topological noise removal. A semi-automatic framework for the correction of such errors is also introduced, significantly reducing the user interaction time with respect to manual correction.

References

1. Aneurist project, `http://www.aneurist.org`
2. Antiga, L.: Patient-Specific Modeling of Geometry and Blood Flow in Large Arteries. Ph.D. thesis, Politecnico di Milano (2002)
3. Bendich, P., Edelsbrunner, H., Kerber, M.: Computing robustness and persistence for images. IEEE Trans. on Vis. and Comp. Graphics 16(6), 1251–1260 (2010)
4. Bogunović, H., Pozo, J.M., Villa-Uriol, M.C., Majoie, C.B.L.M., van den Berg, R., Gratama van Andel, H.A.F., Macho, J.M., Blasco, J., San Román, L., Frangi, A.F.: Automated segmentation of cerebral vasculature with aneurysms in 3DRA and TOF-MRA using geodesic active regions. Med. Phys. 38(1), 210–222 (2011)
5. Caselles, V.: Geometric models for active contours. In: International Conference on Image Processing. vol. 3, pp. 9–12. IEEE (1995)
6. Chen, C., Freedman, D.: Topology noise removal for curve and surface evolution. In: Menze, B., Langs, G., Tu, Z., Criminisi, A. (eds.) MICCAI 2010. LNCS, vol. 6533, pp. 31–42. Springer, Heidelberg (2011)
7. Edelsbrunner, H., Harer, J.: Computational Topology. Amer. Math. Soc. (2010)
8. Friman, O., Hindennach, M., Kühnel, C., Peitgen, H.O.: Multiple hypothesis template tracking of 3D vessel structures. Med. Imag. Anal. 14(2), 160–171 (2010)
9. Lesage, D., Angelini, E.D., Bloch, I., Funka-Lea, G.: A review of 3D vessel lumen segmentation techniques. Med. Imag. Anal. 13(6), 819–845 (2009)
10. Ségonne, F.: Active contours under topology control genus preserving level sets. International Journal of Computer Vision 79(2), 107–117 (2008)
11. Wong, W.C.K., Chung, A.C.S.: Probabilistic vessel axis tracing and its application to vessel segmentation with stream surfaces and minimum cost paths. Med. Imag. Anal. 11(6), 567–587 (2007)
12. Xu, C., Pham, D.L., Prince, J.L.: Image segmentation using deformable models. In: Handbook of Medical Imaging. Medical Image Processing and Analysis, vol. 2, pp. 175–272 (2000)
13. Yureidini, A., Kerrien, E., Cotin, S.: Robust RANSAC-based blood vessel segmentation. In: SPIE Medical Imaging, vol. 8314, p. 8314M. SPIE Press (2012)

Combining Generative Models for Multifocal Glioma Segmentation and Registration

Dongjin Kwon[1], Russell T. Shinohara[2,1],
Hamed Akbari[1], and Christos Davatzikos[1]

[1] Center for Biomedical Image Computing and Analytics, University of Pennsylvania
[2] Department of Biostatistics and Epidemiology, University of Pennsylvania

Abstract. In this paper, we propose a new method for simultaneously segmenting brain scans of glioma patients and registering these scans to a normal atlas. Performing joint segmentation and registration for brain tumors is very challenging when tumors include multifocal masses and have complex shapes with heterogeneous textures. Our approach grows tumors for each mass from multiple seed points using a tumor growth model and modifies a normal atlas into one with tumors and edema using the combined results of grown tumors. We also generate a tumor shape prior via the random walk with restart, utilizing multiple tumor seeds as initial foreground information. We then incorporate this shape prior into an EM framework which estimates the mapping between the modified atlas and the scans, posteriors for each tissue labels, and the tumor growth model parameters. We apply our method to the BRATS 2013 leaderboard dataset to evaluate segmentation performance. Our method shows the best performance among all participants.

1 Introduction

Gliomas are the most common primary brain tumors that arise within the brain parenchyma. They are commonly categorized according to their malignancies, from low-grade to high-grade, but nearly all low-grade gliomas eventually progress to high-grade malignancy [8]. Glioblastoma is the most malignant form of gliomas and has median survival rates of 12-18 months. The standard treatment includes partial or complete resection, chemotherapy, and radiation therapy [14]. Accurate delineation of glioma and edematous parenchyma is helpful for treatment planning and progression monitoring. However, the segmentation of brain gliomas is a challenging task of critical importance in medical image analysis, due to the complex shape and heterogeneous textures of such tumors. Moreover, multifocal gliomas, having 8-10% incidence among gliomas [1], are even more difficult to segment especially for methods assuming a single-focal mass.

To perform this challenging task, many techniques have been proposed. They can be predominantly classified as either discriminative or generative models [10]. Discriminative models extract image features for each voxel and train classifiers using these features guided by annotated training data [15,16]. As these models

P. Golland et al. (Eds.): MICCAI 2014, Part I, LNCS 8673, pp. 763–770, 2014.
© Springer International Publishing Switzerland 2014

directly learn classifiers from image features, they do not require domain-specific knowledge and can concentrate on the specific features relevant to the segmentation. However, their segmentation is restricted to images from the same protocol as the training data, since these models are often carefully fitted to the training data. Generative models incorporate prior information about the appearance and spatial distribution for each tissue type [2,12]. For the prior information, the appearance of tumor and edema are modeled as outliers to the healthy tissue, or tumor growth models are used for localizing tumor structures. However, designing effective prior models requires significant efforts and the performance is limited by the range of domain-specific knowledge employed.

In this paper, we propose a new method for joint segmentation and registration (JSR) of brain gliomas. In order to generate a patient-specific atlas, our method grows tumors on the atlas, with parameters estimated at the same time, and registers the scans to this atlas to infer the segmentation. Differently from the previous JSR framework of [2], we also allow multiple tumor seed points to segment multifocal gliomas. For our method, tumors are grown on each seed using a tumor growth model and combined into the single tumor probability map. Also, we incorporate a tumor shape prior into the framework by introducing an empirical Bayes model [11]. The tumor shape prior is estimated by the random walk with restart [5] using tumor seeds as initial foreground information, which helps the framework to find accurate tumor shapes for difficult cases. Since this shape prior can be considered as another generative model, in principle, our method systematically *combines* two kinds of *generative models*. In the rest of this paper, we describe the atlas generation method for multifocal tumors in Sec. 2 and our JSR framework with shape prior using this atlas in Sec. 3. In Sec. 4, we present our quantitative and qualitative evaluations and conclude the paper in Sec. 5.

2   Atlas Generation for Multifocal Gliomas

In this section, we use a tumor growth model to embed multifocal masses in an atlas of a healthy population. We denote by $\mathcal{T}$ the label map and by t the possible tissue type. Then we denote by '$\mathcal{T}_t|\mathbf{x}$' the tissue type being t at voxel $\mathbf{x}$, namely '$\mathcal{T} = t|\mathbf{x}$'. The atlas p_A is defined as a set of probability maps $p_A(\mathcal{T}_t|\mathbf{x})$ for white matter (WM), gray matter (GM), and cerebrospinal fluid (CSF), i.e. $t \in \{WM, GM, CSF\}$, obtained by averaging aligned segmentations of healthy brains. We adapt the atlas to the subject space by simulating the tumor growth via the diffusion-reaction-advection model of [3].

Unlike most previous methods assuming only a single mass, such as [2], we allow multiple tumor seeds and grow tumors for each given seed location. We then merge each result into the single spatial probability map of tumor (TU). If we assume the subject shows M tumors, then each tumor $i \in \{1, \ldots, M\}$ is characterized by seed location $\mathbf{o}_i$, its size r_i, and other shared tumor parameters including the diffusion coefficient for white matter D_{WM} and the proliferation coefficient p_1. Therefore, each tumor growth is completely defined by the parameters $\mathbf{q}_i \triangleq \{\mathbf{o}_i, r_i, D_{WM}, p_1\}$, and the tumor probability $\mathbf{d}_i$ and its associated

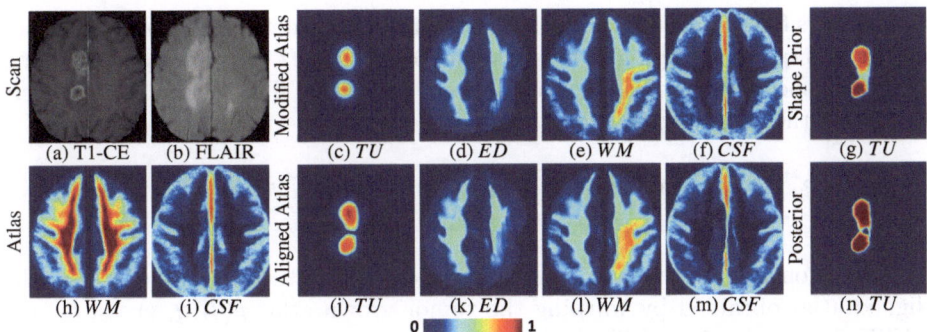

Fig. 1. An example of spatial probabilities for multifocal glioma. We show subject scans in (a)-(b), normal atlas in (h)-(i), spatial probabilities $p(\mathcal{T}_t|\mathbf{q},\mathbf{x})$ obtained by growing tumors on normal atlas in (c)-(f), tumor shape prior in (g), spatial probabilities $p(\mathcal{T}_t|\mathbf{q},\boldsymbol{h},\mathbf{x})$ aligned to the scan in (j)-(m), and tumor posterior $p(\mathcal{T}_{TU}|Y,\mathbf{x})$ in (n).

deformation (mass effect) $\mathbf{u}_i$ are obtained. We also define $\mathbf{q}$ as the set of all tumor parameters $\mathbf{q} = \{\mathbf{q}_1,\ldots,\mathbf{q}_M\}$. The merged tumor probability $p(\mathcal{T}_{TU}|\mathbf{q},\mathbf{x})$ and mass effect $\mathbf{u}(\mathbf{x})$ at voxel $\mathbf{x}$ are simply defined as the sum of each estimation, that is, $p(\mathcal{T}_{TU}|\mathbf{q},\mathbf{x}) \triangleq \min\{\sum_{i=1}^{M} \mathbf{d}_i(\mathbf{x}),1\}$ and $\mathbf{u}(\mathbf{x}) \triangleq \sum_{i=1}^{M} \mathbf{u}_i(\mathbf{x})$. We then construct spatial probability maps for GM and CSF ($t \in \{GM,CSF\}$) by deforming the atlas via the mass effect $\mathbf{u}$ and weighting them with the complement of $p(\mathcal{T}_{TU}|\mathbf{q},\mathbf{x})$:

$$p(\mathcal{T}_t|\mathbf{q},\mathbf{x}) \triangleq p_A(\mathcal{T}_t|\mathbf{u}(\mathbf{x})) \cdot (1 - p(\mathcal{T}_{TU}|\mathbf{q},\mathbf{x})) \, . \tag{1}$$

For the spatial probability map for edema (ED), we model the close proximity of edema to tumor via the Heaviside function $H(\cdot)$ ($H(a) = 0$ for $a \leq 0$ and $H(a) = 1$ for $a > 0$) resulting in

$$p(\mathcal{T}_{ED}|\mathbf{q},\mathbf{x}) \triangleq 0.5 \cdot p_A(\mathcal{T}_{WM}|\mathbf{u}(\mathbf{x})) \cdot (1 - p(\mathcal{T}_{TU}|\mathbf{q},\mathbf{x})) \cdot H(p(\mathcal{T}_{TU}|\mathbf{q},\mathbf{x})) \, , \tag{2}$$

where we multiply 0.5 to avoid preference of edema over WM. The spatial probability for WM is defined by the complement of spatial probability maps of the other tissue types:

$$p(\mathcal{T}_{WM}|\mathbf{q},\mathbf{x}) \triangleq 1 - p(\mathcal{T}_{TU}|\mathbf{q},\mathbf{x}) - p(\mathcal{T}_{ED}|\mathbf{q},\mathbf{x}) - p(\mathcal{T}_{GM}|\mathbf{q},\mathbf{x}) - p(\mathcal{T}_{CSF}|\mathbf{q},\mathbf{x}) \, . \tag{3}$$

After growing tumors on the atlas, a set of tissue type Θ is now defined as $\{TU,ED,WM,GM,CSF\}$. A sample set of the spatial probabilities is shown in Fig. 1 (c)-(f). These spatial probabilities are modified from the atlas shown in Fig. 1 (h)-(i) using the tumor growth model.

3   Joint Segmentation-Registration with Shape Prior

Having defined the spatial probabilities $p(\mathcal{T}_t|\mathbf{q},\mathbf{x})$, we now describe our JSR framework using the atlas we constructed in the previous section as well as shape priors for tumor. The parameters of our JSR framework include the tumor parameters $\mathbf{q}$, the mapping $\boldsymbol{h}$ from the subject space Ω to the atlas space, and the tissue specific means and covariances $\boldsymbol{\Phi}$. We then find optimal parameters by solving the following problem:

$$\{\mathbf{q}^*, \boldsymbol{h}^*, \boldsymbol{\Phi}^*\} \triangleq \arg\max_{\mathbf{q}, \boldsymbol{h}, \boldsymbol{\Phi}} \left\{ \prod_{\mathbf{x} \in \Omega} \sum_{t \in \Theta} p(\mathcal{T}_t | \mathbf{q}, \boldsymbol{h}, \mathbf{x}) \cdot p(Y | \mathcal{T}_t, \boldsymbol{\Phi}, \mathbf{x}) \cdot p(\mathbf{q}, \boldsymbol{h} | \eta^*, \mathbf{x}) \right\},$$
(4)

where Y consists of the subject images, $p(\mathcal{T}_t | \mathbf{q}, \boldsymbol{h}, \mathbf{x}) \triangleq p(\mathcal{T}_t | \mathbf{q}, \boldsymbol{h}(\mathbf{x}))$ is the aligned atlas obtained by warping the tumor grown atlas $p(\mathcal{T}_t | \mathbf{q}, \mathbf{x})$ via $\boldsymbol{h}$, and $p(Y | \mathcal{T}_t, \boldsymbol{\Phi}, \mathbf{x})$ is the image likelihood defined as the multivariate Gaussian for $\boldsymbol{\Phi}$. $p(\mathbf{q}, \boldsymbol{h} | \eta^*, \mathbf{x})$ is the prior function for $\{\mathbf{q}, \boldsymbol{h}\}$ to be used as part of an empirical Bayes approach [11], and we assume the probability distribution of hyperparameters η given Y, i.e. $p(\eta | Y)$, is sharply peaked at η^*. For this prior function, we assume deformed atlas for tumor $p(\mathcal{T}_{TU} | \mathbf{q}, \boldsymbol{h}(\mathbf{x}))$ tends to match the tumor shape prior $p_E(\mathcal{T}_{TU} | \eta^*, \mathbf{x})$ as follows

$$p(\mathbf{q}, \boldsymbol{h} | \eta^*, \mathbf{x}) \triangleq \frac{1}{Z} \exp(-\lambda \cdot ||p(\mathcal{T}_{TU} | \mathbf{q}, \boldsymbol{h}(\mathbf{x})) - p_E(\mathcal{T}_{TU} | \eta^*, \mathbf{x})||^2),$$
(5)

where Z is a normalization constant and λ is a parameter controlling the weight of the shape prior on this function. If $\lambda = 0$, our problem turns into the JSR problem of [2] when a single tumor seed is used. The tumor shape prior $p_E(\mathcal{T}_{TU} | \eta^*, \mathbf{x})$ is inferred directly from images utilizing tumor seed locations using the random walk with restart (RWR) [5]. This method is suitable for estimating heterogeneous tumor regions as it showed strong performance in finding weak boundaries and separating textures in cluttered scenes. Now, we briefly describe the RWR method.

Given subject images Y, let us construct an undirected graph $G = (\mathcal{V}, \mathcal{E})$ with nodes $v \in \mathcal{V}$ and edges $e \in \mathcal{E}$. We assume G is defined on 26-connected neighborhoods. For each edge e_{ij}, we assign the weight w_{ij} which measures the likelihood for having the same label between node v_i and v_j:

$$w_{ij} \triangleq \exp(-||\mathbf{y}_i - \mathbf{y}_j||^2 / \sigma),$$
(6)

where $\mathbf{y}_i$ is a multi-modal intensity vector for node v_i and σ is a constant for normalizing intensity differences. Then we define the adjacency matrix $\mathbf{W} = [w_{ij}]_{N \times N}$, the degree matrix $\mathbf{D} = diag(D_1, \ldots, D_N)$ with $D_j = \sum_{i=1}^{N} w_{ij}$, and the transition matrix $\mathbf{P} = \mathbf{D}^{-1} \times \mathbf{W}$. We also define $\tilde{\mathbf{b}} = [\tilde{b}_i]_{N \times 1}$ as starting locations of the random walker where $\tilde{b}_i = 1$ if v_i is within distance s from tumor seed points and $\tilde{b}_i = 0$ otherwise. The random walker iteratively steps to a neighboring location with the probability proportional to the edge weight. Also, it has a restarting probability c to return to the seed points. Our shape prior for tumors is calculated as the steady-state probability of the random walker for the transition matrix $\mathbf{P}$:

$$[p_E(\mathcal{T}_{TU} | \eta^*, \mathbf{x}_i)]_{N \times 1} \propto c(\mathbf{I} - (1 - c)\mathbf{P})^{-1} \tilde{\mathbf{b}},$$
(7)

where $\mathbf{x}_i$ is a location of a node v_i. In Fig. 1 (g), we show the tumor shape prior obtained using (7) on the subject scan shown in (a)-(b). This shape prior shows high probability values in the tumor region.

Returning to the JSR problem (4), we obtain $\mathbf{q}^*$, $\boldsymbol{h}^*$, and $\boldsymbol{\Phi}^*$ via an implementation of the Expectation Maximization (EM) algorithm [13]. The EM algorithm iteratively determines the solution by computing the posterior

$$p(\mathcal{T}_t|Y,\mathbf{x}) \triangleq p(\mathcal{T}_t|Y,\mathbf{q}',\boldsymbol{h}',\boldsymbol{\Phi}',\mathbf{x}) \propto p(\mathcal{T}_t|\mathbf{q}',\boldsymbol{h}'(\mathbf{x})) \cdot p(Y|\mathcal{T}_t,\boldsymbol{\Phi}',\mathbf{x}) \qquad (8)$$

in the E-Step and updating the parameters in the M-Step by sequentially maximizing the following cost function

$$Q\{(\mathbf{q},\boldsymbol{h},\boldsymbol{\Phi});(\mathbf{q}',\boldsymbol{h}',\boldsymbol{\Phi}')\}$$
$$\triangleq \sum_{\mathbf{x}\in\Omega}\sum_{t\in\Theta} p(\mathcal{T}_t|Y,\mathbf{x}) \cdot \log\Big(p(\mathcal{T}_t|\mathbf{q},\boldsymbol{h},\mathbf{x}) \cdot p(Y|\mathcal{T}_t,\boldsymbol{\Phi},\mathbf{x}) \cdot p(\mathbf{q},\boldsymbol{h}|\eta^*,\mathbf{x})\Big) . \qquad (9)$$

In detail, $\boldsymbol{\Phi}'$ is obtained from $\arg\max_{\boldsymbol{\Phi}} Q\{(\mathbf{q}',\boldsymbol{h}',\boldsymbol{\Phi});(\mathbf{q}',\boldsymbol{h}',\boldsymbol{\Phi}')\}$ using a closed form of [7] and $\boldsymbol{h}'$ is obtained from $\arg\max_{\boldsymbol{h}} Q\{(\mathbf{q}',\boldsymbol{h},\boldsymbol{\Phi}');(\mathbf{q}',\boldsymbol{h}',\boldsymbol{\Phi}')\}$ which iteratively can be solved as in [2]. For updating $\mathbf{q}$, we maximize $Q\{(\mathbf{q},\boldsymbol{h}',\boldsymbol{\Phi}');(\mathbf{q}',\boldsymbol{h}',\boldsymbol{\Phi}')\}$ using a derivative-free pattern search library [4] as there exists no analytical expression for the derivatives of this function with respect to $\mathbf{q}$. We iterate E-Step and M-Step until convergence is achieved. After convergence, we assign $\{\mathbf{q}',\boldsymbol{h}',\boldsymbol{\Phi}'\}$ to $\{\mathbf{q}^*,\boldsymbol{h}^*,\boldsymbol{\Phi}^*\}$, respectively. We show aligned spatial probabilities in Fig. 1 (j)-(m) optimized via the EM algorithm. These spatial probabilities and the tumor posterior (computed using (8)) shown in (n) now fit well to healthy tissue and pathological regions shown in (a)-(b).

4   Experiments

Our method is semi-automatic and requires minimal user inputs including seed point and radius for each tumor to initialize $\mathbf{q}$ and one sample point for each tissue class to initialize means of $\boldsymbol{\Phi}$. For preprocessing, we co-registered all four modalities (T1, T1-CE, T2, and FLAIR), corrected MR field inhomogeneity, and scaled intensities to fit $[0,255]$. We solved the tumor growth model on a lattice of $64\times64\times64$ nodes for efficiency reasons. To differentiate enhancing tumor (ET) and others (NT) including necrosis and non-enhancing core within tumor regions,

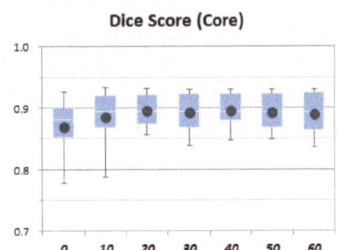

Fig. 2. Box plots of Dice score (core) for varying $\lambda \in [0,60]$

we assume all sub-structures of tumor are equally probable, i.e. $p(\mathcal{T}_{ET}|\mathbf{q},\mathbf{x}) = p(\mathcal{T}_{NT}|\mathbf{q},\mathbf{x}) = p(\mathcal{T}_{TU}|\mathbf{q},\mathbf{x})/2$. In experiments, we substitute TU in Θ as $\{ET,NT\}$. To find best λ in (5), we measured Dice scores for the tumor core region over $\lambda \in [0,60]$ using the training data consisting of 10 subjects having

Table 1. BRATS 2013 Leaderboard Results (Top 4)

Method	Dice whole	core	active	PPV whole	core	active	Sensitivity whole	core	active	Rank whole	core	total
Kwon	0.86	0.79	0.59	0.88	0.84	0.60	0.86	0.81	0.63	**2.00**	**1.33**	**1.89**
Zhao	0.83	0.73	0.55	0.77	0.67	0.46	0.94	0.89	0.78	2.67	3.00	3.67
Tustison	0.79	0.65	0.53	0.83	0.70	0.51	0.81	0.73	0.66	4.33	4.00	4.78
Guo	0.79	0.71	0.50	0.73	0.77	0.50	0.88	0.76	0.60	5.33	2.67	5.56

manual segmentations. As shown in Fig. 2, Dice scores were not significantly different on $\lambda \in [10, 60]$ ($p > 0.1$ using the Wilcoxon signed-rank test) and we chose $\lambda = 40$ for all experiments. For the shape prior in (7), we used $c = 0.0004$ as suggested by [5], $s = 5mm$, and $\sigma = \max_{ij}\{||\mathbf{y}_i - \mathbf{y}_j||^2\}/60$.

We tested our method to the BRATS 2013 leaderboard data via the BRATS online tools [9]. The leaderboard data set is the main data set used for comparing results of participants of BRATS [10] and it consists of 21 high-grade and 4 low-grade glioma subjects. When segmentation results are uploaded to the online tools the performance is measured using manual segmentation labels which are not available for download. The performance measures include Dice scores, positive predictive value (PPV), and sensitivity for three interest regions: whole (complete abnormal regions including tumor and edema), core (tumor regions), and active (enhancing regions of tumor). The top 4 results among 16 participants excerpted from [9] are shown in Table 1. *Zhao* and *Guo* used generative models based on a learned MRF model on supervoxel clusters and active contours with manual initializations, respectively. *Tustison* used a discriminative model based on the decision forest [16]. Note that *Tustison* and *Zhao* are fully-automatic methods and might therefore be at a disadvantage in this comparisons. The details of performance measures and participants' methods are described in [10]. Our method (*Kwon*) performed best among all participants and showed highest average ranks for all regions. The score gap with respect to other participants for the core region is bigger than those of the other regions, which means our method performed especially well for segmenting core regions. The average running time of our method was 85 min on an Intel Core i7 3.4 GHz machine with Windows operating system. Considering it usually takes under 10 min for the user input, the total running time is comparable to *Tustison* [10].

In Fig. 3, segmentation and registration results from our method are displayed. The spatial probabilities aligned to the scan in (d)-(g) show that they fit well to the scan. The tumor shape priors in (h) help to align spatial probabilities for tumor as they initially estimate tumor regions reasonably well. However, our method also showed robust estimation of tumor regions when the shape prior leaked into nearby regions as indicated by arrow in the fourth row of (h). The spatial probabilities for tumor were not expanded to this leaked region as the image likelihood for tumor kept lower values than those of healthy tissues on this region during the EM iterations. As a result, segmentations in (c) show visually reasonable tissue estimation especially for *ET*, *NT*, and *ED* regions.

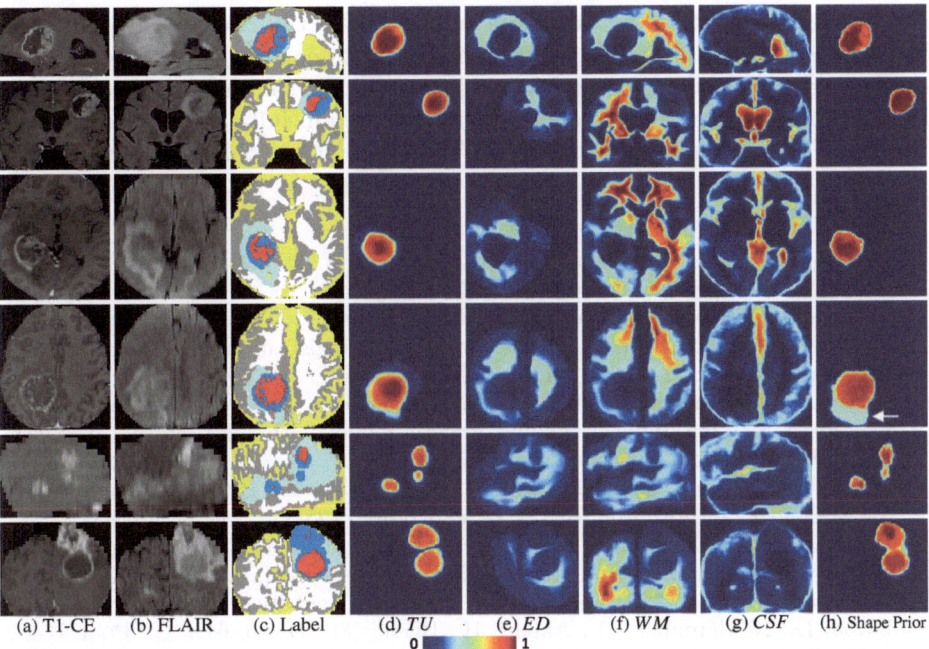

(a) T1-CE   (b) FLAIR   (c) Label   (d) *TU*   (e) *ED*   (f) *WM*   (g) *CSF*   (h) Shape Prior

0 ▬▬▬▬ 1

Fig. 3. Segmentation and registration results for 6 subjects selected from the BRATS 2013 leaderboard data set. The top 4 rows show a single-focal glioma and bottom 2 rows show multi-focal gliomas. We show subject images in (a)-(b), segmentation results in (c) (indicating ET, NT, ED, WM, GM, and CSF in blue, red, cyan, white, gray, and yellow colors, respectively), spatial probabilities $p(\mathcal{T}_t|\mathbf{q}, \boldsymbol{h}, \mathbf{x})$ in (d)-(g), and tumor shape priors in (h).

5   Conclusion

In this paper, we proposed a new joint segmentation and registration method for multifocal glioma images. This method allows multiple tumor seed points to grow each focal mass and combines them to single tumor density for modifying a normal atlas into one with tumors and edema. To perform robustly on tumors having complex shapes and heterogeneous textures, we incorporate a tumor shape prior directly estimated from images into our framework. We then find the optimal solution via the EM algorithm. Our method was evaluated on the BRATS 2013 leaderboard data set and showed the best performance among all participants. Although we only quantitatively validated our segmentation results, our method also produces mappings between a normal atlas and subject scan and simultaneously estimates tumor parameters. These additional results of our method could be used for understanding brain tumor development and for the development of location-based biomarkers. We also expect that our method could improve the registration of pre-operative and post-recurrence brain scans for multifocal gliomas [6].

Acknowledgement. This work was supported by the National Institutes of Health (NIH) under Grant R01 NS042645. Brain tumor image data used in this article were obtained from the MICCAI 2013 Challenge on Multimodal Brain Tumor Segmentation. The challenge database contain fully anonymized images from the Cancer Imaging Archive (TCIA) and the BRATS 2012 challenge.

References

1. Giannopoulos, S., Kyritsis, A.P.: Diagnosis and Management of Multifocal Gliomas. Oncology 79(3-4), 306–312 (2010)
2. Gooya, A., Pohl, K.M., Billelo, M., Cirillo, L., Biros, G., Melhem, E.R., Davatzikos, C.: GLISTR: Glioma Image Segmentation and Registration. IEEE Trans. Med. Imaging 31(10), 1941–1954 (2012)
3. Hogea, C., Davatzikos, C., Biros, G.: An image-driven parameter estimation problem for a reaction-diffusion glioma growth model with mass effects. J. Math. Biol. 56(6), 793–825 (2008)
4. Hough, P.D., Kolda, T.G., Torczon, V.J.: Asynchronous Parallel Pattern Search for Nonlinear Optimization. SIAM J. Sci. Comput. 23(1), 134–156 (2001)
5. Kim, T.-H., Lee, K.M., Lee, S.U.: Generative Image Segmentation Using Random Walks with Restart. In: Forsyth, D., Torr, P., Zisserman, A. (eds.) ECCV 2008, Part III. LNCS, vol. 5304, pp. 264–275. Springer, Heidelberg (2008)
6. Kwon, D., Niethammer, M., Akbari, H., Bilello, M., Davatzikos, C., Pohl, K.M.: PORTR: Pre-Operative and Post-Recurrence Brain Tumor Registration. IEEE Trans. Med. Imaging 33(3), 651–667 (2014)
7. Leemput, K.V., Maes, F., Vandermeulen, D., Suetens, P.: Automated Model-Based Bias Field Correction of MR Images of the Brain. IEEE Trans. Med. Imaging 18(10), 885–896 (1999)
8. Louis, D.N.: Molecular Pathology of Malignant Gliomas. Annu. Rev. Pathol. Mech. Dis. 1, 97–117 (2006)
9. Menze, B.H., et al.: The BRATS Online Tools - Multimodal Brain Tumor Segmentation, BRATS (2013), http://www.virtualskeleton.ch/BRATS/Start2013
10. Menze, B.H., et al.: The Multimodal Brain Tumor Image Segmentation Benchmark, BRATS (2014), http://hal.inria.fr/hal-00935640
11. Morris, C.N.: Parametric Empirical Bayes Inference: Theory and Applications. J. Am. Statist. Assoc. 78(381), 47–55 (1983)
12. Parisot, S., Wells, W., Chemouny, S., Duffau, H., Paragios, N.: Concurrent tumor segmentation and registration with uncertainty-based sparse non-uniform graphs. Med. Image Anal. 18(4), 647–659 (2014)
13. Pohl, K.M., Fisher, J., Grimson, W.E.L., Kikinis, R., Wells, W.M.: A Bayesian model for joint segmentation and registration. NeuroImage 31(1), 228–239 (2006)
14. Sanai, N., Berger, M.S.: Glioma Extent of Resection and Its Impact on Patient Outcome. Neurosurgery 62(4), 753–766 (2008)
15. Verma, R., Zacharaki, E.I., Ou, Y., Cai, H., Chawla, S., Lee, S.K., Melhem, E.R., Wolf, R., Davatzikos, C.: Multiparametric Tissue Characterization of Brain Neoplasms and Their Recurrence Using Pattern Classification of MR Images. Acad. Radiol. 15(8), 966–977 (2008)
16. Zikic, D., Glocker, B., Konukoglu, E., Criminisi, A., Demiralp, C., Shotton, J., Thomas, O.M., Das, T., Jena, R., Price, S.J.: Decision Forests for Tissue-Specific Segmentation of High-Grade Gliomas in Multi-channel MR. In: Ayache, N., Delingette, H., Golland, P., Mori, K. (eds.) MICCAI 2012, Part III. LNCS, vol. 7512, pp. 369–376. Springer, Heidelberg (2012)

Partial Volume Estimation in Brain MRI Revisited

Alexis Roche[1,2,3] and Florence Forbes[4,5]
for the Alzheimer's Disease Neuroimaging Initiative*

[1] Siemens Advanced Clinical Imaging Technology, Lausanne, Switzerland
[2] Department of Radiology, CHUV, Lausanne, Switzerland
[3] Signal Processing Laboratory (LTS5), EPFL, Lausanne, Switzerland
[4] Mistis Project, INRIA, Grenoble, France
[5] Grenoble University, Laboratoire Jean Kuntzmann, Grenoble, France

Abstract. We propose a fast algorithm to estimate brain tissue concentrations from conventional T1-weighted images based on a Bayesian maximum a posteriori formulation that extends the "mixel" model developed in the 90's. A key observation is the necessity to incorporate additional prior constraints to the "mixel" model for the estimation of plausible concentration maps. Experiments on the ADNI standardized dataset show that global and local brain atrophy measures from the proposed algorithm yield enhanced diagnosis testing value than with several widely used soft tissue labeling methods.

1 Introduction

Image-guided diagnosis of brain disease calls for accurate morphometry algorithms, e.g., in order to detect focal atrophy patterns relating to early-stage progression of particular forms of dementia. To date, widely used brain morphometry packages rest upon discrete Markov random field (MRF) image segmentation models [1, 2] that ignore, or do not fully account for *partial voluming*, leading to potentially inaccurate estimation of tissue volumes. Although several partial volume (PV) estimation methods have been proposed in the literature from the early 90's [3–8], none of them seems to be in common use.

One difficulty with PV estimation from a single real-valued image is the necessity to incorporate strong prior knowledge. As already observed in [3], for a number K of tissues, a maximum likelihood approach leads to solving for each voxel one equation with $K - 1$ unknown concentrations, which has multiple solutions when $K > 2$. This is easily understood by considering an example of

---

* Data used in preparation of this article were obtained from the Alzheimer's Disease Neuroimaging Initiative (ADNI) database (adni.loni.ucla.edu). As such, the investigators within the ADNI contributed to the design and implementation of ADNI and/or provided data but did not participate in analysis or writing of this report. A complete listing of ADNI investigators can be found at: http://adni.loni.ucla.edu/wp-content/uploads/how_to_apply/ADNI_Acknowledgement_List.pdf

P. Golland et al. (Eds.): MICCAI 2014, Part I, LNCS 8673, pp. 771–778, 2014.
© Springer International Publishing Switzerland 2014

T1-weighted brain MR image where the mean intensity values of cerebrospinal fluid (CSF), gray matter (GM) and white matter (WM) are, say, 50, 150, and 250, respectively. Any voxel in the brain with intensity 150 could contain either 100% GM, or 50% CSF and 50% WM, or any concentrations of CSF, GM and WM that match an average intensity of 150. A possibility to disambiguate the problem is to use multichannel MR images [3, 9], which have the effect to increase the number of constraints on the unknown concentrations but are only available from specific clinical protocols.

There exist soft labeling methods that compute tissue weights which are sometimes incorrectly interpreted as concentrations. For instance, the variational expectation-maximization (VEM) algorithm for discrete MRF models [1, 10] computes posterior membership probabilities assuming a single tissue per voxel. Tissue weights output by the fuzzy C-mean [11, 12] or random walker [13] algorithms have no clear relation to PV.

Some authors have proposed to estimate PV in the conventional discrete segmentation framework by including labels that represent mixed tissue classes modeled by intensity distributions that may physically reflect PV effects [14], or be computationally more convenient Gaussian distributions [2, 15]. Such approaches have the potential to pinpoint voxels affected by strong PV, but are expected to underestimate PV overall. Another strategy that stays within the framework of discrete MRF models is to perform tissue classification at super-resolution, hence completing a more ambitious task than estimating voxelwise tissue concentrations. This was tackled in [7] using a Monte Carlo variant of the VEM algorithm, which appears to require heavy computation and memory load.

2   A Regularized Tissue Concentration Model

2.1   Bayesian Formulation

We propose to revisit methods that rely on *continuous* MRFs and formulate tissue concentration estimation as a Bayesian maximum a posteriori (MAP) problem following [3, 4, 6, 8]. Let Y denote an input MR image previously submitted to various artifact corrections and skull stripping. We assume the following image appearance model within the intra-cranial mask:

$$y_i = \boldsymbol{\mu}^\top \mathbf{q}_i + \varepsilon_i, \qquad \varepsilon_i \sim N(0, \sigma), \tag{1}$$

where y_i denotes intensity at voxel with index i, $\mathbf{q}_i$ is the associated tissue concentration vector, $\boldsymbol{\mu}$ is the 3-dimensional vector of tissue means corresponding to CSF, GM and WM, respectively, and σ is the noise standard deviation. The assumption of Gaussian noise with constant σ across tissues is justified under large SNR for amplitude images, and more generally for phase array sum-of-squares images, as a first-order approximation to the noncentral chi distributed noise derived from imaging physics [16, 17]. Note that, in discrete labeling models, it is common to assume tissue-dependent variances to account for both acquisition noise and PV effects, however PV effects are modeled deterministically here.

Unknown in (1) are the concentration map $Q = (\mathbf{q}_1, \mathbf{q}_2, \ldots)$ and the global parameters $(\boldsymbol{\mu}, \sigma)$. A maximum likelihood estimation approach would lead to minimize w.r.t. Q, $\boldsymbol{\mu}$ and σ:

$$-2 \log P(Y|Q, \boldsymbol{\mu}, \sigma) = n \log 2\pi\sigma^2 + \frac{1}{\sigma^2} \sum_i (y_i - \boldsymbol{\mu}^\top \mathbf{q}_i)^2, \tag{2}$$

where n is the total number of voxels. As mentioned in the introduction, this is an ill-posed problem. Consider for instance a voxel where the intensity y_i is within the extremal values of $\boldsymbol{\mu}$; we then have an infinity of $\mathbf{q}_i$'s for which $y_i = \boldsymbol{\mu}^\top \mathbf{q}_i$, hence minimizing $(y_i - \boldsymbol{\mu}^\top \mathbf{q}_i)^2$. Moreover, it can be seen that by choosing Q in this fashion, the likelihood becomes infinite for $\sigma = 0$ and $\boldsymbol{\mu}$ with extremal values $\mu_1 = -\infty$ and $\mu_3 = +\infty$. Therefore, maximum likelihood estimators of Q, $\boldsymbol{\mu}$ and σ are both non-unique and physically implausible.

In order to regularize the problem, we add a prior under the form $P(Q, \boldsymbol{\mu}, \sigma) = P(Q)P(\boldsymbol{\mu}, \sigma)$ that expresses three types of knowledge: 1) voxels with mild PV are more frequent than with strong PV; 2) tissue concentration maps are spatially smooth; and 3) mean tissue intensities are bounded. The first two constraints are achieved by:

$$P(Q) \propto e^{-\frac{1}{2}\sum_i \mathbf{q}_i^\top V_\alpha \mathbf{q}_i - \frac{\beta}{2}\sum_{i,j \in \mathcal{N}_i} \|\mathbf{q}_i - \mathbf{q}_j\|^2}, \qquad \text{with} \quad V_\alpha = \begin{pmatrix} 0 & \alpha_1 & \alpha_2 \\ \alpha_1 & 0 & \alpha_3 \\ \alpha_2 & \alpha_3 & 0 \end{pmatrix}, \tag{3}$$

where V_α is a symmetric hollow matrix parametrized by a fixed vector $\boldsymbol{\alpha} \succeq 0$, $\beta > 0$ is another fixed parameter and $\mathcal{N}_i$ stands for the set of neighbors of voxel i in the intra-cranial mask according to a 6-topology in this work. In the limit where $\min \boldsymbol{\alpha} \to \infty$, each term $\mathbf{q}_i^\top V_\alpha \mathbf{q}_i$ becomes infinite unless $\mathbf{q}_i$ concentrates on a single tissue, therefore the prior imposes a hard labeling constraint. The further term weighted by β is a classical interaction potential also used in [3, 4, 8] to favor smooth concentration maps.

As for the global parameters, we choose a prior that prevents an implausibly large gap between mean tissue intensities depending on additional real-valued parameters $\gamma > 0$ and m,

$$P(\boldsymbol{\mu}, \sigma) \propto e^{-\gamma \frac{n}{2\sigma^2} \|\boldsymbol{\mu} - m\mathbf{1}\|^2}, \tag{4}$$

where $\mathbf{1}$ is the vector will all components equal to one. In our implementation, γ is fixed similarly to $\boldsymbol{\alpha}$ and β. Combining the likelihood (2) with the priors (3) and (4), we see that the MAP problem boils down to minimizing the following cost function:

$$C(Q, \boldsymbol{\mu}, \sigma, m) = n \log 2\pi\sigma^2 + \frac{1}{\sigma^2} \sum_i (y_i - \boldsymbol{\mu}^\top \mathbf{q}_i)^2 + \sum_i \mathbf{q}_i^\top V_\alpha \mathbf{q}_i$$

$$+ \beta \sum_{i,j \in \mathcal{N}_i} \|\mathbf{q}_i - \mathbf{q}_j\|^2 + \gamma \frac{n}{2\sigma^2} \|\boldsymbol{\mu} - m\mathbf{1}\|^2. \tag{5}$$

2.2   MAP Tracking Algorithm

It is natural to minimize (5) iteratively by alternating minimization along Q, $(\boldsymbol{\mu}, \sigma)$ and m, yielding three steps:

Step 1. Find the optimal concentration map Q at fixed $(\boldsymbol{\mu}, \sigma)$ and m, which amounts to a quadratic optimization problem subject to linear constraints since Q is restricted to the multidimensional simplex, i.e., $\forall i$, $\mathbf{q}_i \succeq 0$ and $\mathbf{q}_i^\top \mathbf{1} = 1$. This is effectively done by looping over voxels in arbitrary order and solving for each $\mathbf{q}_i$ with all other concentrations held fixed, yielding the following system:

$$\left(\frac{1}{\sigma^2}\boldsymbol{\mu}\boldsymbol{\mu}^\top + V_\alpha + 2\beta n_i \mathbf{I}\right) \mathbf{q}_i - \frac{y_i}{\sigma^2}\boldsymbol{\mu} - 2\beta \sum_{j \in \mathcal{N}_i} \mathbf{q}_j + \lambda \mathbf{1} + \boldsymbol{\nu} = 0,$$

where $n_i = \#\mathcal{N}_i \le 6$ is the number of grid neighbors of voxel i, I is the 3×3 identity matrix, and $(\lambda, \boldsymbol{\nu})$ are Karush-Kuhn-Tucker multipliers satisfying $\boldsymbol{\nu} \succeq 0$ and $\boldsymbol{\nu} \odot \mathbf{q}_i = \mathbf{0}$ that are determined using an active set algorithm [18].

Step 2. Compute the optimal $(\boldsymbol{\mu}, \sigma)$ at fixed Q and m, yielding:

$$\hat{\boldsymbol{\mu}} = \left(n\gamma\mathbf{I} + \sum_i \mathbf{q}_i\mathbf{q}_i^\top\right)^{-1}\left(n\gamma m + \sum_i y_i \mathbf{q}_i\right), \quad \hat{\sigma}^2 = \gamma\|\hat{\boldsymbol{\mu}} - m\mathbf{1}\|^2 + \frac{1}{n}\sum_i (y_i - \hat{\boldsymbol{\mu}}^\top \mathbf{q}_i)^2.$$

Step 3. Compute the optimal m at fixed Q and $(\boldsymbol{\mu}, \sigma)$: $\hat{m} = \boldsymbol{\mu}^\top \mathbf{1}/3$.

The algorithm is initialized with uniform concentrations, i.e. $\forall i$, $\mathbf{q}_i = 1/3$, $\boldsymbol{\mu}$ as the three main histogram modes detected using scale-space analysis [19], and a tiny deviation $\sigma = 10^{-5}$ to ensure that the likelihood term predominates in early iterations. Each iteration requires about 5 seconds using C/Python code for a typical brain MR image on a standard single processor, which could probably be cut down by further code optimization for Step 1.

The algorithm involves fixed parameters $\boldsymbol{\alpha}$, β and γ that were tuned using a BrainWeb simulated T1 image [20] so as to minimize the Hellinger distance w.r.t. the fuzzy tissue volumes provided by BrainWeb, yielding:

$$\boldsymbol{\alpha} = (10.5, 29486, 7)^\top, \qquad \beta = 1.2, \qquad \gamma = 0.005.$$

Note that because α_2 turned out very large, the algorithm optimized in this manner practically proscribes tissue mixing involving both CSF and WM. This helps PV estimation in most brain areas but also creates a systematic artefactual "GM rim" around the ventricles, as seen in Figure 1, which could be avoided using spatially varying priors.

2.3   Comparison with Other Methods

Our MAP formulation (5) generalizes some previously proposed PV estimation algorithms. The case $\boldsymbol{\alpha} = \mathbf{0}$ and $\gamma = 0$ was studied in [3, 4, 8]. The algorithm proposed in [6] corresponds to choosing a uniform $\boldsymbol{\alpha} = (\alpha, \alpha, \alpha)^\top$ and setting

$\beta = \frac{1}{2}\alpha$ and $\gamma = 0$. We observed from visual inspection that these special cases tend to massively overestimate PV on both BrainWeb and real data. Moreover, the γ parameter plays an essential role as it enables estimating intensity parameters μ and σ along with tissue concentrations, preventing convergence towards an absurd solution ($\mu_1 = -\infty$, $\mu_3 = +\infty$ and $\sigma = 0$), an issue that was overlooked in the above cited references.

Another related method, hereafter referred to as the Shattuck/Bach (SB) method [14, 15], relies on labeling voxels according to, e.g., 5 classes that represent pure CSF, GM and WM as well as mixed CSF/GM and GM/WM. This is done in [15] using a VEM algorithm that outputs membership posterior probability maps that are then converted into tissue concentrations using linear fractional content interpolation from adjacent pure tissue intensity means (see [21] for a statistical justification of linear interpolation). Figure 1 illustrates the quantization effect produced by this approach compared to the proposed algorithm.

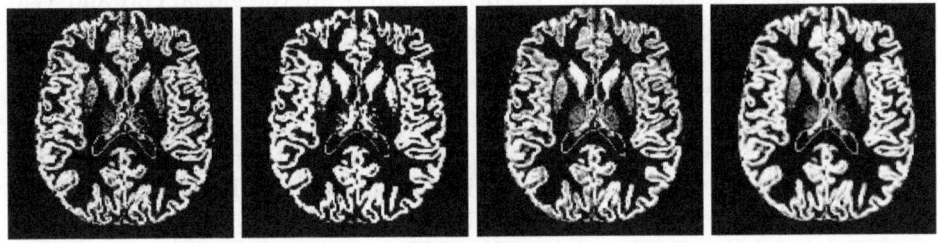

Fig. 1. Gray matter maps estimated from different methods for real data. From left to right, fuzzy C-mean, 3-class VEM, SB method, proposed MAP algorithm

3 Experiments

We evaluated several tissue labeling methods on a *standardized analysis set* [22] from the Alzheimer's Disease (AD) Neuroimaging Initiative (ADNI, adni.loni.ucla.edu) consisting of T1-weighted MR scans with approximately 1 mm³ voxel size, from different 1.5T and 3T acquisition systems. The set comprises 818 subjects, including 229 diagnosed as normal (NL), 401 as mild cognitively impaired (MCI), and 188 as AD. For each subject, we used by default the 1.5T screening scan, or the 3T baseline scan when available (as is the case for 151 subjects), corrected for gradient distortion, B1 inhomogeneity and bias field, as provided by ADNI. All images were further skull-stripped using diffeomorphic registration [23] with an in-house brain MR template, and a crude hippocampus segmentation was performed similarly using a hippocampus mask drawn on the template by a neurologist.

For each ADNI case, we estimated both the global brain tissue ratio (BTR) and the normalized hippocampus volume (NHV) using tissue concentration or pseudo-concentration maps output by four different algorithms: the proposed PV estimation algorithm, the fuzzy C-mean algorithm [11, 12], the VEM algorithm

Table 1. Cross-validated positive and negative likelihood ratios for linear classifiers using respectively age+BTR (top rows) and age+NHV (bottom rows) as features. The largest LR+ and smallest LR- are shown in bold for each comparison.

Marker	Comparison	MAP method		SB method		3-class VEM		Fuzzy C-mean	
		LR$_+$	LR$_-$	LR$_+$	LR$_-$	LR$_+$	LR$_-$	LR$_+$	LR$_-$
	AD vs NL	**2.177**	**0.278**	2.052	0.282	1.994	0.301	1.994	0.351
BTR	MCI vs NL	**1.661**	0.394	1.593	0.407	1.494	**0.385**	1.548	0.419
	AD vs MCI	**1.479**	0.671	1.468	0.679	1.431	0.675	1.463	**0.668**
	AD vs NL	**3.365**	0.165	3.147	0.169	2.865	0.170	3.022	**0.160**
NHV	MCI vs NL	**2.008**	**0.301**	1.911	0.309	1.723	0.347	1.891	0.315
	AD vs MCI	**1.803**	**0.611**	1.746	0.621	1.565	0.664	1.733	0.628

using a conventional 3-class Gaussian mixture model [1, 10], and the SB method using a 5-class model [15], see Section 2.3. The BTR was defined as BTR = $(vol_{GM} + vol_{WM})/vol_{TIV}$, where vol_{GM} and vol_{WM} are the global GM and WM volumes, respectively, and $vol_{TIV} = vol_{CSF} + vol_{GM} + vol_{WM}$ is the total intra-cranial volume. The NHV was defined as NHV = $(vol^*_{GM} + vol^*_{WM})/vol_{TIV}$, where vol^*_{GM} and vol^*_{WM} were the estimated GM and WM volumes within the crude hippocampus mask.

Both the 3-class and SB methods involve a Markov/Potts regularization parameter analogous to β that was optimized using the same BrainWeb matching criterion as for the proposed PV algorithm (see Section 2.2), respectively yielding $\beta = 0.2$ and $\beta = 0.4$ (note that the MAP algorithm was the one achieving the smallest minimal Hellinger distance w.r.t. the BrainWeb fuzzy maps). All algorithms were initialized by the same tissue means found by histogram mode detection [19] and tiny within-class standard deviations 10^{-5}, and run until variations on tissue maps were as small as for the MAP algorithm after 25 iterations. For the SB method, initial CSF/GM and GM/WM means were computed by averaging adjacent histogram modes.

Two-dimensional linear discriminant analysis classifiers using respectively age+BTR and age+NHV as features were implemented for each soft labeling method and cross-validated using a standard leave-one-out procedure in three distinct classification scenarios: AD vs NL, MCI vs NL, and AD vs MCI. Table 1 reports obtained positive and negative likelihood ratios, LR$_+$ = sensitivity/(1 − specificity) and LR$_-$ = (1 − sensitivity)/specificity, which represent post-test disease odds corresponding to even pre-test odds, respectively given a positive and negative test. The proposed PV estimation algorithm achieved the largest correct classification rate, largest LR$_+$ and nearly smallest LR$_-$ in all cases, suggesting its potential to improve diagnostic testing value over conventional atrophy detection methods. McNemar tests [24] were however short of significance, except for comparisons with the 3-class VEM using age+NHV, indicating that the improvement is mild on the simple classification strategies considered here.

4 Conclusion

This work contributes to demonstrate the feasibility of PV estimation from conventional T1-weighted images without resorting to additional image acquisitions. We have extended the "mixel" model originally proposed by Choi *et al* [3] and further developed in [4, 6, 8] so as to alleviate two important drawbacks. First, previous "mixel" models do not enable simultaneous updating of tissue concentration maps and global intensity parameters. Second, they tend to overestimate PV effects as they do not include a tissue homogeneity prior, or use too weak a prior [6].

Our disease classification experiments indicate that the proposed PV estimation algorithm enables more accurate detection of AD and MCI from simple volume biomarkers than conventional brain morphometry methods, thereby confirming the benefit of PV modeling for image-guided diagnosis. While the improvement is mild for the single-biomarker classifiers tested in this work, we anticipate that stronger effects could be seen in multi-dimensional classification using highly localized biomarkers (e.g. voxelwise concentrations), where accurate PV estimation would seem important to detect subtle atrophy patterns.

Extensions of the presented method using atlas-based priors may be needed to correct for systematic errors at the CSF/WM interface, as shown in Figure 1, as well as to tackle estimation of abnormal WM, which is frequent in elderly subjects and is characterized by a drop in WM intensity that makes it appear like GM. The use of atlas-based priors in image-guided diagnosis is however an open research topic as recent work suggests that conventional atlas-based tissue classification methods may lead to reduced population discrimination [25].

References

1. Van Leemput, K., Maes, F., Vandermeulen, D., Suetens, P.: Automated model-based tissue classification of MR images of the brain. IEEE Transactions on Medical Imaging 18(10), 897–908 (1999)
2. Ashburner, J., Friston, K.: Unified segmentation. NeuroImage 26(3), 839–851 (2005)
3. Choi, H.S., Haynor, D.R., Kim, Y.: Partial Volume Tissue Classification of Multichannel Magnetic Resonance Images – A Mixel Model. IEEE Transactions on Medical Imaging 10(3), 395–407 (1991)
4. Nocera, L., Gee, J.C.: Robust partial volume tissue classification of cerebral MRI scans. In: SPIE Medical Imaging. vol. 3034, pp. 312–322. SPIE (1997)
5. Laidlaw, D.H., Fleischer, K.W., Barr, A.H.: Partial-volume Bayesian classification of material mixtures in MR volume data using voxel histograms. IEEE Transactions on Medical Imaging 17(1), 74–86 (1998)
6. Pham, D.L., Prince, J.L.: Unsupervised partial volume estimation in single-channel image data. In: IEEE Workshop on Mathematical Methods in Biomedical Image Analysis (MMBIA), pp. 170–177. IEEE (2000)
7. Van Leemput, K., Maes, F., Vandermeulen, D., Suetens, P.: A Unifying Framework for Partial Volume Segmentation of Brain MR Images. IEEE Transactions on Medical Imaging 22(1), 105–119 (2003)
8. Liang, Z., Wang, S.: An EM Approach to MAP Solution of Segmenting Tissue Mixtures: A Numerical Analysis. IEEE Transactions on Medical Imaging 28(2), 297–310 (2009)

9. Duché, Q., Acosta, O., Gambarota, G., Merlet, I., Salvado, O., Saint-Jalmes, H.: Bi-exponential magnetic resonance signal model for partial volume computation. In: Ayache, N., Delingette, H., Golland, P., Mori, K. (eds.) MICCAI 2012, Part I. LNCS, vol. 7510, pp. 231–238. Springer, Heidelberg (2012)

10. Roche, A., Ribes, D., Bach-Cuadra, M., Krueger, G.: On the Convergence of EM-Like Algorithms for Image Segmentation using Markov Random Fields. Medical Image Analysis 15(6), 830–839 (2011)

11. Brandt, M.E., Bohant, T.P., Kramer, L.A., Fletcher, J.M.: Estimation of CSF, white and gray matter volumes in hydrocephalic children using fuzzy clustering of MR images. Computerized Medical Imaging and Graphics 18(1), 25–34 (1994)

12. Pham, D.L., Prince, J.L.: Adaptive fuzzy segmentation of magnetic resonance images. IEEE Transactions on Medical Imaging 18(9), 737–752 (1999)

13. Grady, L.: Random Walks for Image Segmentation. IEEE Transactions on Pattern Analysis and Machine Intelligence 28(11), 1768–1783 (2006)

14. Shattuck, D., Sandor-Leahy, S., Schaper, K., Rottenberg, D., Leahy, R.: Magnetic resonance image tissue classification using a partial volume model. NeuroImage 13(5), 856–876 (2001)

15. Bach Cuadra, M., Cammoun, L., Butz, T., Cuisenaire, O., Thiran, J.P.: Comparison and validation of tissue modelization and statistical classification methods in T1-weighted MR brain images. IEEE Transactions on Medical Imaging 24(12), 1548–1565 (2005)

16. Gudbjartsson, H., Patz, S.: The Rician Distribution of Noisy MRI Data. Magnetic Resonance in Medicine 34(6), 910–914 (1995)

17. Larsson, E.G., Erdogmus, D., Yan, R., Principe, J.C., Fitzsimmons, J.R.: SNR-optimality of sum-of-squares reconstruction for phased-array magnetic resonance imaging. Journal of Magnetic Resonance 163, 121–123 (2003)

18. Nocedal, J., Wright, S.: Numerical Optimization. Springer, New York (1999)

19. Dauguet, J., Mangin, J.-F., Delzescaux, T., Frouin, V.: Robust inter-slice intensity normalization using histogram scale-space analysis. In: Barillot, C., Haynor, D.R., Hellier, P. (eds.) MICCAI 2004. LNCS, vol. 3216, pp. 242–249. Springer, Heidelberg (2004)

20. Kwan, R.S., Evans, A., Pike, G.: MRI simulation-based evaluation of image-processing and classification methods. IEEE Transactions on Medical Imaging 18(11), 1085–1097 (1999)

21. González Ballester, M.A., Zisserman, A.P., Brady, M.: Estimation of the partial volume effect in MRI. Medical Image Analysis 6, 389–405 (2002)

22. Wyman, B., Harvey, D., Crawford, K., Bernstein, M., Carmichael, O., Cole, P., Crane, P., Decarli, C., Fox, N., Gunter, J., Hill, D., Killiany, R., Pachai, C., Schwarz, A., Schuff, N., Senjem, M., Suhy, J., Thompson, P., Weiner, M., Jack, C.: the Alzheimer's Disease Neuroimaging Initiative: Standardization of analysis sets for reporting results from ADNI MRI data. Alzheimer's & Dementia (2012)

23. Chefd'hotel, C., Hermosillo, G., Faugeras, O.: Flows of diffeomorphisms for multi-modal image registration. In: Proc. IEEE International Symposium on Biomedical Imaging, pp. 753–756 (2002)

24. Bostanci, B., Bostanci, E.: An evaluation of classification algorithms using Mc Nemar's test. In: Bansal, J.C., Singh, P.K., Deep, K., Pant, M., Nagar, A.K. (eds.) Proceedings of Seventh International Conference on Bio-Inspired Computing: Theories and Applications (BIC-TA 2012). AISC, vol. 201, pp. 15–26. Springer, Heidelberg (2013)

25. Ribes, D., Mortamet, B., Bach-Cuadra, M., Jack, C., Meuli, R., Krueger, G., Roche, A.: Comparison of tissue classification models for automatic brain MR segmentation. In: ISMRM, Montreal, Canada (2011)

Sparse Appearance Learning Based Automatic Coronary Sinus Segmentation in CTA

Shiyang Lu[1,3,*], Xiaojie Huang[2,3], Zhiyong Wang[1], and Yefeng Zheng[3]

[1] School of Information Technologies, The University of Sydney, Sydney, Australia
[2] Department of Electrical Engineering, Yale University, New Haven, CT
[3] Imaging and Computer Vision, Siemens Corporation, Corporate Technology, Princeton, NJ
yefeng.zheng@siemens.com

Abstract. Interventional cardiologists are often challenged by a high degree of variability in the coronary venous anatomy during coronary sinus cannulation and left ventricular epicardial lead placement for cardiac resynchronization therapy (CRT), making it important to have a precise and fully-automatic segmentation solution for detecting the coronary sinus. A few approaches have been proposed for automatic segmentation of tubular structures utilizing various vesselness measurements. Although working well on contrasted coronary arteries, these methods fail in segmenting the coronary sinus that has almost no contrast in computed tomography angiography (CTA) data, making it difficult to distinguish from surrounding tissues. In this work we propose a multiscale sparse appearance learning based method for estimating vesselness towards automatically extracting the centerlines. Instead of modeling the subtle discrimination at the low-level intensity, we leverage the flexibility of sparse representation to model the inherent spatial coherence of vessel/background appearance and derive a vesselness measurement. After centerline extraction, the coronary sinus lumen is segmented using a learning based boundary detector and Markov random field (MRF) based optimal surface extraction. Quantitative evaluation on a large cardiac CTA dataset (consisting of 204 3D volumes) demonstrates the superior accuracy of the proposed method in both centerline extraction and lumen segmentation, compared to the state-of-the-art.

1 Introduction

Coronary sinus cannulation is a challenging task in cardiac resynchronization therapy (CRT) for novice interventional cardiologists and low-volume operators. Failure to implant left ventricular lead occurs in up to 12% of the procedures as revealed by large clinical trials [1]. This is often due to inability to cannulate the coronary sinus or unfavorable venous anatomy resulting in the inability to find a stable lead position. Therefore, precisely localizing the coronary sinus becomes an urgent demand and would help interventional cardiologists to utilize prior knowledge of coronary venous anatomy for both the selection of patients suitable for CRT and guidance of lead implantation.

---

* Shiyang Lu and Xiaojie Huang contributed to this work while they were interns at Siemens Corporation, Corporate Technology. They contributed equally to this work.

P. Golland et al. (Eds.): MICCAI 2014, Part I, LNCS 8673, pp. 779–787, 2014.

Several segmentation methods have been proposed to facilitate the identification and localization of coronary venous anatomy from 3D whole-heart acquisitions in computed tomography angiography (CTA) or cardiac magnetic resonance (CMR). In [2], the heart segmentation is achieved automatically but the coronary venous anatomy has to be manually segmented by clinical experts. Sometimes, a few seed points have to be specified by a user to perform a semi-automatic segmentation of the coronary sinus [3,4]. In [5], a 3D cardiac model is applied to extract cardiac chambers and great vessels, including the proximal segment of the coronary sinus. However, the middle and distal segments of the coronary sinus have to be segmented manually. To the best of our knowledge, there is only one study [6] that addresses the fully automatic segmentation of the coronary sinus, which uses the segmented chambers to guide the extraction of coronary sinus.

Quite a few approaches have been proposed for automatic segmentation of coronary arteries in CTA data utilizing various vesselness measurements [7], which potentially can be adapted to segment the coronary sinus. However, most coronary artery segmentation methods are data-driven using no or little high-level prior knowledge, thereby lacking robustness under severe stenosis or low contrast. Recently, Zheng *et al.* [8] present a model-driven approach to predict the initial centerline of a major coronary artery. The initial centerline is further refined using a machine learning based vesselness measurement, which relies on the low-level image intensity features (e.g., it relies on the fact that a coronary artery is brighter than surrounding tissues in CTA). Although this method has achieved excellent robustness on extracting centerlines of coronary arteries (which are contrasted in CTA), it does not work well on coronary sinus because, unlike coronary arteries, the coronary sinus has very weak or no contrast at all in CTA. This presents a big challenge in distinguishing the coronary sinus from surrounding tissues. The problem is further complicated by the large intensity variations inside/outside the coronary sinus.

In this work, rather than modeling the weak discrimination at the low-level intensity, we exploit the flexibility of sparse representation to model the spatial coherence of local appearance inside and outside the coronary sinus. We propose a multiscale sparse appearance learning based approach to estimating a vesselness, which measures the probability of a voxel being at the center of the coronary sinus. Sparse learning has previously been shown to be effective in exploiting spatial coherence in several applications [9]. Here, we employ a multiscale sparse representation model of the local appearance of vessels and background tissues with two series of appearance dictionaries. The appearance dictionaries discriminate image patterns by reconstructing them in the process of sparse learning. We derive an appearance discriminant from the residues as the vesselness measurement score and incorporate the discriminant into a model-driven centerline extraction procedure [8]. After centerline extraction, the original CTA volume is resampled along the extracted centerline for the subsequent boundary detection. The optimal lumen surface is computed by correlating the boundary probabilities with a convex Markov random field (MRF) based graph optimization approach. Experiments on 204 CTA datasets demonstrate that the proposed approach clearly outperforms the state-of-the-art, leading to superior accuracy in both centerline extraction and lumen segmentation.

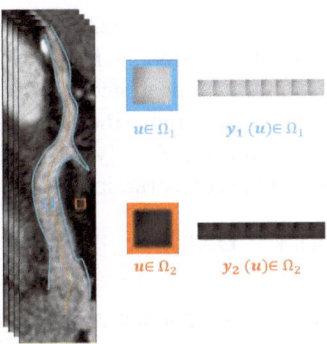

Fig. 1. Construction of appearance vectors for voxels inside (Ω_t^1) and outside (Ω_t^2) of the coronary sinus

2 Coronary Sinus Centerline Extraction

Model-Driven Centerline Extraction. Given an input volume, the heart chambers are segmented using the method presented in [10], and they are then used to predict the initial centerline of the coronary sinus. Afterward, a dynamic programming based optimization is applied to refine the initial centerline path. The initial centerline is represented as a set of evenly sampled points P_i, for $i = 0, 1, \ldots, n-1$. For each point P_i, 41×41 candidate positions P_i^j are uniformly sampled on a plane perpendicular to the centerline path at P_i. The candidates P_i^j are sampled on a regular grid of $20 \times 20\ mm^2$ (with grid spacing of $0.5\ mm$) centered at P_i. We then solve the following shortest path computation problem [8] to select the best position for each point P_i,

$$\bar{P}_0^{J(0)}, \bar{P}_1^{J(1)}, \ldots, \bar{P}_{n-1}^{J(n-1)} = argmin_{P_i^{J(i)}} \sum_{i-0}^{n-1} C(P_i^{J(i)}) + \omega \sum_{i-0}^{n-2} ||P_i^{J(i)} - P_{i+1}^{J(i+1)}||. \quad (1)$$

Here, the first term is the negative of vesselness, penalizing voxels not inside the coronary sinus. The second term is the total length of the path by summing the Euclidean distance between two neighboring points on the path. Free parameter ω, which is used to balance the two terms, is heuristically tuned on a few datasets and then fixed throughout the experiments. In [8], a vesselness measuring the likelihood of a voxel being at the vessel center is learned and estimated via low-level intensity features [11]. To overcome the limitations of this vesselness, in this work, we use a multiscale sparse learning based approach to estimate the likelihood.

Multiscale Sparse Learning for Vesselness Estimation. In cardiac CT images, vessels and background tissues present different appearance in terms of local image patterns. Let Ω denote the 3D image domain. We describe the multiscale local appearance at a voxel $\mathbf{u} \in \Omega$ with a series of appearance vectors $\mathbf{y}^s(\mathbf{u}) \in \mathbb{R}^n$ at different appearance scales $s = 1, \ldots, S$. $\mathbf{y}^s(\mathbf{u})$ is constructed by concatenating orderly the voxels within a block centered at $\mathbf{u}$, as illustrated in Fig. 1. In the following, to simplify the notation, we drop superscript s in $\mathbf{y}^s$ if it does not cause a confusion. Under a sparse model, an appearance vector $\mathbf{y} \in \mathbb{R}^n$ can be represented as a sparse linear combination of the atoms from an appearance dictionary $\mathbf{D} \in \mathbb{R}^{n \times K}$, $K > n$, which encodes the typical patterns of a corresponding appearance class. Different classes of local appearance are modeled with different appearance dictionaries. Learning an overcomplete dictionary $\mathbf{D} \in \mathbb{R}^{n \times K}$ from a training set $\mathbf{Y} = [\mathbf{y}_1, \ldots, \mathbf{y}_M]$ of M appearances is addressed by minimizing the following reconstruction residual error,

$$\min_{\mathbf{D}, \mathbf{X}} ||\mathbf{Y} - \mathbf{D}\mathbf{X}||_2^2, \ s.t., ||\mathbf{X}||_0 \leq T, \tag{2}$$

where $\mathbf{X} = [\mathbf{x}_1, \ldots, \mathbf{x}_K]$ represent the sparse representation of $\mathbf{Y}$ and T is a sparsity factor. We employ the K-SVD algorithm [12] to solve the dictionary learning problem.

For extracting the coronary sinus centerline, we need to discriminate the vessel and the background tissues. Let Ω^1 (the coronary sinus) and Ω^2 (background) denote two local appearance classes, which can be sparsely coded using two appearance dictionaries $\mathbf{D}_1$ and $\mathbf{D}_2$ trained with corresponding samples, respectively [9]. The reconstruction residue of an appearance vector $\mathbf{y}_i$ from class i with respect to dictionary $\mathbf{D}_c$ at the sth scale is defined as

$$\{R(\mathbf{y}_i(\mathbf{u}), \mathbf{D}_c)\}_s = ||\mathbf{y}_i^s(\mathbf{u}) - \{\mathbf{D}_c\hat{\mathbf{x}}_{ic}(\mathbf{u})\}_s||_2, \ \forall i, c \in \{1, 2\}, \tag{3}$$

where $\hat{\mathbf{x}}_{ic}$ is the sparse representation of $\mathbf{y}_i$ obtained via sparse learning (2). Intuitively, an appearance vector from Ω^1 should be reconstructed more accurately using the corresponding dictionary $\mathbf{D}_1$, and vice versa. It is naturally to expect that $\{R(\mathbf{y}_1(\mathbf{u}))\}_s > \{R(\mathbf{y}_2(\mathbf{u}))\}_s$ when $\mathbf{u} \in \Omega^2$, and $\{R(\mathbf{y}_1(\mathbf{u}))\}_s < \{R(\mathbf{y}_2(\mathbf{u}))\}_s$ when $\mathbf{u} \in \Omega^1$. We utilize this local appearance discrimination to estimate the likelihood of a voxel being at the coronary sinus center. By combining the multiscale discriminative information, we obtain a vesselness score for each voxel as

$$p(\mathbf{u}) = \sum_{s=1}^{S} w_s.sgn\{R(\mathbf{y}(\mathbf{u}), \mathbf{D}_2)_s - R(\mathbf{y}(\mathbf{u}), \mathbf{D}_1)_s\}, \tag{4}$$

where w_s is the weighting parameter of the sth appearance scale. This probability indicates the likelihood of voxel $\mathbf{u}$ being at the coronary sinus center, which can be incorporated into the shortest path computation (1) as the cost for a single node.

3   Coronary Sinus Lumen Segmentation

Once the centerline is extracted, the CTA volume is warped and resampled along the centerline path for the subsequent boundary detection. The optimal lumen surface is further computed by correlating the boundary probabilities with a convex Markov random field (MRF) based graph optimization approach [13]. This section describes the necessary steps to segment the coronary sinus lumen surface.

Warping the Volumetric Data.   In the first step of lumen segmentation, a warped and re-sampled version of the image volume is generated. The centerline is resampled to a certain resolution (e.g., $0.1 \ mm$) to get a homogeneous slice distance. For each

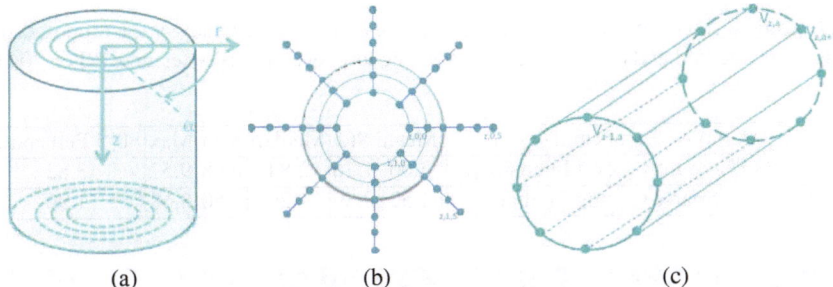

(a)   (b)   (c)

Fig. 2. Coronary sinus lumen segmentation. (a) A cylindrical coordinate space of the warped volume using an extracted centerline; (b) Ray-casting for a discrete sampling; and (c) The tubular MRF graph for lumen surface extraction.

centerline point, an image slice orthogonal to the vessel centerline is extracted where the image is interpolated with bi-linear interpolation at positions between voxels. As illustrated in Fig 2a, the height in the warped volume is expressed by the coordinate z, whereas the angle $\alpha \in [0, 2\pi)$ and the radial distance $r \in \mathbb{R} \geq 0$ uniquely define a point in the other two dimensions, as depicted in Fig. 2a.

Detecting Lumen Boundary. For each slice, R points along each of the T rays are generated. By this way, $T \times Z \times R$ directed candidate boundary points are generated. In this work we utilize the boundary classifier proposed in [10] to calculate boundary probability. Without loss of generality, the predicted boundary probability is a scalar between $[0, 1]$.

Segmenting Lumen Surface. At last, out of all potential boundary candidates we need to select the optimum boundary position as the final segmentation results. The problem is formulated as a first order Markov random field (MRF) with discrete multivariate random variables [13]. A globally optimal configuration for MRFs can be exactly found by calculating the minimal cut in a graph. We thus reduce the surface segmentation task to a network flow problem which can be solved efficiently using the max-flow algorithm.

We firstly re-organize all the boundary candidates in a form such that we can directly incorporate them as the probability distribution of an N_R-label graph-cut problem in the space, $\mathcal{X} = L^V = \{0 \ldots N_R - 1\}^{\{0 \ldots N_S - 1\} \times \{0 \ldots N_A - 1\}}$, where the probabilities of the candidates along with N_R-configurations of ray length are denoted as label assignments $L = \{0 \ldots N_R - 1\}$ for every slice N_S and every ray N_A. The corresponding candidates are denoted as the set of vertices V in MRF notation. Thus, a vertex $v_{z,a} \in V$ of the MRF graph represents one element in the problem domain as z is attached to the corresponding slice and a to the ray angle (see Fig. 2c). A network graph $\hat{G} = (\hat{V}, \hat{E})$ can be constructed with the dimensionality of $N_R \times N_S \times N_A$.

After the graph construction, the max-flow-min-cut algorithm proposed by Boykov and Kolmogorov [14] is utilized to estimate the lumen surface. The minimal "s-t" cut bi-partitions the network graph $\hat{G}$ into two groups S and T along the set of labels L such that each vertex $v_{z,a,i} \in V$ is assigned a unique label $i \in \{0, \ldots, N_R - 1\}$. The lumen surface can then be defined as a set of contours corresponding to the cross-sections.

Table 1. Comparison of the coronary sinus centerline extraction accuracy of the proposed sparse learning based method and previous vesselness using low-level intensity features [8] on 204 CTA datasets

Methods / Error (mm)	Mean	Std	Median	Min	Max	80th Percentile
Vesselness Using Low-Level Intensity [8]	3.00	1.26	2.84	0.98	9.57	3.82
Proposed Sparse Coding Method	1.52	0.89	1.29	0.50	8.68	1.92

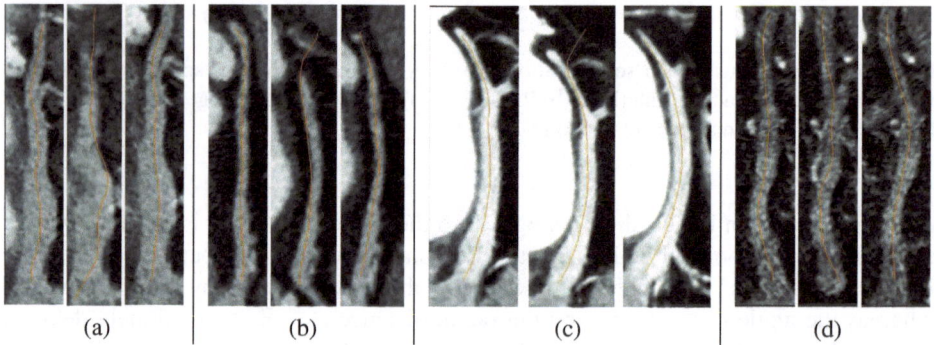

(a)   (b)   (c)   (d)

Fig. 3. Automatically extracted coronary sinus centerlines on four CTA volumes. For each volume, the first column shows the ground truth; the second column shows the centerline extracted using [8]; and the last column shows the centerline extracted using the proposed method.

Each contour is generated by determining the length of the N_A rays, resulting in a set of three-dimensional points that define the contour at a specific cross-section. The third dimension of the contour points is given by the index of the corresponding slice, which is attached to a centerline point. The estimated lumen surface in the warped volume is then transferred back to the original volume space.

4   Experiments

In this section we evaluate the proposed coronary sinus segmentation method on CTA data for both the centerline extraction and lumen segmentation. We collected a total of 204 cardiac CTA volumes and manually annotated coronary sinus centerline and lumen mesh for each volume. In our annotation, the coronary sinus starts from its ostium at the right atrium and ends at the bifurcation to great cardiac vein and left marginal vein. A 10-fold cross-validation is performed to evaluate the segmentation accuracy. We also compare our method with the state-of-the-art coronary artery centerline extraction method [8] re-trained for the coronary sinus.

Centerline Extraction Accuracy.   Two different centerline extraction algorithms are used to generate the centerline. Both algorithms are model-driven and the only difference is on the vesselness used for shortest path computation in (1). The first algorithm [8] utilizes the low-level intensity features to train a vesselness measurement [11]

Table 2. Coronary sinus lumen segmentation accuracy on 204 CTA datasets

Methods / Error (mm)	Mean	Std	Median	Min	Max	80th Percentile
Based on Centerlines Extracted Using [8]	2.10	1.14	1.92	0.44	7.54	2.80
Proposed Method	0.99	0.73	0.81	0.24	6.30	1.29

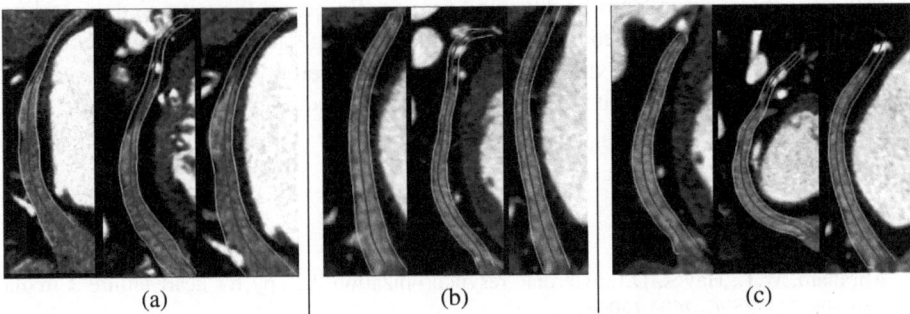

| (a) | (b) | (c) |

Fig. 4. Coronary sinus lumen segmentation results on three CTA datasets. For each volume, the first column shows the ground truth; the second column shows the segmentation based on centerlines extracted using [8]; and the last column shows the segmentation based on centerlines obtained with sparse learning.

and the second algorithm uses the proposed sparse learning based vesselness measurement.

Table 1 shows the centerline accuracy on the evaluation set. The proposed method clearly outperforms the low-level intensity based vesselness [11] with mean error of $1.52\ mm$ vs. $3.00\ mm$. It demonstrates that the multiscale sparse learning based vesselness is more effective in distinguishing the voxels inside and outside the coronary sinus. The maximum centerline error often occurs at the distal end, mainly due to the inaccuracy in determining sinus length. Using a dedicated end-point detector (which is missing in this work) may further improve the centerline accuracy. In Fig. 3, we show centerlines extracted using both approaches on a few representative volumes with various contrast concentration. The proposed method can handle large variation of contrast by the appearance dictionaries learned from a large training set, covering common variations observed in clinical practice. The variations are automatically encoded as different dictionary atoms after training.

Lumen Segmentation Accuracy. In the following experiments, we evaluate the coronary sinus lumen segmentation accuracy. As shown in Table 2, using the proposed method we achieve a mean mesh error of $0.99\ mm$. Since the lumen segmentation is based on the extracted centerline, the centerline accuracy affects the final lumen segmentation quality. Feeding the lumen segmentation module with the centerlines extracted using [8], we obtain a lumen segmentation error as large as $2.10\ mm$. Clearly, the multiscale sparse appearance learning based centerline extraction method is a valuable pre-processing step which leads to superior performance in lumen segmentation. Fig. 4 shows a few examples of the coronary sinus lumen segmentation results.

5   Conclusions

In this work we proposed a novel automatic coronary sinus centerline extraction method combining the advantages of the model-driven approach and multiscale sparse appearance learning. The sparse appearance learning based vesselness can effectively distinguish the coronary sinus from background tissues. Based on the extracted centerline, the lumen surface is segmented using a machine learning based boundary detector and MRF based optimal surface extraction. The proposed method has been evaluated on a large dataset of 204 CTA volumes, showing superior accuracy compared to the state-of-the-art.

References

1. Abraham, W.T., Hayes, D.L.: Cardiac resynchronization therapy for heart failure. Circulation 108(21), 2596–2603 (2003)
2. Ma, Y.L., Shetty, A.K., Duckett, S., Etyngier, P., Gijsbers, G., Bullens, R., Schaeffter, T., Razavi, R., Rinaldi, C.A., Rhode, K.S.: An integrated platform for image-guided cardiac resynchronization therapy. Physics in Medicine and Biology 57(10), 2953–2968 (2012)
3. Garcia, M.P., Toumoulin, C., Haigron, P., Velut, J., Garreau, M., Boulmier, D.: Coronary vein tracking from MSCT using a minimum cost path approach. In: IEEE International Conference on Biomedical Imaging, pp. 17–20 (2010)
4. Ordas, S., Oubel, E., Leta, R., Carreras, F., Frangi, A.F.: A statistical shape model of the heart and its application to model-based segmentation. In: Proc. of SPIE Conf. Medical Imaging, vol. 6511 (2007)
5. Duckett, S.G., Ginks, M.R., Knowles, B.R., Ma, Y., Shetty, A., Bostock, J., Cooklin, M., Gill, J.S., Carr-White, G.S., Razavi, R., Schaeffter, T., Rhode, K.S., Rinaldi, C.A.: Advanced image fusion to overlay coronary sinus anatomy with real-time fluoroscopy to facilitate left ventricular lead implantation in CRT. Pacing and Clinical Electrophysiology 34(2), 226–234 (2011)
6. Ecabert, O., Peters, J., Walker, M.J., Ivanc, T., Lorenz, C., von Berg, J., Lessick, J., Vembar, M., Weese, J.: Segmentation of the heart and great vessels in CT images using a model-based adaptation framework. Medical Image Analysis 15(6), 863–876 (2011)
7. Lesage, D., Angelini, E.D., Bloch, I., Funka-Lea, G.: A review of 3D vessel lumen segmentation techniques: Models, features and extraction schemes. Medical Image Analysis 13(6), 819–845 (2009)
8. Zheng, Y., Tek, H., Funka-Lea, G.: Robust and accurate coronary artery centerline extraction in CTA by combining model-driven and data-driven approaches. In: Mori, K., Sakuma, I., Sato, Y., Barillot, C., Navab, N. (eds.) MICCAI 2013, Part III. LNCS, vol. 8151, pp. 74–81. Springer, Heidelberg (2013)
9. Huang, X., Dione, D.P., Compas, C.B., Papademetris, X., Lin, B.A., Sinusas, A.J., Duncan, J.S.: A dynamical appearance model based on multiscale sparse representation: Segmentation of the left ventricle from 4D echocardiography. In: Ayache, N., Delingette, H., Golland, P., Mori, K. (eds.) MICCAI 2012, Part III. LNCS, vol. 7512, pp. 58–65. Springer, Heidelberg (2012)
10. Zheng, Y., Barbu, A., Georgescu, B., Scheuering, M., Comaniciu, D.: Four-chamber heart modeling and automatic segmentation for 3-D cardiac CT volumes using marginal space learning and steerable features. IEEE Transactions on Medical Imaging 27(11), 1668–1681 (2008)

11. Zheng, Y., Loziczonek, M., Georgescu, B., Zhou, S.K., Vega-Higuera, F., Comaniciu, D.: Machine learning based vesselness measurement for coronary artery segmentation in cardiac CT volumes. In: Proc. of SPIE Medical Imaging. vol. 7962, pp. 1–12 (2011)
12. Aharon, M., Elad, M., Bruckstein, A.: K-SVD: An algorithm for designing overcomplete dictionaries for sparse representation. IEEE Transactions on Signal Processing 54(11), 4311–4322 (2006)
13. Ishikawa, H.: Exact optimization for Markov random fields with convex priors. IEEE Trans. Pattern Anal. Machine Intell. 25(10), 1333–1336 (2003)
14. Boykov, Y., Kolmogorov, V.: An experimental comparison of min-cut/max-flow algorithms for energy minimization in vision. IEEE Transactions on Pattern Analysis and Machine Intelligence 26(9), 1124–1137 (2004)

Optic Cup Segmentation for Glaucoma Detection Using Low-Rank Superpixel Representation

Yanwu Xu[1], Lixin Duan[1], Stephen Lin[2], Xiangyu Chen[1],
Damon Wing Kee Wong[1], Tien Yin Wong[3], and Jiang Liu[1]

[1] Institute for Infocomm Research, Agency for Science, Technology and Research, Singapore
[2] Microsoft Research, P.R. China
[3] Department of Ophthalmology, National University of Singapore, Singapore

Abstract. We present an unsupervised approach to segment optic cups in fundus images for glaucoma detection without using any additional training images. Our approach follows the superpixel framework and domain prior recently proposed in [1], where the superpixel classification task is formulated as a low-rank representation (LRR) problem with an efficient closed-form solution. Moreover, we also develop an adaptive strategy for automatically choosing the only parameter in LRR and obtaining the final result for each image. Evaluated on the popular *ORIGA* dataset, the results show that our approach achieves better performance compared with existing techniques.

1 Introduction

Glaucoma is the second leading cause of blindness worldwide [2], and cannot be cured because the damage to the optic nerve is irreversible. Early detection is thus essential for early treatment and preventing the deterioration of vision.

Among the structural image cues studied for glaucoma diagnosis, the vertical optic cup-to-disc ratio CDR is a major consideration of clinicians [3]. However, clinical assessment by manually annotating the cup and disc for each image is labor-intensive, so automatic methods have been proposed to segment the disc and cup in fundus images. Recently, optic cup segmentation has attracted relatively more attention, since the disc segmentation problem is well-studied in the literature.

Various automated optic cup segmentation methods have been presented, by using traditional image segmentation methods such as level-sets [4] and active shape model (ASM) [5], or using a classification method to identify pixels [6] or regions [7] that are part of the cup or rim (the disc area outside the cup). Comparatively, classification methods show better segmentation accuracy than traditional segmentation methods, by learning prior knowledge from additional training samples. Recently, an interesting superpixel classification framework was proposed in [1], in which superpixel labeling is a key module that pre-learns a linear SVM model from additional samples, or learns a discriminative model on the test image itself using a domain prior in which superpixels near the disc center are always in the cup and ones close to the disc boundary belong to the rim (non-cup). Although the latter method is still a supervised method, no additional training samples are needed. An unsupervised similarity based propagation method is also introduced in [1], but it is lacking in accuracy.

P. Golland et al. (Eds.): MICCAI 2014, Part I, LNCS 8673, pp. 788–795, 2014.

In this work, we employ the same framework [1] of superpixel labeling except that we take an *unsupervised* approach. Based on the domain prior together with the low-rank property of the data, we model the labeling problem from another perspective. Specifically, it is formulated as a low-rank representation (LRR) problem, which can be efficiently solved in closed form. In addition, to avoid manual parameter tuning, an adaptive approach is developed based on analyzing the closed-form solution of the proposed LRR problem. Specifically, we firstly determine with some theoretical guidance a small number of parameter candidates that cover the whole range, and then obtain the final label of each superpixel by fusing the labels corresponding to each candidate parameter by majority voting.

2 Adaptive Low-Rank Reconstruction Based Superpixel Clustering

The superpixel labeling framework proposed in [1] has four major steps as follows:

1. Use the SLIC [8] toolbox to divide an input disc into superpixels;
2. Remove superpixels that lie on blood vessels, since they appear similar whether they lie in the cup or rim;
3. Label each superpixel as belonging either to cup or rim, using different methods;
4. Apply post-processing to obtain a unique ellipse representing the output cup boundary.

In this work, we follow the exact same procedure as in [1] except that we propose a new LRR based unsupervised approach for the major step of superpixel labeling.

2.1 Low-Rank Representation Formulation

Superpixel labeling is essentially a binary clustering problem, in which the two classes correspond to the optic cup and rim, respectively. As illustrated in Fig. 1, superpixels within the optic disc appear similar to each other. Moreover, in an ideal situation where superpixels are similar in the same class but are dissimilar between different classes, the superpixels in each disc image would form only two clusters (corresponding to cup and rim respectively).

Formally, we assume that the given data (feature matrix of superpixels) $\mathbf{X} \in \mathbb{R}^{d \times n}$ come from two linearly independent subspaces, where d is the feature dimension and n is the number of superpixels in a given image. Moreover, the data should have the following self-expressiveness property: each data point (*i.e.* a superpixel) $\mathbf{x}_i$ in the given data (*i.e.* feature matrix of all superpixels in a optic disc) $\mathbf{X}$ can be efficiently represented as a linear combination of all data points, *i.e.* $\mathbf{x}_i = \mathbf{X}\mathbf{z}_i$, where $\mathbf{z}_i \in \mathbb{R}^n$ is the vector of coefficients. Under such an assumption, we seek for an optimal low rank representation $\mathbf{Z} = [\mathbf{z}_1, \ldots, \mathbf{z}_n]$ of all the given data, and finally obtain the partition of the data points into cup or rim via spectral clustering [9] in a manner similar to [10].

In the case that the given data is noise-free and embedded in linear subspaces, the low rank representation $\mathbf{Z}$ can be obtained by solving the following optimization problem [11]:

$$\min_{\mathbf{Z}} \ rank(\mathbf{Z}), \quad s.t. \ \mathbf{X} = \mathbf{X}\mathbf{Z}. \tag{1}$$

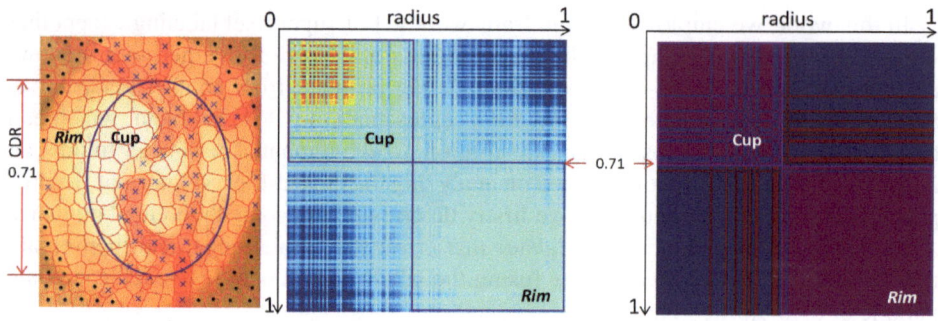

Fig. 1. Illustration of low-rank representation of superpixels in the optic disc. **Left:** 256 super-pixels within the optic disc, where black dots mark superpixels outside of the disc region, blue crosses indicate superpixels lying on blood vessels, and superpixels without dots or crosses are to be labelled. **Middle:** The obtained low rank representation $\mathbf{Z}$ exhibits a block-diagonal structure, in which each column/row corresponds to a superpixel (to be classified) sorted in ascending order of distance from its center to the disc center. Warmer colors indicate higher coefficient values. **Right:** Ncut results with $\mathbf{Z}$, in which most of the superpixels in the cup are classified together in one class, while most of the remaining superpixels are labelled as rim. Purple/blue indicates that two superpixels belong to the same/different class.

However, in real-world cases, data is usually not noise-free. Supposing that the data is corrupted, we penalize the reconstruction error matrix $\mathbf{X} - \mathbf{XZ}$ using the squared Frobenius norm ($\|\cdot\|_F^2$), instead of enforcing the equation constraint in (1). Moreover, since the rank function is non-convex and difficult to optimize, we replace it by the nuclear norm, which is a convex approximation of rank. Accordingly, we arrive at the following low-rank representation (LRR) problem:

$$\min_{\mathbf{Z}} \ \lambda\|\mathbf{Z}\|_* + \|\mathbf{X} - \mathbf{XZ}\|_F^2, \tag{2}$$

where λ is a positive trade-off parameter. A nonlinear version of this problem (2) was dealt with in [12]:

$$\min_{\mathbf{Z}} \ \lambda\|\mathbf{Z}\|_* + \|\Phi(\mathbf{X}) - \Phi(\mathbf{X})\mathbf{Z}\|_F^2, \tag{3}$$

where $\Phi(\mathbf{X}) = [\phi(\mathbf{x})_1,\dots,\phi(\mathbf{x})_n]$, with $\phi(\mathbf{x})_i$ being the nonlinear mapping of $\mathbf{x}_i$, $i = 1,\dots,n$. Using the kernel trick, we introduce a kernel matrix $\mathbf{K} \in \mathbb{R}^{n\times n}$ for which $\mathbf{K}_{i,j} = \phi(\mathbf{x})_i'\phi(\mathbf{x})_j$, so (3) becomes

$$\min_{\mathbf{Z}} \ \lambda\|\mathbf{Z}\|_* + tr((\mathbf{I} - \mathbf{Z})'\mathbf{K}(\mathbf{I} - \mathbf{Z})), \tag{4}$$

where $tr(\cdot)$ is the trace (i.e. the sum of diagonal elements) of a square matrix. For efficient computation, a linear kernel with a low rank approximation of rank 20 is used in our implementation.

2.2 Solution

A nice property of the problem in (4) is that it can be solved in closed form, which only requires a simple process based on singular value decomposition (SVD) of the kernel matrix, as shown in the following lemma:

Lemma 1. *Suppose that the SVD of the kernel matrix $\mathbf{K}$ is $\mathbf{K} = \mathbf{V} diag(\mathbf{s})\mathbf{V}'$, where $\mathbf{s} = [\sigma_1, \ldots, \sigma_n]'$, with $\{\sigma_i\}_{i=1}^{n}$ being the singular values sorted in descending order. The problem (4) is minimized by*

$$\mathbf{Z}_\lambda^* = \mathbf{V} diag(\mathbf{d}_\lambda)\mathbf{V}', \tag{5}$$

where the i-th element of $\mathbf{d}_\lambda$ is $\max(\sigma_i - \lambda, 0)/\sigma_i$.

The proof of this lemma can be found in [12].

2.3 Adaptive Superpixel Clustering

For low-rank representation based methods such as [11], parameter selection is an open problem. In previous works, the reported clustering results are often the one closest to the ground truth after manually tuning the parameters. However, in this work, we propose an adaptive approach to automatically determine candidate values of λ, followed by a majority voting process to obtain the final result based on the clustering results with respect to different candidate values of λ.

Our proposed adaptive approach is based on the following analysis of the closed-form solution in (5). Let $\mathbf{Z}_\lambda^*$ be the optimal solution of problem (4) with the parameter λ, and n_K be the total number of positive singular values of $\mathbf{K}$. We define a set of anchor points $\{\hat{\sigma}_i\}_{i=1}^{n_K+2}$, where $[\hat{\sigma}_1, \ldots, \hat{\sigma}_{n_K+2}] = [\infty, \sigma_1, \ldots, \sigma_n, 0]$. Using these anchor points, we divide the valid range for λ, namely $[0, \infty)$, into $n_K + 1$ intervals $\{\mathcal{S}_i\}_{i=1}^{n_K+1}$ where $\mathcal{S}_i = \{\lambda | \hat{\sigma}_i > \lambda \geq \hat{\sigma}_{i+1}\}$.

Based on the closed-form solution (5), we have the following conclusions: for any $\lambda \in \mathcal{S}_1$, the corresponding optimal solution $\mathbf{Z}_\lambda^*$ is a zero matrix, which provides no useful information for the subsequent clustering process. For any $\lambda \in \mathcal{S}_{n_K+1}$, the corresponding optimal solution is $\mathbf{Z}_\lambda^* = \mathbf{V}_0\mathbf{V}_0'$, where $\mathbf{V}_0 \in \mathbb{R}^{n \times r}$ is obtained by skinny SVD of $\mathbf{K}$, with r being the rank of $\mathbf{K}$. For real-world data which is generally not noise-free, the resultant matrix $\mathbf{Z}_\lambda^*$ may not be desirable for the subsequent clustering process, because it possibly contains too much noise. Therefore, we leave out the λ in the intervals $\mathcal{S}_1$ and $\mathcal{S}_{n_K+1}$.

For each remaining interval $\mathcal{S}_k = \{\lambda | \hat{\sigma}_k > \lambda \geq \hat{\sigma}_{k+1}\}$, where $2 \leq k \leq n_K$, we simply choose $\hat{\sigma}_{k+1}$ as a representative of the values inside this interval. However, under some circumstances, even if λ_1 and λ_2 come from the same interval $\mathcal{S}_{k+1}$, the resultant optimal solutions to (4) may be fairly different from each other. Specifically, we have the following lemma:

Lemma 2. *For any λ_1, λ_2 in the same set $\mathcal{S}_{k+1}$ where $1 < k < n_K$, and the corresponding optimal solutions $\mathbf{Z}_{\lambda_1}^*, \mathbf{Z}_{\lambda_2}^*$ to (4), we have*

$$\frac{\|\mathbf{Z}_{\lambda_1}^* - \mathbf{Z}_{\lambda_2}^*\|_F}{\|\mathbf{Z}_{\lambda_1}^*\|_F} \leq \frac{|\sigma_{k+1} - \sigma_k|\sqrt{\sum_{i=1}^{k} \frac{1}{\sigma_i^2}}}{\sqrt{\sum_{i=1}^{k} \frac{(\sigma_i - \sigma_k)^2}{\sigma_i^2}}}. \tag{6}$$

Proof. Since λ_1, λ_2 are in the same set $\mathcal{S}_{k+1}$, we have $\hat{\sigma}_{k+1} = \sigma_k > \lambda_i \geq \sigma_{k+1} = \hat{\sigma}_{k+2}$, $i = 1, 2$. It can also be easily proved that for any vector $\mathbf{a} \in \mathbb{R}^n$, given that $\mathbf{V}$ is orthogonal, we have $\|\mathbf{V}diag(\mathbf{a})\mathbf{V}'\|_F^2 = \|a\|_F^2 = \sum_{i=1}^n a_i^2$, where a_i is the i-th element of $\mathbf{a}$. Accordingly, considering (5), we have $\|\mathbf{Z}_{\lambda_1}^* - \mathbf{Z}_{\lambda_2}^*\|_F^2 = \|\mathbf{d}_{\lambda_1} - \mathbf{d}_{\lambda_2}\|_F^2 = \sum_{i=1}^k \frac{|\lambda_1 - \lambda_2|^2}{\sigma_i^2}$, and $\|\mathbf{Z}_{\lambda_1}^*\|_F^2 = \sum_{i=1}^k \frac{(\sigma_i - \lambda_1)^2}{\sigma_i^2}$. Therefore, we have

$$\frac{\|\mathbf{Z}_{\lambda_1}^* - \mathbf{Z}_{\lambda_2}^*\|_F}{\|\mathbf{Z}_{\lambda_1}^*\|_F} = \frac{|\lambda_1 - \lambda_2|\sqrt{\sum_{i=1}^k \frac{1}{\sigma_i^2}}}{\sqrt{\sum_{i=1}^k \frac{(\sigma_i - \lambda_1)^2}{\sigma_i^2}}}.$$

Recalling that $\hat{\sigma}_{k+1} = \sigma_k > \lambda_i \geq \sigma_{k+1} = \hat{\sigma}_{k+2}, i = 1, 2$, we have $|\lambda_1 - \lambda_2| \leq |\hat{\sigma}_{k+1} - \hat{\sigma}_k|$ and $\sigma_i - \lambda_1 \geq \sigma_i - \sigma_k$, $i = 1, \ldots, k$, which leads to (6).

Based on Lemma 2, when the bound in (6) (with respect to the interval $\mathcal{S}_{k+1}$) is larger than 10%, we additionally set $0.5(\sigma_{k+1} + \sigma_k)$ as a candidate value of λ. Finally, let $\mathcal{P}$ denote all candidate values for λ.

Given the candidate value set $\mathcal{P}$ for λ, we can efficiently obtain all the corresponding optimal solutions $\{\mathbf{Z}_\lambda^* | \lambda \in \mathcal{P}\}$ by using (5). By performing Ncut [10] based on each $\mathbf{Z}_\lambda^*$, we can obtain a label vector $\mathbf{y}_\lambda \in \{0, 1\}^n$ for all superpixels. Recall that the clustering in our problem is binary, in which the two classes correspond to the cup and rim respectively. For consistent labels $\{\mathbf{y}_\lambda\}$, the class of the central superpixels is assigned as "1" (cup) and the other class as "0" (rim). Therefore, the final clustering label vector $\mathbf{y} \in \{0, 1\}^n$ based on multiple label vectors $\{\mathbf{y}_\lambda\}_{\lambda \in \mathcal{P}}$ can be obtained by majority voting, *i.e.* ,

$$\mathbf{y} = \mathbf{1}\{\frac{1}{|\mathcal{P}|}\sum_{\lambda \in \mathcal{P}} \mathbf{y}_\lambda > 0.5\}, \tag{7}$$

where $\mathbf{1}\{\cdot\}$ is an indicator function, and $|\mathcal{P}|$ is the cardinality of the set $\mathcal{P}$. Therefore, the i-th sample will be assigned to the cup class if the i-th element of $\mathbf{y}$ is equal to 1.

We note that since the candidate values of λ are related to the singular values of $\mathbf{K}$, this scheme *adaptively* selects the candidate values for *each* image.

3   Experiments

To validate the effectiveness of our unsupervised superpixel classification using LRR, the exact same feature representation and experimental settings in [1] are adopted in this work to facilitate comparisons, using the *ORIGA* dataset comprising of 168 glaucoma and 482 normal images. The four labeling methods in [1] are compared, in which only the *pre-learned* method requires a separate training set; for the other three methods, no additional training samples are needed so they can be compared fairly to our proposed approach.

For optic cup segmentation evaluation, we use the same criteria as in [1] and [7], *i.e.*, non-overlap ratio (m_1), absolute area difference (m_2) and absolute CDR error (δ), defined as

Table 1. Performance comparisons on different superpixel labeling methods. Note that our LRR and *refinement only* are unsupervised methods, while the other three are supervised.

Dataset	S_A&S_B			S_C			S_A&S_B&S_C		
Method	m_1	m_2	δ	m_1	m_2	δ	m_1	m_2	δ
LRR	**0.244**	**0.275**	**0.078**	**0.268**	**0.265**	**0.080**	**0.256**	**0.270**	**0.079**
refinement only	0.331	0.341	0.105	0.325	0.318	0.112	0.328	0.329	0.109
intra-image+refinement	0.265	0.313	0.079	0.269	0.267	0.082	0.267	0.290	0.081
intra-image only	0.269	0.324	0.084	0.277	0.283	0.087	0.273	0.303	0.086
pre-learned	0.277	0.314	0.087	0.301	0.285	0.091	0.289	0.300	0.089

$$m_1 = 1 - \frac{area(E_{dt} \bigcap E_{gt})}{area(E_{dt} \bigcup E_{gt})}, \quad m_2 = \frac{|area(E_{dt}) - area(E_{gt})|}{area(E_{gt})},$$
$$\delta = |CDR(E_{dt}) - CDR(E_{dt})|, \tag{8}$$

where E_{dt} denotes a detected cup region, E_{gt} denotes the ground-truth cup region, and $CDR(\cdot)$ calculates the vertical diameter of the cup. Among the three metrics, m_1 is the most commonly used for segmentation.

3.1 Comparison of Different Labeling Methods

Based on the state-of-the-art superpixel framework, using the same domain prior, our proposed LRR method is shown in Table 1 to yield improvements over all the four methods in [1]. The comparison to the unsupervised *refinement only* method shows that our unsupervised method models the problem better with the low-rank property, while the similarity based one does not fully utilize this prior information. The comparison to the other three supervised methods shows that with a proper problem formulation and solution, an unsupervised approach can achieve equal or even better performance than a supervised method, on this specific problem. From some cup segmentation results shown in Fig. 2, one can observe that most failure cases occur when the assumption of LRR does not hold, and some of the failure cases may be caused by the influence of blood vessels that occupy a large area of the cup and are removed early from labeling. This problem will be studied in our future work. For the successful cases that fit the assumption well, the cup regions are very similar with a higher intensity than the rim area.

3.2 Discussion

Validation of Adaptive Parameter Tuning. The results listed in Table 2 are all obtained by using our adaptive clustering scheme, either with or without the use of Lemma 2, to generate additional candidate parameter values. In contrast, the use of additional candidate values achieves better results with an average relative reduction of 1.8%, 2.3% and 2.7% in terms of m_1, m_2 and δ, respectively.

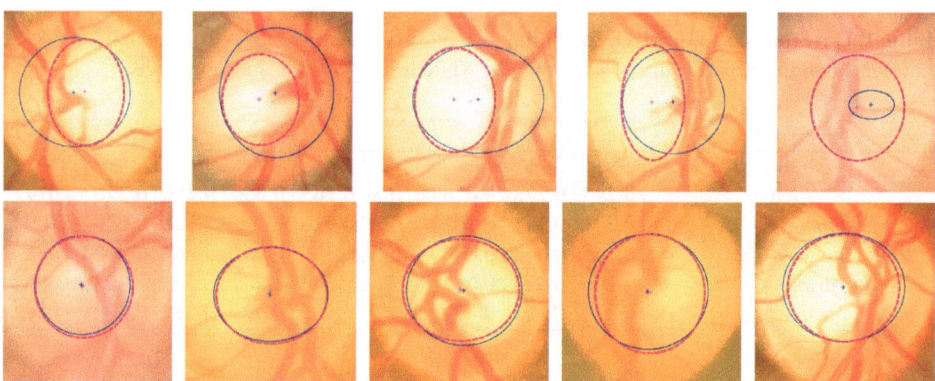

Fig. 2. Some sample results of LRR based cup segmentation with 256 superpixels: failure cases in the top row and successful cases in the bottom row. The cyan × denotes the center of the image, and the red and blue + denote the center of the detected cup and the ground truth, respectively; correspondingly, the red dashed-line ellipse represents the detected cup and the blue solid-line ellipse represents the ground truth.

Table 2. Performance comparisons of our adaptive clustering scheme using different superpixel numbers

Adaptive scheme	Using Lemma 2			Without using Lemma 2		
# superpixels	m_1	m_2	δ	m_1	m_2	δ
2048	0.265	0.271	0.081	0.270	0.276	0.082
1024	0.262	0.274	0.080	0.267	0.280	0.082
512	0.263	**0.270**	**0.079**	0.269	0.277	0.083
256	**0.256**	**0.270**	**0.079**	0.259	0.278	0.081

Influence of Superpixel Number. Every superpixel labelling method in [1] has two to four parameters to be tuned besides the number of superpixels, which is the only parameter that needs to be pre-chosen manually. The cup segmentation errors with different superpixel numbers are listed in Table 2. From the table, a similar conclusion can be made as in [1], that superpixel based results are relatively stable with a proper superpixel size. However, the lowest m_1 is obtained with the smallest number (256) of superpixels per image, and the best result in [1] is obtained with the largest number (2048) of superpixels. A possible explanation is that when dividing an image into very small-sized superpixels, the information contained in each superpixel becomes less discriminative. In contrast, larger-sized superpixels (e.g., when the number of superpixels is 256) preserve more local structure, which may provide more discriminative power.

4   Conclusion

In this work, we deal with the cup segmentation problem for glaucoma detection. We extended the state-of-the-art superpixel framework [1] by modeling the binary superpixel clustering/classification task as a low-rank representation (LRR) problem in which the domain prior and the low-rank property of the superpixels are employed. Moreover, we developed an adaptive strategy to automatically choose the candidate values of the only parameter in the LRR formulation, based on a theoretical analysis of the closed-form solution. In relation to prior art [1] [7], our method yields improved unsupervised segmentation. In addition, the proposed LRR-based unsupervised solution performs as well as or better than the supervised methods presented in [1]. The experimental results also demonstrate the effectiveness of the adaptive parameter selection strategy in producing robust results. For future work, we would like to explore the possibility of developing a similar LRR-based formulation for supervised learning. A supervised or semi-supervised LRR-based solution can benefit from utilizing discriminant information from additional training samples, while offering all the advantages of low-rank representations.

References

1. Xu, Y., Liu, J., Lin, S., Xu, D., Cheung, C.Y., Aung, T., Wong, T.Y.: Efficient Optic Cup Detection from Intra-image Learning with Retinal Structure Priors. In: Ayache, N., Delingette, H., Golland, P., Mori, K. (eds.) MICCAI 2012, Part I. LNCS, vol. 7510, pp. 58–65. Springer, Heidelberg (2012)
2. Kingman, S.: Glaucoma is second leading cause of blindness globally. Bull. World Health Organ. 82(11), 887–888 (2004)
3. Jonas, J., Budde, W., Panda-Jonas, S.: Ophthalmoscopic Evaluation of the Optic Nerve Head. Survey of Ophthalmology 43, 293–320 (1999)
4. Liu, J., Wong, D.W.K., Lim, J., Li, H., Tan, N.M., Zhang, Z., Wong, T.Y., Lavanya, R.: Argali:an automatic cup-to-disc ratio measurement system for glaucoma analysis using level-set image processing. In: IEEE Int. Conf. Engin. in Med. and Biol. Soc (2008)
5. Yin, F., Liu, J., Ong, S.H., Sun, D., Wong, D.W.K., Tan, N.M., Baskaran, M., Cheung, C.Y., Aung, T., Wong, T.Y.: Model-based Optic Nerve Head Segmentation on Retinal Fundus Images. In: IEEE Int. Conf. Engin. in Med. and Biol. Soc., pp. 2626–2629 (2011)
6. Wong, D.W.K., Lim, J.H., Tan, N.M., Zhang, Z., Lu, S., Li, H., Teo, M., Chan, K., Wong, T.Y.: Intelligent Fusion of Cup-to-Disc Ratio Determination Methods for Glaucoma Detection in ARGALI. In: Int. Conf. Engin. in Med. and Biol. Soc., pp. 5777–5780 (2009)
7. Xu, Y., Xu, D., Lin, S., Liu, J., Cheng, J., Cheung, C.Y., Aung, T., Wong, T.Y.: Sliding Window and Regression based Cup Detection in Digital Fundus Images for Glaucoma Diagnosis. In: Fichtinger, G., Martel, A., Peters, T. (eds.) MICCAI 2011, Part III. LNCS, vol. 6893, pp. 1–8. Springer, Heidelberg (2011)
8. Achanta, R., Shaji, A., Smith, K., Lucchi, A., Fua, P., Susstrunk, S.: SLIC Superpixels Compared to State-of-the-art Superpixel Methods. IEEE Transactions on Pattern Analysis and Machine Intelligence (TPAMI) 34(11), 2274–2282 (2012)
9. Cristianini, N., Shawe-Taylor, J., Kandola, J.S.: Spectral kernel methods for clustering. In: Neural Information Processing Systems Conference, NIPS (2001)
10. Shi, J., Malik, J.: Normalized cuts and image segmentation. IEEE Transactions on Pattern Analysis and Machine Intelligence (TPAMI) 22, 888–905 (2000)
11. Liu, G., Lin, Z., Yan, S., Sun, J., Yu, Y., Ma, Y.: Robust recovery of subspace structures by low-rank representation. IEEE Transactions on Pattern Analysis and Machine Intelligence (TPAMI) 35(1), 171–184 (2013)
12. Wang, J., Saligrama, V., Castañón, D.A.: Structural similarity and distance in learning. In: Annual Allerton Conference on Communication, Control, and Computing, Allerton (2011)

3D Prostate TRUS Segmentation Using Globally Optimized Volume-Preserving Prior

Wu Qiu[1], Martin Rajchl[1], Fumin Guo[1], Yue Sun[1], Eranga Ukwatta[2], Aaron Fenster[1], and Jing Yuan[1]

[1] Robarts Research Institute, University of Western Ontario, London, ON, Canada
[2] Department of Biomedical Engineering, Johns Hopkins University, Baltimore, MD, United States

Abstract. An efficient and accurate segmentation of 3D transrectal ultrasound (TRUS) images plays an important role in the planning and treatment of the practical 3D TRUS guided prostate biopsy. However, a meaningful segmentation of 3D TRUS images tends to suffer from US speckles, shadowing and missing edges etc, which make it a challenging task to delineate the correct prostate boundaries. In this paper, we propose a novel convex optimization based approach to extracting the prostate surface from the given 3D TRUS image, while preserving a new global volume-size prior. We, especially, study the proposed combinatorial optimization problem by convex relaxation and introduce its dual continuous max-flow formulation with the new bounded flow conservation constraint, which results in an efficient numerical solver implemented on GPUs. Experimental results using 12 patient 3D TRUS images show that the proposed approach while preserving the volume-size prior yielded a mean DSC of 89.5% $\pm$ 2.4%, a MAD of 1.4 $\pm$ 0.6 mm, a MAXD of 5.2 $\pm$ 3.2 mm, and a VD of 7.5% $\pm$ 6.2% in $\sim$ 1 minute, deomonstrating the advantages of both accuracy and efficiency. In addition, the low standard deviation of the segmentation accuracy shows a good reliability of the proposed approach.

Keywords: Image Segmentation, 3D Prostate TRUS Image, Convex Optimization, Volume Preserving Constraint.

1 Introduction

Prostate adenocarcinoma (PCa) is the most common non-cutaneous malignancy in American men with over 200,000 new cases diagnosed each year [1]. Definitive diagnosis of PCa requires a transrectal ultrasound (TRUS) guided biopsy [2]. Recent developments of biopsy systems using the fusion of 3D prostate TRUS and MR imagesdemonstrated an increased positive yield and greater number of cores with higher Gleason grade [3]. An accurate and efficient automated or semi-automated 3D prostate TRUS segmentation is highly beneficial for the registration of the 3D MR prostate image to TRUS in those systems [4,5,6]. However, the accurate segmentation of 3D TRUS images often suffers from the low quality of TRUS images, as shown in Fig. 1(a), such as US speckles, shadowing

P. Golland et al. (Eds.): MICCAI 2014, Part I, LNCS 8673, pp. 796–803, 2014.

due to calcifications, missing edges or texture similarities between the inner and outer regions of the prostate etc [7], which make it challenging to implement such an automated or semi-automated 3D TRUS segmentation method. The target of this study is to develop an accurate, efficient and reliable 3D prostate TRUS image segmentation approach.

Even though there are extensive studies [8] in delineating prostate boundaries from 3D TRUS images, most of them rely on classifiers, atlas or deformable models. The deformable model based methods typically used a 3D deformable surface as initialization, which is then automatically refined by forces, such as image gradient and smoothness of the surface [9,10,11]. These methods were designed and implemented in a local optimization style, such that the discrete propagation step-size is restricted to be small enough to achieve convergence and it results in low computational inefficiency. In addition, the local optimization based segmentation methods are sensitive to the initialization, and would leak at the locations with weak edges. The direct 3D segmentation methods worked well for the reported applications, but are time consuming and require intensive user interactions that leads to a high observer variability. Classifier based technique, such as support vector machine (SVM), depended on the training datasets [12]; however, the image quality in the datasets significantly varied due to different US machine settings, which prevents this technique from practical clinical applications.

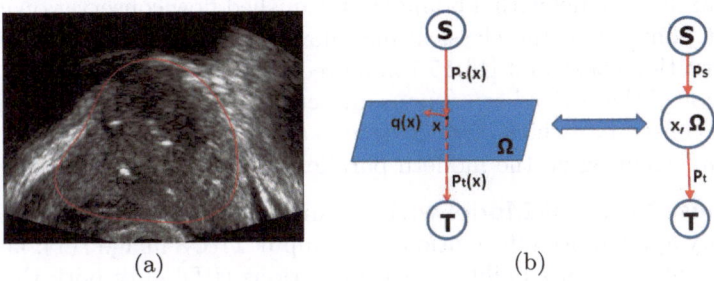

(a)   (b)

Fig. 1. Fig. 1(a) illustrates the typical 2D view of a 3D TRUS image with US speckles, calcifications, weak edge information etc. Fig. 1(b) shows the flow configurations of the proposed continuous max-flow model.

Contributions: In this study, we propose a novel convex optimization based approach to segmenting the prostate from the given 3D TRUS image while enforcing the new global volume-size prior, which is inspired by the work [13]. Such volume-size prior provides a global geometric description for the interesting object region and helps the segmentation procedure avoid suffering from low image quality of TRUS images. We, especially, introduced a non-smooth $L1$ volume prior function (its derivative cannot be directly computed) and employed a continuous convex optimization framework, which yields better efficiency and accuracy while avoiding metrification errors, and results in an efficient numerical solver implemented on GPUs. Promising experimental results demonstrate the advantages of the proposed approach in both accuracy and efficiency, along with a great reliability.

2   Methods

In this section, we introduce a novel global/convex optimization based approach to segmenting an input 3D prostate TRUS image $I(x)$ into the prostate region $\mathcal{R}_P$ and the background region $\mathcal{R}_B$, while imposing a new volume-size prior of the prostate region. Actually, the volume-size information about the interesting object region provides a global geometric description for the image segmentation task; on the other hand, such knowledge can be easily obtained in most applications by learning the given training images or the other information sources. In this work, the prostate volume-size $\mathcal{V}$ of the specified patient is calculated from the pre-segmented 3D prostate T2-weighted MR image of the same patient (see Sec. 3 for more details of the pipeline and initializations). Note: the exact volume-size is not necessary for the proposed approach in this paper and the approximation of the prostate volume could also be obtained from the other image source, for example the 3D prostate CT image.

Especially, we propose a new continuous min-cut formulation with the introduced volume-size preserving prior and solve the challenging combinatorial optimization problem by means of convex relaxation. To this end, a novel continuous max-flow model with a bounded unvanished flow conservation condition, which is in contrast to the classical max-flow models with the exact vanishing flow conservation constraint [14,15,16]; moreover, we show its duality to the convex relaxaion of the studied continuous min-cut formulation with the volume-size preserving constraint, which directly derives an efficient duality-based numerical scheme implementing on the modern parallel computing platforms, e.g. GPUs.

Continuouse Min-Cut Model with Volume-Size Preserving. In this work, the intensity appearance information of the input TRUS image $I(x)$, i.e. the corresponding intensity probability density functions (PDFs) of both the prostate region $\mathcal{R}_P$ and background region R_B, is utilized to assist the prostate TRUS image segmentation task. Such intensity appearance models provide a global descriptor of both regions of prostate and background in image statistics, which can be learned by either sampled pixels or the specified training datasets. Let $\omega^P(I(x))$ be the intensity PDF of the prostate region $\mathcal{R}_P$ appearing on the input image $I(x)$, which actually encodes the probability of each pixel x belonging to the region $\mathcal{R}_P$; and $\omega^B(I(x))$ the PDF of the background region $\mathcal{R}_B$. In consequence, we define the cost function $D_t(x)$ of labeling each pixel x to be in the prostate region $\mathcal{R}_P$, and $D_s(x)$ the labeling cost function w.r.t. the background region $\mathcal{R}_B$, by the log-likelihoods of the respective PDFs, i.e.

$$D_t(x) = -\log\left(\omega^P(I(x))\right), \quad D_s(x) = -\log\left(\omega^B(I(x))\right).$$

Let $u(x) \in \{0,1\}$ be the indicator/labeling function of the prostate region $\mathcal{R}_P$, where $u(x) = 1$ denotes the pixel x inside $\mathcal{R}_P$, and otherwise outside $\mathcal{R}_P$.

With this regard, the classical way to segment the input TRUS image of $I(x)$ is to minimize the min-cut energy function [14,15], e.g. the spatially continuous min-cut model [15]:

$$\min_{u(x)\in\{0,1\}} E(u) := \langle u, D_t \rangle + \langle 1 - u, D_s \rangle + \int_\Omega g(x)\,|\nabla u|\;dx \qquad (1)$$

where $g(x) \geq 0$ stands for the weight function assocaited with image edges, hence the weighted total-variation function measures the weighted area of the prostate region. In this paper, we also enforce preserving the specified volume-size $\mathcal{V}$ in the continuous min-cut model (1) by penalizing the difference between the volume of the prostate region $\mathcal{R}_P$ and $\mathcal{V}$, such that

$$\min_{u(x)\in\{0,1\}} E(u) + \gamma\,|\mathcal{V} - \int_\Omega u\,dx|\,, \qquad (2)$$

where $\gamma > 0$ is a positive parameter to impose a soft volume-size constraint, which is set once for segmenting the whole dataset.

In this work, we solve the introduced challenging combinatorial optimization problem (2) by its convex relaxation, i.e.

$$\min_{u(x)\in[0,1]} E(u) + \gamma\,|\mathcal{V} - \int_\Omega u\,dx| \qquad (3)$$

where the binary labeling constraint $u(x) \in \{0, 1\}$ in (2) is relaxed to the convex set of $u(x) \in [0, 1]$. Given the convex energy function of (3), it results in the convex optimization problem which is much simpler than its original combinatorial optimization model (2) in mathematics.

Continuous Max-Flow Formulation with Bounded Flow Conservation. Now we propose a new *continuous max-flow model* along with the same flow configuration as in [15] (also see Fig. 1(b) for illustration), such that:

$$\max_{p_s,p_t,q,r} \int_\Omega p_s\,dx + r\mathcal{V} \qquad (4)$$

subject to

– *Flow capacity constraints*: the source, sink and spatial flows $p_s(x)$, $p_t(x)$ and $q(x)$ suffice:

$$p_s(x) \leq D_s(x), \quad p_t(x) \leq D_t(x), \quad |q(x)| \leq g(x); \quad \forall x \in \Omega; \qquad (5)$$

– *Bounded flow conservation constraints*: the total flow residue is not vanishing at any pixel $x \in \Omega$ but bounded, *i.e.*

$$(\,\mathrm{div}\,q - p_s + p_t)(x) = r \in [-\gamma, \gamma], \quad \forall x \in \Omega. \qquad (6)$$

Obviously, the proposed continuous max-flow model (4) is distinct from the classical continuous max-flow formulation investigated in [15], in that the flow residue at each pixel x for (4) does not vanish, but is equal to a constant value r which is bounded within the range $[-\gamma, \gamma]$, while a strict flow conservation condition is required for the classical max-flow model of [15]. In addition, the total energy of (4) is evaluated by the total flow streaming from the source plus the total flow residue $r\mathcal{V}$.

Follow the same analysis proposed in [15,16], we can prove

Proposition 1. *The* continuous max-flow model (4) *and the convex relaxation of* volume-preserving continuous min-cut model (3) *are dual (equivalent) to each other, i.e.*

$$(4) \iff (3).$$

The proof is omitted due to the limited space.

Clearly, maximizing the proposed *continuous max-flow model* (4) enjoys great numerical advantages such that it successfully avoids directly tackling the non-linear and non-smooth function terms of the studied *convex relaxed optimization problem* (3). Additionally, it also derives an efficient multiplier-augmented algorithm based on the modern convex optimization theory (see [15] for details), which can be readily implemented on the modern parallel computing platforms, i.e. GPUs, to significantly improve the computational efficiency in practice.

3   Experiments and Results

Image Acquisition: All subjects involved in this study were suspected to have tumors identified by multi-spectral MR imaging. The images were acquired with a rotational scanning 3D TRUS-guided prostate biopsy system, which made use of a commercially available end-firing TRUS transducer (Philips, Bothell WA). The size of each 3D image was $448 \times 448 \times 350$ voxels of size $0.19 \times 0.19 \times 0.19 mm^3$. 12 patient images were tested in this paper.

Implementations: The prostate volume size of each patient used as the volume preserving prior was calculated from the manually pre-segmented prostate T2 weighted MR image of the same patient by three experts. The proposed approach was initialized by a closed surface, which is constructed by the thin-plate spline with positioning ten initial points on the boundary of the prostate (six

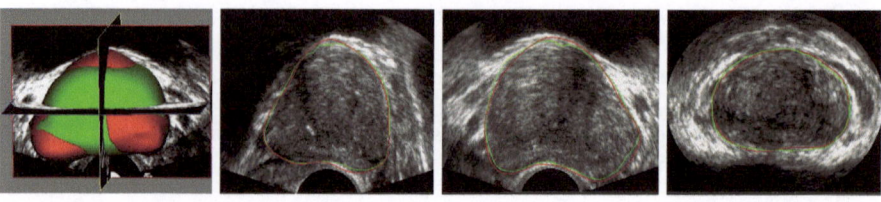

Fig. 2. Segmented ventricles (green contour, DSC: 92.5%) overlapped with manual segmentations (red contour). Left to right: segmented surface, sagittal view, coronal view, and transverse view.

at the transverse view, four at the sagittal view) [17,18]. The inside and outside voxels of the estimated surface are used to generate prior intensity probability density functions (PDFs) for the prostate and background regions, and the cost functions $D_{s,t}(x)$ were calculated by the log-likelihood of the respective intensity PDFs [18]. The closed surface also defines the initial guess of the prostate region and gives the starting value of the labeling function $u(x)$ for the proposed approach. The proposed algorithm was implemented on the parallel computing architecture (CUDA, NVIDIA Corp., Santa Clara, CA) and the user interface in Matlab (Natick, MA). The GPU based algorithm was developed and integrated with the non-optimized Matlab program, which ran on a Windows desktop with an 4-core Intel i7-2600 CPU (3.4 GHz) and a NVIDIA Geforce 5800X GPU.

Evaluation Metrics: A manual segmentation of each image used as the ground truth was compared to the algorithm segmented result, using *volume-based metrics*: Dice similarity coefficient (DSC); *distance-based metrics*: the mean absolute surface distance (MAD) and maximum absolute surface distance (MAXD); and *volume measurement metrics*: absolute volume difference (VD), $|(V_{Manual} - V_{algorithm})/V_{Manual}|$.

Table 1. Segmentation results of 12 patient 3D TRUS images in terms of DSC, MAD, MAXD, and VD, represented as Mean $\pm$ SD, using the continuous max-flow algorithm with (CMF_{VP}) and without (CMF [15]) volume preserving constraint

	DSC (%)	MAD (mm)	MAXD (mm)	VD (%)
CMF_{VP}	89.5 ± 2.4	1.4 ± 0.6	5.2 ± 3.2	7.5 ± 6.2
CMF	78.3 ± 7.4	3.5 ± 1.3	9.4 ± 3.0	15.0 ± 10.2

Accuracy: Figure 2 shows one algorithm segmented prostate (green contours) and manual delineations (red contours) of one patient, visually demonstrating a good agreement. Table 1 shows the mean quantitative segmentation results for 12 patient images using the proposed method. Our approach obtained a mean DSC of 89.5% $\pm$ 2.4%, a MAD of 1.4 ± 0.6 *mm*, a MAXD of 5.2 ± 3.2 *mm*, and a VD of 7.5% $\pm$ 6.2% for the used 12 patient images. More specifically, the proposed continous max-flow algorithm with the volume-preserving prior impoved the accuracy by more than 11% in terms of DSC comparing to the continous max-flow algorithm without priors [15].

Computational Efficiency: The mean segmentation time of the GPU implemented algorithm for one 3D TRUS image, calculated as a mean time using all 3D TRUS images, was 35 ± 5 s in addition to 30 ± 5 s for initialization, hence less than 1.2 minutes for a given 3D TRUS image in avarage.

4   Discussion and Conclusion

This paper proposes an accurate and efficient segmentation algorithm for 3D prostate TRUS images. The experimental results using 12 patient images show that the proposed method yielded a mean DSC of 89.5% ± 2.4%, a MAD of 1.4 ± 0.6 mm, a MAXD of 5.2 ± 3.2 mm, and a VD of 7.5% ± 6.2% within 1.2 minutes compared to manual segmentations. The low standard deviation of the segmentation accuracy in terms of metrics above shows a good consistency during all the segmentations, which is an important aspect in clinic. We compared our proposed approach with the prostate segmentation algorithms using 3D TRUS images, which used similar evaluation metrics and provided best segmentation accuracy in a literature reviewing paper [8]. The mean DSC of 89.5% obtained by our method are comparable to a volume overlap of 83.5% obtained by Tutar et al. [9] and 86.4% obtained by Garnier et al. [11], and a volume overlap error of 6.63% obtained by Mahdavi et al. [10]. The mean MAD of 1.4 mm obtained by our method is comparable to 1.26 mm obtained by Tutar et al. [9]. In addition, the computational time of 35 seconds of our method excluding initialization time is less than 1-4 minutes obtained by Tutar et al. [9]. Although Mahdavi et al. [10] reported 14 seconds for one image segmentation in their experiments, their method required additional 1-3 minutes for modification. The method by Garnier et al. [11] required 26 seconds, but it was implemented in C language and the computation was limited in an user defined ROI. Note that the computation of the energy formulations $E(u)$ in (1) including the data cost functions $D_{s,t}(x)$ and the image edge weight function $g(x)$ were developed using a Matlab code and run on CPU, which could be parallelized or converted to the C program to speed up computation.

In conclusion, this paper proposed a novel globally optimized volume-preserving segmentation approach for 3D TRUS images. The quantitative validation results using different metrics (DSC, MAD, MAXD, and VD) showed that it is capable of delineating the prostate surface accurately and efficiently. Its performance results suggest that it may be suitable for the clinical use involving the image guided prostate biopsy procedures.

Acknowledgments. The authors are grateful for the funding support from the Ontario Research Fund (OFC) and the Canada Research Chairs (CRC) Program.

References

1. Jemal, A., Siegel, R., Xu, J., Ward, E.: Cancer statistics, 2010. CA Cancer J. Clin. 60(5), 277–300 (2010)
2. Qiu, W., Yuchi, M., Ding, M., Tessier, D., Fenster, A.: Needle segmentation using 3D hough transform in 3D TRUS guided prostate transperineal therapy. Med. Phy. 40(4), 042902–1–13 (2013)
3. Leslie, S., Goh, A., Lewandowski, P.M., Huang, E.Y.H., de Castro Abreu, A.L., Berger, A.K., Ahmadi, H., Jayaratna, I., Shoji, S., Gill, I.S., Ukimura, O.: Contemporary image-guided targeted prostate biopsy better characterizes cancer volume, gleason grade and its 3d location compared to systematic biopsy. The Journal of Urology 187(suppl. 4), e827 (2050)

4. Sonn, G.A., Natarajan, S., Margolis, D.J., MacAiran, M., Lieu, P., Huang, J., Dorey, F.J., Marks, L.S.: Targeted biopsy in the detection of prostate cancer using an office based magnetic resonance ultrasound fusion device. The Journal of Urology 189(1), 86–92 (2013)
5. Qiu, W., Yuan, J., Ukwatta, E., Yue, S., Rajchl, M., Fenster, A.: Prostate segmentation: An efficient convex optimization approach with axial symmetry using 3d trus and mr images. IEEE Trans. Med. Imag. 33(4), 947–960 (2014)
6. Litjens, G., Toth, R., van de Ven, W., Hoeks, C., Kerkstra, S., van Ginneken, B., Vincent, G., Guillard, G., Birbeck, N., Zhang, J., et al.: Evaluation of prostate segmentation algorithms for mri: the promise12 challenge. Med. Imag. Anal. 18(2), 359–373 (2014)
7. Qiu, W., Yuan, J., Ukwatta, E., Tessier, D., Fenster, A.: 3D prostate segmentation using level set with shape constraint based on rotational slices for 3D end-firing TRUS guided biopsy. Med. Phy. 40(7), 072903–1–12 (2013)
8. Ghose, S., Oliver, A., Martí, R., Lladó, X., Vilanova, J., Freixenet, J., Mitra, J., Sidibé, D., Meriaudeau, F.: A survey of prostate segmentation methodologies in ultrasound, magnetic resonance and computed tomography images. Computer Methods and Programs in Biomedicine 108(1), 262–287 (2012)
9. Tutar, I.B., Pathak, S.D., Gong, L., Cho, P.S., Wallner, K., Kim, Y.: Semiautomatic 3D prostate segmentation from TRUS images using spherical harmonics. IEEE Trans. Med. Imaging 25(12), 1645–1654 (2006)
10. Mahdavi, S.S., Moradi, M., Wen, X., Morris, W.J., Salcudean, S.E.: Evaluation of visualization of the prostate gland in vibro-elastography images. Med. Imag. Anal. 15(4), 589–600 (2011)
11. Garnier, C., Bellanger, J.J., Wu, K., Shu, H., Costet, N., Mathieu, R., de Crevoisier, R., Coatrieux, J.L.: Prostate segmentation in HIFU therapy. IEEE Trans. Med. Imag. 30(3), 792–803 (2011)
12. Akbari, H., Fei, B.: 3D ultrasound image segmentation using wavelet support vector machines. Med. Phys. 39(6), 2972–2984 (2012)
13. Gorelick, L., Schmidt, F.R., Boykov, Y., Delong, A., Ward, A.: Segmentation with non-linear regional constraints via line-search cuts. In: Fitzgibbon, A., Lazebnik, S., Perona, P., Sato, Y., Schmid, C. (eds.) ECCV 2012, Part I. LNCS, vol. 7572, pp. 583–597. Springer, Heidelberg (2012)
14. Boykov, Y., Veksler, O., Zabih, R.: Fast approximate energy minimization via graph cuts. IEEE Trans. Patt. Anal. Mach. Intel. 23(11), 1222–1239 (2001)
15. Yuan, J., Bae, E., Tai, X.: A study on continuous max-flow and min-cut approaches. In: Davis, L., Malik, J. (eds.) IEEE CVPR, San Francisco, USA, pp. 2217–2224 (2010)
16. Yuan, J., Bae, E., Tai, X.-C., Boykov, Y.: A continuous max-flow approach to potts model. In: Daniilidis, K., Maragos, P., Paragios, N. (eds.) ECCV 2010, Part VI. LNCS, vol. 6316, pp. 379–392. Springer, Heidelberg (2010)
17. Yuan, J., Qiu, W., Ukwatta, E., Rajchl, M., Sun, Y., Fenster, A.: An efficient convex optimization approach to 3D prostate MRI segmentation with generic star shape prior. In: Ayache, N., Delingette, H., Golland, P., Mori, K. (eds.) Prostate MR Image Segmentation Challenge, MICCAI, vol. 7512. Springer (2012)
18. Qiu, W., Yuan, J., Ukwatta, E., Sun, Y., Rajchl, M., Fenster, A.: Dual optimization based prostate zonal segmentation in 3D MR images. Med. Imag. Anal. 18(4), 660–673 (2014)

Lung Segmentation from CT with Severe Pathologies Using Anatomical Constraints

Neil Birkbeck[1], Timo Kohlberger[1], Jingdan Zhang[1],
Michal Sofka[1], Jens Kaftan[2], Dorin Comaniciu[1], and S. Kevin Zhou[1,⋆]

[1] Imaging & Computer Vision, Siemens Corporate Technology, Princeton, NJ, USA
[2] Molecular Imaging, Siemens Healthcare, Oxford, UK

Abstract. The diversity in appearance of diseased lung tissue makes automatic segmentation of lungs from CT with severe pathologies challenging. To overcome this challenge, we rely on contextual constraints from neighboring anatomies to detect and segment lung tissue across a variety of pathologies. We propose an algorithm that combines statistical learning with these anatomical constraints to seek a segmentation of the lung consistent with adjacent structures, such as the heart, liver, spleen, and ribs. We demonstrate that our algorithm reduces the number of failed detections and increases the accuracy of the segmentation on unseen test cases with severe pathologies.

1 Introduction

Healthy lung tissue is easily distinguishable from surrounding soft tissue in CT images due to its high air content. In contrast, pathologies like tumors, interstitial lung diseases (ILD), and plural effusion [1], may dramatically alter both the appearance and texture of the lung and its surroundings (see Fig. 1). Due to this variability, automatic methods for segmenting healthy lung that rely on appearance alone, such as region growing or registration, are inappropriate for segmenting lungs from CT with severe pathologies [7].

In order to account for specific pathologies, such as ILD, some existing methods focus on utilizing texture cues [4,10], or for tumors, robust statistical shape models can be used [9]. In order to robustly segment diseased lung parenchyma, other researchers have identified the need to use other nearby anatomical context. For example, the curvature of nearby ribs [6] or the distance to spine [2] can be used in addition to appearance information, or stable landmarks that take into account neighboring ribs can be used to better align a statistical shape model on the lung [8].

⋆ Zhou is corresponding author. Birkbeck and Kohlberger are with Google, Zhang with Microsoft, and Sofka with Cisco. All work was done while they were with Siemens.

[1] Pleural effusion is an accumulation of pleural fluid between the parietal and visceral pleura, and thus part of the pleural cavity, but not of the actual lung. It is a common cause for decreased lung function and only affects the lungs directly. For this reason, we include both the lung and the pleural cavity in our segmentation.

P. Golland et al. (Eds.): MICCAI 2014, Part I, LNCS 8673, pp. 804–811, 2014.
© Springer International Publishing Switzerland 2014

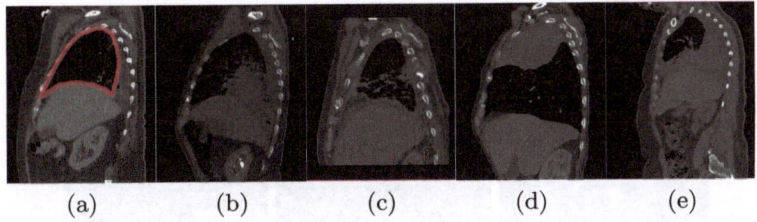

(a)   (b)   (c)   (d)   (e)

Fig. 1. Examples of pathological lungs. In (a), the boundary between low/high intensity gives rise to a lung-like shape (red), making it hard to rely solely on a shape prior to segment pathologies.

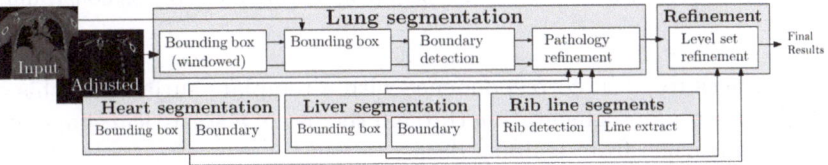

Fig. 2. The proposed pathological lung segmentation pipeline

However, none of these methods utilize all available anatomical context surrounding the lung regions. We propose a learning-based algorithm capable of segmenting lung from CT scans with several pathologies. To be robust against pathologies, we rely on context external to the lung for each phase of the pipeline, including detection, coarse segmentation, and fine-scale refinement. For the segmentation, we use region-specific anatomical constraints such as distance to ribs or adjacent organs (e.g. liver and heart).

2 Methods

The lung is bounded by the ribs on the outside surface, the heart on the mediastinum side, and, e.g., the right lung is bounded by the liver on the bottom. In order to use these adjacent structures, our algorithm starts by automatically detecting them (e.g., lung, heart, liver & spleen §2.1) and rib segments (§2.2) using statistical classifiers. The lung mesh is then deformed using appearance cues and neighboring structures as geometric constraints (§2.3). A final refinement balances the need for a fine-scale geometry while maintaining proximity to adjacent structures and ensuring no overlap between segmentations (§2.5). This final refinement maintains the integrity of the segmentation in the presence of pathologies by constraining the refined solution to lie close to the detected solution. The algorithm components and data flow are outlined in Fig. 2.

2.1 Organ Detection

A central assertion in our approach is that we can apply region-specific geometric constraints to the segmentation. In order to apply such constraints, we need our

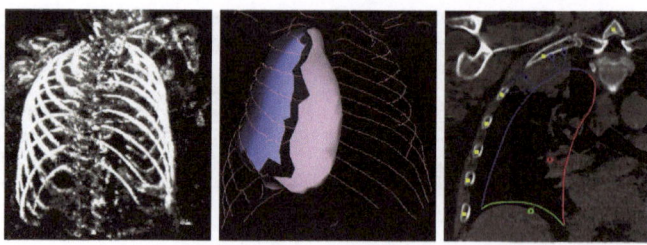

Fig. 3. Examples of rib lines (left), the 3D region parts for the right lung (middle), and region specific geometric constraints (right). The lung surface is divided into three partitions: the rib region (blue), the heart/mediastinum region (red) and the bottom region (green). Each region of the surface uses neighboring anatomy as constraints.

detected surfaces to be in correspondence with a template surface. To this end, we initialize our organ segmentation through the use of a statistical shape model that has been learned from training data.

Let $\mathcal{C} = (\mathcal{V}, \mathcal{T})$ be a mesh with vertices $\mathcal{V} = \{\mathbf{v}_i = (x_i, y_i, z_i)\}_{i=1}^n$ and triangles $\mathcal{T}$. We model shape variation with a point-distribution model [1] using a low-dimensional set of M shape modes, $\mathbf{U}_j = \{\mathbf{u}_{ij}\}_{i=1}^n$, and a mean vector $\bar{\mathbf{v}}_i$: $\mathbf{v}_i = \bar{\mathbf{v}}_i + \sum_{j=1}^M \lambda_j \mathbf{u}_{ij}$, where $\{\lambda_j\}_{j=1}^M$ is a shape coefficient vector defining the shape. Given a transformation, $T(\mathbf{v}; \theta)$ parameterized by θ, e.g., a similarity transform, the initial organ detection seeks the most probable configuration given the input image, I:

$$\mathcal{C}^0 = \mathrm{argmax}_{\mathcal{C}} \; P(\mathcal{C}|I, \{\bar{\mathbf{v}}_i\}, \{\mathbf{u}_{ij}\}) = \mathrm{argmax}_{\mathcal{C}} \; P(\theta, \{\lambda_j\}_{j=1}^M | I, \{\bar{\mathbf{v}}_i\}, \{\mathbf{u}_{ij}\}). \quad (1)$$

This problem is solved with the discriminative method marginal space learning [11], and it is used to reliably estimate an initial object segmentation of the lungs, $\mathcal{C}_{\mathrm{llung}}^0 \& \mathcal{C}_{\mathrm{rlung}}^0$, heart, $\mathcal{C}_{\mathrm{heart}}^0$, spleen, $\mathcal{C}_{\mathrm{spleen}}^0$, and liver, $\mathcal{C}_{\mathrm{liver}}^0$, (e.g., [5]).

For the lungs, to avoid failed detection on large effusions with dramatically different appearance, we first estimate the shape on a contrast adjusted input image, $I_{win} = \max(0, \min(1, (I - 80)/496))$, where I is in Hounsfield unit (HU).

2.2 Rib Points Extraction

In order to extract points on the ribs to be used as constraints, discriminative classifiers are used to identify likely rib points. These likely rib points are then grouped into short segments, and unlikely segments are culled (Figure 3).

First, a per-voxel rib probability map, $I_{rib}(\mathbf{x})$, is obtained from a two-level cascade of discriminative classifiers,

$$I_{rib}(\mathbf{x}) = P_{2mm}^{\mathrm{rib}}(+1|I_{2mm}, \mathbf{x})\pi[P_{2mm}^{\mathrm{rib}}(+1|I_{2mm}, \mathbf{x}) > \tau_2]\pi[P_{4mm}^{\mathrm{rib}}(+1|I_{4mm}, \mathbf{x}) > \tau_1]$$

$$(2)$$

where $\pi[.]$ is an indication function, P^{rib} are rib point classifiers trained using Haar-like features, τ_1 is a threshold used to limit computation in the 2nd level

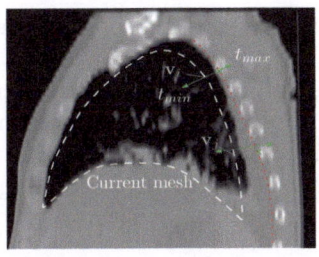 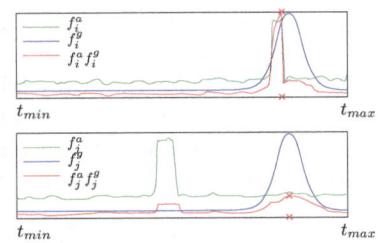

Fig. 4. Two points on the current mesh surface. $\mathbf{v}_i$ is a healthy point, so the appearance term is reliable, and the geometric term has little effect as indicated by the response curves as a function of depth. On the other hand, $\mathbf{v}_j$ is a pathological point and the appearance term is misleading. The product of appearance and geometry gives the correct displacement.

(2mm) to highly likely voxels, and τ_2 [2] is used to further threshold the 2mm classifier response. I_{4mm} and I_{2mm} are volumes that have been isotropically resampled to the corresponding resolution.

From the rib probability map I_{rib}, connected components of the thresholded mask are obtained. Each segment is grown to a maximum of size of $s_{max} = 9000mm^3$. Components less than $s_{min} = 2000mm^3$ are pruned. The remaining segments should be like bent cylinders. To prune candidate segments that are not like bent cylinders, a final test on the sizes of the segment along its principle directions is performed. Let $\alpha_1 > \alpha_2 > \alpha_3$ denote the sizes of the segment in its three principle directions. Remaining segments are pruned if $\frac{\alpha_1}{\alpha_2} < 2.5$ or $\frac{\alpha_2}{\alpha_3} > 3$.

Finally, the center points of each segment are extracted by traversing along its principal direction and intersecting a fixed number of planes with the segment.

2.3   Pathological Lung Surface Refinement

The key component of the pathological boundary detector is to combine image appearance cues with spatially dependent anatomical constraints that come from the ribs and organs detected using methods in the previous sections. The mesh initialization from §2.1 is already in correspondence with a known atlas. Also, the indices, $\mathcal{I} = \{1 \le i \le n\}$ of the mean mesh vertices are partitioned into 3 subsets: $\mathcal{I} = \mathcal{I}_{ribs} \bigcup \mathcal{I}_{heart} \bigcup \mathcal{I}_{bottom}$, each subset corresponding to one anatomical region. During boundary refinement, each vertex independently is deformed to $\mathbf{v}_i \leftarrow \mathbf{v}_i + t_i \mathbf{n}$, where

$$t_i = \mathrm{argmax}_{t \in [t_{\min}, t_{\max}]} P_i(t|I), \tag{3}$$

with the search being locally constrained within a range $[t_{\min}, t_{\max}]$. The resulting displaced mesh is regularized by projection onto the shape subspace, and the process is repeated for a few iterations.

The per-vertex score in (3) is computed as a combination of appearance, $f_i^a(t)$, and structural cues, $f_i^g(t)$, $P_i(t|I) = f_i^a(t) f_i^g(t)$. We assume $f_i^a(t)$ is the

---

[2] In practice, we tune τ_1 and τ_2 through the ROC curve and the final performance is insensitive to small changes in these parameters.

best model to use assuming no pathology. However, the opposite is true for pathological surfaces, where appearance cues are misleading, and we rely on $f_i^g(t)$. Figure 4 illustrates how the geometric term helps in the case of a pathology.

Unlike previous methods that model the appearance term with an image gradient (e.g., [9]), or region-based term, we instead use a discriminative model for the appearance in the form of a classifier that is learned from training data [5]:

$$f_i^a(t) = P(+1|\mathbf{v}_i + t\mathbf{n}_i, I). \tag{4}$$

The classifier, $P(+1|\mathbf{v}_i + t\mathbf{n}_i, I)$, measures the probability that the displaced point $\mathbf{v}_i + t\mathbf{n}_i$ belongs to the surface of the lung. To model this posterior, we use a probabilistic boosting tree with steerable features [11].

The anatomical term, $f_i^g(t)$, penalizes the surface from being far away from the adjacent structure using a Gaussian kernel mixed with a uniform prior:

$$f_i^g(t) = \exp\left(-\frac{(t - (\mathbf{y}_{\text{struct}}(\mathbf{v}_i) - \mathbf{v}_i)^T \mathbf{n}_i - \tau_i)^2}{2\sigma_i^2}\right) + \frac{\alpha}{t_{max} - t_{min}}, \tag{5}$$

where $\mathbf{y}_{\text{struct}}(\mathbf{v})$ is the closest point on the adjacent relevant structure from the source point $\mathbf{v}$. The per-vertex τ_i parameter allows for a spatially varying offset between the adjacent structure and the lung surface being segmented. These spatially varying parameters account for errors in mesh correspondence and unreliability of geometric constraints, e.g., on regions close to the spine. Adding the uniform prior reduces the influence of the geometric in the case that $\mathbf{y}_{\text{struct}}(\mathbf{v})$ is far away from $\mathbf{v}_i$.

We estimate the spatial varying $\{\tau_i\}$ and $\{\sigma_i\}$ from a given set of K training instances. We first compute for each vertex i an estimate of τ_i as the average distance to the neighboring structure from that point: $\bar{\tau}_i = \frac{1}{K}\sum_k^K \tau_{i,k}$, with $\tau_{i,k}$ being the distance estimated for training sample k. The standard deviation can be used as an estimate for σ_i. To ensure these values vary smoothly over the surface, we perform a weighted smoothing operation over the surface of the mesh, $\tau_i = (\bar{\tau}_i + mean_{j \in N(i)}(\bar{\tau}_j))/2$, where $N(i)$ are neighbors of vertex i.

2.4 Identifying Pathological Lungs

To make our pipeline capable of also efficiently handling healthy lung cases, we only apply the pathological boundary processing if the initialization from the basic pipeline is determined to be pathological. Determining if a case is healthy or pathological also uses anatomical constraints. A lung is determined as pathological when either the anatomical constraints between the lung/rib surface and lung/bottom organ surface are not satisfied. (Fig. 5).

For the lung/rib surface, first, we sample the rib probability image above the surface of the lung attached to the rib and take the maximum value of I_{rib} at values of 2mm, 4mm, and 6mm above the lung surface. We then produce a binary function on the lung surface for regions of the lung surface that are confidently close to a rib as $\chi(\mathbf{v}) = (\max_{t=2,4,6} I_{rib}(\mathbf{v} + nt)) > 0.67$. If any part of the rib-adjacent lung surface is more than 25mm from a point with $\chi(\mathbf{v}) = 1$,

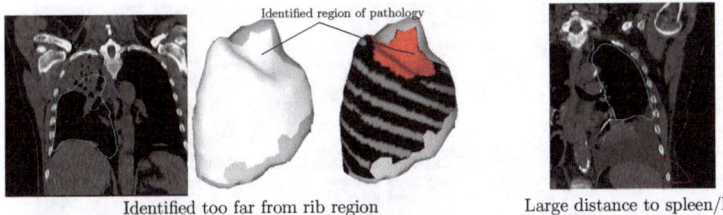

Identified too far from rib region   Large distance to spleen/liver

Fig. 5. If lung regions adjacent to the rib surface are too far from the ribs, the input is identied as pathological. For the bottom region, the pathological pipeline will be activated if the surface is not close enough to the adjacent organ (e.g., liver or spleen).

then we declare that the lung is a pathology. Figure 5 illustrates the regions of the surface near a rib, as well as the red region farther than 25mm.

To identify cases where the bottom region is pathological, the vertices on the bottom region that are closely coupled to the bottom organ are identified as $A = \{\mathbf{v}_i : i \in \mathcal{I}_{bottom}, \sigma_i \leq 5\}$. If too many vertices in A (e.g., 15%) are far from the bottom organ (say beyond $3\sigma_i$), we perform the pathological processing.

2.5 Final Refinement

Although the explicit mesh-based representation above allowed us to easily define region-specic anatomical constraints that were necessary to segment pathological lungs, the mesh-based surface representation is inadequate in obtaining voxel-level fine-scale detail. In order to obtain a more precise segmentation, we convert the initialized mesh surfaces into an implicit formulation and perform a fine-scale refinement using level sets [3]. The level set representation allows us to integrate appearance-based data terms with anatomical constraints (such as non-overlapping constraints) between neighboring organs. See [3] for details.

3 Experiments

Our lung detectors and related parameters have been trained on a total of 185 right lung and 196 left lung cases. Using the percentage of ground truth lung volume with values greater than 512 HU as an indicator of the severity of the pathology, the majority of our training examples are from healthy lungs: only 7 (resp. 2) left (resp. right) lung cases had between 25%-50% unhealthy tissue. We test our pipeline on a set of CT images containing 17 left and 33 right lung pathologies having an average dimension of $465 \times 448 \times 328$ and spacing of $1.11 \times 1.11 \times 2.61$mm. Our cases have 12 left lungs with greater than 25% unhealthy tissue, 5 of which are greater than 50%. There are 21 right lung cases with greater than 25% unhealthy tissue and 10 cases with greater than 50% unhealthy tissue. The average run time for our test cases is 64s, including processing time for lung, liver, heart, and spleen, and ribs. All training and test data sets are manually annotated by experts.

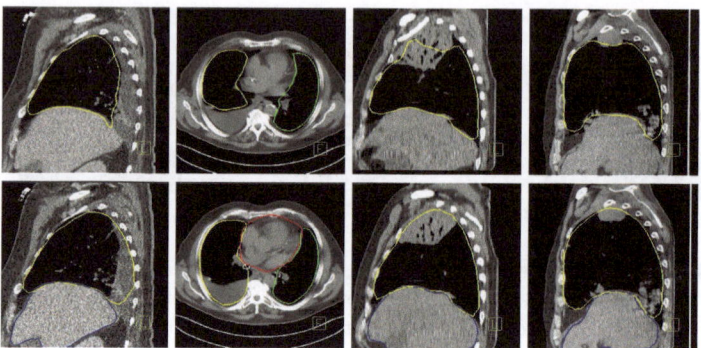

Fig. 6. Lung segmentation without (top) and with anatomical constraints (bottom) using the heart (red) and liver (blue). Errors decrease from 8.55mm to 4.49mm, 22.26mm to 6.16mm, 4.7mm to 3.3mm, and 3.2mm to 2.57mm.

Table 1. Average surface-to-surface error (Mean, median, and 80% highest error in mm) & volumetric stats (Dice Coeff and Relative Volume Difference) on unseen cases.

	Mean(STD)	Median	80%	Dice Coeff	Rel.Vol.	Fail
L.Lung Basic	4.76(2.47)	4.23	7.18	0.84	-0.14	3
L.Lung Path.	3.44(0.96)	3.84	4.25	0.89	-0.06	0
L.Lung LevSet	2.49(1.14)	2.19	3.69	0.91	0.01	0
R.Lung Basic	5.72(3.96)	4.02	8.25	0.85	-0.19	5
R.Lung Path.	3.64(1.21)	3.36	4.31	0.91	-0.06	0
R.Lung LevSet	2.23(0.97)	2.01	2.69	0.94	0.06	0

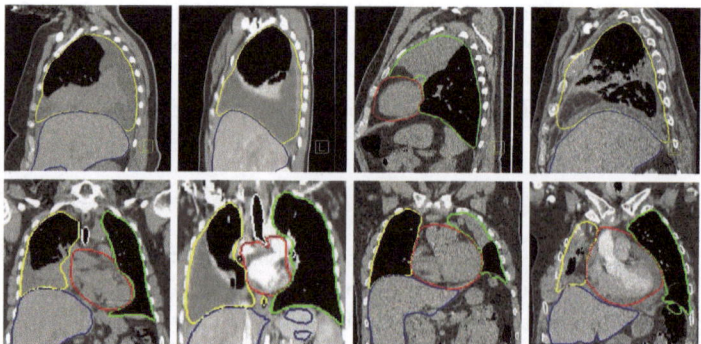

Fig. 7. Qualitative results of the hard cases used in the experimental analysis

The basic detection pipeline that relies on the input image only to detect the bounding box fails on 3/17 and 5/33 cases for left and right lung respectively (i.e., bounding box fails to return a box with high enough confidence). Table 1 illustrates statistics on mean surface-to-surface distance error (in mm) and volumetric statistics for the unseen test set. The error was only computed on the non-failure cases. In the table, the mean and median errors decrease after using the pathological pipeline. But as pathologies may only occupy a small region of the surface, the error measure between the basic detection and pathological detection may only decrease slightly. In the case of large tumors and effusions, the use of the anatomical constraints is essential to providing a geometric consistent lung segmentation. This is better illustrated with examples (Fig. 6). The geometric constraints give a segmentation that hugs the rib boundary regardless of appearance. The final refinement causes a decrease in surface error on all regions (including healthy regions), further boosting the performance. Fig. 7 shows the final level set refinement on several challenging cases.

4   Conclusions

The lung image appearance is affected by large changes due to pathologies. We have shown that structural constraints are necessary to accurately segment pathological lungs, when combined with statistical learning. Future improvements include more accurate rib segmentation, better correspondence in shape models, or other anatomical constraints say from the aorta.

References

1. Cootes, T., Taylor, C., Cooper, D., Graham, J.: Active shape models-their training and application. Computer Vision and Image Understanding 61(1), 38–59 (1995)
2. Hua, P., Song, Q., Sonka, M., Hoffman, E., Reinhardt, J.: Segmentation of pathological and diseased lung tissue in ct images using a graph-search algorithm. ISBI (March 2011)
3. Kohlberger, T., Sofka, M., Zhang, J., Birkbeck, N., Wetzl, J., Kaftan, J., Declerck, J., Zhou, S.K.: Automatic multi-organ segmentation using learning-based segmentation and level set optimization. In: Fichtinger, G., Martel, A., Peters, T. (eds.) MICCAI 2011, Part III. LNCS, vol. 6893, pp. 338–345. Springer, Heidelberg (2011)
4. Korfiatis, P., Kalogeropoulou, C., Karahaliou, A., Kazantzi, A., Skiadopoulos, S., Costaridou, L.: Texture classification-based segmentation of lung affected by interstitial pneumonia in high-resolution CT. Medical Physics 35, 5290 (2008)
5. Ling, H., Zhou, S.K., Zheng, Y., Georgescu, B., Suehling, M., Comaniciu, D.: Hierarchical, learning-based automatic liver segmentation. CVPR, 1–8 (2008)
6. Prasad, M., Brown, M., Ahmad, S., Abtin, F., Allen, J., da Costa, I., Kim, H., McNitt-Gray, M., Goldin, J.: Automatic segmentation of lung parenchyma in the presence of diseases based on curvature of ribs. Acad. Radiol. 15, 1173–1180 (2008)
7. Sluimer, I., Prokop, M., van Ginneken, B.: Toward automated segmentation of the pathological lung in ct. TMI 24(8), 1025–1038 (2005)
8. Sofka, M., Wetzl, J., Birkbeck, N., Zhang, J., Kohlberger, T., Kaftan, J., Declerck, J., Zhou, S.K.: Multi-stage learning for robust lung segmentation in challenging CT volumes. In: Fichtinger, G., Martel, A., Peters, T. (eds.) MICCAI 2011, Part III. LNCS, vol. 6893, pp. 667–674. Springer, Heidelberg (2011)
9. Sun, S., McLennan, G., Hoffman, E.A., Beichel, R.: Model-based segmentation of pathological lungs in volumetric ct data. In: The Third International Workshop on Pulmonary Image Analysis (2010)
10. Wang, J., Li, F., Li, Q.: Automated segmentation of lungs with severe interstitial lung disease in CT. Medical Physics 36, 4592 (2009)
11. Zheng, Y., Barbu, A., Georgescu, B., Scheuering, M., Comaniciu, D.: Fast automatic heart chamber segmentation from 3D CT data using marginal space learning and steerable features. In: ICCV. pp. 1–8. IEEE (2007)

Erratum: Iterative Most Likely Oriented Point Registration

Seth Billings and Russell Taylor

Johns Hopkins University, Department of Computer Science, Baltimore, MD, USA
{sbillin3,rht}@jhu.edu

P. Golland et al. (Eds.): MICCAI 2014, Part I, LNCS 8673, pp. 178–185, 2014.
© Springer International Publishing Switzerland 2014

DOI: 10.1007/978-3-319-10404-1_101

Errata List

Page Corrections

180   Algorithm 1, Line 5: The denominator term in the expression for estimating σ^2 should be $3n$ rather than n, i.e., σ^2 is the average square residual distance of the match positions divided by the spatial dimensionality:

$$\sigma^2 = \frac{1}{3n} \sum_{i=1}^{n} \|\boldsymbol{y}_{\mathrm{p}i} - T(\boldsymbol{x}_{\mathrm{p}i})\|_2^2$$

184   Figure 2: Please see below for the corrected version of this figure. A bug in the script used to generate the original figure resulted in mis-plotting the values corresponding to the IMLOP algorithm. Note that the corrected figure strengthens the conclusions of the paper, i.e., the registration accuracy of IMLOP is better than previously shown and IMLOP detects the inaccurate registration outcomes more robustly than previously shown.

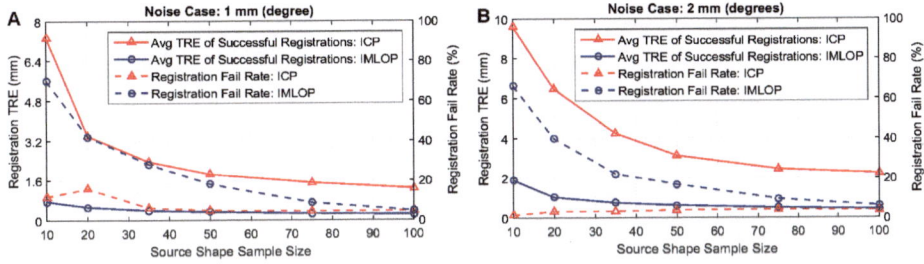

Fig. 2. Corrected version of Figure 2

The original online version for this chapter can be found at
http://dx.doi.org/10.1007/978-3-319-10404-1_23

Author Index